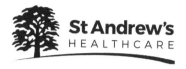

St Andrew's
HEALTHCARE

SPEAKING VOLUMES

To be returned on or before the date marked below

St. Andrews Hospital, Billing Road, Northampton, NN1 5DG
You can contact the Patient Library on x6447

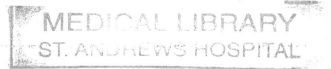

DSM-IV SOURCEBOOK

VOLUME 2

Edited by

Thomas A. Widiger, Ph.D.
Allen J. Frances, M.D.
Harold Alan Pincus, M.D.
Ruth Ross, M.A.
Michael B. First, M.D.
Wendy Wakefield Davis, Ed.M.

Published by the American Psychiatric Association
Washington, DC

Note: The authors have worked to ensure that all information in this book concerning drug dosages, schedules, and routes of administration is accurate as of the time of publication and consistent with standards set by the U.S. Food and Drug Administration and the general medical community. As medical research and practice advance, however, therapeutic standards may change. For this reason and because human and mechanical errors sometimes occur, we recommend that readers follow the advice of a physician who is directly involved in their care or the care of a member of their family.

The findings, opinions, and conclusions of this report do not necessarily represent the views of the officers, trustees, all members of the task force, or all members of the American Psychiatric Association. The views expressed are those of the authors of the individual chapters. Task force reports are considered a substantive contribution of the ongoing analysis and evaluation of problems, programs, issues, and practices in a given area of concern.

Copyright © 1996 American Psychiatric Association

ALL RIGHTS RESERVED

Manufactured in the United States of America on acid-free paper

First Edition

99 98 97 96   4 3 2 1

American Psychiatric Association

1400 K Street, N.W., Washington, DC   20005

Library of Congress Cataloging-in-Publication Data

(Revised for vol. 2)

DSM-IV sourcebook.

   Developed by the DSM-IV Task Force of American
Psychiatric Association.

   Includes bibliographical references and index.

   1. Diagnostic and statistical manual of mental
disorders.   2. Mental illness—Classification.
3. Mental illness—Diagnosis.   I. Widiger, Thomas A.
II. American Psychiatric Association. Task Force on
DSM-IV.   III. Title: DSM-4 sourcebook.   [DNLM: 1. Mental
Disorders—classification.   2. Psychiatry—nomenclature.
WM 15 D277 1994]

RC455.2.C4D754 1994   616.89′075   93-48304

ISBN 0-89042-065-3 (v. 1)

ISBN 0-89042-069-6 (v. 2)

British Library Cataloguing in Publication Data

A CIP record is available from the British Library.

Contents

SECTION I
MOOD DISORDERS

SECTION II
LATE LUTEAL PHASE DYSPHORIC DISORDER

SECTION III
ANXIETY DISORDERS

SECTION IV
PERSONALITY DISORDERS

SECTION V
PSYCHIATRIC SYSTEM
INTERFACE DISORDERS

SECTION VI
SEXUAL DISORDERS

Contributors

Jules Angst, M.D. Professor of Psychiatry and Head, Research Department, Psychiatrische Universitätsklinik Zürich, Zurich, Switzerland

Jacqueline Lalive Aubert, M.D. Service de Psychiatrie I, Department of Psychiatry, University of Geneva, Geneva, Switzerland

Lee Baer, Ph.D. Director of Research, Obsessive-Compulsive Unit, Harvard University, Boston, Massachusetts

James C. Ballenger, M.D. Professor and Chairman, Department of Psychiatry, Medical University of South Carolina, Charleston, South Carolina

David H. Barlow, Ph.D. Distinguished Professor of Psychology and Co-Director, Center for Stress and Anxiety Disorders, University at Albany, State University of New York, Albany, New York

Mark S. Bauer, M.D. Associate Professor, Department of Psychiatry and Human Behavior, Brown University; Department of Veterans Affairs Medical Center, Providence, Rhode Island

David Bear, M.D. Professor of Psychiatry, University of Massachusetts at Worcester, Worcester, Massachusetts

Gale Beardsley, M.D. Clinical Assistant Professor of Psychiatry, Brown University Program in Medicine, Providence, Rhode Island

Deborah C. Beidel, Ph.D. Associate Professor of Psychiatry and Behavioral Sciences, Medical University of South Carolina, Charleston, South Carolina

David P. Bernstein, Ph.D.   Assistant Professor of Psychiatry, Mount Sinai School of Medicine; Clinical Psychologist, Bronx VA Medical Center, New York, New York

Arthur S. Blank, M.D.   Psychiatry Service, VA Medical Center, Minneapolis, Minnesota

T. D. Borkovec, Ph.D.   Professor of Psychology, Pennsylvania State University, University Park, Pennsylvania

John Bradford, M.D.   Director, Forensic Program and Sexual Behaviors Clinic, Royal Ottawa Hospital, Ottawa, Ontario, Canada

Elizabeth A. Brett, Ph.D.   Associate Clinical Professor of Psychiatry (Psychology), Yale University School of Medicine, New Haven, Connecticut

Etzel Cardeña, Ph.D.   Assistant Professor, Department of Psychiatry, Uniformed Services University of the Health Sciences, Bethesda, Maryland

David M. Clark, Ph.D.   Department of Psychiatry, University of Oxford, Warneford Hospital, Oxford, United Kingdom

Lee Anna Clark, Ph.D.   Professor, Department of Psychology, University of Iowa, Iowa City, Iowa

C. Robert Cloninger, M.D.   Wallace Renard Professor of Psychiatry, Washington University Medical School, St. Louis, Missouri

Elizabeth M. Corbitt, Ph.D.   Research Fellow, Western Psychiatric Institute and Clinic, Pittsburgh, Pennsylvania

Guylaine Côté, Ph.D.   Center for Stress and Anxiety Disorders, University at Albany, State University of New York, Albany, New York

Michelle G. Craske, Ph.D.   Associate Professor, Psychology Department, University of California, Los Angeles, California

George C. Curtis, M.D.   Professor of Psychiatry, Director of Anxiety Disorders Program, Psychiatry Department, The University of Michigan, Ann Arbor, Michigan

Jonathan Davidson, M.D.   Professor of Psychiatry, Director of Anxiety and Traumatic Stress Program, Duke University Medical Center, Durham, North Carolina

Wendy Wakefield Davis, Ed.M.   Editorial Coordinator, DSM-IV, American Psychiatric Association, Washington, DC

Peter A. DiNardo, Ph.D.   Center for Stress and Anxiety Disorders, University at Albany, State University of New York, Albany, New York

David L. Dunner, M.D.   Professor, Department of Psychiatry; Director, Outpatient Psychiatry; Co-Director, Center for Anxiety and Depression; Vice-Chairman for Clinical Services, University of Washington, Seattle, Washington

Jean Endicott, Ph.D.   Professor of Clinical Psychology, Department of Psychiatry, College of Physicians and Surgeons, Columbia University, New York, New York

Cecile Ernst, M.D.   Psychiatrische Universitätsklinik Zürich, Zurich, Switzerland

John Fairbank, Ph.D.   Adjunct Associate Professor of Medical Psychology, Department of Psychiatry; Research Scholar, Department of Psychology, Social and Health Sciences, Duke University, Durham; Senior Research Clinical Psychologist, Center for Social Research and Policy Analysis, Research Triangle Institute, Research Triangle Park, North Carolina

Susan J. Fiester, M.D.   Private practice, Chevy Chase, Maryland

Ivan Vasconcelos Figueira, M.D.   Assistant Professor of Psychiatry, Federal University of Rio de Janeiro, Rio de Janeiro, Brazil

Max Fink, M.D.   Professor of Psychiatry and Neurology, Department of Psychiatry and Behavioral Sciences, School of Medicine, State University of New York at Stony Brook, Long Island, New York

Michael B. First, M.D.   Assistant Professor of Clinical Psychiatry, Columbia University, New York, New York

Edna B. Foa, Ph.D.   Professor and Director of the Center for the Treatment and Study of Anxiety in the Department of Psychiatry, The Medical College of Pennsylvania, Philadelphia, Pennsylvania

David G. Folks, M.D.   Professor and Chair, Department of Psychiatry, Creighton-Nebraska Universities, Omaha, Nebraska

Allen J. Frances, M.D.   Chairman, Department of Psychiatry, Duke University Medical Center, Durham, North Carolina; and Chair, Task Force on DSM-IV, American Psychiatric Association

Ellen Frank, Ph.D.   Professor of Psychiatry and Psychology, Department of Psychiatry, University of Pittsburgh School of Medicine, Pittsburgh, Pennsylvania

George Fulop, M.D.   Associate Professor of Psychiatry, Division of Behavioral Medicine and Consultation Psychiatry, Mount Sinai School of Medicine, New York, New York

Abby J. Fyer, M.D.   Professor of Clinical Psychiatry, College of Physicians and Surgeons, Columbia University, New York, New York

Martha L. Rhodes, M.D. (Martha Gay)   Adult Psychiatry, Park Nicollet Medical Center, Bloomington, Minnesota

Jeffrey Geller, M.D.   Director of Public Sector Psychiatry, University of Massachusetts Medical School, Worcester, Massachusetts

Mark S. George, M.D.   Senior Staff Fellow, Biological Psychiatry Branch, National Institute of Mental Health, Bethesda, Maryland

Judith H. Gold, M.D., F.R.C.P.C.   Private practice, Halifax, Nova Scotia, Canada

Michael G. Goldstein, M.D.   Associate Professor of Psychiatry and Human Behavior, Brown University Program in Medicine, Providence, Rhode Island

Wayne Goodman, M.D.   Professor of Psychiatry, University of Florida College of Medicine, Gainesville, Florida

Bonnie L. Green, Ph.D.   Professor of Psychiatry, Georgetown University Medical School, Washington, DC

John Gunderson, M.D. Associate Professor of Psychiatry, Harvard Medical School, Boston; Director of Psychosocial Research, McLean Hospital, Belmont, Massachusetts

Robert E. Hales, M.D. Chair, Department of Psychiatry, California Pacific Medical Center; Clinical Professor of Psychiatry, University of California, San Francisco, San Francisco, California

Wilma M. Harrison, M.D. Associate Professor of Clinical Psychiatry, Department of Psychiatry, College of Physicians and Surgeons, Columbia University, New York, New York

Richard G. Heimberg, Ph.D. Professor of Psychology, University at Albany, State University of New York, Albany, New York

Judith L. Herman, M.D. Associate Clinical Professor of Psychiatry, Harvard Medical School; Director of Training in the Victims of Violence at Cambridge Hospital, Boston, Massachusetts

Elizabeth M. Hill, Ph.D. Director of Biometrics Division, Psychiatry Department, The University of Michigan, Ann Arbor, Michigan

Joseph A. Himle, M.S.W. Senior Social Worker and Lecturer, Psychiatry Department, The University of Michigan, Ann Arbor, Michigan

Robert M. A. Hirschfeld, M.D. Titus Harris Professor and Chairman, Department of Psychiatry and Behavioral Sciences, University of Texas Medical Branch, Galveston, Texas

Eric Hollander, M.D. Vice-Chairman and Associate Professor of Psychiatry and Director of Clinical Psychopharmacology, Mt. Sinai School of Medicine and Queens Hospital Center, New York, New York

Craig S. Holt, Ph.D. Assistant Professor, Department of Psychiatry and Psychology, University of Iowa, Iowa City, Iowa

Robert H. Howland, M.D. Assistant Professor of Psychiatry, Western Psychiatric Institute and Clinic, Department of Psychiatry, University of Pittsburgh School of Medicine, Pittsburgh, Pennsylvania

Emily B. Hoyer, B.A. Genetic Epidemiology Research Unit, Yale University School of Medicine, New Haven, Connecticut

Michael Jenike, M.D. Harvard University, Boston, Massachusetts

Russell Joffe, M.D. Clarke Institute of Psychiatry, Toronto, Ontario, Canada

Oren Kalus, M.D. Staff Psychiatrist, Ulster County Mental Health, Kingston, New York

Wayne Katon, M.D. University of Washington School of Medicine, Seattle, Washington

Terence M. Keane, Ph.D. Director of National Center for PTSD, Boston VA Medical Center; Professor of Psychiatry, Tufts University School of Medicine, Boston, Massachusetts

Martin B. Keller, M.D. Mary E. Zucker Professor and Chairman, Department of Psychiatry and Human Behavior, Brown University; Psychiatrist-in-Chief, Butler Hospital; Executive Psychiatrist-in-Chief, Brown Affiliated Hospitals, Providence, Rhode Island

Dean L. Kilpatrick, Ph.D. Professor of Clinical Psychology, Department of Psychiatry and Behavioral Science, Medical University of South Carolina; Director of the National Crime Victims Research and Treatment Center, Charleston, South Carolina

Steven A. King, M.D. Associate Professor and Director, Division of Pain Medicine, Department of Psychiatry, Temple University School of Medicine, Philadelphia, Pennsylvania

Cassandra L. Kisiel, B.A. Research Assistant, Psychosocial Research Program, McLean Hospital, Belmont, Massachusetts

Donald F. Klein, M.D. Professor of Psychiatry, College of Physicians and Surgeons, Columbia University, New York, New York

Michael J. Kozak, Ph.D. Associate Professor of Psychiatry, Center for the Treatment and Study of Anxiety, Medical College of Pennsylvania, Philadelphia, Pennsylvania

John E. Kurtz, Ph.D. Research Fellow, Rehabilitation Institute of Michigan, Detroit, Michigan

Yue-Joe Lee, M.D. Department of Psychiatry, Taiwan University, Taipei

Henry R. Lesieur, Ph.D. Chairman, Department of Criminal Justice Services, Illinois State University, Normal, Illinois

James Levenson, M.D. Professor of Psychiatry, Medicine, and Surgery, Medical College of Virginia, Richmond, Virginia

Andrew P. Levin, M.D. Assistant Professor of Clinical Psychiatry, College of Physicians and Surgeons, Columbia University, New York, New York

Julie A. Lewis, B.A. Psychiatry Department, The University of Michigan, Ann Arbor, Michigan

Roberto Lewis-Fernández, M.D. Fellow, Harvard University Medical School, Boston, Massachusetts

Michael R. Liebowitz, M.D. Professor of Clinical Psychiatry, College of Physicians and Surgeons, Columbia University; New York State Psychiatric Institute, New York, New York

R. Bruce Lydiard, M.D., Ph.D. Professor of Psychiatry, Medical University of South Carolina, Charleston, South Carolina

Wolfgang Maier, M.D. Psychiatrische Klinik und Poliklinik, Johannes Gutenberg-Universität Mainz, Mainz, Germany

Salvatore Mannuzza, Ph.D. Associate Professor of Clinical Psychology, Columbia University, New York, New York

John S. March, M.D., M.P.H. Assistant Professor of Psychiatry, Duke University Medical Center, Durham, North Carolina

Lynn Y. Martin, R.N., M.S., C.S. Research Coordinator, Anxiety and Mood Disorders Clinic, New York Hospital, Cornell University Medical Center, White Plains, New York

Ronald L. Martin, M.D.   Professor and Chairman, Department of Psychiatry and Behavioral Sciences, University of Kansas School of Medicine-Wichita, Wichita, Kansas

Patrick J. McGrath, M.D.   Associate Professor of Clinical Psychiatry, Department of Psychiatry, College of Physicians and Surgeons, Columbia University, New York, New York

Richard J. McNally, Ph.D.   Associate Professor, Department of Psychology, Harvard University, Boston, Massachusetts

M. Eileen McNamara, M.D.   Assistant Professor of Psychiatry and Human Behavior, Brown University Program in Medicine, Providence, Rhode Island

Kathleen Ries Merikangas, Ph.D.   Associate Professor of Psychiatry and Epidemiology; Director, Genetic Epidemiology Research Unit, Yale University School of Medicine, New Haven, Connecticut

Theodore Millon, Ph.D.   Professor of Psychology in Psychiatry, Harvard Medical School, Boston, Massachusetts; Professor, Department of Psychology, University of Miami, Miami, Florida

Michael Moran, M.D.   Associate Professor of Psychiatry, University of Colorado School of Medicine, Denver, Colorado

Karla Moras, Ph.D.   Assistant Professor of Psychology in Psychiatry; Director, Assessment Unit, Center for Psychotherapy Research, University of Pennsylvania, Philadelphia, Pennsylvania

Leslie C. Morey, Ph.D.   Associate Professor, Department of Psychology, Vanderbilt University, Nashville, Tennessee

A. Egido Nardi, M.D.   Assistant Professor of Psychiatry, Federal University of Rio de Janeiro, Rio de Janeiro, Brazil

Jeffrey Newcorn, M.D.   Associate Professor of Psychiatry and Pediatrics, Division of Child and Adolescent Psychiatry, Mount Sinai School of Medicine, New York, New York

Raymond Niaura, Ph.D.   Associate Professor of Psychiatry and Human Behavior, Brown University Program in Medicine, Providence, Rhode Island

Tracy O'Leary, M.D.   Center for Stress and Anxiety Disorders, University at Albany, State University of New York, Albany, New York

Lars-Goran Öst, Ph.D.   Psychiatric Research Center, University of Uppsala, Ulleraker Hospital, Uppsala, Sweden

Isabel Pakianathan, M.D.   Department of Psychiatry, Stanford University, Stanford, California

Barbara L. Parry, M.D.   Associate Professor of Psychiatry, University of California, San Diego, California

David Pauls, Ph.D.   Associate Professor, Yale University School of Medicine, Child Study Center, New Haven, Connecticut

Bruce Pfohl, M.D.   Professor of Psychiatry, University of Iowa College of Medicine, Iowa City, Iowa

Katharine A. Phillips, M.D.   Chief, Outpatient Services, and Director, Body Dysmorphic Disorder Clinic, Butler Hospital; Assistant Professor of Psychiatry, Brown University School of Medicine, Providence, Rhode Island

Harold Alan Pincus, M.D.   Deputy Medical Director and Director, Office of Research, American Psychiatric Association, Washington, DC

Roger K. Pitman, M.D.   Clinical Investigator and Coordinator for Research and Development, VA Medical Center, Manchester, New Hampshire; Associate Professor of Psychiatry, Harvard Medical School, Boston, Massachusetts

Daniel Purnine, M.S.   Western Psychiatric Institute and Clinic, Pittsburgh, Pennsylvania

Frederic M. Quitkin, M.D.   Professor of Clinical Psychiatry, Department of Psychiatry, College of Physicians and Surgeons, Columbia University, New York, New York

Judith G. Rabkin, Ph.D.   Professor of Clinical Psychology in Psychiatry, Department of Psychiatry, College of Physicians and Surgeons, Columbia University, New York, New York

Ronald Rapee, Ph.D.   School of Behavioral Sciences, Macquarie University, Sydney, Australia

Steven A. Rasmussen, M.D.   Department of Psychiatry, Brown University School of Medicine, Providence, Rhode Island

Heidi S. Resnick, Ph.D.   Associate Professor, Department of Psychiatry and Behavioral Science, Medical University of South Carolina, Charleston, South Carolina

John Riskind, Ph.D.   Associate Professor, Department of Psychology, George Mason University, Fairfax, Virginia

Elsa Ronningstam, Ph.D.   Instructor in Psychology, Harvard Medical School, Boston, Massachusetts

Richard Rosenthal, M.D.   Assistant Clinical Professor of Psychiatry, Department of Psychiatry, University of California, Los Angeles, California

Ruth Ross, M.A.   Science Writer, DSM-IV

Barbara O. Rothbaum, Ph.D.   Assistant Professor in Psychiatry, Department of Psychiatry and Behavioral Sciences, Emory University School of Medicine, Atlanta, Georgia

Anthony J. Rothschild, M.D.   Department of Psychiatry, Harvard Medical School; Affective Disease Program, McLean Hospital, Boston, Massachusetts

Peter Roy-Byrne, M.D.   University of Washington School of Medicine, Seattle, Washington

A. John Rush, M.D.   Betty Jo Hay Distinguished Chair in Mental Health, Department of Psychiatry, Mental Health Clinical Research Center, University of Texas Southwestern Medical Center, Dallas, Texas

Cordelia W. Russell, B.A.   Boston University, Boston, Massachusetts

Paul M. Salkovskis, Ph.D. Psychiatry Department, University of Oxford, Warneford Hospital, Oxford, United Kingdom

Alan F. Schatzberg, M.D. Chairman, Department of Psychiatry and Behavioral Sciences, Stanford University School of Medicine, Stanford, California; Department of Psychiatry, Harvard Medical School, Boston, Massachusetts; Affective Disease Program, McLean Hospital, Boston, Massachusetts

Raul C. Schiavi, M.D. Professor of Psychiatry, Director Human Sexuality Program, Mount Sinai School of Medicine, New York, New York

Chester W. Schmidt, Jr., M.D. Chief, Department of Psychiatry, Johns Hopkins Bayview Medical Center, Baltimore, Maryland

Franklin R. Schneier, M.D. Associate Professor of Clinical Psychiatry, College of Physicians and Surgeons, Columbia University, New York, New York

Leslie R. Schover, Ph.D. Staff Psychologist, Center for Sexual Function, The Cleveland Clinic Foundation, Cleveland, Ohio

R. Taylor Segraves, M.D. Professor of Psychiatry, Case Western Reserve University; Interim Chair, Department of Psychiatry, Metrohealth Medical Center, Cleveland, Ohio

Sally K. Severino, M.D. Associate Professor of Clinical Psychiatry, New York Hospital–Cornell Medical Center, Westchester Division, White Plains, New York

M. Tracie Shea, Ph.D. Associate Professor, Department of Psychiatry and Human Behavior, Brown University Medical School; Veterans Administration Medical Center, Providence, Rhode Island

Larry J. Siever, M.D. Professor of Psychiatry, Mount Sinai School of Medicine; Director of Outpatient Division, Bronx Veterans Administration Medical Center/Mount Sinai Medical Center, New York, New York

Jeremy M. Silverman, Ph.D. Assistant Professor of Psychiatry, Mount Sinai School of Medicine; Clinical Psychologist, Bronx Veteran's Administration Medical Center, New York, New York

Lauren E. Smith, B.A. Research Assistant, Psychosocial Research Program, McLean Hospital, Belmont, Massachusetts

David Spiegel, M.D. Professor, Department of Psychiatry, Stanford University, Stanford, California

Robert L. Spitzer, M.D. Professor of Psychiatry, College of Physicians and Surgeons, Columbia University, New York, New York

Jonathan W. Stewart, M.D. Associate Professor of Clinical Psychiatry, Department of Psychiatry, College of Physicians and Surgeons, Columbia University, New York, New York

Nada Stotland, M.D. Associate Professor, Departments of Psychiatry and Obstetrics and Gynecology, University of Chicago, Chicago, Illinois

Alan Stoudemire, M.D. Professor of Psychiatry, Emory University School of Medicine, Atlanta, Georgia

James J. Strain, M.D. Director, Division of Behavioral Medicine and Consultation Psychiatry; Professor, Department of Psychiatry, Mount Sinai School of Medicine, New York, New York

Richard P. Swinson, M.D., F.R.C.P. Clinical Director, University of Toronto, Clarke Institute of Psychiatry, Toronto, Ontario, Canada

K. M. Talbot, B.S. Research Assistant, Department of Psychiatry and Behavioral Sciences, University of Texas Medical Branch, Galveston, Texas

Diana Roscow Terrill, M.A. National Institute of Mental Health, Bethesda, Maryland

Michael E. Thase, M.D. Associate Professor of Psychiatry, Department of Psychiatry, Western Psychiatric Institute and Clinic, University of Pittsburgh School of Medicine, Pittsburgh, Pennsylvania

Joseph Triebwasser, M.D. Assistant Psychiatrist, Harvard Medical School, McLean Hospital, Boston, Massachusetts

Samuel M. Turner, Ph.D. Professor of Psychiatry and Behavioral Sciences, Medical University of South Carolina, Charleston, South Carolina

Thomas W. Uhde, M.D. Professor and Chairman, Department of Psychiatry, Wayne State University School of Medicine, Detroit, Michigan

David Useda, B.A. Doctoral Candidate, Department of Psychology, University of Missouri, Columbia, Missouri

Marcio Versiani, M.D. Professor of Psychiatry, Federal University of Rio de Janeiro, Rio de Janeiro, Brazil

Hilary M. C. Warwick, B.M., M.R.C.Psych. Department of Psychiatry, University of Oxford, Warneford Hospital, Oxford, United Kingdom

David Watson, Ph.D. Department of Psychology, University of Iowa, Iowa City, Iowa

Jan E. Weissenburger, M.A. Psychological Associate II, Department of Psychiatry and Mental Health Clinical Research Center, University of Texas Southwestern Medical Center, Dallas, Texas

Peter C. Whybrow, M.D. Professor and Chairman, Department of Psychiatry, University of Pennsylvania, Philadelphia, Pennsylvania

Thomas A. Widiger, Ph.D. Professor, Department of Psychology, University of Kentucky, Lexington, Kentucky

Michael Wise, M.D. Clinical Professor of Psychiatry, Louisiana State University Medical School and Tulane University Medical School, New Orleans, Louisiana

Thomas N. Wise, M.D. Professor of Psychiatry, Georgetown University School of Medicine, Washington, DC; Chair, Department of Psychiatry, Fairfax Hospital, Falls Church, Virginia

Dennis Wolf, M.D. Division of Behavioral Medicine and Consultation Psychiatry, Mount Sinai School of Medicine, New York, New York

Mary C. Zanarini, Ed.D. Assistant Professor of Psychology, Harvard Medical School, Boston, Massachusetts

Preface

DSM-IV Sourcebook: Volumes 1–3—Literature Reviews

For more than 5 years, the Task Force on DSM-IV and members of the DSM-IV Work Groups participated in a comprehensive effort of empirical review leading to the publication of the fourth edition of the American Psychiatric Association's *Diagnostic and Statistical Manual of Mental Disorders* (DSM-IV). The *DSM-IV Sourcebook* chronicles these efforts and their results, documenting the rationale and empirical support for the text and criteria sets presented in DSM-IV. The major emphasis in the DSM-IV process has been on empirical review and documentation, and the *Sourcebook,* published in four to five volumes, is an important means of presenting that documentation. The first three volumes contain the DSM-IV literature reviews and summarize the DSM-IV Work Groups' efforts that led to the publication of the *DSM-IV Options Book* in 1991. The fourth volume will contain the results of the DSM-IV data reanalyses, and the fifth volume will contain the results of the DSM-IV field trials. (If possible, the fourth and fifth volumes will be collapsed into one volume.)

The *DSM-IV Sourcebook* is the culmination of a process that began in September 1987, when the American Psychiatric Association (APA) Committee on Psychiatric Diagnosis and Assessment met to explore possible timetables for the publication of DSM-IV. Because of the work already proceeding on the 10th edition of the International Classification of Diseases (ICD-10) by the World Health Organization (1992), the Committee concluded that work should also begin on DSM-IV to allow for mutual influence and convergence of the two systems (Frances et al. 1989). From the outset, the Committee recommended that review of the empirical evidence on diagnostic issues—often stimulated by the publication of DSM-III (American Psychiatric Association 1980) and DSM-III-R (American Psychiatric Association 1987)—be the centerpiece for the development of DSM-IV.

In May 1988, the Board of Trustees of APA appointed a task force to undertake the preparation of DSM-IV. Thirteen Work Groups were formed, each chaired by a member of the Task Force. These Work Groups covered the Anxiety Disorders;

Child and Adolescent Disorders; Eating Disorders; Late Luteal Phase Dysphoric Disorder; Mood Disorders; the Multiaxial system; Delirium, Dementia, and Amnestic and Other Cognitive ("Organic") Disorders; Personality Disorders; Psychiatric System Interface Disorders (consisting of Somatoform, Factitious, Dissociative, Impulse Control, and Adjustment Disorders); Psychotic Disorders; Sexual Disorders; Sleep Disorders; and Substance-Related Disorders.

Two conferences were held to develop the process by which DSM-IV would be constructed. These conferences were attended by representatives of the DSM-IV Task Force, the various Work Groups, and expert consultants on the design, analysis, and review of empirical research. The first Methods Conference was held in August 1988 to discuss procedures for gathering and analyzing data from different studies to achieve a comprehensive and objective consideration of the empirical literature. The second Methods and Applications Conference was held in November 1988 to discuss in more detail procedures for reviewing research, for selecting validators for existing and proposed items, for conducting field trials, and for resolving the various issues that would be addressed by the respective Work Groups. It was decided that the development of DSM-IV should proceed through three interactive stages of empirical review and documentation: 1) literature reviews, 2) reanalyses of existing data sets, and 3) focused field trials (Widiger et al. 1991). The goal of this process was to maximize the impact of empirical research on the deliberations and decisions of the DSM-IV Work Groups and Task Force and to document the empirical support for the resulting recommendations and proposals (Frances et al. 1990).

For any substantial revision of, addition to, or deletion from DSM-III-R to be considered for DSM-IV, it had to be accompanied by a review of the empirical and clinical literature (Widiger et al. 1990). Those conducting the reviews were to function as if they were consensus scholars (persons with no preconceptions who are fully aware of the clinical and research literature) (Cooper 1984). The reviews were not to be position papers arguing for particular proposals but rather systematic, comprehensive, and objective overviews of the most relevant empirical research. These literature reviews are presented in the first three volumes of the *DSM-IV Sourcebook*.

The literature reviews also served to identify gaps and inadequacies within the literature on questions of crucial importance to the DSM-IV Work Groups. Fortunately, in many such instances, relevant existing data sets were available that had not yet been analyzed in a fashion that would provide useful answers. Therefore, the second stage of the DSM-IV development process was to obtain and reanalyze multiple data sets to address questions not answered in the published literature. This also allowed us to generate and pilot new proposals for criteria sets for DSM-IV (Widiger et al. 1991). These efforts were funded in part by the John D. and

Catherine T. MacArthur Foundation, and the results will be presented in Volume 4 of the *DSM-IV Sourcebook.*

The culmination of the literature review and data reanalysis process was the publication of the *DSM-IV Options Book* (American Psychiatric Association 1991). The purpose of the *Options Book* was both to present the major diagnostic issues, and options for dealing with them, that had been identified by the Task Force on DSM-IV and to encourage review, comments, and the contribution of additional available data. Summaries describing how the information from the literature reviews and data reanalyses aided the Task Force and Work Groups in developing these options are presented in the *Sourcebook.* It is hoped that the publication of this information will provide an explanation and documentation for the decisions made in DSM-IV.

The third stage of the DSM-IV development process was to perform focused field trials to assess the extent to which proposed revisions would actually improve the reliability and/or validity of criteria sets and to address the issues identified by the literature reviews. The field trials allowed the DSM-IV Work Groups to compare alternative options (usually DSM-III, DSM-III-R, ICD-10 research criteria, and the various proposals for DSM-IV that had been generated during the first two steps) and to study the possible impact of any suggested changes. Funding for the field trials was obtained from the National Institute of Mental Health in collaboration with the National Institute on Drug Abuse and the National Institute on Alcohol Abuse and Alcoholism. The results of the focused field trials and the rationale for the final decisions of the Work Groups and Task Force will be presented in Volume 5 (or Volume 4) of the *DSM-IV Sourcebook.*

The culmination of this final stage in the DSM-IV development process was the publication of the *DSM-IV Draft Criteria* (American Psychiatric Association 1993). The purpose of this document was to invite review and comment on the proposed criteria before they appeared in DSM-IV. Readers were asked to help identify any mistakes, inconsistencies, oversights, unforeseen problems, potential for misuse, or boundary confusions.

In the rest of this Preface, we detail the organization and format of the literature reviews presented in the first three volumes of the *DSM-IV Sourcebook.* Separate introductions to Volume 4 and Volume 5 will deal with issues specific to the data reanalyses and field trials, respectively.

The DSM-IV literature reviews are divided into three volumes, organized with respect to shared concerns and issues. Volume 1 presents the reviews for Substance-Related Disorders; Delirium, Dementia, and Amnestic and Other Cognitive Disorders (including a review on Mental Disorders Due to a General Medical Condition); Schizophrenia and Other Psychotic Disorders; Medication-Induced Movement Disorders; and Sleep Disorders. Volume 2 presents the reviews for the Mood

Disorders, Late Luteal Phase Dysphoric Disorder, Anxiety Disorders, Personality Disorders, Psychiatric System Interface Disorders (consisting of Somatoform, Factitious, Dissociative, Impulse Control, and Adjustment Disorders), and Sexual Disorders. Volume 3 presents the reviews for Childhood Disorders, Eating Disorders, Family-Relational Issues, Multiaxial Issues, and Cultural Issues. The section for each group of disorders begins with an introductory chapter that provides an executive summary of the material contained within that section as well as an overview of the activities and procedures of the Work Group. This is followed by the individual literature reviews dealing with the specific questions addressed by the Work Group.

Experts on the methodology of literature review provided guidelines for performing systematic, objective, and comprehensive evaluation of the available clinical research literature (Cooper 1984). The authors of the reviews were encouraged to follow an explicit format for conducting the review and presenting its findings. Successive drafts of each review were distributed widely to the advisers to each Work Group, who were specifically chosen to include individuals who represented a wide range of viewpoints on any given issue. Many of the reviews have also been published in revised form in professional and scientific journals and presented at conferences and meetings. We have encouraged the authors to publish and present their findings and interpretation to receive as much peer review and critical commentary as possible. This iterative process and the explicit format have been very helpful in identifying the various inadequacies, gaps, and biases that occurred in earlier drafts (e.g., failure to cover an important issue, a bias in the selection of studies, gaps in the coverage or presentation of the literature, disagreements concerning the interpretation of empirical findings, and failure to consider alternative options).

Each review contains the following sections: Statement of the Issues, Significance of the Issues, Methods, Results, Discussion, and Recommendations (Widiger et al. 1990). The "Statement of the Issues" section outlines explicitly the issues being addressed in the review and keeps the review focused on the pertinent nosological questions. This section informs the reader of the focus and scope of the review.

The "Significance of the Issues" section frames the importance of the issues and discusses their clinical and/or empirical significance.

The "Methods" section ensures replicability of the review and documents the extent to which the reviews were systematic and comprehensive in their coverage of the literature. This section indicates the types of studies that were considered and the ways they were identified with any explicit inclusion or exclusion criteria (e.g., requirements with respect to the populations sampled, the criteria sets used, how recently the study was conducted, and other methodological features). Authors were instructed to conduct computerized literature searches, to review specified journals systematically, and to solicit input from all the leading researchers in the field to minimize bias in the identification and consideration of studies that might result from the authors' own perspective on the literature.

The "Results" section provides an objective and thorough, yet succinct, summary of the findings most relevant to the issues. To facilitate a balanced presentation of the findings, the authors were discouraged from presenting their own conclusions or recommendations in this section.

The "Discussion" section addresses the implications of the clinical research findings for DSM-IV. Authors were encouraged to delineate and discuss all meaningful options for resolving the issues (including those they might not favor) and to outline the advantages and disadvantages of each option.

In the "Recommendations" section, the authors present their own recommendations for DSM-IV based on their review of the literature. In a few instances, these recommendations were not shared by the respective Work Group. In such cases, the recommendations were revised or the authors were requested to be explicit regarding their disagreements and to indicate the advantages and disadvantages of the various options. Authors were also encouraged to make suggestions for future research that would be helpful to the authors of DSM-V.

It is unlikely that readers will agree with all the recommendations presented in these reviews. Many of the issues do not have clear or obvious solutions, and more or less plausible arguments can often be made for a variety of alternative viewpoints. Our efforts have been directed toward achieving solutions that provide an optimal balance between false positives and false negatives in the diagnostic process. The advance of fundamental understanding of mental disorders will undoubtedly provide much clearer (and probably often very different) answers to the questions raised here.

In preparing the first three volumes of the *DSM-IV Sourcebook,* we have kept in mind that not all readers will be interested in all the fine points concerning every issue. For this reason, the chair of each Work Group prepared an introductory section for each group of disorders, including an executive summary of the important points in each review. For those interested in pursuing a subject in more detail, the individual reviews discuss the questions at hand in much greater depth and provide extensive reference sections.

Thomas A. Widiger, Ph.D.
Allen J. Frances, M.D.
Harold Alan Pincus, M.D.
Michael B. First, M.D.
Ruth Ross, M.A.
Wendy Wakefield Davis, Ed.M.

References

American Psychiatric Association: Diagnostic and Statistical Manual of Mental Disorders, 3rd Edition. Washington, DC, American Psychiatric Association, 1980

American Psychiatric Association: Diagnostic and Statistical Manual of Mental Disorders, 3rd Edition, Revised. Washington, DC, American Psychiatric Association, 1987

American Psychiatric Association: DSM-IV Options Book: Work in Progress 9/9/91. Washington, DC, American Psychiatric Association, 1991

American Psychiatric Association, Task Force on DSM-IV: DSM-IV Draft Criteria 3/1/93. Washington, DC, American Psychiatric Association, 1993

Cooper HM: The Integrative Research Review: A Systematic Approach, Vol 2. Beverly Hills, CA, Sage, 1984

Frances AJ, Widiger TA, Pincus HA: The development of DSM-IV. Arch Gen Psychiatry 46:373–375, 1989

Frances AJ, Pincus HA, Widiger TA, et al: DSM-IV: work in progress. Am J Psychiatry 147:1439–1448, 1990

Widiger TA, Frances AJ, Pincus HA, et al: DSM-IV literature reviews: rationale, process, and limitations. Journal of Psychopathology and Behavioral Assessment 12:189–202, 1990

Widiger TA, Frances AJ, Pincus HA, et al: Toward an empirical classification for the DSM-IV. J Abnorm Psychol 100:280–288, 1991

World Health Organization: The ICD-10 Classification of Mental and Behavioral Disorders: Clinical Descriptions and Diagnostic Guidelines. Geneva, World Health Organization, 1992

Acknowledgments

DSM-IV has been a team effort, with more than 1,000 people (and numerous professional organizations) helping us in its preparation. The Task Force on DSM-IV and Work Group members have worked hard and cheerfully throughout the demanding process of developing DSM-IV. Without their energy and expertise, this project would not have been possible.

Bob Spitzer has our thanks for his untiring efforts and unique perspective. Norman Sartorius, Michael Rutter, Darrel Regier, Lewis Judd, Fred Goodwin, and Chuck Kaelber were instrumental in facilitating a mutually productive interchange between the American Psychiatric Association (APA) and the World Health Organization. Dennis Prager, Peter Nathan, and David Kupfer helped us in developing a novel data reanalysis strategy that has been supported with funding from the John D. and Catherine T. MacArthur Foundation.

There are several individuals within APA who deserve special recognition. Mel Sabshin's special wisdom and grace made even the most tedious tasks seem worth doing. The APA Committee on Diagnosis and Assessment (chaired by Layton McCurdy) provided valuable direction and counsel. We also thank the APA Presidents (Drs. Fink, Pardes, Benedek, Hartmann, English, and McIntyre) and Assembly Speakers (Drs. Cohen, Flamm, Hanin, Pfaehler, and Shellow), who helped with the planning of our work. Carolyn Robinowitz and her staff in the APA Medical Director's office provided valuable assistance in the organization of the project.

The energy, intelligence, and scholarship of the authors of the DSM-IV literature reviews have surpassed our highest demands and expectations. Each review was read and commented on by many authorities in the field. Reviews often went through as many as half a dozen revisions. We would like to thank all those who contributed to this tremendous effort (in particular, the Work Group chairs, literature review authors, and commentators) for their unflagging efforts and good nature throughout this effort.

Excellent administrative and editorial support was provided by Myriam Kline, Gloria Miele, Sarah Tilly, Willa Hall, Kelly MacKinney, Helen Stayna, Nina Rosenthal, Susan Mann, Joanne Mas, Nancy Vettorello, Nancy Sydnor-Greenberg, Cindy Jones, Rebekah Brown, and Stacey Tipp, without whose help these volumes would have been impossible. Finally, we thank Ron McMillen, Claire Reinburg, and Pam Harley for their expert production and editorial assistance.

We thank our patient readers. We hope that our efforts are useful to you.

Allen J. Frances, M.D.
Chair, Task Force on DSM-IV

Harold Alan Pincus, M.D.
APA Deputy Medical Director

Michael B. First, M.D.
Editor, DSM-IV Text and Criteria

Thomas A. Widiger, Ph.D.
Research Coordinator

Wendy Wakefield Davis, Ed.M.
Editorial Coordinator

Ruth Ross, M.A.
Science Writer

Section I

Mood Disorders

Introduction to Section I

Mood Disorders

A. John Rush, M.D.

This introduction provides an executive summary of the proceedings of the DSM-IV Mood Disorders Work Group through the stage of defining the options proposed in the DSM-IV Options Book (American Psychiatric Association 1991). What follows highlights the issues that were identified for each disorder and the rationale for each proposed option. Resolution of the options rests on field trial results and data reanalyses, which will be presented in later volumes of the DSM-IV Sourcebook, as well as logical consistency, ease of use, responses from the field, and efforts to avoid minor discrepancies between DSM-IV and ICD-10 (World Health Organization 1992).

Development of the Options

The Mood Disorders Work Group defined a list of relevant areas for potential revision based on one or more of the following rationales: 1) substantial data relevant to diagnostic reliability or validity had accumulated since DSM-III (e.g., rapid cycling bipolar disorder); 2) clinical and research reports had used diagnostic concepts or terms not operationalized in DSM-III (e.g., atypical symptom features, postpartum depression, bipolar II disorder); 3) new potential "entities" were recently reported (e.g., recurrent brief depression) or viewed as common in some settings (e.g., minor depression); 4) substantial debate surrounded either the definition or clinical relevance of an existing condition (e.g., melancholia, schizoaf-

Supported in part by NIMH Grant MH-41115 to the Department of Psychiatry, UT Southwestern Medical Center.

I thank Donna Shafer and David Savage for secretarial assistance and Kenneth Z. Altshuler, M.D., Stanton Sharp Distinguished Chair and Chairman for administrative support. Special thanks to the members of the DSM-IV Mood Disorders Work Group, to those who conducted the literature reviews, and to our many correspondents.

fective disorder); 5) previous operationalizations appeared to be logically muddled or clinically confusing (e.g., dysthymia); 6) if certain options under discussion were to be selected, certain entities would need clarification (e.g., should cyclothymic disorder be revised if bipolar II is adopted?); and 7) the "entity" was new in DSM-III-R (e.g., seasonal pattern) so that recent research should be reviewed to determine whether revisions were indicated.

Other issues, not specifically reviewed, were discussed and put forth as options by the Work Group based on feedback from practitioners (e.g., changing the term *major depression* to *major depressive disorder;* considering descriptors of course of illness as an alternative to diagnosing multiple mood disorders). Specific operational questions were also addressed by data reanalyses, logic, and/or clinical consensus (e.g., should there be a duration requirement for manic or hypomanic episodes?).

To resolve some issues, field trials and data reanalyses are being conducted (e.g., How long is a hypomanic episode? Can course descriptors be reliably used?). In other instances, a judgment call based on the literature reviews that appear in the following chapters, along with comments from the field and logical consistency, will form the basis for the decision. In most cases, we adhered to the principle of "do not change without an empirical basis" to resolve options. In some instances, data were available for DSM-III categories or criteria items but fewer or no data were available for DSM-III-R categories or criterion items. When there was little dissatisfaction with DSM-III-R, no options were proposed. When, based on clinical experience, DSM-III-R was generally viewed as less satisfactory than DSM-III, and data were available on DSM-III but not DSM-III-R, the option of returning to DSM-III was proposed (e.g., adding irritability, along with sadness, to the criterion mood symptom for major depression).

Given that the area of mood disorders is of substantial interest to many researchers and virtually all practitioners, the price of frivolous, cosmetic, or poorly documented changes is perhaps higher than for other areas in which research is only beginning and for which, therefore, clinical experience, logical consistency, and ease of use per se are the essential bases for revision. In some areas, the fact that there are few clear-cut data using DSM-III-R criteria, the current dissatisfaction of some clinicians and researchers (e.g., with the definition of seasonal depression), and the substantial data gathered by others (e.g., the study of seasonal affective disorder by Rosenthal et al. 1984) combine with the relative newness of the category or modifier (e.g., with seasonal pattern) to pose a philosophical debate on whether and how to revise. Ease of use or apparent utility of terms or concepts (e.g., for major depressive disorder) forms another relevant basis for proposing options, especially when "data" are not likely ever to be collected.

Another principle involved in selecting options was that the changes should not heighten the disparity between entities found in children, adolescents, and adults. If anything, changes should reduce disparity to facilitate use (e.g., including *irritable* as an alternative to *sad mood* in the mood item for major depression). The Work Group also recognizes that changes based solely on a single data reanalysis or field trial are on shaky scientific ground (i.e., a single study does not create a scientific fact without replication).

Furthermore, to facilitate comparison of data, minor wording changes in criteria may result from attempts to be compatible with ICD-10 and vice versa, where consensus can be obtained without violating the concept captured by the category. Conversely, when the concept itself is affected, options were generally not put forth, because they would have required substantial data not available at the time. For example, ICD-10 allows mild major depressive episodes to have fewer of the requisite nine symptoms than moderate or severe episodes of the same condition. DSM-IV does not present this as an option. In this case, the logical and conceptual bases for the DSM-IV option were discussed with the ICD-10 group, but a compromise was not feasible.

A final principle for an option to be considered was that new "categories" required substantial data, whereas modifiers of potential clinical relevance (not coded at the four-digit level) could be proposed with less, but still substantial, data as to clinical relevance. For example, cross-sectional symptom features (e.g., atypical, melancholic, psychotic) may be quite relevant to treatment selection and therefore of clinical value, even if the "entities" with different cross-sectional symptom features have identical etiologies. In addition, course modifiers (e.g., recurrent with good or poor interepisode recovery, with postpartum onset, with seasonal pattern) may have prognostic value and, therefore, implications for prophylactic treatment even though the entities do not have established etiological distinctions. In fact, current mood disorder diagnoses are still at the syndromal level, so that multiple etiologies are likely for even classical entities and a single etiology may apply to different entities.

Terminology Options

The Work Group and a number of other experts were polled to discuss adding the term *disorder* to the DSM-III-R mood entities because it helps clarify for patients, families, and society at large that these are disorders, not just bad moods of varying intensity or length, grumbling, or complaining. Thus, the options of renaming *major depression* as *major depressive disorder, dysthymia* as *dysthymic disorder,* and *depression not otherwise specified* (NOS) as *depressive disorder not otherwise specified,* are proposed.

Organizational Options

The major mood categories, including major depressive and dysthymic disorders and depressive disorder NOS, bipolar and cyclothymic disorders and bipolar disorder NOS, will be retained in DSM-IV. The group termed *organic mood disorders* in DSM-III-R will be retained, but an option is proposed to rename these as secondary mood disorders and move them into the mood disorders section to facilitate clinical use when considering the differential diagnoses of mood syndromes or symptoms. It is also proposed that mood syndromes induced by either prescribed medications or substances of abuse be identified as substance-induced mood disorders and be listed within the mood disorders section for similar reasons.

Bipolar II, recurrent hypomanic and major depressive episodes in the absence of manic episodes, is now subsumed under bipolar disorder NOS in DSM-III-R. An option for DSM-IV is to designate this as a category either under major depressive disorder, recurrent, or as a distinct bipolar category, bipolar II disorder.

Major depression will continue to be classified with single and recurrent episodes. An option for dysthymia is to narrow it so that if clear-cut major depressive episodes occur in the course of a chronic "dysthymic level" of symptoms, then major depressive disorder with antecedent dysthymic disorder could be diagnosed. Alternatively, dysthymic disorder may be modified specifically to include "pure" dysthymic disorder (without major depressive episodes) and dysthymic disorder with major depressive episodes. The reason for these options is that the term *dysthymia* currently refers to patients 1) without major depressive episodes, 2) with major depressive episodes, and 3) with prior major depressive episodes in prolonged but partial remission (albeit an incorrect usage). A clearer specification of course of illness has implications for continuation and maintenance treatment planning. Furthermore, different courses of similar symptomatic conditions may have implications for differential treatment selection or even for etiology (e.g., rapid cycling versus non–rapid cycling bipolar disorder). Because there is controversy regarding the reliability of such course descriptors and their prognostic value, both a field trial and a data reanalysis are under way to shed light on these issues.

An option for depressive disorder NOS may be to provide text examples or additional categories to include minor depression, recurrent brief depressive disorder, and/or mixed anxiety/depression (see below). The reasons for these options are 1) the high incidence of "less than major" symptoms in epidemiological and primary care populations, 2) their apparent clinical relevance (prognostic, treatment planning, health service use rate), and 3) the need to provide tentative definitions for research purposes. Conversely, whether these are "valid" disorders has not yet been fully agreed on. The premature creation of new disorders limits research concerning other equally plausible definitions. In addition, classifying patients as "disordered" when they experience only transient symptoms potentially increases both the cost and stigma associated with these illnesses.

Course Modifier Options

An option for DSM-IV is to further emphasize the prior course of illness for various diagnoses (including the mood disorders) because prior course of illness assists in 1) prediction of the course of a disorder in a patient over time (e.g., postpartum onset of mania or severe [psychotic] depression may herald a bipolar disorder), 2) planning continuation or maintenance treatments, 3) selection of acute treatment (e.g., light therapy for a seasonal pattern; anticonvulsants for rapid cycling bipolar disorder), or 4) distinguishing etiologically distinct disorders from each other (e.g., probands with highly recurrent major depressive episodes are more likely found in pedigrees with either recurrent major depressive or bipolar disorder) (Goodwin and Jamison 1990).

Symptom Feature Options

In DSM-III-R, some symptom features can be designated by a fifth digit (mild, moderate, severe, psychotic, etc.) or by the modifier *melancholic*. A third possibility is to add the modifier *atypical*. The following provides the background for evaluating each of these cross-sectional symptom feature groupings.

In DSM-III-R, psychotic symptoms (i.e., hallucinations or delusions) are specified as part of the severity descriptor for major depressive episodes for both bipolar and major depressive disorders. Psychotic features can now be, and in DSM-IV will continue to be, divisible into those that are mood congruent and mood incongruent, because the latter appear associated with a poorer prognosis and therefore a greater likelihood for extended neuroleptic treatment.

One option being considered is whether to make psychotic depressions a separate entity not on a severity continuum, because some data reveal that those with milder depressive symptoms can have psychotic features. On the other hand, breaking psychotic features from the severity continuum would likely cause a loss of fifth-digit coding and put such an entity on equal footing with other symptom modifiers (e.g., atypical) for which there may currently be less persuasive data.

Compared with DSM-III, DSM-III-R broadened the melancholic symptom features category and moved it to an unnumbered modifier status. The controversy concerns whether melancholic features have any relevance to treatment selection and whether they were optimally defined in DSM-III-R. Options being considered are 1) returning to the DSM-III listing but requiring *either* pervasive anhedonia *or* unreactive mood rather than both or 2) noting the key symptoms in the text while retaining the DSM-III-R definition. The rationale for retaining this modifier is that it predicts a positive response to electroconvulsive therapy (ECT) (Abou-Saleh and Coppen 1983; Crow et al. 1984; Gibbons et al. 1982; Mendels and Cochran 1968; Rao and Coppen 1979) and to tricyclic medication in some (Bielski and Friedel 1977; Prusoff and Paykel 1977; Prusoff et al. 1980; Simpson et al. 1988) but not all (Coryell and Turner 1985; Georgotas et al. 1987; Paykel et al. 1988) studies. When defined narrowly, these features are associated with a positive family history (Leckmann et al. 1984; McGuffin et al. 1987; von Knorring 1987); when defined more broadly, they are not (Andreasen et al. 1986; Zimmerman et al. 1985).

With regard to atypical symptom features, the definition varies among the groups studying them. Symptoms include overeating, oversleeping, weight gain, reactive mood, interpersonal rejection sensitivity, leaden paralysis, marked anxiety, sleep onset insomnia, and phobic symptoms. Two types, A (anxious) and V (vegetative), have been proposed (Liebowitz et al. 1984, 1988).

The rationale for the option to consider atypical symptom features as a modifier or category for DSM-IV is based on the potential clinical utility of identifying patients for whom tricyclic antidepressants are not particularly effective compared with monoamine oxidase inhibitors (MAOIs). This finding has been reported by some (Davidson et al. 1982; Himmelhoch et al. 1991; Klein 1989; Liebowitz et al. 1984, 1988; Quitkin et al. 1988, 1989, 1990; Thase et al. 1992;) but not all (Paykel et al. 1983; Ravaris et al. 1980) groups. Thus, the major argument for the atypical modifier is that tricyclic medications are not particularly effective in these patients, whereas MAOIs appear to be.

The argument against this grouping is that it is unknown whether this is a distinct entity. For example, do depressions with these symptom features run in families? Do they repeat across depressive episodes in individuals, or do they simply represent a phase of an illness that can change over time? Are depressions with atypical features associated with an identifiable, unique biology? What is the relationship between atypical and melancholic symptom features during an episode and over the course of the illness? Some preliminary follow-up data (Akiskal et al. 1978) suggest that atypical symptoms may be more likely to appear earlier in the course of major depressive disorder, whereas melancholic features are more likely to appear later. Finally, the optimal definition is yet to be agreed on, and reliability is not fully established.

Finally, catatonic features are seen with mood, schizophrenic, and general medical conditions, and thus, their presence does not imply an automatic diagnosis of schizophrenia. Therefore, the options to be considered include 1) noting the differential diagnosis under schizophrenia, 2) creating a listing of catatonic symptom features for each disorder grouping (i.e., mood disorders, schizophrenia, and psychiatric disorders due to general medical conditions) that is either a) a distinct list for each grouping or b) a common list to be noted as a modifier in all three groups, or 3) creating a stand-alone syndrome of catatonia and noting that the etiological basis may include any one of several disorder groupings.

The benefit of including a catatonic symptom modifier would be to alert practitioners to this presentation in each relevant section, because treatment selection is affected by the presence of these features. A separate and distinct catatonic symptom listing for each grouping would not only make clinical practice complex, but the data on which to generate such a list are very sparse. The option of including a stand-alone category for catatonic symptoms would require that such a syndrome exist independently of other recognized mental disorder groups, at least in a reasonable number of cases. Evidence for the latter is not abundant.

Options Among Bipolar Disorders

Bipolar Disorder

One option for bipolar disorder is to return to the DSM-III duration requirement for the minimum duration of a manic episode (e.g., 7 days) (except when patients are so severely ill that intervention is required before 7 days have elapsed). The argument for this option is that a display of manic symptoms for a day or less seems to lack clinical face validity. Furthermore, without a time frame for mania, rapid cycling is logically difficult to define. On the other hand, some patients (a minority) do in fact have episodes that last for less than 7 days. If the 7-day duration requirement is implemented, these patients would fall under bipolar disorder NOS, because they never experienced a manic episode that met the duration criterion. This will be resolved based on clinical impressions and compatibility with ICD-10.

Mixed-Phase Episode

The concept of a mixed-phase episode may logically require revision, especially if the rapid cycling course modifier (see below) is adopted. Currently, mixed phase has two related but potentially different clinical referents: 1) patients who switch or alternate quickly between short, severe depressive and manic episodes with no euthymic intervals or 2) patients with a mood episode during which (even within the same 24-hour period) symptoms meet criteria for both manic and major depressive episodes simultaneously without obvious shifts of polarity. If both the rapid cycling course modifier and the minimal duration criterion for a manic episode are adopted, then mixed phase would logically refer only to cases in which there is a simultaneous presentation that included both manic and major depressive symptoms. When there are rapid alternations between poles, this would be considered either rapid cycling bipolar I disorder (in which the 7- and 14-day requirements, respectively, for mania and for depressive episodes are met) or as bipolar disorder NOS.

Bipolar Disorder, Single Episode (Versus Recurrent)

The option of including bipolar disorder, single episode in DSM-IV is proposed to increase ICD-10 compatibility, to identify patients with a single manic episode and to preserve the unipolar-bipolar dichotomy. With the introduction of substance- and treatment-induced mood syndromes, it is logical not to change the diagnosis from major depressive disorder to bipolar when a patient has experienced a manic or hypomanic episode only when induced by prescription medications or substances of abuse, although the text may alert the reader to a higher risk of bipolar diathesis in some such patients, if the induction was treatment with a tricyclic or MAOI.

Bipolar II Disorder

Bipolar II disorder, recurrent major depressive and hypomanic episodes (Dunner et al. 1970, 1976a, 1976b), is not specifically identified in DSM-III-R, instead falling under the rubric of bipolar disorder NOS. If one or more manic episodes occur, the diagnosis is changed to bipolar I disorder. The rationale for the option of including bipolar II disorder as a specific category in DSM-IV includes the following: 1) bipolar II disorder has prognostic relevance (Coryell et al. 1989; Dunner 1983, 1987; Dunner et al. 1976a, 1976b); 2) family studies indicate that first-degree relatives of probands with bipolar II disorder have a higher incidence of bipolar II disorder than those of unipolar or bipolar I probands (Andreasen et al. 1987; Coryell et al. 1984; Endicott et al. 1985; Fieve et al. 1984; Gershon et al. 1982); 3) it signals a cautionary note in the use of antidepressant medication (although how common tricyclic-induced rapid cycling is in bipolar II disorder is not well established) (see Chapter 13, by Bauer and Whybrow, this volume); 4) it may raise the notion of lithium maintenance more strongly than for recurrent unipolar depression according to some (Dunner et al. 1982; Fieve et al. 1976) but not others (Kane et al. 1982); and 5) most adult patients with a bipolar II diagnosis do not develop bipolar I disorder over a 5-year follow-up (Coryell et al. 1989). This probably differs in children and adolescents, however (Carlson 1990).

To ensure that cases of recurrent major depressive disorder are not inappropriately converted into a bipolar disorder, however, a duration criterion (e.g., 3–7 days) for hypomanic episodes would be added. In addition, two options designed to reduce false positives are proposed: 1) including a stricter specification of a hypomanic episode as being distinctly different from the individual's usual self in a way that is observable by others and 2) possibly requiring more than one clear-cut hypomanic episode.

Another option is to place bipolar II disorder within the major depression, recurrent grouping, as proposed in ICD-10 (perhaps with a modifier *with hypomanic episodes*). Favoring this option is the evidence that family members of bipolar II probands have a high incidence of major depression. Against this option is the potential for confusion when practitioners encounter a bipolar course classified within a unipolar grouping. The final decision will rest on logical analysis and clinical input.

If a separate category for bipolar II disorder is adopted, bipolar disorder NOS would consist of various bipolar conditions with presentations that are insufficiently clear-cut to qualify for either formal bipolar I or II disorder. Examples include single or recurrent hypomanic episodes without interepisode subsyndromal depressive symptoms (which might lead to a diagnosis of cyclothymic disorder) or without major depressive episodes (which if present, would call for the diagnosis of bipolar II disorder). Further, a patient with bipolar disorder NOS might meet severity but not duration criteria for all previous and current major depressive or manic episodes.

Cyclothymic Disorder

To diagnose cyclothymia, DSM-III-R requires at least 2 years of mood symptoms with both "poles" observable and with few, if any, euthymic periods. Those with cyclothymic disorder often have multiple hypomanic episodes but, by definition, do not enter full major depressive episodes for a least the first 2 years. If bipolar II disorder is adopted, then an option for DSM-IV is for those with cyclothymic disorder who develop a major depressive episode to change their diagnosis to bipolar II disorder rather than carrying two mood disorder diagnoses. Favoring this option are logic, simplicity, and evidence that some individuals with cyclothymic disorder have a "bipolar" diathesis. Against it is a concern that those with a labile personality style and a "garden variety" major depressive episode may be incorrectly recruited into the bipolar II group. The use of higher thresholds (see above) for hypomania is proposed to protect against these potential false positives. Decisions will be based on logic, simplicity, and clinical consensus.

Course Modifiers

Bipolar disorders can exhibit seasonal or rapid cycling patterns, and the postpartum period may be a period of higher risk for the onset or exacerbation of these disorders. Seasonal patterns (especially fall onset, spring offset) have been reported for depressive episodes in both bipolar I and II disorders (the latter seem far more frequent). DSM-IV will likely continue the seasonal pattern modifier for bipolar disorders. The options are to retain the current DSM-III-R definition or to "expand the window" to only require three, rather than two, episodes and to allow greater clinical latitude in estimating the relationship between onset and offset of the depressive episode and season (i.e., to avoid the "pseudospecificity" that is inherent in specifying a 90-day window in onset/offset). Finally, some have reported summer-based rather than winter-based depressive episodes. Although it would seem logical to also designate these episodes as seasonal, there is a danger of creating, by chance alone, an extremely high incidence of seasonal episodes. In addition, light therapy has not been tested for efficacy in such "summer" episodes (i.e., the clinical value of identifying such episodes is not apparent).

The rapid cycling course modifier, an option for DSM-IV, could apply to bipolar I or II disorder or to bipolar disorder NOS. For bipolar I and II, it would require at least four mood (manic, hypomanic, or major depressive) episodes within the last year. For bipolar disorder NOS, a rapid cycling pattern could describe cases with four or more manic or major depressive episodes defined by symptom severity that did not meet duration requirements for these episodes within the preceding year.

In favor of the rapid cycling modifier are the following: 1) a disproportionate incidence of women has been found among rapid cyclers compared with nonrapid cyclers in most (Bauer et al. 1990; Dunner and Fieve 1974; Tondo et al. 1981; Wehr et al. 1988) but not all (Joffe et al. 1987) studies; 2) lithium alone appears less effective (Dunner and Fieve 1974; Prien et al. 1984; Wehr et al. 1988); 3) anticonvulsants may be particularly effective (Kishimoto et al. 1983; Okuma et al. 1981; Post 1988; Post et al. 1989); 4) prognosis is poorer (Dunner and Fieve 1974; Roy-Bryne et al. 1985; Wehr et al. 1988); 5) high-dose thyroid may be effective (Bauer and Whybrow 1990; Gjessing 1976; Stancer and Persad 1982); 6) thyroid axis disorders may cause rapid cycling (Bauer et al. 1990; Cowdry et al. 1983; Wehr et al. 1988); and 7) antidepressant medications contribute to a rapid cycling pattern in some people (Wehr and Goodwin 1979a, 1979b, 1979c; Wehr et al. 1988). Therefore, the course modifier would have relevance to treatment selection, prognosis, and the nature of the initial medical evaluation of such patients. Conversely, rapid cycling appears to be a phase in the course of bipolar disorder (i.e., at times patients display rapid cycling patterns, whereas at other times they do not) (Coryell et al. 1989), which suggests a lack of etiological differentiation at least in some cases.

Bipolar disorders usually have interepisode periods that are largely symptom free. The onset is typically precipitous (i.e., without antecedent psychopathology), although sometimes the initial episode of mania or depression is heralded by subsyndromal symptomatology (e.g., cyclothymic disorder, subsyndromaldepressive symptoms) (Goodwin and Jamison 1990).

Other options are for course modifiers to specify mood-related psychopathology before the first episode of mania, hypomania, or major depression and/or between formal mood episodes (e.g., with or without interepisode recovery). Favoring this option is the idea that antecedent mood symptomatology, if untreated, predicts subsequent degrees of interepisode recovery. The level of interepisode residual symptomatology may have prognostic value and logically provides a baseline by which to judge overall treatment efficacy. For example, when patients who have not previously exhibited interepisode symptomatology while not on antidepressant medication develop such symptoms on medication, they may need a medication change. Against this option are the following: 1) the prognostic value of such descriptors is not well established; 2) the system is complex; and 3) clinicians often use such information without a need for formal categories.

Another course modifier option is to specify whether manic or depressive episodes were precipitated in the postpartum period, which appears to be a high-risk period for those with an established or a newly expressed bipolar condition. Favoring this notation is the finding that episodes are likely to repeat in subsequent postpartum periods (Davidson and Robertson 1985; Paffenbarger et al. 1961; Protheroe 1969). The option is to provide a modifier "with postpartum onset" for major depressive and manic episodes in bipolar I or II disorders, for major depressive episodes in the course of major depressive disorder, and for acute psychotic episodes that have a postpartum onset, given the implications for prognosis and prophylaxis. Against the option is complexity and lack of etiological distinction and the ability to alert those using the manual to these findings in the text.

Schizoaffective Disorder

The definition of schizoaffective disorder in DSM-III-R is somewhat ambiguous and may mislabel some patients as having schizoaffective disorder who actually have schizophrenia or postpsychotic depressions. In addition, questions have been raised concerning the prevalence of this category and its performance in relation to longitudinal course, given the more narrow definition that followed as a consequence of allowing mood incongruent psychotic features. Finally, whether this diagnostic entity would be better characterized by a description of longitudinal course than by a diagnosis based only on the current episode was evaluated. The placement of schizoaffective disorder within the mood disorder or schizophrenia grouping was evaluated by reviewing the literature on prognosis, treatment, and familial loadings. The concern was to provide a clearer description of the condition itself that would ultimately facilitate clinical utility.

Options for Depressive Disorders

Few symptom or duration criteria options are proposed for major depressive disorder, which will continue to be classified as single episode or recurrent. Based on ongoing field trials, a higher threshold for the number of symptoms required (e.g., 6 or 7 of the 9 DSM-III-R criterion symptoms of major depression) could evolve. Alternatively, another option is adding a requirement of significant functional impairment, as in the Research Diagnostic Criteria (RDC) (Spitzer et al. 1978), that may better differentiate a troubled time (e.g., situational adjustment reaction or grief) from major depression. The issue concerns the possibility of falsely diagnosing major depression when transient adjustment disorder is present. The difficulty is whether impairment, symptom numbers, or even duration are sufficient to correct the problem. Clinical consensus, field trial results, and a conservative position (no data, no change) will contribute to the resolution.

Dysthymic disorder was reevaluated for the reasons noted above. In addition, the issue was raised whether symptoms specific to dysthymia (as opposed to major depression) could be identified, thereby providing for a greater differentiation between these two categories. There was concern that dysthymia might be excluding some who should be included or that major depression was including some for whom a diagnosis of dysthymia would be more appropriate.

The options included adding course modifiers for major depression and/or clarifying the symptom features. How to differentiate chronic major depression from dysthymia will be examined. The clinical and epidemiological issue here is that many dysthymic patients have episodes of major depression, whereas many patients have recurrent major depression with antecedent dysthymia, usually with poor interepisode recovery (i.e., a return to the baseline, antecedent dysthymic symptom level). How to optimally conceptualize and define these two disorders (or these two variants of the same disorder) is at question. The answers will rest on logic, consistency, ease of use, clinical consensus, and field trial findings.

No criteria are to be specified for depressive disorder NOS in DSM-IV, because its greatest clinical utility is in the identification of unclear cases. Case examples may be provided in the text. Another option is for some of these examples to become additional formal categories in and of themselves (either in DSM-IV itself or in an appendix). Three "less than major" groupings are under discussion.

Minor depression was defined by RDC as symptoms of major depression and other noncriterion symptoms of major depression that fluctuate over time but that are present for at least 2 weeks at a time. That is, minor depression is like major depression in duration and possibly course but not in severity. It may or may not have the chronic multiyear pattern seen in dysthymic disorder. Based on epidemiological studies, substantial short-term morbidity is associated with such "subsyndromal" depressive symptoms. Treatment responses, familial aggregation, biological findings, and relationship to personality disorders are yet to be clarified. Favoring the adoption of this category is epidemiological prominence and cost in terms of health care. Against such a move is the lack of validating data noted above and the lack of a full, general medical, and psychiatric evaluation of those identified as having minor depression by epidemiological interview methods.

A second entity, recurrent, brief depression, is characterized by recurrent (6–10 times/year), brief episodes (usually 3–7 days) that meet severity but not duration criteria for a major depressive episode. It occurs more often in females, is unrelated to the menstrual cycle, and is associated with a family history of mood disorders and substantial morbidity (Angst et al. 1990). The treatment implications for this category are under investigation. Favoring adoption of this option are 1) apparent epidemiological prominence, 2) the need for additional research in the area, and 3) compatibility with ICD-10. Against it are the lack of biological and treatment-response data; its relatively recent appearance on the research scene; lack of clarity about its relationship to personality disorders, particularly borderline personality; and substantial comorbidity with other mood and anxiety disorders.

Mixed anxiety/depression is an option being considered for DSM-IV. This entity would consist of some depressive and anxiety symptoms of the type found in major depressive and generalized anxiety disorders that do not meet and have not previously met criteria for other formal mood or anxiety disorders (e.g., major depressive, panic, or generalized anxiety disorders). Some practitioners feel that such patients are commonly encountered in primary care settings. Whether this is a distinct entity based on course, familial pattern, treatment response, and prognostic or biological findings has not been evaluated.

Turning to course modifiers, seasonal pattern for recurrent major depressive and bipolar disorders will be retained in DSM-IV because it has 1) implications for selecting phototherapy (Terman et al. 1989) and 2) prognostic significance (i.e., it repeats more often than not from year to year). Whether such a seasonal pattern is familial, is associated with a unique biology, predicts a good or poor response to specific antidepressant medications, or ultimately evolves into a nonseasonal or more chronic pattern are unanswered questions. The only debate (which has resulted in the proposed options) is whether the DSM-III-R window (60 versus 90 days) and the requisite number of prior seasonal episodes (3 versus 2) is too restrictive. In favor of broadening the criteria are the following considerations: 1) most research on light therapy has used the 90-day window and the two-episode requirement, and 2) there is a need for reimbursement availability for phototherapy without waiting for a third episode. Against it is 1) a concern that the broadened criteria will be too inclusive, causing an epidemic of light-box sales; 2) there are insufficient data to determine the epidemiological effect of changing the case definitions; and 3) there is continued skepticism by some concerning the efficacy of light therapy.

Major depressive episodes may display complete or only partial interepisode remission. In the latter case, 1) the likelihood of a subsequent episode is higher (Prien and Kupfer 1986), 2) the need for additional treatment may be indicated, and 3) the prognosis following subsequent episodes is for continuing incomplete interepisode recovery. For these reasons, an option for DSM-IV is to specify *with partial or with complete interepisode recovery* for major depression. Favoring this option is evidence that antecedent dysthymia is associated with poorer interepisode recovery, its potential use in planning continuation or maintenance treatment, and greater familial loading in this group. Against it is complexity, the ability to cover this issue with a second diagnosis (dysthymia), and the lack of etiological, biological, or treatment selection distinctness. The issue will be resolved by clinical consensus, response from the field, and field trial results.

Summary

A wide range of options for DSM-IV mood disorders have been proposed. The rationale for the specific options are detailed in the following chapters. A major concern is to strike a balance in selecting among the options so that clinicians and patients are optimally served. Judgments as to greater or lesser clinical relevance must be made based on data and consensus (e.g., Does treatment selection count more heavily than prognostic value? How much data are sufficient for a new category? How much data are sufficient for a change in criteria?). Ultimately, both science and clinical judgment must be combined to resolve these clinically relevant controversies. Obviously, the DSM-IV mood disorders section will not close the book on the classification of these disorders but will hopefully strike a balance between what is now known with reasonable certainty and what experienced clinicians find practical and useful.

References

Abou-Saleh MT, Coppen AP: Classification of depression and response to antidepressive therapies. Br J Psychiatry, 143:601–603, 1983

Akiskal HS, Bitar A, Puzantian V, et al: The nosological status of neurotic depression. Arch Gen Psychiatry 35:756–766, 1978

American Psychiatric Association: DSM-IV Options Book: Work in Progress. Washington, DC, American Psychiatric Association, 1991

Andreasen NC, Scheftner W, Reich T, et al: The validation of the concept of endogenous depression: a family study approach. Arch Gen Psychiatry 43:246–251, 1986

Andreasen NC, Rice J, Endicott J, et al: Familial rates of affective disorder. Arch Gen Psychiatry 44:461–489, 1987

Angst J, Merikangas K, Scheidegger P, et al: Recurrent brief depression: a new subtype of affective disorder. J Affect Disord 19:87–98, 1990

Bauer M, Whybrow P: Rapid cycling bipolar affective disorder, II: treatment of refractory rapid cycling with high dose thyroxine, a preliminary study. Arch Gen Psychiatry 47:434–440, 1990

Bauer M, Whybrow P, Winokur A: Rapid cycling bipolar affective disorder, I: association with grade I hypothyroidism. Arch Gen Psychiatry 47:427–432, 1990

Bielski RJ, Friedel RP: Subtypes of depression: diagnosis and medical management. West J Med 126:347–352, 1977

Carlson GA: Child and adolescent mania: diagnostic considerations. J Child Psychol Psychiatr 31:331–341, 1990

Coryell W, Turner R: Outcome with desipramine therapy in subtypes of nonpsychotic major depression. J Affect Disord 9:149–154, 1985

Coryell W, Endicott J, Reich T: A family study of bipolar II disorder. Br J Psychiatry 145:49–54, 1984

Coryell W, Keller M, Endicott J, et al: Bipolar II illness: course and outcome over a five-year period. Psychol Med 19:129–141, 1989

Cowdry R, Wehr T, Zis A, et al: Thyroid abnormalities associated with rapid cycling bipolar illness. Arch Gen Psychiatry 40:414–420, 1983

Crow TJ, Deakin JFW, Johnston EC, et al: The Northwick Park ECT trial: predictors of response to real and simulated ECT. Br J Psychiatry 144:227–237, 1984

Davidson J, Robertson E: A follow-up study of postpartum illness. Acta Psychiatr Scand 71:451–457, 1985

Davidson J, Miller R, Turnbull C, et al: Atypical depression. Arch Gen Psychiatry 39:527–534, 1982

Dunner DL: Subtypes of bipolar affective disorder with particular regard to bipolar II. Psychiatr Dev 1:75–86, 1983

Dunner DL: Stability of bipolar II affective disorder as a diagnostic entity. Psychiatr Ann 17:18–20, 1987

Dunner DD, Fieve R: Clinical factors in lithium carbonate prophylaxis failure. Arch Gen Psychiatry 30:229–233, 1974

Dunner DL, Gershon ES, Goodwin FK: Heritable factors in the severity of affective illness. Am J Psychiatry 123:187–188, 1970

Dunner DL, Fleiss DL, Fieve RR: The course of development of mania in patients with recurrent depression. Am J Psychiatry 133:905–908, 1976a

Dunner DL, Gershon ES, Goodwin FK: Heritable factors in the severity of affective illness. Biol Psychiatry 11:31–42, 1976b

Dunner DL, Stallone F, Fieve RR: Prophylaxis with lithium carbonate: an update (letter to editor). Arch Gen Psychiatry 39:1344–1345, 1982

Endicott J, Nee J, Andreasen N, et al: Bipolar II: combine or keep separate? J Affect Disord 8:17–28, 1985

Fieve RR, Kumbaraci T, Dunner DL: Lithium prophylaxis of depression in bipolar I, bipolar II and unipolar patients. Am J Psychiatry 133:925–929, 1976

Fieve RR, Go R, Dunner DL, et al: Search for biological/genetic markers in a long-term epidemiological and morbid risk study of affective disorders. J Psychiatr Res 18:425–445, 1984

Georgotas A, McCue RE, Cooper T, et al: Clinical predictors of response to antidepressants in elderly patients. Biol Psychiatry 22:733–740, 1987

Gershon ES, Hamovit J, Guroff JJ, et al: A family study of schizoaffective, bipolar I, bipolar II, unipolar and normal control probands. Arch Gen Psychiatry 39:1157–1167, 1982

Gibbons RD, Clark DC, David JM: A statistical model for the classification of imipramine response in depressed inpatients. Psychopharmacology 78:185–189, 1982

Gjessing R: Rhythm and periodicity, in Contribution to the Somatology of Periodic Catatonia. Edited by Gjessing L, Jenner A. Oxford, Pergamon, 1976

Goodwin FK, Jamison KR: Manic-Depressive Illness. New York, Oxford University Press, 1990

Himmelhoch JM, Thase ME, Mallinger AG, et al: Tranylcypromine versus imipramine in anergic bipolar depression. Am J Psychiatry 148:910–916, 1991

Joffe R, Kutcher S, MacDonald C: Thyroid function and bipolar affective disorder. Psychiatry Res 25:117–121, 1987

Kane JM, Quitkin FM, Rifkin A, et al: Lithium carbonate and imipramine in the prophylaxis of unipolar and bipolar II illness. Arch Gen Psychiatry 39:1065–1069, 1982

Kishimoto A, Ogura C, Hazama H, et al: Long-term prophylactic effects of carbamazepine in affective disorders. Br J Psychiatry 43:327–332, 1983

Klein DF: The pharmacological validation of psychiatric diagnosis, in Validity of Psychiatric Diagnosis. Edited by Robins L, Barrett J. New York, Raven, 1989

Leckmann JF, Weissman MM, Prusoff BA, et al: Subtypes of depression: family study perspective. Arch Gen Psychiatry 41:833–838, 1984

Liebowitz M, Quitkin F, Stewart J, et al: Phenelzine v imipramine in atypical depression: a preliminary report. Arch Gen Psychiatry 41:669–677, 1984

Liebowitz M, Quitkin F, Stewart J, et al: Antidepressant specificity in atypical depression. Arch Gen Psychiatry 45:129–137, 1988

McGuffin P, Katz R, Bebbington P: Hazard, heredity and depression: a family study. J Psychiatr Res 21:365–375, 1987

Mendels J, Cochran C: The nosology of depression: the endogenous-reactive concept. Am J Psychiatry 124:1–11, 1968

Okuma T, Inanaga K, Otsuki S, et al: A preliminary double-blind study of the efficacy of carbamazepine in prophylaxis of manic-depressive illness. Psychopharmacology 73:95–96, 1981

Paffenbarger RS, Steinmatz CH, Pooler BG, et al: The picture puzzle of the postpartum psychoses. J Chronic Dis 13:161–173, 1961

Paykel ES, Rowan PR, Rao B, et al: Atypical depression: nosology and response to antidepressants, in Treatment of Depression: Old Controversies and New Approaches. Edited by Clayton P, Barrett J. New York, Raven, 1983

Paykel ES, Hollyman JA, Freeling P, et al: Predictors of therapeutic benefit from amitriptyline in mild depression: a general practice placebo-controlled trial. J Affect Disord 14:83–95, 1988

Post R: Approaches to treatment-resistant bipolar affectively ill patients. Clin Neuropharmacol 11:93–104, 1988

Post R, Rubinow D, Uhde T, et al: Dysphoric mania: clinical and biological correlates. Arch Gen Psychiatry 46:353–358, 1989

Prien R, Kupfer DJ: Continuation drug therapy for major depressive episodes: how long should it be maintained? Am J Psychiatry 143:18–23, 1986

Prien R, Kupfer DJ, Mansky P, et al: Drug therapy in the prevention of recurrences in unipolar and bipolar affective disorders: report of the NIMH Collaborative Study Group comparing lithium carbonate, imipramine, and lithium carbonate-imipramine combination. Arch Gen Psychiatry 41:1096–1104, 1984

Protheroe C: Puerperal psychosis: a long-term study, 192–961. Br J Psychiatry 115:9–30, 1969

Prusoff BA, Paykel ES: Typological prediction of response to amitriptyline: a replication study. Int Pharmacopsychiatry 12:153–159, 1977

Prusoff BA, Weissman MM, Klerman GL, et al: Research diagnostic criteria subtypes of depression. Arch Gen Psychiatry 37:796–801, 1980

Quitkin F, Stewart J, McGrath P, et al: Phenelzine versus imipramine in the treatment of probable atypical depression: defining syndrome boundaries of selective MAOI responders. Am J Psychiatry 145:306–311, 1988

Quitkin F, McGrath P, Stewart J, et al: Phenelzine and imipramine in mood reactive depressives: further delineation of the syndrome of atypical depression. Arch Gen Psychiatry 45:787–793, 1989

Quitkin FM, McGrath PJ, Stewart JW, et al: Atypical depression, panic attacks, and response to imipramine and phenelzine. Arch Gen Psychiatry 47:935–941, 1990

Rao VAR, Coppen A: Classification of depression and response to amitriptyline therapy. Psychol Med 9:321–325, 1979

Ravaris C, Robinson D, Ives J, et al: Phenelzine and amitriptyline in the treatment of depression. Arch Gen Psychiatry 37:1075–1080, 1980

Rosenthal NE, Sack DA, Gillin JC, et al: Seasonal affective disorder: a description of the syndrome and preliminary findings with light therapy. Arch Gen Psychiatry 41:72–80, 1984

Roy-Bryne P, Post R, Uhde T, et al: The longitudinal course of recurrent affective illness: life chart data from research patients at the NIMH. Acta Psychiatr Scand Suppl 71:3–34, 1985

Simpson GM, Pi EH, Gross L, et al: Plasma levels and therapeutic response with trimipramine treatment in endogenous depression. J Clin Psychiatry 49:113–116, 1988

Spitzer RL, Endicott J, Robins E: Research Diagnostic Criteria: rationale and reliability. Arch Gen Psychiatry 35:773–782, 1978

Stancer H, Persad E: Treatment of intractable rapid-cycling manic-depressive disorder with levothyroxine: clinical observations. Arch Gen Psychiatry 39:311–312, 1982

Terman M, Terman JS, Quitkin FM, et al: Light therapy for seasonal affective disorder: a review of the efficacy. Neuropsychopharmacology 2:1–22, 1989

Thase ME, Mallinger AG, McKnight D, et al: Treatment of imipramine-resistant depression, IV: a double-blind, cross-over study of tranylcypromine in anergic bipolar depression. Am J Psychiatry 149:195–198, 1992

Tondo L, Laddomada P, Serra G: Rapid cyclers and antidepressants. Int Pharmacopsychiatry 16:119–123, 1981

von Knorring L: Morbidity risk for psychiatric disorders in relatives of patients with neurotic-reactive depression, in Anxious Depression: Assessment and Treatment. Edited by Racagni G, Smeraldi E. New York, Raven, 1987

Wehr T, Goodwin FK: Rapid cycling between mania and depression caused by maintenance tricyclics. Psychopharmacol Bull 15:17–19, 1979a

Wehr T, Goodwin FK: Rapid cycling in manic-depressives induced by tricyclic antidepressants. Arch Gen Psychiatry 36:555–559, 1979b

Wehr T, Goodwin FK: Tricyclics modulate frequency of mood cycles. Chronobiologia 6:377–385, 1979c

Wehr T, Sack D, Rosenthal N, et al: Rapid cycling affective disorder: contributing factors and treatment response on 51 patients. Am J Psychiatry 145:179–184, 1988

World Health Organization: The ICD-10 Classification of Mental and Behavioural Disorders: Clinical Descriptions and Diagnostic Guidelines. Geneva, World Health Organization, 1992

Zimmerman M, Coryell W, Stangl D: Iowa discriminant index for endogenous depression: family history correlates. Psychiatry Res 16:45–59, 1985

Chapter 1

Dysthymia

Martin B. Keller, M.D., and Cordelia W. Russell, B.A.

Statement of the Issues

The history of dysthymia in the nomenclature reveals a number of issues that continue to be questioned in regard to the criteria for diagnosing dysthymia. A literature review was compiled as part of the work of the DSM-IV Mood Disorders Work Group. Based on this review, several issues were selected as the basis for a field trial that is currently taking place. The questions that addressed regarding dysthymia in DSM-IV deal with 1) the need for further differentiation between dysthymia and major depression, 2) the role heterogeneity plays in the diagnosis of dysthymia, 3) whether there is an excess of dysthymia diagnoses, 4) the differentiation between dysthymia and personality disorders, and 5) the differentiation of dysthymia as it occurs in children/adolescents and adults.

Significance of the Issues

The significance of these issues for the diagnosis of dysthymia can be seen by their reappearance as controversial issues in the development of the term *dysthymia*. The following history highlights the changes in the diagnosis from Schneider's (1958) "dysthymic psychopaths" to the current DSM-III-R definition of dysthymia (American Psychiatric Association 1987).

We acknowledge the help of the following people who provided information on their research and added insight into this literature review: Drs. Hagop Akiskal, Jules Angst, David Barlow, James Barrett, Aaron Beck, Gabrielle Carlson, David Clark, Paul Chodoff, David Dunner, Allen Frances, Ellen Frank, Michael First, John Gunderson, Robert Hirschfeld, R.E. Kendall, Daniel Klein, Donald Klein, Gerald Klerman, James Kocsis, Peter Lewinsohn, Michael Liebowitz, John Markowitz, James McCullough, Ivan Miller, Katharine Phillips, Edward Rhoads, Norman Rosenthal, John Rush, William Sanderson, Tracie Shea, Robert Spitzer, Jonathan Stewart, Svenn Torgersen, Herman van Praag, and Myrna Weissman.

History and Significance of Dysthymia in the Nomenclature

Growing dissatisfaction with the use of the term *neurotic depression,* which was the most commonly diagnosed affective disorder in the DSM-II (American Psychiatric Association 1968; National Institute of Mental Health Biometrics Division Report 1975), led to the introduction of a number of alternative diagnostic categories in the literature, and finally, the DSM-II category "neurotic depression" was replaced by the DSM-III classification of dysthymia (American Psychiatric Association 1980; Silverstein et al. 1982). The main reason for this change was the belief that it was primarily the chronic "characterological" tendency to dysphoria that was the most meaningful dimension of neurotic depressions that were otherwise nosologically heterogeneous (Akiskal et al. 1978). Furthermore, the goal of having a more atheoretical and phenomenologically based definition led to classifying dysthymia under the affective disorders while recognizing that the affective components may be secondary to an underlying personality disorder (Akiskal et al. 1983).

Although dysthymia has been in the literature since it was coined by Karl Ludwig Kahlbaum (1828–1899), the term *dysthymic disorder* was rarely used until it was included in the psychiatric nomenclature in DSM-III in 1980 to categorize chronic depressions that were of a long duration but less severe than major depressive episodes. It was used to replace the DSM-II concept of neurotic depression. This revision arose as a result of studies showing substantial heterogeneity in neurotic depression (Akiskal et al. 1978; Kendall 1976; Kiloh et al. 1972; D. F. Klein 1974; Klerman et al. 1979; Paykel 1971) and a decision to create a diagnostic category based purely on phenomenology (Spitzer et al. 1980). An important aspect of this change is that, in DSM-III, dysthymic disorder is included on Axis I as an affective disorder, and there is no category for chronic depression in the personality disorder section of DSM-III. This basic structure has been maintained in DSM-III-R (American Psychiatric Association 1987), although there have been several important modifications from the DSM-III criteria.

Two precursors to the reintroduction of the term *dysthymic disorder* are *neurotic depression* in DSM-II and *depressive personality* (Chodoff 1972; Kahn 1975). These terms emphasize the temperamental traits of dysphoria, the repetitive neurotic tendency toward gloomy despair, and the nebulous distinction between depression (state) and personality (trait) in the chronic course of these low-grade depressions (Akiskal 1983a; Yerevanian and Akiskal 1979).

Two other terms used to describe chronic depression are *minor depression of at least 2 years duration* and *intermittent depression.* Both terms were defined in the Research Diagnostic Criteria (RDC) originally published in 1978 (Spitzer et al. 1978). These terms are very similar to the DSM-III and DSM-III-R diagnosis of dysthymia. The definitions require a depressed mood that is present most or all of the time for at least 2 years, which may be interrupted by brief periods of normal mood. The course and associated symptoms of dysthymia are of insufficient severity to meet the criteria for major depressive episode. Since 1978, the RDC categories of chronic minor and intermittent depression have been used in several investigations (Keller and Shapiro 1982; Rounsaville et al. 1980).

The substitution of dysthymia, a concept with strong affective connotations, for a psychological condition that was in the domain of neurotic pathology was criticized in articles by several prominent theoreticians and researchers (Cooper and Michels 1981; Frances 1980). The essence of their concern was that the inclusion of dysthymia as an affective disorder should have required criteria for the presence of vegetative symptoms. This essential criterion would have further classified the disorder and allowed a nonvegetative chronic depression to appear in the personality disorder section (Frances 1980). Their opinion was that this change illustrated the inevitability of theory in nosology and assumed that all affective disorders have biological characteristics in common (Cooper and Michels 1981). The proportion of psychiatrists who agree with this position is unknown.

Method

In the following sections, we attempt to review all literature reporting data bearing on the validity of dysthymia as a diagnostic entity and of the criteria for meeting the diagnosis. When possible, unpublished data sets were reviewed and summarized (with the authors' permission) if their data were relevant and were based on research studies that were methodologically rigorous. Finally, an attempt is made to synthesize these data and to propose recommendations for change in the DSM-IV criteria of dysthymia. The general principle is to only change the definition if data exist to support a change.

Studies of dysthymia conducted after 1980 have used criteria from both DSM-III and DSM-III-R to define the disorder. Criteria from both DSM-III and DSM-III-R are included to specifically document the changes made after 1980. DSM-III-R has only been in use since 1987; therefore, the majority of published studies reviewed made the diagnosis of dysthymia with DSM-III criteria.

Results

Definition

DSM-III.   Dysthymic disorder (or depressive neurosis) is defined in the DSM-III (1980) as a persistently depressed mood or a loss of pleasure. This is present, with periods of normal mood lasting no longer than a few months, for at least 2 years

(1 year for children) but is not of sufficient severity to warrant a diagnosis of major depression. During this episode, by definition, there are no delusions or hallucinations, and the episode has a chronic course with no clear onset.

The DSM-III criteria state that at least 3 of the following 13 symptoms must be present during the depressive episode: insomnia or hypersomnia; chronic tiredness or low energy level; feelings of inadequacy, loss of self-esteem, or self-deprecation; decreased effectiveness or productivity at school, work, or home; decreased attention, concentration, or ability to think clearly; social withdrawal; loss of interest in or enjoyment of pleasurable activities; irritability or excessive anger (in children, expressed toward parents or caretakers); inability to respond with apparent pleasure to praise or rewards; less active or talkative than usual or feels slowed down or restless; pessimistic attitude toward the future, brooding about past events; feeling sorry for oneself; tearfulness or crying; recurrent thoughts of death or suicide (DSM-III, p. 223).

Impairment for this disorder is considered mild or moderate unless there is a suicide attempt or a superimposed major depressive episode. Complications that do arise are considered similar to those of a major depression. If there is a superimposed major depressive disorder, the individual is likely to remain in a dysthymic disorder when recovered from the major depressive disorder. In the case of a major depressive disorder in partial remission for a period of 2 years, dysthymic disorder becomes an alternative diagnosis to major depressive disorder in partial remission.

This disorder, according to DSM-III, is considered more common in females, with onset usually occurring in early adult life. Some cases may begin in childhood or adolescence with predisposing factors of attention deficit disorder, conduct disorder, mental retardation, a severe specific developmental disorder, or a chaotic environment. For adults, predisposing factors include chronic psychosocial stressors, chronic physical disorders, or mental disorders such as personality disorders or unremitted affective disorders.

Other factors that may suggest dysthymic disorder when associated with depressive symptoms are obsessive-compulsive disorder, alcohol dependence, or chronic depressive disorder. Dysthymia may only be diagnosed if it is clearly different from the individual's normal mood. For children, dysthymic disorder may be superimposed on attention deficit disorder, organic mental disorder, or specific developmental disorder (DSM-III).

DSM-III-R: definitions and changes from DSM-III. The revised version of the DSM-III was published in 1987. As mentioned earlier, the basic structure of dysthymia remained unchanged in DSM-III-R, although there were several important modifications.

In DSM-III-R, dysthymic disorder is similarly defined as the presence of a persistently depressed mood that lasts most of the day or is present more often than it is absent over a 2-year period. One major difference in this revised diagnosis is the choice of symptoms to be reported on. In DSM-III, 3 of 13 symptoms were required for a diagnosis of dysthymia. For the DSM-III-R diagnosis, a patient must report at least 2 of the following 6 symptoms: poor appetite or overeating, insomnia or hypersomnia, low energy or fatigue, low self-esteem, poor concentration or difficulty making decisions, and pessimism. The symptoms of appetite and concentration were not present in the DSM-III diagnosis. Further changes require that a patient can never be without these symptoms for more than 2 months at a time.

Exclusion criteria for dysthymia in DSM-III-R include the presence of a major depressive episode during the first 2 years of the disturbance, a manic or hypomanic episode at any time in the patient's life, psychotic symptoms or the residual phase of schizophrenia, and/or the mood being sustained by a specific organic factor or substance. With the exclusion of psychotic symptoms, the exclusion criteria for the DSM-III-R are new additions to the diagnosis. In DSM-III, there is reference to such mental disorders as obsessive-compulsive disorder and alcohol dependence, stating that dysthymia can be clearly distinguished from these. This statement does not appear in the DSM-III-R criteria.

DSM-III-R also requires the specification of primary/secondary type and early/late onset (D. N. Klein et al. 1988b). The primary type indicates that the dysthymia did not occur exclusively during the course of another chronic nonmood Axis I or Axis III disorder; the secondary specification implies the converse. Early onset describes an onset before age 21 years, whereas late onset describes an onset age of 21 years or older. The age at onset specification has been proposed in DSM-III-R because of evidence suggesting that early onset characterizes a more homogeneous group.

The distinction between early and late onset was added to the DSM-III-R as a useful hypothesis to be studied. In 1988, a study was published that provided data to support the validity of the distinction between early- and late-onset dysthymia in DSM-III-R (D. N. Klein et al. 1988b). This study found that the early-onset group was more severe at the follow-up, had more prior episodes of major depression, and had a higher family prevalence of affective disorders, thus supporting a distinction. Other studies have been published that have not been able to substantiate the distinction between early and late onset, and some feel that early onset did not represent a qualitatively different state (Akiskal et al. 1980, 1981; McCullough et al. 1988; Miller et al. 1986).

The symptoms of dysthymia are similar to those of major depression. The two diagnoses differ only in severity and duration. In clinical practice, randomized clinical trials, and naturalistic studies, subjects diagnosed with dysthymia were most commonly seeking treatment for a superimposed major depression.

In cases where dysthymia follows directly after a major depression, the diagnosis is major depression in partial remission. If there has been a full remission from a major depressive episode for at least 6 months, before the development of dysthymia, then dysthymia can be diagnosed.

To date, we have not found any data that support the 6-month requirement.

ICD-10. The tenth revision of the International Classification of Diseases (ICD-10; World Health Organization 1989 draft) defines dysthymia as "a period of at least 2 years of constant or constantly recurring depression" that would include at least three of nine symptoms. These symptoms are a reduction in energy or activity, insomnia, loss of self-confidence or feelings of inadequacy, difficulty concentrating, often in tears, loss of interest or enjoyment in sex and other pleasurable activities, feeling of hopelessness and despair, a perceived inability to cope with routine responsibilities of everyday life, and pessimism about the future or brooding about the past. The ICD-10 definition of dysthymia differs from the DSM-III-R definition in severity. ICD-10 refers to a "constant or constantly recurring depression," whereas DSM-III-R refers to a depressed mood that is present "more days than not." The two diagnoses also differ in the number of symptoms that are possible for a diagnosis, and ICD-10 does not mention the diagnoses that cannot be superimposed onto dysthymia.

One of the main differences between ICD-10 and the DSM-III-R is that ICD-10 clearly differentiates between research and clinical guidelines for its diagnoses (Farmer and McGuffin 1989).

Epidemiology. The epidemiology of dysthymia (*chronic depression* in the earlier research) has been studied by surveying the lifetime prevalence of the disorder among various groups (Bland et al. 1988; Karno et al. 1987; Myers et al. 1984; Robins et al. 1984; Weissman et al. 1988a, 1988b). Chronic depression has been found to be common in these studies of community samples, with 2.7%–4.3% being diagnosed with dysthymia.

For the majority of these studies, the instrument used was the Diagnostic Interview Schedule (DIS) (Robins et al. 1981), whose reliability for the diagnosis of dysthymia has been questioned. In one study, dysthymia had a sensitivity of 20%, a specificity of 78%, and a kappa of .03 (Eaton and Kessler 1985, p. 186). The studies cited in support of the DIS are weakest in defending the assessment of dysthymia, because this diagnosis was changed to major depression in two evaluative trials (Robins et al. 1981, 1982). Neither report provided kappa statistics, sensitivity, or specificity for dysthymia. Epidemiologic studies of dysthymia in children and adolescents have not yet been conducted.

Clinical Description

Age at onset.   Until the late 1970s, depressive disorders, including dysthymia, were usually overlooked in children because they were thought to be changes that occur during adolescence. Two subclassifications of dysthymia that include an early age at onset have been proposed by Akiskal (1983a)—character spectrum disorder and subaffective dysthymia. Akiskal postulates a distinction in the developmental and symptomatological pictures of these disorders, with parental acrimony/divorce and parental loss in childhood being thought to provide the developmental roots of the characterological disturbance, and passivity, pessimism, self-reproach, and conscientiousness being manifest as part of the long-standing personality of subaffective dysthymic individuals (Akiskal 1983b).

A significant amount of research on early-onset dysthymia has been provided by Kovacs et al. (1984a, 1984b). The results have suggested that dysthymia has an earlier age at onset than major depression in children. The age range for the onset of dysthymia in school-age depressed children ranges from 6 to 13 years, and frequently precedes episodes of major depression (Kovacs et al. 1984b). Kovacs et al. (1984a) also report that a younger age at onset predicts a more prolonged episode of dysthymia.

In conclusion, Kovacs states that, although dysthymia and major depression are related, they represent separate disorders in school-age children. "Dysthymia may 'weaken' the [child] and prepare the ground for major depression" (Kovacs et al. 1984b, p. 648).

Roy et al. (1985) focused their study on patients who had met DSM-III criteria for dysthymia since adolescence. This study concerned the neuroendocrine and personality variables in dysthymic disorder. These dysthymic patients had significantly higher neuroticism scores and lower self-esteem, higher self-criticism, delusional guilt, and hostility. The dysthymic patients also had considerable impairment and maladjustment as suggested by rates of unemployment and neuroticism and hostility scores. These results substantiate the diagnosis of children and adolescents with early onset of dysthymia.

A recent study conducted by D. N. Klein et al. (1988c) concluded that there was a close relationship between primary early-onset dysthymia and major affective disorder. The study indicates that early-onset dysthymia may be a more severe form of affective illness.

Currently, no data have been collected that support a change in the criteria.

"Double depression."   One controversy in the classification of dysthymia stems from the overlap often found between dysthymia and major depression—"double depression" (Keller and Shapiro 1982). In a study conducted by Akiskal et al.

(1981), 90% of 137 outpatients originally diagnosed with dysthymic disorder were found to be complicated by major affective episodes. Perry (1985) found that all 23 of his subjects, who had been diagnosed with a definite personality disorder (who did not have an antisocial personality disorder) had been depressed for more than 50% of the time for 2 years or more. In this study, Perry found that 87% of borderline personality disorder patients who had dysthymic disorder also had a major depression and that 93% of patients with antisocial personality disorder who had a dysthymic disorder also had a major depression. Further research has shown that a high majority of those from a clinical population diagnosed with dysthymia go on to develop a major depression (Keller and Lavori 1984). In a prospective study of children, it was found that more than 70% of those originally diagnosed with dysthymia developed a major depression over a 5-year follow-up (Kovacs et al. 1984a, 1984b). "The use of the term `double depression' [was not meant] to denote a distinct disease entity which will have a unique pattern of familial aggregation" (Keller and Lavori 1984, p. 402). Rather it has been used to clarify phenomenology and assessment of course, particularly recovery and relapse.

The diagnostic term *"pure" dysthymia* has been used to distinguish individuals who develop dysthymia but do not go on to develop a superimposed major depression. Cases of pure dysthymia have been studied; however, the subjects are hard to find in clinical samples (Keller and Lavori 1984).

Comorbidity with disorders other than depression.   A modest amount of data have been collected since the publication of DSM-III that report that a high proportion of patients with dysthymia have comorbid disorders (Akiskal et al. 1981; D. N. Klein et al. 1988c; Markowitz et al. 1992; Weissman et al. 1988a, 1988b). Questions have been raised as to whether dysthymia occurs as a distinct disorder or merely as a complication of other primary mental disorders. On the other hand, the most frequent comorbid conditions (major depressive disorders, anxiety disorders, and cluster C personality disorders) share many defining criteria with dysthymic disorders. Therefore, much of the "comorbidity" may be artifactual. Finally, some of the comorbid conditions may represent either aspects of the dysthymic state (e.g., generalized anxiety, eating disorders) or complications (e.g., substance abuse) (Ross et al. 1988).

Follow-Up Studies

Duration of dysthymic episode.   In children, the average length of a dysthymic episode is significantly longer than a major depression, with 3 years being the average length for dysthymia and 32 weeks for a major depressive episode (Kovacs et al. 1984a). The duration can range from 2 to 20 years in an overall age study of dysthymia (Rounsaville et al. 1980). In these patients, the median duration is approximately 5 years (Keller and Shapiro 1982; Rounsaville et al. 1980). This is partly expected based on the definition of the criteria.

The choice of a 1-year duration for adolescents/children and 2 years for adults requires validation. One study has provided data supporting the 1-year duration of dysthymia in adolescents (Lewinsohn et al. 1993). In the adolescent sample in this study, 46 subjects had a lifetime diagnosis of dysthymia in which 47.5% had episode duration of less than 2 years. The mean episode duration was 2.8 years, with a standard deviation of 0.29 years (the mode of the distribution was 1 year).

Recovery.   It is important to diagnose both major depression and dysthymia to assess outcome (Keller and Shapiro 1982). A 2-year follow-up study by Keller and Lavori (1984) found that 97% of the patients studied had recovered from their major depressive disorder. Only 39% had recovered from the underlying acute and chronic phases of dysthymia. Thus, subjects with dysthymia are more likely than subjects with major depression (and no dysthymia) to continue to have depressive symptoms after 2 years of prospective follow-up.

A 2-year follow-up in a naturalistic study (Barrett 1984) found that 63% of the subjects claimed no improvement and, in some cases, reported a more severe illness. After 2 years, 61% of the patients with double depression had not recovered from the underlying dysthymic disorder (Keller et al. 1983).

These results substantiate the term *double depression* and support the inclusion of dysthymia as a separate diagnosis from major depression.

Relapse/recurrence.   Keller et al. (1983) studied a group of 66 patients, originally diagnosed with double depression, who had recovered from their major depression. These patients were studied at 6-month intervals over a 1-year period to determine the amount of relapse found in cases of double depression.

Overall, during the year, 25 (38%) of the patients recovered from chronic minor depression, 24 (36%) relapsed into an RDC major affective disorder, and 17 (26%) remained in a state of chronic minor depression. In the first 6 months of the first year of recovery, 20 patients (30%) recovered from their chronic minor depression, 12 (18%) relapsed into a major affective disorder, and 34 (52%) remained in a chronic depression. During the second 6-month interval, 34 patients remained in a chronic minor depression, 5 (15%) recovered from their chronic minor depression, and 12 (35%) relapsed into a major affective disorder.

This study indicates that over a 1-year period after recovery from major depression, patients with double depression have an increased chance of relapsing into a major affective episode and a decreased chance of recovering from a chronic minor depression.

Delineation From Other Disorders: Exclusion Criteria

Primary/secondary dysthymia. The primary/secondary subtype of major depression was originated by the Washington University Group (Robins and Guze 1972). As mentioned earlier, this distinction has been published by Friedman et al. (1982) in relation to dysphoria. The results indicate that, in general, the presence of a prior nonaffective disorder and the presence of a concurrent disorder (also known as comorbidity) predicts a more pernicious course for the affective disorder. This does not validate primary/secondary as separate "diseases" but does provide a meaningful prognostic distinction for research and clinical practice. The evidence for the validity or "usefulness" of this classification of dysthymia needs to be investigated.

Chronic major depression and dysthymia. The following distinctions between chronic major depression and dysthymia are conceptual statements by researchers in the field that are not yet supported by data.

Some researchers in the field feel that it would be best to define dysthymia (relative to major depression) in terms of severity and chronicity differences rather than qualitative differences. The most typical course would consist of an insidious onset of symptoms at an early age followed by a fluctuating or progressive course that will often meet current diagnostic criteria for major depression. This may represent a more severe and malignant form of typical recurrent unipolar affective disorder than the episodic type, as suggested by the reports of increased family rates of affective illness and poor outcome. Some of these cases, however, seem highly responsive to treatment with antidepressant medication. The differences are quantitative based on severity and chronicity and not qualitative. One suggestion is the possibility of a category of unipolar depressive disorder that includes major depression and dysthymia and that chronicity and severity be the fourth-digit modifier.

The feeling, therefore, is that whenever dysthymia and major depression coexist, regardless of which came first, there is a unitary phenomenon that can only be differentiated on a severity and chronicity continuum.

The information listed above is open to many interpretations and does not lead to unequivocal conclusions on this issue. However, the data do substantiate the need for further research into this issue.

Depressive personality. Depressive personality in DSM-I and DSM-II was defined under the category of neurotic depression. In addition to depressive personality, this category also included depressions that were not endogenous, psychotic, or manic depressive. As mentioned earlier, this term was deleted from DSM-III in 1980 when the diagnosis of dysthymia was established.

The proposal has been made to include the diagnosis of depressive personality disorder in DSM-IV (see Phillips et al., Chapter 33, this volume). The argument is that the diagnosis of dysthymia is broad in the way it is currently formulated, and it does not serve as a depressive personality disorder. "Dysthymia as a concept connotes that the depression is merely long-standing, not characterological."

Another notable difference between the two types of diagnoses is that the features of the Axis I diagnosis of dysthymia are more somatic than cognitive. The only cognitive symptoms are lowered self-esteem and hopelessness. The proposal for a depressive personality disorder states three requirements for a depressive personality that would distinguish it from dysthymia. These requirements are an early-onset/lifelong pattern, features that are part of a personality structure or character, and features that are more cognitive and interpersonal than somatic.

Data are being gathered in the DSM-IV field trial on mood disorders to determine whether there is empirical evidence to distinguish depressive personality from dysthymia.

Generalized anxiety disorder.   D. N. Klein et al. (1988c) reported a lifetime prevalence of 56% for anxiety disorders in a sample of 32 early-onset dysthymic patients (types of anxiety disorders were not reported). Alnaes and Torgersen (1988) reported a strong overlap between dysthymia and generalized anxiety disorder.

Discussion

As a result of this review, various proposals were put forward for the diagnosis of dysthymia. This review indicates that there would be value in further differentiating the criteria for dysthymia, major depression, and depressive personality disorder. For this reason, the proposals originally put forward further emphasized the distinctive qualities of dysthymia that have been found in the research over the past 10 years. The symptom list was expanded, and the overall definition of the disorder was revised in these original proposals. The definition of dysthymia that the Work Group is aiming for is one that further distinguishes dysthymia from major depression.

Three other changes have been suggested to further clarify and classify the diagnosis of dysthymia (Kocsis and Frances 1987). The first suggestion is to make a further distinction in severity threshold between dysthymia and major depression. The current diagnostic system may be creating a high prevalence of double depression because of the close relationship of symptoms in the two disorders. One proposal is to increase the severity of the criteria for major depression, thus decreasing the number of individuals with dysthymia and increasing the distinction between major depression and dysthymia.

A second suggestion that has been made after a review of the changes in symptoms between DSM-III and DSM-III-R is that cognitive and functional symptoms are the most characteristic of dysthymic disorder and should be included in the diagnostic system (Kocsis and Frances 1987).

As mentioned earlier, Cooper and Michels (1981) suggested the inclusion of vegetative symptoms to further classify dysthymia as an affective disorder.

Recommendations

Based on the studies that have been reviewed and the comments from clinicians in the field, the following proposal of optional changes for the diagnosis for dysthymia has been put forward.

The number of symptoms possible for the diagnosis of dysthymia were shortened between DSM-III and DSM-III-R. It is felt that these symptoms may not accurately represent the disorder. The DSM-IV mood disorders field trial is in the process of testing the presence and accuracy of the DSM-III, DSM-III-R, and ICD-10 symptoms of dysthymia to determine the most representative set of symptoms for the disorder.

Another option for DSM-IV is to diagnose only pure dysthymic patients and exclude patients with a superimposed major depression. One other option is to either keep the subtypes of primary versus secondary and early- versus late-onset dysthymia, or substitute for these subtypes a criterion stating that dysthymia is a disorder with an insidious or indistinct onset of depressed mood (e.g., "my whole life," "since I can remember").

These options are being tested in the DSM-IV mood disorders field trial. After analysis from data obtained through the field trial, final decisions will be made for dysthymia in DSM-IV.

References

Akiskal HS: Dysthymic disorder: psychopathology of proposed chronic depressive subtypes. Am J Psychiatry 140:11–21, 1983a

Akiskal HS: Dysthymic and cyclothymic disorders: a paradigm for high risk research in psychiatry, in The Affective Disorders. Edited by Davis JM, Mass JW. Washington, DC, American Psychiatric Press, 1983b, pp 211–231

Akiskal HS, Bitar AH, Puzantian MD, et al: The nosologic status of major depression: a prospective three- to four-year follow-up examination in light of the primary-secondary distinction and unipolar bipolar dichotomies. Arch Gen Psychiatry 35:756–766, 1978

Akiskal HS, Rosenthal TL, Haykel RF, et al: Characterological depressions: clinical and sleep EEG findings separating "subaffective dysthymia" from "character spectrum disorders." Arch Gen Psychiatry 37:777–783, 1980

Akiskal HS, King D, Rosenthal TL, et al: Chronic depression, part I: clinical and familial characteristics in 137 probands. J Affect Disord 3:297–315, 1981

Akiskal HS, Hirschfeld RMA, Yerevanian BI: The relationship of personality to affective disorders: a critical review. Arch Gen Psychiatry 40:801–810, 1983

Alnaes R, Torgersen S: DSM-III symptom disorders (Axis I) and personality disorders (Axis II) in an outpatient population. Acta Psychiatr Scand 78:348–353, 1988

American Psychiatric Association: Diagnostic and Statistical Manual of Mental Disorders, 2nd Edition. Washington, DC, American Psychiatric Association, 1968

American Psychiatric Association: Diagnostic and Statistical Manual of Mental Disorders, 3rd Edition. Washington, DC, American Psychiatric Association, 1980

American Psychiatric Association: Diagnostic and Statistical Manual of Mental Disorders, 3rd Edition, Revised. Washington, DC, American Psychiatric Association, 1987

Barrett J: Naturalistic change over two years in neurotic depressive disorders (RDC categories). Compr Psychiatry 25(4):404–418, 1984

Bland RC, Orn H, Newman SC: Lifetime prevalence of psychiatric disorders in Edmonton. Acta Psychiatr Scand 77:24–32, 1988

Chodoff P: The depressive personality: a critical review. Arch Gen Psychiatry 27:665–673, 1972

Cooper AM, Michels R: Book review, American Psychiatric Association: Diagnostic and Statistical Manual of Mental Disorders, 3rd Edition. Am J Psychiatry 138:128–129, 1981

Eaton WW, Kessler LG (eds): Epidemiologic Field Methods in Psychiatry: The Epidemiologic Catchment Area Program. New York, Academic Press, 1985

Farmer A, McGuffin P: Annotation: the classification of the depressions: contemporary confusions revisited. Br J Psychiatry 155:437–443, 1989

Frances AJ: The DSM-III personality disorders section: a commentary. Am J Psychiatry 137:1050–1054, 1980

Friedman R, Clarkin J, Lorn R, et al: DSM-III and affective pathology in hospitalized adolescents. J Nerv Ment Dis 170(9):511–521, 1982

Kahn E: The depressive character. Folia Psychiatrica et Neurologica Japonica 29:290–303, 1975

Karno M, Hough RL, Burnam AM, et al: Lifetime prevalence of specific psychiatric disorders among Mexican Americans and non-Hispanic whites in Los Angeles. Arch Gen Psychiatry 44:695–701, 1987

Keller MB, Lavori PW: Double depression, major depression and dysthymia: distinct entities or different phases of a single disorder? Psychopharmacol Bull 20(3):399–402, 1984

Keller MB, Shapiro RW: "Double depression": superimposition of acute depressive episodes on chronic affective disorders. Am J Psychiatry 139(4):438–442, 1982

Keller MB, Lavori PW, Endicott J, et al: "Double depression": two year follow-up. Am J Psychiatry 140(6):689–694, 1983

Kendell RE: The classification of depression: a review of contemporary confusion. Br J Psychiatry 129:15–28, 1976

Kiloh LG, Andrews G, Neilson M, et al: The relationship of the syndromes called endogenous and neurotic depression. Br J Psychiatry 121:183–196, 1972

Klein DF: Endogenomorphic depression: a conceptual and terminological revision. Arch Gen Psychiatry 31:447–454, 1974

Klein DN, Clark DC, Dansky L, et al: Dysthymia and the offspring of parents with primary unipolar affective disorder. J Abnorm Psychol 97(3):265–274, 1988a

Klein DN, Taylor EB, Dickstein S, et al: The early-late onset distinction in DSM-III-R dysthymia. J Affect Disord 14:25–33, 1988b

Klein DN, Taylor EB, Dickstein S, et al: Primary early-onset dysthymia: comparison with primary nonbipolar nonchronic major depression on demographic, clinical, familial, personality, and socioenvironmental characteristics and short-term outcome. J Abnorm Psychol 97:387–398, 1988c

Klerman GL, Endicott J, Spitzer R, et al: Neurotic depressions: systematic analysis of multiple criteria and meanings. Am J Psychiatry 136:57–61, 1979

Kocsis JH, Frances AJ: A critical discussion of DSM-II dysthymic disorder. Am J Psychiatry 144(12):1534–1542, 1987

Kovacs M, Feinberg TL, Crouse-Novak M, et al: Depressive disorders in childhood: I. Arch Gen Psychiatry 41:229–237, 1984a

Kovacs M, Feinberg TL, Crouse-Novak M, et al: Depressive disorders in childhood: II. Arch Gen Psychiatry 41:643–649, 1984b

Lewinsohn PM, Hops H, Roberts RE, et al: Adolescent psychopathology, I: prevalence and incidence of depression and other DSM-III-R disorders in high school students. J Abnorm Psychol 102:133–144, 1993

Markowitz JC, Moran ME, Kocsis JH, et al: Prevalence and co-morbidity of dysthymic disorder among psychiatric outpatients. J Affect Disord 24:63–71, 1992

McCullough JP, Kasnetz MD, Braith JA, et al: A longitudinal study of an untreated sample of predominantly late onset characterological dysthymia. J Nerv Ment Dis 176(11):658–667, 1988

Miller IW, Normal WH, Dow MG: Psychosocial characteristics of "Double Depression." Am J Psychiatry 143(8):1042–1044, 1986

Myers JM, Weissman MM, Tischler GL, et al: Six-month prevalence of psychiatric disorders in three communities, 1980–1982. Arch Gen Psychiatry 41:959–967, 1984

National Institute of Mental Health Biometrics Division Report, 1975

Paykel ES: Classification of depressed patients: a cluster analysis derived grouping. Br J Psychiatry 118:275–288, 1971

Perry JP: Depression in borderline personality disorder: lifetime prevalence at interview and longitudinal course of symptoms. Am J Psychiatry 142(1):15–21, 1985

Robins E, Guze SB: Classification of affective disorders: the primary-secondary, the endogenous, and the neurotic-psychotic concepts, in Recent Advances in the Psychobiology of Depressive Illness. Edited by Williams TA, Katz MM, Sheild JA. Washington, DC, Department of Health, Education and Welfare, 1972

Robins LN, Helzer JE, Croughan J, et al: National Institute of Mental Health diagnostic interview schedule: its history, characteristics and validity. Arch Gen Psychiatry 38:381–389, 1981

Robins LN, Helzer JE, Ratcliff KS, et al: Validity of diagnostic interview schedule, version II: DSM-III diagnoses. Psychol Med 12:855–870, 1982

Robins LN, Helzer JE, Weissman MM, et al: Lifetime prevalence of specific psychiatric disorders in 3 sites. Arch Gen Psychiatry 41:949–958, 1984

Ross HE, Glaser FB, Germanson T: The prevalence of psychiatric disorders in patients with alcohol or other drug problems. Arch Gen Psychiatry 45:1023–1031, 1988

Rounsaville BJ, Shokomskas D, Prusoff BA: Chronic mood disorders in depressed outpatients: diagnosis and response to pharmacotherapy. J Affect Disord (2):72–88, 1980

Roy A, Sutton M, Pickar D: Neuroendocrine and personality variables in dysthymic disorder. Am J Psychiatry 142:94–97, 1985

Schneider K: Psychopathic Personalities, translated by MW Hamilton. London, Cassell, 1958

Silverstein ML, Warren RA, Harrow M, et al: Changes in diagnosis from DSM-II to Research Diagnostic Criteria and DSM-III. Am J Psychiatry 139(3):366–368, 1982

Spitzer RL, Endicott J, Robins E: Research Diagnostic Criteria: rationale and reliability. Arch Gen Psychiatry 35:773–782, 1978

Spitzer RL, William JBW, Skodol AE: DSM-III: the major achievements and an overview. Am J Psychiatry 137:151–164, 1980

Weissman MM, Leaf PJ, Bruce ML, et al: The epidemiology of dysthymia in five communities: rates, risks, co-morbidity and treatment. Am J Psychiatry 145:815–819, 1988a

Weissman MM, Leaf PJ, Tischler GL, et al: Affective disorders in five United States communities. Psychol Med 18:141–153, 1988b

World Health Organization: ICD-10 Chapter V. Diagnostic Criteria for Research. Mental and Behavioral Disorders (Including Disorders of Psychological Development). World Health Organization, Geneva, 1989 draft for field trials

Yerevanian BI, Akiskal HS: "Neurotic," characterological, and dysthymic depression. Psychiatr Clin North Am 2:595–617, 1979

Chapter 2

Cyclothymic Disorder

Robert H. Howland, M.D., and Michael E. Thase, M.D.

Statement of the Issues

The DSM-III-R (American Psychiatric Association 1987) criteria for cyclothymia specify that there be no clear evidence of a major depressive or manic episode during the first 2 years of the mood disturbance, thus distinguishing it from the residual symptoms of a bipolar disorder in partial remission. An important issue, however, is whether such patients without an initial major affective episode will continue to have subsyndromal mood symptoms or will later develop the more severe symptoms of bipolar disorder. A proposal for DSM-IV suggests that patients with cyclothymic disorder should never meet the criteria for a major affective episode rather than restricting this exclusionary criteria to the first 2 years of the disorder. Patients with cyclothymic symptoms who have ever had a major affective episode would be classified as having a subtype of bipolar disorder, thus leaving a more homogeneous group of patients with subsyndromal (cyclothymic) symptoms. In this chapter, the current concept of cyclothymia is reviewed, which permits an examination of the relationship between cyclothymia and other specific affective disorders and helps clarify the diagnostic validity of cyclothymic disorder within the classification of affective disorders.

Significance of the Issues

Over the past decade, chronic subsyndromal affective disorders, such as cyclothymic disorder, have been the subject of increasing clinical and research interest

Completion of this manuscript was supported in part by NIMH Grant MH-30915 (MHCRC) and a Young Investigator Award from the National Alliance for Research on Schizophrenia and Depression. We thank Lisa Stupar for assistance in preparation of the manuscript.

(Howland 1992). One reason for this interest is a growing awareness that these conditions are not rare, yet they have received little formal attention from both clinicians and researchers. Another reason is the renewed controversy about such conditions and whether they are personality disorders or affective disorders. This controversy was sharpened in 1980, when chronic mild affective conditions were removed from the category of personality disorders or neuroses where they had been placed in DSM-II (American Psychiatric Association 1968) and placed within the section on affective disorders in DSM-III (American Psychiatric Association 1980). This change resulted in the classification of cyclothymia as a subsyndromal variant of bipolar disorder. An important unresolved issue, however, is the possible heterogeneity of cyclothymia and its relationship to diagnostically similar disorders.

Resolving this issue is important to the clinician because the diagnosis may have a significant impact on the choice of treatment. Also, for the researcher, diagnostic sensitivity and specificity are important because they will help identify a group of patients who have a more homogeneous disorder that can then be studied to better understand the pathophysiology and treatment of the illness. Thus, the proposal by the DSM-IV Work Group to distinguish between cyclothymic patients with and without any major affective episodes at any time during their mood disturbance is an attempt to define a homogeneous disorder with subsyndromal cyclothymic symptoms that is distinct from bipolar disorder and can be studied in its own right.

Method

Establishing diagnostic validity is a process that requires attention not only to descriptive clinical variables but also to data from laboratory studies, family history, treatment response, and longitudinal course. In this chapter, the concept of cyclothymia is reviewed in this framework (Howland and Thase 1993). This helps to clarify the diagnostic validity of cyclothymic disorder within the larger domain of affective disorders and to determine the extent of the heterogeneity that exists in the current definition of cyclothymia, in light of the DSM-IV Work Group's proposal to limit it to a more homogeneous subsyndromal condition. This review primarily includes literature on the clinical phenomenology, family history, biology, and treatment of cyclothymia published during the past 15 years, because formal diagnostic criteria have only been available during this time. In addition, the relationship of cyclothymic disorder to dysthymic disorder, personality disorders, and bipolar II and rapid cycling bipolar disorders is examined.

Results

Clinical Phenomenology

Cyclothymic disorder is a chronic biphasic disorder manifesting brief and/or mild episodes of hypomania and depression. The types of individual symptoms do not appear to distinguish cyclothymic disorder from other affective disorders, although the depressive episodes may be marked by psychomotor retardation and hypersomnia, which is more characteristic of bipolar depression (Akiskal et al. 1977; Depue et al. 1981; Jelliffe 1911). Despite general agreement regarding the use of typical hypomanic and depressive symptoms in the diagnostic criteria for cyclothymic disorder, there is significant diversity in the literature regarding how these symptoms are defined and used by researchers to distinguish cyclothymic disorder from normal mood states and from more severe conditions such as bipolar I and bipolar II disorders (Coryell 1982; Dunner et al. 1982). These diagnostic problems make it difficult to compare clinical data regarding cyclothymic disorder from different studies. They also make it difficult to assess the longitudinal course and outcome of cyclothymic disorder, which is important for understanding the relationship between cyclothymic disorder and bipolar disorder.

The onset of cyclothymic disorder is early in life (Akiskal et al. 1977; Dunner et al. 1982) and may not be significantly different from that of bipolar disorder (Peselow et al. 1982a). In contrast to the relatively equal sex distribution found in bipolar disorder, many studies have reported a predominance of females among patients with cyclothymic disorder (Akiskal et al. 1977; Depue et al. 1981; Dunner et al. 1982), but this was not found in a larger epidemiological study (Weissman and Myers 1978). Prevalence rates for cyclothymic disorder, cyclothymic personality, or cyclothymic temperament range from 0.4% to 9.2% (Akiskal et al. 1977, 1979; Depue et al. 1981; Kraepelin 1921; Weissman and Myers 1978; Wetzel et al. 1980), which can be compared to the approximate 1% lifetime prevalence of bipolar disorder.

Despite the importance of understanding the course and outcome of cyclothymic disorder, there has been very little systematic study of this issue. Many early writers believed cyclothymia (or cyclothymic temperament) frequently developed into manic-depressive psychoses, but this was not inevitable in all patients (Jelliffe 1911). Kraepelin (1921) determined that only 53% of his patients with a cyclothymic temperament developed manic-depressive psychoses; it is not clear from his work how many patients with manic-depressive psychoses had evidence of premorbid cyclothymia. In a prospective follow-up study of 50 patients with cyclothymic disorder, Akiskal et al. (1979) found that 36% developed bipolar disorder over a 1- to 2-year period. The same research group prospectively followed

10 cyclothymic children and adolescents who were first-degree relatives of bipolar probands over a 3-year period and reported that 7 subsequently developed a bipolar disorder (Akiskal et al. 1985). Finally, Waters (1979) retrospectively reviewed 33 cases of bipolar disorder and found that 33% manifested premorbid behaviors that were consistent with cyclothymic disorder.

Some of the clinical and demographic features of cyclothymic disorder are summarized in Table 2–1. These studies all support a strong clinical pheno-menological association between bipolar disorder and at least one subtype of cyclothymic disorder. Together with the findings that cyclothymic disorder may be more prevalent and have a more uneven sex distribution than bipolar disorder, these results suggest that cyclothymic disorder is clinically heterogeneous and is neither a necessary nor a sufficient condition for the later development of bipolar disorder (Wetzel et al. 1980). More systematic and long-term follow-up studies are needed to further clarify this relationship and define other possible clinical subtypes of cyclothymic disorder (Howland and Thase 1993).

Family History

Compared with clinical and follow-up studies, there have been a far greater number of family history studies of cyclothymic disorder. Historical accounts indicate that many cases of cyclothymia were familial, and many relatives manifested similar symptoms (Jelliffe 1911). More recent studies have confirmed a genetic relationship between cyclothymic disorder and bipolar disorder (Akiskal et al. 1977; Dunner et al. 1976a, 1982; Gershon et al. 1982; Klein et al. 1985, 1986), although other nonbipolar affective disorders are also found in these families (Gershon et al. 1975). Also, Klein et al. (1988) did not find an increased familial prevalence of cyclothymia

Table 2–1.   Clinical phenomenology of cyclothymic disorder

	Cyclothymic disorder	Bipolar disorder
Age at onset (years)	<30	<30
Course	Chronic, fluctuating, indefinite affective episodes	Classically definite affective episodes
Mania/depression	30%–70% at follow-up	100%
Hypersomnia	±	+
Psychomotor retardation	±	+
Percentage female	50%–75%	50%
Prevalence	0.4%–9.2%	1.2%

Note.   + = present. ± = possibly present. − = absent.

in unipolar probands compared with medical and control subjects, suggesting that the genetic aspects of cyclothymia are more specifically associated with bipolar, rather than unipolar, pedigrees. The family history studies of cyclothymia are summarized in Table 2–2.

The findings from family history studies of probands with cyclothymic or bipolar disorder are very similar, because the familial risk for both bipolar and unipolar disorders is increased, whereas family studies of unipolar probands suggest the risk of unipolar disorder is much greater than that of bipolar disorder. This suggests a stronger genetic association between cyclothymic disorder and bipolar disorder. However, it is uncertain from these data whether cyclothymia may "breed true" as a subsyndromal disorder, because cyclothymia has not been evaluated as an independent variable and is often included in this research as a "fringe" or "borderline" affective condition.

Biological Studies

Research literature on the biology of cyclothymia is extremely limited. Two studies have examined neuroendocrine function in patients with cyclothymic disorder. Depue et al. (1985) found cortisol hypersection and poor regulation of cortisol levels in response to experimental stress in their subjects with cyclothymic disorder compared with control subjects, which is similar to that seen in other major affective disorders. Beck-Friis et al. (1985) included 4 patients with cyclothymic disorder among 32 acutely ill patients with major depressive disorder in a study investigating serum melatonin and the dexamethasone suppression test (DST). Serum melatonin levels were not significantly different between cyclothymic patients and control subjects, but there was a nonsignificant trend for increased melatonin levels in cyclothymic patients compared with noncyclothymic patients. In addition, two of the cyclothymic subjects were DST nonsuppressors, which was not significantly different from the rate in noncyclothymic subjects. Clearly, there is a great need for additional neurochemical and neuroendocrine studies in cyclothymic disorder, especially in comparison to bipolar disorder.

Sleep disturbances are common in patients with cyclothymic disorder (Akiskal et al. 1979) but have not been formally evaluated with the use of sleep EEG techniques. Papousek (1975) postulated a circadian rhythm abnormality as the fundamental genetic disturbance in cyclothymic disorder, but there has not been any research to test this hypothesis. In an interesting case report of identical twins, one of whom had cyclothymic disorder, Lange and Waldmann (1971) found quantitative differences in the 24-hour EEG between these subjects. Wager et al. (1990) performed a study of cholinergic rapid eye movement (REM) sleep induction in 10 patients with atypical depression, including 5 patients who also met criteria for DSM-III atypical bipolar disorder or cyclothymia. They reported that

Table 2–2. Family history studies of cyclothymic disorder

Author	Proband (N)	Familial morbid risk (%)			
		Bipolar	Unipolar	Cyclothymic	Dysthymic
Dunner et al.	Bipolar I (29)	5.4[a]	13[b]	9[c]	
1976a	Bipolar II (16)	14.7[a]	9.1	2.9	
	Unipolar (23)	0	9.8[b]	2.7	
	Normal (28)	0	1.5	0	
Klein et al.	Bipolar (24)	3	3	24[d]	8
1985	Nonaffective (14)	0	5	0	0
Gershon et al.	Bipolar I	8.6[b]	14[b]	2.7[e]	4.2
1982	Bipolar II	7.1[b]	17.3[b]	2.6[e]	4.2
	Unipolar	3	16.6[b]	0	8.4
	Normal	0.5	5.8	0.8	5.3
Gershon et al.	Bipolar (54)	3.82[b]	6.75[b]	2.64[b]	
1975	Unipolar (16)	2.09[b]	11.49[b]	2.09[b]	
	Normal (75)	0.19	0.58	0	
Akiskal et al.	Bipolar (50)	26[d]	22		
1977	Cyclothymic (46)	30[d]	15		
	Nonaffective (50)	2	10		
Dunner et al. 1982	Bipolar other (42)	19.6	10.7		
Klein et al.	Unipolar (24)	4	9[g]	2	17[g]
1988	Medical (19)	0	0	0	0
	Normal (18)	0	0	0	0
Depue et al.				Affective disorder	
1981	Bipolar (5)			80%[f]	
	Cyclothymic (30)			43%[f]	
	Nonaffective (33)			3%[f]	

[a] Significantly different from unipolar and normal.
[b] Significantly different from normal.
[c] Significantly different from normal only. Percentages represent cyclothymia and dysthymia together, but cyclothymia was found only in bipolar probands.
[d] Significantly different from nonaffective.
[e] Nonsignificant trend compared with unipolar and normal.
[f] Percentages expressed are the proportion of probands having at least one relative with an affective disorder.
[g] Significantly different from medical and normal.

patients with these additional diagnoses were not distinguishable from the group as a whole on the basis of REM sleep induction. Finally, Lenhart (1985) examined electrodermal activity in cyclothymic subjects and control subjects. He was able to distinguish between these groups because of a reduced skin conductance response in the cyclothymic subjects, but not all measures of electrodermal activity were significantly different.

The available biological studies are too few to be conclusive but do suggest that some biological disturbances will be found to be associated with cyclothymic disorder in future investigations. Whether these biological abnormalities will define cyclothymic subtypes awaits future research.

Treatment Studies

Several studies regarding the treatment of cyclothymic disorder have appeared in the literature, but these include patients with other comorbid conditions. Ananth et al. (1979) found that premorbid cyclothymic personality was a positive predictor of lithium response in bipolar patients. In a study of 20 patients with anergic depression, Neubauer and Bermingham (1976) reported that 8 also had cyclothymia; all responded with dramatic improvement when lithium was added to their treatment regimen. In a treatment study of premenstrual tension, the only subjects who responded to lithium were 3 with cyclothymic disorder (Steiner et al. 1980). Finally, an open trial of lithium in 14 cocaine abusers was conducted by Gawin and Kleber (1986); the only patients responding to treatment were the 9 who also had cyclothymic disorder.

In addition to these studies of lithium efficacy in patients with cyclothymic disorder and other disorders, additional studies have investigated its use in pure patient populations. These studies are summarized in Table 2–3. In a prospective study of 104 cyclothymic patients, Rosier et al. (1974) reported that successful prophylaxis against affective episodes occurred in 97% of the cases. Dunner et al. (1976b) treated 4 "bipolar other" patients (i.e., similar to cyclothymic disorder) with lithium and 4 with placebo, but the number of cases was too small to make any meaningful comparisons. Akiskal et al. (1979) found that 9 of 15 cyclothymic patients treated openly with lithium significantly improved, compared to only 2 of 10 psychiatric control subjects. Finally, Peselow and colleagues retrospectively evaluated the prophylactic effects of lithium in cyclothymic disorder alone (Peselow et al. 1981) and compared with unipolar and bipolar II disorders (Peselow et al. 1982b) using life-table analysis. The authors suggested that lithium exerted some prophylactic effects against depressive episodes, which were greatest in the bipolar II group, least in the cyclothymic group, and intermediate in the unipolar group.

Considered together, these studies provide some evidence to support the efficacy of lithium in cyclothymic disorder, although the response rate may be less

Table 2–3. Lithium treatment in cyclothymic disorder

Author	Diagnosis (N)	Treatment response (%)	Follow-up
Rosier et al. 1974	Cyclothymic (104)	97[a]	2.5–3 years prospective, uncontrolled
Dunner et al. 1976b	Bipolar II (32)	[b]	Average 16 months prospective, placebo control
	Bipolar other (8)	[c]	
Akiskal et al. 1979	Cyclothymic (15)	60[d]	Average 1 year prospective,
	Nonaffective (10)	20	uncontrolled
Peselow et al. 1982b	Bipolar II (102)	42–55[e]	2 years retrospective,
	Unipolar (43)	31–42	life table uncontrolled
	Cyclothymic (69)	26–36	

[a]Percentage having favorable prophylaxis against affective episodes.
[b]Significant reduction in mean number of hypomanic episodes but not depressive episodes with lithium compared with placebo.
[c]No significant difference in mean affective episodes between lithium and placebo.
[d]Percentage having significant clinical improvement during lithium treatment.
[e]Percentage probability of remaining free of depression after 2 years of treatment.

than for other bipolar disorders. These findings are consistent with the idea that cyclothymic disorder is heterogeneous, consisting of a lithium-responsive bipolar subgroup and an ill-defined nonbipolar subgroup that is not responsive to lithium. Of particular interest regarding this possibility are the results from an additional analysis of the data of Peselow et al. (1982b). They divided their cyclothymic patients into groups having a positive or negative family history for affective illness and found a nonsignificant trend for better lithium response in the patients with a positive family history. Future studies of lithium and other drugs, such as anticonvulsants, are needed to identify additional factors that may predict response to treatment (Howland and Thase 1993).

Relationship to Other Disorders

Bipolar II disorder. From a clinical perspective, cyclothymic disorder differs from bipolar II disorder only in the severity of the depressive periods, a distinction that may be both arbitrary and difficult to make reliably with a retrospective history. This raises the issue of whether cyclothymic disorder is more closely related to bipolar II disorder than to the fully symptomatic bipolar I disorder. In a 1- to 2-year follow-up of their patients with cyclothymic disorder, Akiskal et al. (1979) reported that 6% could be reclassified as having bipolar I disorder and 30% as having bipolar II disorder. However, this follow-up period may be too short to adequately assess the ultimate outcome of cyclothymic disorder. In contrast, Endicott et al. (1985) did not find a significant difference in the lifetime rate of cyclothymic disorder between patients with bipolar I and bipolar II disorders. In their study of the age at onset for subtypes of bipolar disorder, which was defined by the age at first psychiatric treatment, Peselow et al. (1982a) found a nonsignificant trend for an earlier age at onset in "bipolar other" (i.e., cyclothymic) patients compared with bipolar II patients, suggesting a clinical difference between these groups. The same research group also reported differences in the response to lithium between groups with cyclothymic disorder and bipolar II disorder (Peselow et al. 1982b).

Family history studies also may provide valuable information regarding the relationship between cyclothymic disorder and bipolar II disorder. Three studies have compared the family histories of probands with bipolar I and bipolar II disorders. There was no difference in the morbid risk for cyclothymic disorder in two of the studies (Endicott et al. 1985; Gershon et al. 1982). In the third study, the morbid risk for minor affective disorder, including cyclothymic disorder, was increased in the relatives of bipolar I patients (Dunner et al. 1976a). Dunner et al. (1982) found that the rate of bipolar II disorder in the first-degree relatives of "bipolar other" (i.e., cyclothymic) patients was approximately twice that of bipolar I disorder, but there was no control group for comparison. Finally, Klein et al. (1985) found 9 cases of cyclothymic disorder and only 1 case of bipolar II disorder in 37 adolescent offspring of parents with bipolar disorder, although the full clinical expression of their disorder would not be expected at such a young age, and their diagnoses may change over time.

These clinical and family history studies do not provide sufficient evidence to support a specific relationship between cyclothymic disorder and bipolar II disorder. It is quite possible that some types of cyclothymic disorder can progress to bipolar II and, ultimately, bipolar I disorder, but the clinical and biological factors that may better define this progression await discovery in long-term prospective studies of cyclothymic subgroups.

Rapid cycling bipolar disorder. Rapid cycling bipolar disorder is characterized by four or more episodes of depression and/or mania per year (Dunner et al. 1977). Using this definition, cyclothymic disorder can be considered to be a rapid cycling disorder because of the typically short and frequent affective episodes, although it is not usually conceptualized in this way. Therefore, it is important to consider the relationship between cyclothymic disorder and "typical" rapid cycling bipolar disorder.

Rapid cycling patients do not differ symptomatically from other bipolar patients. Females account for 70% or more of rapid cycling cases (Dunner et al. 1977; Kukopulos et al. 1983; Wehr et al. 1988), which is a higher percentage of females than is seen in most cyclothymic populations (Akiskal et al. 1979; Weissman and Myers 1978). Like cyclothymic disorder, rapid cycling may be less responsive to lithium treatment (Dunner et al. 1977).

In a study of "bipolar other" (i.e., cyclothymic) patients, Dunner et al. (1982) found rapid cycling in approximately 28%, a rate somewhat higher than is typically seen among all bipolar patients, but there were no control groups for comparison. In an earlier study, these investigators also reported a nonsignificant trend for a lower prevalence of "bipolar other" patients, compared with bipolar I and bipolar II patients, among a group of rapid cyclers (Dunner et al. 1977). Nurnberger et al. (1988) conducted a family study of rapid cycling bipolar probands and found no significant difference in the risk for cyclothymic personality between families of rapid cyclers and non–rapid cyclers. In contrast to these studies, Kukopulos et al. (1983) did report an association between cyclothymic temperament and rapid cycling bipolar disorder. They noted that the majority of their subjects developed rapid cycling late in the course of their illness (rather than from the outset), and most had bipolar II disorders. Of particular interest, a premorbid cyclothymic temperament was found in 44% of their patients. Furthermore, a cyclothymic temperament was found in 66% of the patients with an early-onset rapid cycling pattern but only 36% of those with a late-onset rapid cycling pattern.

Despite the intriguing findings of Kukopulos et al. (1983), there is not sufficient evidence to support a strict relationship between cyclothymic disorder and rapid cycling bipolar disorder. Clearly, not all patients with cyclothymic disorder will develop rapid cycling and not all patients with rapid cycling have premorbid cyclothymia. If confirmed, the data of Kukopulos et al. (1983) suggest that rapid cycling is a heterogeneous condition, perhaps with early-onset forms associated with cyclothymia and late-onset forms associated with pharmacological induction.

Dysthymic disorder.   Akiskal (1981) has suggested that dysthymic disorder can be considered a variant of cyclothymic disorder because of its early age at onset, intermittent course, typical symptoms of anergia and hypersomnia, family history of bipolar disorder in some patients, and increased incidence of pharmacological hypomania. An increased family history of bipolar disorder, but not cyclothymic disorder, has been reported in dysthymic probands compared with unipolar probands (Howland and Thase 1991). Likewise, in another study, the prevalence of dysthymic, but not cyclothymic, disorder was increased in the offspring of unipolar patients compared with control subjects (Klein et al. 1988). However, Akiskal et al. (1985) found a similar number of cases of cyclothymic disorder and dysthymic disorder in 68 children and siblings of bipolar patients. Although modest, these findings do support the possibility that some patients with dysthymic disorder are similar to cyclothymic patients. Because of the well-recognized underdiagnosis of mild hypomanic states (Coryell 1982), it is conceivable that, after a careful history and an assessment of affective symptoms are obtained, many of these dysthymic patients could be reclassified as cyclothymic. Nevertheless, this relationship may only apply to a certain subgroup of patients with dysthymic disorder. Additional treatment and biological and follow-up studies are needed to clarify this issue (Howland 1991; Howland and Thase 1991).

Personality disorders.   Many studies have found various personality traits, temperaments, and disorders in association with cyclothymic disorder (Akiskal 1981; Alnaes and Torgensen 1989; Jelliffe 1911; Wetzel et al. 1980). Moreover, socially problematic behaviors such as marital discord, promiscuity, poor work performance, and substance abuse, which many clinicians consider to be indicative of a primary characterological disturbance, also can be recognized as psychosocial complications of an underlying affective disorder (Akiskal et al. 1979; Jelliffe 1911) and may often respond to appropriate treatment.

Thus, accurate clinical assessment of these patients may be difficult, especially when they manifest affective instability among other symptoms. It is probable that a subgroup of patients with cyclothymic disorder (who do not have a significant family history of affective disorder, manifest "typical" cyclothymic symptoms, or respond to lithium) may in fact have a nonbipolar disorder. For example, patients with borderline personality disorder frequently manifest a variety of affective symptoms, which makes it difficult to distinguish between an affective and nonaffective disorder. Indeed, Akiskal (1981) has suggested many of these patients may have unrecognized, and hence undertreated, affective disorders. Others have also recognized the comorbidity of borderline personality disorder and affective disorders (Fyer et al. 1988). These findings emphasize the clinical heterogeneity of and similarity between conditions such as cyclothymic disorder and borderline personality disorder. Such a diagnostic distinction may not be easy to make, and further research is needed to help clarify this issue.

Discussion

Several important conclusions regarding cyclothymic disorder can be drawn from this review. First, there is a subgroup of patients with cyclothymic disorder whose clinical characteristics, longitudinal course, family history, and treatment response place them firmly in the category of bipolar disorder. Cyclothymic disorder may thus represent the earliest manifestation of bipolar illness in these patients. Some patients with cyclothymic disorder may develop symptoms of bipolar II disorder or rapid cycling, but these probably represent stages in the progression to bipolar disorder in most cases. Identification of a bipolar cyclothymic subtype suggests that this particular subgroup of patients should be treated like patients with bipolar disorder. How or whether treatment affects the natural course of this cyclothymic subtype (e.g., altering the progression to bipolar disorder) is unknown. Furthermore, evidence for a strict correlation between the characteristics of this bipolar cyclothymic subtype (e.g., bipolar family history, longitudinal course) and treatment response is lacking. Therefore, whether or how well cyclothymic patients without these characteristics respond to pharmacological treatment is unknown. More research is needed to establish the clinical and biological correlates of treatment response in all subtypes of cyclothymic disorder.

A second conclusion from this review is that cyclothymic disorder is a heterogeneous condition. Although cyclothymic disorder is strongly associated with bipolar disorder, not all patients necessarily have a family history of bipolar disorder, respond to lithium treatment, or progress to a fully symptomatic bipolar illness. However, it is not clear clinically which patients have a truly chronic subsyndromal affective condition and which of them have another condition that merely resembles the clinical phenomenology of cyclothymic disorder (e.g., borderline personality disorder). DSM-III and DSM-III-R use the category of cyclothymia to describe an affective disorder that is consistent with the subtype described above, but this use does not adequately represent the clinical heterogeneity seen in practice. Thus, the DSM-IV Mood Disorders Work Group proposal that cyclothymic patients who have ever had any major depressive or manic episode be reclassified as having a subtype of bipolar disorder would help reduce this heterogeneity. Nevertheless, some of the remaining group of patients with subsyndromal cyclothymic symptoms may later manifest full affective episodes during long-term longitudinal follow-up.

Recommendations

Because of the clinical heterogeneity of cyclothymia and its strong association with affective disorders, we support the recommendation of the DSM-IV Mood Disorders Work Group to revise the criteria for cyclothymic disorder so that these patients never meet criteria for a major depressive or manic episode. Patients who have such episodes should be reclassified as having a subtype of bipolar disorder. This reclassification clarifies and stresses the linkage between "subbipolar" cyclothymic disorder and bipolar disorder. The remaining group of cyclothymic patients, which is heterogeneous and does not have a clear association with bipolar affective disorder, should continue to be classified as having cyclothymic disorder, reflecting both the mild mood symptoms and the separation from other more clearly defined affective disorders. This reformulation would help to define a more homogeneous group of patients with cyclothymic disorder for additional research. In particular, long-term prospective follow-up studies, biological investigations, and well-controlled treatment trials are needed to further clarify this diagnostic group and better understand its relationship to affective disorders and other nonaffective psychiatric conditions.

References

Akiskal HS: Subaffective disorders: dysthymic, cyclothymic and bipolar II disorders in the "borderline" realm. Psychiatr Clin North Am 4:25–26, 1981

Akiskal HS, Djenderedjian AH, Rosenthal RH, et al: Cyclothymic disorder: validity criteria for inclusion in the bipolar affective group. Am J Psychiatry 134:1227–1233, 1977

Akiskal HS, Khani MK, Scott-Strauss A: Cyclothymic temperamental disorders. Psychiatr Clin North Am 2:527–554, 1979

Akiskal HS, Downs J, Jordan P, et al: Affective disorders in referred children and younger siblings of manic-depressives. Arch Gen Psychiatry 42:996–1003, 1985

Alnaes R, Torgensen S: Personality and personality disorders among patients with major depression in combination with dysthymic or cyclothymic disorders. Acta Psychiatr Scand 79:363–369, 1989

American Psychiatric Association: Diagnostic and Statistical Manual of Mental Disorders, 2nd Edition. Washington, DC, American Psychiatric Association, 1968

American Psychiatric Association: Diagnostic and Statistical Manual of Mental Disorders, 3rd Edition. Washington, DC, American Psychiatric Association, 1980

American Psychiatric Association: Diagnostic and Statistical Manual of Mental Disorders, 3rd Edition, Revised. Washington, DC, American Psychiatric Association, 1987

Ananth J, Engelsmann F, Kiriakos R, et al: Prediction of lithium response. Acta Psychiatr Scand 60:279–286, 1979

Beck-Friis J, Kjellman BF, Aperia B, et al: Serum melatonin in relation to clinical variables in patients with major depressive disorder and a hypothesis of a low melatonin syndrome. Acta Psychiatr Scand 71:319–330, 1985

Coryell W: Hypomania. J Affect Dis 4:167–171, 1982

Depue RA, Slater JF, Wolfstetter-Kausch H, et al: A behavioral paradigm for identifying persons at risk for bipolar depressive disorder: a conceptual framework and five validation studies. J Abnorm Psychol 90:381–437, 1981

Depue RA, Kleiman RM, Davis P, et al: The behavioral high-risk paradigm and bipolar affective disorder, VII: serum free cortisol in nonpatient cyclothymic subjects selected by the general behavior inventory. Am J Psychiatry 142:175–181, 1985

Dunner DL, Gershon ES, Goodwin FK: Heritable factors in the severity of affective illness. Biol Psychiatry 11:31–42, 1976a

Dunner DL, Stallone F, Fieve RR: Lithium carbonate and affective disorders. Arch Gen Psychiatry 33:117–120, 1976b

Dunner DL, Patrick V, Fieve RR: Rapid cycling manic depressive patients. Compr Psychiatry 18:561–566, 1977

Dunner DL, Russek FD, Russek B, et al: Classification of bipolar affective disorder subtypes. Compr Psychiatry 23:186–189, 1982

Endicott J, Nee J, Andreasen N, et al: Bipolar II: combine or keep separate? J Affect Disord 8:17–28, 1985

Fyer MY, Frances AJ, Sullivan T, et al: Comorbidity of borderline personality disorder. Arch Gen Psychiatry 45:348–352, 1988

Gawin F, Kleber H: Pharmacologic treatments of cocaine abuse. Psychiatr Clin North Am 9:573–583, 1986

Gershon ES, Mark A, Cohen N, et al: Transmitted factors in the morbid risk of affective disorders: a controlled study. J Psychiatr Res 12:283–299, 1975

Gershon ES, Hamovit J, Guroff JJ, et al: A family study of schizoaffective, bipolar I, bipolar II, unipolar, and normal control probands. Arch Gen Psychiatry 39:1159–1167, 1982

Howland RH: Pharmacotherapy of dysthymia: a review. J Clin Psychopharmacol 11:83–92, 1991

Howland RH: Dysthymic disorder. Directions in Psychiatry 12(2):1–8, 1992

Howland RH, Thase ME: Biological studies of dysthymia. Biol Psychiatry 30:283–304, 1991

Howland RH, Thase ME: A comprehensive review of cyclothymic disorder. J Nerv Ment Dis 181:485–493, 1993

Jelliffe SE: Cyclothymia: the mild forms of manic-depressive psychoses and the manic-depressive constitution. Am J Insanity 67:661–676, 1911

Klein DN, Depue RA, Slater JF: Cyclothymia in the adolescent offspring of parents with bipolar affective disorder. J Abnorm Psychol 94:115–127, 1985

Klein DN, Depue RA, Slater JF: Inventory identification of cyclothymia, IX: validation in offspring of bipolar I patients. Arch Gen Psychiatry 43:441–445, 1986

Klein DN, Clark DC, Dansky L, et al: Dysthymia in the offspring of parents with primary unipolar affective disorder. J Abnorm Psychol 97:265–274, 1988

Kraepelin E: Manic-Depressive Insanity and Paranoia. Edinburgh, Livingston, 1921

Kukopulos A, Caliari B, Tundo A, et al: Rapid cyclers, temperament, and antidepressants. Compr Psychiatry 24:249–258, 1983

Lange H, Waldmann H: The importance of circadian rhythm for bioelectrical brain activity and psychopathological symptoms in cyclothymia (English abstract), in The Nature of Sleep. Edited by Jovanovic UJ. Stuttgart, Gustav Fischer Verlag, 1971, pp 187–190

Lenhart RE: Lowered skin conductance in a subsyndromal high-risk depressive sample: response amplitudes versus tonic levels. J Abnorm Psychol 94:649–652, 1985

Neubauer H, Bermingham P: A depressive syndrome response to lithium. J Nerv Ment Dis 163:276–281, 1976

Nurnberger J, Guroff JJ, Hamovit J, et al: A family study of rapid-cycling bipolar illness. J Affect Dis 15:87–91, 1988

Papousek M: Chronobiological aspects of cyclothymia (English summary). Fortschr Neurol Psychiatr 43:381–440, 1975

Peselow ED, Dunner DL, Fieve RR, et al: Prophylactic effect of lithium against depression in cyclothymic patients: a life-table analysis. Compr Psychiatry 22:257–264, 1981

Peselow ED, Dunner DL, Fieve RR, et al: Age of onset of affective illness. Psychiatr Clin 15:124–132, 1982a

Peselow ED, Dunner DL, Fieve RR, et al: Lithium prophylaxis of depression in unipolar, bipolar II, and cyclothymic patients. Am J Psychiatry 139:747–752, 1982b

Rosier YA, Broussolle P, Fontang M: Lithium gluconate: systematic and factorial analysis of 104 cases observed for 2 1/2 to 3 years among patients regularly followed up and presenting cyclothymias or periodic dysthymias (English abstract). Ann Med Psychol 132:389–397, 1974

Steiner M, Haskett RF, Osmun JN, et al: Treatment of premenstrual tension with lithium carbonate. Acta Psychiatr Scand 61:96–102, 1980

Wager S, Robinson D, Goetz R, et al: Cholinergic REM sleep induction in atypical depression. Biol Psychiatry 27:441–446, 1990

Waters BGH: Early symptoms of bipolar affective psychosis. Can Psychiatr Assoc J 2:55–60, 1979

Wehr TA, Sack DA, Rosenthal NE, et al: Rapid cycling affective disorder: contributing factors and treatment responses in 51 patients. Am J Psychiatry 145:179–184, 1988

Weissman MM, Myers JK: Affective disorders in a US urban community. Arch Gen Psychiatry 35:1304–1311, 1978

Wetzel RD, Cloninger CR, Hong B, et al: Personality as a subclinical expression of the affective disorders. Compr Psychiatry 21:197–205, 1980

Chapter 3

Bipolar Depression With Hypomania (Bipolar II)

David L. Dunner, M.D.

Statement of the Issue

The purpose of this review is to determine whether patients with depression and hypomania, commonly referred to as bipolar II, should be more distinctly classified in DSM-IV than they have been in DSM-III (American Psychiatric Association 1980) or DSM-III-R (American Psychiatric Association 1987). Patients who had been classified as bipolar II were included in DSM-III as atypical bipolar disorder and in DSM-III-R as bipolar disorder not otherwise specified (NOS). In the descriptors of these classifications, specific reference was made to patients who were bipolar II. The basis for the review is to determine whether bipolar II patients could be separated from bipolar I and unipolar depressive patients on the basis of the Robins and Guze criteria (1970) for validation of psychiatric illness.

Significance of the Issue

The rationale for the work group to address this topic relates to the clinical use of bipolar II. The separation of patients with depression and hypomania as a somewhat distinct illness may be useful in planning treatment for such patients. In addition, the status of such patients in the nomenclature as a residual category has several implications. First, if bipolar II patients have a clinically separate syndrome, then grouping them with atypical patients would obscure the identity of a clinically useful syndrome. Second, the inclusion of bipolar II in an NOS category means that

We appreciate the assistance of Dr. Thomas Widiger in providing the literature search. Material presented in this chapter has also appeared in Dunner (1993).

phases of the illness could not be separately and distinctly coded by using fifth-digit modifiers.

From a historical perspective, the concept of subdividing bipolar disorders was initiated by Dunner and colleagues (1970, 1976c) through research at the National Institute of Mental Health (NIMH). The collaborative depression project evaluated a classification of bipolar disorder equivalent to the bipolar I group described by Dunner et al. (1970, 1976c): bipolar disorder with mania and a separate group, bipolar disorder with hypomania, which would be equivalent to both bipolar II as defined by Dunner et al. (1970, 1976c) and cyclothymic disorder as described by Akiskal et al. (1977, 1979). In DSM-III, the diagnosis of bipolar disorder relied on a definition of mania that was symptom based without any severity measures. Thus, patients who had 1 week of manic or hypomanic symptoms could meet the criteria for bipolar disorder. The effect of DSM-III was to merge bipolar II patients and bipolar I patients into a single bipolar category. In DSM-III-R, bipolar disorder was more clearly differentiated from the other hypomanic subtypes by having a severity criterion. Bipolar II patients were grouped with the bipolar not otherwise specified group, and cyclothymic disorder was largely unchanged from DSM-III.

Method

The method was a literature search in which articles that compared subgroups of bipolar and unipolar patients were reviewed. To be included in the review, the article had to be data-based and include data related to clinical description, family history, laboratory studies, or follow-up studies. The article also had to compare bipolar II patients with bipolar I patients, unipolar patients, or both. Additional articles were obtained by reviewing references and data collected by me. The initial draft of the review was distributed for comments among investigators in the field and the work group itself.

Results

Clinical Differentiation

Using DSM-III-R criteria, bipolar II and unipolar patients both meet criteria for major depressive disorder. In contrast to unipolar patients, bipolar II patients also have symptoms of mania that meet the same criteria for manic episode as bipolar I patients, except that the episodes of mania have never been sufficiently severe to cause hospitalization or impairment in occupational functioning. Thus, the symptoms and duration of symptoms (i.e., a distinct period of three symptoms of mania) are the same for bipolar I and bipolar II patients, with the difference being that bipolar II patients do not have manic symptoms severe enough to result in significant social role disruption or hospitalization. For many bipolar II patients, the hypomanic symptoms lead to a period of creativity and productivity. The depressive phase of bipolar II meets criteria for major depressive disorder and can be differentiated from unipolar illness not on the basis of depressive symptoms, but rather on the basis of the course of illness (i.e., the presence of hypomania).

Initial studies (Dunner et al. 1970, 1976c) supported the distinction of bipolar II from both bipolar I and unipolar patients on the basis of clinical criteria. Bipolar II patients had an intermediate age at onset compared with bipolar I and unipolar patients. Bipolar II patients also had a higher frequency of suicide attempts than either of the other groups of patients, and their propensity to suicide after hospital discharge was also disproportionately high.

Additional studies of bipolar I, bipolar II, and unipolar disorder also supported making this distinction. Bipolar II patients have consistently shown either an intermediate age at onset between bipolar I or unipolar patients or an earlier onset of illness compared with bipolar I patients (Angst 1978; Ayuso-Guittierrez and Ramos-Brieva 1982; Endicott et al. 1985; Keeler and Othmer 1987).

Some studies show a difference in sex ratio by diagnosis. Thus, Angst's study (1978) showed a fairly equal sex distribution for bipolar I patients but a preponderance of women among bipolar II patients.

Differences in the course of illness can also be demonstrated. A greater frequency of episodes as evidenced by rapid cycling has been shown among bipolar II and bipolar I patients compared with unipolar patients (Dunner et al. 1977b). Ayuso-Guitterrez and Ramos-Brieva (1982) found that bipolar I patients tend to have an equal percentage of manic and depressive episodes, whereas bipolar II patients tend to have more depressive than hypomanic episodes and a greater frequency of episodes. Giles et al. (1986) also noted that, in the population they were studying, the number of episodes of illness was greater in bipolar II than in unipolar patients, although bipolar I patients had the highest number of episodes. Endicott et al. (1985) showed that bipolar I and bipolar II patients had a similar age at onset compared with unipolar patients. Haag et al. (1987) did not find a difference in pattern of onset of illness (whether depression, mania, or hypomania occurred initially) when comparing bipolar I and bipolar II patients. Peselow et al. (1982) also found differences in age at onset of illness among bipolar I, bipolar II, and unipolar patients, with bipolar I patients having the earliest age at onset and unipolar patients the latest age at onset.

Several studies have shown a preponderance of bipolar II disorder among patients with seasonal affective disorder (Rosenthal et al. 1984; Thompson and

Issacs 1988; Wirz-Justice et al. 1986). Stallone et al. (1980) replicated the finding of an increased frequency of suicide attempts in bipolar II patients compared with bipolar I and unipolar patients.

Dunner et al. (1976a) found that bipolar I patients were more likely to have psychomotor retardation during depression than bipolar II or unipolar patients. Assessment of severity of depression by nurse ratings was different for the three patient groups. For example, bipolar I patients were rated as more depressed by the nurses than by patient self-ratings, and the same was true for the unipolar patients. However, for bipolar II patients, the nurses rated the depression as less than the patients' self-ratings, suggesting that bipolar II patients feel more depressed than they exhibit to others.

In summary, bipolar II patients differ from bipolar I and unipolar patients on a number of clinical variables including age at onset, sex ratio, course of illness, symptom pattern during the illness, and frequency of suicide attempts.

Familial and Genetic Studies

The early differentiation of bipolar and unipolar patients was based on clinical and familial data. The study by Dunner et al. (1970, 1976c) suggested that bipolar II patients had a higher familial prevalence of suicide than bipolar I or unipolar patients.

In the 1970s, three large-scale family studies of affective disorders were undertaken (Coryell et al. 1984; Fieve et al. 1984; Gershon et al. 1982). These studies used similar, although not entirely identical, diagnostic criteria and methodologies. The core methodology involved patients who were prospectively ascertained and who were diagnosed using fairly rigorous criteria, whereas their relatives were directly interviewed using structured instruments. There was general agreement about how to diagnose mania in the relatives of the patients. The studies differed mainly in the criteria used to diagnose depression among relatives. Fieve et al. (1984) required relatives to be treated for depression to be counted as ill. The NIMH collaborative study required relatives to meet Research Diagnostic Criteria (RDC) (Andreasen et al. 1987; Coryell et al. 1984; Endicott et al. 1985; Spitzer and Endicott 1978). Gershon et al. (1982) required relatives to have social incapacitation from mood disorder to be counted as ill.

Findings from these three studies are quite similar. First, all the studies found a higher morbid risk of bipolar I disorder among relatives of bipolar I patients compared with other subtypes. Second, all the studies showed an elevation in bipolar I in relatives of bipolar II patients compared with unipolar patients or control subjects. Third, all the studies showed a higher rate of unipolar disorder among relatives of patients of any subtype. Fourth, all the studies showed a consistent elevation of bipolar II among relatives of bipolar II patients. Higher rates of suicide were not demonstrated among relatives of bipolar II patients (Fieve et al. 1984).

In summary, the family data support several conclusions: 1) bipolar II disorder is more similar to bipolar I disorder than to unipolar disorder, in that relatives of both have an increased risk for mania compared with relatives of unipolar patients; and 2) these studies support the notion that bipolar II patients may be somewhat distinct from both bipolar I and unipolar patients, because the highest morbid risk for bipolar II is found among relatives of bipolar II probands.

Biological and Pharmacological Differentiation

The early studies of biological differentiation showed similarities between bipolar II and bipolar I patients and differences from unipolar patients with regard to average evoked response (Buschbaum et al. 1971). Corticosteroid excretion in the urine was lower in bipolar I patients during depression than in unipolar and bipolar II patients (Dunner et al. 1972). Subsequent studies of biological factors have not clearly separated bipolar I from bipolar II or unipolar patients. In many of these studies, the numbers of subjects evaluated have been quite small.

Studies of sleep have shown variable results. Ansseau et al. (1984, 1985) showed greater variability of night-to-night rapid eye movement (REM) latency in bipolar II compared with bipolar I and unipolar subjects, but this was based on a sample of only four bipolar I and two bipolar II patients. Giles et al. (1986), in a study that was controlled for age, showed that bipolar II patients were similar to bipolar I patients, but differed from unipolar patients regarding the percentages of patients with hypersomnia, REM latency, and non-REM time.

The dexamethasone suppression test (DST) showed a higher DST nonsuppression rate in bipolar I patients than in unipolar and bipolar II patients, but only five bipolar I and three bipolar II patients were studied (Zisook et al. 1985). In another study, there was a higher DST nonsuppression rate among both bipolar I and II patients than inpatients with unipolar depression. However, when studied alone, bipolar II patients were not significantly associated with DST nonsuppression (Asnis et al. 1982). Again this study involved only small numbers of subjects. Lithium red blood cell plasma ratio was studied by Rihmer et al. (1983), Dunner et al. (1978), and Kim et al. (1978), and no significant differences were found. The activity of platelet monoamine oxidase was studied by several groups (Fieve et al. 1980; Samson et al. 1985), and no significant differences were found comparing bipolar I, bipolar II, and unipolar patients. Erythrocyte catechol-O-methyltransferase activity did not differ among depressive subtypes (Dunner et al. 1977a). Goodnick et al. (1982) measured the half-life of elimination of lithium in euthymic patients after they had been stabilized with lithium treatment. Half-lives of lithium in plasma and erythrocytes were considerably longer for bipolar I and bipolar II patients than for unipolar patients. Plasma lithium levels, age, and sex distribution were similar for the three groups.

Pharmacological studies have not clearly separated bipolar II from unipolar or bipolar I patients. Donnelly et al. (1978) studied lithium response in acute depression. Their findings suggested that lithium response was similar in bipolar I and bipolar II patients and somewhat higher than in unipolar patients, but the results were not statistically different. Other pharmacological studies of maintenance therapy against depression (Kane et al. 1982) showed that maintenance therapy against depression was not significantly statistically different for patients with recurrent unipolar depression than for patients with bipolar II disorder. Fieve et al. (1976) and Dunner et al. (1982) showed that lithium treatment did prevent recurrence of depression in bipolar II patients if studied for a long enough time. Although there was no hypomania in the lithium-treated group compared with the placebo-treated patients, the effect of lithium on hypomania was not statistically better than placebo, perhaps because of the small number of subjects studied.

An earlier study by Gershon et al. (1971) showed a differential response rate to L-dopa administration to depressed patients for bipolar I, II, and unipolar subjects. L-Tryptophan administration did not result in improvement in unipolar patients, whereas 50% of a small number of depressed bipolar I and bipolar II patients responded (Farkas et al. 1976).

There is no clear biological marker for depression; thus, attempts to show differences between bipolar and unipolar patients have not generally been replicated with regard to biological factors, and there is no useful marker for studying bipolar II patients and their relationship to other depressed patient groups. The average evoked-response data suggest that bipolar II patients are more similar to patients with bipolar I disorder than to patients with unipolar depression. Identification of a meaningful biological marker would be important in furthering the understanding of the relationship between bipolar II disorder and other depressive disorders. Although pharmacological differences appear to differentiate these subtypes of depression, many of the studies have involved small numbers of subjects.

Stability of Illness Over Time (Follow-Up Studies)

It is clear that many patients who later become bipolar I begin with depression or with histories of hypomania. Thus, patients with bipolar II illness may at some point develop a significant manic episode and become bipolar I. Dunner et al. (1976b) studied a large group of patients who were bipolar I to determine their course of illness. The majority of bipolar I patients were hospitalized for mania during their initial manic episode or had a depressive episode immediately followed by significant mania. Thirty-two bipolar I patients experienced one or more depressive episodes before becoming manic. An analysis of these data suggested that the development of mania in patients with recurrent depression was related both to the number of depressive episodes and to time. The majority of these patients became bipolar I after three depressive episodes and within 10 years of their first depressive episode. Prospective data from a group of unipolar and bipolar II patients suggested a 5% probability that such patients would ultimately become manic. These patients had not been treated with maintenance pharmacotherapy.

In a sample of the Iowa 500 series, 9 of 225 unipolar patients became manic during follow-up from 1 month to 20 years after the index hospitalization for depression (Winokur and Morrison 1973). Thus, there was less than a 5% chance of becoming bipolar in this sample. Another study of the Iowa 500 revealed that 11%–17% of unipolar patients became bipolar on follow-up (Tsuang et al. 1981). These data were obtained by actually interviewing subjects 10–40 years after their initial hospitalization. In a 5-year follow-up study from the NIMH collaborative study (Coryell et al. 1989), 11% of bipolar II and 4% of unipolar patients developed mania on follow-up. However mania was determined by RDC and did not necessarily imply that the patients were hospitalized.

In summary, patients with bipolar II illness tend to have a stable lifetime course. A percentage of such patients will develop mania, and their diagnosis will be converted from bipolar II to bipolar I over time. The percentage of conversion seems to vary from 5% to perhaps 17% on follow-up for up to 30 years, with a few of the studies supporting the lower conversion rate.

Reliability of the Diagnosis of Bipolar II

It is clear that the diagnosis of bipolar II and its differentiation from unipolar disorder depends largely on recognition of the history of hypomania. In Fieve's group, similar interviewing styles and diagnostic criteria were employed and the kappa for two-rater agreement for diagnosis of bipolar II was quite high (0.85; Dunner, unpublished data).

This relatively high degree of interrater reliability was based on clinical interviews. Lower reliability is usually obtained with structured interviews (such as the SADS-L [Spitzer and Endicott 1978]). Mazure and Gershon (1979) reinterviewed 47 affective disorder patients with a structured interview and found that 2 of the 3 patients originally diagnosed as bipolar II were correctly diagnosed at the second interview and that none of the patients with unipolar depression were diagnosed as bipolar II on the reinterview. Rice et al. (1986) reinterviewed 50 relatives of probands from the NIMH collaborative depressive study 5 years after the first interview. They found that 6 of the 7 patients who were positive for hypomania at the first interview were negative at the reinterview (kappa = .09). However, Rice et al. also concluded that the low base rate of hypomania in that sample suggested that hypomania was a valid diagnosis with low sensitivity.

Clinicians are likely to agree on a diagnosis of hypomania if they obtain the history. However, the milder the hypomania, the more difficult it is to distinguish this state from true unipolar disorder and thus to differentiate bipolar II from unipolar disorder.

In summary, hypomania may be difficult to diagnose by history and is certainly more difficult to elicit than manic states. However, it is also clear that, at some threshold of severity, hypomania is reasonably apparent to most investigators, even those using structured interviews, because such a condition has been found by a number of researchers over the years.

Discussion

Studies from several areas report the separation of bipolar II from other affective disorders, notably, bipolar I and unipolar depression (Dunner 1983; Fieve and Dunner 1975). By applying the Robins and Guze (1970) criteria, bipolar II can be considered distinct from unipolar (major depressive) disorder and bipolar I (bipolar) disorder. Thus, one appropriate option would be to categorize bipolar II (bipolar depression with hypomania) as a distinct subtype in the nomenclature. The advantages of this addition include the ability to subtype the depressive phase of such patients, to assist the clinician in recognizing the potential for suicide among such patients, and to clarify diagnostic issues for research. The disadvantages include the addition of a subtype where there may be diagnostic disagreement among interviewers.

A second option would be to add the modifier "with hypomania" to major depressive disorder. The advantage of this option is that it involves a simpler change in the nomenclature. The disadvantages include obscuring the bipolar-unipolar distinction. Furthermore, this option would make further subtyping difficult.

Recommendations

Several options have been recommended by the DSM-IV Mood Disorders Work Group. The first option is to separate bipolar II from bipolar disorder and from bipolar disorder NOS. Thus, the bipolar spectrum would include bipolar disorder with mania (bipolar I), bipolar disorder with hypomania (bipolar II), cyclothymic disorder, and bipolar disorder NOS. The second option is to indicate the presence of a history of hypomania by adding a modifier to major depressive disorder.

References

Akiskal HS, Djenderedjian AH, Rosenthal RH, et al: Cyclothymic disorder: validating criteria for inclusion in the bipolar affective group. Am J Psychiatry 134:1227–1233, 1977

Akiskal HS, Khani MK, Scott-Strauss A: Cyclothymic temperamental disorders. Psychiatr Clin North Am 2:527–554, 1979

American Psychiatric Association: Diagnostic and Statistical Manual of Mental Disorders, 3rd Edition. Washington, DC, American Psychiatric Association, 1980

American Psychiatric Association: Diagnostic and Statistical Manual of Mental Disorders, 3rd Edition, Revised. Washington, DC, American Psychiatric Association, 1987

Andreasen NC, Rice J, Endicott J, et al: Familial rates of affective disorder. Arch Gen Psychiatry 44:461–489, 1987

Angst J: The course of affective disorders, II: topology of bipolar manic-depressive illness. Arch Psychiatr Nervenkr 226:65–73, 1978

Ansseau M, Kupfer DJ, Reynolds CF, et al: REM latency distribution in major depression: clinical characteristics associated with sleep onset REM periods. Biol Psychiatry 19:1651–1666, 1984

Ansseau M, Kupfer DJ, Reynolds CF: Internight variability of REM latency in major depression: implications for the use of REM latency as a biological correlate. Biol Psychiatry 20:489–505, 1985

Asnis GM, Halbreich U, Nathan RS, et al: The dexamethasone suppression test in depressive illness: clinical correlates. Psychoneuroendocrinology 7:295–301, 1982

Ayuso-Guittierrez JL, Ramos-Brieva JA: The course of manic-depressive illness: a comparative study of bipolar I and bipolar II patients. J Affect Disord 4:9–14, 1982

Buschbaum M, Goodwin FK, Murphy DL, et al: Average evoked response in affective disorders. Am J Psychiatry 128:19–25, 1971

Coryell W, Endicott J, Reich T, et al: A family study of bipolar II disorder. Br J Psychiatry 145:49–54, 1984

Coryell W, Keller M, Endicott J, et al: Bipolar II illness: course and outcome over a five-year period. Psychol Med 19:129–141, 1989

Donnelly EF, Goodwin FK, Waldman IN, et al: Prediction of antidepressant responses to lithium. Am J Psychiatry 135:552–562, 1978

Dunner DL: Subtypes of bipolar affective disorder with particular regard to bipolar II. Psychiatric Developments 1:75–86, 1983

Dunner DL: A review of the diagnostic studies of "bipolar II" for the DSM-IV Work Group on mood disorders. Depression 1:2–10, 1993

Dunner DL, Gershon ES, Goodwin FK: Heritable factors in the severity of affective illness. Scientific Proceedings of the American Psychiatric Association 123:187–188, 1970

Dunner DL, Gershon ES, Goodwin FK, et al: Excretion of 17-hydroxycorticosteroids in unipolar and bipolar depressed patients. Arch Gen Psychiatry 26:360–363, 1972

Dunner DL, Dywer T, Fieve RR: Depressive symptoms in patients with unipolar and bipolar affective disorder. Compr Psychiatry 17:447–451, 1976a

Dunner DL, Fleiss DL, Fieve RR: The course of development of mania in patients with recurrent depression. Am J Psychiatry 133:905–908, 1976b

Dunner DL, Gershon ES, Goodwin FK: Heritable factors in the severity of affective illness. Biol Psychiatry 11:31–42, 1976c

Dunner DL, Levitt M, Kambaraci T, et al: Erythrocyte catechol-O-methyltransferase activity in primary affective disorder. Biol Psychiatry 12:237–244, 1977a

Dunner DL, Patrick V, Fieve RR: Rapid cycling manic depressive patients. Compr Psychiatry 18:561–566, 1977b

Dunner DL, Meltzer HL, Fieve RR: Clinical correlates of the lithium pump. Am J Psychiatry 135:1062–1064, 1978

Dunner DL, Stallone F, Fieve RR: Prophylaxis with lithium carbonate: an update. Arch Gen Psychiatry 39:1344–1345, 1982

Endicott J, Nee J, Andreasen N, et al: Bipolar II: combine or keep separate? J Affect Disord 8:17–28, 1985

Farkas T, Dunner DL, Fieve RR: L-Tryptophan in depression. Biol Psychiatry 11:295–302, 1976

Fieve RR, Dunner DL: Unipolar and bipolar affective states, in The Nature and Treatment of Depression. Edited by Flack FF, Draghi SC. New York, Wiley, 1975, pp 145–166

Fieve RR, Kumbaraci T, Dunner DL: Lithium prophylaxis of depression in bipolar I, bipolar II and unipolar patients. Am J Psychiatry 133:925–929, 1976

Fieve RR, Kumbaraci T, Kassir S, et al: Platelet monoamine oxidase activity in affective disorder. Biol Psychiatry 15:473–478, 1980

Fieve RR, Go R, Dunner DL, et al: Search for biological/genetic markers in a long-term epidemiological and morbid risk study of affective disorders. J Psychiatr Res 18:425–445, 1984

Gershon ES, Bunney WE Jr, Goodwin FK, et al: Catecholamines and affective illness: studies with L-dopa and alpha-methyl-para-tyrosine, in Brain Chemistry and Mental Disease. Edited by Ho BT, McIssac WM. New York, Plenum, 1971, pp 135–161

Gershon ES, Hamovit J, Guroff JJ, et al: A family study of schizoaffective, bipolar I, bipolar II, unipolar and normal control probands. Arch Gen Psychiatry 39:1157–1167, 1982

Giles DE, Rush AJ, Roffwarg HP: Sleep parameters in bipolar I, bipolar II, and unipolar depressions. Biol Psychiatry 21:1340–1343, 1986

Goodnick PJ, Meltzer HL, Fieve RR, et al: Differences in lithium kinetics between bipolar and unipolar patients. J Clin Psychopharmacol 2:48–50, 1982

Haag H, Heidorn A, Haag M, et al: Sequence of affective polarity and lithium response: preliminary report on Munich sample. Prog Neuropsychopharmacol Biol Psychiatry 11:205–208, 1987

Kane JM, Quitkin FM, Rifkin A, et al: Lithium carbonate and imipramine in the prophylaxis of unipolar and bipolar II illness. Arch Gen Psychiatry 39:1065–1069, 1982

Keeler LL, Othmer E: Atypical bipolar disorder: Is it a distinct entity? Psychiatric Annals 17:21–27, 1987

Kim YB, Dunner DL, Gross H, et al: Lithium erythrocyte: plasma ratio in primary affective disorder. Compr Psychiatry 19:123–134, 1978

Mazure K, Gershon ES: Blindness and reliability in lifetime psychiatric diagnosis. Arch Gen Psychiatry 36:521–525, 1979

Peselow ED, Dunner DL, Fieve RR, et al: Age of onset of affective illness. Psychiatr Clin 15:124–132, 1982

Rice JP, McDonald-Scott P, Endicott J, et al: The stability of diagnosis with an application to bipolar II disorder. Psychiatry Res 19:285–296, 1986

Rihmer Z, Arato M, Szentistrany I, et al: Red blood cell/plasma lithium ratio in manic-depressive, schizoaffective, and schizophrenic patients. Psychiatrica Clin 16:405–410, 1983

Robins E, Guze SB: Establishment of diagnostic validity in psychiatric illness: its application to schizophrenia. Am J Psychiatry 126:983–987, 1970

Rosenthal, NE, Sack RA, Gillin JC, et al: Seasonal affective disorder: a description of the syndrome and preliminary findings with light therapy. Arch Gen Psychiatry 41:72–80, 1984

Samson JA, Gudeman JE, Schatzberg AF, et al: Toward a biochemical classification of depressive disorders, VIII: platelet monoamine oxidase activity in subtypes of depressions. J Psychiatr Res 19:547–555, 1985

Spitzer RL, Endicott J: Schedule for Affective Disorders and Schizophrenia (Lifetime Version), 3rd Edition. New York, New York State Psychiatric Institute, 1978

Stallone F, Dunner DL, Ahearn J, et al: Statistical predictions of suicide in depressives. Compr Psychiatry 21:381–387, 1980

Thompson C, Isaacs G: Seasonal affective disorder: a British sample. J Affect Disord 14:1–11, 1988

Tsuang MT, Woolson RF, Winokur G, et al: Stability of psychiatric diagnosis: schizophrenia and affective disorders followed up over a 30 to 40 year period. Arch Gen Psychiatry 38:535–539, 1981

Winokur G, Morrison J: The Iowa 500: follow-up of 225 depressives. Br J Psychiatry 123:543–548, 1973

Wirz-Justice A, Bucheli C, Graw P, et al: Light treatment of seasonal affective disorder in Switzerland. Acta Psychiatr Scand 74:193–204, 1986

Zisook S, Janowsky DS, Overall JE, et al: The dexamethasone suppression test and unipolar/bipolar distinctions. J Clin Psychiatry 46:461–465, 1985

Chapter 4

Schizoaffective Disorder

Jacqueline Lalive Aubert, M.D., and A. John Rush, M.D.

Statement of the Issues

A number of questions about the definition of schizoaffective (SA) disorder remain open. The first issue we focus on in this chapter is the delineation of both affective and psychotic features, as they are used as inclusion and exclusion criteria. The second issue we deal with concerns the implications of the temporal relationship between symptoms (i.e., the overlap and separation of mood and psychotic symptoms during episodes). The third question we address concerns the validity and clinical utility of adding new criteria for defining a course based on interepisode recovery.

Significance of the Issues

Is SA disorder a form of schizophrenia with a better prognosis? Naturalistic follow-up studies from the beginning of the century to the late 1960s, as reviewed by Maj (1984b), point out that acuteness of onset and the presence of mood features are associated with less severe clinical forms of psychosis (Hoch 1921; Hunt and Appel 1936; Kant 1940; Kasanin 1933; Kirby 1913; Langfeldt 1937, 1956; Rachlin 1935; Vaillant 1963, 1964), even if the condition falls within the group of Bleulerian schizophrenias (American Psychiatric Association 1952, 1968). Studies in the late 1960s and 1970s, commonly based on Research Diagnostic Criteria (RDC) (Spitzer et al. 1975, 1978), emphasize the importance of mood features. For RDC, SA disorder includes manic or depressive syndromes, during which more or less brief periods with Schneiderian first-rank symptoms (FRS) occur (Schneider 1959). RDC defined subtypes of SA, based on course of illness, with the implication that

This review was supported in part by Grant MH-41115. We appreciate the secretarial support of David Savage and Fast Word, Inc., of Dallas.

the more acute episodes were associated with a better prognosis. Studies based on RDC suggest that SA disorder is a heterogeneous group that occupies an intermediate position between schizophrenia and mood disorders (Abrams and Taylor 1976; Clayton et al. 1968; Fowler et al. 1972; Taylor and Abrams 1973; Tsuang and Dempsey 1979; Winokur et al. 1969).

The International Classification of Diseases (ICD-8, ICD-9, and ICD-10) (World Health Organization 1968, 1977, 1992) lists SA psychosis under schizophrenia. SA psychosis presents with pronounced affective features intermingled with schizophrenic features, tending to remission but prone to recur. ICD-10 includes various types of SA psychosis: SA manic type, other acute or transient psychosis, and reactive psychosis, all of which are defined as episodic psychotic disorders with prominent affective and schizophrenic symptoms. All remain classified under schizophrenia.

DSM-III (American Psychiatric Association 1980) lists SA disorder under psychotic disorders not otherwise specified (295.7) to include cases for which the differential diagnosis between affective and schizophreniform disorder or schizophrenia is uncertain, without defining criteria. For DSM-III, mood-incongruent psychotic features are allowed to be part of mood disorders. DSM-III-R (American Psychiatric Association 1987) emphasizes the temporal relationship of schizophrenic and mood symptoms and provides the following diagnostic criteria: a major depressive or manic syndrome concurrent at some time with symptoms meeting Criterion A for schizophrenia and, during at least one episode, delusions or hallucinations are present for at least 2 weeks when mood symptoms are not prominent. Consequently, the DSM-III-R proviso that psychotic symptoms be present for at least some time without mood symptoms provides a narrower definition of SA disorder than ICD-9 or RDC.

In this chapter, we focus on recent studies encompassing symptomatic features, treatment response, and biological, familial, and course data associated with SA disorder, either to compare them with schizophrenic and mood disorders or to assign characteristics depending on SA types. A review of the literature provides a basis for determining whether changes in the criteria or in the placement of SA disorder should be recommended for DSM-IV.

Method

The literature search on SA disorder was conducted with MEDLARS (1980 to January 1989) and Medline computer databases (1980 to October 1991). The search was keyed on the following areas: first, review articles including historical developments of diagnostic criteria and controversies about diagnostic systems, and second, operationalized clinical and laboratory studies, based on the following diagnostic systems: Feighner criteria for affective disorders and schizophrenia (Feighner et al. 1972), RDC, DSM-III and DSM-III-R, ICD-8 and ICD-9, and Vienna Research Criteria (VRC), characterized by the presence/absence of a schizoaxial syndrome (i.e., formal thought disorder and defect symptomatology) (Berner and Simhandl 1983).

Results

Most relevant data are provided in the tables. The text includes comments on the main results and conclusions pertinent to each issue.

Symptom Features

Four of the eight studies reviewed used RDC (see Table 4–1). Moldin et al. (1987) studied a pool of probands and relatives of patients, who were diagnosed with schizophrenia, SA disorder, unipolar (UP) disorder, or bipolar (BP) disorder using the Minnesota Multiphasic Personality Inventory (Hathaway and McKinley 1970) and the RDC. They found some familial and symptomatic overlap between SA disorder and both schizophrenic and mood disorders. They suggested that SA may be located on a genetic continuum between schizophrenia and mood disorders.

Rosenthal et al. (1980) pointed out that bipolar I patients, presenting either with FRS (Schneider 1959) or without FRS, had similar rates for transmission of affective disorders and treatment response but that those with FRS had an earlier age at onset. They pointed out that SA disorder, particularly manic type, may be a variant of affective disorders. Pope et al. (1980) concluded that SA disorder, particularly SA manic, should be included in the group of affective disorders when compared with schizophrenia, BP, and SA patients with two or more mood-incongruent symptoms. BP and SA patients had similar clinical and social outcome. Welner et al. (1979) studied the long-term course of schizophrenic probands and their relatives, who presented with affective, schizophrenic, or SA syndrome (60%). Course and outcome were globally better in the relatives of the SA group, but Welner suggested that *undiagnosed schizophrenia* could be a more appropriate term than *SA disorder* when considering the long-term course of these relatives.

Two studies using ICD-8 suggested that SA disorder is not a separate entity. Angst et al. (1983) evaluated the relationship between various symptom clusters and the diagnosis of SA disorder. They found that SA disorder was associated with various symptom clusters and concluded that SA disorder was a transitional diagnosis between schizophrenia and affective psychosis. Jensen (1984) found that, in consecutive hospitalizations, patients who were diagnosed at least once as having

Table 4–1. Symptom feature studies

Study	Sample	Method	Results	Comments
Moldin et al. 1987	14 schizophrenic, 17 schizo-affective, 13 unipolar, and 12 bipolar (RDC) patients; 118 normal	Comparison of diagnosis with MMPI profiles	Psychometric measures converged with RDC phenotypes	Schizoaffective disorder is on a continuum between schizophrenia and affective disorders
Rosenthal et al. 1980	71 bipolar I patients (by RDC and SADS)	Comparison between RDC positive and negative symptoms	74% of bipolar I were RDC positive at least once during an acute phase; RDC-positive bipolar I had a younger onset; no difference in response to lithium between RDC positive and negative; RDC-positive and -negative bipolar I had 24% family transmission of affective disorders	Schizoaffective disorder is a variant of affective disorder, more in manic than in depressed phases
Pope et al. 1980	219 RDC schizophrenic, affective, and schizo-affective patients (schizo-affective manic with 2 or more mood-incongruent symptoms)	Comparison between schizo-phrenic, manic, and schizo-affective manic patients	Except for short-term response to treatment (weaker in schizo-affective patients), schizoaffective manics and manics did not differ on symptoms and social outcome (0.5- to 5-year follow-up); schizo-affective manic and manic patients did not differ in family transmission	Schizoaffective manic patients are within manic group. Psychotic symptoms are not specific for differentiat-ing between diagnostic subgroups
Welner et al. 1979	20 RDC schizophrenic patients; 30 relatives with affective, schizophrenic, or both symptoms	Comparison between symptoms and course of probands and relatives	Probands had a 90% chronic course with 75% deterioration; relatives had a 70% chronic course with 50% deterioration; 60% met schizo-affective diagnosis at some time	Schizoaffective disorder is an undiagnosed psychosis resembling schizophrenia

Study	Sample	Design	Results	Conclusion
Angst et al. 1983	143 schizophrenic, 40 schizoaffective, and 89 affective psychosis (by ICD-8 and PSE) patients	Compared correspondence between diagnosis and symptoms	Schizoaffective psychosis is combined with different symptom clusters	Schizoaffective psychosis may be a transitional diagnosis
Jensen 1984	114 patients with at least one ICD-8 schizoaffective diagnosis	Compared the combination of diagnosis on consecutive hospitalizations	In longitudinal studies, schizoaffective disorder was combined with schizophrenia and bipolar psychoses	A schizoaffective diagnosis has a descriptive value only for current episodes
Winokur 1989	604 unipolar nonpsychotic, 100 bipolar nonpsychotic, 76 unipolar mood-congruent, 113 bipolar mood congruent, 60 unipolar mood-incongruent, and 80 bipolar mood-incongruent patients by DSM-III	Five subgroup comparisons: 1) unipolar nonpsychotic vs. bipolar nonpsychotic; 2) unipolar mood congruent vs. bipolar mood congruent; 3) unipolar mood incongruent vs. bipolar mood incongruent; 4) unipolar mood congruent vs. bipolar mood incongruent; 5) unipolar mood incongruent vs. bipolar mood congruent	Nonpsychotic bipolar and mood-congruent bipolar have acute and earlier onset vs. nonpsychotic unipolar and mood-congruent unipolar; incongruent bipolar vs. incongruent unipolar are in the same direction; unipolar are more likely female, regardless of symptom profile; acute schizoaffective bipolar and unipolar vs. acute bipolar and unipolar are similar for number of hospitalizations, outcome, and relapse data	Results suggest that acute schizoaffective disorder is on the affective continuum and not on the schizophrenic continuum
Shanda et al. 1984	90 delusional psychotic patients (by Schneiderian FRS, RDC, ICD-8, DSM-III, and VRC)	Compared the ability of various diagnostic systems to predict episodic or chronic course	DSM-III, RDC, and VRC allowed definition of a delusional/psychotic subgroup, which had significantly better prognosis	6- to 9-year follow-up confirmed the correspondence between episodic course and affective components

Note. FRS = first rank symptoms. MMPI = Minnesota Multiphasic Personality Inventory. PSE = Present State Examination. RDC = Research Diagnostic Criteria. SADS = Schedule for Affective Disorders and Schizophrenia. VRC = Vienna Research Criteria.

SA disorder were, over time, also diagnosed as having schizophrenia, bipolar disorder, or reactive psychotic episodes.

Winokur (1989) compared the course of illness in six subgroups of DSM-III patients: nonpsychotic UP and BP, mood-congruent psychotic UP and BP, and mood-incongruent psychotic UP and BP. He noted that the presence of psychotic features did not modify the expected differences between UP and BP.

Shanda et al. (1984) used a variety of diagnostic systems to determine which could predict course of illness in patients with delusional psychoses. DSM-III, RDC and VRC (but not ICD-8) for SA disorder identified a psychotic affective subgroup, with an episodic course and a better prognosis.

Treatment-Response Studies

The seven studies cited in Table 4–2 compared the efficacy of lithium treatment as either an acute-phase or maintenance-phase treatment.

Carman et al. (1981) compared the acute-phase treatment response of RDC schizophrenic and SA manic or SA depressed patients who were randomly assigned to a neuroleptic treatment in combination with either lithium or placebo. Predictors of good response to lithium were a higher initial severity, presence of affective symptoms, and an episodic course. Lithium was more frequently effective in the SA group, but some schizophrenic patients also improved.

Mattes and Nayak (1984) found a poor response to lithium treatment in RDC SA (mainly schizophrenic) disorder patients, when they compared 1 year of lithium treatment with 1 year of fluphenazine treatment. These findings confirm the poor response to lithium when schizophrenic features are prominent. In another study (Romeo et al. 1985), patients with DSM-III acute purely affective disorders (SA manic and BP manic) were treated for 2 years with slow-release lithium. Results revealed that quality of response to prophylactic treatment was proportional to purity of affective features. Conversely, lithium had no effect on mood-incongruent psychotic symptoms. A long-term prophylactic lithium treatment (more than 3 years) in BP, UP, and SA outpatients led to a better response (fewer relapses and rehospitalizations) in DSM-III BP than in SA patients, and in both of them compared with UP patients (Bouman et al. 1986). These results suggest that BP disorder could be a variant of affective disorders and SA disorder a variant of schizophrenic disorder.

Furthermore, ICD-9 SA patients without VRC schizoaxial syndrome responded better to 5 years of lithium treatment than SA patients with schizoaxial syndrome (Küfferle and Lenz 1983). When patients were rediagnosed by RDC, VRC, or Kendell and Perris's criteria and treated with lithium for 2 years, Maj (1984a) found that ICD-9 SA patients had fewer relapses under treatment (except for the VRC patients with schizoaxial syndrome), whereas RDC and Kendell criteria

Table 4–2. Treatment-response studies

Study	Sample	Method	Results	Comments
Carman et al. 1981	11 RDC chronic schizophrenic, 7 schizoaffective (5 manic type) inpatients	Compared the efficacy of 4 weeks of treatment with neuroleptics/lithium (<0.6 mEq/L) and neuroleptics/placebo; clinical assessment by BPRS and composite score (psychosis, depression, arousal) derived from the BPRS	Favorable response to lithium on arousal (10 patients), psychosis (5 patients), and depression (5 patients); good responders evidenced initial severity, affective symptoms, and an episodic course	Lithium treatment (with neuroleptics) may also help some poor-prognosis schizophrenic patients
Mattes and Nayak 1984	14 RDC schizoaffective (primarily schizophrenic) outpatients	Compared the efficacy of combined lithium (<0.6 mEq/L)/placebo and fluphenazine/placebo treatment for 1 year	At 1-year follow-up, 6 patients on lithium and 1 on fluphenazine had relapsed (3 had schizophrenic, 3 had schizoaffective, and 1 had manic episodes); 2 patients on fluphenazine dropped out	Schizoaffective (mainly schizophrenic) patients are poor responders to lithium treatment
Romeo et al. 1985	29 DSM-III acute affective inpatients, 15 "pure affective" and 14 either schizoaffective or bipolar manic with mood-incongruent psychotic features	Compared the effects of a 2-year slow-release lithium treatment (0.5–0.6 mEq/L); global evaluation scored from 0 (worst) to 4 (best)	Mean score was 2.73 for pure affective patients, 3.05 for bipolars, 1.33 for schizoaffective, and 3.15 for bipolar with mood incongruent psychotic symptoms	Lithium effectiveness is proportional to the purity of the affective component, which seems independent of mood incongruent psychotic symptoms
Bouman et al. 1986	104 affective disorder (Feighner criteria), 56 bipolar (DSM-III), 28 schizoaffective (DSM-III), 9 schizomanic, 3 schizo-depressed (Kendell criteria), and 20 unipolar patients	Controlled lithium prophylaxis treatment	Mean duration of treatment was 44 months, with 1.0 episode and 0.2 hospitalizations; probability of no relapse during treatment and worsened course after lithium discontinuation was higher for bipolar and schizoaffective patients; the more episodes before treatment, the most effective treatment was on rate of rehospitalizations	Lack of effectiveness of lithium prophylaxis on unipolar

(continued)

Table 4–2. Treatment-response studies *(continued)*

Study	Sample	Method	Results	Comments
Küfferle and Lenz 1983	60 ICD-9 schizo-affective patients, rediagnosed according to VRC (schizoaxial syndrome)	Compared the efficacy of 5 years of lithium treatment on number of episodes and hospitalizations, according to presence/absence of schizoaxial syndrome	Patients with schizoaxial syndrome had 2.12 episodes and 1.82 admissions before lithium treatment, compared to 2.06 episodes and 1.41 admissions during the same period; patients without schizoaxial syndrome had 3.02 episodes and 2.02 admissions before lithium treatment, compared to 1.66 episodes and 1.12 admissions during the same period	Schizoaffective disorder with schizoaxial syndrome had a poorer lithium response and may be a variant of schizophrenia; schizo-affective disorder without schizoaxal syndrome had better lithium response and may be a variant of affective disorder
Maj 1984a	38 ICD-9 schizo-affective patients, rediagnosed according to RDC, VRC, Kendell and Perris's criteria (cycloid psychosis)	Compared clinical course and characteristics of outcome in responders and nonresponders according to diagnostic criteria after 2 years of lithium treatment (0.6–1.0 mEq/L)	The number of episodes decreased in all patients except the group with schizoaxial syndrome; RDC and Kendell's schizomanic patients had a better outcome than the schizo-depressed; a personal and/or family history of affective disorders was predictive of good response, contrary to personal and/or family history of schizophrenic episodes; biological parameters are not predictive of treatment response	There may be two variants of schizoaffective disorder: one more schizophrenic, the other more affective
Maj 1988	49 ICD-9 schizo-affective patients	Efficacy of lithium treatment on broadly defined schizoaffective disorder (by ICD) in a 2-year prospective study	Lithium is not effective on schizophrenic symptoms or schizodepressive episodes; a previous course predicted a good response to lithium	A subgroup of schizo-affective disorder is similar to bipolar disorder with regard to treatment response

Note. BPRS = Brief Psychiatric Rating Scale. VRC = Vienna Research Criteria. RDC = Research Diagnostic Criteria.

SA manic patients had a better outcome than did the SA depressed patients. In a prospective 2-year study with the same sample, Maj (1988) confirmed that the SA depressed patients had a poorer prognosis, whereas a previous BP course predicted a good treatment response.

Laboratory Test Findings

All the studies in Table 4–3 are based on RDC, and some also included a polydiagnostic approach. One group of studies used neurological tests to differentiate SA disorder patients from affective and schizophrenic patients. The Hoffman reflex recovery curves (Goode and Manning 1988) revealed that both SA and affective disorder patients evidenced symmetrical recovery curves in both legs, whereas they were asymmetrical in schizophrenic patients. Neuromorphological measures (mean sulcal width, global cerebellar atrophy, mean white matter density with left-right asymmetry) did not significantly differentiate schizophrenic from chronic SA disorder patients (Smith et al. 1987). Ventricular size and cortical and cerebellar atrophy measures obtained by computed tomography (CT) scan (Rieder et al. 1983) did not reveal significant differences between SA, BP, and schizophrenic patients. The rates of middle ear muscle activity during rapid eye movement (REM) sleep were higher in half of the schizophrenic patients compared with patients with major depression and control subjects, whereas these rates were below normal in the patients with SA disorder (Benson and Zarcone 1982). Shorter REM latency as measured by the sleep EEG did not differentiate schizophrenic and SA disorder patients (Zarcone et al. 1987). Moreover, oculomotor stereognosis examinations showed that right-left identification abnormalities were more marked in schizophrenic than in SA and affective disorder patients (Walker 1981).

The following studies, also based on RDC, evaluated neuroendocrine function in different diagnostic groups. Based on RDC, Coccaro et al. (1985) found more nonsuppressors on the dexamethasone suppression test (DST) in those with psychotic affective disorders than in those with SA disorder. When rediagnosed by DSM-III criteria, the SA patients fell into an intermediate position between depressed patients with psychotic symptoms and nondepressed psychotic patients. Maj (1986) found the same trend, with 40% DST nonsuppression in those with major depression, compared to a 25% nonsuppression rate in the SA depressed group. Hubain et al. (1986) studied the DST in affective and psychotic disorders and found that presence of psychotic features was associated with more nonsuppression but only in the group with affective illness. Psychosis per se was not clearly the cause of nonsuppression. Moreover, a blunted response of thyroid-stimulating hormone (TSH) to thyrotropin-releasing hormone (TRH) was higher in those with endogenous major depression and SA disorder, depressed phase, than in those with SA disorder, manic phase, or acute schizophrenia (Sauer et al. 1984). These results

Table 4–3. Laboratory test findings

Study	Sample	Method	Results	Comments
Goode and Manning 1988	16 schizophrenic, 19 affective disorder, and 19 schizoaffective disorder patients by RDC	Hoffman reflex recovery curves with measures in both legs	Recovery of both legs was correlated in affective and schizoaffective patients but not in schizophrenic patients	Schizoaffective disorder equals affective disorder but not schizophrenia
Smith et al. 1987	31 schizophrenic and 8 chronic schizoaffective patients by RDC; 32 schizophrenic, 2 schizophreniform, and 3 schizoaffective patients by DSM-III	Neuromorphological measures including CT scan, BPRS, and NHSI twice weekly	No correlation between BPRS + NHSI and neuromorphology measures	Schizoaffective disorder equals schizophrenia
Rieder et al. 1983	28 chronic schizophrenic, 15 chronic schizoaffective, and 19 bipolar patients by RDC	CT scan: VBR values, sulcal ratings, cerebellar ratings	No significant difference between diagnostic groups for ventricular size, cortical atrophy, or cerebellar atrophy; each group included some subjects with some abnormalities	Schizoaffective disorder equals bipolar equals schizophrenia
Benson et al. 1982	11 schizophrenic, 8 schizoaffective, 10 major depressed, and 13 controls by RDC	Tympanic acoustic impedance during REM sleep + EMG + EOG using ZDS and STAS measures	MEMA was higher for schizophrenic than for schizoaffective, depressed, and control patients; schizoaffective patients had lower rates than depressed and control patients; no difference between depressed and control patients	Schizoaffective did not equal schizophrenic, depressed, or controls; schizophrenic does not equal depressed or controls; depressed equals controls
Zarcone et al. 1987	12 schizophrenic, 12 major depressed, 8 schizoaffective, and 18 control by RDC	10 sleep measures: sleep latency (strict and lenient definitions), waking after onset, total sleep, slow-wave sleep, REM and % REM sleep, mean period	Compared with controls, REM latency was shorter in any diagnostic group; no interdiagnostic group comparisons showed any significant difference REM length, REM latency	Schizoaffective equals schizophrenia

Study	Subjects	Method	Results	Comments
Walker 1981	15 schizophrenic, 15 schizoaffective, and 15 affective disorder patients by RDC	(strict and lenient definitions), average and lowest values; Neuromotor examinations: stereognosis + mirror movement + movement regularity + right/left identification + oculomotor function + attentional assessment	Schizophrenic patients showed more oculomotor stereognosis, right-left identification abnormalition, more errors or omissions on the attentional task under distraction	Schizoaffective equals affective but not schizophrenic
Coccaro et al. 1985	10 psychotic depressed, 9 schizoaffective depressed, and 12 functional psychosis (not depressed) by RDC and DSM-III	DST nonsuppression (>5 µg/dl)	Nonsuppression occurred in 90% of psychotic depressed, 20% schizoaffective depressed, and 17% of nondepressed psychotic patients; cortisol values were greater in the psychotic depressed group; rediagnosed by DSM-III criteria, nonsuppression occurred in 75% of depressed, 40% of schizoaffective depressed, and 14% of nondepressed psychotic patients	DST may help to distinguish patients with primary depressive disorders with psychotic symptoms from patients with coexisting depressed and psychotic features
Maj 1986	52 major depressive and 20 schizoaffective depressed patients	DST accompanied by assessment with BPRS and HRSD	DST nonsuppression occurred in 40% of major depressive and 25% of schizoaffective depressed patients; no difference between schizoaffective depressed suppressors and nonsuppressors with regard to symptoms, severity of illness, and family history	

(continued)

Table 4–3. Laboratory test findings (*continued*)

Study	Sample	Method	Results	Comment
Hubain et al. 1986	65 RDC (Feighner criteria) major depressive (21 bipolar; 44 unipolar), 15 minor depressive, 10 schizoaffective, and 22 schizophrenic patients	Compared the predictive value of DST response for typing homogeneous subgroups of affective disorder	Best predictive value of DST for primary endogenous unipolar depression (96%) decreased to 27.4% for psychotic vs. nonpsychotic depression	Psychotic symptoms, in addition to major depression, may dysregulate the HPA axis
Sauer et al. 1984	18 schizoaffective depressed, 12 schizo-affective manic, 30 endogenous depressed, and 20 acute schizo-phrenic patients by RDC	DST + TRHST (blunting = <5 μg/ml) and assessment with BPRS and HDSD	DST nonsuppression occurred in 89% of schizoaffective depressed, 57% of endogenous depressed; and of 25% schizophrenic; blunted TSH response higher in endogenous depressed than in schizoaffective manic and schizo-phrenic but not different from schizoaffective depressed	The high rate of nonsuppres-sion in schizoaffective may be due to the strictness of RDC and the severity of depression; coupling of DST nonsuppression and TRHST blunting may define a major depressive subgroup with-out mood-incongruent psychotic features
Wahby et al. 1988	14 schizoaffective depressed, 23 schizophrenic, 41 unipolar depressive patients by RDC	TSH test in addition to assessment with HRSD; one-half of patients on anti-depressant medication and/ or neuroleptics	No difference in delta TSH maximum among schizoaffective, schizophrenic, and control; mean delta TSH maximum lower in unipolar depressive patients; blunting rate of TSH response was higher in unipolar depressive patients	TSH response to TRH in schizoaffective depressed patients is closer to that in schizophrenic than in unipolar depressive patients
Wahby et al. 1990	Same sample as above	Prolactin response to TRH	No significant difference between delta maximum prolactin in schizo-affective, schizophrenic, and control subjects; prolactin response to TRH significantly lower in unipolar depressive patients	Schizoaffective depressed are closer to schizophrenic than to unipolar depressive in prolactin response to TRH, as for TSH response to TRH

Study	Patients	Method	Results	Conclusion
Kiriike et al. 1988	10 schizoaffective manic, 9 manic, and 27 schizophrenic patients by RDC	DST + TRHST in addition to assessment with BPRS	No difference in rate of TRHST blunting and DST nonsuppression in schizoaffective manic and manic; both were higher than in schizophrenic group	Schizoaffective manic and manic patients have more disturbance in both endocrinological axes than do schizophrenic patients
Langer et al. 1986	114 patients: 73 major depressive, 10 minor depressive, 17 schizophrenic, 12 schizoaffective (4 depressed, 8 manic), 2 manic, and 24 normal	Compared diagnostic repartition, response to treatment, and outcome of normal vs. blunted responders to TRHST	Blunted TSH response was 39% in depressed, 35% in psychotic, and 7% in normal; blunted TSH response predicted a better response to antidepressants or neuroleptics than a normal TRH response; blunted TSH response showed a 29% relapse rate at 2 months, 59% at 12 months under treatment maintenance vs. 15% and 36% in normal TSH response	TRHST might be a state marker that helps predict treatment response

Note. BPRS = Brief Psychiatric Rating Scale. CT = computed tomography. DST = dexamethasone suppression test. HPA = hypothalamic-pituitary-adrenal. HRSD = Hamilton Rating Scale for Depression. MEMA = middle ear muscle activity. NHSI = New Haven Schizophrenia Index. PSE = Present State Examination. REM = rapid eye movement. RDC = Research Diagnostic Criteria. SADS = Schedule for Affective Disorders and Schizophrenia. STAS = State-Trait Anxiety Scale. TRH = thyrotropin-releasing hormone. TSH = thyroid-stimulating hormone. VRC = Vienna Research Criteria. ZDS = Zung Depression Scale. TRHST = thyrotropin-releasing hormone stimulation test. VBR = ventricular brain ratio.

contradict Wahby et al.'s (1988) findings that the response to TRH of patients with SA disorder, depressed phase, was closer to that of the schizophrenic than the unipolar depressed group. In the same sample of SA depressed male patients, the prolactin responses to TSH were also closer to values of schizophrenic patients than to those with major depression, even if the results were lacking in specificity (Wahby et al. 1990). Kiriike et al. (1988) found a higher TSH blunting rate in patients with both SA disorder, manic phase, and bipolar disorder, manic phase, than in schizophrenic patients. Langer et al. (1986) found that a blunted TSH response predicted a better response to medication and less risk of relapse, both for affective and psychotic patients.

Family Studies

Sixteen family studies that focused on the familial transmission of schizophrenic, atypical psychotic, major mood, and SA disorders were found. Detailed results are provided in Table 4–4.

The first group of studies are based on RDC. Coryell and Zimmerman (1988) concluded that there is a separate transmission of psychotic and nonpsychotic affective disorders and pointed out that probands with SA disorder had a high likelihood of having relatives with schizophrenia and SA disorder, whereas those with major depression had a high likelihood of having relatives with SA disorder. Gershon et al. (1988) suggested that there may be two variants of SA disorder, one transmitted with BP disorder and the other with schizophrenia and unipolar depression. Baron et al. (1982) found that SA (mainly schizophreniform) probands had a higher incidence of schizophrenia and had SA disorder (mainly schizophrenic) relatives, whereas SA (mainly affective) probands had more BP, UP, and SA (mainly affective) disorder relatives. They suggested that SA disorder (mainly schizophreniform) was a variant of schizophrenia, whereas SA (mainly affective) was a variant of affective disorders, and that SA manic and SA depressed may have different familial transmission.

Furthermore, according to Maj (1989), SA disorder with full affective and schizophrenic syndromes was associated with schizophrenia, affective disorders, and SA disorders, but when SA disorder met criteria for "bouffée delirante", the morbid risk for schizophrenia was null. Thus, he suggested that SA disorder was a heterogeneous entity. DeLisi et al. (1987) compared the observed versus expected concordance of diagnosis and symptoms in families with two or more siblings with chronic psychosis. The distribution of diagnoses among the pairs resulted in the significant segregation of chronic schizophrenia and SA disorder within families and more concordant pairs than expected. Conversely, there was no significant concordance between symptom distribution in sibling pairs. Shanda et al. (1986) rediagnosed probands who presented with mood-incongruent psychosis by RDC

Table 4–4. Family studies

Study	Probands	Relatives (morbid risk, generally in %, age corrected)			
Coryell and Zimmerman 1988	RDC	**573 relatives**			
		% Schizophrenia	% Major depressed	% Schizoaffective-D	% Schizophrenic spectrum
	21 S	1.4	0.0	2.3	5.6
	29 major depressed	0.0	25.2	22.5	1.9
	47 SA	2.0	1.9	5.3	5.6
	38 never ill	0.0	10.9	2.5	2.5
Gershon et al. 1988	48 RDC chronic psychosis	**237 relatives**			
		% Schizophrenia	% Affective	% Schizoaffective	% not ill
	Chronic S	All psychosis: 6.2	BP/UP = 2.2/14.7	Acute: 5.0	71.9
	Chronic AD	All psychosis: 11.7	BP/UP = 9.6/9.3	Acute: 0.0	69.4
	30 control	All psychosis: 2.0	BP/UP = 0.8/6.7	Acute: 0.3	90.1
Baron et al. 1982	RDC	% Schizophrenia	% Affective	% Schizoaffective	
	50 S	7.9	BP/UP = 0.6/4.5	SA-S/SA-A = 1.7/0.0	
	40 BP	0.7	BP/UP = 14.5/16.3	SA-S/SA-A = 0.0/1.4	
	45 UP	0.0	BP/UP = 2.2/17.7	SA-S/SA-A = 0.8/3.0	
	28 SA-S	4.1	BP/UP = 0.0/10.9	SA-S/SA-A = 0.7/0.0	
	22 SA-A	0.0	BP/UP = 1.6/26.5	SA-S/SA-A = 0.0/3.2	
Maj 1989	RDC	**259 relatives**			
		% Schizophrenia	% Affective	% Schizoaffective	
	20 SA = full S & A syndromes	6.1	6.6	2.2	
	18 SA = bouffée delirante	0.0	4.5	4.5	
	25 S	9.0	3.8	1.9	
	25 BP	0.0	13.2	1.9	

(continued)

Table 4-4. Family studies (continued)

Study	Probands	Relatives (morbid risk, generally in %, age corrected)		
DeLisi et al. 1987	RDC illness in 123 siblings	53 sets of siblings with chronic psychosis		
	57 chronic S	Concordant pairs	n observed	n expected
	8 chronic SA-M	Chronic S/chronic S	17	12.75
	2 nonchronic SA-M	SA chronic/nonchronic	3	13.75
	36 chronic SA-D	SA chronic/chronic	15	
	2 nonchronic SA-D	Total	35	26.5
	16 chronic SA mixed			
	2 nonchronic SA mixed	Discordant pairs		
		Chronic S/SA-M nonchronic	1	
		Chronic S/SA-D nonchronic	2	
		Chronic S/SA mixed nonchronic	0	26.25
		Chronic S/SA-M chronic	2	
		Chronic S/SA-D chronic	9	
		Chronic S/SA mixed chronic	4	
		Total	18	26.25
Shanda et al. 1986	67 delusional psychosis	419 relatives		
		% Schizophrenia	% Affective-D	% Schizoaffective-D
	32 S-RDC	1.9	0.0	0.0
	17 S-VRC	5.4	0.0	0.0
	5 A-RDC	0.0	7.9	2.6
	13 A-VRC	0.0	5.3	—
	RDC psychosis	2.6	0.9	0.2
	VRC psychosis	2.6	1.4	0.0

		% Schizophrenia	% Affective	% Schizoaffective	Sform/atypical/paranoid
Kendler et al. 1985	DSM-III				
	159 S/723 relatives	3.7	UP/BP = 6.0/1.2	1.4	0.1/2.5/0.9
	261 control/1,056 relatives	0.2	UP/BP = 7.6/0.3	0.1	0.1/0.3/0.0
Kendler et al. 1986	DSM-III				
	24 SA-S/91 relatives	3.6	6.9	0.1	0.0/1.5/0.0
	42 SA/149 relatives	5.6	11.0	2.7	2.2/1.8/1.0
	19 AD/50 relatives	4.3	20.0	0.0	0.0/2.9/0.0
	201 control/1,056 relatives	0.2	6.8	0.1	0.0/0.3/0.0
				(O/E = observed/expected)	
Faraone and Tsuang 1988	DSM-III, 510 S probands	% S relatives	% Atypical S relatives		
	S	O/E = 3.7/3.4	O/E = 4.9/4.8		
	Atypical S	O/E = 4.9/4.4	O/E = 5.3/7.3		
	Control	O/E = 0.2/0.3	O/E = 0.4/0.3		
Mendlewicz et al. 1980	DSM-III	% Schizophrenia	% Affective		
	55 S	16.9	BP/UP = 1.4/7.4		
	55 BP	1.8	BP/UP = 18.7/20.6		
	55 UP	3.2	BP/UP = 2.1/27.2		
	55 SA	10.8	BP/UP = 13.1/22.4		
Maj et al. 1991	DSM-III-R	% Schizophrenia	% Affective		
	28 S	8.8	1.7		
	28 MDD with MIC symptoms	3.8	6.5		
	19 MDD with MC symptoms	2.2	12.3		
	27 not psychotic	0.0	16.9		
	21 SA depressive type	8.7	2.4		
	18 control	0.0	2.6		

(continued)

Table 4–4. Family studies *(continued)*

Study	Probands	Relatives (morbid risk, generally in %, age corrected)			
Winokur et al. 1985	ICD-8 probands				
	Probands(140 S, 40 SA, 30 BP, 59 UP)	Relatives			
		No psychotic symptoms	**Psychotic symptoms**		
	No psychotic symptoms	0.52	0.48		
	Psychotic symptoms	0.32	0.68		
	Instances of psychosis in family pairs	P/R = Proband/Relatives −/+ = absence/presence			
		P−/R−	**P−/R+**	**P+/R−**	**P+/R+**
	169 S	6	3	53	107
	95 SA	3	7	33	50
	94 UP	28	25	22	19
	43 BP	11	12	12	8
	Family comparisons				
	73 S	2	2	14	55
	30 SA	0	2	5	23
	35 UP	10	10	7	8
	15 BP	2	6	4	3
	50 UP + BP	12	16	11	11
Angst et al. 1979a, 1979b	150 ICD-8 SA	1,004 relatives			
		% Schizophrenia	**% Affective**	**% Schizoaffective**	**% Unspecified psychosis**
	41 SA males	male/female 6.5/6.3	male/female 2.6/6.7	male/female 1.9/3.1	9.4
	109 SA females	male/female 4.6/5.2	male/female 5.2/9.0	male/female 2.8/4.0	
	97 SA manic	5.9	BP/UP 0.9/5.9	4.0	
	53 SA nonmanic	4.6	BP/UP 1.1/5.1	1.1	
	72 S dominant SA	5.9	5.8	3.3	
	73 A dominant SA	4.6	7.9	2.9	

Scharfetter and Nüssperli 1980	269 ICD-8 functional psychosis		
	% Schizophrenia	1,577 relatives % Affective	% Schizoaffective
33 hebephenic (H)	H 4.7; C 1.9; P 0.9	—	—
38 catatonic (C)	H 4.5; C 5.8; P 1.9	BP/UP = 2/2	0.6
69 paranoid (P)	H 1.0; C 0.7; P 4.5	BP/UP = 0.5/1	0.3
59 BP	H 1.5; C -; P -	BP/UP = 2.2/7.7	—
30 UP	H 0.3; C 1.9; P 0.6	BP/UP = 2.1/9.0	0.3
40 SA	H 3.0; C 7.0; P 1.5	BP/UP = 4.4/4.4	2.5

Stassen et al. 1988	248 ICD-8 functional psychosis		
	n Schizophrenia	350 relatives n Affective	n Schizoaffective
136 S	48	D/BP = 43/15	2
49 D	24	D/BP = 73/17	2
42 BP	23	D/BP = 46/16	4
21 SA-BP	38	D/BP = 49/11	—

Cluster characterization	Probands	Relatives
Nonpsychotic depressive syndrome	14	93
MC psychotic nonsuicidal depressive syndrome		22
MC psychotic suicidal depressive syndrome	35	38
BP nonpsychotic manic-depressive syndrome	9	27
BP psychotic manic-depressive syndrome	24	28
BP-MC psychotic manic–depressive syndrome, suicidal	9	
S-BP MC and MIC psychotic syndrome, suicidal	27	9
S syndrome, thought disorder, MIC-affect, delusions, hallucinations	136	116

Note. A = affective. AD = affective disorder. BP = bipolar disorder. D = depressed. UP = unipolar disorder. MDD = major depressive disorder. MC = mood congruent. MIC = mood incongruent. RDC = Research Diagnostic Criteria. S = schizophrenia. SA = schizoaffective disorder. SA-A = schizoaffective disorder, affective. SA-S = schizoaffective disorder, schizophreniform. SA-D = schizoaffective disorder, depressed. SA-M = schizoaffective disorder, manic. VRD = Vienna Research Critieria.

and VRC and found that RDC mood-incongruent probands had relatives with schizophrenia, affective disorder, and SA disorder, whereas VRC mood-incongruent patients were prone to transmit only schizophrenia and affective disorders.

The next series of studies were based on DSM-III. Kendler et al. (1985) examined the morbid risk (MR) in relatives of schizophrenic probands included in the Iowa 500 study who fulfilled the Feighner criteria. Their risk was 18 times higher for schizophrenia compared with relatives of control subjects and 3 times higher compared with all nonaffective psychoses. MR was also higher for SA disorder, paranoid disorder, and atypical psychosis. Kendler et al. (1986) also studied the familial transmission of illnesses in probands who did not meet Feighner criteria for schizophrenia (Iowa non-500) but who had schizophreniform, SA, or psychotic affective disorders. Their results showed that atypical psychotic patients were aggregated in families of probands with DSM-III nonchronic schizophrenia. Their results also revealed that the presence of affective features in schizophrenic-like syndromes did not indicate a family predisposition to transmit affective disorders. Rediagnosed by RDC, probands with SA or affective disorders had the same patterns of transmission for affective disorders as probands diagnosed with affective disorder by DSM-III. With the same sample of probands, Faraone and Tsuang (1988) applied a two-threshold model for family transmission both of schizophrenia and atypical schizophrenia. They found that, even if atypical schizophrenia were a clinically less severe form of schizophrenia, the MR for the relatives of subjects with atypical schizophrenia was more severe, both for schizophrenia and for atypical schizophrenia. Mendlewicz et al. (1980) studied MR for schizophrenia and affective illness in relatives of schizoaffective probands and possible linkage with X chromosome markers for protanopia and deuteranopia. Results indicated that some SA syndromes may also be transmitted through the X chromosome.

To assess the validity of the DSM-III-R definitions, Maj et al. (1991) studied families of probands with schizophrenia or major affective disorders. They found that SA disorder patients, depressed phase, had a high familial incidence of schizophrenia, that probands with mood-congruent, psychotic major depression had families as loaded for mood disorder as those with nonpsychotic major depression. On the other hand, mood-incongruent psychotic depression seemed to be a heterogeneous disorder.

The next four studies used ICD-8 diagnoses. Winokur et al. (1985) studied whether transmission of psychotic symptoms, either mood congruent or incongruent, was dependent on the illness itself. They paired probands and relatives according to the presence or absence of these symptoms and studied the familial transmission of the disorders. For BP and UP probands, there was no evidence of any excess pairing for psychotic and nonpsychotic symptoms. The presence or absence of psychosis in probands and relatives was mainly due to schizophrenic and SA disorders. These results are consistent with the idea that a large number of SA disorder patients are, in fact, schizophrenic.

Angst et al. (1979a, 1979b) compared morbid risk according to sex and types of SA disorder. The probands with SA disorder had more SA and affective disorders in female than male relatives. The probands with SA disorder, manic, had more affective, SA, and unspecified psychotic disorders in relatives than did the probands with SA disorder, depressed. Probands with SA disorder, largely schizophreniform type, had more relatives with schizophrenia and fewer relatives with affective disorder than the probands with SA disorder, largely affective. There was no difference in the familial risk for disorder between these two types of SA disorder.

Scharfetter and Nüssperli (1980), in the Zurich study, compared the risk of transmission for schizophrenic, affective, and SA disorders. Psychotic illnesses were present in up to a quarter of the relatives of the probands with SA disorder, which suggested a combination of two genetic dispositions, one for schizophrenic and one for affective psychotic illnesses in these relatives. Using the same study, Stassen et al. (1988) addressed the question of phenotypal equivalence in proband and relative groups, using symptom clusters analysis and syndrome correspondence. Results revealed clear syndromal patterns, with good agreement between probands and relatives. When the phenotypes of proband were compared with the phenotypes of relatives (independently from index cases), the results revealed an important syndromal overlap between the two major psychoses, with an intermediate position for schizobipolar subjects.

Course of Illness

Longitudinal follow-up studies allow a comparison between cross-sectional symptom features and the longitudinal course of illness, including the type and degree of remission between episodes of illness (Table 4–5).

Three studies used DSM-III or DSM-III-R criteria. Marneros et al. (1988a, 1988b, 1988c) found that half of the probands with SA disorder had an acute onset. In more than half, the first episode met criteria for SA disorder based on symptom features. The majority had a polymorphous course with bipolar-type episodes. Most episodes had mood-incongruent psychotic features. At outcome, half of the sample was in full remission, whereas fewer than 10% continued to have severe residual symptoms. Opjordsmoen (1989) compared the course and outcome of SA, major depressive, and schizophrenic disorder cases. Most of the SA patients remained monomorphous (depressed), except for some who evidenced shifts to mania or schizomania when treated with antidepressant medication. The SA disorder, depressed-phase-group evidenced a course intermediate between major depression and schizophrenia for all variables including types of episodes, quality of interepisode recovery, phasic versus gradual course, trends to improvement

Table 4–5. Course of illness

Study	Sample/method	Onset	Course	Outcome
Marneros et al. 1988a, 1988b, 1988c	72 schizoaffective patients (mean follow-up = 25 years) evaluated using DSM-III, DSM-III-R, PSE, GAS, and DAS	49% acute, 30% subacute, 21% insidious first episode, 2/3 SA (50% SA-D), 13% schizo-phrenic, 14% affective, 7% noncharacteristic; life event before the first episode 54%	Syndrome shifts: polymorphous = 61% (bipolar = 68%); mono-morphous = 29% (unipolar = 82%); schizoaffective = 66%; mood-incongruent symptoms = 94%; inactivity of illness (>3 years) = 52%, longer for unipolar schizoaffective	Residuum: 50% full remission; 6%–8% severe residuum (GAS: 51% = 91–100, 25% = 51–90, 24% 0–50) (DAS: 51% = good, 40% = sufficient, 8% = poor)
Opjordsmoen 1989	33 schizoaffective depressed, 50 major depressed, 94 schizo-phrenic (mean follow-up = 22 years) evaluated using DSM-III, SADS, GAS	Psychotic symptoms before index admission: 3m in major depression and schizoaffective depressed, 10m in manic: index episode acute in 46% major depression, 27% schizoaffective depressed, 7% schizophrenic	92% major depression = only unipolar; 88% schizoaffective de-pressed = only schizodepressive; 4% of major depression treated with antidepressants had mania or schizomanic shift; acute with full remission was 46% in major depression, 27% in schizoaffective, and 7% schizophrenic: acute (more than one episode) was 46% in major depression; 55% in schizo-affective; 9% in schizophrenic *Improved:* 3% schizoaffective, 2% schizophrenic *Deteriorated:* 3% schizoaffective, 9% schizophrenic *Gradually improved, mild defect:* 3% schizoaffective disorder; 6% schizophrenic Gradually improved, moderate defect: 3% schizoaffective, 28% schizophrenic *Steady psychotic:* 10% schizophrenic *Uncertain:* 1% schizophrenic	Better for major depression than for schizoaffective disorder; better for schizo-affective disorder than for schizophrenia; much better for major depression than for schizophrenia GAS: major depression = 73, schizoaffective = 67, schizophrenic = 47 *% of healthy:* major depression = 66%, schizoaffective = 42%, schizophrenic = 10% *% psychotic:* major depression = 18% schizoaffective = 36%, schizophrenic = 48%

Berg et al. 1983	20 male patients with affective disorder (FRS). 30-year follow-up (by DSM-III)	Acute (<3 weeks) $n = 6$; subacute (3–6 weeks) $n = 11$; insidious (>6 weeks) $n = 3$	*Length of hospitalization:* <1 year, $n = 19$ >6 months, $n = 17$ *After first discharge:* recovered $n = 16$, improved $n = 3$, unimproved $n = 1$	*Last diagnosis:* 3 bipolar, 5 schizoaffective, 9 schizophrenic, 3 alcoholic *End of study:* recovered = 5 (3 bipolar, 2 schizo-affective); improved = 3 (1 schizoaffective, 2 alco-holic); unimproved = 12
Maj and Perris 1990	77 schizoaffective (30 manic, 47 major depressed) by RDC 10-year retrospective study with 3-year prospective follow-up. Assessment with CPRS, DAS, Strauss Carpenter Scale	*Episodes:* Schizoaffective disorder had 30% affective (10% manic, 20% depressed), 50% schizo-affective (17 manic, 32 depressed),12% schizophrenic, 8% other episodes. Affective disorder had 55% depression, 34% mania, 2% schizoaffective manic, 4% schizoaffective depressed, 1% schizophrenia	4% had other episodes; polymorphous course: 60% schizoaffective-depressed, 17% affective disorder	Symptomatic interepisodes were more frequent in schizoaffective than in affective disorder (by CPRS) Strauss Carpenter Scale mean global score lower for schizo-affective, significantly lower for schizoaffective depressed Poorer outcome for schizo-affective disorder with mono-morphous course and schizo-affective disorder with affective and schizophrenic episodes
Grossman et al. 1991	41 RDC schizoaffective, 20 bipolar-manic (82% psychotic), 20 major depressed (20% psychotic), 20 schizo-phrenic). 2-year and 4- to 5-year prospective follow-up using Strauss Carpenter Scale	2-year follow-up: very poor out-come (43% schizoaffective, 35% bipolar, 10% unipolar, 55% schizophrenic)	34% schizoaffective with clear psychotic symptoms, 27% with mood-incongruent symptoms Second-year follow-up: slight improvement for schizoaffective but not for schizophrenic Trend in bipolar toward less psychosis than in schizoaffective. Rehospital-ization average = 3 months (much lower for unipolar)	No significant difference between diagnostic groups, but better social outcome for unipolar; general trend toward worsening

(continued)

Table 4–5. Course of illness *(continued)*

Study	Sample/method	Onset	Course	Outcome
Koehler 1983	26 RDC schizoaffective (20 depressed, 6 manic); 30-year follow-up assessed with Strauss-Carpenter Scale	53.9% schizoaffective with FRS at first admission		Schizoaffective with FRS outcome score = 5.29; schizoaffective without any FRS means outcome score = 3.58 FRS symptoms weight = no significant predictive value
Armbruster et al. 1983	113 schizoaffective assessed with RDC and ICD-Angst criteria (schizophreniform and cycloid psychosis); mean follow-up = 22.4 years	Catatonic or depressive first episode = better prognosis	Paranoid hallucinatory form = less favorable prognosis	Kasanin schizoaffective had 55% noncharacteristic and 5% characteristic residuum. RDC and schizophreniform schizoaffective had 47% non-characteristic, 11, 5% characteristic residuum. Angst schizoaffective had 59% noncharacteristic, 11% schizophrenic residuum; cycloid psychosis had 38% residuum
Angst et al. 1980	150 schizoaffective and 95 bipolar depressed inpatients.18-year retro-spective and 13-year prospective follow-up. Assessed with Angst-modified ICD criteria	Schizoaffective mean age = 31.8, vs. 34.7 for bipolar disorder	Schizoaffective vs. bipolar depressed: relapse free at 1 year, 18% vs. 27%; 1 to 5 years, 45% vs. 57%; >5 years: 37% vs. 17%; mean duration of illness = 22 vs. 24 years	Schizoaffective vs. bipolar disorder: full remission, 27% vs. 36%; partial remission, 38% vs. 27%, chronic course: 2% vs. 0%; ongoing episodes: 15% vs. 13%

Note. DAS = Disorder Assessment of Symptoms. FRS = first-rank symptoms. GAS = Global Assessment Scale. PSE = Present State Examination. RDC = Research Diagnostic Criteria. SADS = Schedule for Affective Disorders and Schizophrenia.

versus deterioration, and quality of social outcome. Berg et al. (1983) studied 20 male patients initially diagnosed with SA disorder by DSM-III who presented with both an affective disorder and Schneiderian FRS. At the end of the study, three-quarters of the sample had changed diagnoses, 3 to bipolar disorder with an episodic course and good interepisode recovery, 9 to schizophrenia (generally chronic), and 3 to alcoholism. For the 5 who continued to be diagnosed with SA disorder, 2 recovered, 2 were unimproved, and 1 was improved.

Three follow-up studies used RDC to define SA disorder. Maj and Perris (1990) compared SA and affective disorder patients and found that a polymorphous course was more frequent in SA disorder. For SA disorder patients, 50% of the episodes had SA symptoms (with twice as many depressed- as manic-type episodes), 30% had affective symptoms, and 12% had schizophrenic symptoms. For affective disorder patients, over 50% of the episodes were depressed, one third were manic, and very few of the episodes were SA or schizophrenic type. Continuing symptoms between episodes of illness were more likely in SA than in affective disorder patients. Global outcome was significantly poorer for SA (depressed type) patients than for those with major depressive disorder. Grossman et al. (1991) compared patients with SA disorder, patients with BP disorder (most of whom had an initial mood-incongruent psychotic episode), patients with major depressive disorder (few with initial psychotic mood-incongruent symptoms), and schizophrenic patients. They concluded that, at follow-up, SA patients had outcomes that were intermediate between the outcomes for schizophrenic and affective disorder patients. The global outcomes for SA patients were poor, similar to those for schizophrenic patients, but they evidenced a nonsignificant tendency to better functioning. Compared with BP patients, SA patients showed mixed or confusing results, whereas the UP depressed patients had a clearly better outcome. For all patients, mood-incongruent schizophrenic-like symptoms in the acute phase predicted a bad outcome, even when affective symptoms were present. Koehler (1983) investigated the relevance of FRS symptoms to outcome in RDC SA disorder patients and came to the opposite conclusion. Results revealed that the presence or absence of FRS at the index admission did not predict Global Assessment Scale (GAS) global outcome score, either individually or globally.

Armbruster et al. (1983) isolated cases from the Marneros (1988a, 1988b, 1988c) studies that met diagnostic criteria for SA disorder according to Kasanin, RDC, Angst-modified ICD (Angst et al. 1979a, 1979b), and Scandinavian schizophreniform psychosis. Outcome was assessed in terms of schizophrenic residual symptoms and residual symptoms that were not schizophrenic in nature. Results revealed that, compared with the global FRS schizophrenic group, SA disorder patients had a better prognosis, less schizophrenic residua, more complete remissions, and more noncharacteristic residua. Differences between outcome among patients with SA disorder, defined by various symptomatic criteria, suggest that subgroups of SA can be identified based on course rather than relying solely on cross-sectional symptom features. This idea is consistent with the findings of Angst et al. (1980), who compared the course and outcome of SA and BP disorder patients and found that SA and BP disorders were similar for many course and outcome variables but that SA patients were less likely to achieve full remissions than BP patients.

Discussion

When different diagnostic systems (e.g., RDC, DSM-III, DSM-III-R, ICD-9, and VRC) are compared, and when cross-sectional symptom features for a single episode of illness are the sole basis for the diagnosis, heterogeneous findings result. When the same diagnostic system is used, results are somewhat more consistent with regard to types of SA disorder (e.g., acute versus chronic, SA manic, SA depressed, and SA BP). The relationship between symptom clusters and ICD diagnosis (Angst et al. 1983) revealed that SA disorder overlapped with both affective and schizophrenic disorders, suggesting that SA disorder could not be defined as a clearly separate entity.

The distinctions between mood-congruent and mood-incongruent psychotic symptoms, the presence or absence of FRS, and the presence or absence of schizo-axial syndrome provide some basis for subdividing the types of SA disorder, although these distinctions seem more relevant to predicting outcome. Moreover, the presence or absence of mood-congruent or mood-incongruent psychotic symptoms do not contribute to a better distinction between UP, SA, and major affective disorders (Winokur 1989).

The presence of both psychotic and affective symptoms intermingled in a single episode of illness creates a broad definition of SA disorder. Placing patients with mood-incongruent psychotic symptoms within the mood disorder group appropriately narrows the SA disorder group. However, consideration of other dimensions, such as treatment response, laboratory test findings, familial studies, and course of illness, may provide a basis for further limiting heterogeneity.

Treatment response to lithium alone, or lithium combined with neuroleptics, either in acute or long-term treatment, revealed that the more acute and the more manic the onset features in those with SA disorder, the better the response to lithium. That is, response to lithium will be better for mainly affective SA disorder than for mainly schizophrenic SA disorder and better for SA manic-phase than for SA depressed-phase patients. Lithium was not effective for psychotic symptoms per se. These conclusions hold for DSM-III criteria (Romeo et al. 1985), in which the efficacy of lithium was proportional to the prominence of affective symptoms. They also pertain when ICD criteria or VRC are used to define SA disorder. Thus, there may be two variants of SA disorder, one more schizophrenic and the other more affective in terms of treatment response.

Laboratory studies using neurological and neuromorphological measures either found no difference between SA, schizophrenic, and affective disorders or found that SA disorder was closer to schizophrenic than to affective disorders. These studies, however, found little correspondence between these measures and clinical affective and schizophrenic symptom features.

Neuroendocrine studies of SA disorder revealed dysregulation of the hypothalamic-pituitary-adrenal (HPA) axis. DST and TSH response of TRH were more like those in affective than schizophrenic disorders, particularly for the "mainly affective" versus "mainly schizophrenic" SA disorder groups and more so for the schizomanic than for the schizodepressed groups. These findings were particularly clear when studies used RDC to define SA disorder, probably because RDC includes more patients with psychotic affective disorders than the DSM-III or DSM-III-R SA disorder groups.

Family studies revealed heterogeneous results with regard to the risk of schizophrenic, affective, other atypical psychotic, and SA disorders, depending on how SA disorder was defined. Overall, SA disorder was not common among relatives compared with either major affective or schizophrenic disorders. Second, SA disorder did not seem to be directly transmitted as a separate entity. SA "mainly affective" disorder (and more so for the manic than depressed type) had high family loading for affective disorders (BP more than UP). SA disorder (mainly schizophrenic or depressed type) was associated with higher familial loadings for schizophrenia. Family studies revealed that family risk differed depending on how SA disorder was defined. DSM-III-R SA disorder, depressive type, was more likely to be associated with greater familial risk for schizophrenia, whereas probands with mood incongruent psychotic major depression had higher family loadings for affective disorder (Maj et al. 1991). Thus, the DSM-III-R requirement of temporal overlap between affective and psychotic symptoms, as well as the presence of a period with psychotic symptoms without prominent mood symptoms, appears to appropriately narrow the SA disorder definition.

Studies of course and outcome of SA disorder suggest that course descriptors or modifiers might assist not only in prognosis but also in treatment selection. A poorer degree of interepisode recovery and the presence of a characteristic schizophrenic residua were associated with greater global deterioration and functional impairment. Overall, an episodic course with a good interepisode recovery was usually associated with a good outcome and a predominance of affective (often manic) features. A chronic course was associated with prominent schizophrenic symptoms and a poor outcome. An episodic course with residual psychotic symptoms between full episodes was associated with an intermediate outcome.

Recommendations

SA disorder has had an evolving history. There are multiple definitions. Some rests solely on cross-sectional symptom features; others include symptoms related to the course of illness. None rest solely on course of illness (e.g., episodic, episodic with poor interepisode recovery, chronic). The RDC definition of SA disorder is broad and includes patients with UP and BP mood disorders, especially those with psychotic, mood-incongruent features and those with psychotic periods that do not meet criteria for schizophrenia. These findings led to an appropriate narrowing of SA disorder in DSM-III and DSM-III-R. The decision is supported by studies of family history, course, biological tests, and treatment response. The DSM-III and DSM-III-R definition of SA disorder is more likely than the RDC definition to identify a group that is more closely related to schizophrenia. Whether course modifiers would be a useful addition by which to better gauge prognosis or treatment selection for SA disorder as defined by DSM-III-R is not fully resolved.

References

Abrams R, Taylor MA: Mania and schizoaffective disorder manic type: a comparison. Am J Psychiatry 133:1445–1449, 1976

American Psychiatric Association: Diagnostic and Statistical Manual: Mental Disorders. Washington, DC, American Psychiatric Association, 1952

American Psychiatric Association: The Diagnostic and Statistical Manual of Mental Disorders, 2nd Edition. Washington, DC, American Psychiatric Association, 1968

American Psychiatric Association: The Diagnostic and Statistical Manual of Mental Disorders, 3rd Edition. Washington, DC, American Psychiatric Association, 1980

American Psychiatric Association: The Diagnostic and Statistical Manual of Mental Disorders, 3rd Edition, Revised. Washington, DC, American Psychiatric Association, 1987

Angst J, Felder W, Lohmeyer B: Schizoaffective disorders: results of genetic investigation, I. J Affect Disord 1:139–153, 1979a

Angst J, Felder W, Lohmeyer B: Are schizoaffective psychoses heterogeneous? results of genetic investigation, II. J Affect Disord 1:155–165, 1979b

Angst J, Felder W, Lohmeyer B: Course of schizoaffective psychoses: results of a followup study. Schizophr Bull 6:579–585, 1980

Angst J, Scharfetter C, Stassen HH: Classification of schizo-affective patients by multidimensional scaling and cluster analysis. Psychiatr Clin 16:254–264, 1983

Armbruster B, Gross G, Hüber G: Long-term prognosis and course of schizo-affective, schizophreniform, and cycloid psychoses. Psychiatr Clin 16:156–168, 1983

Baron M, Gruen R, Asnis L, et al: Schizoaffective illness, schizophrenia, and affective disorders: morbidity, risk and genetic transmission. Acta Psychiatr Scand 65:253–262, 1982

Benson KL, Zarcone VP Jr: Middle ear muscle activity during REM sleep in schizophrenic, schizoaffective, and depressed patients. Am J Psychiatry 139:1474–1476, 1982

Berg E, Lindelius R, Petterson U, et al: Schizoaffective psychoses: a long-term follow-up. Acta Psychiatr Scand 67:389–398, 1983

Berner P, Simhandl C: Approaches to an exact definition of schizoaffective psychoses for research purposes. Psychiatr Clin 16:245–253, 1983

Bouman TK, Niemantsverdriet-Van-Kampen JG, Ormel J, et al: The effectiveness of lithium prophylaxis in bipolar and unipolar depressions and schizo-affective disorders. J Affect Disord 11:275–280, 1986

Carman JS, Bigelow LB, Wyatt RJ: Lithium combined with neuroleptics in chronic schizo-phrenic and schizoaffective patients. J Clin Psychiatry 42:124–128, 1981

Clayton PJ, Rodin L, Winokur G: Family history studies, III: schizoaffective disorder, clinical and genetic factors including one- to two-year follow-up. Compr Psychiatry 9:31–49, 1968

Coccaro E, Prudic J, Rothpearl A, et al: The dexamethasone suppression test in depressive, non-depressive and schizoaffective psychosis. J Affect Disord 9:107–113, 1985

Coryell W, Zimmerman M: The heritability of schizophrenia and schizoaffective disorder: a family study. Arch Gen Psychiatry 45:323–327, 1988

DeLisi LE, Goldin LR, Maxwell ME, et al: Clinical features of illness in siblings with schizophrenia or schizoaffective disorder. Arch Gen Psychiatry 44:891–896, 1987

Faraone SV, Tsuang MT: Familial links between schizophrenia and other disorders: appli-cation of the multifactorial polygenic model. Psychiatry 51:37–47, 1988

Feighner JP, Robins E, Guze SB, et al: Diagnostic criteria for use in psychiatric research. Arch Gen Psychiatry 26:57–63, 1972

Fowler RC, McCabe MS, Cadoret RJ, et al. The validity of good prognosis schizophrenia. Arch Gen Psychiatry 26:182–185, 1972

Gershon ES, Delisi LE, Hamovit J, et al: A controlled family study of chronic psychoses, schizophrenia and schizoaffective disorder. Arch Gen Psychiatry 45:328–336, 1988

Goode DJ, Manning AA: Specific imbalance of right and left sided motor neuron excitability in schizophrenia. J Neurol Neurosurg Psychiatry 51:626–629, 1988

Grossman LS, Harrow M, Goldberg JF, et al: Outcome of schizoaffective disorder at two long-term follow-ups: comparisons with outcome of schizophrenia and affective dis-orders. Am J Psychiatry 10:1359–1365, 1991

Hathaway SR, McKinley JC: Minnesota Multiphasic Personality Inventory, Revised. Min-neapolis, University of Minnesota, 1970

Hoch A: Benign Stupors: A Study of a New Manic-Depressive Reaction Type. New York, Macmillan, 1921

Hubain PP, Simonnet MP, Mendlewicz J: The dexamethasone suppression test in affective illness and schizophrenia: relationship with psychotic symptoms. Neuropsychobiology 16:57–60, 1986

Hunt R, Appel K: Prognosis in the psychoses lying midway between schizophrenia and manic-depressive psychoses. Am J Psychiatry 93:313–339, 1936

Jensen LB: "Schizophrenia, schizo-affective type" a useful diagnosis? ten years experience from Danish psychiatric hospitals. Arch Psychiatr Neurol Sci 234:285–289, 1984

Kant O: Types and analyses of the clinical pictures of recovered schizophrenics. Psychiatr Q 14:676–700, 1940

Kasanin J: The acute schizoaffective psychoses. Am J Psychiatry 13:97–126, 1933

Kendler KS, Gruenberg AM, Tsuang MT: Psychiatric illness in first-degree relatives of schizophrenic and surgical control patients: a family study using DSM-III criteria. Arch Gen Psychiatry 42:770–779, 1985

Kendler KS, Gruenberg AM, Tsuang MT: A DSM-III family study of the nonschizophrenic psychotic disorders. Am J Psychiatry 143:1098–1105, 1986

Kirby GH: The catatonic syndrome and its relation to manic depressive insanity. J Nerv Ment Dis 40:694–704, 1913

Kiriike N, Izumiya Y, Nishiwaki S, et al: TRH test and DST in schizoaffective mania, mania and schizophrenia. Biol Psychiatry 24:415–422, 1988

Koehler K: Prognostic prediction in RDC schizo-affective disorder on the basis of first-rank symptoms weighted in terms of outcome. Psychiatr Clin 16:186–197, 1983

Küfferle B, Lenz G: Classification and course of schizo-affective psychoses: follow-up of patients treated with lithium. Psychiatr Clin 16:169–177, 1983

Langer G, Koinig G, Hatzinger R, et al: Response of thyrotropin to thyrotropin-releasing hormone as predictor of treatment outcome. Arch Gen Psychiatry 43:861–868, 1986

Langfeldt G: The prognosis in schizophrenia and the factors influencing the course of the disease. Acta Psychiatr Neurol Scand Suppl 13:1–128, 1937

Langfeldt G: The prognosis in schizophrenia. Acta Psychiatr Scand Suppl 13:1–66, 1956

Maj M: Effectiveness of lithium prophylaxis in schizoaffective psychosis: application of a polydiagnostic approach. Acta Psychiatr Scand 70:228–234, 1984a

Maj M: Evolution of the American concept of schizoaffective psychosis. Neuropsychobiology 11:7–13, 1984b

Maj M: Response to the dexamethasone suppression test in schizoaffective disorder depressed type. J Affect Disord 11:63–68, 1986

Maj M: Lithium prophylaxis of schizoaffective disorders: a prospective study. J Affect Disord 14:129–136, 1988

Maj M: A family study of two subgroups of schizoaffective patients. Br J Psychiatry 154:640–643, 1989

Maj M, Perris C: Patterns of course in patients with a cross-sectional diagnosis of schizoaffective disorder. J Affect Disord 20:71–77, 1990

Maj M, Starace F, Pirozzi R: A family study of DSM-III-R schizoaffective disorder, depressive type, compared with schizophrenia and psychotic and nonpsychotic major depression. Am J Psychiatry 148:612–616, 1991

Marneros A, Deister A, Rohde A, et al: Long-term course of schizoaffective disorders, part I: definitions, methods, frequency of episodes and cycles. Eur Arch Psychiatry Neurol Sci 237:264–275, 1988a

Marneros A, Rohde A, Deister A, et al: Long-term course of schizoaffective disorders, part II: length of cycles, episodes and intervals. Eur Arch Psychiatry Neurol Sci 237:276–282, 1988b

Marneros A, Rohde A, Deister A, et al: Long-term course of schizoaffective disorders, Part III: onset, type of episodes, and syndrome shift, precipitating factors, suicidality, seasonality, inactivity of illness and outcome. Eur Arch Psychiatry Neurol Sci 237:283–290, 1988c

Mattes JA, Nayak D: Lithium versus fluphenazine for prophylaxis in mainly schizophrenic schizo-affectives. Biol Psychiatry 19:445–450, 1984

Mendlewicz J, Linkowski P, Wilmotte J: Relationship between schizoaffective illness and affective disorders or schizophrenia: morbidity risk and genetic transmission. J Affect Disord 2:289–302, 1980

Moldin SO, Gottesman II, Erlenmeyer-Kimling L: Psychometric validation of psychiatric diagnoses in the New York high-risk study. Psychiatry Res 22:159–177, 1987

Opjordsmoen S: Long-term course and outcome in unipolar affective and schizoaffective psychoses. Acta Psychiatr Scand 79:317–326, 1989

Pope HG, Lipinskii JF, Cohen BM, et al: Schizo-affective disorder: an invalid diagnosis? a comparison of schizo-affective disorder, schizophrenia, and affective disorder. Am J Psychiatry 137:921–926, 1980

Rachlin HL: A follow-up study of Hoch's benign stupor cases. Am J Psychiatry 92:531–558, 1935

Rieder RO, Mann LS, Weinberger DR, et al: Computed tomographic scans in patients with schizophrenia, schizoaffective, and bipolar affective disorder. Arch Gen Psychiatry 40:735–739, 1983

Romeo R, Bastinello S, Janiri L, et al: Slow-release lithium in treatment of schizoaffective syndromes. Int J Clin Pharmacol Res 5:205–212, 1985

Rosenthal NE, Rosenthal LN, Stallone E, et al: Towards the validation of RDC schizo-affective disorder. Arch Gen Psychiatry 37:804–810, 1980

Sauer H, Koehler KG, Hornstein C, et al: The dexamethasone suppression test and thyroid stimulating hormone response to TRH in RDC schizoaffective patients. Eur Arch Psychiatr Neurol Sci 234:264–267, 1984

Scharfetter C, Nüssperli M: The group of schizophrenias, schizoaffective psychoses, and affective disorders. Schizophr Bull 6:586–591, 1980

Schneider K: Clinical Psychopharmacology. Translated by Hamilton MW, Anderson EW. New York, Grune and Stratton, 1959, pp 89–114

Shanda H, Thau K, Küfferle B, et al: Heterogeneity of delusional syndromes: diagnostic criteria and course prognosis. Psychopathology 17:280–287, 1984

Shanda H, Lieber A, Küfferle B, et al: Delusional psychoses genetic findings as a critical variable for the validation of diagnostic criteria. Psychopathology 19:259–266, 1986

Smith RC, Baumgartner R, Ravichandran GK, et al: Cortical atrophy and white matter density in the brains of schizophrenics and clinical response to neuroleptics. Acta Psychiatr Scand 75:11–19, 1987

Spitzer RL, Endicott J, Robins E: Research Diagnostic Criteria (RDC) for a Selected Group of Functional Disorders, 2nd Edition. New York, Biometrics Research Institute, 1975

Spitzer RL, Endicott J, Robins E: Research Diagnostic Criteria: rationale and reliability. Arch Gen Psychiatry 35:773–782, 1978

Stassen HH, Scharfetter C, Winokur G, et al: Familial syndrome patterns in schizophrenia, schizoaffective disorder, mania, and depression. Eur Arch Psychiatry Neurol Sci 237:115–123, 1988

Taylor MA, Abrams R: The phenomenology of mania: a new look at some old patients. Arch Gen Psychiatry 29:520–522, 1973

Tsuang MT, Dempsey M: Long-term outcome of major psychoses, II: schizoaffective disorder compared with schizophrenia, affective disorders, and a surgical control group. Arch Gen Psychiatry 36:1302–1304, 1979

Vaillant GE: The natural history of the remitting schizophrenias. Am J Psychiatry 120:367–376, 1963

Vaillant GE: Prospective prediction of schizophrenic remission. Arch Gen Psychiatry 38:509–518, 1964

Wahby VS, Ibrahim GA, Giller EL, et al: Thyrotropin response to thyrotropin-releasing hormone in RDC schizodepressed men. J Affect Disord 15:81–85, 1988

Wahby VS, Ibrahim GA, Chuy IL, et al: Prolactin response to thyrotropin-releasing hormone in schizoaffective depressed compared to depressed and schizophrenic men and healthy controls. Schizophr Res 3:277–281, 1990

Walker E: Attentional and neuromotor functions of schizophrenics, schizoaffectives and patients with other affective disorders. Arch Gen Psychiatry 38:1355–1358, 1981

Welner A, Welner Z, Fishman R: The group of schizoaffective and related psychoses, IV: a family study. Compr Psychiatry 20:21–26, 1979

Winokur G: The schizoaffective continuum: Euclid's second axiom. Ann Clin Psychiatry 1:19–42, 1989

Winokur G, Clayton PJ, Reich T: Manic-Depressive Insanity. St. Louis, MO, Mosby, 1969

Winokur G, Scharfetter C, Angst J: A family study of psychotic symptomatology in schizophrenia schizoaffective disorder unipolar depression and bipolar disorder. Eur Arch Psychiatry Neurol Sci 234:295–298, 1985

World Health Organization: Manual of the International Statistical Classification of Diseases, Injuries and Causes of Death, 8th revision (ICD-8). Geneva, World Health Organization, 1968

World Health Organization: Manual of the International Statistical Classification of Diseases, Injuries and Causes of Death, 9th revision (ICD-9). Geneva, World Health Organization, 1977

World Health Organization: Manual of the International Statistical Classification of Diseases and Related Health Problems, 10th revision (ICD-10), Volume 1. Geneva, World Health Organization, 1992

Zarcone VP Jr, Benson KL, Berger PA: Abnormal rapid eye movement latencies in schizophrenia. Arch Gen Psychiatry 44:45–48, 1987

Chapter 5

Minor Depression

Kathleen Ries Merikangas, Ph.D., Cecile Ernst, M.D.,
Wolfgang Maier, M.D., Emily B. Hoyer, B.A., and
Jules Angst, M.D.

Statement and Significance of the Issues

The primary question regarding minor depression is whether any separate diagnosis is warranted. That is, is it possible to increase the sensitivity of the diagnostic classification without diminishing its specificity? It is clear from the data on treatment rates of individuals with minor depression that there is a significant level of impairment and distress caused by depressive symptoms, even if there are too few of them to qualify for a diagnosis of major depression. Minor depression has also been shown to be particularly relevant in the diagnoses of people suffering from medical illness and people over age 65 years. Criteria for this disorder have also been shown to cover a significant proportion of undiagnosed treated cases of depression, which indicates that the inclusion of this disorder in the nosology would serve to alleviate this apparent gap. Data concerning this disorder are relatively sparse; few studies have employed specific criteria for minor depression. More information is essential, especially in the area of treatment response and familial patterns of this disorder. However, the evidence as it stands indicates that this illness warrants serious consideration for inclusion in DSM-IV.

Method

The literature covered in this review includes published work regarding only those studies meeting the following requirements: 1) the studies must employ *specific*

This research was supported by the Research Scientist Development Award MH00499 from the Alcohol, Drug Abuse, and Mental Health Administration of the United States Public Health Service to Dr. Merikangas and by the Swiss National Foundation Grant 3.873.0.88 to Dr. Angst.

standardized diagnostic criteria based on direct clinical interviews; and 2) the authors must report the source and method of recruitment of the sample and provide evidence of systematic ascertainment.

A search via computer (Medline and Index Medicus programs) of the holdings of the National Library of Medicine for work published in the last 26 years regarding depression and minor subtypes thereof yielded a list of approximately 220 abstracts, roughly 180 of which were eliminated due to the above restrictions, leaving a total of about 40 articles for consideration in this review. The bibliographies from these papers were then reviewed thoroughly and methodically to provide an additional source for relevant articles. Direct contact with several investigators with data or relevant information on minor depression was also helpful in directing and refining this review.

Results

Validity and Utility

Several sources of evidence have been employed to study the utility and the validity of the category of minor depression. The aspect of coverage of minor depression (i.e., the proportion of undiagnosed treated cases of depression that would have received the diagnosis of minor depression) was investigated in the Zurich Cohort Study of Young Adults. In this study, there were 138 subjects who had received treatment for depression, of whom 51% did not meet diagnostic criteria for a DSM-III-R (American Psychiatric Association 1987) affective disorder. After applying the category of recurrent brief depression (Angst et al. 1990), which covered 77% of the treated nondiagnosed subjects, the use of the concept of minor depression permitted 80% of the remaining undiagnosed individuals with a history of treatment (an additional 18%) to be thus classified.

The concept of minor depression has been found to be particularly relevant in two groups, elderly subjects in community or primary care settings and patients with physical diseases (Blazer 1991). Minor depression was cited more often in studies of physical diseases than in any other context. The illnesses that appeared to be most strongly associated with minor depression in the literature were stroke, cancer, and diabetes. However, the nature of the relationship between minor depression and these conditions has not been established. As Cassem (1990) notes, it is difficult to draw distinctions between symptoms related to the impairment of the medical illness and those that can be attributed to the depression itself.

Does the stroke patient with five of nine positive symptoms differ from a patient with only depressed mood and intact interest, energy, concentration, appetite, and motor and sleep patterns? We know that the first requires antidepressant medication, does the second? Is minor depression a useful category to retain? The assumption about pathophysiology again appears here: namely, secondary depression is "psychogenic," whereas induced depression is organic. (pp. 600–601)

Cassem also recommended (pp. 602–603) that an epidemiological study be conducted that would focus on a random sample of medically ill inpatients and outpatients and generate data similar to the data from the National Institute of Mental Health (NIMH) Epidemiological Catchment Area (ECA) studies of primary psychiatric disorders.

The Zurich Cohort Study examined the validity of the category of minor depression according to family history of affective disorders (Angst, in press). Similar proportions of subjects with minor depression and major depression had a positive family history of depression and treatment for depression among their first-degree relatives. The lack of differential family history of affective disorder between patients with major and minor depression provides evidence for the validity of the category of minor depression.

Four studies have examined the longitudinal course of minor depression (Angst, in press; Coryell et al. 1991; Wing and Sturt 1978; Wing et al. 1981). As described below, all of these studies demonstrated that minor depression was associated with continued expression of depression over time. However, there was little longitudinal stability of the concept of minor depression itself.

Broadhead (1990) studied the validity of the construct of minor depression in the elderly by investigating the amount of time during the prior 3 months in which the respondent was unable to maintain his or her routine activities. The results revealed that the number of days of impairment (mean ± SD 6.06 ± 4.37) associated with minor depression was significantly greater than found among asymptomatic elderly adults (mean ± SD 1.97 ± 10.7).

Reliability

Despite the large number of reliability studies of the major categories of psychiatric disorders, none of the studies investigated the reliability of the assessment or classification of minor depression. Similarly, the studies of the reliability of family history information did not systematically examine the category of minor depression, with the exception of the study by Gershon and Guroff (1984), which indirectly investigated the reliability of this category. In a comparison between the interview diagnosis of an index case and a relative report, about 60% of those with either minor depression or depressive personality were characterized as affected by relative report.

Definitional Features

Minor depression was first operationalized in the Research Diagnostic Criteria (RDC) (Spitzer et al. 1978) (Table 5–1). A 2-week duration of 2 of the 16 symptoms is required for a definite diagnosis of minor depression. A broader array of symptoms is required for minor depression than for major depression. The former category is comprised of a combination of depressive symptoms and those associated with personality traits. Moreover, impairment is also essential. In this respect, RDC minor depression is a precursor to the current concept of dysthymia.

Table 5–1.   Research Diagnostic Criteria for minor depression

Depressed mood, characterized by two or more of the symptoms below[*]:
1) Poor appetite or weight loss or increased appetite or weight gain (change of 1 lb. per week over several weeks or 10 lb. per year when not dieting)
2) Sleep difficulty or sleeping too much
3) Loss of energy, fatiguability, or tiredness
4) Psychomotor agitation or retardation (but not mere subjective feeling of restlessness or being slowed down)
5) Loss of interest or pleasure in usual activities, including social contact or sex (do not include if limited to a period when delusional or hallucinating)
6) Feelings of self-reproach or excessive or inappropriate guilt (either may be delusional)
7) Complaints or evidence of diminished ability to think or concentrate, such as slowed thinking, or indecisiveness (do not include if associated with obvious formal thought disorder)
8) Recurrent thoughts of death or suicide, or any suicidal behavior
9) Nonverbal manifestations of depression such as tearfulness or sad face
10) Pessimistic attitude
11) Brooding about past or current unpleasant events
12) Preoccupation with feelings of inadequacy
13) Resentful, irritable, angry, or complaining mood or behavior
14) Demandingness or clinging dependency
15) Self-pity
16) Excessive somatic concern

Duration of episode must be **at least 1 week** for probable and 2 weeks for definite diagnosis.

Exclusion criteria: Major depressive disorder; schizophrenia; schizoaffective disorder, manic or depressed type; Briquet's disorder (somatization disorder); unspecified functional psychosis; manic disorder; cyclothymic personality; labile personality; or intermittent depressive disorder.

[*]Work or social **impairment** is required.

Source.   Adapted from Spitzer et al. 1978.

In recent studies considered in this review, the category of minor depression is introduced to cover subthreshold cases of major depression. Therefore, the definition employed here is identical to that of major depression in terms of duration and specific symptoms but with fewer symptoms required than are needed to meet DSM-III (American Psychiatric Association 1980) or DSM-III-R criteria.

Although ICD-10 (World Health Organization 1991) does not include a specific category for minor depression, the category of "depressive episode" is graded for severity according to the number of criteria symptoms (i.e., for severe, 8 of 10 symptoms; for moderate, 6 of 10; and for mild, 4 of 10).

Clinical Studies

Surveys of minor depression in primary care settings that use structured diagnostic interviews have yielded remarkably stable findings across studies. Table 5–2 shows the point prevalence of minor depression in primary care studies. The average point prevalence of minor depression was 3.7%, with a range from 3.4% to 4.7% (Barrett et al. 1988; Blacker and Clare 1987; Hoeper et al. 1979; Ormel et al. 1991).

Elevated rates of minor depression were found in the samples that were screened for psychopathology with a symptom checklist before the administration of a diagnostic interview. Sireling et al. (1985) in London, England, and Winter et al. (1991) in Mainz, Germany, reported point prevalence rates of 25.9% and 32.9%, respectively.

Blazer (1991) reported that approximately 20% of elderly persons in institutional settings suffer clinically significant depressive symptoms that are not covered by the diagnostic category of major depression. The inclusion of minor depression substantially reduces the number of otherwise undiagnosed elderly adults with depressed mood in these settings.

Table 5–2.   Minor depression: primary care studies—point prevalence of minor depression in primary care settings

	N	Point prevalence (%)
General primary care study		
Hoeper et al. 1979	247	3.4
Blacker and Clare 1987	1,091	3.4
Barrett et al. 1988	260	3.6
Ormel et al. 1991	179	4.7
Subjects screened for depression or treatment		
Sireling 1985	143	25.9
Winter et al. 1991	49	32.9

Minor depression has been an important construct in categorizing depression among individuals with major physical illnesses. The most frequent application of minor depression has been in the classification of depression associated with stroke. All forms of depression are more prevalent in individuals with illnesses affecting the central nervous system (Cassem 1990). Robinson et al. (1984) reported that 20% of poststroke patients meet criteria for minor depression. Eastwood et al. (1989) reported even higher rates: 40% of the poststroke cases in their study met criteria for minor depression, whereas only 10% of the sample met criteria for major depression. Robinson et al. (1984, 1987) used RDC criteria for minor depression to study poststroke depression and found that patients meeting four of eight or five of nine criteria (i. e., major depression criteria) spontaneously remitted between 1 and 2 years after the stroke, whereas those meeting only two of eight or three of nine had not yet recovered at the 2-year follow-up. Cassem's (1990) review of depression and anxiety secondary to medical illness concluded that

> a full nosological classification should account for at least five categories of depressive syndromes found clinically in medical patients: *major depression,* requiring five of nine criteria; *minor depression,* requiring three of nine criteria; *adjustment disorder with depressed mood,* signifying a more pure psychological reaction to the illness (such as the patient who cannot tolerate the dependency of hospitalization and regresses); *organic mood syndrome,* such as the patient who becomes dysphoric after receiving a beta blocker; and *uncomplicated bereavement,* the normal response to serious illness, which always inflicts a narcissistic injury. (p. 606)

The major difficulty in classifying depression associated with physical disease is distinguishing between symptoms of the disease or its treatment and those of depression, which may be independent of the disease or may be a psychological reaction to the impending disability or death associated with the illness. Because of possible error in the attribution of symptoms to the disease, Cassem (1990) recommends that all symptoms of depression be counted, regardless of their purported derivation.

Treatment response of persons with depression secondary to medical illness has been superior to that of persons with depression secondary to psychiatric disorders. This suggests that minor depression should not only be diagnosed in persons with medical illness, particularly those most strongly associated with depression, including stroke, cancer, epilepsy, Parkinson's disease, and multiple sclerosis, but the usual treatment modalities for major depression should be considered as well.

Treatment Studies

There have been only three studies that reported the results of antidepressant treatment of patients with RDC-defined minor depression (Davidson et al. 1988; Paykel et al. 1988; Stewart et al. 1983, 1985). Davidson et al. (1988) assessed isocarboxazid versus placebo in a 6-week trial. Paykel et al. (1988) examined the difference between amitriptyline and placebo in a 6-week trial. Stewart et al. (1983, 1985) compared desipramine and placebo in a 6-week trial that included only seven subjects with "pure" minor depression. No difference between active treatment and placebo was reported in any of the three studies.

In summary, the treatment data are too sparse to provide any conclusive evidence regarding the validity of the diagnostic category of minor depression.

Family Studies

There are very few family studies of affective disorders that have systematically examined the transmission of minor depression among probands and their relatives. Moreover, no adoption or twin study specifically addressed the affective subtype of minor depression.

The controlled family studies (Table 5–3) that employed RDC criteria for minor depression are the Yale University-NIMH Collaborative Family Study of Depression (Weissman et al. 1982, 1984), the NIMH Collaborative Study (Andreasen et al. 1986, 1987), and the Mainz Family Study of Depression (Maier et al. 1992). Data from these studies indicated that minor depression was not associated with bipolar disorder. There was a mild elevation in the rates of minor depression among the relatives of persons with nonbipolar major depression (Gershon et al. 1982; Grove et al. 1987; Maier et al. 1992; Weissman et al. 1982). The latter study presented the results of classifying minor depression according to the presence or absence of the application of a hierarchical system with other affective disorders, with such disorders as bipolar and major depression taking precedence over the category of minor depression. Thus, the family studies suggest that there is an increased risk of minor depression among the relatives of probands with major depression.

In an uncontrolled family study, Andreasen et al. (1986, 1987) and Grove et al. (1987) examined whether persons with the melancholic subtype of depression or persons with primary as opposed to secondary depression had differential rates of positive family histories for depression. They reported that the rates of minor depression among the relatives of probands did not differ according to the proband's subtype of depression.

Follow-Up Studies

Two early studies of the course of minor affective disorder in the community found that persons with minor depression tend to exhibit affective symptoms over 1 year

Table 5–3. Minor depression: family studies of depression—rate (%) of minor depression in relatives of probands

| | | | Proband diagnosis | | | |
| | | | Nonbipolar | | | |
Study	Schizoaffective	Bipolar	All	Primary/secondary	Melancholic/nonmelancholic	Normal control
Gershon et al. 1982	1.2	3.7	8.4			5.3
Weissman et al. 1984						
No hierarchy		5.3	9.7			6.0
Hierarchy		4.5	5.3			2.5
Andreasen et al. 1986					11.4/10.3	
Grove et al. 1987				11.5/9.0		
Maier et al. 1992			6.6			4.0

(Wing and Sturt 1978; Wing et al. 1981). There was only one prospective follow-up study that examined the longitudinal stability of minor depression. A 6-year follow-up of subjects who met RDC criteria for minor depression among the spouses and relatives of 616 affectively ill probands, compared to age- and sex-matched control subjects, was conducted by Coryell et al. (1991). The study found that individuals with minor depression at the index evaluation exhibited greater illness recurrence over time than did those without a history of minor depression. The rate of relapse was found to be 33.3% for those with three depressive symptoms, 42.5% for those with four symptoms, and 50.0% for those with five symptoms (i.e., those who meet criteria for major depression). In contrast, the follow-up study of poststroke patients cited above revealed no association between the number of depressive symptoms and the severity of the course of depression (Robinson et al. 1984, 1987).

Epidemiological Studies

We conducted an exhaustive review of all the major epidemiological studies of affective disorders. Only a small proportion of the nearly 40 studies of this type employed specific diagnostic criteria for minor depression. Although several studies investigated subthreshold symptom-level depression, anxiety was usually included, and minor depression could not be distinguished from manifestations of anxiety syndromes (e.g., Bebbington et al. 1989).

Lifetime prevalence. Epidemiological studies have consistently yielded lifetime rates of minor depression of approximately 10% (Table 5–4). Weissman and Myers (1978) employed the RDC definition of minor depression derived from a Schedule for Affective Disorders and Schizophrenia (SADS-L; Endicott and Spitzer 1978) interview in a sample of 500 adults from the New Haven community. The lifetime prevalence of minor depression was 9.2%.

The rates of RDC minor depression among the relatives of the normal probands in the above-cited family studies may also be used as an estimate of population prevalence. The lifetime rates of RDC minor depression ranged from 4.0% to 6.0% in the four family studies utilizing those criteria.

The sample in which the Zurich study (Angst, in press) was conducted is limited to a single age cohort; the data are thus not comparable to those of epidemiological studies of adults across all ages. The study used DSM-III-R criteria for major depression but lowered the threshold number of symptoms from five to three or four of nine; in 20- to 30-year-old residents of the Canton of Zurich, Switzerland, the weighted lifetime prevalence of "pure" minor depression was found to be 7.4% (no sex difference was noted); this rate excluded subjects who, over the 10-year span of the study, were ever diagnosed as having a more severe type of depression. The weighted prevalence rose to 10.9% when all subjects who had been diagnosed at least once with minor depression, without regard to comorbidity, were included.

Data from the Zurich Study (Angst, in press) also indicated that the mean age at onset was the same for minor depression as for other more severe depressive subtypes. The expression of minor depression tended to begin in late adolescence, between the ages of 15 and 19 years. In contrast to more severe depressive syndromes, there was an equal sex ratio for "pure" minor depression.

Another study of a Swiss population (Wacker et al. 1990) using ICD-10 criteria for mild depression revealed a lifetime rate of 9.5%.

Point prevalence.   In the four stages of interviews in the Zurich study (Angst, in press), the 1-year weighted prevalences were 5.7%, 3.9%, 1.4%, and 2.5%, respectively; the decreasing rate may be partially attributed to the fact that about 40% of the subjects having minor depression at ages 19–21 years progressed later into other more severe categories of depression.

Faravelli and Incerpi (1985) used RDC criteria for minor depression and found a 1-year prevalence of 4.5% among the general population of Florence, Italy. Weissman et al. (1978), using the same criteria, found a point prevalence of 2.5% in New Haven, Connecticut.

Table 5–4.   Minor depression: epidemiological studies—prevalence rates (%) of minor depression in epidemiological surveys

Study	Criteria	Sample	Lifetime	1 year	Point
Weissman and Myers 1978	RDC	New Haven, CT	9.2		
Weissman et al. 1984	RDC	New Haven, CT			2.5
Faravelli and Incerpi 1985	RDC	Florence, Italy		4.5	
Wacker et al. 1990	ICD-10, DSM-III-R	Basel, Switzerland	9.5		
Blazer 1991	DSM-III-R modified	U.S. adults, age ±65 years	4.5		
Angst, in press	DSM-III-R modified	Zürich, Switzerland, adults, ages 20–30 years	7.5 pure, 10.9 all	1979: 5.7 1981: 3.9 1986: 1.4 1988: 2.5	

Note.   RDC = Research Diagnostic Criteria.

The lifetime prevalence of RDC-defined minor depression in the New Haven community survey (Weissman et al. 1978) was higher in 20- to 45-year-old females ($P \leq .05$) than in males of the same age. The results of the New Haven community survey indicated that 15.4% of subjects with a current diagnosis of minor depression also had other (RDC) diagnoses and that 50% of subjects with a lifetime diagnosis of minor depression had other past or current diagnoses. Results from the Zurich study (Angst, in press) also revealed associations between minor depression and other disorders; hypomania and dysthymia were associated with a longitudinal diagnosis of minor depression to the same degree as other affective syndromes, including major depression. Minor depression was also found to be associated with a lifetime treatment rate of 35%. The frequency of social phobia and neurasthenia in subjects with minor depression was higher than that in nondepressed control subjects and lower than that in subjects with major depression. Unlike more severe types of depression, Angst's (in press) definition of minor depression was not associated with panic disorder, agoraphobia, or suicide attempts.

Blazer (1991) investigated the prevalence and expression of minor depression in elderly Americans (i.e., age 65 years or older) from the general population, as well as from institutional settings (as described earlier). He noted that between 4% and 12% of Americans report depressive symptoms not easily classified into the usual DSM-III or DSM-III-R categories such as major depression, dysthymia, or adjustment disorder with depressed mood. However, by the use of the category of minor depression in which the threshold number of symptoms was reduced, a large proportion of these subjects could be appropriately classified. The lifetime prevalence of minor depression in this sample was 4.5%, three times greater than that of major depression. Moreover, in contrast to those of every other DSM-III-R Axis I disorder, rates of minor depression were greater in elderly than in younger adults. There were no differences in the rates of minor depression within the older American sample by race or marital status, and the sex ratio only moderately favored females (1.3:1.0).

Discussion and Recommendations

The results of the study domains reviewed here are inconsistent with respect to evidence of the validity and utility of the category of minor depression. Epidemiological and primary care studies indicate that although the absolute rates of "pure" minor depression are quite low, the application of this diagnostic category results in the classification of up to 40% of individuals who would currently be diagnosed as having depression not otherwise specified (NOS). Philipp et al. (1992)

report that the addition of the minor depressive subtype would reduce the cases of NOS depression by more than 80%. This construct is particularly useful in characterizing depression in elderly subjects and in those with medical illness.

There are several sources of information that support the validity of the category of minor depression. The results of a single longitudinal study provide strong evidence of the importance of the category in predicting recurrence in depression over the longitudinal course. Family history data among patients with minor depression reveal equal lifetime prevalence rates of affective disorder and rates of treatment for affective disorder among patients with minor depression (Angst, in press). Moreover, the family study data provide weak evidence of mildly increased rates of minor depression among the relatives of subjects with major depression. Rates of impairment among minor depressive patients have been shown to be significantly greater than those of dysthymic patients and control subjects.

The only sources of evidence that may counter claims concerning the validity of this diagnosis are two treatment studies that did not demonstrate efficacy of antidepressant treatment in a very small sample of minor depressive patients.

The need for more systematic studies of the validity of this category is strongly indicated by this review. However, the evidence at this time converges to suggest that minor depression, as defined above, should be included in the DSM-IV.

References

American Psychiatric Association: Diagnostic and Statistical Manual of Mental Disorders, 3rd Edition. Washington, DC, American Psychiatric Association, 1980

American Psychiatric Association: Diagnostic and Statistical Manual of Mental Disorders, 3rd Edition, Revised. Washington, DC, American Psychiatric Association, 1987

Andreasen NC, Scheftner W, Reich T, et al: The validation of the concept of endogenous depression: a family study approach. Arch Gen Psychiatry 43:246–251, 1986

Andreasen NC, Rice J, Endicott J, et al: Familial rates of affective disorder: a report from the National Institute of Mental Health Collaborative Study. Arch Gen Psychiatry 44:461–469, 1987

Angst J: Minor depression and recurrent brief depression, in Chronic Diseases and Their Treatment. Edited by Akiskal HS, Cassano GB. New York, Guilford (in press)

Angst J, Merikangas K, Scheidegger P, et al: Recurrent brief depression: a new subtype of affective disorder. J Affect Disord 19:87–98, 1990

Barrett JE, Barrett JA, Oxman TE, et al: The prevalence of psychiatric disorders in a primary care practice. Arch Gen Psychiatry 45:1100–1106, 1988

Bebbington PJ, Katz R, McGuffin P, et al: The risk of minor depression before age 65: results from a community survey. Psychol Med 19:393–400, 1989

Blacker CVR, Clare AW: Depressive disorder in primary care. Br J Psychiatry 150:737–751, 1987

Blazer DG: Epidemiology of depressive disorders in late life, in Program and Abstracts: National Institutes of Health Consensus Development Conference on the Diagnosis and Treatment of Depression in Late Life, November 4–6, 1991, p 18

Broadhead WE, Blazer DG, George LK, et al: Depression, disability days, and days lost from work in a prospective epidemiological survey. J Am Med Assoc 264:2524–2528, 1990

Cassem EH: Depression and anxiety secondary to medical illness. Psychiatr Clin North Am 13(4):597–612, 1990

Coryell W, Endicott J, Keller MB: Predictors of relapse into major depressive disorder in a nonclinical population. Am J Psychiatry 148:1353–1358, 1991

Davidson JRT, Giller EL, Zisook S, et al: An efficacy study of isocarboxazid and placebo in depression and its relationship to depressive nosology. Arch Gen Psychiatry 45:120–124, 1988

Eastwood MR, Rifat SL, Nobbs H, et al: Mood disorder following cerebrovascular accident. Br J Psychiatry 154:195–200, 1989

Endicott J, Spitzer RL: A diagnostic interview: the Schedule for Affective Disorders and Schizophrenia. Arch Gen Psychiatry 35:837–844, 1978

Faravelli G, Incerpi G: Epidemiology of affective disorders in Florence. Acta Psychiatr Scand 72:331–333, 1985

Gershon ES, Guroff JJ: Information from relatives: diagnosis of affective disorders. Arch Gen Psychiatry 41:173–180, 1984

Gershon ES, Hamovit J, Guroff JJ, et al: A family study of schizoaffective, bipolar I, bipolar II, unipolar, and normal control probands. Arch Gen Psychiatry 39:1157–1167, 1982

Grove WM, Andreasen NC, Winokur G, et al: Primary and secondary affective disorders: unipolar patients compared on familial aggregation. Compr Psychiatry 28:113–126, 1987

Hoeper EW, Nycz GR, Cleary PD, et al: Estimated prevalence of RDC mental disorder in primary medical care. Int J Mental Health 8:6–15, 1979

Maier W, Lichtermann D, Minges J, et al: The risk of minor depression in families of probands with major depression: sex differences and familiality. Eur Arch Psychiatry Clin Neurosci 242:89–92, 1992

Ormel J, Koeter MWJ, van den Brink W, et al: Recognition, management, and course of anxiety and depression in general practice. Arch Gen Psychiatry 48:700–706, 1991

Paykel ES, Hollyman JA, Freeling P: Predictors of therapeutic benefit from amitriptyline in mild depression: a general practice placebo-controlled trial. J Affect Disord 14:83–95, 1988

Philipp M, Delmo CD, Buller R, et al: Differentiation between major and minor depression. Psychopharmacology 106:S75–S78, 1992

Robinson RG, Starr LB, Price TR: A two-year longitudinal study of mood disorders following stroke: prevalence and duration at six months follow-up. Br J Psychiatry 144:256–262, 1984

Robinson RG, Bolduc P, Price TR: A two-year longitudinal study of post-stroke depression: diagnosis and outcome at one- and two-year follow-up. Stroke 18:837–843, 1987

Sireling LI, Paykel ES, Freeling P, et al: Depression in general practice: case thresholds and diagnosis. Br J Psychiatry 147:113–119, 1985

Spitzer RL, Endicott J, Robins E: Research Diagnostic Criteria for a Selected Group of Functional Disorders, 3rd Edition. New York, New York State Psychiatric Institute, Biometrics Research, 1978

Stewart JW, Quitkin FM, Liebowitz MR, et al: Efficacy of desipramine in depressed outpatients. Arch Gen Psychiatry 40:202–207, 1983

Stewart JW, McGrath PJ, Quitkin FM, et al: Relevance of DSM-III depressive subtype and chronicity of antidepressant efficacy in atypical depression. Arch Gen Psychiatry 46:1080–1087, 1985

Wacker HR, Battegay R, Müllejans R, et al: Using the CIDI-C in the general population, in Psychiatry: A World Perspective. Edited by Stefanis CN, Rabavilas AD, Soldatos CR. Amsterdam, Elsevier, 1990

Weissman MM, Myers JK: Affective disorders in a United States urban community: the use of Research Diagnostic Criteria in an epidemiological survey. Arch Gen Psychiatry 35:1304–1314, 1978

Weissman MM, Myers JK, Harding PS: Psychiatric disorder in a U.S. urban community 1975–1976. Am J Psychiatry 135:459–462, 1978

Weissman MM, Kidd KK, Prusoff BA: Variability in rates of affective disorders in relatives of depressed and normal probands. Arch Gen Psychiatry 39:1397–1403, 1982

Weissman MM, Gershon ES, Kidd KK, et al: Psychiatric disorders in relatives of probands with affective disorders. Arch Gen Psychiatry 41:13–21, 1984

Wing JK, Sturt E: The PSE-ID-CATEGO system: a supplementary manual. London, Institute of Psychiatry (mimeo), 1978

Wing JK, Bebbington P, Hurry J, et al: The prevalence in the general population of disorders familiar to psychiatrists in hospital practice, in What Is a Case? The Problem of Definition in Psychiatric Community Surveys. Edited by Wing JK, Bebbington P, Robins L. London, Grant McIntyre, 1981, pp 45–61

Winter P, Philipp M, Buller R, et al: Identification of minor affective disorders and implications for psychopharmacotherapy. J Affect Disord 22:125–134, 1991

World Health Organization: International Classification of Diseases, Tenth Revision (ICD-10): Clinical Descriptions and Diagnostic Guidelines, Chapter V (Categories F00–F99). Geneva, World Health Organization, Division of Mental Health, 1991

Chapter 6

Recurrent Brief Depression

Kathleen Ries Merikangas, Ph.D., Emily B. Hoyer, B.A., and
Jules Angst, M.D.

Statement and Significance of the Issues

Longitudinal course has been recognized as an important aspect of psychiatric disorders, one that may enable predictions of the outcome of subjects, validations of diagnostic categories, and classifications of subtypes of disorders, since the work of Falret (1851), Kahlbaum (1874), and Kraepelin (1899). Consideration of course has had a broad impact on the study of affective disorders. Questions and issues arising from the possibilities presented by the investigation of the progress of a disorder across time are preeminent among the concerns of researchers and clinicians to this day (e.g., Akiskal 1983; Angst and Wicki 1991; Jablensky 1987; Keller et al. 1983, 1986; Schneider 1958; Standage 1979; Zimmerman et al. 1986; Zis and Goodwin 1979).

During the past decade, there has been considerable progress in the development of diagnostic criteria for major depression. However, there are no widely accepted standards for defining the course and outcome of depression. Moreover, the data on the long-term course of depression are highly variable and thus inadequate. The course of affective disorders is generally characterized according to two major features: the duration of particular episodes and the recurrence of such episodes over a defined period. Both features may be seen as continua on which depressive severity ranges from the time-limited and infrequent expression of the normal human emotion of depression at one end to the full and severe expression of chronic and incapacitating depression at the other end. Placement of the threshold for distinguishing normal variation in mood from depressive disorder

This research was supported by the Research Scientist Development Award MH00499 from the Alcohol, Drug Abuse and Mental Health Administration of the United States Public Health Service to Dr. Merikangas and by the Swiss National Foundation Grant 3.873.0.88 to Dr. Angst.

has generally been based on duration (which has arbitrarily ranged from 1 week for minor depression in the Research Diagnostic Criteria [RDC] [Spitzer et al. 1978] to 4 weeks in the Feighner criteria [Feighner et al. 1972]) in most systems of standardized diagnostic criteria.

Cases involving subjects with episodes of depression of brief duration are not new. Paskind (1929) commented in an introduction that, "although descriptions of manic-depressive depression are numerous, there are few reports of a form of the disease which is common and significant. I refer to attacks lasting from a few hours to a few days." He also reported that "[he was convinced that] these miniature attacks are the disorder recognized as manic-depressive depression. The symptoms are exactly like those of longer attacks. . . . That the brief and the long attacks are the same disorder is further indicated by their occurrence in the same person, the only essential difference being the time factor" (p. 125). Most brief depressive episodes noted today are associated with bipolar disorder, which is described in DSM-III-R (American Psychiatric Association 1987) as one or more manic episodes usually accompanied by one or more major depressive episodes.

Recurrence has also been employed to define cases of depression in the major diagnostic systems but, like duration, has primarily been applied to the classification of bipolar rather than unipolar disorder. Both the RDC and DSM-III-R specify criteria for mood disorders that are based on both duration and recurrence of depressive episodes. More recently, ICD-10 has incorporated categories for recurrent depression of both brief and extended duration.

Recurrent episodes of major depression are associated with greater severity in terms of clinical features, suicide attempts, impairment, biological factors (e.g., reduced rapid eye movement [REM] latency), and poorer treatment response than nonrecurrent depression (Akiskal et al. 1989; Frank et al. 1989; Giles et al. 1987; Keller 1985). Moreover, probands with recurrent depression exhibit greater familial loading for depression than those without recurrent depression (Bland et al. 1986; Weissman et al. 1986).

The discrete subtype of depression under consideration in this review, recurrent brief depression (RBD), was first described by Angst and Dobler-Mikola (1985), whose innovative combination of duration and recurrence criteria is listed below. Clayton et al. (1980) had previously described a syndrome of very brief depression, which they observed in a study of affective disorders among professional women. Very brief depression was characterized by depressed mood of 3–7 days' duration with three depressive symptoms and a change in mood or personality that was recognized by others. Clayton et al. stressed that the episodes were not systematically associated with the premenstrual phase in females, a finding borne out by Angst et al. (1990).

The Zurich group (Angst and Dobler-Mikola 1985) found that a substantial proportion of a cohort of young adults in Zurich, Switzerland, failed to meet diagnostic criteria for depression yet reported significant impairment and distress from depressive symptoms. Angst and Dobler-Mikola (1985) proposed a set of criteria "identical to the [DSM-III] diagnostic criteria for major depression concerning mood and number of symptoms," with associated recurrence and occupational impairment but with a lower threshold for duration than the RDC or DSM-III (American Psychiatric Association 1980) criteria.

1. The subject must experience dysphoric mood or loss of interest or pleasure.
2. Four of eight symptoms of depression (significant weight loss or gain; insomnia or hypersomnia; psychomotor agitation or retardation; loss of interest in usual activities or decrease in sexual drive; loss of energy or fatigue; feelings of worthlessness or guilt; diminished ability to think, concentrate, or make decisions; recurrent suicidal ideation or attempt at suicide or thoughts of death) causing impairment in usual occupational activities are required to constitute an episode.
3. The episode must last less than 1 week according to Angst's revisions (formerly less than 2 weeks).
4. Episodes must occur once or twice per month for 1 year.

The aims of this chapter are to review the evidence regarding RBD as a subtype of affective disorder, to clarify the diagnostic issues arising from that information, and to evaluate (to the degree possible) whether the inclusion of RBD in the DSM-IV is warranted.

Method

The literature covered in this review includes published work from only those studies that met the following requirements: 1) the studies used standardized diagnostic criteria based on direct clinical interviews, and 2) the authors reported the source and method of recruitment of the sample and provide evidence of systematic ascertainment.

A search via computer (Medline and Index Medicus programs) of the holdings of the National Library of Medicine for published work on depression and recurrent or brief subtypes of depression yielded a list of approximately 150 abstracts, roughly 110 of which were eliminated because of the above restrictions, leaving a total of about 40 articles for consideration in this review. The bibliographies from these papers were then thoroughly and methodically reviewed to provide an additional source for relevant articles. Direct contact with several investigators with data or relevant information on recurrent depression was also helpful in directing and refining this review.

Results

Validity and Utility

In the Zurich study (Angst et al. 1990), the validity of the RBD subtype was tested according to symptomatology, impairment, subjective distress, family history, and course. RBD was distinguished from the control group on all of these criteria and showed less overlap with dysthymia than did major depression. Validation criteria did not discriminate between RBD and major depression either cross-sectionally or longitudinally. RBD, according to data on impairment, did not appear to be a milder subtype of affective disorder than major depression. The methods and results of this study are described in more detail below.

Reliability

As mentioned earlier, data on recurrent brief depressive episodes are highly variable. Because studies with which one might validate or modify criteria for the RBD subtype have not been replicated, conclusions drawn from these data are neither convincing nor salient. However, the completion of a large study by the World Health Organization (WHO) that includes as an instrument a structured interview on RBD (Lecrubier and Lépine, unpublished interview in current use, 1990) is expected at the end of 1991; the data from WHO and the results from other investigations provoked by the inclusion of RBD in ICD-10 may corroborate or contradict the evidence gathered so far.

Definitional Features

The criteria used in the Zurich study for RBD were revised by Montgomery et al. (1989) in the following manner: the Zurich group (Angst 1988) proposed that depressive episodes should recur monthly for 1 year, which Montgomery et al. found to exclude several subjects with severe impairment whose episodes, although greater than 12 per year, return sporadically (thus their use of the term *intermittent brief depressions* or *3-day depressions*). Data from this study also indicated that 25% of subjects have at least one interval of more than 4 weeks. Montgomery et al. also shortened the length of time for retrospective assessments of episodes from 1 year to 3 months, in the hope that increased precision and accuracy of memory would aid in ensuring greater reliability for these assessments. These criteria also included more specific and extensive requirements for severity of impairment and allowed for the separate diagnosis of superimposed major depression and for specification of the subject's history of major depression.

Although this abbreviated period of assessment will enhance the reliability of the symptom data, a 3-month period may be too brief to be relevant for cases ascertained in the community. The issues surrounding these diagnostic choices and the data on which they are based are described in more detail in the "Discussion and Recommendations" section.

ICD-10

The criteria first suggested for field trials for the ICD-10 (World Health Organization 1987) included recurrent depressive disorders (mild, severe, and variable). For recurrent severe depressive disorder, these criteria require two severe depressive episodes (defined as a period of depression with an unspecified number of symptoms with biological impairment, such as weight loss, sleep disturbance, etc., in addition to dysphoria and social impairment) of at least 2 weeks duration separated by at least 6 months of normal mood. For recurrent mild depressive disorder, repeated episodes of depressed mood, the majority of which constitute mild depressive episodes (characterized by symptoms similar to, but less severe than, those for severe depressive episode, and excluding the distinguishing and more severe features of a severe episode) are required. The onset of this disorder may be acute or insidious and may occur at any age. Duration of individual episodes may vary from a few weeks to several months. Because these criteria, which are similar to the DSM-III-R criteria for major depressive episode, do not concern brief episodes of depressive symptoms, they are of little use in the project of fitting brief depressive episodes into classification systems.

The second draft of the ICD-10 criteria for field trials (World Health Organization 1989) included recurrent brief depressive disorder. The complete ICD-10 was recently released (World Health Organization 1991) and reflects this change; it includes criteria for recurrent brief depressive disorder.

Although recurrent depressive symptoms associated with the menstrual cycle are excluded from the category of recurrent brief depression, data from the Zurich study (Angst et al. 1990) and from Clayton et al. (1980) demonstrated fairly conclusively that RBD was unrelated to premenstrual syndrome. Angst et al. emphasized that "both the high frequency of RBD among males and the lower rate of premenstrual and menstrual depressive symptoms among subjects with RBD are at variance with [the hormonal cycle] explanation."

Clinical Studies

Stout et al. (1986) conducted a study of the lifetime psychiatric diagnoses of women seeking treatment for premenstrual syndrome, the results of which suggested a great degree of overlap between symptoms associated with premenstrual syndrome and those related to certain affective, anxiety, and substance use disorders. For example, the rate of suicide attempts among subjects in this sample who did not meet criteria for major depression seems to indicate a weakness in the classification system.

> The discrepancy between the low number of women meeting DIS/DSM-III criteria for major depressive episode and the high number of women reporting suicidal ideation and suicide attempts suggests that women seeking treatment for premenstrual syndrome may be more likely than women in the community to experience shorter periods of depressive symptoms than required to meet criteria for major depressive episode, but that the shorter duration symptoms can be intense and severe . . . [T]he number of previous suicide attempts in this group of women whose premenstrual symptoms are disruptive enough to cause them to seek treatment at a specialty clinic certainly indicates that they constitute a high-risk group. These indices of severity . . . warrant further exploration of premenstrual depressive symptoms and affective disorders despite the small percentage of women meeting criteria for a major depressive disorder. (p. 520)

Clayton's studies (Clayton et al. 1980; Welner et al. 1979) did not indicate that the brief depressive episodes suffered by subjects were related to premenstrual syndrome, nor did the Zurich study (Angst et al. 1990), which revealed a high rate of RBD among male subjects and a decreased rate of premenstrual and menstrual depressive symptoms among subjects with RBD. Rather than casting doubt on the results of Stout et al., these data may instead underscore the stated point that more research needs to be done regarding recurrent brief depression and its comorbidity with other disorders.

Treatment Studies

Montgomery et al. (1990) conducted a placebo-controlled study of low-dose flupenthixol or mianserin in subjects who did not have major depression to test the efficacy of the treatment in reducing suicidal behavior. A relationship between brief depression and suicide attempts was evident from previous studies (Montgomery et al. 1979, 1983) in which the occurrence of recurrent depressive episodes with durations of less than 2 weeks predicted future suicidal behavior in a group of patients with prior histories of suicide attempts. The mianserin/placebo comparison study demonstrated that six items—reduced sleep, reduced appetite, lassitude, suicidal thoughts, inability to feel, and pessimistic thoughts—from the Montgomery and Asberg Depression Rating Scale (MADRS) (Montgomery and Asberg 1979) each predicted subsequent suicidal behavior ($P < .05$). In the combined placebo groups from the flupenthixol/placebo and mianserin/placebo studies, each of six items—suicidal thoughts, reduced appetite, reduced sleep, apparent sadness, lassitude, and reported sadness—predicted subsequent suicidal acts in a 6-month treatment period ($P < .05$). According to Montgomery et al. (1990),

> These results suggest that brief episodes of depression lasting less than 2 weeks are associated with suicidal behavior in a group of recurrent suicidal attempters in whom DSM-III major depression had been excluded. Furthermore these data identify which symptoms reflect the greatest risk of suicidal behavior in recurrent brief depression and suggests [sic] that it is the depression itself which recurs and produces the suicide attempt. (p. 730)

Other treatment-outcome studies have been carried out on subjects with borderline personality disorder (Cowdry and Gardner 1988; Goldberg et al. 1986; Montgomery et al. 1979), but as Montgomery et al. (1989) make clear, the lack of quantification of such variables as duration of prior symptoms or prior affective stability in subjects precludes the possibility of generalizing from the findings of the studies.

Family Studies

Because the RBD category has only recently been introduced, there were no family studies of this depressive subtype in the literature. In the article cited in detail below, Angst et al. (1990) presented family history data of unspecified depressive disorders according to different subtypes of affective disorders in the cohort. The results showed that family history of treatment for depression was approximately twice as high among the depressive groups as among the control groups. There was no difference in the rates of positive family history between the depressive subgroups (major depression and RBD).

Follow-Up Studies

Montgomery et al. (1989) conducted a follow-up study of 20 patients with a history of suicidal behavior who did not meet criteria for major depression. Some of the subjects satisfied criteria (DSM-III) for borderline personality disorder and mixed personality disorder. The severity and duration of their episodes of depression were measured every 2 weeks for 4–6 months.

The severity of 70% of the episodes was recorded as moderate or severe on the MADRS (Montgomery and Asberg 1979); 30% were classified as mild (MADRS scores under 24). The episodes recurred at erratic intervals, and those not lasting more than 2 weeks had a mean length of 3.4 days (97% of the patients with episodes under 2 weeks in duration had episodes lasting 1 week or less; 81%, 4 days or less). Except for the duration requirement, the episodes of depression included symptomatology sufficient to meet DSM-III major depression criteria.

The results of this study indicate that suicidal behavior in patients without major depression is perhaps related to "intermittent short-lived depressions" or "3-day depressions" and that perhaps treatment with appropriate pharmacotherapy designed to reduce the frequency and severity of these depressions would reduce suicidal behavior.

Epidemiological Studies

Evidence for the validity of RBD was systematically investigated by Angst et al. (1990) at the 7 year follow-up of the original sample on which RBD was defined. The standard used for validity was that of Robins and Guze (1970), which requires four elements to be present: inclusion criteria, delimitation from other disorders, family history, and longitudinal course.

The subjects for the Zurich study were selected according to their scores on the Hopkins Symptom Checklist (SCL-90-R) (Derogatis 1977) in 1978. Two-thirds of the sample was comprised of subjects with scores above the 85th percentile. The remaining third of the subjects were randomly selected from those scoring below the 85th percentile on the Hopkins instrument. There were four waves of interviews: 1979, 1981, 1986, and 1988. The number of subjects completing all four interviews was 356 (192 females and 164 males); the number completing both the 1979 and 1986 interviews was 457 (232 females and 225 males). All 591 initial subjects participated in the 1979 interview, 456 of whom were reinterviewed in 1981; 457 subjects, some of whom did not participate in 1981, were reinterviewed in 1986. Of the subjects who participated in the 1986 interview, 90% were interviewed again in 1988.

The SPIKE, a semistructured diagnostic instrument developed for epidemiological studies (Angst et al. 1984), was used to collect information about the subjects regarding childhood characteristics, treatment history, symptoms, duration and frequency of symptoms, subjective degree of suffering, treatment, social consequences, previous history, family history of psychiatric and somatic syndromes, and use and abuse of substances. The SPIKE is not based on a particular diagnostic system but yields data that can fit multiple diagnostic systems and algorithms. Diagnoses from the 1986 and 1988 interviews were made according to DSM-III criteria for most of the major diagnostic categories. The diagnosis of major depression was made according to each of the following systems: Feighner, RDC, DSM-III, and DSM-III-R.

To test the validity of RBD as a subtype of depression, subgroups of depressive patients (i.e., RBD only, major depression only, major depression and RBD, and no depression) were compared on clinical severity, subjective distress, social and occupational impairment, and treatment-seeking behavior. The RBD group was nearly identical to the group with major depression on all of the features listed above; the RBD group also reported a degree of subjective distress equivalent to that of those with major depression. Subjects reporting the combination of the two syndromes manifested significantly greater severity on all of the above clinical validators, which suggests that recurrence is an important criterion in grading the severity of major depression.

Of 23 depressive symptoms measured by the SPIKE, only 1 symptom, difficulty in thinking, which was more elevated in the major depression group, distinguished the RBD group from the major depression group. Neither the mean number of DSM-III symptomatic criteria for depression nor the mean total number of symptoms differentiated the RBD group from the subjects with major depression. The group with both RBD and major depression, on the other hand, reported greater frequencies of inhibition, guilt, anxiety about everyday tasks, and being tired of living than either of the two other groups. Additionally, the mean total number of depressive symptoms was greater in the combined group than in either the major depression or the RBD group. These findings indicate a higher level of severity among subjects with both RBD and major depression. The total score and the mean scores on the subscales of the SCL-90 (Derogatis 1977) did not differ significantly between the subtypes. In addition, although the depressive groups displayed approximately twice the rate of family history of treatment for depression compared with the control group, there was no difference in the rates of positive family history between the depressive subgroups. One interesting difference between the groups was in lifetime history of suicide attempts: the RBD group had a higher rate than the major depression group, and nearly one-third of the combined group had a history of suicide attempts.

The stability of the subtypes was established across a 10-year period; the proportions of subjects who continued to manifest the same depressive subtypes over the longitudinal course were equal for the RBD and major depression subjects according to the original (1979) classification of depressive subtype ($\chi^2 = 0.276$; $df = 2$; NS). Similar proportions of the major depression and RBD samples developed the other subtype or a combination of both; this suggests that RBD cannot solely be an early manifestation of or a residual form of major depression. These data suggest that severity of depression is more appropriately measured by a combination of standardized symptoms and recurrence rather than merely by the duration of a depressive episode.

In summary, the validity of RBD was demonstrated according to symptomatology, impairment, subjective distress, family history, and course. The group with RBD was shown to be distinct from the control group on all of these criteria. Validation criteria did not discriminate between RBD and major depression either cross-sectionally or longitudinally. RBD, according to the data, did not appear to be a milder form of affective disorder than major depression. This was emphasized by the twofold increase in the number of suicide attempts (which Montgomery et al. [1983] had shown to be associated with recurrent depression) in the group with major depression and RBD compared with the major depression group (the 1988 rates of suicide attempts were as follows: major depression, 13.8; RBD, 14.6; major depression + RBD, 32.1). This seems to indicate that the classification of RBD would allow researchers and clinicians to distinguish subgroups of major depressive disorders with markedly different risks of suicidal behavior. Recurrent brief depression was also shown to be distinct from dysthymia; in fact, there was a more substantial degree of overlap between major depression and dysthymia than between RBD and dysthymia.

Discussion

The primary issue regarding recurrent depressive disorders is whether any separate diagnosis for recurrent depression is warranted. If so, specific criteria for RBD, criteria with optimal reliability, coverage, and clinical implications, need to be tested systematically. Because the criteria are used to determine who will receive treatment for a specific disorder, the importance of a thorough understanding of course becomes more obvious, especially in light of the potentially fatal outcome (due to suicide) of mood disorders for some subjects (Montgomery et al. 1989; Welner et al. 1979). As noted in a recent abstract ("Recurrent Brief Depression and Anxiety (Editorial)" 1991), the time limits used to distinguish diagnoses are based on questionable reasoning. For example, although a diagnosis of major depressive episode requires a 2-week period of depressive symptoms, the diagnosis of generalized anxiety disorder, the anxiety disorder corresponding to major depressive episode, requires that symptoms be present for almost all of a 6-month period to meet criteria. Suicide rates demonstrate that subthreshold conditions such as these brief and recurrent episodes of depression must be taken seriously (Angst et al. 1990); if those patients who make recurrent suicide attempts were diagnosed with RBD and given antidepressant treatment prophylactically, prevention of suicide might be achieved with greater success (Montgomery and Montgomery 1982; Montgomery et al. 1983). Despite the lack of consensus regarding classification of recurrent depressive disorders, there is a little empirical data on which to base appropriate thresholds and boundaries for recurrent depression.

The following points have been raised regarding the inclusion of RBD in DSM-IV:

1) Recurrent depressive disorders should be included in the classification system under (DSM-III-R) borderline personality disorder, because of the brief and episodic nature of the expression of symptoms, particularly suicidal ideation,

depression, and anxiety, among persons with borderline personality ("Recurrent Brief Depression and Anxiety (Editorial)" 1991; Standage 1979). In addition, Montgomery's data (1989) on RBD were based on a sample of persons with borderline personality disorder.

Although the simultaneous manifestation of Axis I and Axis II disorders may present a complicated clinical picture, there is no a priori evidence regarding the nature of the interaction of the expression of depressive symptoms in individuals with borderline personality disorder. Therefore, to be consistent with the DSM-IV goal (as described in Frances et al. 1990) of avoiding the use of inferences in developing hierarchical associations between disorders, RBD should not be subsumed under the category of borderline personality disorder. At this time, conclusions regarding the nature of the association between RBD and the personality disorders are precluded by the lack of longitudinal data on RBD. The relatively young age of the cohort from which RBD was identified did not permit assessment of whether the disorder may constitute an early manifestation of bipolar disorder or may later become major depression. As Montgomery et al. (1989) point out, this distinction may be more complex than it first appears.

> Some of the features which characterize this group who have repeated suicidal attempts are included in the criteria for borderline personality disorders. An individual with acute depressions which recur unpredictably every 2–3 weeks might understandably be described as having affective instability, one of the diagnostic features of borderline personality disorder.
>
> Other diagnostic criteria of borderline personality disorder which may be misleading include suicidal attempts, impulsivity, avoiding being alone, inappropriate control of anger, and a pattern of unstable relationships. These can all be viewed either as direct depressive symptoms or the by-product of a long-term recurring illness. It seems as if the DSM-III diagnostic system has incorporated some behavioral consequences of a recurrent depressive illness under the personality disorder Axis II dimension. This has the unfortunate effect of implying that individuals with these acute episodes have long-standing character defects, with the expectation of a poor prognosis, rather than having a primary depressive illness which may well be responsive to treatment. (pp. 129–130)

2) The inclusion of subthreshold depressive disorders may create false positives. The evidence of both Angst et al. (1990) and Montgomery et al. (1990) suggests that this is not the case. Lifetime treatment rates among those with RBD approximated (Angst et al. 1990) those among persons with major depression (i.e., 50%). Without the classification of RBD, 30% of the subjects who had been treated for depression would be classified as having depressive disorder not otherwise specified in DSM-III-R. This information indicates that RBD fills an important gap in the nosology.

Additionally, course and outcome data (Angst et al. 1990; Clayton et al. 1980; Montgomery and Montgomery 1982; Montgomery et al. 1983; Stout et al. 1986; Welner et al. 1979) indicate that the severity of impairment suffered by those with recurrent brief depressive episodes is comparable to the severity of impairment due to major depression. More than two-thirds of the cases in the Zurich study who did not meet criteria for major depression or dysthymia received a diagnosis of recurrent brief depression (Angst 1990b). As noted above, the prevalence of suicide attempts was twice as high (Angst et al. 1990) in those with both RBD and major depression as in those with RBD or major depression alone. In addition, the ICD-10 has included RBD, maintaining severity and symptom requirements in the criteria while abbreviating the duration requirements, thus further emphasizing that the severity of the disorder does not appear to decrease with the duration. Although this evidence may suggest nothing more than that younger populations experience and respond to psychiatric disorders in a different fashion than older populations, the fact remains that many cases of depression go undiagnosed due to course requirements, and the cost in human suffering, and, sometimes, human life, may be reduced by instituting a more responsive diagnostic system.

3) Reliability of recall of brief episodes over a 1-year period is likely to be poor (Angst 1988; Brown and Harris 1982; Jenkins et al. 1979; Montgomery et al. 1989). Recall bias may indeed make course-based diagnostic discriminations very difficult, and the criteria may likewise be difficult to apply in a cross-sectional manner, thus making the results less applicable to the general population. Data on the reliability of recall of brief versus longer episodes of depression, or recurrent episodes, are insufficient to conclude that RBD may be assessed reliably.

Recommendations

Ample clinical data and the validation data provided by the Zurich study suggest that RBD is an important subtype of affective disorder, at least in young adults. Failure to consider recurrent but brief episodes of depression may lead to drastic underestimates of major depression, as well as leaving a large proportion of cases that involve young adults with severe depression and its consequences without a diagnostic category.

However, the lack of replicated data with which to study the validity of this subtype, aside from the findings of the investigators who first introduced this concept to the nomenclature (Angst 1988, 1990a; Angst and Dobler-Mikola 1985; Angst and Wicki 1991; Angst et al. 1984, 1990; Merikangas et al. 1994) and those of another investigator who studied recurrent brief episodes of depression in a clinical sample of patients with borderline personality disorder (Montgomery et al.

1979), is a serious obstacle to its inclusion in diagnostic classification systems. The reliability of the data, which has yet to be replicated, has not been proven to a degree sufficient to warrant the inclusion of RBD as a DSM-IV subtype at this time.

Systematic probes for RBD have been added to a structured interview (Lecrubier and Lépine, unpublished interview in current use, 1990) now in use in studies being conducted under the auspices of WHO at several sites including France, Germany, Italy, and the United Kingdom. These data, in conjunction with those provoked by the inclusion of RBD as a subtype of mood disorder in ICD-10, should elucidate the issues surrounding the diagnosis and classification of RBD with greater depth and success than could be provided in this review. In light of the above situation, and because the completion of the WHO studies is anticipated by the end of 1991, it is recommended that RBD be included in the DSM-IV appendix for disorders needing further study and that a final decision be delayed until the data from WHO and other studies are examined thoroughly. Clearly there is a need for more research regarding recurrent depressive episodes of brief duration in older cohorts to fully validate the inclusion of this subtype in diagnostic systems. Data are also scarce concerning the relation of these episodes to the personality disorders, possible treatment options and their relative efficacy, degree and method of possible familial transmission of this disorder, comorbidity of RBD with other psychiatric disorders, long-term course and outcome of this disorder (i.e., is RBD a precursor or early stage of another mood disorder?) as well as its short-term course (i.e., true prospective data collected over short intervals are needed), the incidence of this disorder among samples ascertained from nontreatment settings, and the true prevalence of this disorder in the general population.[1]

References

Akiskal HS: Dysthymic disorder: psychopathology of proposed chronic depressive subtypes. Am J Psychiatry 140:11–20, 1983

Akiskal HS, Cassano GB, Musetti L, et al: Psychopathology, temperament, and past course in primary major depressions, I: review of evidence for a bipolar spectrum. Psychopathology 22:268–277, 1989

---

[1]Since the preparation of this review, several clinical, epidemiological, and biological studies have provided evidence for the magnitude and clinical significance of this subtype of depression. The largest of these studies, an international multicenter study of primary care settings, revealed a high prevalence of RBD in general practice (Weiler E, Boyer P, Lépine J-P, et al: Prevalence of recurrent brief depression in primary care. *Eur Arch Psychiatry Clin Neurosci* [in press]).

American Psychiatric Association: Diagnostic and Statistical Manual of Mental Disorders, 3rd Edition. Washington, DC, American Psychiatric Association, 1980

American Psychiatric Association: Diagnostic and Statistical Manual of Mental Disorders, 3rd Edition, Revised. Washington, DC, American Psychiatric Association, 1987

Angst J: Clinical course of affective disorders, in Depressive Illness: Prediction of Course and Outcome. Edited by Helgason T, Daly RJ. Berlin, Springer-Verlag, 1988, pp 1–48

Angst J: Natural history and epidemiology of depression: results of community studies, in Current Approaches: Prediction and Treatment of Recurrent Depression. Edited by Cobb J, Goeting NLM. Duphar Medical Relations, 1990a, pp 1–11

Angst J: Recurrent brief depression: a new concept of depression. Pharmacopsychiatry 23:63–66, 1990b

Angst J, Dobler-Mikola A: The Zurich study: a prospective epidemiological study of depressive, neurotic, and psychosomatic syndromes, IV: recurrent and nonrecurrent brief depression. Eur Arch Psychiatry Neurol Sci 234:408–416, 1985

Angst J, Wicki W: The Zurich study: a prospective epidemiological study of depressive, neurotic, and psychosomatic syndromes, XI: is dysthymia a separate form of depression? results of the Zurich cohort study. Eur Arch Psychiatry Clin Neurosci 240:349–354, 1991

Angst J, Dobler-Mikola A, Binder J: The Zurich study: a prospective epidemiological study of depressive, neurotic, and psychosomatic syndromes, I: problem, methodology. Eur Arch Psychiatry Neurol Sci 234:13–20, 1984

Angst J, Merikangas K, Scheidegger P, et al: Recurrent brief depression: a new subtype of affective disorder. J Affect Disord 19:87–88, 1990

Bland RC, Newman SC, Orn H: Recurrent and nonrecurrent depression: a family study. Arch Gen Psychiatry 43:1085–1089, 1986

Brown GW, Harris T: Fall-off in the reporting of life events. Soc Psychiatry 17:23–28, 1982

Clayton PJ, Marten S, Davis MA, et al: Mood disorder in women professionals. J Affect Disord 2:37–46, 1980

Cowdry RW, Gardner DL: Pharmacotherapy of borderline personality disorder. Arch Gen Psychiatry 45:111–119, 1988

Derogatis LR: SCL-90: Administration, Scoring and Procedures Manual for the R (Revised) Version and Other Instruments of the Psychopathology Rating Scales Series. Baltimore, MD, Johns Hopkins University School of Medicine, 1977

Falret JP: De la folie circulaire ou forme de maladie mentale caracterisée par l'alternative regulière de la manie et de la melancolie. Bulletin de l'Académie Nationale de Medecine (Paris), 1851

Feighner JP, Robins E, Guze SB, et al: Diagnostic criteria for use in psychiatric research. Arch Gen Psychiatry 26:57–63, 1972

Frances A, Pincus HA, Widiger TA, et al: DSM-IV: work in progress. Am J Psychiatry 147:1439–1448, 1990

Frank E, Kupfer DJ, Perel JM: Early recurrence in unipolar depression. Arch Gen Psychiatry 46:397–400, 1989

Giles DE, Jarrett RB, Roffwarg HP, et al: Reduced REM latency: a predictor of recurrence in depression. Neuropsychopharmacology 1:33–39, 1987

Goldberg SC, Schulz SC, Schulz PM, et al: Borderline and schizotypal personality disorders treated with low-dose thiothixene vs. placebo. Arch Gen Psychiatry 43:680–686, 1986

Jablensky A: Prediction of the course and outcome of depression. Psychol Med 17:1–9, 1987

Jenkins CD, Hurst MW, Rose RM: Life changes: do people really remember? Arch Gen Psychiatry 36:379–384, 1979

Kahlbaum J: Die Katatonie oder das Spannungsirresein. Eine klinische Form psychischer Krankheiten. Berlin, Hirschwald, 1874

Keller MB: Chronic and recurrent affective disorders: incidence, course, and influencing factors, in Chronic Treatments in Neuropsychiatry. Edited by Kemali D, Racagni G. New York, Raven, 1985, pp 111–120

Keller MB, Lavori PW, Lewis CE, et al: Predictors of relapse in major depressive disorder. J Am Med Assoc 250:3299–3304, 1983

Keller MB, Lavori PW, Rice J, et al: The persistent risk of chronicity in recurrent episodes of nonbipolar major depressive disorder: a prospective follow-up. Am J Psychiatry 143:24–28, 1986

Kraepelin E: Psychiatrie: Ein Lehrbuch fur Studierende und Aerzte, 6th Edition. Leipzig, Barth, 1899

Merikangas K, Wicki W, Angst J: Heterogeneity of depression: classification of depressive subtypes by longitudinal course. Br J Psychiatry 164:342–348, 1994

Montgomery SA, Asberg M: A new depression scale designed to be more sensitive to change. Br J Psychiatry 134:382–389, 1979

Montgomery S, Montgomery D: Pharmacological prevention of suicidal behaviour. J Affect Disord 4:291–298, 1982

Montgomery S, Montgomery D, McAuley R, et al: Maintenance therapy in repeat suicidal behaviour: a placebo controlled trial, in Proceedings of the 10th International Congress for Suicide Prevention and Crisis Intervention, 1979, pp 227–229

Montgomery SA, Roy D, Montgomery DB: The prevention of recurrent suicidal acts. Br J Clin Pharmacol 15:183S–188S, 1983

Montgomery SA, Montgomery D, Baldwin D, et al: Intermittent 3-day depressions and suicidal behaviour. Neuropsychobiology 22:128–134, 1989

Montgomery SA, Montgomery D, Baldwin D, et al: The duration, nature, and recurrence rate of brief depressions. Prog Neuropsychopharmacol Biol Psychiatry 14:729–735, 1990

Paskind H: Brief attacks of manic-depressive depression. Archives of Neurological Psychiatry (Chicago) 22:123–134, 1929

Recurrent brief depression and anxiety (editorial). Lancet 337:586–587, 1991

Robins E, Guze SB: Establishment of diagnostic validity in psychiatric illness: its application to schizophrenia. Am J Psychiatry 126:983–987, 1970

Schneider K: Psychopathic Personalities. Translated by Hamilton MW. London, Cassell, 1958

Spitzer RL, Endicott J, Robins E: Research Diagnostic Criteria: rationale and reliability. Arch Gen Psychiatry 35:773–782, 1978

Standage KF: The use of Schneider's typology for the diagnosis of personality disorder: an examination of reliability. Br J Psychiatry 135:238–242, 1979

Stout AL, Steege JF, Blazer DG, et al: Comparison of lifetime psychiatric diagnoses in premenstrual syndrome clinic and community samples. J Nerv Ment Dis 174:517–522, 1986

Weissman MM, Merikangas KR, Wickramaratne P, et al: Understanding the clinical heterogeneity of major depression using family data. Arch Gen Psychiatry 43:430–434, 1986

Welner A, Marten S, Wochnik E, et al: Psychiatric disorders among professional women. Arch Gen Psychiatry 36:169–173, 1979

World Health Organization: ICD-10 1986 Draft of Chapter V Categories F00–F99: Mental, Behavioral, and Developmental Disorders: Clinical Descriptions and Diagnostic Guidelines (1986 draft for field trials). Geneva, World Health Organization, 1987

World Health Organization: ICD-10 1988 Draft of Chapter V Categories F00–F99: Mental, Behavioral, and Developmental Disorders: Clinical Descriptions and Diagnostic Guidelines (1988 draft for field trials). Geneva, World Health Organization, 1989

World Health Organization: International Classification of Diseases, 10th Edition (ICD-10): Clinical Descriptions and Diagnostic Guidelines. Geneva, World Health Organization, 1991

Zimmerman M, Coryell W, Pfohl B: Validity of familial subtypes of primary unipolar depression. Arch Gen Psychiatry 43:1090–1096, 1986

Zis AP, Goodwin FK: Major affective disorder as a recurrent illness: a critical review. Arch Gen Psychiatry 36:835–839, 1979

Chapter 7

Psychotic (Delusional) Major Depression: Should It Be Included as a Distinct Syndrome in DSM-IV?

Alan F. Schatzberg, M.D., and Anthony J. Rothschild, M.D.

Statement of the Issues

In recent years, considerable attention has been paid to psychotic or delusional depression as a distinct subtype of depression. This disorder is quite common, representing some 14% of subjects with major depression in the community (Johnson et al. 1991) and 25% of consecutively admitted depressed patients (Coryell et al. 1984b). In DSM-III-R (American Psychiatric Association 1987), it is generally referred to as major depression with psychotic features. In this chapter, we review data from studies on clinical characteristics, biology, familial transmission, treatment response, and course that relate to whether such a designation should be included in DSM-IV as a distinct syndrome (Feighner et al. 1972). We propose that there are sufficient data and clinical reasons to designate major depression with psychotic features as a distinct depressive syndrome in DSM-IV.

The text of this chapter is reprinted with permission of the *American Journal of Psychiatry* (Schatzberg and Rothschild 1992).

Supported in part by grants from NIMH (MH38675 and MH47457), the Poitras Charitable Foundation, the Ruth Rothstein Greif Fund, and a National Alliance for Research on Schizophrenia and Depression Young Investigator Award. Patti Brown, Linda Messier, Meghan Bessette, and Gertrud Cory assisted in the preparation of this manuscript.

Significance of the Issues

Delusional or psychotic depression is a severe form of mood disorder characterized by delusions or hallucinations. The view that delusional depression is a distinct disorder was largely born out of the psychopharmacological era (Kantor and Glassman 1977), and the renewed interest in this disorder rests heavily with observations made by Glassman et al. (1977) in their classic imipramine plasma level studies. The history of this syndrome has been reviewed in detail by Kantor and Glassman (1977), as well as by our group (Rothschild 1985). The significance of psychotic symptoms as predictors of outcome was explored in early studies (i.e., before the introduction of electroconvulsive therapy [ECT]). In these studies, patients with what today would be called psychotic major depression (PMD) often did more poorly than their counterparts with nonpsychotic (major) depression (NPMD), but the presence of delusions itself was "not a clear predictor of outcome" (Kantor and Glassman 1977). Patients with delusions without prominent mood symptoms, however, generally did poorly.

After the introduction of ECT, interest in psychotic depression waned considerably when a number of early studies (in the 1950s and 1960s) reported that delusions predicted neither good nor poor response to ECT (Kantor and Glassman 1977). PMD and NPMD patients both responded well (approximately 80% response rate) to this powerful treatment (Kantor and Glassman 1977). (Note, however, that several later studies have questioned these earlier findings; see below.) The introduction of tricyclic antidepressants (TCAs) led to a renewed interest in psychotic depression, as it had with other disorders such as panic disorder. However, in contrast to panic disorder or agoraphobia with panic attacks, which were noted to be highly responsive to imipramine, psychotic depression was in a sense reborn as a syndrome because it responded unexpectedly poorly to TCAs. This lack of response has led to numerous recent studies on clinical characteristics, biological measures, course, and family history, many of which have argued that psychotic depression is a distinct subtype of depression and should be designated as such.

There has, however, been a long-standing debate as to whether psychotic depression is indeed a distinct syndrome or merely represents a severe depressive subtype. In the European literature, *psychotic depression* generally has been used to indicate a syndrome characterized by pronounced neurovegetative signs and symptoms, with or without a thought disorder. This approach was carried over into DSM-II (American Psychiatric Association 1968), in which patients with psychotic depressive reactions were those who demonstrated severe depressive episodes in response to one or more identifiable stressors. Delusions or hallucinations were not required for this diagnosis. In DSM-III and DSM-III-R (American Psychiatric Association 1980, 1987), the dimensional qualifier "with psychotic features," as part of the fifth-digit severity code, denotes a thought disorder, (i.e., the presence of hallucinations or delusions) that primarily reflects the severity of the depressive disorder rather than a distinct characteristic. However, data reviewed in this chapter may suggest a predictive validity for PMD (as demonstrated in responses to treatment, outcome, family history, and biological measures) that is more consistent with PMD as a categorical entity than one merely defined by being positioned at one end of a severity dimension. Moreover, the finding that (unlike NPMD) PMD does not respond particularly well to TCAs but does respond to other treatment approaches underscores the importance for careful assessment of this disorder.

Methods

We reviewed all English language studies available (as of 1991) on delusional (psychotic) major depression. Computerized searches (Medline, Index Medicus) were used to help identify studies. Emphasis is placed on those studies that directly compared samples of delusional and nondelusional major depressed patients.

Results

Characteristics

The hallmark feature separating PMD from NPMD patients is the occurrence of delusions or hallucinations in the former. Delusions can be classified broadly as guilty, paranoid, or somatic. Hallucinations are divided into auditory, visual, and somatic types. Generally, delusions are viewed as mood congruent if they reflect lowered mood and/or underlying nihilistic, overly self-deprecatory, or guilty beliefs. Table 7–1 summarizes data from studies in which PMD and NPMD patients were compared on specific clinical features. Psychotic depressions are often severe in nature, with patients demonstrating relatively high total Hamilton Depression Rating Scale (HDRS) (Hamilton 1960) scores (Lykouras et al. 1986b; Spiker et al. 1985) that are often significantly higher than for NPMD comparison groups (Coryell et al. 1984b; Frances et al. 1981; Glassman and Roose 1981; Lykouras et al. 1986b; Nelson et al. 1984). Although these observations could be interpreted as supporting the notion that psychotic depression is merely a more severe variant of depression, a number of investigators have argued that psychotic depression is indeed a separate disorder. For one, studies of depressed patients have identified NPMD patients with total HDRS scores in the range seen in PMD patients (Glass-

Table 7–1. Characteristics of patients with delusional and nondelusional major depression

Study	Diagnostic instrument/ classification system	Diagnoses (n)	Prospective study (Y/N)	Findings
Nelson and Bowers 1978	None/RDC	27 primary unipolar inpatients: 14 with delusions and 13 without	N	All 14 delusional patients demonstrated a psychomotor disturbance, in contrast to 7 of 13 nondelusional patients ($P < .05$); although more delusional patients demonstrated self-reproach and suicidal ideation, differences did not attain significance; there were no differences in frequency of sleep or appetite disturbance, decreased energy, loss of interest, or poor concentration.
Frances et al. 1981	SADS/RDC	64 unipolar, endogenous major depressive disorder: 30 psychotic and 34 nonpsychotic; all inpatients	Y	On 24-item HDRS, psychotic patients demonstrated significantly greater feelings of guilt, early insomnia, agitation, paranoid symptoms, hopelessness, and total scores. No other differences were noted.
Charney and Nelson 1981	Delusional distinctions based on SADS/RDC-type criteria were used	120 primary unipolar major depression: 54 delusional, 66 nondelusional; all inpatients	N	Delusional patients showed significantly higher percentages of agitation, referential thinking, ruminative thinking, self-reproach, retardation, energy, and anxiety; formal ratings were not used.
Glassman and Roose 1981	Delusional definition based on SADS/RDC	63 RDC unipolar major depressed patients: 21 delusional and 42 nondelusional; all inpatients	Y	Delusional patients demonstrated higher scores on items of a modified HDRS: personal appearance, negative self-esteem, negative expectations; difficulty in functioning, guilt, hypochondriasis, anxiety, psychomotor retardation, depressed mood, and total HDRS scores; when 28 patients were matched for age, sex, and total HDRS score, delusional patients demonstrated greater psychomotor retardation and agitation scores.

Study	Instrument	Sample		Findings
Frangos et al. 1983	None/RDC	264 RDC primary unipolar major depressed patients: 145 psychotic and 119 nonpsychotic; all inpatients	N	No differences between the two groups in incidence of suicide attempts; psychotic patients demonstrated a significantly greater number of episodes of agitation.
Roose et al. 1983	None/RDC and DSM-III	Chart review of 14 unipolar endogenously depressed inpatients who committed suicide; 10 of 14 were delusional	N	Delusionally depressed patients were 5 times more likely to commit suicide than were nondelusionally depressed patients.
Nelson et al. 1984	None/RDC and DSM-III	25 patients with RDC major depressive disorder, endogenous subtype: 13 with DSM-III delusions and 12 without; all inpatients	Y	On 21-item HDRS, delusional patients demonstrated significantly higher total scores and subscale scores for suicidal ideation and delusions but not for depressed mood or other subscales. Individual item data not presented.
Coryell et al. 1984b	None/DSM-III	235 DSM-III unipolar or bipolar patients with depression: 55 with psychotic features	Y	On 17-item HDRS, delusional patients had significantly higher total scores, but this was due primarily to higher scores on guilt, hypochondriasis, and insight; psychotic patients also demonstrated significantly greater depressed mood and retardation.
Lykouras et al. 1986b	Athens University Instrument/ DSM-III	DSM-III major depressive disorders; 22 delusional and 36 nondelusional; all inpatients	Y	On 21-item HDRS, delusional patients demonstrated significantly higher total scores and scores on the following items: depressed mood, guilt, initial insomnia, middle insomnia, retardation, agitation, and paranoid symptoms.
Lykouras et al. 1986a	None/DSM-III	95 DSM-III unipolar major depressed patients: 55 delusional and 40 nondelusional; all inpatients	N	Dependent personality traits were more common in nondelusional patients; no differences were observed in other personality traits (e.g., compulsive, passive-aggressive, narcissistic). No differences were observed in frequency of significant retardation or agitation. *(continued)*

Table 7–1. Characteristics of patients with delusional and nondelusional major depression *(continued)*

Study	Diagnostic instrument/ classification system	Diagnoses (*n*)	Prospective study (Y/N)	Findings
Rothschild et al. 1989b	SADS/DSM-III	DSM-III major depressed patients: 15 delusional and 15 nondelusional; 22 unipolar; all inpatients	Y	Delusional patients did significantly worse for both left and right hands on m's and n's test (frontal lobe) and on the drawing quality test (frontal and temporal lobe).
Rothschild et al. 1989a	SCID/DSM-III-R	54 DSM-III-R major depressed patients: 45 unipolar, 9 bipolar NOS; 13 delusional and 14 nondelusional	Y	Delusional patients had significantly higher total HDRS ($P = .005$) and BPRS ($P = .000$) scores than nondelusional patients. Delusional patients had significantly higher HDRS factor scores on retardation ($P = .012$) and cognitive disturbance ($P = 005$) but not on anxiety/somatization, weight, diurnal variation, and sleep disturbance compared with NPMD patients. Delusional patients had higher BPRS factor scores on thinking disturbance ($P = .02$), withdrawal/retardation ($P = .02$), and hostile/suspiciousness ($P = .009$) but not anxious/depression compared with NPMD patients.
Parker et al. 1991	Parker Core/DSM-III, RDC, and ICD-9	137 patients who met endogenous or melancholia criteria on DSM-III, RDC, or ICD-9; 35 were delusional; inpatients and outpatients	Y	Delusional endogenous patients demonstrated significantly greater frequencies of severe psychomotor disturbance, absence of diurnal variation, sustained and fixed depressive context, and constipation.
Johnson et al. 1991	DIS/DSM-III	DSM-III unipolar major depressed patients: 114 delusional and 662 nondelusional	Y	Delusional patients demonstrated more suicide attempts, more frequent reoccurrences, greater disability, more hospitalizations, and greater chronicity but overall were not more symptomatic.

Note. BPRS = Brief Psychiatric Rating Scale. HDRS = Hamilton Depression Rating Scale. RDC = Research Diagnostic Criteria. SADS = Schedule for Affective Disorders and Schizophrenia. SCID = Structured Clinical Interview for DSM-III-R. NOS = not otherwise specified. NPMD = nonpsychotic major depression.

man and Roose 1981). Thus, the development of delusions must rest with risk factors or biological processes other than severity. Moreover, in studies reporting greater overall severity in PMD patients, they do not appear to demonstrate greater severity on all symptoms. Rather, differences between PMD and NPMD patients appear to occur primarily in particular symptoms or symptom clusters. For example, as indicated in Table 7–1, our group has reported that PMD patients have significantly higher total HDRS scores than NPMD patients ($P = .005$) (Rothschild et al. 1989a). This was primarily due to the PMD patients having significantly greater HDRS factor scores on retardation ($P = .012$) and cognitive disturbance ($P = .005$) than NPMD patients. The HDRS factor scores of anxiety/somatization, weight, diurnal variation, and sleep disturbance were not significantly different between PMD and NPMD patients. On the Brief Psychiatric Rating Scale (BPRS), PMD patients had a greater mean total score than NPMD patients ($P = .001$) and higher factor scores of thinking disturbance ($P = .02$), withdrawal/retardation ($P = .02$), and hostile/suspiciousness ($P = .009$) than NPMD patients. The two groups did not differ on the factor score of anxious/depression.

In regard to specific symptoms, patients with PMD demonstrate significantly more severe or more common psychomotor disturbances (retardation or agitation) than do NPMD patients (Charney and Nelson 1981; Coryell et al. 1984b; Frances et al. 1981; Glassman and Roose 1981; Lykouras et al. 1986b; Nelson and Bowers 1978). Some studies have reported greater agitation in PMD (Charney and Nelson 1981; Frances et al. 1981; Nelson and Bowers 1978), whereas others have reported greater retardation (Glassman and Roose 1981). At least two studies have reported both greater agitation and retardation (Charney and Nelson 1981; Lykouras et al. 1986b). Only one (retrospective) study failed to find significant differences in either retardation or agitation (Lykouras et al. 1986a). Greater agitation or retardation in PMD does not appear to be due to increased severity. Glassman and Roose (1981) reported that when patients with PMD and NPMD were matched for total HDRS scores, PMD patients still demonstrated significantly greater psychomotor retardation or agitation scores. Similar data were reported by Lykouras et al. (1986b) (see below). Several investigators have also reported significantly greater feelings of guilt in PMD than in NPMD (Charney and Nelson 1981; Coryell et al. 1984b; Frances et al. 1981; Glassman and Roose 1981; Lykouras et al. 1986b), but at least one study failed to confirm this finding (Frangos et al. 1983).

A number of other symptoms have been reported to be more pronounced in PMD than in NPMD: depressed mood (Coryell et al. 1984b; Glassman and Roose 1981; Lykouras et al. 1986b), paranoid symptoms (Frances et al. 1981; Lykouras et al. 1986b), hopelessness (Frances et al. 1981), hypochondriasis (Coryell et al. 1984b; Glassman and Roose 1981), anxiety (Charney and Nelson 1981; Glassman and Roose 1981), early insomnia (Frances et al. 1981; Lykouras et al. 1986b), and middle insomnia (Lykouras et al. 1986b). However, the data in support of each of these being more pronounced in PMD are less robust and less consistent than are the data in support of psychomotor disturbance or guilt (see above). Lykouras et al. (1986b) reported a number of differences between PMD and NPMD patients on specific symptoms (e.g., insomnia). However, after covarying out for overall severity, only depressed mood, psychomotor retardation, and paranoid symptoms remained significantly higher in PMD patients.

Risk for completing suicide has been reported to be greater in hospitalized PMD patients than in their NPMD counterparts (Roose et al. 1983), and suicidal ideation has also been reported to be significantly greater in PMD than in NPMD patients (Nelson et al. 1984). However, other studies comparing the two groups on suicidal ideation or attempts have failed to find statistically significant differences between them (Charney and Nelson 1981; Coryell et al. 1984b; Frances et al. 1981; Frangos et al. 1983; Glassman and Roose 1981; Nelson and Bowers 1978). These data suggest that most somatic depressive symptoms and suicidal ideation/behavior cannot be used to consistently separate PMD and NPMD patients but that psychomotor disturbance, guilt, and psychotic symptoms do appear to separate PMD and NPMD patients.

Although psychomotor agitation and guilt appear to help separate PMD from NPMD even after covarying out for overall severity, one may argue that these symptoms are merely separating endogenous or melancholic major depressive patients from their nonendogenous counterparts. Although few studies have specifically examined an "endogenous" dimension separately from one of severity, one could argue that a high proportion of severely ill, hospitalized NPMDs would also meet criteria for endogenous depression and that these various symptoms are in fact separating psychotic major endogenous depression from nonpsychotic major endogenous depression. Without applying specific endogenous criteria to define the nonpsychotic sample, however, this question is moot.

Recently, Parker et al. (1991) reported on symptom differences between delusional and nondelusional patients, all of whom met criteria for both DSM-III melancholia and Research Diagnostic Criteria (RDC; Spitzer et al. 1978) definite endogenous syndromes. In contrast to endogenous NPMD patients, endogenous PMD patients significantly demonstrated a more frequent psychomotor disturbance, an absence of diurnal variation in mood, a fixed depressive content, and constipation. Indeed, the authors used latent class analyses and reported that psychotic features (i.e., hallucinations or delusions) were sufficient but not necessary to characterize individual patients as being "psychotic." These data suggest that psychosis is a separate dimension from endogenicity and that psychomotor disturbances are not merely separating endogenous and nonendogenous patients.

Cognitive impairment, determined by objective/quantitative measures, has been less well studied than specific symptom characteristics. Rothschild et al. (1989b) reported that PMD patients demonstrated greater impairment on neuro-psychological testing than did NPMD patients, partialing out for severity as measured by total HDRS score. We have hypothesized that cognitive deficits in psychotic (and in some nonpsychotic) depressive patients reflect significantly increased cortisol activity (Rothschild et al. 1989b) (see below). Studies on neuro-psychological performance may provide greater specificity in separating PMD from NPMD patients than do specific symptoms.

The studies described above have frequently compared clinical populations in tertiary/academic settings, and, in several studies, populations were identified retrospectively. Such approaches have a number of limitations, particularly potential selection bias of more refractory or more severe patients. The Epidemiological Catchment Area Study (Johnson et al. 1991) recently reported that PMD patients were not more symptomatic overall than were NPMD patients and that the two groups did not differ in symptom patterns other than the presence of a thought disorder. (Specific depression rating scales were not employed in this study, however.) PMD patients did, however, differ significantly from NPMD patients in demonstrating greater morbidity at 1 year, including more frequent suicide attempts (see "Course and Outcome" section below for further discussion).

Biological Studies

Hypothalamic-pituitary-adrenal (HPA) axis activity.   There is now abundant evidence for specific abnormalities in PMD on measures of HPA axis activity (Table 7–2A). Many centers have reported that patients with PMD demonstrate among the highest rates of dexamethasone nonsuppression and that patients with PMD have markedly elevated postdexamethasone cortisol levels (Asnis et al. 1982; Caroff et al. 1983; Carroll et al. 1976, 1980; Coryell et al. 1982a; Evans et al. 1983; Mendlewicz et al. 1982; Rihmer et al. 1984a; Rothschild et al. 1982; Rudorfer et al. 1982; Schatzberg et al. 1983), although not all studies are in agreement (Ayuso-Gutierrez et al. 1985; Coryell et al. 1984b; Kocsis et al. 1985; Nelson et al. 1984). Significant differences between PMD and NPMD patients have been observed on 24-hour measures of urinary free cortisol (Anton 1987). Although patients with other affective psychoses such as mania show high nonsuppression rates (Arana et al. 1983), patients with nonaffective psychoses such as schizophrenia do not (Arana et al. 1983; Rothschild et al. 1982).

The elevated cortisol levels after dexamethasone administration in PMD patients are not merely due to greater severity of depressive illness or to the presence of endogenous symptoms. For example, Evans et al. (1983) did not find significant differences in the rates of dexamethasone nonsuppression between NPMD patients

Table 7–2A. Biological studies: HPA axis activity

Study	Diagnostic instrument/ classification system	Diagnoses (n)	Prospective study (Y/N)	Findings
Carroll et al. 1976	None/Feighner	6 endogenomorphic delusionally depressed inpatients	Y	100% of delusional patients had abnormal response to dexamethasone.
Carroll et al. 1980	None/RDC and Feighner	14 primary psychotic endogenous unipolar depressed patients	Y	11 of 14 delusional patients (79%) exhibited nonsuppression on DST.
Coryell et al. 1982a	None/DSM-III and Feighner	103 major depressed inpatients: 18 delusional and 75 non-delusional	Y	Delusional patients were more likely to exhibit nonsuppression on DST than nondelusional patients (7 of 18 and 14 of 75, respectively), although differences were not significant.
Asnis et al. 1982	SADS/RDC	40 endogenously major depressed inpatients: 26 unipolar & 14 bipolar; 10 delusional and 30 nondelusional	Y	7 of 10 delusional patients (70%) were non-suppressors on DST (2 mg) vs. 7 of 30 nondelusional patients ($P = .012$).
Mendlewicz et al. 1982	None/RDC	95 inpatients with major depressive disorder: 54 primary (29 unipolar, 25 bipolar) and 41 secondary; 37 delusional and 58 nondelusional	Y	4 P.M. postdexamethasone cortisol plasma levels were significantly higher ($P < .001$) in delusional patients compared with nondelusional patients.
Rothschild et al. 1982	None/DSM-III	40 delusional inpatients: 14 DSM-III unipolar major depressed, 8 bipolar depressed, 14 schizo-phrenic, 4 atypical, 31 controls	N	Mean postdexamethasone cortisol levels for unipolar delusionally depressed patients significantly higher than for delusional bipolar depressives ($P < .05$), psychotic schizophrenics ($P < .05$), atypical psychotics ($P < .05$), or control subjects ($P < .05$).
Rudorfer et al. 1982	None/RDC and Feighner	31 unipolar, primary, endogenously depressed inpatients: 15 delusional and 16 nondelusional	Y	Delusional patients had higher frequency of DST nonsuppression than nondelusional patients. Whereas 10 of 15 (67%) delusional patients were DST nonsuppressors, only 3 of 16 (19%) non-delusionals were DST nonsuppressors ($P < .01$).

Evans et al. 1983	None/DSM-III	47 depressed inpatients, 30 meeting DSM-III criteria for unipolar major depression: 10 delusional and 30 nondelusional	Y	Delusional patients had DST nonsuppression rate of 100%, which was significantly greater ($P < .005$) than the other depressed patients.
Schatzberg et al. 1983 (overlap with Rothschild et al. 1982)	None/DSM-III	45 unipolar major depressed: 14 delusional and 31 nondelusional	N	Of the 9 major depressed patients with plasma cortisol levels of 15 μg/dl or more, 7 showed delusional features. In contrast, of the 36 patients with major depression with plasma cortisol levels less than 15 μg/dl, only 7 showed delusional features ($P < .001$). All 6 patients with plasma cortisol levels greater than 17 μg/dl were delusional.
Caroff et al. 1983	None/DSM-III	29 major depressed inpatients with melancholia: 26 unipolar and 3 bipolar; 11 delusional and 18 nondelusional	Y	Significantly more delusional patients (7 of 11, 64%) than nondelusional patients (3 of 18, 17%; $P = .013$) exhibited DST nonsuppression at 8 A.M.
Coryell et al. 1984a	None/DSM-III	232 major depressed inpatients, unipolar and bipolar: 55 delusional and 177 nondelusional	Y	No significant differences in nonsuppression rates at 8 A.M. or 4 P.M. between delusional and non-delusional patients. At 8 A.M., trend difference ($P < .09$) for delusional patients to more frequently demonstrate cortisol values of ≥10 μg/dl.
Nelson et al. 1984	None/RDC	25 patients with major depressive episode: 13 delusional and 12 nondelusional; all inpatients	Y	Using 2-mg DST, delusional patients exhibited a trend ($P < .07$) toward a higher frequency (85%) of nonsuppression compared with nondelusional patients (50%). No significant differences in UFC or plasma cortisol.
Rihmer et al. 1984a	None/RDC	93 female primary endogenous major depressed inpatients: 27 delusional and 66 nondelusional; 45 unipolar and 48 bipolar	Y	Delusional patients had significantly higher ($P < .001$) frequency (89%) of DST nonsuppression than did nondelusional patients (59%).

(continued)

Table 7–2A. Biological studies: HPA axis activity (*continued*)

Study	Diagnostic instrument/ classification system	Diagnoses (*n*)	Prospective study (Y/N)	Findings
Ayuso-Gutierrez et al. 1985	None/DSM-III	73 unipolar major depressed inpatients: 26 delusional and 47 nondelusional	Y	No significant differences between delusional and nondelusional patients on DST.
Kocsis et al. 1985	RDC/SADS	132 patients: 85 unipolar and 47 bipolar; 25 delusional and 107 nondelusional	Y	No significant differences between delusional and nondelusional patients on any HPA measure except hypersecretion of UFC, which was present in a smaller percentage of the psychotic subjects ($P < .02$).
Anton 1987	None/DSM-III	32 male DSM-III major depressed inpatients: 25 unipolar and 7 bipolar; 18 delusional and 14 nondelusional	Y	Subgroup of delusional patients with UFC >90 μg/24 hours. Whereas 6 of 17 delusional patients (35%) had UFC (>90 μg/24 hours, only 1 of 14 nondelusional patients (7%) exhibited UFC >90 μg/24 hours.
Brown et al. 1988	None/DSM-III	93 DSM-III unipolar major depressed patients: 25 delusional and 68 nondelusional	Y	Delusionality predicted 34% of the variance in in morning postdexamethasone cortisol levels. Agitation predicted 22% and melancholia predicted 27%.

Note.   DST = dexamethasone suppression test. HPA = hypothalamic-pituitary-adrenal axis. RDC = Research Diagnostic Criteria. SADS = Schedule for Affective Disorders and Schizophrenia. UFC = urinary free cortisol.

with melancholia and NPMD patients without melancholia. The two groups also did not differ on mean postdexamethasone cortisol levels. Yet both groups had significantly lower mean postdexamethasone cortisol levels than did PMD patients. Rihmer et al. (1984a) reported significantly higher rates of DST nonsuppression in psychotic endogenously depressed inpatients than in their nonpsychotic endogenous counterparts. Furthermore, Brown et al. (1988) used a stepwise multiple regression analysis to examine for the effects of severity, agitation, delusions, melancholic subtype, age, and weight loss on postdexamethasone cortisol levels in 93 unipolar major depressed patients. They reported that agitation predicted 22%, melancholia 27%, and delusionality 34% of the variance in morning postdexamethasone cortisol levels. Severity of illness, age, and weight loss added no further significant predictive value and did not affect cortisol levels when examined separately from the other variables.

In summary, the vast majority of studies point to significantly greater HPA axis activity in PMD than in NPMD patients, although not all studies agree. Specific differences in patient samples (e.g., relative proportion of unipolar versus bipolar patients [Coryell et al. 1984b; Schatzberg et al. 1983], drug free status) could help account for the lack of consistency. The literature does not support the notion that the increased HPA activity seen in patients with PMD is merely the result of increased severity of depression, presence of endogenous features, or the psychosis per se but rather is related to the interaction between the affective disorder and the psychosis. Our group has hypothesized that the development of delusions in depressed patients is due to the effects of hypercortisolemia on dopaminergic systems (Schatzberg et al. 1985) because glucocorticoids increase dopamine (DA) levels in human plasma (Rothschild et al. 1984) and rat brain (Rothschild et al. 1985) and homovanillic acid (HVA) levels in rat brain (Wolkowitz et al. 1986) and human cerebrospinal fluid (CSF) (Banki et al. 1983).

Dopaminergic activity. Several studies have demonstrated that patients with PMD have an activation of the dopaminergic system that is not seen in NPMD patients (Table 7–2B). PMD patients demonstrated significantly higher levels of unconjugated plasma DA both before and after administration of dexamethasone than did NPMD patients (Rothschild et al. 1987). Studies measuring the DA metabolite, HVA, have also reported higher levels in PMD patients than in NPMD patients. Sweeney et al. (1978) reported that the probenecid-induced accumulation of CSF HVA was higher in PMD than in NPMD patients. Furthermore, Aberg-Wistedt et al. (1985) reported that PMD patients had significantly higher concentrations of CSF HVA compared to NPMD patients. Higher CSF levels of 5-hydroxyindoleacetic acid (5-HIAA) were also found in the PMD patients compared with the NPMD patients (Aberg-Wistedt et al. 1985) (see

Table 7–2B. Biological studies: dopaminergic activity

Study	Diagnostic instrument/ classification system	Diagnoses (n)	Prospective study (Y/N)	Findings
Sweeney et al. 1978	None/RDC	15 female unipolar depressed in-patients: 7 delusional and 8 nondelusional	Y	Delusional group had significantly higher ($P = .03$) CSF HVA than nondelusional group.
Aberg–Wistedt et al. 1985	None/RDC	50 unipolar endogenous major depressive disorder inpatients: 8 delusional and 42 nondelusional	Y	CSF HVA in delusional patients was significantly higher ($P < .001$) than in nondelusional patients.
Devanand et al. 1985	None/DSM-III and Feighner	29 unipolar major depressed inpatients: 11 delusional and 18 nondelusional	Y	Female delusional patients had significantly higher ($P < .02$) plasma HVA levels than controls, whereas nondelusional patients did not.
Mazure et al. 1987	None/DSM-III	33 unipolar major depressed inpatients: 8 delusional and 25 nondelusional	Y	Female delusional patients had significantly higher ($P < .01$) plasma HVA levels than nondelusional patients.
Rothschild et al. 1987	None/DSM-III and RDC	22 patients with major depression: 13 unipolar, 6 bipolar, and 3 with dysthymic disorder; 16 inpatients and 6 outpatients; 4 delusional and 18 nondelusional	Y	Plasma dopamine levels in the delusional subgroup were significantly higher ($P < .001$) both before and after dexamethasone than those in the nondelusional group.
Lykouras et al. 1988	None/DSM-III	40 DSM-III unipolar major depressed patients: 18 delusional and 22 nondelusional; all inpatients	Y	No differences were found in urinary HVA between delusional patients and nondelusional groups.
Wolkowitz et al. 1989	SADS-L/DSM-III and RDC	27 major depressed patients: 17 unipolar and 10 bipolar; 8 delusional and 19 nondelusional	Y	Significant decrease ($P < .06$) in plasma HVA after dexamethasone administration in delusional patients.

Note. CSF = cerebrospinal fluid. HVA = homovanillic acid. RDC = Research Diagnostic Criteria. SADS-L = Schedule for Affective Disorders and Schizophrenia, Lifetime Version.

"Measures of Serotonin Function" section below).

Studies of plasma HVA also indicate that PMD patients have greater activation of dopaminergic systems than do NPMD patients. Devanand et al. (1985) reported that plasma HVA was significantly elevated in PMD women compared with NPMD women. Mazure et al. (1987) reported that plasma HVA levels were significantly higher in PMD patients than in melancholic NPMD patients, who in turn had higher plasma HVA levels than nonmelancholic NPMD patients. Finally, Wolkowitz et al. (1985, 1989) have demonstrated a relative blunting (trend significance) of the plasma HVA response to dexamethasone in PMD patients compared with patients with NPMD. One study (Lykouras et al. 1988) reported no baseline differences in urinary levels of HVA in PMD versus NPMD. Overall, the data indicate that PMD can be distinguished biologically from NPMD on measures of dopaminergic activity. Although studies have generally emphasized the possible role of severity rather than that of endogenicity, data from Mazure et al. (1987) suggested that elevated plasma HVA levels in PMD are not due to the presence of endogenous features.

Enzyme studies.   Evidence has been growing for specific biochemical enzyme abnormalities that may be specific for PMD (Table 7–2C). Previous studies have shown that unipolar PMD patients have lower serum dopamine-beta-hydroxylase (DBH) activity (Meltzer et al. 1976; Mod et al. 1986), and unipolar NPMD patients have higher serum DBH activity (Matuzas et al. 1982; Mod et al. 1986) than do healthy control subjects. The low levels of serum DBH activity in unipolar PMD patients have been hypothesized to be a potential marker of relative risk for developing pronounced increases in DA levels in the face of chronic elevation of cortisol levels (Schatzberg et al. 1985).

Computed tomography (CT) scans.   Several studies have reported differences on CT scans between PMD and NPMD patients (Table 7–2D). Targum et al. (1983) studied 38 melancholic depressed hospitalized patients (unipolar and bipolar) and found that the mean ventricle-to-brain ratio (VBR) of the PMD patients was greater (although not significantly) than of NPMD patients or neurological control subjects. Of the 20 PMD patients, 5 (25%) had VBRs greater than 2 standard deviations from the mean of the 26 neurological control subjects, in contrast to none of the 18 NPMD patients. Luchins and Meltzer (1983) examined VBR in 18 depressed patients. Five of the 9 PMD (56%) but only 1 of the 9 NPMD (11%) patients had a VBR 1 standard deviation outside the control mean (Fischer exact p). However, there was no difference in mean VBRs between groups. Subsequently, Schlegel and Kretzschmar (1987) reported that PMD patients had significantly greater mean VBRs than did control subjects, and NPMD patients did not.

Table 7–2C. Biological studies: enzyme studies

Study	Diagnostic instrument/ classification system	Diagnoses (*n*)	Prospective study (Y/N)	Findings
Meltzer et al. 1976	None/RDC	33 unipolar depressed inpatients: 22 delusional and 11 nondelusional	Y	Delusional patients had significantly lower DBH levels than controls.
Matuzas et al. 1982	None/RDC	29 definite, primary major depressed outpatients, all unipolar nondelusional, and 34 healthy controls	Y	Nondelusional patients had significantly greater (*P* < .025) DBH activity than controls.
Mod et al. 1986	None/RDC	208 primary endogenous depressed patients: 93 unipolar and 115 bipolar; 63 delusional and 145 nondelusional	Y	DBH activity was significantly lower (*P* < .001) in delusional unipolar patients than in nondelusional patients.

Note. DBH = dopamine-beta-hydroxylase. RDC = Research Diagnostic Criteria.

Table 7–2D. Biological studies: computed tomography scans

Study	Diagnostic instrument/ classification system	Diagnoses (n)	Prospective study (Y/N)	Findings
Luchins and Meltzer 1983	None/RDC	18 patients with major depression: 11 unipolar and 7 bipolar; 9 delusional and 9 nondelusional	Y	5 of 9 delusional patients (56%) but only 1 of 9 nondelusional patients (11%) had VBR 1 standard deviation outside the control mean ($P < .05$).
Targum et al. 1983	SADS-L/DSM-III	38 inpatients with major depression with melancholia: 29 unipolar and 9 bipolar; 20 delusional and 18 nondelusional	Y	VBR of delusional patients was greater ($P < .10$) than in nondelusional patients; 5 of 20 of the delusional patients (25%) had VBRs greater than 2 standard deviations from the mean of the neurological controls, in contrast to none of the 18 nondelusional patients.
Schlegel and Kretzschmar 1987	None/DSM-III and RDC	60 inpatients who met DSM-III criteria for unipolar major depression ($n = 33$), manic ($n = 5$), depressive bipolar disorder ($n = 17$), and RDC schizo-affective ($n = 5$); 22 delusional and 38 nondelusional	Y	Delusional patients had significantly greater VBRs than controls, while nondelusional patients did not.
Rothschild et al. 1989b	SADS/DSM-III	DSM-III major depressed patients: 15 delusional and 15 nondelusional; 22 unipolar; all inpatients	Y	Unipolar delusional patients had significantly larger ($P < .05$) anterior pole and cella media VBRs and significantly greater ($P < .05$) left and right inferior parietal brain atrophy than nondelusional patients.

Note. RDC = Research Diagnostic Criteria. SADS-L = Schedule for Affective Disorders and Schizophrenia, Lifetime Version. VBR = ventricular brain ratio.

We (Rothschild et al. 1989b) reported on VBRs in a sample of unipolar delusional and nondelusional depressed patients. Statistically significant differences between PMD and NPMD patients were observed in VBR, as well as in ratings of inferior parietal atrophy. Unipolar PMD patients had significantly greater mean anterior pole and cella media VBRs and more left and right inferior parietal brain atrophy than did their unipolar NPMD counterparts (Rothschild et al. 1989b). The enlarged VBRs and greater inferior parietal brain atrophy in the unipolar PMD patients correlated with poorer performance on neuropsychological testing (Rothschild et al. 1989b). Interestingly, the enlarged VBRs seen in unipolar PMD patients were also associated with higher levels of plasma cortisol in this study (Rothschild et al. 1989b) and others (Rao et al. 1989). The possible effects of endogenous symptoms generally have not been explored in these studies. Still the data overall do suggest an association in unipolar major depressed patients between symptoms of psychosis and enlarged VBRs. This is in contrast to psychotic schizophrenic patients, in whom positive symptoms (delusions and hallucinations) have been associated with smaller ventricles (Andreasen et al. 1982; Luchins et al. 1984).

Electroencephalographic (EEG) sleep profiles. Comparisons of EEG sleep profiles in PMD and NPMD patients have also indicated differences between the two groups (Table 7–2E). PMD patients exhibit significantly diminished slow-wave sleep, poorer sleep efficiency, and reduced percentage of rapid eye movement (REM) sleep time compared with NPMD patients (Kupfer and Foster 1975; Kupfer et al. 1978, 1980; Mendels and Hawkins 1968). However, these findings may have reflected sample differences in age, severity, and agitation between the two groups (Thase et al. 1986a). In a study that specifically controlled for the effects of age, severity, agitation, and other clinical characteristics, patients with PMD were found to have increased wakefulness, a higher percentage of stage one sleep, a decreased percentage of REM sleep, and decreased REM activity compared with NPMD patients (Thase et al. 1986b). A more recent study (Kupfer et al. 1989) found an increased percentage of intermittent wakefulness in the PMD patients compared with the NPMD patients. When EEG spectral analysis was used, more specific, significant differences between PMD and NPMD patients emerged. PMD patients had increased power in the higher bandwidths or "microarousals" (Kupfer et al. 1989) that could not be attributed to actual awake time differences, because manually scored records could not validate that awake time was significantly different between the two patient groups. The increased power observed in the higher bandwidths in the PMD patients (Kupfer et al. 1989) suggested that the arousal level in these patients may be a potentially distinguishing feature of PMD patients. PMD patients also appeared more likely to have extremely short sleep-onset REM latencies than NPMD patients (Kupfer et al. 1989). One study

Table 7–2E. Biological studies: EEG sleep profile

Study	Diagnostic instrument/ classification system	Diagnoses (n)	Prospective study (Y/N)	Findings
Mendels and Hawkins 1968	None/DSM-III	21 depressed inpatients: 4 psychotic and 17 neurotic	Y	Psychotic patients spent significantly less ($P < .01$) time sleeping, significantly more ($P < .01$) time awake, were more drowsy ($P < .05$), and had more stage 1 sleep ($P < .01$) than neurotic patients. Psychotic patients spent less time in stage 4 ($P < .01$).
Kupfer et al. 1978	None/RDC	95 major depressed patients: 66 inpatients and 29 outpatients; 47 primary (17 delusional, 30 nondelusional), and 48 secondary	Y	Delusional patients had significantly greater early-morning awakening ($P < .05$), significantly less time spent asleep ($P < .05$), decreased percentage of delta sleep ($P < .05$), and decreased percentage of REM sleep ($P < .05$) than nondelusional patients.
Kupfer et al. 1980	SADS/RDC	29 primary major depressed delusional inpatients	Y	Patients with delusions of guilt or sin demonstrated both increased sleep discontinuity and decreased REM sleep, whereas patients with somatic delusions showed increased REM activity.
Thase et al. 1986	SADS/RDC	106 major depressed inpatients: 27 delusional and 79 nondelusional; 86 unipolar, 8 bipolar I, and 12 bipolar II	Y	Delusional patients had increased wakefulness ($P < .05$), increased stage 1 percentage ($P < .05$), decreased REM percentage ($P < .01$), and decreased REM activity ($P < .05$).
Kupfer et al. 1989	SADS/RDC	12 unipolar depressed inpatients: 6 delusional and 6 nondelusional	Y	Delusional patients had increased percentage of intermittent wakefulness, increased "microarousals," and shorter sleep-onset REM latencies than nondelusional patients.
Hudson et al. 1992	None/DSM-III-R	19 unipolar major depressed inpatients: 5 delusional and 14 nondelusional	Y	No statistically significant differences between delusional and nondelusional patients in mean values of polysomnographic variables or in prevalence of sleep-onset REMs.

Note. RDC = Research Diagnostic Criteria. REM = rapid eye movement. SADS = Schedule for Affective Disorders and Schizophrenia.

(Hudson et al. 1992) did not find any statistically significant differences between PMD and NPMD patients on sleep profiles.

The diminished generation of REM sleep seen in PMD patients may indicate a functional hyperactivity of central dopaminergic systems, because administration of dopaminergic agonists to control subjects results in increased arousal and considerable suppression of REM sleep (Gillin et al. 1978). It is also of interest that a 1-mg dose of dexamethasone results in a 20% reduction of REM sleep in NPMD patients (Kupfer et al. 1984), a reduction of about the same magnitude of difference observed between PMD and NPMD patients (Thase et al. 1986b). Thus, the decreased generation of REM sleep seen in PMD patients may be secondary to corticosteroid-dopamine interactions (see previous section). In any case, sleep EEG studies provide further evidence for considering PMD as a distinct subtype of major depression.

Measures of serotonin function.   Differences between PMD and NPMD patients on measures of serotonin function have also been reported (Table 7–2F). Healy et al. (1986) reported on measures of platelet serotonin uptake in a group of 28 endogenously depressed patients. Delusional and nondelusional patients differed in absolute values for serotonin uptake rate into platelets (Healy et al. 1986). In addition, delusional patients did not show the lowering of serotonin uptake rate compared with endogenously depressed patients as a whole. The difference between the PMD and NPMD groups was maintained after treatment was started but was not present after clinical recovery, suggesting a state rather than trait phenomenon (Healy et al. 1986).

PMD patients demonstrate higher CSF 5-HIAA levels than do NPMD patients (Aberg-Wistedt et al. 1985). In the study of Aberg-Wistedt et al. (1985), a strong positive correlation between CSF 5-HIAA and CSF HVA levels was observed. They noted that the higher HVA/5-HIAA ratio in their PMD patients suggested a primary problem in dopaminergic neurotransmission and a secondary effect on serotonergic neurons (Aberg-Wistedt et al. 1985). The higher HVA/5-HIAA ratio in the PMD patients is consistent with another study that found that hallucinations in depressed patients were strongly associated with higher HVA/5-HIAA ratios (Agren and Terenius 1985). In contrast, one study (Sweeney et al. 1978) did not find that PMD and NPMD patients differed on measures of CSF 5-HIAA, and another study did not observe differences between PMD and NPMD patients in urinary 5-HIAA (Lykouras et al. 1988). Overall, however, there do appear to be differences in serotonin transmission between PMD and NPMD patients, but it is difficult at this point to determine whether this is independent of a disturbance in dopaminergic neurotransmission.

Table 7–2F. Biological studies: serotonin measures

Study	Diagnostic instrument/ classification system	Diagnoses (n)	Prospective study (Y/N)	Findings
Sweeney et al. 1978	None/RDC	15 female unipolar depressed inpatients: 7 delusional and 8 nondelusional	Y	CSF 5-HIAA did not differ between delusional and nondelusional groups.
Aberg-Wistedt et al. 1985	None/RDC	50 unipolar endogenous major depressive disorder inpatients: 8 delusional and 42 nondelusional	Y	CSF 5-HIAA in delusional patients was significantly higher ($P < .001$) than in nondelusional patients.
Agren and Terenius 1985	SADS/RDC	118 inpatients with major depression: 77 unipolar, 9 bipolar I, and 32 bipolar II; 21 delusional and 97 nondelusional	Y	Hallucinations in depressed patients were strongly associated with higher CSF HVA/5-HIAA ratios.
Healy et al. 1986	None/ICD-9	28 endogenously depressed patients: 18 unipolar and 10 bipolar; 8 delusional and 20 nondelusional	Y	Delusional and nondelusional patients differed in absolute values for 5-HT uptake rate into platelets. Delusional patients did show lowering of 5-HT uptake rate compared with endogenously depressed patients as a whole.
Lykouras et al. 1988	None/DSM-III	40 DSM-III unipolar major depressed patients: 18 delusional and 22 nondelusional; all inpatients	Y	No differences were found in urinary 5-HIAA between delusional and nondelusional groups.

Note. CSF = cerebrospinal fluid. 5-HIAA = 5-hydroxyindoleacetic acid. 5-HT = serotonin. HVA = homovanillic acid. RDC = Research Diagnostic Criteria. SADS = Schedule for Affective Disorders and Schizophrenia.

Summary.   In summary, a growing body of evidence from studies of the HPA axis, dopaminergic activity, enzyme studies, CT and magnetic resonance imaging (MRI) scans, EEG sleep profiles, and measures of serotonergic function all point to distinct biological abnormalities in PMD compared with NPMD. Although many of the studies did not explore the possible effects of endogenous states on specific differences, several did, and these results suggest that biological differences between PMD and NPMD are not due to differences in relative endogenicity (Evans et al. 1983; Kocsis et al. 1985; Mazure et al. 1987; Rihmer et al. 1984b).

Family Studies

As indicated in Table 7–3, first-degree relatives of PMD patients demonstrate higher rates of depression (Leckman et al. 1984; Nelson et al. 1984) and higher rates of the psychotic subtype (Leckman et al. 1984) than do the family members of NPMD patients, although not all studies are in agreement (Coryell et al. 1982b). In addition, the relatives of PMD patients are significantly (six times) more likely to have bipolar disorder than are the relatives of NPMD patients (Weissman et al. 1984). In some ways, limited family data are less compelling than are data from other categories, and further studies are needed to confirm and extend these findings. The higher incidence of bipolar disorder in the families of PMD patients is intriguing in light of the association of bipolar illness with young-onset PMD (Akiskal et al. 1983; Strober and Carlson 1982).

Course and Outcome

One-year follow-up.   The course, prognosis, and outcome of PMD and NPMD patients differ (Table 7–4). Several studies have noted poorer short-term outcome in PMD than in NPMD. In a prospective study, Robinson and Spiker (1985), found that significantly more patients with PMD followed a chronically ill pattern during the first posthospitalization year. They compared 52 unipolar PMD patients with 52 unipolar NPMD patients matched for sex, age at index episode of depression, and age at first episode of depression. In a 1-year retrospective follow-up after discharge from inpatient treatment, patients with PMD had a significantly higher rate of episodes of major depression lasting longer than 9 months than did NPMD patients (Robinson and Spiker 1985). PMD patients also were more likely to be in a major depressive episode at 1-year follow-up than were NPMD patients. Consistent with the poorer clinical response of the patients with PMD, there was a trend for the PMD patients to have a higher total number of hospitalizations over the 1-year follow-up period than the NPMD patients (Robinson and Spiker 1985). Murphy (1983) also reported a poorer 1-year outcome for geriatric patients with PMD than for those with NPMD. Kettering et al. (1987) found that the course of

Table 7–3. Family studies

Study	Diagnostic instrument/classification system	Diagnoses (n)	Prospective study (Y/N)	Findings
Coryell et al. 1982b	None/Feighner and DSM-III	221 patients with primary unipolar depressions: 108 delusional and 113 nondelusional	N	Morbid risks for affective disorder in first-degree relatives of delusional and nondelusional probands were not significantly different.
Leckman et al. 1984	SADS-L/RDC and DSM-III	133 unipolar major depressed patients: 21 delusional and 112 nondelusional	Y	Rates of major depression were highest for relatives of probands with delusional depression. Depressed relatives of depressed probands with the delusional subtype were more likely to have the delusional subtype than the depressed relatives of nondelusional probands.
Nelson et al. 1984	None/RDC	25 inpatients with major depressive disorder, endogenous subtype: 13 delusional and 12 nondelusional	Y	11 of 13 delusional patients (85%) had a family history of depression, in contrast to only 3 of 12 nondelusional patients (25%) ($P < .01$). Non-delusional patients had a greater (67%), although not statistically significant, prevalence of alcoholism in the family as compared with delusional patients (39%).
Weissman et al. 1984	SADS-L/RDC and DSM-III	810 first-degree relatives of 133 probands with unipolar major depression (21 delusional, 112 nondelusional)	Y	Prevalence of bipolar disorder was nearly 6 times as high among the relatives of delusional probands as among relatives of nondelusional probands.

Note. RDC = Research Diagnostic Criteria. SADS-L = Schedule for Affective Disorders and Schizophrenia, Lifetime Version.

Table 7–4. Course and outcome

Study	Diagnostic instrument/ classification system	Diagnoses (n)	Prospective study (Y/N)	Findings
Nelson and Bowers 1978	None/RDC	27 primary unipolar inpatients: 14 delusional and 13 nondelusional	N	Episodes of depressive illness in delusionally depressed patients were characterized by similar symptomatology, including specific delusional content from episode to episode.
Charney and Nelson 1981	None; delusional distinction based on SADS/RDC	120 primary unipolar major depression; all inpatients	N	In delusional patients, 89% of prior depressive episodes were delusional, compared to only 12% in the nondelusional group ($P < .001$). Delusions tended to be of similar form and content from episode to episode.
Coryell and Tsuang 1982	None/Feighner and DSM-III	225 patients with primary unipolar major depression: 117 delusional and 108 nondelusional	N	At 1-year follow-up, 27 of 48 nondelusional patients (56%) had recovered, in contrast to only 36 of 129 delusional patients (28%) ($P < .05$). At 4-year follow-up, no differences were observed.
Strober and Carlson 1982	SADS/RDC	60 adolescent primary unipolar inpatients	Y	Bipolar outcome was associated with symptom cluster of mood-congruent psychotic features, rapid symptom onset, and psychomotor retardation.
Akiskal et al. 1983	None/Feighner	82 primary unipolar outpatients: 41 with bipolar outcome and 41 with unipolar outcome	Y	17 of 41 patients with bipolar outcome were delusionally depressed at baseline, in contrast to only 6 of 41 who remained unipolar ($P < .01$).
Murphy 1983	PSE/Feighner and SPAS	30 geriatric, first-episode primary depressed unipolar patients	Y	At 1-year follow-up, only 1 of 10 delusional patients (10%) had a good outcome, in contrast to 14 of 20 nondelusional patients (70%)($P < .01$).
Robinson and Spiker 1985	None/RDC	104 unipolar major depressed inpatients: 52 delusional and 52 nondelusional	N	At 1-year follow-up, delusional patients had a significantly higher rate of major depression lasting longer than 9 months and a higher total number of hospitalizations in the past year.

Coryell et al. 1987	SADS/RDC	506 unipolar major depressed patients followed up at 2 years: 55 delusional and 451 nondelusional; 379 inpatient and 127 outpatient	N	Delusional patients were more psychosocially impaired at 6 months, but not at 2 years, compared with nondelusional patients.
Kettering et al. 1987	SADS/RDC	59 unipolar depressed inpatients: 31 delusional and 28 nondelusional		14 months after hospital discharge, delusional patients showed significantly ($P < .05$) more moodincongruent delusions and fewer depressive ($P < .10$) and anxiety ($P < .05$) symptoms as compared with nondelusional patients.
Coryell et al. 1990	SADS, GAS, LIFE, LIFE-II/RDC	73 delusional major depressed patients: 62 unipolar and 11 bipolar	Y	48 of 73 delusional patients (66%) rated as psychosocially impaired at 5 years.
Rothschild et al. 1990	SCID/DSM-III-R	54 DSM-III-R major depressed patients: 45 unipolar and 9 bipolar NOS; 13 delusional and 41 nondelusional	Y	Delusional patients did not differ from nondelusional patients on measures of depressive, anxious, or psychotic symptoms at 1 year. Delusional patients demonstrated significantly ($P < .05$) poorer functioning than nondelusional patients at 1 year.
Johnson et al. 1991	DIS/DSM-III	DSM-III unipolar major depressed patients: 114 delusional and 662 nondelusional	Y	Delusional patients had increased risk of multiple episodes, greater economic impairment, higher lifetime risk of psychiatric hospitalization, and increased risk of hospitalization for medical reasons than nondelusional patients.

Note. DIS = Diagnostic Interview Schedule. GAS = Global Assessment Scale. LIFE = Longitudinal Interview Follow-Up Evaluation. NOS = not otherwise specified. PSE = Present State Examination. RDC = Research Diagnostic Criteria. SADS = Schedule for Affective Disorders and Schizophrenia. SCID = Structured Clinical Interview for DSM-III-R. SPAS = Survey Psychiatric Assessment Schedule.

psychotic and affective symptoms in PMD differs from that seen in NPMD. In their study of PMD and NPMD patients 1 year after discharge, affective and anxiety symptoms were less persistent and provided a smaller contribution to the total clinical picture in PMD patients compared with NPMD patients. However, PMD patients were more likely to demonstrate mood-incongruent delusions at 1 year.

Recently, our group (Rothschild et al. 1990) reported that, at 1-year follow-up, patients diagnosed as PMD at baseline did not differ from NPMD patients on measures of depressive, anxious, or psychotic symptoms. However, those patients who had originally met PMD criteria demonstrated significantly poorer functioning at 1 year, as measured by the Social Adjustment Scale (SAS) (Weismann et al. 1978). In our sample, significant correlations were observed between cortisol levels at 1 year and measures of functioning at 1 year (Rothschild et al. 1990). Higher urinary free cortisol (UFC) levels at 1 year correlated with poorer overall functioning at 1 year, as measured by the total SAS score.

Recent data from the Epidemiological Catchment Area Study (Johnson et al. 1991) provide further evidence for a different course of PMD when compared with NPMD. Patients with PMD had an increased risk of multiple episodes of depression compared with NPMD patients (73.7% versus 61.9%, $P < .05$). In addition, patients with PMD also had significantly greater economic impairment (Johnson et al. 1991). More patients with PMD were receiving public assistance (17.5% versus 7.2%, $P < .01$) and/or disability payments (15.9% versus 6.7%, $P < .01$) than NPMD patients. PMD was not associated with significantly more reports of economic impairment because of emotional, alcohol, or drug problems when compared with NPMD (5.7% versus 3.6%, NS) (Johnson et al. 1991). Patients with PMD also had a higher lifetime rate of psychiatric hospitalization (22.8% versus 14.7%, $P < .05$) and an increased risk of hospitalization for medical reasons in the last year compared with NPMD patients (Johnson et al. 1991). At 1-year follow-up, patients with PMD were more likely to be currently depressed (last month, 18.7% versus 11.1%, $P < .05$) and to continue to be financially dependent (27.4% versus 11.2%, $P < .01$) than were NPMD subjects (Johnson et al. 1991).

Longer-term (2+ years) follow-up.   In the Iowa 500 study, Coryell and Tsuang (1982) found that the initial presence of delusions predicted a poorer short-term (2- to 5-year) outcome, whereas a 40-year follow-up with structured interviews found no consistent trends distinguishing PMD from NPMD on marital, occupational, residential, or symptomatic outcome ratings. In the Depression Collaborative Study, Coryell et al. (1987) reported that despite substantially greater levels of impairment during the 5 years preceding intake into the study, patients with unipolar PMD were as likely to recover as were patients with unipolar NPMD during a 2-year follow-up period. Patients with PMD were more psychosocially impaired at 6 months, but these differences resolved during the ensuing 18 months (Coryell et al. 1987). In a 5-year follow-up of the patients reported previously by Coryell et al. (1984a, 1987), significantly greater social impairment, but not depression, was observed in PMD patients (Coryell et al. 1990).

Bipolar outcome. PMD with onset in adolescence or young adulthood appears to be related to bipolar disorder. Akiskal et al. (1983) reported on the follow-up of a cohort of depressed patients who had not had a history of mania at the time of index study (i.e., were unipolar). The incidence of baseline psychotic depression (42%) was significantly greater ($P < .01$) in patients who became bipolar during follow-up than in those who had not (15%). Similarly, Strober and Carlson (1982) reported that a bipolar outcome in adolescents originally studied when depressed was predicted by a depressive symptom cluster comprising mood-congruent psychotic features, rapid symptom onset, and psychomotor retardation. These data suggest that PMD in a young adult may often prove to be the first episode of a bipolar disorder.

Recurrent psychotic episodes. Studies have demonstrated a remarkable consistency in the clinical presentation of patients with PMD over time. Charney and Nelson (1981), reporting on 54 PMD and 66 NPMD unipolar patients, found that for the PMD patients, 89% of all prior depressive episodes were psychotic, compared to only 12% for the NPMD group ($P < .001$). In addition, examination of the prior depressive episodes of the PMD patients indicated that delusions in these patients tended to be of similar form and content from episode to episode (Charney and Nelson 1981). An earlier study (Nelson and Bowers 1978) of 14 unipolar PMD patients also found that, within patients, episodes of depressive illness in PMD patients were characterized by similar symptomatology, including specific delusional content.

Treatment

The patterns of response to somatic therapies in PMD patients are quite different from those seen in NPMD patients. (For reviews of this area, see Anton and Burch 1990; Chan et al. 1987; Glassman and Roose 1981; Kantor and Glassman 1977; Nelson and Bowers 1978; Rothschild 1985; Spiker et al. 1985.) Although most reports on somatic therapy of PMD have been the result of open trials or retrospective reviews, the past few years have witnessed a few double-blind studies (Tables 7–5A through D). Overall, the literature points to a number of reasonable conclusions regarding the somatic treatment of PMD.

1. PMD responds poorly to placebo. Placebo response rates appear higher in NPMD.

Table 7–5A. Treatment: tricyclic antidepressants (TCAs)

Study	Diagnostic instrument/ classification system	Diagnoses (*n*)	Prospective study (Y/N)	Treatment	Findings
Angst 1961	Not specified/Stenstedt classification of endogenous depression	200 depressed patients; 150 inpatients with endogenous depression and depressive-schizo-phrenic mixed psychoses admitted to hospital; 105 inpatients and 50 outpatients with en-dogenous depression; 24 with depressive-schizo-phrenic mixed psychoses	Y	Day 1: 4 intramuscular injections of Tofranil, 25 mg each; day 2: 4 injections, 50 mg each; treated 1–3 or 4–8 weeks; not blinded	In endogenous and depressive-schizophrenic mixed psychosis, Tofranil was successful in approxi-mately two-thirds of cases; patients treated 4–8 weeks responded better; hypochondriacal delusions, ideas of poverty, and agitation predicted poor response.
Hordern et al. 1963	None/none	137 primarily depressed patients; all inpatients; 27 delusional	Y	Random assignment to amitriptyline or imipramine; 150 mg/ day for 1 week, followed by 200 mg/day for 3–5 weeks; double blind vis-à-vis specific TCA	52 of 59 nondelusional patients did well on amitriptyline, in contrast to 4 of 10 delusional patients; 37 of 51 nondelusional patients did well on imipramine, in contrast to 0 of 17 delusional patients.
Glassman et al. 1975	None/none	13 delusional and 21 nondelusional inpatients	Y	1-week placebo washout followed by imipramine at 3.5 mg/kg/day; average daily dose for men was 250 mg and for women was 200 mg; 4 weeks of active treatment	3 of 13 delusional patients responded. in contrast to 14 of 21 nondelusional patients (*P* < .05); differences between groups remained significant after con-trolling for severity; 9 of the 10 del-usional nonresponders to imipramine subsequently responded to ECT.

Simpson et al. 1976	Depression Questionnaire— Patient and Psychiatrist Forms/DSM-II	51 newly admitted depressed patients: 35 endogenous (15 delusional) and 16 depressive neurosis; 35 women and 16 men	Y	Double-blind comparison of 150 mg vs. 300 mg/ day of imipramine; 4-week trial.	Improvement in the overall sample with both dosages, although greater and more consistent improvement was noted in the 300-mg group; delusional depressive patients responded less well than nondelusional, although 50% of delusional did respond to treatment; 7 of 15 delusional patients failed to respond (5 of these received 150 mg/day), in contrast to onlt 3 of 20 endogenous depressive patients (1 received 150 mg/day).
Glassman et al. 1977	None/Research Psychiatrist Screening	60 depressed nonschizo-phrenic patients: 42 women and 18 men; bipolar, unipolar non-delusional, and unipolar delusional subgroups	Y	3.5 mg/kg/day of impira-mine hydrochloride for 28 days	Patients with steady-state plasma levels above median do better clinically than those with lower levels; 6 of 17 unipolar delusionals responded, in contrast to 18 of 30 nondelusionals; plasma level attained was important for nondelusional but not for delusional patients.
Davidson et al. 1977	None/Feighner criteria	5 delusional and 5 non-delusional patients; primarily unipolar	Y	Double-blind comparison of 90 mg/dayphenelzine or 150 mg/day imip-ramine for 3 weeks; placebo washout	Significantly greater reduction in HDRS and BDS total scores in nondelusional patients.

(continued)

Table 7–5A. Treatment: tricyclic antidepressants (TCAs) *(continued)*

Study	Diagnostic instrument/ classification system	Diagnoses (*n*)	Prospective study (Y/N)	Treatment	Findings
Quitkin et al. 1978 (based on Klein 1967)	Lorr Multidemension Scale for Rating Psychiatric Patients	34 major depressive disorder–like; no unipolar vs. bipolar distinction; 13 psychotic and 21 nonpsychotic; all inpatients	Y	6-week comparison of imipramine vs. placebo; 300 mg/day of imipramine (max dose), 13 treated with placebo and 21 with imipramine	Main effect for drug; no interaction of drug effect and pretreatment psychotic state; study has been criticized for its retrospective definition of psychosis.
Avery and Lubrano 1979	None/European-based system	437 patients; 181 delusional, 97 typical and 84 atypical delusions; 256 nondelusional; all inpatients	Y	Imipramine 200 mg/day to a maximum of 350 mg/day for at least 25 days; not blinded	72 of 181 delusional patients responded, in contrast to 174 of 256 non-delusional patients (*P* < .001).
Charney and Nelson 1981	See Table 7–1	49 RDC major depressive episode inpatients; 9 delusional and 40 nondelusional	N	TCAs; at least 250 mg for a minimum of 3 weeks, except for 2 patients whose delusional thinking worsened	2 of 9 delusional patients responded, in contrast to 32 of 40 nondelusional patients (*P* < .01); 6 of 7 delusional patients who failed to respond to TCAs alone responded to TCA in combination with an antipsychotic.
Frances et al. 1981	See Table 7–1	See Table 7–1	N	TCAs alone; details not specified	3 of 18 psychotic patients responded to TCAs alone, vs. 17 of 23 nonpsychotic patients (*P* < .001); significantly longer overall treatment was required for psychotic patients; TCAs combined with antipsychotics and ECT were effective for psychotic patients.

Study	Criteria	Sample		Method	Results
Glassman and Roose 1981	See Table 7–1	See Table 7–1	Y	Placebo for 7 days; preliminary to imipramine study; single blind.	18 of 60 nondelusional depressed patients responded, in contrast to 0 of 21 delusional patients ($P < .02$).
Brown et al. 1982	SADS/RDC	64 unipolar major depressed patients; all inpatients	N	At least 3 weeks of 150 mg/day of amitriptyline or equivalent; max dose was 300 mg/day	3 of 18 psychotic patients responded to antidepressants alone, in contrast to 17 of 23 nonpsychotic patients; both groups responded equally to ECT; 0 of 3 psychotic patients responded to combined TCA/AP treatment.
Nelson et al. 1984	None/RDC	25 patients with major depressive episode; 13 delusional and 12 nondelusional; all inpatients	Y	Double-blind, random assignment to 150 mg imipramine or amitriptyline for 4 weeks	2 of 13 delusional patients fully recovered (HDRS <8), in contrast to 7 of 12 nondelusionals ($P < .05$); differences at 4 weeks were due to persistent depressive symptoms rather than delusions.
Howarth and Grace 1985	None/Feighner criteria for affective disorder and own definition for delusions	56 met Feighner criteria for at least a diagnosis of probable primary affective disorder; 34 delusional and 22 nondelusional; all inpatients	N	Various TCAs in 10- to 60-day trials.	21 of 34 delusional patients responded, in contrast to 9 of 22 nondelusional patients; delusional patients responded over a 9-week period; nondelusional patients responded over initial 3 weeks.
Chan et al. 1987	None/RDC	16 psychotic and 59 nonpsychotic depressives; all inpatients	N	Various TCAs; dosage and duration were not specified; 2- to 4-week pretreatment washout;	4 of 16 psychotic patients showed good to excellent responses to TCAs, in contrast to 40 of 59 nonpsychotic; 0 of 16 psychotic patients demonstrated *(continued)*

Table 7–5A. Treatment: tricyclic antidepressants (TCAs) *(continued)*

Study	Diagnostic instrument/classification system	Diagnoses (n)	Prospective study (Y/N)	Treatment	Findings
Chan et al. 1987 *(continued)*				19 of 59 nonpsychotic patients responded during washout, in contrast to 3 of 16 psychotic; degree of response was also less in psychotic patients	excellent responses, in contrast to 26 of 59 nonpsychotic patients; differences did not appear due to unipolar/bipolar distinction, age, or psychomotor disturbance; study reviewed other studies as well; authors combined these results with a review of other studies; including patients in this report, 127 of 363 psychotic patients (35%) responded in contrast to 464 of 691 nonpsychotic patients (67%)—highly significant.
Kocsis et al. 1990	SADS/RDC	132 patients; 85 unipolar and 47 bipolar; 25 psychotic and 107 nonpsychotic	Y	Double-blind treatment with amitriptyline or imipramine up to 250 mg/day for 4 weeks; 2-week drug-free washout	67% of 49 moderately depressed patients had good outcome, *vs.* 39% of 38 nonpsychotic severely depressed, *vs.* 32% of 19 psychotic; response of nonpsychotic severe and psychotic patients did not differ significantly; both response rates were worse than in group of nonpsychotic moderately depressive.

Note. BDS = Beck Depression Scale. ECT = electroconvulsive therapy. HDRS = Hamilton Depression Rating Scale. RDC = Research Diagnostic Criteria. SADS = Schedule for Affective Disorders and Schizophrenia.

For additional studies, see Table 7–5B for Avery and Winokur (1977), Minter and Mandel (1979a, 1979b), and Lykouras et al. (1986) and Table 7–5C for Minter and Mandel (1979a, 1979b), Moradi et al. (1979), Kaskey et al. (1980), and Spiker et al. (1985).

Table 7–5B. Treatment: electroconvulsive therapy (ECT)

Study	Diagnostic instrument/ classification system	Diagnoses (*n*)	Prospective study (Y/N)	Treatment	Findings
Davidson et al. 1977	See Table 7–5A	See Table 7–5A	Y	ECT, number not specified.	4 of 4 psychotic unipolar depressives who failed to respond to imipramine or phenelzine responded to ECT.
Avery and Winokur 1977	None/Feighner et al. (1972) research criteria for probable primary depression or RDC schizo-affective disorder, depressive type	519 individuals with 609 hospitalizations with DSM-I or DSM-II depression diagnosis between 1959 and 1969	N	ECT, adequate if 5 or 7 treatments given; adequate dose of anti-depressants (imipramine, amitriptyline, desipramine, or nortriptyline)—for 4 weeks, with at least 2 weeks at 150 mg or more; protriptyline or phenelzine—4 weeks at least 45 mg for 2 weeks; tranylcypromine or isocarboxazid—4 weeks at least 30 mg for 2 weeks	1) Nonsignificant trend for greater marked response rate among delusionals to ECT (30%) than to antidepressants (9%) in 1959–1960 and 1967–1968 samples; 2) combining unipolar, schizoaffective patients who had nondepressed hallucinations or delusions with the group of delusional patients resulted in an increased difference in rates of delusional patients who responded to ECT (42%) vs. those who responded to TCAs (18%), $P < .05$.
Avery and Lubrano 1979	See Table 7–5A	See Table 7–5A	Y	8–10 ECT treatments after trial of imipramine (200–350 mg/day for 30 days) failed	In the overall group, 137 of 190 (72%) responded to ECT; response rates in subgroups were endogenous, 93 of 109 (85%); severe, 91 of 110 (83%); delusional, 91 of 109 (83%); neurotic/reactive, 8 of 31 (26%).

(continued)

Table 7–5B. Treatment: electroconvulsive therapy (ECT) *(continued)*

Study	Diagnostic instrument/ classification system	Diagnoses (*n*)	Prospective study (Y/N)	Treatment	Findings
Minter and Mandel 1979a	None/none	54 inpatients; probable or definite psychotic major depressive disorder; psychosis defined as delusions, hallucinations, or depressive stupor	N	TCAs alone—3 weeks at 150 mg/day or more; antipsychotic—2 weeks at 300 mg/day or more; tricyclics and antipsychotics; ECT—10 treatments in the 1 failure	Poor response in 8 of 11 patients treated with antidepressants alone; all other treatments had more responders than nonresponders; good and partial responders to antidepressants alone vs. good and partial responders to all other treatments (*P* < .001, Fisher exact); ECT group, 9 of 11 good response; excellent responses of depression and psychotic elements to ECT, ECT with antipsychotic medication, plus antidepressant and antipsychotic medication.
Minter and Mandel 1979b	None/RDC	11 patients with psychotic major depressive disorder; all inpatients	Y	ECT trial—at least 6 treatments; TCA—3 weeks at maximal tolerated dose	0 of 3 responded to TCA alone; 4 of 4 responded to neuroleptics alone; 2 of these 4 showed improvement in psychosis but no change in depression—these 2 responded to ECT; 3 of 3 responded to ECT; 3 of 4 responded to ECT-neuroleptic combination; 2 of 2 responded to TCA-neuroleptic combination.

| Charney and Nelson 1981 | See Table 7–5A | See Table 7–5A | N | For TCAs, all non-responders received 250 mg/day for a minimum of 3 weeks | 1) 2 of 9 delusional patients responded to TCAs alone, in contrast to 32 of 40 nondelusional ($P < .01$); 8 of 26 delusional patients responded to neuroleptics alone, in contrast to 0 of 1 nondelusional patient ($P = $ NS); 25 of 37 delusional patients responded to TCA-neuroleptic combination, in contrast to 9 of 10 nondelusional patients ($P = $ NS); 9 of 11 delusional patients responded to ECT, in contrast to 1 of 4 nondelusional patients ($P = $ NS); 2) 6 of 7 delusional patients failed to respond to TCAs alone: 3 responded to TCA-neuroleptic combination, and 3 responded to ECT; 3) 15 of 18 delusional patients who failed to respond to neuroleptics alone responded to addition of a TCA; 12 delusional patients showed a partial response to TCA-neuroleptics; 7 of 8 of these patients responded to ECT. |

(continued)

Table 7–5B. Treatment: electroconvulsive therapy (ECT) *(continued)*

Study	Diagnostic instrument/ classification system	Diagnoses (*n*)	Prospective study (Y/N)	Treatment	Findings
Brown et al. 1982	See Frances et al. 1981, Tables 7–1 and 7–5A	64 inpatients with major depression: 30 psychotic and 34 nonpsychotic; all unipolar	N	6 or more ECT treatments; adequate TCA trial was 150 mg/day amitriptyline	6 of 7 psychotic patients responded to ECT, and 6 of 6 nonpsychotics responded, 17 of 23 nonpsychotic patients responded to TCAs, in contrast to 3 of 18 psychotics (*P* < .01); psychotic patients responded better to ECT than to TCAs (*P* < .01); no difference in nonpsychotics between ECT and TCA response rates.
Rich et al. 1984 (overlap with Rich et al. 1986)	None/RDC and DSM-III	44 inpatients; 38 with RDC major depressive disorder, 10 of whom were psychotic; 6 with schizoaffective disorder; 41 with DSM-III major depressive disorder, of whom 13 were psychotic; organic affective syndrome (*n* = 3)	Y	3 times/week; generally unilateral; 8% of treatments were bilateral	Psychotic patients did not respond preferentially to ECT over other subtypes.
Rich et al. 1986	None/DSM-III and RDC	30 patients with primary unipolar depressive disorder: 9 psychotic and 21 nonpsychotic; all inpatients	Y	ECT 3 times a week with a single seizure each; frequency and number of treatments decided by patient and treating M.D.; decision about	75% of psychotic and nonpsychotic groups improved; two-thirds of each group had concomitant drug therapy (antidepressants, antipsychotics, or both).

| Lykouras et al. 1986 | None/DSM-III | 58 major depressive episode inpatients: 22 delusional and 36 nondelusional | Y | stopping/continuing antidepressant medications made by treating psychiatrist | Mean number of ECT treatments was 8.3/patient | 7 delusional patients did not respond to initial treatment with antidepressants, 6 responded to ECT and 1 to the addition of neuroleptics; 2 delusional patients who failed to respond to TCA-neuroleptic combination responded to ECT. |

Note. RDC = Research Diagnostic Criteria. TCA = tricyclic antidepressant.

Table 7–5C. Treatment: tricyclic antidepressants (TCAs)/neuroleptics

Study	Diagnostic instrument/ classification system	Diagnoses (*n*)	Prospective study (Y/N)	Treatment	Findings
Nelson and Bowers 1978	None/RDC	13 delusional unipolar depressives	N	Antipsychotic and TCAs (either amitriptyline or imipramine); average oral dose of TCA = 2.5 mg/kg.	12 of 13 responded; of the 12, 5 had complete alleviation of symptoms and 7 were clearly less depressed, nonpsychotic, and able to resume usual level of functioning.
Minter and Mandel 1979a	See Table 7–5B	See Table 7–5B	N	See Table 7–5B	16 of 16 patients treated with antidepressant in combination with antipsychotics responded; 14 of 15 patients treated with antipsychotics responded; 3 of 11 patients treated with antidepressant alone responded.
Moradi et al. 1979	None/SADS-type diagnoses	13 male VA inpatients with depression, accompanied by delusions consistent with depression	N	TCAs alone—150 mg/day for 2 weeks to 4 months; neuroleptic doses not given	0 of 7 improved on TCAs alone (2 became worse) vs. 5 of 5 improved with neuroleptics (*P* < .001); 12 of 13 only improved when neuroleptic was given or added, 2 of whom received ECT with neuroleptics.
Kaskey et al. 1980	None/DSM-III/ RDC	23 psychotically depressed inpatients; schizoaffective— 3, unipolar—16, bipolar—4	N	TCA—100 mg of imipramine/day or equivalent; neuroleptic—200 mg of chlorpromazine/day or its equivalent; or the combination of two treatments; all nonresponders exceeded minimum criteria	7 of 7 (100%) treated with neuroleptics plus TCAs were classified as responders, vs. 2 of 6 (33%) with neuroleptic alon,e vs. 3 of 10 (30%) with TCA alone (*P* < .01).

| Spiker et al. 1985 | SADS/RDC | Y | All inpatients with major depressive disorder primary subtype; psychotic subtype based on delusions (ambiguous cases dropped); 54 subjects, 36 women and 22 men; 51 completed the trial | 7-day placebo washout; perphenazine ($n = 17$)—50 mg/day; amitriptyline ($n = 19$)—218 mg/day; amitriptyline and perphenazine ($n = 22$)—170 mg and 54 mg/day, respectively; 35 days of active treatment | 14 of 18 (78%) assigned to amitriptyline plus perphenazine responded, vs. 7 of 17 (41%) with amitriptyline alone, vs. 3 of 16 (19%) with perphenazine alone; amitriptyline plus perphenazine significantly more effective; $P < .01$. Response = no longer delusional. |

Note. RDC = Research Diagnostic Criteria. SADS = Schedule for Affective Disorders and Schizophrenia.
For additional studies, see Table 7–5A for Charney and Nelson (1981) and Frances et al. (1981) and Table 7–5D for Anton and Bruch (1990).

Table 7–5D. Treatment: amoxapine

Study	Diagnostic instrument/ classification system	Diagnoses (n)	Prospective study (Y/N)	Treatment	Findings
Anton and Burch 1990	None/DSM-III	46 inpatients with major depression with psychotic features	Y	Double blind; 21 patients received amoxapine 100–400 mg/day; 25 patients received amitriptyline 50–200 mg/day and perphenazine 8–32 mg/day (dosages increased over first 4 days to maximum value given); 5-day placebo washout	38 patients completed trials; 17 in amoxapine group and 21 in amitriptyline-perphenazine group; 82% of amoxapine group showed improvement, vs. 85% of amitriptyline-perphenazine group; amitriptyline-perphenazine group had significantly more extrapyramidal side effects; tendency for amitriptyline-perphenazine group to have higher global response rate.
Anton and Sexauer 1983	None/DSM-III	4 male inpatients with major depression with psychotic features	N	200 mg amoxapine daily	3 of 4 patients showed elevated serum prolactin levels, suggesting postsynaptic dopamine blockage; 4 of 4 patients showed marked mood and functional improvement.

2. In contrast to NPMD, PMD responds poorly (or at best very slowly) to TCAs when they are administered alone.

3. PMD patients respond better to the combination of a TCA with a neuroleptic than to a TCA alone.

4. PMD patients respond equally well to amoxapine (a four-ringed tricyclic-like antidepressant with serotonin-2 receptor blocking properties and a neuroleptic metabolite) or to the combination of a neuroleptic and a TCA.

5. PMD patients who fail to respond to TCAs often respond to ECT. However, ECT may not be more effective in PMD patients than in NPMD patients.

Placebo. Glassman and Roose (1981) reported that PMD patients did not demonstrate responses to placebo. The placebo washout was an initial phase of protocols designed to explore the relationship of imipramine plasma levels to antidepressant response. Of 60 NPMD patients, 18 (30%) responded to placebo, in contrast to 0 of 21 PMD patients. In a recent study, Anton and Burch (1990) reported that 10% of PMD patients responded during placebo washout. Unfortunately, these studies were single blind during the placebo phase, making definitive conclusions difficult. In another study, Chan et al. (1987) reported that 19 of 59 nonpsychotic patients responded during a 2-week washout period, in contrast to 3 of 16 PMD patients. These 3 PMD patients only demonstrated partial responses.

TCAs alone. Early studies on TCA therapy in depression noted depressed patients with psychotic features responded poorly to imipramine or amitriptyline (Angst 1961; Friedman et al. 1961; Hordern et al. 1963). These observations were largely overlooked until the imipramine plasma level studies of Glassman et al. (1975, 1977). They administered fixed milligram per kilogram doses of imipramine to both PMD and NPMD patients and also observed that PMD patients responded more poorly to imipramine than did NPMD patients (Glassman et al. 1975). Specifically, 3 of 13 (23%) PMD patients responded, in contrast to 14 of 21 (67%) NPMD patients. This difference attained statistical significance and was not due to severity of illness (more severely depressed patients did not respond more poorly to imipramine). (See below for further discussion of severity issue.)

In a landmark study, DeCarolis administered imipramine to 437 depressed patients (Avery and Lubrano 1979). Patients were treated with 200–300 mg/day for at least 25 days, and nonresponders after 30 days were treated with ECT (see below). PMD patients did more poorly on imipramine (40% response rate) than did endogenous or neurotic-reactive depressive patients (61% and 60%, respectively). Subsequently, a number of studies (many of them retrospective reviews) have again confirmed that PMD patients respond more poorly to TCAs alone than do NPMD patients (Chan et al. 1987; Charney and Nelson 1981; Frances et al. 1981). Indeed, in their recent report, Chan et al. (1987) reviewed response data on over 1,000 depressed patients from 12 studies including their own (Avery and Lubrano 1979; Avery and Winokur 1977; Brown et al. 1982; Chan et al. 1987; Charney and Nelson 1981; Davidson et al. 1977; Friedman et al. 1961; Glassman et al. 1977; Hordern et al. 1963; Howarth and Grace 1985; Nelson et al. 1984; Simpson et al. 1976). They calculated that 127 of 363 (35%) PMD patients responded to TCA therapy, in contrast to 464 of 891 (67%) NPMD patients ($\chi^2 = 104.2$, $df = 1$, $P < 2 \times 10^{-24}$) of these studies are summarized in Table 7–5A. As indicated in this table, these results do not appear to be due to a general pattern of underdosing.

We have identified two additional studies that were not included in Chan's summary; one appeared before the Chan study (Frances et al. 1981), the other after (Kocsis et al. 1990). They both reported lower response rates to TCAs in PMD than in NPMD patients. Frances et al. (1981), in a retrospective chart review, reported that 3 of 18 PMD patients responded to TCAs, in contrast to 17 of 23 patients with NPMD ($\chi^2 = 10.8$, $df = 1$, $P < .001$). In the Extramural Depression Collaborative Study, imipramine or amitriptyline was administered for 4 weeks to 132 patients (Kocsis et al. 1990). We recalculated the tricyclic response rates of PMD and NPMD patients in this study, which was lower (albeit of trend significance, $P = .06$) in PMD (32%) than in NPMD (55%) patients. In addition to all these reports that have compared PMD and NPMD patients, there are several other reports that PMD patients respond poorly to TCAs (see Minter and Mandel 1979a, 1979b, Table 7–5B; Kaskey et al. 1980, Table 7–5C).

There are two notable exceptions to the finding that PMD patients respond more poorly to TCAs than do NPMD patients. Quitkin et al. (1978) reanalyzed a previous study of Klein (1967) that had compared 6 weeks of treatment with imipramine versus placebo in depressed patients. They concluded that delusions did not predict poor response to imipramine and argued that PMD patients often required treatment for prolonged periods and at higher dosages. (Most studies have employed 4 weeks of treatment with TCAs.) This reanalysis has been criticized for its retrospective definition of psychotic and nonpsychotic groups, using the F factor of the Lorr Multidimensional Scale (Lorr et al. 1955) for psychiatric patients. The F factor includes nondelusional items (e.g., poor orientation and hostile impulses), raising questions about the accuracy of the retrospectively performed diagnoses (Chan et al. 1987; Frances et al. 1981; Glassman and Roose 1981). In a retrospective review of patients treated for up to 9 weeks, Howarth and Grace (1985) reported that PMD patients responded significantly better to tricyclic/tetracyclic antidepressants than did NPMD patients. Of 34 psychotic patients, 21 (62%) responded, in contrast to 9 of 22 (41%) nonpsychotic patients. PMD patients, however, responded more slowly to treatment, with the authors estimating that over 40% may require treatment for at least 4–9 weeks. Again many of the other previous studies had used shorter treatment periods (e.g., 4 weeks). These data indicate that the nature of response to tricyclics differs in the two groups but that some delusional patients may do well on TCAs if they are prescribed for sufficient periods.

Several studies have explored whether the poorer responses observed with TCA therapy were due to the effects of severity or endogenicity. Glassman et al. (1977) noted slightly lower response rates (56%) in more severe NPMD (total HDRS score 27) than in less severe NPMD patients (75%); however, this difference did not attain statistical significance. Chan et al. (1987) reported that degree of incapacitation or endogenous status failed to predict poor response to TCAs, in contrast to delusional status, which did.

On the other hand, in the Extramural Depression Collaborative Study (Kocsis et al. 1990), the response rate to TCA therapy differed significantly among PMD patients, moderately depressed NPMD patients (defined as a total HDRS score of 26 or less), and severely depressed NPMD patients (HDRS score of 27 or greater). Severely depressed NPMD patients did not differ significantly from PMD patients in their response rates (39% and 32%, respectively). Total HDRS scores in severely depressed NPMD patients were similar to those seen in the PMD patients, suggesting general severity could be a factor in why PMD patients do poorly on TCAs. Moderately depressed NPMD patients did significantly better than did the combined group of PMD and severely depressed NPMD patients. There are a number of caveats regarding this study. It combined unipolar and bipolar patients in contrast to most of the other studies. In addition, the severely ill psychotic group was significantly older than the moderately ill nonpsychotic group or those patients with psychotic depression.

The DeCarolis study (Avery and Lubrano 1979) also suggested that severity may predict poor response. As indicated above, PMD patients did more poorly on imipramine (40% response rate) than did endogenous or neurotic-reactive depressive patients (61% and 60%, respectively). However, patients designated as being severely depressed also did poorly (35% response rate). Because patients in this study may not have been placed into discrete categories for analyses (i.e., the same patients were probably classified as both delusional and severe), it is difficult to comment on the relative effects of severity on treatment response. The data from this study suggest, however, that the poorer responses to imipramine in PMD patients are not merely due to endogenous symptoms. The role of severity in determining poor responsivity of PMD patients to TCAs requires further study.

ECT.   A number of lines of investigation suggest that ECT is an effective treatment for PMD. Many retrospective clinical reports point out that PMD patients who are poor responders to TCAs do well when subsequently treated with ECT (Brown et al. 1982; Charney and Nelson 1981; Davidson et al. 1977; Frances et al. 1981;

Glassman et al. 1975; Lykouras et al. 1986; Minter and Mandel 1979a, 1979b; Moradi et al. 1979) (see Table 7–5B). For example, Glassman et al. (1975) reported that 9 of the 10 PMD patients who had failed to respond in their prospective imipramine study responded well to ECT. This finding was perhaps most dramatic in the DeCarolis study (Avery and Lubrano 1979). As discussed above, in that study, only 40% of the PMD patients responded to initial treatment with imipramine. However, 83% of the failures responded to ECT. A high response rate to ECT was also observed in severely depressed patients who had responded poorly to imipramine, although here again there may have been great overlap between the psychotic and severely depressed groups of patients. In contrast, neurotic-reactive depressions responded well to imipramine, and patients who failed to respond to imipramine generally did not respond to ECT.

Avery and Winokur (1977) reviewed hospital records of 59 depressed patients hospitalized at Psychopathic Hospital in Iowa City, Iowa, between 1959 and 1969. Of depressed patients with delusions, 42% responded to ECT, in contrast to only 18% who responded to adequate antidepressant trials ($P < .05$). The delusional group included some patients with nondepressive hallucinations or delusions (i.e., schizoaffective), making comparison of this study with others somewhat difficult.

Four studies have compared response to ECT in PMD versus NPMD patients. Rich et al. (1984, 1986) and Brown et al. (1982) found ECT to be equally effective in PMD and NPMD patients. However, Charney and Nelson (1981) reported that response to ECT was better in PMD patients than in their NPMD counterparts (Table 7–5B). Taken together, these data suggest ECT is an effective treatment for psychotic depression, although it may not be more effective in PMD than in severely depressed NPMD patients.

TCA-neuroleptic combination.   The combination of TCA-neuroleptics has been reported to be an effective treatment for PMD in both retrospective and prospective studies (see Table 7–5C). Several groups have reported that patients who had failed to respond to TCAs alone went on to respond to the combination of a TCA with a neuroleptic (Charney and Nelson 1981; Frances et al. 1981; Minter and Mandel 1979a).

Spiker et al. (1985) compared the combination of amitriptyline plus perphenazine, amitriptyline alone, and perphenazine alone in the treatment of PMD patients. Mean daily doses were: 218 mg amitriptyline alone, 50 mg perphenazine alone, and the combination of 170 mg of amitriptyline and 54 mg of perphenazine. The protocol called for 35 days of active treatment. Fourteen of 18 (78%) patients treated with the combination responded, in contrast to 7 of 17 (41%) amitriptyline-treated patients or 3 of 16 (19%) patients treated with perphenazine. Of the 13 patients who failed to respond to perphenazine, 7 were not psychotic at completion of the study but were still depressed. A high proportion of patients who had failed to respond to either amitriptyline or perphenazine alone responded when the other drug was added. Differences in responses to the combination over each ingredient alone were not due to one compound raising the blood level of the other. This study included both bipolar and unipolar patients with psychotic depression.

Amoxapine.   Anton and Burch (1990) reported that in psychotic depression, amoxapine, a four-ring compound that is related to the antipsychotic loxapine, was comparable to the combination of amitriptyline with perphenazine. This study was undertaken after open trials suggested 60%–80% response rates to amoxapine in PMD patients (Anton and Sexauer 1983). After a single-blind, 5-day placebo washout, patients were randomized to receive amoxapine or the combination of amitriptyline-perphenazine under double-blind conditions. The maximum daily doses were 400 mg of amoxapine and 200 mg of amitriptyline and 32 mg of perphenazine for the combination. In this study, 82% of the amoxapine group and 85% of the amitriptyline-perphenazine group demonstrated moderate to marked improvement. The combination produced significantly more extrapyramidal side effects, and there was a tendency for the combination to produce more in the way of anticholinergic side effects. The authors noted that the ratio of serotonin-2/dopamine-2 receptor blockade of amoxapine was similar to a number of atypical neuroleptics, suggesting a possible mechanism of action for the antipsychotic effect of this compound (Table 7–5D).

Summary.   In summary, studies on psychotic depression indicate the condition responds 1) infrequently to placebo, 2) poorly (or, at best, very slowly) to TCAs alone, 3) well to treatment with amoxapine alone or the combination of a TCA with a neuroleptic, and 4) well to ECT. In contrast, NPMD patients demonstrate higher response rates to both placebo and TCAs alone than do PMD patients. The relative contribution of severity as a factor in lowering responsivity to TCA therapy still requires further study.

Discussion and Recommendations

The major efforts expended in recent decades toward developing clinically valid classification systems have resulted in the inclusion of a large number of syndromes in DSM-III-R, for many of which there are relatively limited data on those key dimensions (e.g., biology and treatment response) needed to validate their designation as distinct disorders. Indeed, some investigators have argued that many DSM-III-R disorders would be better classified under a broader rubric of affective disorder (Hudson and Pope 1990). In contrast, the data reviewed in this chapter strongly suggest that unipolar major depression with psychotic features is a disorder that can be differentiated from unipolar major depression without psychotic features on a number of important dimensions, in particular, symptoms, biological characteristics, course/outcome, and treatment response.

Still a number of questions can and should be raised about a separate designation. First, could the so-called differentiating characteristics of PMD versus NPMD merely be separating a more severe from a less severe disorder rather than demarcating a truly distinct syndrome? As indicated in detail above, severity alone did not appear to account for the differences between PMD and NPMD. For example, in regard to symptom characteristics, Coryell et al. (1984) reported significantly higher total 17-item HDRS scores in PMD than in NPMD patients, but these differences were mainly due to three delusional items. In that study, psychomotor disturbance was the only somatic symptom to separate the two groups. PMD patients did not demonstrate significantly greater scores on the remaining neurovegetative symptoms. The differences in HPA activity (Brown et al. 1988), sleep (Thase et al. 1986), and treatment response (Chan et al. 1987; Glassman et al. 1977) between PMD and NPMD patients also did not appear to be due to differences in severity. However, particularly in regard to treatment, further prospective investigation is required, because some studies have also reported poor responses to TCAs in severely ill NPMD patients (Avery and Lubrano 1979; Kocsis et al. 1990).

Could the differences between PMD and NPMD be due to differences in endogenicity? This is an important issue because guilt and psychomotor disturbance are clearly endogenous symptoms. A few studies explored the specific role of endogenicity, and these also failed to demonstrate that PMD versus NPMD differences were due to more intense endogenous-type symptoms in the former. Indeed, the recent study by Parker et al. (1991) of a well-defined group of patients who met RDC criteria for endogenous depression and DSM-III criteria for melancholic depression clearly indicates that the differentiating symptoms are not merely separating endogenous from nonendogenous (or more endogenous from less endogenous) patients. Moreover, data from a number of studies on HPA activity (Brown et al. 1988; Evans et al. 1983; Rihmer et al. 1984b) and treatment response (Avery and Lubrano 1979; Chan et al. 1987) also failed to substantiate that differences were due to endogenicity and not to psychosis.

The findings that young PMD patients are at high risk for developing bipolar disorder (Akiskal et al. 1983; Strober and Carlson 1982) and that there is increased familial risk for bipolar disorder in PMD (Weissman et al. 1984) could suggest that PMD should be classified as a bipolar disorder. There are a number of arguments against this designation. For one, the relatively high risk for a switch into mania has been described in adolescent, but not older, patients. Thus, only in younger patients does PMD potentially signify the first episode of a bipolar disorder. Although the prevalence of PMD is higher in bipolar than unipolar patients (Coryell et al. 1984b), this observation does not negate the observations that unipolar PMD and NPMD disorders can be differentiated. One could argue that PMD/NPMD differences merely reflect the differentiation of a form-fruste bipolar psychotic depression from unipolar NPMD. However, data from our group and others point to differences between unipolar PMD and bipolar PMD patients on cortisol (Schatzberg et al. 1983) and dopamine-beta-hydroxylase (Mod et al. 1986; Rihmer et al. 1984b) activity. Although further studies are required, the limited data gathered to date suggest that unipolar PMD differs from bipolar PMD.

An argument can be made that there is little to be gained from having another DSM-IV category rather than continuing a dimensional designation for psychosis. Although many technical issues (Grayson 1987) regarding a categorical versus dimensional designation of PMD have not been explored, data on morbidity and treatment response point to the practical need for clearer separation of this disorder. Furthermore, the difficulty in making the diagnosis results in its frequently being missed in the clinical setting and in patients' receiving less than optimal treatment and having poorer outcomes (Dubovsky 1991). A separate designation with clear criteria would assist both patients and practitioners alike. Although we believe a separate designation would be beneficial, further research on potentially demarcating symptoms and other key dimensions (e.g., biology, treatment response) are required to develop an optimal set of criteria and to resolve lingering questions about severity, endogenicity, bipolarity, and optimal treatment.

The DSM-IV Work Group on Mood Disorders, chaired by Dr. A. John Rush, carefully considered the evidence provided in this review. They concurred that the clinical relevance of specifically designating patients with psychotic major depression is high. Two options (listed in the *DSM-IV Options Book: Work in Progress* [Task Force on DSM-IV 1991]) were provided.

The first option was to continue the system as is (i.e., psychosis would be designated by a qualifying decimal point under the severity code). The advantage of this approach is that it ensures that the syndrome has a specific numerical code. The disadvantage is that it still implies psychosis is the end of a severity continuum. If this option is adopted, the text would be used to note that psychotic symptoms do occur in the less severely depressed.

The second option is to designate the syndrome with a separate modifier "major depressive disorder with psychotic features." The advantage of this option is that it avoids the implication that psychosis is on a continuum with severity. The disadvantage is that for administrative reasons, the syndrome might not receive its own numerical code, which would then limit the practicality of any such designation, and the crosswalk to ICD-10 (World Health Organization 1990) would be made impractical. After much deliberation, the Work Group recommended the first option, although it recognized that it was less than optimal.

References

Aberg-Wistedt A, Wistedt B, Bertilsson L: Higher CSF levels of HVA and 5-HIAA in delusional compared to nondelusional depression. Arch Gen Psychiatry 42:925–926, 1985

Agren H, Terenius L: Hallucinations in patients with major depression: interactions between CSF monoaminergic and endorphinergic indices. J Affect Disord 9:25–34, 1985

Akiskal HS, Walker P, Puzantian VR, et al: Bipolar outcome in the course of depressive illness: phenomenologic, familial, and pharmacologic predictors. J Affect Disord 5:115–128, 1983

American Psychiatric Association: Diagnostic and Statistical Manual of Mental Disorders, 2nd Edition. Washington, DC, American Psychiatric Association, 1968

American Psychiatric Association: Diagnostic and Statistical Manual of Mental Disorders, 3rd Edition. Washington, DC, American Psychiatric Association, 1980

American Psychiatric Association: Diagnostic and Statistical Manual of Mental Disorders, 3rd Edition, Revised. Washington, DC, American Psychiatric Association, 1987

Andreasen NC, Olsen SA, Dennert JW, et al: Ventricular enlargement in schizophrenia: relationship to positive and negative symptoms. Am J Psychiatry 139:297–301, 1982

Angst J: A clinical analysis of the effects of Tofranil in depression. Psychopharmacologia 2:381–407, 1961

Anton RF: Urinary free cortisol in psychotic depression. Biol Psychiatry 2:24–34, 1987

Anton RF Jr, Burch EA Jr: A comparison study of amoxapine versus amitriptyline plus perphenazine in the treatment of psychotic depression. Am J Psychiatry 147:1203–1208, 1990

Anton RF, Sexauer JO: Efficacy of amoxapine in psychotic depression. Am J Psychiatry 140:1344–1347, 1983

Arana GW, Barreira PJ, Cohen BM, et al: The dexamethasone suppression test in psychotic disorders. Am J Psychiatry 140:1521–1523, 1983

Asnis GM, Halbreich U, Nathan RS, et al: The dexamethasone suppression test in depressive illness: clinical correlates. Psychoneuroendocrinology 7:295–301, 1982

Avery O, Lubrano A: Depression treated with imipramine and ECT: the DeCarolis study reconsidered. Am J Psychiatry 136:559–562, 1979

Avery O, Winokur G: The efficacy of electroconvulsive therapy and antidepressants in depression. Biol Psychiatry 12:507–523, 1977

Ayuso-Gutierrez JL, Almoguera MI, Garcia-Camba E, et al: The dexamethasone suppression test in delusional depression: further findings. J Affect Disord 8:147–151, 1985

Banki CM, Arato M, Papp A: Cerebrospinal fluid biochemical examinations: do they reflect clinical or biological differences? Biol Psychiatry 18:1033–1044, 1983

Brown RP, Frances A, Kocsis JH, et al: Psychotic vs. nonpsychotic depression: comparison of treatment response. J Nerv Ment Dis 170:635–637, 1982

Brown RP, Stoll PM, Stokes PE, et al: Adrenocortical hyperactivity in depression: effects of agitation, delusions, melancholia, and other illness variables. Psychiatry Res 23:167–178, 1988

Caroff S, Winokur A, Rieger W, et al: Response to dexamethasone in psychotic depression. Psychiatry Res 8:59–64, 1983

Carroll BJ, Curtis GC, Mendels J: Neuroendocrine regulation in depression, II: discrimination of depressed from nondepressed patients. Arch Gen Psychiatry 33:1051–1058, 1976

Carroll BJ, Greden JF, Feinberg M, et al: Neuroendocrine dysfunction in genetic subtypes of primary unipolar depression. Psychiatry Res 2:251–258, 1980

Chan CH, Janicak PG, Davis JM, et al: Response of psychotic and nonpsychotic depressed patients to tricyclic antidepressants. J Clin Psychiatry 48:197–200, 1987

Charney DS, Nelson JC: Delusional and nondelusional unipolar depression: further evidence for distinct subtypes. Am J Psychiatry 138:328–333, 1981

Coryell W, Tsuang MT: Primary unipolar depression and the prognostic importance of delusions. Arch Gen Psychiatry 39:1181–1184, 1982

Coryell W, Gaffney G, Burkhardt PE: The dexamethasone suppression test and familial subtypes of depression: a naturalistic replication. Biol Psychiatry 17:33–40, 1982a

Coryell W, Tsuang MT, McDaniel J: Psychotic features in major depression: is mood congruence important? J Affect Disord 4:227–236, 1982b

Coryell W, Lavori P, Endicott J, et al: Outcome in schizoaffective, psychotic, and nonpsychotic depression. Arch Gen Psychiatry 41:787–791, 1984a

Coryell W, Pfohl B, Zimmerman M: The clinical and neuroendocrine features of psychotic depression. J Nerv Ment Dis 172:521–528, 1984b

Coryell W, Endicott J, Keller M: The importance of psychotic features to major depression: course and outcome during a 2-year follow-up. Acta Psychiatr Scand 75:78–85, 1987

Coryell W, Keller M, Lavori P, et al: Affective syndromes, psychotic features and prognosis, I: depression. Arch Gen Psychiatry, 47:651–657, 1990

Davidson JRT, McLeod MN, Kurland AA, et al: Antidepressant drug therapy in psychotic depression. Br J Psychiatry 131:493–496, 1977

Devanand DP, Bowers MB, Hoffman FJ, et al: Elevated plasma homovanillic acid in depressed females with melancholia and psychosis. Psychiatry Res 15:1–4, 1985

Dubovsky SL: What we don't know about psychotic depression. Biol Psychiatry 30:533–536, 1991

Evans DL, Burnett G, Nemeroff CB: The dexamethasone suppression test in the clinical setting. Am J Psychiatry 140:586–589, 1983

Feighner JP, Robins E, Guze SB, et al: Diagnostic criteria for use in psychiatric research. Arch Gen Psychiatry 26:57–73, 1972

Frances A, Brown RP, Kocsis JH, et al: Psychotic depression: a separate entity? Am J Psychiatry 138:831–833, 1981

Frangos E, Athanassenas G, Tsitourides S, et al: Psychotic depressive disorder: a separate entity? J Affect Disord 5:259–265, 1983

Friedman C, Bowbray MS, Hamilton VJ: Imipramine (Tofranil) in depressive states. J Mental Sci 107:948–953, 1961

Gillin JC, Mendelson WB, Sitaram N, et al: The neuropharmacology of sleep and wakefulness. Annu Rev Pharmacol Toxicol 18:563–569, 1978

Glassman AH, Roose SP: Delusional depression: a distinct clinical entity? Arch Gen Psychiatry 38:424–427, 1981

Glassman AH, Kantor SJ, Shostak M: Depression, delusions, and drug response. Am J Psychiatry 132:716–719, 1975

Glassman AH, Perel JM, Shostak M, et al: Clinical implications of imipramine plasma levels for depressive illness. Arch Gen Psychiatry 34:197–204, 1977

Grayson DA: Can categorical and dimensional views of psychiatric illness be distinguished? Br J Psychiatry 151:355–361, 1987

Hamilton M: A rating scale for depression. J Neurol Neurosurg Psychiatry 23:56–62, 1960

Healy D, O'Halloran A, Carney PA, et al: Platelet 5-HT uptake in delusional and nondelusional depressions. J Affect Disord 10:233–239, 1986

Hordern A, Holt NF, Burt CG, et al: Amitriptyline in depressive states: phenomenology and prognostic considerations. Br J Psychiatry 109:815–825, 1963

Howarth BG, Grace MGA: Depression, drugs and delusions. Arch Gen Psychiatry 42:1145–1147, 1985

Hudson JI, Pope HG Jr: Affective spectrum disorder: does antidepressant response identify a family of disorders with a common psychophysiology? Am J Psychiatry 147:552–564, 1990

Hudson JI, Lipinski JF, Keck PE, et al: Polysomnographic characteristics of young manic patients: comparison with unipolar depressed patients and normal control subjects. Arch Gen Psychiatry 49:378–383, 1992

Johnson J, Horwath E, Weissman MM: The validity of major depression with psychotic features based on a community study. Arch Gen Psychiatry 48:1075–1081, 1991

Kantor SJ, Glassman AH: Delusional depressions: natural history and response to treatment. Br J Psychiatry 131:351–360, 1977

Kaskey GB, Nasr S, Meltzer HY: Drug treatment in delusional depression. Psychiatry Res 1:267–277, 1980

Kettering RL, Harrow M, Grossman L, et al: The prognostic relevance of delusions in depression: a follow-up study. Am J Psychiatry 144:1154–1160, 1987

Klein DF: Importance of psychiatric diagnosis in prediction of clinical drug effects. Arch Gen Psychiatry 16:118–126, 1967

Kocsis JH, Davis JM, Katz MM, et al: Depressive behavior and hyperactive adrenocortical function. Am J Psychiatry 142:1291–1298, 1985

Kocsis JH, Croughan JL, Katz MM, et al: Response to treatment with antidepressants of patients with severe or moderate nonpsychotic depression and of patients with psychotic depression. Am J Psychiatry 147:621–624, 1990

Kupfer DJ, Foster FG: The sleep of psychotic patients: does it all look alike? in Biology of the Major Psychoses. Edited by Freedman OX. New York, Raven, 1975

Kupfer DJ, Foster FG, Coble PA, et al: The application of EEG sleep for the differential diagnosis of affective disorders. Am J Psychiatry 135:69–74, 1978

Kupfer DJ, Broudy D, Coble PA, et al: EEG sleep and affective psychosis. J Affect Disord 2:17–25, 1980

Kupfer DJ, Jarrett DB, Frank E: The effects of dexamethasone administration on EEG sleep in depressed patients. J Affect Disord 7:93–98, 1984

Kupfer DJ, Reynolds CF, Elders CL: Comparison of EEG sleep measures among depressive subtypes and controls in older individuals. Psychiatry Res 27:13–21, 1989

Leckman JF, Weissman MM, Prusoff BA, et al: Subtypes of depression: family study perspective. Arch Gen Psychiatry 41:833–838, 1984

Lorr M, Jenkins RL, OConnor JP: Factors descriptive of psychopathology and behavior of hospitalized psychotics. J Abnorm Soc Psychol 50:78–86, 1955

Luchins DJ, Meltzer HY: Ventricular size and psychosis in affective disorder. Biol Psychiatry 10:1197–1198, 1983

Luchins DJ, Levine RJ, Meltzer HY: Lateral ventricular size, psychopathology, and medication response in the psychoses. Biol Psychiatry 19:29–44, 1984

Lykouras E, Malliaras GN, Christodoulou GM, et al: Delusional depression: phenomenology and response to treatment. Psychopathology 19:157–164, 1986a

Lykouras E, Malliaras O, Christodoulou GN, et al: Delusional depression: phenomenology and response to treatment: a prospective study. Acta Psychiatr Scand 73:324–329, 1986b

Lykouras E, Markianos M, Malliaras O, et al: Neurochemical variables in delusional depression. Am J Psychiatry 145:214–217, 1988

Matuzas W, Meltzer HY, Uhlenhuth EH, et al: Plasma dopamine-B-hydroxylase in depressed patients. Biol Psychiatry 17:1415–1424, 1982

Mazure CM, Bowers MB, Hoffman F, et al: Plasma catecholamine metabolites in subtypes of major depression. Biol Psychiatry 22:1469–1472, 1987

Meltzer HY, Cho HW, Carroll BJ, et al: Serum dopamine-B-hydroxylase activity in the affective psychoses and schizophrenia. Arch Gen Psychiatry 33:585–591, 1976

Mendels J, Hawkins DR: Sleep and depression: further considerations. Arch Gen Psychiatry 19:445–452, 1968

Mendlewicz J, Charles G, Franckson JM: The dexamethasone suppression test in affective disorder: relationship to clinical and genetic subgroups. Br J Psychiatry 141:464–470, 1982

Minter RE, Mandel MR: A prospective study of the treatment of psychotic depression. Am J Psychiatry 136:1470–1472, 1979a

Minter RE, Mandel MR: The treatment of psychotic major depressive disorder with drugs and electroconvulsive therapy. J Nerv Ment Dis 167:726–733, 1979b

Mod L, Rihmer Z, Magyar I, et al: Serum DBH activity in psychotic vs. nonpsychotic unipolar and bipolar depression. Psychiatry Res 19:331–333, 1986

Moradi SR, Muniz CE, Belar CO: Male delusional depressed patients: response to treatment. Br J Psychiatry 135:136–138, 1979

Murphy E: The prognosis of depression in old age. Br J Psychiatry 142:111–119, 1983

Nelson JC, Bowers MB: Delusional unipolar depression. Arch Gen Psychiatry 35:1321–1328, 1978

Nelson WH, Khan A, Orr WW: Delusional depression, phenomenology, neuroendocrine function and tricyclic antidepressant response. J Affect Disord 6:297–306, 1984

Parker G, Hadzi-Pavlovic D, Hickie I, et al: Distinguishing psychotic and nonpsychotic melancholia. J Affect Disord 22:135–148, 1991

Quitkin F, Rifkin A, Klein DF: Imipramine response in deluded depressive patients. Am J Psychiatry 135:806–811, 1978

Rao VP, Krishnan RR, Goli V, et al: Neuroanatomical changes and hypothalamic-pituitary-adrenal axis abnormalities. Biol Psychiatry 26:729–732, 1989

Rich CL, Spiker DG, Jewell SW, et al: DSM III, RDC, and ECT: depressive subtypes and immediate response. J Clin Psychiatry 45:14–18, 1984

Rich CL, Spiker DG, Jewell SW, et al: ECT response in psychotic versus nonpsychotic unipolar depressives. J Clin Psychiatry 47:123–125, 1986

Rihmer Z, Arato M, Szadoczky E, et al: The dexamethasone suppression test in psychotic vs. nonpsychotic endogenous depression. Br J Psychiatry 145:508–511, 1984a

Rihmer Z, Bagdy G, Arato M: Serum dopamine beta-hydroxylase activity in female manic-depressive patients. Biol Psychiatry 19:423–427, 1984b

Robinson DG, Spiker DG: Delusional depression: a one year follow-up. J Affect Disord 9:79–83, 1985

Roose SP, Glassman AH, Walsh BJ: Depression, delusions, and suicide. Am J Psychiatry 140:1159–1162, 1983

Rothschild AJ: Delusional depression: a review of the literature and current perspectives. McLean Hosp J 2:68–83, 1985

Rothschild AJ, Schatzberg AF, Rosenbaum AH, et al: The dexamethasone suppression test as a discriminator among subtypes of psychotic patients. Br J Psychiatry 141:471–474, 1982

Rothschild AJ, Langlais PJ, Schatzberg AF, et al: Dexamethasone increases plasma free dopamine in man. J Psychiatr Res 3:217–223, 1984

Rothschild AJ, Langlais PJ, Schatzberg AF, et al: The effects of a single acute dose of dexamethasone on monoamine and metabolite levels in rat brain. Life Sci 36:2491–2501, 1985

Rothschild AJ, Schatzberg AF, Langlais PJ, et al: Psychotic and nonpsychotic depressions, I: comparison of plasma catecholamines and cortisol measures. Psychiatry Res 20:143–153, 1987

Rothschild AJ, Samson JA, Schildkraut JJ, et al: Biochemical abnormalities in psychotic depression. Continuing Medical Education Syllabus and Scientific Proceedings in Summary Form, American Psychiatric Association Annual Meeting, 1989a, p 174

Rothschild AJ, Benes F, Hebben N, et al: Relationships between brain CT scan findings and cortisol in psychotic and nonpsychotic depressed patients. Biol Psychiatry 26:565–575, 1989b

Rothschild AJ, Schatzberg AF, Samson JA, et al: Cortisol and outcome in depression. New Research Program and Abstracts, American Psychiatric Association Annual Meeting, MR 409, 1990

Rudorfer MV, Hwu H-G, Clayton PJ: Dexamethasone suppression test in primary depression: significance of family history and psychosis. Biol Psychiatry 17:41–48, 1982

Schatzberg AF, Rothschild AJ: Psychotic (delusional) major depression: should it be included as a distinct syndrome in DSM-IV? Am J Psychiatry 149:733–745, 1992

Schatzberg AF, Rothschild AJ, Stahl JB, et al: The dexamethasone suppression test: identification of subtypes of depression. Am J Psychiatry 140:88–91, 1983

Schatzberg AF, Rothschild AJ, Langlais PJ, et al: A corticosteroid/dopamine hypothesis for psychotic depression and related states. J Psychiatr Res 19:57–64, 1985

Schlegel S, Kretzschmar K: Computed tomography in affective disorders, part I: ventricular and sulcal measurements. Biol Psychiatry 22:4–14, 1987

Simpson GM, Lee JH, Cuculic Z, et al: Two dosages of imipramine in hospitalized endogenous and neurotic depressives. Arch Gen Psychiatry 33:1093–1103, 1976

Spiker DG, Weiss JC, Dealy RS, et al: The pharmacological treatment of delusional depression. Am J Psychiatry 142:430–436, 1985

Spitzer RL, Endicott J, Robins E: Research Diagnostic Criteria: rationale and reliability. Arch Gen Psychiatry 35:773–782, 1978

Strober M, Carlson G: Bipolar illness in adolescents with major depression: clinical, genetic, and psychopharmacologic predictors in a three- to four-year prospective follow-up investigation. Arch Gen Psychiatry 39:549–555, 1982

Sweeney D, Nelson C, Bowers M, et al: Delusional versus nondelusional depression: neurochemical differences. Lancet 2:100–101, 1978

Targum SD, Rosen LN, DeLisi LE, et al: Cerebral ventricular size in major depressive disorder: association with delusional symptoms. Biol Psychiatry 18:329–336, 1983

Task Force on DSM-IV: DSM-IV Options Book: Work in Progress. American Psychiatric Association, 1991

Thase ME, Kupfer DJ, Ulrich RF: Current status of EEG sleep in the assessment and treatment of depression, in Advances in Human Psychopharmacology, Vol 4. Edited by Burrows GO, Werry JS. Greenwich, CT, JTI Press, 1986a

Thase ME, Kupfer DJ, Ulrich RF: Electroencephalographic sleep in psychotic depression: a valid subtype? Arch Gen Psychiatry 43:886–893, 1986b

Weissman MM, Prusoff BA, Thompson WD, et al: Social adjustment by self-report in a community sample and in psychiatric outpatients. J Nerv Ment Dis 166:317–326, 1978

Weissman MM, Prusoff BA, Merikangas KR: Is delusional depression related to bipolar disorder? Am J Psychiatry 141:892–893, 1984

Wolkowitz OM, Sutton ME, Doran AR, et al: Dexamethasone increases plasma HVA but not MHPG in normal humans. Psychiatry Res 16:101–109, 1985

Wolkowitz OM, Sutton M, Loula M, et al: Chronic corticosterone administration in rats: behavioral and biochemical evidence of increased central dopaminergic activity. Eur J Pharmacol 122:329–338, 1986

Wolkowitz OM, Doran A, Breier A, et al: Specificity of HVA response to dexamethasone in psychotic depression. Psychiatry Res 29:177–186, 1989

World Health Organization: ICD-10 Chapter V: Mental and Behavioral Disorders: Diagnostic Criteria for Research. Geneva, Switzerland, World Health Organization, 1990

Chapter 8

Catatonia

Max Fink, M.D.

Statement of the Issues

The purpose of this chapter is to summarize the literature and research that is relevant to the question of whether catatonia should be included as a modifier for a mood disorder diagnosis.

Significance of the Issues

Catatonia is a motor syndrome associated with disturbances in affect, mood, and thought, classified in DSM-III (American Psychiatric Association 1980) and DSM-III-R (American Psychiatric Association 1987) as a subtype of schizophrenia (Table 8–1). It was once defined as a rare phenomenon but has been increasingly diagnosed in the past two decades, often in association with diverse psychiatric diagnoses (Bush et al., unpublished data, 1993; Gelenberg 1976; Pataki et al. 1992; Rogers 1985). The main reasons for reviewing the evidence for catatonia are that catatonic features have been described more often in association with affective disorders than with schizophrenia (Abrams and Taylor 1976; Abrams et al. 1979), and successful treatment is not associated with the application of conventional interventions for schizophrenia, as in the use of neuroleptic drugs affecting dopaminergic systems.

This review considers the validity of the syndrome of catatonia from the vantage points of criteria used to validate syndromes in psychiatry. Is the syndrome of catatonia distinct enough to define a reasonable number of cases not accounted

Aided in part by the International Association for Psychiatric Research, Inc., P.O. Box 457, St. James, New York 11780-0457.

I am indebted to my associates, Drs. Andrew Francis, George Bush, George Petrides, Yiannis Zervas, Jolie Pataki, and Gregory Fricchione, and to my former collaborators Michael Taylor and Richard Abrams, for stimulating my interest in catatonia.

Table 8–1.   DSM-III-R diagnostic criteria for 295.2x schizophrenia, catatonic type

A type of schizophrenia in which the clinical picture is dominated by any of the following:

(1)   catatonic stupor (marked decrease in reactivity to the environment and/or reduction in spontaneous movements and activity) or mutism

(2)   catatonic negativism (an apparently motiveless resistance to all instructions or attempts to be moved)

(3)   catatonic rigidity (maintenance of a rigid posture against efforts to be moved)

(4)   catatonic excitement (excited motor activity, apparently purposeless and not influenced by external stimuli)

(5)   catatonic posturing (voluntary assumption of inappropriate or bizarre postures)

---

for by present syndromes? Is catatonia associated with a particular prognosis? Is catatonia associated with a specific epidemiology? Is catatonia associated with a specific family history? Is catatonia associated with a specific biology? Is catatonia associated with specific treatment strategies?

Method

We have been acquainted with the world literature on catatonia for almost a decade. For our recent reviews and studies, we read the report of Kahlbaum in translation (1873/1973) and the literature cited over the past five decades as found in *Index Medicus* and the recent Medline databases. For this review, selected articles are cited, with an emphasis on recent research reports.

Results

History of the Concept of Catatonia

The syndrome of catatonia was initially described as a distinct disorder by Kahlbaum in 1873. In his work *Die Katatonie oder das Spannungirresein*, as translated by Mora (1973), Kahlbaum wrote,

> Catatonia is a brain disease with a cyclic, alternating course, in which mental symptoms are, consecutively, melancholy, mania, stupor, confusion, and eventually dementia. One or more of these symptoms may be absent from the complete series of psychic "symptom complexes." In addition to the mental symptoms, locomotor neural processes with the general character of convulsions occur as typical symptoms. (Kahlbaum 1873/1973, p. 83)

His contemporary, Kraepelin (1904), grouped patients who exhibited the signs of catatonia within the class of dementia praecox, although his descriptions of patients identified as suffering from manic-depressive insanity included many with the signs of catatonia. This formulation was adopted by Bleuler (1924) in his concept of schizophrenia and remained the standard view that was incorporated in DSM-III in 1980 with catatonia listed *only* as a subtype of schizophrenia (295.3x). Based on DSM-III or DSM-III-R criteria, the signs of catatonia compel the diagnosis of schizophrenia, regardless of the longitudinal history, associated findings, or comorbid diagnoses. The term *catatonia* is not indexed in DSM-III-R; the term *catatonic type, schizophrenia* is the only term in the DSM-III-R index (p. 557) that refers to catatonia under the letter *C*. The actual description of catatonia is also limited (Table 8–1).

This state of affairs conflicts with two sets of recent data: 1) literature that describes systemic disorders in which the signs of catatonia are prominent and 2) a response pattern to interventions that are ordinarily not reported to be useful in patients with schizophrenia. These data compel consideration of catatonia in conditions other than schizophrenia in DSM-IV (Fink and Taylor 1991).

Conditions other than schizophrenia in which catatonic features have been recognized include the idiosyncratic appearance of lethal (pernicious) catatonia (Stauder 1934), the neuroleptic malignant syndrome (Caroff 1980; Delay and Deniker 1960), periodic catatonia (Kraepelin 1904), and manic excitement (Bell 1849). These conditions are not directly associated with either the life course or the neurological aberrations commonly found in schizophrenia.

Among patients with mental disorders, catatonic features are prominent in patients with severe affective disorders, particularly in the manic phases of illness (Abrams and Taylor 1976; Barnes et al. 1986). For example, in a prospective study of 55 consecutive patients who satisfied criteria for catatonia, only 4 met criteria for schizophrenia, whereas 34 were bipolar, manic phase (Abrams and Taylor 1976). The relationship with mania has repeatedly been reported (Abrams et al. 1979; Bonner and Kent 1936; Kirby 1913). Patients with a bipolar disorder may exhibit manic excitement with confusion, described as manic delirium (Bell 1849), which is indistinguishable from catatonic excitement or catatonic furor. A retrospective review of the experience in a university psychiatric service found that catatonic features were more common over time in patients with discharge diagnoses of affective disorders (63%) than in patients with schizophrenia (37%) (Pataki et al. 1992). A prospective study in the same institution found catatonic features in diversely diagnosed patients, with 11% diagnosed as schizophrenia or schizoaffective disorder, 11% major depressive disorder, 18% organic affective disorders, and 39% manic disorders (Bush et al., unpublished data, 1993).

Rogers (1985, 1992) has studied the motor disorders seen in severe psychiatric illnesses and has found that motor disorders are frequent in those with severe mental illness but that these signs are ignored by psychiatrists, especially those who are enamored of psychological factors. His argument is that the motor expressions, be they catatonia, neuroleptic malignant syndrome, dystonia, or parkinsonism, are reflections of coarse brain diseases that underlie these behavioral (and motor) disorders. This view is also well expressed by Taylor (1990, 1993).

Abrams et al. (1979) suggested two subtypes within the typical description of catatonia: a retarded type characterized by mutism, negativism, and stupor and an excited type characterized by stereotypy, catalepsy, and automatic cooperation. The former was unrelated to prognosis, but the latter was associated with a favorable response to treatment and a better longitudinal prognosis.

Catatonic features are also found in patients with systemic illnesses, particularly neurological disorders, or they may result from drug toxicity (Fricchione 1985; Fricchione et al. 1990; Gelenberg and Mandel 1977). The syndrome of rigidity, fever, autonomic instability, and stupor associated with the use of neuroleptic drugs is identified as the *neuroleptic malignant syndrome* (NMS) (Caroff 1980). It has many characteristics of catatonia, particularly lethal or pernicious catatonia. Many authors argue that these syndromes have a similar pathogenesis (Casey 1987; Devanand 1989; Fleischhacker et al. 1990; Mann et al. 1990; Tan and Ong 1991). NMS can be lethal, although the syndrome is now better recognized, and treatment (withdrawal of neuroleptics, supportive measures, treatment with dantrolene or bromocriptine, or ECT) has markedly improved prognosis (Davis et al. 1991; Ebadi et al. 1990; Mann et al. 1986; Philbrick and Rummans 1994).

Kraepelin (1904) described *periodic catatonia,* characterized by periods of excitement followed by stupor with catatonic features. Gjessing (1938) believed that the problem was in nitrogen metabolism and reported the successful treatment of the disorder with desiccated thyroid. Others identified periodic catatonia as a form of motility psychosis (Astrup 1979), and more recently, Taylor (1984) suggested that periodic catatonia was a variant of bipolar affective disorder. An acute clinical form, labeled *lethal catatonia,* may present with high fever, rigidity, and extreme hyperactivity and/or stupor. Lethal catatonia is not always fatal, which has led some authors to suggest *pernicious catatonia* as a more descriptive name (Kalinowsky 1987).

Some authors note that the incidence of catatonia has declined since the beginning of the century (Mahendra 1981; Silva et al. 1989). Although the frequency of catatonia in psychiatric settings is not established (Rosebush et al. 1990), many are impressed that its recognition is increasing. Pataki et al. (1992) identified 20 patients with catatonic features admitted to a university inpatient psychiatric service over a 6-year period. Considering a psychiatric admission rate of 408 (SD = 49.9) cases per year, the incidence of catatonia was 0.5% per year. This number underrepresents the incidence of catatonia, because Pataki et al. only looked at charts where the syndrome of catatonia had already been recognized as a primary or secondary diagnosis and had been recorded as being within the DSM-III category of schizophrenia, catatonic type (295.2). Charts that carried the diagnosis but had inadequate substantiation were excluded. Because short-lasting or abortive forms of the syndrome are more likely to be undocumented when they do not become a main focus of treatment or occur in the context of another primary diagnosis, many instances may not have been recorded and detected.

My colleagues and I at University Hospital at Stony Brook have identified catatonia a few times each year, often in patients who are not suffering from schizophrenia (Pataki et al. 1992). More recently, a prospective study was undertaken in the same hospital unit, and 15 cases with at least two features of catatonia were identified from 215 cases that were screened, an incidence of 7% (Bush et al., unpublished data, 1993).

Definition of Catatonia

Catatonia is a motor syndrome that occurs in association with affective, intrinsic brain and metabolic disorders, in drug-induced syndromes, and schizophrenia. As elucidated by Taylor (1990), catatonia is a state phenomenon resulting from dysfunction of the brain's motor regulation centers. It is not the result of permanent structural changes and, regardless of co-occurring symptoms, resolves quickly with treatment. Despite the wide range of disorders in which it has been identified, it is the commonality of features and its complete resolution with treatment that compels its consideration as a separate identifiable syndrome.

Catatonia appears in many guises and is often difficult to recognize. It is characterized by motor abnormalities and by periods of motor hyperactivity or hypoactivity. Mutism and negativism are prominent and are often accompanied by posturing, waxy flexibility, and stereotyped movements (Figure 8–1). Stupor, posturing, and negativism comprise the syndrome most often identified as catatonia. These more dramatic features are relatively uncommon, encouraging the belief that catatonia has become rare.

Diagnosis

Authors disagree on the number of signs and symptoms that should be considered necessary and/or sufficient to support the diagnosis of catatonia. Taylor (1990) proposed the presence of two or more classical symptoms, although he implied that he would be satisfied by one alone. In a systematic screening study of 215 consecutive admissions, 192 had no sign of catatonia, 8 had one sign, none had two signs, and 15 had three or more signs (Bush et al., unpublished data, 1993). In examining motor disorders in psychiatric patient populations, others describe different ways

Standardized Examination for Catatonia

- The method described here is used to complete the 23-item Bush-Francis Catatonia Rating Scale (BFCRS) and the 14-item Bush-Francis Catatonia Screening Instrument (BFCSI). Item definitions on the two scales are the same. The BFCRS measures the severity of 23 signs on a 0–3 continuum, whereas the BFCSI measures only the presence or absence of the first 14 signs.
- Ratings are to be made based solely on observed behaviors during the examination, with the exception of completing the items for "withdrawal" and "autonomic abnormality," which may be based on directly observed behavior and/or chart documentation.
- As a general rule, rate only items that are clearly present. If uncertain as to the presence of an item, rate the item as 0.

Procedure:	Examines:
1) Observe patient while trying to engage in a conversation.	Activity level Abnormal movements Abnormal speech
2) Examiner scratches head in exaggerated manner.	Echopraxia
3) Examine arm for cogwheeling. Attempt to reposture, instructing patient to "keep arm loose"—move arm with alternating lighter and heavier force.	Rigidity Negativism Waxy flexibility Gegenhalten
4) Ask patient to extend arm. Place one finger beneath hand and try to raise slowly after stating, "Do NOT let me raise your arm."	Mitgehen
5) Extend hand stating, "Do NOT shake my hand."	Ambitendence
6) Reach into pocket and state, "Stick out your tongue. I want to stick a pin in it."	Automatic obedience
7) Check for grasp reflex.	Grasp reflex

- -

8) Check chart for reports of previous 24-hour period. Especially check for oral intake, vital signs, and any incidents.

9) Attempt to observe patient indirectly, at least for a brief period each day.

Figure 8–1. Bush-Francis Catatonia Rating Scale. Use the presence or absence of items 1–14 for screening. Use the 0–3 scale for items 1–23 to rate severity.
Source. Derived from Bush et al., unpublished data, 1993.

Bush-Francis Catatonia Rating Scale

Patient:
Date:
Time:
Examiner:

1. **Excitement:** Extreme hyperactivity, constant motor unrest that is apparently nonpurposeful Not to be attributed to akathisia or goal-directed agitation
   0 = Absent
   1 = Excessive motion, intermittent
   2 = Constant motion, hyperkinetic without rest periods
   3 = Full-blown catatonic excitement, endless frenzied motor activity

2. **Immobility/stupor:** Extreme hypoactivity, immobile, minimally responsive to stimuli
   0 = Absent
   1 = Sits abnormally still, may interact briefly
   2 = Virtually no interaction with external world
   3 = Stuporous, nonreactive to painful stimuli

3. **Mutism:** Verbally unresponsive or minimally responsive
   0 = Absent
   1 = Verbally unresponsive to majority of questions; incomprehensible whisper
   2 = Speaks less than 20 words/5 minutes
   3 = No speech

4. **Staring:** Fixed gaze, little or no visual scanning of environment, decreased blinking
   0 = Absent
   1 = Poor eye contact, repeatedly gazes less than 20 seconds between shifting of attention, decreased blinking
   2 = Gaze held longer than 20 seconds, occasionally shifts attention
   3 = Fixed gaze, nonreactive

5. **Posturing/catalepsy:** Spontaneous maintenance of posture(s), including mundane (e.g., sitting/standing for long periods without reacting)
   0 = Absent
   1 = Greater than 1 minute
   2 = Greater than 1 minute, less than 15 minutes
   3 = Bizarre posture, or mundane maintained more than 15 minutes

6. **Grimacing:** Maintenance of odd facial expressions
   0 = Absent
   1 = Less than 10 seconds
   2 = Less than 1 minute
   3 = Bizarre expression(s) or maintained more than 1 minute

7. **Echopraxial/echolalia:** Mimicking of examiner's movements/speech
   0 = Absent
   1 = Occasional
   2 = Frequent
   3 = Constant

8. **Stereotypy:** Repetitive, non-goal-directed motor activity (e.g., finger play, repeatedly touching, patting or rubbing self); abnormality not inherent in act but in its frequency
   0 = Absent
   1 = Occasional
   2 = Frequent
   3 = Constant

9. **Mannerisms:** Odd, purposeful movements (hopping or walking tiptoe, saluting passersby, or exaggerated caricatures of mundane movements); abnormality inherent in act itself
   0 = Absent
   1 = Occasional
   2 = Frequent
   3 = Constant

10. **Verbigeration:** Repetition of phrases or sentences (like a scratched record)
    0 = Absent
    1 = Occasional
    2 = Frequent, difficult to interrupt
    3 = Constant

11. **Rigidity:** Maintenance of a rigid position despite efforts to be moved, exclude if cog-wheeling or tremor present
    0 = Absent
    1 = Mild resistance
    2 = Moderate
    3 = Severe, cannot be repostured

(continued)

12. **Negativism:** Apparently motiveless resistance to instructions or attempts to move/examine patient. Contrary behavior, does exact opposite of instruction
    0 = Absent
    1 = Mild resistance and/or occasionally contrary
    2 = Moderate resistance and/or frequently contrary
    3 = Severe resistance and/or continually contrary

13. **Waxy flexibility:** During reposturing of patient, patient offers initial resistance before allowing himself or herself to be repositioned, similar to that of a bending candle
    0 = Absent
    3 = Present

14. **Withdrawal:** Refusal to eat, drink, and/or make eye contact
    0 = Absent
    1 = Minimal PO intake/interaction for less than 1 day
    2 = Minimal PO intake/interaction for more than 1 day
    3 = No PO intake/interaction for 1 day or more

15. **Impulsivity:** Patient suddenly engages in inappropriate behavior (e.g., runs down hallway, starts screaming, or takes off clothes) without provocation. Afterward can give no or only a facile explanation
    0 = Absent
    1 = Occasional
    2 = Frequent
    3 = Constant or not redirectable

16. **Automatic obedience:** Exaggerated cooperation with examiner's request or spontaneous continuation of movement requested
    0 = Absent
    1 = Occasional
    2 = Frequent
    3 = Constant

17. **Mitgehen:** "Anglepoise lamp" arm raising in response to light pressure of finger, despite instructions to the contrary
    0 = Absent
    3 = Present

18. **Gegenhalten:** Resistance to passive movement that is proportional to strength of the stimulus, appears automatic rather than willful
    0 = Absent
    3 = Present

19. **Ambitendency:** Patient appears motorically "stuck" in indecisive, hesitant movement
    0 = Absent
    3 = Present

20. **Grasp reflex:** Per neurological examination
    0 = Absent
    3 = Present

21. **Perseveration:** Repeatedly returns to same topic or persists with movement
    0 = Absent
    3 = Present

22. **Combativeness:** Usually in an undirected manner, with no or only a facile explanation afterward
    0 = Absent
    1 = Occasionally strikes out, low potential for injury
    2 = Frequently strikes out, moderate potential for injury
    3 = Serious danger to others

23. **Autonomic abnormality:** Circle: temperature, blood pressure, pulse, respiratory rate, diaphoresis
    0 = Absent
    1 = Abnormality of 1 parameter (exclude preexisting hypertension)
    2 = Abnormality of 2 parameters
    3 = Abnormality of 3 or more parameters

to assess and define catatonia (Gelenberg 1976; Lohr and Wisniewski 1987; Morrison 1975; Rogers 1985; Rosebush et al. 1990; Taylor 1990). Bush et al. (unpublished data, 1993) developed a provisional rating scale and a guide to the examination for catatonic features. The clinical features associated with catatonia and their definition are shown in Figure 8–1 (derived from Bush et al., unpublished data, 1993). Based on the analyses by Taylor (1990) and Bush et al. (unpublished data, 1993) the presence of two or more signs of catatonia would be sufficient to make a provisional diagnosis of the syndrome.

There are no specific tests to verify the diagnosis of catatonia. Some authors note that a marked change in brain function, induced by sedative (barbiturates, benzodiazepines) or stimulant (amphetamine, methamphetamine) drugs is often accompanied by a transient recovery from mutism, negativism, stupor, or excitement. Such responses are inconsistent, however, occurring in half the catatonic cases identified (McCall 1992; McCall et al. 1992). The administration of amobarbital to a mute patient may allow the clinician to obtain more information regarding mental status and also facilitate feeding and toileting. A similar reduction in motor symptoms follows the intravenous administration of lorazepam (Fricchione 1985; Rosebush et al. 1990).

There are no data as to family occurrence of the syndrome and no epidemiological studies other than the institutional surveys already cited (Abrams and Taylor 1976; Bush et al., unpublished data, 1993; McCall et al. 1992; Pataki et al. 1992; Rosebush et al. 1990). There are no specific biological studies of the syndrome, other than those examining the effects of sedative drugs, although recent abstracts cite studies of dopamine metabolism (Northoff et al. 1993a, 1993b).

Treatment Implications of Catatonic Features

The treatment of catatonia has unique characteristics. Sedation by barbiturates or benzodiazepines is often associated with relief of the syndrome. Recent reports by Fricchione (1985) and Rosebush et al. (1990) emphasize that the relief with intravenous lorazepam is often persistent. In a prospective study by Bush et al. (unpublished data, 1993), 21 patients with at least three signs of catatonia were treated with lorazepam at doses of 4–8 mg/day for up to 5 days, with relief of catatonia in 16 patients. The remaining 5 patients were successfully treated with ECT. In the Pataki et al. (1992) retrospective review, 11 of 19 patients received ECT, with successful resolution of catatonia in 8 patients.

The differential diagnosis of catatonia has critical treatment implications. In patients with schizophrenia, neuroleptic drugs are usually the preferred intervention. The administration of neuroleptics to patients with the catatonia syndrome may, in fact, be hazardous, because catatonia is a risk factor for the development of NMS (White and Robins 1991), and NMS is a potential effect of all neuroleptics, including clozapine (DeGupta and Young 1991; Miller et al. 1991). In cases of malignant catatonia, early intervention with ECT is associated with favorable prognosis (Mann et al. 1990; Philbrick and Rummans 1994).

Discussion and Recommendations

A review of recent reports on catatonic symptoms finds that such features do not occur exclusively in the context of schizophrenia. Indeed, patients identified in four disorder groupings can present with catatonic features: mood disorders (especially mania), systemic disorders secondary to medications and toxic agents, and schizophrenia; catatonic features, although not common, occur often enough among the severely ill so that they should not be ignored. The prognostic implications, biological and family features, and incidence deserve further study. Finally, catatonic features have specific treatment implications. Taken together, our findings argue that clinicians be alerted to both the various conditions that may present with catatonic features and to their treatment implications.

Therefore, based on this review, we recommend that DSM-IV recognize the possibility that the syndrome of catatonia may be prominent in patients with mood disorders and include a subtype "with catatonia" for mood disorders, thus encouraging practitioners to identify the syndrome.

References

Abrams R, Taylor MA: Catatonia, a prospective clinical study. Arch Gen Psychiatry 33:579–581, 1976

Abrams R, Taylor MA, Stolurow KA: Catatonia and mania: patterns of cerebral dysfunction. Biol Psychiatry 14:111–117, 1979

American Psychiatric Association: Diagnostic and Statistical Manual of Mental Disorders, 3rd Edition. Washington, DC, American Psychiatric Association, 1980

American Psychiatric Association: Diagnostic and Statistical Manual of Mental Disorders, 3rd Edition, Revised. Washington, DC, American Psychiatric Association, 1987

Astrup C: The Chronic Schizophrenias. Oslo, Universitetsforlaget, 1979

Barnes MP, Saunders M, Walls TJ, et al: The syndrome of Karl Ludwig Kahlbaum. J Neurol Neurosurg Psychiatry 49:991–996, 1986

Bell LV: On a form of disease resembling some advanced stages of mania and fever. Am J Insanity 6:97–127, 1849

Bleuler E: Textbook of Psychiatry. New York, Macmillan, 1924

Bonner CA, Kent GH: Overlapping symptoms in a catatonic excitement and manic excitement. Am J Psychiatry 92:1311–1322, 1936

Breakey WR, Kala AK: Typhoid catatonia responsive to ECT. BMJ 2:357–359, 1977

Bush G, Fink M, Petrides G, et al: A rating scale for catatonic signs, I: prospective study of prevalence and phenomenology, II: use in monitoring response to lorazepam and electroconvulsive therapy. Unpublished data, 1993

Caroff SN: The neuroleptic malignant syndrome. J Clin Psychiatry 41:79–83, 1980

Casey DA: Electroconvulsive therapy in the neuroleptic malignant syndrome. Convulsive Ther 3:278–283, 1987

Davis JM, Janicak PG, Sakkas P, et al: Electroconvulsive therapy in the treatment of the neuroleptic malignant syndrome. Convulsive Ther 7:111–120, 1991

DeGupta K, Young A: Clozapine-induced neuroleptic malignant syndrome. J Clin Psychiatry 52:105–107, 1991

Delay J, Deniker P: Apport de la clinique à la connaissance de l'action des neuroleptiques. Revue Canadienne de Biologie 20:397–423, 1960

Devanand DP: Clinical differentiation between lethal catatonia and neuroleptic malignant syndrome. Am J Psychiatry 146:1240–1241, 1989

Ebadi M, Pfeiffer RF, Murrin LC: Pathogenesis and treatment of neuroleptic malignant syndrome. Gen Pharmacol 21:367–386, 1990

Fink M, Taylor MA: Catatonia: a separate category for DSM-IV? Integrative Psychiatry 7:2–10, 1991

Fleischhacker WW, Unterweger B, Kane JM, et al: The neuroleptic malignant syndrome and its differentiation from lethal catatonia. Acta Psychiatr Scand 81:3–5, 1990

Fricchione GL: Neuroleptic catatonia and its relationship to psychogenic catatonia. Biol Psychiatry 20:304–313, 1985

Fricchione GL, Kaufman LD, Gruber BL, et al: Electroconvulsive therapy and cyclophosphamide in combination for severe neuropsychiatric lupus with catatonia. Am J Med 88:442–443, 1990

Gelenberg AJ: The catatonic syndrome. Lancet 2:1339–1341, 1976

Gelenberg AJ, Mandel MR: Catatonic reactions to high potency neuroleptic drugs. Arch Gen Psychiatry 34:947–950, 1977

Gjessing R: Disturbances in somatic function in catatonia with a periodic course and their compensation. J Ment Sci 84:608–621, 1938

Kahlbaum KL: Die Katatonie oder das Spannungirresein (1873). Translated as Catatonia by Mora. Baltimore, MD, Johns Hopkins University Press, 1973

Kalinowsky LB: Lethal catatonia and neuroleptic malignant syndrome (letter). Am J Psychiatry 144:1106, 1987

Kirby GH: The catatonic syndrome and its relationship to manic depressive insanity. J Nerv Ment Dis 40:694–704, 1913

Kraepelin E: Lectures on Clinical Psychiatry. Translated by Johnstone J. London, Bailliere, Tindall & Cox, 1904

Lohr JB, Wisniewski AA: Movement Disorders: A Neuropsychiatric Approach. New York, Guilford, 1987

Mahendra B: Where have all the catatonics gone? Psychol Med 11:669–671, 1981

Mann SC, Caroff SN, Bleier HR, et al: Lethal catatonia. Am J Psychiatry 143:1374–1381, 1986

Mann SC, Caroff SN, Bleier HR, et al: Electroconvulsive therapy of the lethal catatonia syndrome. Convulsive Ther 6:239–247, 1990

McCall WV: The response to an amobarbital interview as a predictor of outcome in patients with catatonic mutism. Convulsive Ther 8:174–178, 1992

McCall WV, Shelp FE, McDonald WM: Controlled investigation of the amobarbital interview for catatonic mutism. Am J Psychiatry 149:202–206, 1992

Miller DD, Sharafuddin MJ, Kathol RG: A case of clozapine-induced neuroleptic malignant syndrome. J Clin Psychiatry 52:99–101, 1991

Morrison JR: Catatonia: diagnosis and treatment. Hosp Community Psychiatry 26:91–94, 1975

Northoff G, Demisch L, Pflug B: Neuroleptics and dopamine in catatonia (abstract). Pharmacopsychiatry 26:182, 1993a

Northoff G, Wenke J, Demish L, et al: Plasma dopamine metabolites HVA and DOPAC in catatonia (abstract). Pharmacopsychiatry 26:182, 1993b

Pataki J, Zervas IM, Jandorf L: Catatonia in a university in-patient service (1985–1990). Convulsive Ther 8:163–173, 1992

Philbrick KL, Rummans TA: Malignant catatonia. J Neuropsychiatry Clin Neurosci 6:1–13, 1994

Rogers D: The motor disorders of severe psychiatric illness: a conflict of paradigms. Br J Psychiatry 147:221–232, 1985

Rogers D: Motor Disorder in Psychiatry. Chichester, UK, John Wiley, 1992

Rosebush PI, Hildebrand AM, Furlong BG, et al: Catatonic syndrome in a general psychiatric population: frequency, clinical presentation, and response to lorazepam. J Clin Psychiatry 51:357–362, 1990

Silva H, Jerez S, Catenacci M, et al: Disminucion de la esquizofrenia catatonica en pacientes hospitalizados en 1984 respecto de 1964 (Decrease of catatonic schizophrenia in patients hospitalized in 1984 compared to 1964). Acta Psiquiatr Psicol Am Lat 35(3–4):132–138, 1989

Stauder KH: Die tödliche katatonia. Arch Psychiatr Nervenkr 102:614–634, 1934

Tan TKS, Ong SH: Catatonia and NMS (letter). Br J Psychiatry 158:858, 1991

Taylor MA: Schizoaffective and allied disorders, in Neurobiology of Mood Disorders. Edited by Post RM, Ballenger JC. Baltimore, MD, Williams & Wilkins, 1984, pp 136–156

Taylor MA: Catatonia: a review of the behavioral neurologic syndrome. Neuropsychiatry Neuropsychol Behav Neurol 3:48–72, 1990

Taylor MA: The Neuropsychiatric Guide to Modern Everyday Psychiatry. New York, Free Press, 1993

White DAC, Robins AH: Catatonia: harbinger of the neuroleptic malignant syndrome. Br J Psychiatry 158:419–421, 1991

Chapter 9

Melancholic Symptom Features

A. John Rush, M.D., and Jan E. Weissenburger, M.A.

Statement and Significance of the Issues

Historical Perspective on the Concept of Melancholia

Jackson (1986) provides the most thorough historical review of the concept of melancholia, covering 2,500 years from Hippocrates (4th and 5th centuries B.C.) to the present day. *Melancholia* is the Latin transliteration from Greek. The Greeks used the term to describe a mental disorder involving prolonged fear and depression. The Greek *melaina chole* translated into Latin as *atra bilis* and into English as black bile. Melancholia was thought to be one of a group of disorders (melancholic diseases) caused by black bile.

The notion of "without cause" was introduced in the 6th and 7th centuries. The inclusion of guilt in the description of melancholia began in the 16th century with the Reformation. The segregation of hypochondriasis from melancholia with physical symptoms (e.g., pain, gastrointestinal disturbances) was advanced by the works of Willis, Sydenham, and Boeihave. Melancholia with and without delusions was separated in the 19th century. The entry of the term into the popular language and the associated romanticization of the notion (e.g., love-melancholy, nostalgia) occurred in the late 18th century.

The further evolution of melancholia in the 19th century has been reviewed by Berrios (1988). The 19th century built six theoretical principles into our present concept of manic-depressive illness (Kraepelin's rejoining of melan-

Supported in part by a grant from the National Institute of Mental Health (MH-41115) to the Department of Psychiatry, UT Southwestern Medical Center.

We thank David Savage for secretarial assistance and Kenneth Z. Altshuler, M.D., Stanton Sharp Professor and Chairman, for administrative support. Special thanks to the members of the DSM-IV Mood Disorders Work Group, those who conducted the literature reviews, as well as to our many correspondents.

cholic and manic episodes [Kraepelin 1904]): 1) it was a "primary" disorder of affect rather than of intelligence or cognition (Bolton 1908), 2) it had a stable psychopathology (Foville 1882), 3) it had brain representation (Ritti 1876), 4) it was periodic in nature (Baillarger 1854; Falret 1854), 5) it was genetic (Foville 1882), and 6) it tended to appear in individuals with recognizable personality predispositions (Ritti 1876). The real causes of the episodes were endogenous in nature (Chaslin 1912).

The 20th century has witnessed both an evolution of the concept (melancholia/endogenous) and the development of a large number of measurement systems by which the notion may be operationalized. Of particular note is the fact that few investigators have actually concluded that the concept should be discarded. Rather, the debate has centered over measurement. For example, Kendell (1976) reviews the contemporary confusion in the classification of depression and concludes, "there is widespread agreement on the need to distinguish the two" (psychotic-endogenous and neurotic-reactive), and "it is increasingly clear that the former is more soundly based than the latter" (p. 25), a conclusion also reached by Mendels and Cochrane (1968) and echoed by Parker et al. (1989).

The early 20th century witnessed initial progress toward social acceptance of those with psychopathology. The term *depression* replaced *melancholia, alienists* became *psychiatrists,* and *very disturbed psychopathological states* became *reactions to life events* (Jackson 1986, pp. 195–202). During this social evolution, the diagnostic terms underwent a variety of changes. In 1896, Kraepelin, noted for his descriptive work, coined the term *manic-depressive psychosis* (Kraepelin 1904). He accepted Mobius's (1893) etiological classification of "exogenous" illnesses caused by bacterial, chemical, or other toxins and "endogenous" illnesses arising from degenerative or hereditary diseases. In 1913, Kraepelin wrote, "the principal demarcation in etiology is, above all, between internal and external causes. The two major groups of diseases, exogenous and endogenous, are thus naturally divided" (Kraepelin 1913, as cited in Mendels and Cochrane 1968, p.2)

This was in part the source of the nature/nurture split in the conceptualization of psychiatric disorders. This unfortunate link between phenomenology and etiology (bypassing the syndrome notion of Sydenham) has contributed to contemporary diagnostic controversy. Lange (1926, 1928) expanded this dichotomization by stating that endogenous (manic-depressive psychosis) depression, exogenous depression, and mixed forms could occur. Those endogenous depressions that followed some environmental stress were termed *reactive.*

In 1926, Mapother, the ultimate "lumper," stated that "in manic depressive psychosis, we are dealing with a merely quantitative deviation from normal (different only in prolongation or disastrous in its degree)." He included anxiety neuroses with depression, which resulted in much debate (Partridge 1949).

Mapother's view was based on three papers (his own M.D. thesis of 1929 and two papers by Lewis [1934, 1936]). He found the differential diagnostic task difficult in practice as well.

Gillespie (1929) was one of the very few to provide research data on this dispute. He divided 25 depressed patients into three groups: reactive or psychoneurotic, autonomous, and involutional. There was no difference in the occurrence of precipitating antecedents between the reactive and autonomous groups. The main difference was reactivity. The reactive patients showed emotional responses to environmental changes, whereas the autonomous group did not (i.e., reactivity of mood). Gillespie made no etiological inferences, but when his views were integrated with Kraepelin's, the mood-autonomous group was equated with the endogenous (manic-depressive psychosis) group (due to internal causes) and the mood-reactive group was equated with the exogenous group (due to external causes). Again, etiological and descriptive concepts were confused.

Lewis (1934) found 51 of 61 depressed patients had a history of a precipitating situation and concluded that reactive and endogenous depressions could not be separated. Note that 10 patients actually had no such precipitant, and others apparently had subsyndromal pathology before the precipitating event. Thus, Lewis' own data (without a control group) argue for some subdivision based on historical features (precipitant versus no precipitant).

The need to conceptually separate nosology from etiology was argued most strongly by Cattell (1943), who pointed out that "nosology necessarily precedes etiology." That is, a phenomenological separation is an essential first step by which to isolate subgroups of syndromes that can then be tested against various potential validators (family history, course, treatment response, genetics, biological tests, etc.) and in predicting response to electroconvulsive therapy (ECT).

The endogenous/reactive debate continued to confuse phenomenology with etiology until the late 1950s and early 1960s. With the advent of antidepressant medication and the recognition of the key role of ECT in severe depressions, researchers began to search for predictors of treatment response (clinical feature predictors, biological test predictors).

Throughout the 1960s and 1970s, a plethora of descriptive systems evolved that were based on descriptive statistical studies or on treatment prediction efforts. Notably, nearly all included a melancholic-like factor or subtype (e.g., Roth 1959 [endogenous depression]; van Praag et al. 1965 [vital depression]; Pollitt 1965 [physiological depression]; Overall et al. 1966 [retarded depression]; Paykel 1971 [psychotic depression]; Blinder 1966a, 1966b [physiological retarded depression]; Kendell 1968 [psychotic depression]; Winokur et al. 1988 [primary depression]; Kielholz 1972 [endogenous depression, including cyclic, periodic, involutional, and schizophrenic depression]).

The first specific diagnostic criteria in American psychiatry, the St. Louis criteria (Feighner et al. 1972), did not include a melancholic or endogenous subtype, although the subsequent Research Diagnostic Criteria (RDC) (Spitzer et al. 1978) did include a description of endogenous signs and symptoms.

By the late 1970s, the separation of life events from phenomenology per se had occurred. This resulted in the creation of an Axis IV diagnosis for DSM-III (American Psychiatric Association 1980). For Americans, the terms *endogenous* (RDC) or *melancholic* (DSM-III) had come to mean a constellation of signs and symptoms seen cross-sectionally in patients at the nadir of their episode without reference to the presence or absence of precipitating life events. However, in recent publications, one often finds bipolar, depressed-phase patients included "by definition" in a group with endogenous (RDC or DSM-III melancholic) unipolar patients, a throwback to the historical confounding of presumed etiology and cross-sectional phenomenology.

Klein (1974) attempted to separate stress and phenomenology. He combined endogenous (nonprecipitated) and endogenous (precipitated) into a new category termed *endogenomorphic,* hypothesizing a central defect in the pleasure/reward system and distinguished it from reactive depressions. Specific predictions were made with regard to medication-placebo differences in these two groups. Furthermore, a conceptual distinction between precipitating factors and symptom features was attained. One prediction is that nonendogenomorphic depressive patients should have a higher placebo response rate, which has been borne out (see below).

Historically, the concept of melancholic or endogenous features is longstanding. Until recently, however, conceptual confounding of etiology and phenomenology have been present. In the 1950s and 1960s, the term also began to imply a positive response to ECT and to antidepressant medication.

In this chapter, we update this historical picture using data from studies published between 1975 and 1992. Issues concerning the operationalization of the concept, the logical construction of items relevant to the concept, and validation attempts using treatment response, laboratory tests, family history, course of illness, and other "validators" are discussed in separate sections below.

Current Questions

In this chapter, we use the term *melancholic* (endogenous) to refer to patients who meet a set of descriptive criteria aimed at defining a categorical subdivision within the population of patients who are at the nadir of an episode of major depression. A number of different meanings (Hirschfeld and Katz 1978; Klerman 1980) have been attributed to the terms *endogenous* and *melancholic*. These terms may describe those depressions that 1) are not precipitated by stress, 2) are biological in etiology,

3) are unresponsive to environmental events, 4) are responsive to biological treatments, 5) occur in patients without personality pathology, and 6) exhibit a particular pattern of symptomatology. As noted above, the last approach was taken by both the RDC and DSM-III, in which patients were classified by a set of criteria, with the resulting classification expected to correspond to some or all of the other "endogenous" characteristics (1–6), thus providing external validation of the criteria or category.

In preparing this chapter, we addressed two specific questions: 1) Is there sufficient evidence for the validity of this subtype to support its continued inclusion in DSM-IV? and 2) What are the optimal operational clinical criteria by which to define melancholia?

Method

The first problem encountered in this review is the diversity of schemes by which the concept has been or is now being defined. Although historical evidence provides strong grounds for supposing that there is such an entity (clinicians seem to recognize melancholia when they see it), there is no coherent consensus regarding its specific definition. To address the question of validation, therefore, we have chosen reports that use a stated, explicit scheme for defining this category, whether it be ICD-9 (World Health Organization 1978), RDC, DSM-III, etc. Therefore, we begin this review with a comparison of the commonly used schemes for defining melancholia. We also logically cross-compare these schemes with an eye toward three clinically relevant questions: 1) Is melancholia just more severe depression? 2) What is a reasonably small number of signs and symptoms needed to define the category? and 3) Assuming that having different criteria for different age groups is simply not feasible, which of the various items used to define the endogenous/ melancholic category are most easily applied and are of the most utility in depressed children and adolescents?

We then examine the validity of the endogenous/melancholic subtype with regard to 1) internal validity of clinical descriptive information; 2) prediction of treatment response; 3) laboratory tests, including the dexamethasone suppression test (DST), polysomnogram (PSG), thyrotropin-releasing hormone (TRH) stimulation test (TRHST), and others; 4) the repetition of endogenous/melancholic features across episodes in patients with recurrent depression; 5) its relation to family history; and 6) its relation to a particular course of illness. The chapter concludes with an outline of strategic options for DSM-IV.

Results

A Logical Assessment of Current Operational Schemes

Over the last 30 years, a variety of operational definitions of the melancholic, endogenous, endogenomorphic concept have been put forth. They include 1) major depression with melancholia (DSM-III), 2) major depression with melancholic features (DSM-III-R) (American Psychiatric Association 1987), 3) endogenous depression (RDC), 4) World Health Organization (WHO) Depression Scale (Bech et al. 1980), 5) definite endogenous depression (Newcastle Scale Version I [NCS1]) (Bech et al. 1980; Carney et al. 1965), 6) definite endogenous depression (Newcastle Scale Version II [NCS2]) (Bech et al. 1980; Roth et al. 1983), 7) Hamilton Rating Scale for Depression (HRSD) (Hamilton 1960) Endogenomorphic Subscale (Kovacs et al. 1981; Thase et al. 1983), 8) definite endogenous depression (Michigan Discrimination Index [MDI] [Feinberg and Carroll 1982]), and 9) endogenous depression (Chicago Medical School Index [CMSI] [Taylor et al. 1981]).

Table 9–1 shows the criteria included in each of these nine systems. It illustrates the heterogeneity and the overlap across systems. We have divided the criteria into those that are based on signs and symptoms and those that are based on other characteristics, such as course of illness.

Psychomotor retardation is included in all nine systems. It is defined as behavior that is observed by the clinician (usually) or by family and/or patient. A threshold for declaring retardation present is usually not specified in the system. Rather, clinician judgment is required. How this sign/symptom relates to children and adolescents is unclear, although a few reports do indicate that it is found in this population.

Late insomnia is included in seven of the nine systems. Because this symptom may occur alone in transient situational disturbances (e.g., jet lag), some delimiting words are probably needed. Late insomnia appears more often in older than in younger adults. Its applicability to children and adolescents remains unclear. It is confounded with overall severity.

Early-morning worsening is included in seven of the nine systems. It is not included in the MDI or NCS1, both of which are statistically derived schemes. The applicability of the symptom to children also remains unclear. It is not confounded with the severity of depression.

Significant weight loss is included in seven of the nine systems. It is not included in NCS2 or the MDI. If weight loss is sudden, it may falsely include transient, situational adjustment reactions (e.g., being divorced, getting fired). It may be significant if it occurs over a longer period. This symptom is confounded with the overall severity of depression.

Table 9–1. Diagnostic criteria for "melancholic" depression according to nine major classification systems

Criterion items	Diagnostic system									Total
	DSM-III	DSM-III-R	RDC	WHO	NCS1	NCS2	HRSD	MDI	CHI	
Symptoms										
Psychomotor retardation	X	X	X	X	X	X	X	X	X	9
Late insomnia	X	X	X	X		X	X		X	7
A.M. worsening	X	X	X	X		X	X		X	7
Weight loss	X	X	X	X			X	X	X	7
Psychomotor agitation		X	X		X		X	X	X	6
Guilt	X		X		X		X		X	5
Anhedonia	X	X	X		X					4
Distinct quality	X		X	X	X					4
Appetite loss	X	X	X					X		4
Delusions				X	X	X		X		4
Unreactivity	X	X	X							3
Loss of interest			X				X	X		3
Middle insomnia			X				X			2
Hopelessness							X			1
Suicidal thoughts/behavior									X	1
Sad, anxious, dysphoric									X	1
Course features										
No personality disturbance		X		X	X				X	4
No precipitants				X	X			X		3
Recurrent course				X	X					2
Sudden onset				X		X				2
Duration of illness				X		X				2
Persistent depression				X		X				2
Pyknic body type					X					1
Complete interepisode recovery		X								1
Previous somatic treatment response		X								1

Psychomotor agitation is included in six of the nine systems. It is not included in DSM-III, WHO, or NCS2. It must be observed to count as positive. It may be highly related to delusions. It is less constantly present than psychomotor retardation and occurs relatively infrequently.

Guilt is included in five of the nine systems. It is not included in DSM-III-R, WHO, NCS2, or the HRSD. This symptom is difficult to distinguish from self-blame. Pathological guilt is infrequent in Westernized (Nelson and Charney 1980) and underdeveloped (Marsella 1987) countries. It may be difficult to elicit in children. It is confounded with severity.

Distinct quality to mood is included in four of the nine systems (DSM-III, RDC, WHO, NCS1). It needs both a threshold and specific definition. It requires the patient to have had prior experience with a major loss and therefore may be difficult to elicit in children. It is not confounded with severity.

Anhedonia is included in four of the nine systems (DSM-III, DSM-III-R, RDC, MDI). All American systems include this symptom. The threshold needs to be defined. In theory, it is one of the core features of melancholia. It is also found in children. If the item reduced interest/pleasure in major depression became only reduced interest, anhedonia would not be confounded with overall severity.

Appetite loss is included in four of the nine systems (DSM-III, DSM-III-R, RDC, MDI). It has a high likelihood of occurrence if there is weight loss. Weight loss without appetite loss should exclude weight loss as a positive symptom, because it suggests the presence of another disease.

Delusions are included in four of the nine systems (WHO, NCS1, NCS2, MDI). They are infrequent overall (Nelson and Chaney 1980) and are very rare in outpatients. Three of the four systems including this symptom are European. It is included as part of the severity scaling in DSM-III and DSM-III-R systems and therefore is confounded with severity. Parenthetically, current evidence would argue somewhat against delusional depression being a variation on severity. Delusions 1) repeat across episodes, 2) predict differential response to tricyclics alone, 3) predict a positive response to ECT, 4) run in families, 5) are separable from anhedonic psychomotor retarded depression (Nelson and Charney 1980), and 6) were historically separated out in the 1880s.

Unreactivity of mood is included in three of the nine systems (DSM-III, DSM-III-R, RDC). All systems including this symptom are American. It may be difficult to separate from anhedonia. It has a theoretical basis for inclusion. It is not confounded with overall severity. The threshold is not well specified, however (e.g., half-way to normal mood for how many minutes?).

Loss of interest is included in three of the nine systems (RDC, HRSD, MDI). This symptom is very nonspecific. It is found in many other diseases and in nearly all depressions and is therefore likely to produce a high percentage of false positives. It is confounded with severity.

Middle insomnia is included in two of the nine systems (RDC, HRSD). If it is present without late insomnia, it probably identifies false positives. It is important to distinguish middle insomnia from late insomnia with operational criteria. It is confounded with overall severity.

Hopelessness, suicidal, and dysphoric are each included in one of the nine systems. They are all nonspecific. Many systems include other features that go beyond signs or symptoms. Their inclusion partly reflects the diversity of meanings of the term, as well as attempts to improve prognostication or treatment selection using the endogenous/melancholic concept. As these systems have evolved, there has been an unevenness in the introduction of these items that are not symptoms or signs. In some cases, the introduction has been based on statistical study (e.g., NCS1), whereas in others (e.g., DSM-III-R, CHI) clinical consensus formed the basis for the changes.

No personality disorder is included in four of the nine systems (DSM-III-R, WHO, NCS1, CHI). This is difficult to assess during a depressive episode. Logically, there is no reason to expect that a personality disorder would protect an individual from developing a melancholic depression. It is not likely to be predictive of biological responsiveness. The diagnosis of an Axis II disorder continues to be relatively unreliable.

No precipitant is included in three of the systems (WHO, NCS1, MDI). This feature is reported to be rare because much empirical evidence suggests that melancholic features often occur in the presence of precipitants (Leff et al. 1970). In DSM-IV, it will only confound Axes I and IV.

Recurrent course is included in two of the nine systems (WHO, NCS1). There are data suggesting that a recurrent course does not differentiate RDC endogenous from nonendogenous depressions (Rush et al. 1989a). Furthermore, seasonal affective disorder is recurrent but is unlikely to have endogenous/melancholic features (i.e., this fact increases false positives). The first episode of depression can be melancholic based on symptom features, but by requiring a recurrent course, such cases would be less likely to be so labeled. Many nonmelancholic (nonendogenous) depressions are also episodic.

Sudden onset is included in two of the nine systems (WHO, NCS2). Because situational adjustment reactions are also often sudden in onset, inclusion of this feature would logically increase false positives. A negative rating for slow onset is difficult to employ clinically.

Duration of illness is included in two of the nine systems (WHO, NCS2). It is defined as positive if the duration of the current episode is greater than 3 months. To our knowledge, there are no empirical data to support or refute this notion. The interest here may be to reduce the likelihood of including situational adjustment reaction with insomnia and weight or appetite loss. It hinges on the notion that course and symptoms/signs are strongly related.

Persistence of depression (depressed mood) is included in two of the nine systems (WHO, NCS2). It is defined as positive in NCS2 if the depressed mood is present every day without remission. In WHO, it is defined as positive if the reduction in the HRSD score at the end of the placebo period is 39% or less from the baseline score. The degree to which this overlaps with unreactivity of mood is unclear. It is probably addressing a similar clinical notion. Note that this feature is European, whereas unreactive mood is American. If we equate the two, then five of nine systems (three American and two European) contain this feature. It is not confounded with severity. It has a long history, beginning with Gillespie (1929).

Pyknic body type is only included in NCS1. It is a vintage feature with no empirical evidence to support its relationship to melancholia.

Good interepisode recovery is only included in DSM-III-R. This feature also applies to seasonal affective disorders and nonendogenous depressions (see Rush et al. 1989a). In fact, the degree of interepisode recovery does not distinguish endogenous from nonendogenous depression (Giles et al. 1987; Rush et al. 1989a). It is difficult for the patient to rate this feature while depressed. Recovery may depend on both medication and natural history. This feature can, by definition, only be rated for recurrent depressions; therefore, it may be more difficult to apply equally to children, who are less likely to have had prior episodes of depression. Finally, the reliability of patient recall involving prior history may be reduced during an episode.

Positive response to biological treatment is only included in DSM-III-R. This feature eliminates patients with treatment-resistant depression, many of whom have melancholic features, who do not respond to ECT. Not all patients are exposed to such treatment. Positive response to somatic therapy assumes a degree of specificity for melancholia that may be untrue (depending on how melancholia is defined); therefore, it can bias the sample and create false positives (i.e., some melancholic depressions respond to tricyclics and many nonendogenous depressions respond to placebo alone). It is difficult to apply in children, who have had less of an opportunity for exposure to biological treatments for depression.

Can Patients With Melancholic Features Be Differentiated From Those Without Melancholic Features Based on Clinical/Descriptive Studies?

Farmer and McGuffin (1989) review the current status of the classification debate. A variety of multivariate statistical techniques have been applied to the examination of subtypes of depression over the past 20 years. Although some have argued against their use in the study of classification (Kendell 1974; Maxwell 1971; Paykel 1981), these have primarily included factor and principal component analyses of the signs and symptoms commonly associated with depression, as well as cluster and latent class analyses applied to persons having depressive diagnoses (Paykel 1971). Parker et al. (1989) have recently provided an extensive review of this literature. They present a summary regarding the results relevant to the endogenous/melancholic subtype. This review focuses on the nine major factor analytically based studies that confirm the endogenous construct. Parker et al. (1989) did not examine the literature based on latent class and cluster analytic methods in their review. Such a review was prevented, in the case of latent class analyses, by the small number of studies available and their inconsistent results. Results of studies using cluster analytic techniques are also inconsistent and are plagued by theoretical disagreements about what is the appropriate type of clustering method to use.

Parker et al. (1989) used several quantitative analyses to examine the consistencies in results of the nine major studies they reviewed. They sought to assess both the extent to which the studies identified a consistent set of endogenous features and the relative importance of the identified features to the diagnosis of endogenous depression. Studies included were limited to those sampling clinical groups of patients with diagnoses of primary depression. Because only studies that reported finding an endogenous factor were included, they differ somewhat from the set of studies reviewed earlier by Nelson and Charney (1980) and Mendels and Cochrane (1968). Symptom features analyzed by Parker et al. (1989) were those that had been included in at least three of the nine studies reviewed.

Indices of consistency revealed a moderate to high degree of agreement in the factor loadings between most studies, with lower agreement for only three studies. This suggests that the studies, in general, identified similar sets of endogenous features. The features occurring most regularly included severity, psychomotor retardation, lack of a precipitant, nonreactivity, older age, not immature/hysterical, adequate personality, not hypochondriacal, distinct quality of mood, nondiurnal variability, delusions/paranoid features, and guilt. Features less consistently related to the endogenous factor across studies include terminal insomnia, agitation, diurnal variation, weight loss, and obsessional symptoms and personality. In summary, the results suggest that endogenous depression is most consistently associated with normal personality, lack of a clear precipitant, nonreactivity to environmental events, severe depression, and a small number of clinical features, which are fewer in number than what had previously been suggested by Rosenthal and Klerman (1966). This difference may be related to the restrictive criteria for inclusion of studies and variables in the review by Parker et al. (1989).

In an important latent class analysis of 788 patients from the National Institute of Mental Health (NIMH) Collaborative Study of the Psychobiology of Depression (77% inpatients, 24% bipolar, 17% psychotic), Young et al. (1986) found two endogenous/melancholic subtypes, anhedonic and vegetative, based on the Schedule for Affective Disorders and Schizophrenia (SADS) (Endicott and Spitzer 1978) data. The anhedonic subtype was characterized by unreactive mood, whereas the distinctive feature in the vegetative subtype was weight loss. Both subtypes evidenced lack of pleasure, distinct quality to mood, and psychomotor retardation. The vegetative subtype by itself was rare (5%), whereas the combination of the two subtypes was common (51.6%). The anhedonic subtype alone was present in 25% of cases, and 20% lacked both subtypes. The anhedonic subtype is akin to Klein's (1974) endogenomorphic depression and to Nelson and Charney's (1980) autonomous depression. Consistent with Young et al. (1986), Hibbert et al. (1984) reported that anhedonic and vegetative symptoms did not covary over time. Waldman (1982) found that diurnal variation with morning worsening is less common in more severe depression.

Young et al. (1986) rarely found vegetative symptoms in depressive patients who were not anhedonic and suggested two distinct types. Bebbington et al. (1988) and McGuffin et al. (1988a, 1988b) failed to show any differences in antecedent adversity between endogenous and nonendogenous based on the CATEGO classification system (Wing et al. 1974).

Do Melancholic Features Predict Treatment Response?

The sedation threshold, with endogenous depressions having a lower threshold, separates endogenous psychotic from neurotic depressive patients in most (Boudreau 1958; Nymgaard 1959; Shagass and Jones 1958) but not all (Roberts 1959a, 1959b) studies. Busfield et al. (1961) and Strongin and Hinsie (1939) found less salivary secretion in endogenous and nonendogenous depressions. Roberts (1959a, 1959b) and Monro and Conitzer (1950) found that neurotic depressions improved with a single intravenous methylamphetamine challenge, whereas endogenous depressions actually worsened.

With the advent of antidepressant medications and the recognition of the efficacy of ECT in severe depressions, a search for predictors of ECT response (clinical features, biological tests, etc.) was initiated. Hobson (1953) found a good outcome with sudden onset, good insight, self-reproach, short duration, and obsessional personality. Roth (1959) and Sargent (1961) also found ECT better in endogenous than nonendogenous depressions. Others also reported that endogenous depressions respond more favorably than nonendogenous depressions to ECT (Carney et al. 1965; Cook 1944; Mendels 1965, 1967; Rose 1963; Sands 1946; Sargent and Slater 1946). In fact, there have been no negative studies to date in this regard. There has been a report that nonendogenous depressions may be made worse with ECT (Sargent 1961). Crow et al. (1984) compared fictitious versus real ECT in 70 inpatients (62 subjects completed a total of eight treatments). Differences between the two treatments were significant for the delusional and retarded groups but not for the other groups. A similar finding has been noted more recently with sleep deprivation. These findings are notable because, if endogenous depression is simply a more severe form of nonendogenous depression, then a treatment that is effective for the more severe form should not make the milder form of the illness worse. Similar differential predictions of treatment response to imipramine (Kiloh et al. 1962) and to phenelzine (Harrington and Imlah 1960) have been noted.

Mendels and Cochrane (1968) summarized seven factor analytic studies, finding a common endogenous feature factor consisting of retardation, deep depression, unreactive mood, severe loss of interest, and visceral (gastrointestinal) symptoms. For these, there was a high loading across all seven studies. Moderate loading (.30–.40) was associated with lack of a precipitant, middle insomnia, and lack of self-pity. Fair agreement across studies included weight loss, early-morning awakening, guilt, and normal personality.

Brown et al. (1982), in a retrospective chart review of 64 inpatients with RDC major depression, found that 6 of 7 psychotic patients responded to ECT, whereas only 3 of 18 responded to tricyclic antidepressants.

Riesby et al. (1977) found a negative correlation between end-of-treatment HRSD (day 35) and imipramine plus desipramine steady-state levels for the endogenous (but not for the nonendogenous) group. Gibbons et al. (1982), in a reanalysis of the data, found that pretreatment psychomotor retardation and decreased libido clearly differentiated treatment responders from nonresponders. Abou-Saleh and Coppen (1983) reported that those in the middle range on the Newcastle diagnostic scale responded best to ECT ($n = 78$) and to antidepressant medication ($n = 122$), replicating prior reports by Rao and Coppen (1979) and Millin and Coppen (1980). With inpatients, the endogenous subtype may be predictive of response to S-adenosylmethionine (SAM) (Carney et al. 1986).

Turning to outpatient studies, the issue of prediction remains unclear. Simpson et al. (1988) found an 85% response rate to trimipramine in 20 RDC endogenous outpatients (no control group), although the rate is higher than expected (60%–70%) for mixed outpatient groups. Prusoff and Paykel (1977) studied four outpatient subgroups (psychotic, anxious, hostile, and young with personality disorder; $N = 143$) who were treated with amitriptyline and found that the psychotic patients responded best and the anxious group fared least well.

Prusoff et al. (1980) found that patients with RDC endogenous depression did poorly with interpersonal psychotherapy (IPT) (Klerman et al. 1984) alone, and best with the combination of IPT and amitriptyline (IPT alone was no more effective than unscheduled treatment in RDC endogenous depression). Patients with RDC nonendogenous depression did best with IPT alone, a finding that was not replicated in the more recent report of the NIMH Treatment of Depression

Collaborative Research Program (Elkin et al. 1989).

Paykel et al. (1988) studied 141 outpatients (100 with major depression and 41 with minor depression by RDC) who were treated with antidepressants by general practitioners and found no differential response prediction based on melancholic features. Georgatos et al. (1987) found no differences in response rates by endogenous/nonendogenous or melancholic/nonmelancholic subtypes in older (over 55 years of age) depressed outpatients following a 7-day placebo washout. However, the small sample size may have precluded a definitive answer.

Coryell and Turner (1985) reported that RDC endogenous or nonendogenous depression did not predict differential response in 42 outpatients treated with desipramine. Given the small number of RDC endogenous completers ($n = 12$), however, interpretations are tentative. Rush et al. (1989b) also failed to find a preferential response for the RDC endogenous/nonendogenous subtype in a sample of 42 outpatients treated with desipramine or amitriptyline.

Conversely, endogenous/melancholic outpatients appear to have a poorer placebo response than their nonmelancholic counterparts. Davidson et al. (1988), in a three-center study of 174 outpatients, found a low placebo response rate in RDC endogenous, NCS1 endogenous, and DSM-III melancholic subtypes. This is consistent with other reports in outpatients (Fairchild et al. 1986) and inpatients (Nelson et al. 1990).

The relatively better predictions obtained with inpatients versus outpatients based on the melancholic/endogenous features may be due to 1) a higher placebo response rate in the nonendogenous outpatient than in the nonendogenous inpatient groups noted above, 2) poor specificity/sensitivity of the definitions used for endogenous (e.g., the category is too restrictive), or 3) the relative diagnostic selectivity of ECT versus tricyclics in remediating various forms of depression.

Do Melancholic Features Relate to Laboratory Test Findings?

Research evidence addressing the differential discrimination of a distinct melancholic subtype of depression based on biological functioning is reviewed for 1) the DST, 2) sleep PSG characteristics, 3) TRHST, and 4) other laboratory tests.

Dexamethasone suppression test (DST).   Much research has examined the DST in relation to endogenous or melancholic subtypes. The major work in this area is summarized in Tables 9–2 through 9–5. Only studies involving a minimum of 40 patients were included. Five of seven inpatient studies that compared the DST to the RDC endogenous/nonendogenous dichotomy were positive, Stokes et al. (1984) and Zimmerman et al. (1985a) being the only negative studies (Table 9–2). Zimmerman et al. (1985a) did not report a normal control sample, and some patients were diagnosed without a structured interview. The Stokes et al. (1984)

Table 9–2. Dexamethasone suppression test studies comparing Research Diagnostic Criteria endogenous versus nonendogenous

Author	Interview method	Dose (mg)	Sample time	Threshold (μg/dl)	Patient status	Subjects	N	% NS
Brown and Shuey 1980	Clinical	2.0	8 A.M., 4 P.M., 11:30 P.M.	6.0	Inpatient	Endogenous	6	67
						Nonendogenous	43	16
Carroll et al. 1981	Clinical/ SADS (73%)	1.0	8 A.M., 4 P.M., 11:30 P.M.	5.0	Inpatient	Endogenous	54	67
						Nonendogenous + other	22	4
Rush et al. 1983	SADS-L	1.0	8 A.M., 4 P.M., 11 P.M.	4.0	Inpatient	Endogenous (UP + BP)	46	48
						Nonendogenous (UP)	11	9
Davidson et al. 1984	Clinical	1.0	4 P.M.	5.0	Inpatient	Endogenous	40	40
						Probable endogenous + nonendogenous	9	10
Stokes et al. 1984	SADS	1.0	8:30 A.M.	5.0	Inpatient	Definite + probable endogenous	94	29
						Nonendogenous	17	47
Zimmerman et al. 1985a	Clinical/SADS	1.0	8 A.M., 4 P.M.	5.0	Inpatient	Endogenous (UP + BP)	107	36
						Probable endogenous (UP + BP)	31	32
						Nonendogenous (UP + BP)	21	33
Kumar et al. 1986	SADS	1.0	4 P.M., 11 P.M.	5.0	Inpatient	Endogenous (UP + BP)	46	61
						Probable endogenous	23	52
						Nonendogenous	4	0
Carroll et al. 1980	Clinical/ SADS	1.0	4 P.M.	6.0	Outpatient	Endogenous	38	42
						Probable endogenous	21	14
						Nonendogenous	13	8
Giles and Rush 1982	SADS-L	1.0, 2.0	4 P.M.	4.0	Outpatient	Endogenous	55	44
						Nonendogenous	95	4

(continued)

Table 9–2. Dexamethasone suppression test studies comparing Research Diagnostic Criteria endogenous versus nonendogenous *(continued)*

Author	Interview method	Dose (mg)	Sample time	Threshold (µg/dl)	Patient status	Subjects	N	% NS
Rush et al. 1982	SADS-L	1.0, 2.0	4 P.M.	4.0	Outpatient	Endogenous	32	41
						Nonendogenous	38	5
Peselow et al. 1983	Clinical	1.0	4 P.M.	4.0	Outpatient	Endogenous	52	33
						Nonendogenous	36	22
Rabkin et al. 1983	Clinical	1.0, 2.0	4 P.M.	5.0	Outpatient	Endogenous	33	18
						Nonendogenous	21	14
Calloway et al. 1984	Clinical	1.0	4 P.M.	5.0	Outpatient	Endogenous	34	56
						Probable endogenous	15	47
						Nonendogenous	23	26
Giles et al. 1987	SADS-L	1.0	4 P.M.	4.0	Outpatient	Endogenous	37	41
						Nonendogenous	58	15
Peselow et al. 1987	Clinical/SADS	1.0	4 P.M.	5.0	Outpatient	Endogenous	73	36
						Nonendogenous	54	13

Note. SADS = Schedule for Affective Disorders and Schizophrenia. SADS-L = Schedule for Affective Disorders and Schizophrenia, Lifetime Version (Endicott and Spitzer 1978). BP = bipolar. NS = nonsuppression. UP = unipolar.

Table 9–3. Dexamethasone suppression test studies comparing Newcastle endogenous versus neurotic

Author	Interview method	Dose (mg)	Sample time	Threshold (µg/dl)	Patient status	Subjects	N	% NS
McIntyre et al. 1981	Clinical	1.0	8 A.M., 4 P.M.	5.0	Inpatient	Endogenous	70	51
						Neurotic	27	4
Coppen et al. 1983	Clinical	1.0	3–4 P.M.	5.0	Inpatient	Endogenous	78	81
						Neurotic	41	49
Holden 1983	Clinical	1.0	4 P.M., 11 P.M.	4.0	Inpatient	Endogenous	22	73
						Neurotic	19	11
Kasper and Beckmann 1983	Clinical	1.0	8 A.M.	4.0	Inpatient	Endogenous	41	53
						Neurotic	26	23
Ames et al. 1984	Clinical	1.0	4 P.M.	5.0	Inpatient	Endogenous	28	39
						Neurotic	62	31
Davidson et al. 1984	Clinical	1.0	4 P.M.	5.0	Inpatient	Endogenous	27	48
						Neurotic	19	11
Zimmerman et al. 1985a	Semistructured interview	1.0	8 A.M., 4 P.M.	5.0	Inpatient	Endogenous	59	48
						Neurotic	100	28
Holsboer et al. 1980	Clinical	2.0	4 P.M.	5.0	Outpatient	Endogenous	37	30
						Neurotic	56	14
Calloway et al. 1984	Clinical	1.0	4 P.M.	5.0	Outpatient	Endogenous	36	47
						Neurotic	36	42

Note. NS = nonsuppression.

Table 9–4. Dexamethasone suppression test studies comparing DSM-III melancholic versus nonmelancholic

Author	Interview method	Dose (mg)	Sample time	Threshold (µg/dl)	Patient status	Subjects	N	% NS
Coryell et al. 1982	Chart review + interview	1.0	8 A.M., 4 P.M.	5.0	Inpatient	Melancholic	34	27
						Nonmelancholic	17	35
Arana et al. 1983	Clinical	1.0	4 P.M.	4.5	Inpatient	Melancholic	15	40
						Nonmelancholic	14	57
Johnson et al. 1984	Clinical	1.0	8 A.M., 4 P.M.	5.0	Inpatient	Melancholic	14	43
						Nonmelancholic	42	38
Stokes et al. 1984	SADS	1.0	8:30 A.M.	5.0	Inpatient	Melancholic	37	24
						Nonmelancholic	74	35
Zimmerman et al. 1985a	Clinical/SADS	1.0	8 A.M., 4 P.M.	5.0	Inpatient	Melancholic	70	44
						Nonmelancholic	89	28
Cook et al. 1986	Clinical	1.0	4 P.M.	5.0	Inpatient	Melancholic	19	58
						Nonmelancholic	50	6
Rubin et al. 1987	Clinical/SADS	1.0	7 A.M., 3 P.M., 11 P.M.	3.5	Inpatient	Melancholic	16	44
						Nonmelancholic (endogenous)	24	33
Brown et al. 1988	Clinical	1.0	9 A.M.	5.0	Inpatient	Melancholic	73	84
						Nonmelancholic	17	24
Gitlin et al. 1984	Clinical + chart review	1.0	4 P.M.	5.0	Outpatient	Melancholic	86	38
						Nonmelancholic	23	35

Note. SADS = Schedule for Affective Disorders and Schizophrenia. SADS-L = Schedule for Affective Disorders and Schizophrenia, Lifetime Version (Endicott and Spitzer 1978). NS = nonsuppression.

sample contained only 17 nonendogenous patients, the sample was not consecutive, and only the 8:00 A.M. serum cortisol determination was used.

Six of the eight outpatient studies comparing the DST to the RDC endogenous/nonendogenous dichotomy were positive (Table 9–2). Neither of the two negative studies utilized a structured interview method. In summary, the majority of studies using RDC (11 of 15) have found significantly higher rates of DST nonsuppression among RDC endogenous compared with nonendogenous patients.

Similarly, six of nine studies using the NCS1 or NCS2 found higher DST nonsuppression rates among endogenous patients (Table 9–3). With the NCS, six of seven inpatient studies were positive, whereas neither of the two outpatient studies were positive. Given this split between inpatient and outpatient studies, it may be that the NCS1 and NCS2 are a bit restrictive in relation to the DST.

Conversely, only three of nine studies comparing DSM-III melancholic and nonmelancholic subtypes found significantly higher DST nonsuppression rates among the melancholic group. Notable is the consistently higher incidence of DST nonsuppression in the DSM-III nonmelancholic versus the RDC nonendogenous group, which may account for the failure to differentiate DSM-III melancholic and nonmelancholic groups. These data suggest that the DSM-III classification of melancholia is too restrictive to provide discrimination based on the DST. That is, the DSM-III nonmelancholic group in most of these studies contained large percentages of DST nonsuppressors. This notion was recently tested by Kraemer and Rush (unpublished data, 1994) in a set of 487 depressed patients. The RDC endogenous/nonendogenous, but not the DSM-III melancholic/nonmelancholic,

Table 9–5. Summary of results on dexamethasone suppression test (DST) and depressive subtypes

	Inpatient			Outpatient		
System	Positive studies	N	% DST NS	Positive studies	N	% DST NS
RDC	5/7			6/8		
Endogenous		393	50		354	39
Nonendogenous		127	16		338	13
DSM-III	3/8			0/1		
Melancholic		278	45		86	38
Nonmelancholic		327	32		23	35
Newcastle	6/7			0/2		
Endogenous		325	56		73	38
Neurotic		294	22		92	28

dichotomy related significantly to DST status. There are currently no studies of the DST in relation to DSM-III-R melancholic features.

Polysomnogram (PSG). Four distinct, but not pathognomic, PSG abnormalities have been consistently found in studies of symptomatic depressed patients.

The first, disturbed sleep continuity, includes prolonged sleep latency, mid-nocturnal awakenings, multiple stage changes, and terminal insomnia (Gillin et al. 1984). Sleep continuity disturbances may be related to a lower threshold for arousal to sound (Zung 1969). They tend to be more severe in older patients (Gillin et al. 1981). The overall effect of these disturbances is that sleep in depressed patients is inefficient (i.e., a smaller portion of time spent in bed is actually spent sleeping). Sleep efficiency may be especially low in psychotically depressed patients (Kupfer et al. 1978).

Second, depressed patients demonstrate reduced or absent deeper stages of sleep (stages 3 and 4), whereas more stage 1 sleep may be found. Although delta sleep decreases with age in both depressed patients and normal individuals, it is consistently lower at every age in depressed patients (reviewed by Gillin et al. 1984).

Third, and perhaps the most widely accepted and replicable abnormality, is the presence of a reduced first non–rapid-eye-movement (REM) period, with a sub-sequent early appearance of the first REM period following sleep onset. This reduced REM latency, although not unique to depression, is consistently found in all published studies of depressed patients. A REM latency threshold of less than 60 minutes distinguished endogenous from nonendogenous depressed outpa-tients, with a diagnostic confidence of 83% (Rush et al. 1982). PSG findings in bipolar disorder, depressed phase, are similar to those found in unipolar depres-sion, especially in unipolar endogenous depression (Duncan et al. 1979; Giles et al. 1986) (see Reynolds and Shipley 1985 for a review). There may be a relationship between the severity of illness and REM latency in that more severely depressed patients may demonstrate an even shorter REM latency than the less severely depressed (Kupfer and Foster 1972).

The fourth finding in the PSG of depressed patients is an altered temporal distribution of REM sleep. REM sleep appears to be shifted so that more occurs toward the beginning of the night, which is partly accounted for by reduced REM latency. However, a relatively normal REM-to-REM cycle length is maintained. Finally, there is an increased REM density in the first one to three REM periods (Kupfer and Thase 1983).

Within major depression, the RDC primary/secondary dichotomy appeared to be a valid categorical distinction based on early PSG studies. For example, Kupfer (1976) and Coble et al. (1976) discriminated primary from secondary major depressive disorder with a greater than 80% accuracy, based on REM latency and

REM density. Gillin et al. (1979) reported that reduced REM latency was characteristic of 64% of patients with primary major depression. Akiskal (1981) successfully distinguished patients with primary depression, patients with secondary depression, and healthy control subjects with 90% accuracy, using a REM latency threshold of less than 70 minutes on two consecutive nights of PSG recording.

Most (Feinberg et al. 1982; Giles et al. 1987; Rush et al. 1982, 1983), but not all (Berger et al. 1983), recent reports that have evaluated the RDC endogenous/nonendogenous distinction have found validation by the PSG. In fact, the preponderance of RDC endogenous depressions are found in the group with primary depression. That is, the RDC endogenous/nonendogenous distinction rather than the RDC primary/secondary dichotomy was validated by the PSG. In fact, some patients with depressive syndromes "secondary" to other psychiatric disorders such as substance abuse, obsessive-compulsive disorder, generalized anxiety disorder, subaffective dysthymia, and schizophrenia also evidence reduced REM latency (Gillin et al. 1984; Reynolds and Kupfer 1987).

As noted above, the DST provides information about the functional integrity of the hypothalamic-pituitary-adrenal (HPA) axis. The PSG and DST have been combined in five studies that relate either or both findings to descriptive diagnostic subtypes. Rush et al. (1982) studied 70 adult patients with RDC nonpsychotic, unipolar major depression using both the PSG and the DST. In this largely outpatient sample, the DST was both specific (95%) and accurate (confidence interval 87%), although its sensitivity was low (41%). A REM latency of less than 62 minutes provided a more sensitive (66%), but less specific (79%), indicator of RDC endogenous versus nonendogenous depression. DST nonsuppression was nearly always accompanied by a significant reduction in REM latency (only one DST nonsuppressor evidenced a mean REM latency of greater than 62 minutes). This finding has been replicated by Feinberg et al. (1982), Giles et al. (1987), Mendelwicz et al. (1984), Rush et al. (1983; unpublished data, 1994b). Conversely, over 40% of RDC endogenous outpatients showed neither DST nor PSG abnormality, although they were equivalent in symptom severity as measured by the 17-item HRSD.

Mendelwicz et al. (1984) found that the DST provided 100% specificity and 67% sensitivity, whereas REM latency showed a lower specificity of 78% and a higher sensitivity of 85% in 39 depressed inpatients compared to 9 normal control subjects. Kerkhofs et al. (1986) compared 27 age-matched DST suppressors to 27 DST nonsuppressors. The DST nonsuppressors had significantly shorter REM latency, less slow-wave sleep, and more awake time than did DST suppressors. All had diagnoses of RDC endogenous major depression. The groups were similar with regard to depressive symptom severity as measured by the HRS-D. Not Rush et al. (1982), Mendelwicz et al. (1984), or Kerkhofs et al. (1986) reported a difference in REM density between DST suppressors and nonsuppressors.

In a subsequent larger replication, Giles et al. (1987) found that the incidence of both DST nonsuppression and reduced REM latency was higher in a sample of 103 patients with RDC endogenous depression. In addition, patients with probable RDC endogenous depression were not different from RDC nonendogenous in this study. A REM latency of less than 65 minutes provided a sensitive (68%) and a somewhat specific (58%) indicator of endogenous versus nonendogenous depression. Again, the vast majority of DST nonsuppressors evidenced reduced REM latency.

In summary, all five available studies relating both the PSG and DST to the endogenous subtype have similar findings; namely, both reduced REM latency and DST nonsuppression are more likely in the endogenous subtype, and about half of those with reduced REM latency also evidence DST nonsuppression (Feinberg et al. 1982; Giles et al. 1987; Mendelwicz et al. 1984; Rush et al. 1982, 1983, unpublished data, 1994b). Conversely, over 40% of RDC endogenous outpatients evidenced neither DST nor PSG abnormalities, although they had equivalent symptom severity, whereas the vast majority of DST nonsuppressors evidenced reduced REM latency.

As recently reviewed (Debus and Rush 1990; Kryger et al. 1989), PSG abnormalities generally provide validation of the RDC endogenous/nonendogenous dichotomy (Feinberg et al. 1982; Giles et al. 1987; Rush et al. 1982, 1983). Estimates of the sensitivity of reduced REM latency in detecting endogenous/melancholic depression lie in the area of 60%–80%. In the only study to date that examined specific symptoms, Giles et al. (1986) reported a significant association between reduced REM latency and the RDC endogenous symptoms of terminal insomnia, pervasive anhedonia, unreactive mood, and appetite loss in an almost exclusively outpatient sample of 103 endogenously depressed patients. To our knowledge, there are no negative studies relating the PSG to the RDC endogenous/nonendogenous subdivision.

Thyrotropin-releasing hormone stimulation test (TRHST). Despite early indications that the TSH response to TRH may be a specific marker of biological alterations in endogenous depression (Loosen and Prange 1982), recent studies are not consistent in this regard. The possible confounding effects of age and gender have brought some results into question (Baumgartner et al. 1986; Cuttelod et al. 1974; Olsen et al. 1978; Snyder and Utiger 1972; Wenzel et al. 1974). In addition, lack of specificity has limited the usefulness of the TRHST as a discriminator of endogenous/melancholic depression (Baumgartner et al. 1986; Kirkegaard et al. 1978; Langer et al. 1984; Rubin et al. 1987). Overall, the sensitivity of the TRHST for endogenous/melancholic depression is approximately 25%–35% (Aggernaes et al. 1983; Kirkegaard and Faber 1981; Rush et al. 1983). The greater incidence of

DST nonsuppression than TRHST blunting among endogenous/melancholic patients suggests that an underlying dysfunction in the HPA system may be more central to this type of depression. Studies examining both the DST and TRHST in the same patients have generally found substantial noncorrespondence between results of the two tests (Asnis et al. 1981; Dam et al. 1984; Extein et al. 1981; Kupfer et al. 1984; Larsen et al. 1985; Rubin et al. 1987). This noncorrespondence may in part be due to a liberal threshold for declaring the TRHST abnormal or blunted, however. In a recent comparison, Rush et al. (unpublished data, 1994a) used a threshold of 5.0 IU/ml (as based on a large normal control study [Schlesser et al. 1983]) and found that the vast majority of TRHST blunters were also DST nonsuppressors, whereas many DST nonsuppressors had normal TRHSTs. Furthermore, the TRHST significantly differentiated RDC endogenous from nonendogenous depression.

The substantial rate of abnormal blunting to TRHST in nondepressed psychiatric groups (alcoholism, anorexia nervosa, and borderline personality disorder) suggests that these diagnostic groups may share a common biological alteration that is detected by the TRHST (Loosen 1985; Loosen and Prange 1982).

Only two studies (Rush et al. 1983, unpublished data, 1994a) have contrasted the PSG and TRHST and endogenous/melancholic subtypes. Because Rush et al. (unpublished data, 1994a) include the sample reported in Rush et al. (1983), only the latter study is discussed. In this report, the TRHST significantly differentiated RDC unipolar endogenous (22 of 87, 25%) from nonendogenous (4 of 46, 9%). Bipolar, depressed-phase patients also evidenced a significant rate of TRHST blunting (12 of 27, 44%). Most with a blunted TRHST also evidenced DST nonsuppression (26 of 38, 68%).

In 67 "endogenous" patients (16 bipolar, depressed phase; 51 unipolar endogenous), all three laboratory tests were obtained and were contrasted with all three tests in 28 RDC unipolar nonendogenous patients. In this subset, the TRHST differentiated the endogenous (13 of 67, 19%) and nonendogenous (2 of 28, 7%) groups, as did the DST (42% versus 18%) and reduced REM latency (61% versus 36%). Nearly all of the endogenous group (69%) who evidenced a blunted TRHST also evidenced reduced REM latency (less than 65 minutes). Given the other studies indicating that a blunted TRHST differentiates RDC endogenous from nonendogenous depressions, and given the overlap with the PSG that also differentiates these two groups, one can conclude that independent corroboration of the PSG's relationship with the RDC endogenous/nonendogenous dichotomy exists.

Other biological tests.   Several other biological abnormalities have occasionally been related to melancholic/endogenous depression. They have not been examined to as great an extent as the preceding three tests, however. These other biological abnormalities include salivary cortisol, growth hormone response, and urinary 3-methoxy-4-hydroxyphenylglycol (MHPG) levels. The utility of salivary cortisol in identifying endogenous/melancholic depression is in question. Most studies suggest that it provides good discrimination between endogenous/melancholic and other types of depression (Ansseau et al. 1984; Cook et al. 1986; Hanada et al. 1985), although some do not (Copolov et al. 1985, 1989). ^{3}H-imipramine binding has been the subject of 17 studies. Those depressed patients who show reduced binding are largely more severely depressed. Whether they are endogenous/melancholic per se has not been carefully evaluated.

Do Melancholic Symptom Features Predictably Repeat Across Recurrent Episodes?

The phenomenological expression of mood disorder may change over time: "today's dysthymic may well become tomorrow's major depressive." Major depression may also become bipolar disorder. A subtype that may have treatment selection implications may or may not repeat itself from episode to episode. If it does not repeat, then what does the form it takes over the longitudinal course tell us about the nature of the condition?

In the case of endogenous versus nonendogenous depression, age is related to the probability of the diagnosis, because older depressed patients are more likely to present with endogenous than nonendogenous symptoms (Parker et al. 1991). This may simply be the result of different neurobiological substrates in the older versus younger patients, or it may represent the ever-clearer clinical expression of the *forme fruste* of the condition itself.

In a retrospective chart review for patients seen between 1964 and 1969, Kendell (1974) found that 47% of 101 endogenous depressions received the same subtype diagnosis at a subsequent admission. Similarly, Paykel et al. (1976) reported a correlation of 0.42 between initial and subsequent scores on an empirically derived endogenous versus neurotic factor scale in 33 patients who relapsed during an 8-month follow-up. Young et al. (1987), in a report from the NIMH Collaborative Study, concluded that reliable diagnoses of the RDC endogenous subtype were stable across subsequent depressive episodes in only a small number of cases. Although the stability across episodes was greater than expected by chance, the absolute amount of agreement was small. However, of the original sample, only 13 (11%) were RDC nonendogenous, 72 (60%) were RDC endogenous, and 34 (29%) were RDC probable endogenous. Of the 13 nonendogenous patients, 9 went on to become RDC probable endogenous ($n = 5$) or RDC endogenous ($n = 4$). Of the original 34 RDC probable endogenous, 14 (41%) repeated as probable endogenous, and 11 (32%) went on to develop endogenous depression. If one combines the probable and the definite endogenous groups, assuming that further observation would allow evolution of the disorder, then of 106 original endogenous depressions, 78 (73%) repeated, whereas of 13 original nonendogenous depressions, 4 repeated and 9 went on to develop the endogenous subtype. These data are consistent with the idea that nonendogenous depressions may, over time, become endogenous and that, once established, most melancholic major depressive episodes repeat. However, none of the few available studies fully answers this question.

Are Melancholic Features Associated With a Higher Incidence of Mood Disorders in First-Degree Relatives?

Early reports suggested that endogenous/melancholic features were associated with a higher likelihood of a family history of depression, whereas nonendogenous/ nonmelancholic depressions were more likely to be associated with a family history of psychopathic states (Buzzard 1930; Gillespie 1926, 1929; Strauss 1930). More recent studies have suggested the association of alcoholism, but not depression, with families of nonendogenous/nonmelancholic depressed patients (Andreasen and Grove 1982; Perris et al. 1983; Winokur 1983; Winokur and Pitts 1964). In addition, two studies using DSM-III to diagnose melancholic/nonmelancholic depression confirmed higher rates of alcoholism in family members of nonmelancholic probands (Price et al. 1984; Zimmerman et al. 1986).

In another study, Zimmerman et al. (1985b) used a discriminant index derived from the RDC for diagnosing endogenous depression. In a large sample of 257 depressed inpatients, the morbid risks of depression in first-degree relatives were equivalent for both the endogenous/melancholic ($n = 138$ or 16.8%) and nonendogenous/nonmelancholic ($n = 113$ or 17.7%). The morbid risk rates for alcoholism and antisocial personality were significantly higher for relatives of patients with nonendogenous/nonmelancholic depression, with a risk of 15.3% for RDC alcoholism and 3.1% for RDC antisocial personality. Relatives of the endogenous/melancholic patients had risk rates of 9.5% for alcoholism and 1.4% for antisocial personality. These more recent studies, along with several other earlier reports, suggest that the endogenous/melancholic and nonendogenous/nonmelancholic dichotomy is distinguished by a higher family incidence for nonmood disorders in the nonendogenous/nonmelancholic group.

Leckman et al. (1984) found that relatives of probands with "autonomous" and delusional types of depression had higher rates of major depression than did relatives of either control subjects or patients with nonendogenous forms of depression. A post hoc data analysis revealed an increased rate of major depression among family members with the endogenous symptoms of appetite reduction and guilt. The incidence of major depression in relatives of probands with appetite reduction was 16.5%, whereas only 9.5% of relatives without an appetite disturbance were so affected. Similarly, in the probands with guilt, 16.2% of relatives were affected, compared to only 8.9% of relatives of probands without guilt. Endogenous symptoms that were not associated with differential familial incidence of depression included delusions, psychomotor agitation and retardation, loss of interest, depressive severity, lack of reactivity, early-morning awakening, morning worsening, loss of interest in sex, and middle insomnia. Leckman et al. (1984) speculate that excessive guilt may lie on a continuum with delusional depression, and specifically with depressions accompanied by delusions of guilt.

Von Knorring (1987) has presented data on the morbidity risk for depression, alcoholism, and schizophrenia in patients diagnosed with either neurotic/reactive or unipolar affective disorders. The category of neurotic/reactive included patients meeting criteria for DSM-III diagnoses of major depression, atypical depression, dysthymia, and adjustment disorder with depressed mood. When classified by ICD-9, the same group of patients also met criteria for diagnoses of neurotic depression (approximately 70% of the sample), brief depressive reaction (20%), manic-depressive psychoses, and affective psychoses. The primary criteria used for diagnosing patients as neurotic/reactive included a clear-cut depressive symptomatology of a neurotic, nonpsychotic dimension that arose as a reaction to external events or represented an acute breakdown in patients with an unstable personality and a tendency to react with depressive, anxious, or psychosomatic symptoms when under stress. The morbidity risk for depression in first-degree family members of neurotic/reactive patients ($n = 390$) was 9.1%, compared to a significantly greater 17.4% risk in relatives of patients with unipolar affective disorders ($n = 420$). The risk rate of alcoholism was 2.5% for families of patients with neurotic/reactive depression and 0.8% for families of those with unipolar affective disorders (not statistically significant). These results are similar to those of Zimmerman et al. (1986), who found the risk of depression in relatives of patients with unipolar affective disorder (17.4%) to be similar to the rates found in relatives of patients with both endogenous (16.8%) and nonendogenous (17.7%) depression. The lower rate (9.1%) of depression in first-degree relatives of von Knorring's (1987) neurotic/reactive patients compared with the 17.7% rate in the Zimmerman et al. (1986) study may result from the more heterogeneous nature of this group (e.g., it includes patients with dysthymic and adjustment disorders). Conversely, both Zimmerman et al. (1986) and von Knorring (1987) found higher rates of alcoholism in families of nonendogenous/nonmelancholic probands than in the families of endogenous/melancholic probands.

In a review of family, twin, and adoption studies, von Knorring et al. (1985) concluded that there was no strong support for a specific genetic factor in neurotic/reactive depression. These studies have generally contrasted patients with neurotic/reactive or unspecified types of depression with individuals having no psychiatric disorder, leaving the issue of genetic transmission in endogenous/melancholic depression unresolved.

In a separate study, von Knorring et al. (1985) assessed the risk of affective disorders in family members of depressed probands with different levels of platelet monoamine oxidase (MAO) activity. First-degree relatives of low-platelet MAO probands had an increased risk for both neurotic/reactive depression and alcoholism. Relatives of probands with abnormally high platelet MAO levels showed an increased risk for bipolar affective disorder. Platelet MAO seems to be under genetic control (Murphy 1976; Pandey et al. 1979; Rice et al. 1982; Winter et al. 1978). Parents of probands with low-platelet MAO have lower-platelet MAO than parents of probands with high-platelet MAO (Puchall et al. 1980). Low-platelet MAO is found in adjustment disorders with depressed mood (von Knorring et al. 1985) and in alcoholic subjects (Major and Murphy 1978; Pandey et al. 1980; von Knorring and Oreland 1978; Wieberg et al. 1977). In a 2-year follow-up study, Coursey et al. (1982) found more mental health problems (depression, alcoholism, suicide) in relatives of probands with low-platelet MAO. Thus, low-platelet MAO may be a clue to poor adaptation to stress. The platelet MAO studies suggest that the endogenous/melancholic, nonendogenous/nonmelancholic dichotomy may be valid.

Failde et al. (1987) conducted a family study in which the neurotic/reactive category was subdivided into two component types of neurotic and reactive depression and examined separately. Their results suggested that there was a significantly lower risk (1.1%) of affective disorder in the parents of the neurotic group than in the parents of the reactive group (13.3%). However, the reactive group was quite small ($n = 12$). The results suggested that there may be a reduced risk of depression in family members of patients with neurotic depression. In this context, neurotic refers to a depressed mood that is seen as part of a chronic personality disorder. Note that the 13.3% risk in parents of reactive depressed patients approximates the 17% rate for all first-degree relatives of probands with major depressive disorder reported by Zimmerman et al. (1986). This suggests that the neurotic/reactive group is heterogeneous. Those with chronic neurotic personality disorders have a much lower incidence of depression in first-degree relatives. Those with reactive depression (many of whom met RDC and DSM-III criteria for major depression) had much higher rates of familial depression.

Researchers have at times failed to find any increase in depression among relatives of patients with endogenous versus nonendogenous illness. A large study by Andreasen et al. (1986) confirmed the lack of an association between familial depression and the endogenous/melancholic subtype. These investigators assessed the incidence of depression in 2,942 first-degree relatives of 566 patients with unipolar major depression. Relatives of patients with endogenous/melancholic depression, as defined by four diagnostic systems, did not have higher rates of depression than relatives of nonendogenous/nonmelancholic patients. The four diagnostic systems used in this study for diagnosing endogenous/melancholic included the NCS, RDC, DSM-III, and an "autonomous" depression scale developed by investigators at Yale University. This study found generally much higher rates of depression (30%–35% for major depression) in relatives of both endogenous/melancholic and nonendogenous/nonmelancholic patients than have been reported by others (e.g., von Knorring et al. 1985; Zimmerman et al. 1986). This finding may relate to the use of the SADS-L (Endicott and Spitzer 1978) with the family members themselves rather than an assessment based on the perhaps incomplete knowledge and impression of pathology provided by the depressed proband. The rates of alcoholism in families of endogenous and nonendogenous groups were found to differ only when RDC was used to diagnose the relatives. In this case, the familial alcoholism rates were 18.4% for the nonendogenous/nonmelancholic group and 13.3% for the endogenous/melancholic group. These rates are somewhat higher, but the pattern of differences is quite similar to that found in the Zimmerman et al. (1986) study, using an RDC-based discriminant index to diagnose endogenous/nonendogenous subtypes in depressed probands.

In contrast to these results, McGuffin et al. (1987) found the morbid risk of severe depression in relatives of endogenous/melancholic depressed probands (14.7%) to be approximately twice the risk in relatives of probands with nonendogenous/nonmelancholic depression (7.9%). Subgroups were identified with neurotic and psychotic/endogenous depression by the CATEGO classification system (Wing et al. 1974). These results are not as surprising or discrepant as they may initially seem. When the risk of depression in family members was expanded to include either a moderate or severe level, both groups were equivalent (23.7% morbid risk in neurotic and 25.7% in endogenous probands). As the authors state, the results "demonstrate that variability in rates of illness among relatives are as much a function of the chosen diagnostic criteria as they are of the proband characteristics." Except with a very narrow definition of illness, both endogenous and nonendogenous forms had equal familiality (McGuffin et al. 1988a, 1988b). There was no inverse relationship between presence of family depression and reactivity to stress in the proband (McGuffin et al. 1988b).

In summary, the RDC endogenous versus nonendogenous dichotomy does not predict a differential loading for mood disorders in the families of either subgrouping. Relatives of the nonendogenous/nonmelancholic probands, however, do appear in most studies to have a higher incidence of alcoholism, sociopathy, or other nonmood difficulties than do relatives of endogenous/melancholic probands. Andreasen et al. (1986) also found a significant association between endogenous/melancholic subtypes and recurrent episodes in the proband and a history of a recurrent course of illness in family members. Whether this was based on age corrections is unclear, however.

Relevant to this issue is Winokur's (1987) conclusion that the term *neurotic* depression is used in two basic ways: 1) to refer to depression secondary to personality disorders, neuroses, or substance abuse disorders and 2) to refer to primary depression with a family history of alcoholism. He thus equates the neurotic subtype of depression with an increased risk for familial alcoholism, based on previous data that have suggested such an association (Pfohl et al. 1984; Winokur 1985).

Note that a failure to validate a phenomenological subdivision by family history methods or by family studies must be carefully interpreted. Either endogenous/melancholic is not genetic, or it is neither more nor less genetic than the nonendogenous/nonmelancholic subtype. Given the potential relationship between platelet MAO activity (high versus low) and subtype, as well as other evidence of biological abnormalities in the nonendogenous/nonmelancholic group and its association with impulse regulation (alcoholism, sociopathy), it is entirely reasonable that both subtypes run in families. Whether the subtype breeds true is as yet unclear.

Are Melancholic Features Associated With a Unique Course of Illness?

In a 15-year follow-up study of 145 patients who were hospitalized for depressive disorders between 1966 and 1970, Kiloh et al. (1988) found that patients who had initial diagnoses of endogenous depression were more likely to have been rehospitalized than those with an index diagnosis of neurotic depression. The endogenous group at initial admission was older (64% over age 50 years) and remained in the hospital longer (4–6 weeks). Patients with endogenous depression had a higher readmission rate than the nonendogenous group; 50% of the endogenous group for whom the index admission was not the first were readmitted within 2 years. For the complete endogenous group, a 50% readmission risk was present at 4.3 years, versus 17 years for the nonendogenous group. These results are very similar to the Lee and Murray (1988) 18-year follow-up study that found rates of 3.5 years and 20 years, respectively.

However, patients with endogenous depression had as poor an overall outcome as the nonendogenous group (Kiloh et al. 1988). The patients included in the endogenous depressed group in this study met DSM-III criteria for either unipolar major depression, melancholic and/or psychotic type, or bipolar disorder. The patients included in the neurotic group fell into the DSM-III categories of major depression without melancholic and/or psychotic features, or dysthymic disorder or adjustment disorder with depressed mood. The endogenous and neurotic groups were equivalent when outcome was classified into three categories: recovery and continued wellness, partial or complete recovery with a recurrence and continued incapacitation, or suicide. None of the 69 patients with an initial diagnosis of endogenous depression subsequently developed other psychiatric disorders, which suggests that once this subtype is expressed, it remains diagnostically stable. In contrast, 7 of 76 patients (10%) initially diagnosed with neurotic depression developed other psychiatric illnesses (4 with subsequent melancholic depression). An in-depth retrospective examination of the index admission data confirmed that these patients were not just mild cases of endogenous depression at initial admission. Thus, some cases of neurotic depression subsequently develop into the endogenous type. In general, it may be more likely that nonendogenous episodes are followed by endogenous ones than vice versa. The suggested association between increasing age and endogenous depression provides indirect support for this hypothesis (Parker et al. 1989).

A 6.5-year follow-up of a heterogeneous sample of depressed patients by Brockington et al. (1982) found that nonpsychotic depressive patients at the index episode ($n = 45$) were very likely to have a course of illness free from psychotic symptoms and social complications. In contrast, patients with psychotic depression (mood congruent and incongruent) differed from each other and from schizophrenic patients in general outcome measures and in the symptoms exhibited at subsequent admissions. The mood-incongruent patients continued to show schizophrenic symptoms during the 6-year follow-up period. The mood-congruent group (6 of 11) had a tendency to evidence a manic-depressive course in their illness.

Parker et al. (1989) provide a summary of factor loadings for the variable of previous episodes of illness in six factor analytic studies of depression (Carney et al. 1965; Garside et al. 1971; Kiloh and Garside 1963; Kiloh et al. 1971; Mendels and Cochrane 1968; Paykel et al. 1971). None of these studies provide evidence that episodic course is highly related to endogenous depression.

Several studies have examined the prediction of outcome based on depressive symptoms. Chaturvedi and Sarmukaddam (1986) reported that total negative symptom scores on the Scale for Assessment of Negative Symptoms (SANS) (Andreasen 1982) had a higher negative correlation with global improvement (Spearman's $r = -.46$, $P = .001$) in a sample of 34 outpatients with RDC definite endogenous major depression. Negative symptom subscales measuring poverty of speech, affective flattening, and avolition-apathy and individual negative symptom items measuring inability to feel emotions, feelings of emptiness in thinking, and feelings of avolition were significantly related to poor outcome. Outcome was measured after 1 year with a global 5-point Clinical Global Impression (GCI) (Guy 1976) scale (recovered, moderate improvement, minimal improvement, no improvement, and worsened). The negative symptoms examined in this study are common among the list of endogenous/melancholic features included in the major diagnostic systems. Results suggest that endogenous depression with many of these negative features is particularly treatment resistant or vulnerable to early relapse.

Life Events and Melancholic Features

The role of antecedent life events has been reviewed by Paykel (1974). Only a few studies have related life events to depressive phenomenological subtypes. Leff et al. (1970) and Thomson and Hendrie (1972) found no differences for life events in endogenous and nonendogenous outpatient groups. Hirschfeld (1981) found no differences in life events between situational and nonsituational depressions. Brown et al. (1979) and Paykel (1974; Paykel et al. 1971) found that presence or absence of life events had little relation to psychotic (endogenous) versus neurotic subtypes. Roy et al. (1985) reported a higher rate of life events in DSM-III melancholic patients (all inpatients) ($n = 20$) but not in DSM-III nonmelancholic patients ($n = 20$) compared with matched control subjects ($n = 41$). This finding is similar to Perris (1984a, 1984b). According to Winokur et al. (1988), the classical dichotomy between a spontaneously occurring endogenous depression and nonendogenous depression associated with a significant precipitating life event has not received much validating empirical support. Winokur et al. (1988) suggest that a differentiation between the concepts of "neurotic" and "reactive" depressions may be useful. They propose that neurotic depression occurs in the course of a long-standing illness marked by personality problems, conflicts, and neurotic symptoms. In contrast, reactive depressions are experienced as a response to one or more significant life events. In their study of patients with secondary depression, Winokur et al. (1988) found that patients with depression secondary to psychiatric disorders such as somatoform, anxiety, and personality disorders were similar to the type they proposed as "neurotic" depression, whereas the patients with depression secondary to physical illnesses fit the "reactive" group.

In an examination of improvement among 43 nonendogenous patients, Parker et al. (1985) found that baseline factors of depressive severity, a recent breakup of an intimate relationship, and weight loss were associated with better improvement after 20 weeks. Positive life events occurring after assessment were associated with improvement at both 6 and 20 weeks. Similarly, resolution of a negative life event predicted improvement at 20 weeks. Treatment consisted of psychotherapy and counseling for an open-ended period. One might suggest, based on the classical distinction between endogenous and reactive depression, that the relationship between life events and clinical improvement in this nonendogenous sample was accentuated by the high rate of negative life events in this subtype of depression. Perris (1984a, 1984b) and Roy et al. (1985) found that patients with nonendogenous/nonmelancholic depression experience a significantly greater number of negative life events than do patients with endogenous/melancholic depressions. Other researchers, however, have not found a difference in the number of negative life events reported by patients with endogenous and nonendogenous depression (Leff et al. 1970; Thomson and Hendrie 1972).

Which Melancholic Features Are Found in Depressed Children and Adolescents?

Melancholic/endogenous features as defined by the RDC do occur in the depressive episodes of children and adolescents. The frequency varies widely and may depend on age, patient status, and sensitivity. Thus, melancholic symptoms are rare in preschoolers (Kashani and Carlson 1987), for whom major depression itself is uncommon, and occur at least in mild forms in about half of prepubescent and adolescent patients with major depression (Ryan et al. 1987). Although the rates of specific endogenous symptoms differ between prepubescent children and adolescents (Carlson and Kashani 1988), when a principal components factor analysis of 187 young people (ages 6–17 years) was conducted by Ryan et al. (1987), an endogenous factor emerged. Items loading on this factor included anhedonia, fatigue, psychomotor retardation, social withdrawal, depressed mood, anorexia, decreased weight, diurnal variation (with morning worsening), and hypersomnia.

The most recent comprehensive review of DST results in children and adolescents does not specifically address subtypes of major depression (Casat et al. 1989). Those individual studies in which the endogenous/melancholic subtype was described do not suggest much predictive validity. Moreover, no significant differences were found in cortisol secretion in prepubescent children with major depression compared with nonpsychiatric or normal control subjects, nor were there differences in the endogenously depressed subgroup (Puig-Antich et al. 1989a).

The few familial aggregation studies that have been conducted using children/adolescents do validate the endogenous subtype, albeit not strongly. The RDC endogenous subtype was associated with a significantly higher prevalence of major depression (.10 versus .03, $P < .03$) and suicide attempts (.04 versus .00, $P < .03$) in second-degree relatives of child probands with major depression (Puig-Antich et al. 1989b). In two studies of adolescent populations, Weissman (personal communication, July 1990) found no differences in rates of parental depression and Strober (personal communication, August 1990) found lower familial rates of alcoholism, drug abuse, and antisocial personality in the relatives of adolescents hospitalized for RDC endogenous depression.

Kovacs et al. (1984) did not address the impact of the endogenous subtype on the course of illness in their sample of 8- to 13-year-old children. Weissman (personal communication, July 1990) found that melancholic (versus nonmelancholic) children in her sample had lower C-GAS scores (50.7 versus 57.2) and, not surprisingly, more depressive symptoms. Strober (1983) found melancholia to be associated with a longer time to recovery during the index episode and increased probability of relapse during a 3- to 5-year follow-up. It is noteworthy, however, that many endogenously depressed adolescents were also psychotically depressed. Data from both Strober and Carlson (1982) and Akiskal et al. (1985) show a high probability of subsequent manic episodes in adolescents whose depressions are characterized by psychomotor retardation, hypersomnia, and psychotic symptoms.

Results from double-blind studies of antidepressant medication in children and adolescents have been inconclusive with regard to definite therapeutic efficacy in this age group. The high rate of placebo response and the difficulty in getting substantial numbers of subjects to undertake and complete a drug trial have complicated the research in this area. There is no evidence, however, that children and adults with endogenous depression respond differently from those with nonendogenous depression.

In conclusion, as with adults, there is some support for the melancholic subtype in children and adolescents. Whether the clustering of symptoms represents a difference of degree or kind from nonendogenous depression remains unclear. At least as defined by the RDC, predictive validity is not robust. Conversely, the course modifiers included in DSM-III-R, namely episode recovery and response to biological treatment, are useless in first-episode depressions. This, of course, has particular impact in the case of children and adolescents. Whether there is merit in including preexisting personality disorders is also unclear. The data supporting such a suggestion in adults are slim and, in children and adolescents, in whom many personality disorders are excluded by definition, the data are presently absent. Therefore, the recommendation is that the course modifiers be eliminated altogether, at least for those age 18 years and younger.

Discussion and Recommendations

In summary, melancholic features have a long history. These features present with or without psychotic symptoms (hallucinations/delusions). The descriptive clinical studies that best separate melancholic from nonmelancholic subgroups are those that use both symptom features (usually at the nadir of the episode), course of illness, and other clinical features (e.g., the Newcastle Scale). Cluster, factor, and latent class analytic studies of these descriptive features provide overlapping findings. Melancholic symptom features included most consistently are psychomotor retardation, anhedonia, unreactive mood, and distinct quality to mood. Associated, but not always present, are the classic vegetative symptoms and diurnal variation.

Melancholic features predict good response to ECT and poor response to placebo. Melancholic features may predict a good response to S-adenosylmethionine. Such features are associated with a poor response to alprazolam according to some (Goldberg et al. 1986; Lenox et al. 1984; Rush et al. 1985) but not all (Feighner et al. 1983; Rickels et al. 1985) investigators.

Melancholic features are less predictive of a positive response to tricyclic antidepressants in outpatients, although surprisingly few studies are available. Melancholic features (as defined by RDC and Newcastle Scale but not ICD or DSM-III) relate to DST nonsuppression. Reduced REM latency relates to the endogenous features in nearly all studies to date.

Although melancholic features do not reliably repeat across episodes, current data support the notion that with repeated episodes (or with increasing age, because they are related), nonmelancholic episodes are more likely to become melancholic episodes than the converse. No data are available to determine whether melancholic features breed true in families, although psychotic depressions do run in families and appear to repeat over episodes (Schatzberg and Rothschild 1992). Melancholic probands seem more likely to have a first-degree relative with severe depression. Melancholic features are not associated with a unique course of illness, although the melancholic episodes may be briefer than nonmelancholic episodes (Parker et al. 1991), whereas the DSM-III melancholic category may be too restrictive (Zimmerman and Spitzer 1989). The RDC and Newcastle systems broaden the group, which explains the apparent confirmation by both DST and PSG for these groups.

There are several options for DSM-IV: 1) continue to use the DSM-III-R definition, 2) return to the DSM-III definition, 3) move toward a Newcastle definition, 4) move to RDC, or 5) create yet another definition.

Against continuing the DSM-III-R definition unchanged are the facts that 1) we have little data relevant to the validity of DSM-III-R, 2) DSM-III-R includes features not included in any other system (e.g., good interepisode recovery, no personality disorder, good response to biological treatment), and 3) DSM-III-R features are likely to be less applicable to children or adolescents, because they may not have had many prior episodes or biological treatment.

A return to DSM-III would not recognize the need for a broader category, as evidenced by DST, PSG, and course-of-illness studies. Furthermore, DSM-III criteria (as is true of other criteria) confound severity with the "category" and symptom threshold definitions are lacking (e.g., how unreactive must the mood be?).

A third option is to modify the criteria to better fit the Newcastle definition. Although the evidence for validity is present for several validators, the list is too long for easy clinical use, and it includes course-of-illness variables that are not yet well supported by the existing research.

A fourth option, the RDC, is supported by some of the validation studies above, but the RDC definition is confounded with severity, and it requires a list of 10 items that are clinically difficult to apply.

A final option, to redefine the category once again, trying to broaden the DSM-III category with a shorter list of symptoms, is logical. However, whether a new list would have the predictive value (e.g., ECT response) or be validated by laboratory tests is unstudied. The "core" symptoms of psychomotor retardation, anhedonia, unreactive mood, and distinct quality to mood would constitute such a list. Evidence for this listing of signs/symptoms is that they 1) relate to reduced REM latency (Giles et al. 1987), 2) recur across factor/cluster analytic studies, 3) relate to a positive response to ECT or tricyclic antidepressants, and 4) run in families. Specific operational definitions (as specified by Bech and Allerup 1986) would have to be developed for each item on this list. However, without additional data, the optimal choice among these options would rest more on opinion than empirical data. This area remains fertile ground for new research.

References

Abou-Saleh MT, Coppen A: Classification of depression and response to antidepressive therapies. Br J Psychiatry 143:601–603, 1983

Aggernaes H, Kirkegaard C, Krog-Meyer I, et al: Dexamethasone suppression test and TRH test in endogenous depression. Acta Psychiatr Scand 67:258–264, 1983

Akiskal HS: Subaffective disorders: dysthymic, cyclothymic and bipolar II disorders in the "borderline" realm. Psychiatr Clin North Am 4:25–26, 1981

Akiskal HS, Downs J, Jordan P, et al: Affective disorders in referred children and younger siblings of manic-depressives. Arch Gen Psychiatry 42:996–1004, 1985

American Psychiatric Association: Diagnostic and Statistical Manual of Mental Disorders, Third Edition. Washington, DC, American Psychiatric Association, 1980

American Psychiatric Association: Diagnostic and Statistical Manual of Mental Disorders, Third Edition, Revised. Washington, DC, American Psychiatric Association, 1987

Ames D, Burrows G, Davies B, et al: A study of the dexamethasone suppression test in hospitalized depressed patients. Br J Psychiatry 144:311–313, 1984

Andreasen NC: Negative symptoms in schizophrenia: definition and reliability. Arch Gen Psychiatry 39:784–788, 1982

Andreasen NC, Grove WM: The classification of depression: traditional views versus mathematical approaches. Am J Psychiatry 139:45–52, 1982

Andreasen NC, Scheftner W, Reich T, et al: The validation of the concept of endogenous depression: a family study approach. Arch Gen Psychiatry 43:246–251, 1986

Ansseau M, Scheyvaerts M, Doumont A, et al: Concurrent use of REM latency, dexamethasone suppression, clonidine, and apomorphine tests as biological markers of endogenous depression: a pilot study. Psychiatry Res 12:261–272, 1984

Arana GW, Barreira PJ, Cohen BM, et al: The dexamethasone suppression test in psychotic disorders. Am J Psychiatry 140:1521–1523, 1983

Asnis GM, Sachar EJ, Halbreicht U, et al: Endocrine responses to thyrotropin-releasing hormone in major depressive disorders. Psychiatry Res 5:205–215, 1981

Baillarger JGF: De la folie à double-forme. Annales Medico-Psychologiques 6:367–391, 1854

Baumgartner A, Hahnenkamp L, Meinhold H: Effects of age and diagnosis on thyrotropin response to thyrotropin-releasing hormone in psychiatric patients. Psychiatry Res 17:285–294, 1986

Bebbington P, Brugha T, McCarthy B, et al: The Camberwell Collaborative Depression Study, I: depressed probands: adversity and the form of depression. Br J Psychiatry 152:754–765, 1988

Bech P, Allerup A: A categorical approach to depression by a three-dimensional system. Psychopathology 19:327–339, 1986

Bech P, Gram LF, Reisby N, et al: The WHO Depression Scale: relationship to the Newcastle scales. Acta Psychiatr Scand 62:140–155, 1980

Berger M, Lund R, Bronisch T, et al: REM latency in neurotic and endogenous depression and the cholinergic REM induction test. Psychiatry Res 10:113–123, 1983

Berrios GE: Depressive and manic states during the 19th century, in Handbook of Affective Disorders. Edited by Gorgotas D, Cancro T. New York, Elsevier, 1988, pp 13–25

Blinder MG: Differential diagnosis and treatment of depressive disorders. JAMA 195:8–12, 1966a

Blinder MG: The pragmatic classification of depression. Am J Psychiatry 123:259–269, 1966b

Bolton JS: Maniacal-depressive insanity. Brain 31:301–318, 1908

Boudreau D: Evaluation of the sedation threshold test. Arch Neurol Psychiatry 80:771–775, 1958

Brockington IF, Helzer JE, Hillier VF, et al: Definitions of depression: concordance and prediction of outcome. Am J Psychiatry 139:1022–1027, 1982

Brown G, Ni Bhrolchain M, Harris T: Psychotic and neurotic depression. J Affect Disord 1:195–211, 1979

Brown RP, Frances A, Kocsis JH, et al: Psychotic vs nonpsychotic depression: comparison of treatment response. J Nerv Ment Dis 170:635–637, 1982

Brown RP, Stoll PM, Stokes PE, et al: Adrenocortical hyperactivity in depression: effects of agitation, delusions, melancholia and other illness variables. Psychiatry Res 23:167–178, 1988

Brown WA, Shuey I: Response to dexamethasone and subtype of depression. Arch Gen Psychiatry 37:747–751, 1980

Busfield BL, Wechsler H, Barnum WJ: Studies of salivation in depression, II: physiological differentiation of reactive and endogenous depression. Arch Gen Psychiatry 5:472–477, 1961

Buzzard EF: Discussion on the diagnosis and treatment of the milder forms of the manic-depressive psychosis. Proc R Acad Med 23:881–882, 1930

Calloway SP, Dolan RJ, Fonagy P, et al: Endocrine changes and clinical profiles in depression, I: the dexamethasone suppression test. Psychol Med 14:749–758, 1984

Carlson GA, Kashani JH: Phenomenology of major depression from childhood through adulthood: analysis of three studies. Am J Psychiatry 145:1222–1225, 1988

Carney MWP, Roth M, Garside RF: The diagnosis of depressive syndromes and the prediction of ECT response. Br J Psychiatry 111:659–674, 1965

Carney MWP, Reynolds EH, Sheffield BF: Prediction of outcome in depressive illness by the Newcastle diagnosis scale: its relationship with the unipolar/bipolar and DSM-III systems. Br J Psychiatry 150:43–48, 1986

Carroll BJ, Feinberg M, Greden JF, et al: Diagnosis of endogenous depression: comparison of clinical, research and neuroendocrine criteria. J Affect Disord 2:177–194, 1980

Carroll BJ, Feinberg M, Greden JF, et al: A specific laboratory test for the diagnosis of melancholia: standardization, validation and clinical utility. Arch Gen Psychiatry 38:15–22, 1981

Casat CD, Arana GW, Powell K: The DST in children and adolescents with major depressive disorder. Am J Psychiatry 146:503–507, 1989

Cattell RB: The description of personality, I: foundations of trait measurement. Psychol Rev 50:559–594, 1943

Chaslin P: Elements de Semiologie et Clinique Mentales. Paris, Asselin et Houzeau, 1912

Chaturvedi SK, Sarmukaddam SB: Prediction of outcome in depression by negative symptoms. Acta Psychiatr Scand 74:183–186, 1986

Coble P, Foster FG, Kupfer DJ: Electroencephalographic sleep diagnosis of primary depression. Arch Gen Psychiatry 33:1124–1127, 1976

Cook LC: Convulsive therapy. J Ment Sci 90:435–464, 1944

Cook N, Harris B, Walker R, et al: Clinical utility of the dexamethasone suppression test assessed by plasma and salivary cortisol determinations. Psychiatry Res 18:143–150, 1986

Copolov DL, Rubin RT, Mander AJ et al: Pre- and postdexamethasone salivary cortisol concentrations in major depression. Psychoneuroendocrinology 10:461–467, 1985

Copolov DL, Rubin RT, Stuart GW, et al: Specificity of the salivary cortisol dexamethasone suppression test across psychiatric diagnoses. Biol Psychiatry 25:879–893, 1989

Coppen A, Abou-Saleh M, Millin P, et al: Dexamethasone suppression test in depression and other psychiatric illness. Br J Psychiatry 142:498–504, 1983

Coryell W, Turner R: Outcome with desipramine therapy in subtypes of nonpsychotic major depression. J Affect Disord 9:149–154, 1985

Coryell W, Gaffney G, Burkhardt PE: DSM-III melancholia and the primary-secondary distinction: a comparison of concurrent validity by means of the dexamethasone suppression test. Am J Psychiatry 139:120–122, 1982

Coursey RD, Buchsbaum MS, Murphy DL: Two-year follow-up of subjects and their families defined as at risk for psychopathology on the basis of platelet MAO activities. Neuropsychobiology 8:51–56, 1982

Crow TJ, Deakin JFW, Johnstone EC, et al: The Northwick Park ECT trial: predictors of response to real and simulated ECT. Br J Psychiatry 144:227–237, 1984

Cuttelod S, Lemarchand-Beraud T, Magnenat P, et al: Effect of age and role of kidneys and liver on thyrotropin in man. Metab Clin Exp 23:101–113, 1974

Dam H, Mellerup ET, Rafaelsen OJ: Diurnal variation of total plasma trytophan in depressive patients. Acta Psychiatr Scand 69:190–196, 1984

Davidson J, Turnbull C, Strickland R, et al: Comparative diagnostic criteria for melancholia and endogenous depression. Arch Gen Psychiatry 41:506–511, 1984

Davidson JRT, Giller EL, Zisook S, et al: An efficacy study of isocarboxazid and placebo in depression, and its relationship to depressive nosology. Arch Gen Psychiatry 45:120–127, 1988

Debus JR, Rush AJ: Sleep EEG findings in depression, in Depression: New Directions in Theory, Research and Practice. Edited by McCann CD, Endler NS. Toronto, Wall & Emerson, 1990, pp 337–360

Duncan WC, Jr, Pettigrew KD, Gillin JC: REM architecture changes in bipolar and unipolar depression. Am J Psychiatry 136:1424–1427, 1979

Elkin I, Shea MT, Watkins JT, et al: National Institute of Mental Health Treatment of Depression Collaborative Research Program: general effectiveness of treatments. Arch Gen Psychiatry 46:971–982, 1989

Endicott J, Spitzer RL: A diagnostic interview: the Schedule for Affective Disorders and Schizophrenia—Lifetime Version. Arch Gen Psychiatry 35:837–844, 1978

Extein I, Pottash ALC, Gold MS: Relationship of thyrotropin-releasing hormone test and dexamethasone suppression test abnormalities in unipolar depression. Psychiatry Res 4:49–53, 1981

Failde M, Eisemann M, Perris C: Psychiatric morbidity among relatives of different subgroups of neurotic depression. Acta Psychiatr Scand 75:487–490, 1987

Fairchild CJ, Rush AJ, Vasavada N, et al: Which depressions respond to placebo? Psychiatry Res 18:217–226, 1986

Falret JP: Memorie sur la folie circulaire. Bulletin de l'Académie de Medicine 19:382–415, 1854

Farmer A, McGuffin P: The classification of the depressions: contemporary confusion revisited. Br J Psychiatry 155:437–443, 1989

Feighner JP, Robins E, Guze SB, et al: Diagnostic criteria for use in psychiatric research. Arch Gen Psychiatry 26:57–63, 1972

Feighner JP, Meredith CH, Frost NR, et al: A double-blind comparison of alprazolam vs. imipramine and placebo in the treatment of major depressive disorders. Acta Psychiatr Scand 68:223–233, 1983

Feinberg M, Carroll BJ: Separation of subtypes of depression using discriminant analysis, I: separation of unipolar endogenous depression from nonendogenous depression. Br J Psychiatry 140:384–391, 1982

Feinberg M, Gillin JC, Carroll BJ, et al: EEG studies of sleep in the diagnosis of depression. Biol Psychiatry 17:305–316, 1982

Foville A: Folie a double-forme. Brain 5:288–323, 1882

Garside RF, Kay DWK, Wilson IC, et al: Depressive symptoms and the classification of patients. Psychol Med 1:333–338, 1971

Georgotas A, McCue RE, Cooper T, et al: Clinical predictors of response to antidepressants in elderly patients. Biol Psychiatry 22:733–740, 1987

Gibbons RD, Clark DC, Davis JM: A statistical model for the classification of imipramine response in depressed inpatients. Psychopharmacology 78:185–189, 1982

Giles DE, Rush AJ: Relationship of dysfunctional attitudes and dexamethasone response in endogenous and nonendogenous depression. Biol Psychiatry 17:1303–1314, 1982

Giles DE, Rush AJ, Roffwarg HP: Sleep parameters in bipolar I, bipolar II and unipolar depression. Biol Psychiatry 21:1340–1343, 1986

Giles DE, Schlesser MA, Rush AJ, et al: Polysomnographic findings and dexamethasone nonsuppression in unipolar depression: a replication and extension. Biol Psychiatry 22:872–882, 1987

Gillespie RD: Discussion on manic-depressive psychosis. BMJ 2:878–879, 1926

Gillespie RD: The clinical differentiation of types of depression. Guy's Hosp Rep 9:306–344, 1929

Gillin JC, Sitaram N, Duncan WC: Muscarinic supersensitivity: a possible model of the sleep disturbances of primary depression. Psychiatry Res 1:17–22, 1979

Gillin JC, Duncan WC, Murphy DL, et al: Age-related changes in sleep in depressed and normal subjects. Psychiatry Res 4:73–78, 1981

Gillin JC, Sitaram N, Wehr T, et al: Sleep and affective illness, in Neurobiology of Mood Disorders. Edited by Post RM, Ballenger JC. Baltimore, MD, Williams & Wilkins, 1984

Gitlin MJ, Gwirtzman H, Fairbanks L, et al: Dexamethasone suppression test and treatment response. J Clin Psychiatry 45:387–389, 1984

Goldberg SC, Ettigi P, Schulz PM, et al: Alprazolam versus imipramine in depressed out-patients with neurovegetative signs. J Affect Disord 11:139–145, 1986

Guy W: ECDEU Assessment Manual for Psychopharmacology Research. DHEW Publication No. (ADM) 76-338. Superintendent of Documents, U.S. Government Printing Office, Washington, DC, 1976

Hamilton M: A rating scale for depression. J Neurol Neurosurg Psychiatry 23:56–62, 1960

Hanada K, Yamada N, Kazutaka S, et al: Direct radioimmunoassay of cortisol in saliva and its application to the dexamethasone suppression test in affective disorders. Psychoneuroendocrinology 10:193–201, 1985

Harrington J, Imlah NW: A preliminary evaluation of phenelzine in a neurosis unit, in Final Report of the Symposium on Depression. Royal College of Surgeons, May 24, 1960

Hibbert GA, Teasdale JD, Spencer P: Covariation of depressive symptoms over time. Psychol Med 14:451–455, 1984

Hirschfeld R: Situational depression: validity of the concept. Br J Psychiatry 139:297–305, 1981

Hirschfeld RMA, Katz MM: Phenomenology and classification of depression, in Psychopharmacology: A Generation of Progress. Edited by Lipton MA, DiMascio A, Killiam KF. New York, Raven, 1978

Hobson RF: Prognostic factors in electric convulsive therapy. J Neurol Neurosurg Psychiatry 16:275–281, 1953

Holden NL: Depression and the Newcastle Scale: their relationship to the dexamethasone suppression test. Br J Psychiatry 142:505–507, 1983

Holsboer F, Bender W, Benkert O, et al: Diagnostic value of dexamethasone suppression test in depression (letter). Lancet 2:706, 1980

Jackson SW: Melancholia and Depression: From Hippocratic Times to Modern Times. New Haven, CT, Yale University Press, 1986

Johnson GF, Hunt G, Kerr K, et al: Dexamethasone suppression test (DST) and plasma dexamethasone levels in depressed patients. Psychiatry Res 13:305–313, 1984

Kashani JH, Carlson GA: Seriously depressed preschoolers. Am J Psychiatry 144:348–350, 1987

Kasper S, Beckmann H: Dexamethasone suppression test in a pluridiagnostic approach: its relationship to psychopathological and clinical variables. Acta Psychiatr Scand 68:31–37, 1983

Kendell RE: The classification of depressive illnesses. Maudsley Monograph No. 18. London, Oxford University Press, 1968

Kendell RE: The stability of psychiatric diagnoses. Br J Psychiatry 124:352–356, 1974

Kendell RE: The classification of depressions: a review of contemporary confusion. Br J Psychiatry 129:15–28, 1976

Kerkhofs M, Missa J, Mendlewicz J: Sleep electroencephalographic measures in primary major depressive disorder: distinction between DST suppressor and nonsuppressor patients. Biol Psychiatry 21:225–228, 1986

Kielholz P: Diagnostic aspects in the treatment of depression, in Depressive Illness: Diagnosis, Assessment, Treatment. Edited by Kielholz P. Berne, Hans Huber, 1972

Kiloh LG, Garside RF: The independence of neurotic depression and endogenous depression. Br J Psychiatry 109:451–463, 1963

Kiloh LG, Ball JRB, Garside RF: Prognostic factors in treatment of depressive states with imipramine. BMJ 1:1225–1229, 1962

Kiloh LG, Andrews G, Neilson M, et al: The relationship of the syndromes called endogenous and neurotic depression. Br J Psychiatry 121:183–196, 1971

Kiloh LG, Andrews G, Neilson M: The long-term outcome of depressive illness. Br J Psychiatry 153:752–757, 1988

Kirkegaard C, Faber J: Altered serum levels of thyroxin, triiodothyronines and diodothyronines in endogenous depression. Acta Endocrinol 96:199–207, 1981

Kirkegaard C, Bjorum N, Cohn D, et al: Thyrotropin-releasing hormone (TRH) stimulation test in manic-depressive illness. Arch Gen Psychiatry 35:1017–1021, 1978

Klein DF: Endogenomorphic depression: a conceptual and terminological revision. Arch Gen Psychiatry 31:447–454, 1974

Klerman GL: Overview of affective disorders, in Comprehensive Textbook of Psychiatry. Edited by Kaplan HI, Freedman AH, Sadock BJ. Baltimore, MD, Williams & Wilkins, 1980

Klerman GL, Rounsaville BJ, Weissman MM, et al: Interpersonal Psychotherapy for Depression. New York, Basic Books, 1984

Kovacs M, Rush AJ, Beck AT, et al: Depressed outpatients treated with cognitive therapy and pharmacotherapy: a one-year follow-up. Arch Gen Psychiatry 38:33–39, 1981

Kovacs M, Feinberg TL, Crouse-Novak MA, et al: Depressive disorders in childhood, I: a longitudinal prospective study of characteristics and recovery. Arch Gen Psychiatry 41:229–237, 1984

Kraemer HC, Rush AJ: The dexamethasone suppression test in patients with affective disorders: extension of results with signal detection methods. Unpublished data, 1994

Kraepelin E: Lectures on Clinical Psychiatry. London, Bailliere, Tindall & Cox, 1904

Kraepelin E: Manic-depressive insanity and paranoia, from Textbook of Psychiatry, 8th Edition. Translated by Barclay RM. Edinburgh, E & S Livingstone, 1921

Kryger MH, Roth T, Dement WC: Principals and Practice of Sleep Medicine. Philadelphia, PA, WB Saunders, 1989

Kumar A, Alcser K, Grunhaus L, et al: Relationships of the dexamethasone suppression test to clinical severity and degree of melancholia. Biol Psychiatry 21:436–444, 1986

Kupfer DJ: A psychobiologic marker for primary depressive disease. Biol Psychiatry 11:159–174, 1976

Kupfer DJ, Foster FG: Interval between onset of sleep and rapid eye movement sleep as an indicator for depression. Lancet 2:684–686, 1972

Kupfer DJ, Thase ME: The use of the sleep laboratory in the diagnosis of affective disorders, in Psychiatric Clinics of North America. Edited by Akiskal H. Philadelphia, PA, WB Saunders, 1983

Kupfer DJ, Foster FG, Coble P, et al: The application of EEG sleep for the differential diagnosis of affective disorders. Am J Psychiatry 135:68–74, 1978

Kupfer DL, Jarrett DB, Frank E: Relationship among selected neuroendocrine and sleep measures in patients with recurrent depression. Biol Psychiatry 19:1525–1536, 1984

Lange J: Uber melancholie. Z Ges Neurol Psychiatr 101:293, 1926. Cited in Rogerson CH: Differentiation of neuroses and psychoses, with special reference to states of depression and anxiety. J Nerv Ment Sci 86:632–644, 1940

Lange J: Die endogenen und reaktiven gemutserkrankungen, in Handbuch der Geisteskrankheiten. Edited by Bumke O. Berlin, J. Springer, 1928

Langer G, Resch L, Aschauer H, et al: TSH-response patterns to TRH stimulation may indicate therapeutic mechanisms of antidepressant and neuroleptic drugs. Neuropsychobiology 11:213–218, 1984

Larsen JK, Bjorum N, Kirkegaard C, et al: Dexamethasone suppression test, TRH test and Newcastle II depression rating in the diagnosis of depressive disorders. Acta Psychiatr Scand 71:499–505, 1985

Leckman JF, Caruso KA, Prusoff BA, et al: Appetite disturbance and excessive guilt in major depression. Arch Gen Psychiatry 41:839–844, 1984

Lee AS, Murray RM: The long-term outcome of Maudsley depressives. Br J Psychiatry 153:741–751, 1988

Leff MJ, Roatch JR, Bunney WE Jr: Environmental factors preceding the onset of severe depression. Psychiatry 33:293–301, 1970

Lenox RH, Shipley JE, Peyser JM, et al: Double-blind comparison of alprazolam versus imipramine in the inpatient treatment of major depressive illness. Psychopharmacol Bull 20:79–82, 1984

Lewis A: Melancholia: a clinical survey of depressive states. J Ment Sci 80:277–378, 1934

Lewis A: Prognosis in the manic-depressive psychoses. Lancet 2:997–999, 1936

Loosen PT: The TRH-induced TSH response in psychiatric patients: a possible neuroendocrine marker. Psychoneuroendocrinology 10:237–260, 1985

Loosen PT, Prange AJ Jr: Serum thyrotropin response to thyrotropin-releasing hormone in psychiatric patients: a review. Am J Psychiatry 139:405–416, 1982

Major LF, Murphy DL: Platelet and plasma amine oxidase activity in alcoholic individuals. Br J Psychiatry 132:548–554, 1978

Mapother E: Discussion on manic-depressive psychosis. BMJ 2:872–879, 1926

Marsella AJ: The measurement of depressive experience and disorder across cultures, in The Measurement of Depression. Edited by Marsella AJ, Hirschfeld RMA, Katz MM. New York, Guilford, 1987

Maxwell AE: Multivariate statistical methods and classification problems. Br J Psychiatry 119:121–127, 1971

McGuffin P, Katz R, Bebbington P: Hazard, heredity and depression: a family study. J Psychiatr Res 21:365–375, 1987

McGuffin P, Katz R, Aldrich J, et al: The Camberwell Collaborative Depression Study, II: investigation of family members. Br J Psychiatry 152:766–774, 1988a

McGuffin P, Katz R, Bebbington P: The Camberwell Collaborative Depression Study, III: depression and anxiety in the relatives of depressed probands. Br J Psychiatry 152:775–782, 1988b

McIntyre IM, Norman TR, Burrows GD, et al: Letter to editor. BMJ 283:1609–1610, 1981

Mendels J: Electroconvulsive therapy and depression. Br J Psychiatry 3:675–690, 1965

Mendels J: The prediction of response to electroconvulsive therapy. Am J Psychiatry 124:153–159, 1967

Mendels J, Cochrane C: The nosology of depression: the endogenous-reactive concept. Am J Psychiatry 124:1–11, 1968

Mendlewicz J, Kerkhofs M, Hoffmann G, et al: Dexamethasone suppression test and REM sleep in patients with major depressive disorder. Br J Psychiatry 145:383–388, 1984

Millin P, Coppen A: Who responds to amitriptyline? Lancet 1:763–764, 1980

Mobius PJ: Ariss der Lehre von den Nervenkrankheiten. Leipzig, Abel, 1893

Monro AB, Conitzer H: A comparison of desoxyephedrine (Methedrine) and electroshock in the treatment of depression. J Ment Sci 96:1037–1042, 1950

Murphy DL: Clinical, genetic, hormonal, and drug influences on the activity of human platelet monoamine oxidase, in Monoamine Oxidase and Its Inhibition. Edited by Wolstenholme GEW, Knight J. Amsterdam, Elsevier/Excerpta Medica/North-Holland, 1976

Nelson JC, Charney DS: Primary affective disorder criteria and the endogenous-reactive distinction. Arch Gen Psychiatry 37:787–793, 1980

Nelson JC, Mazure CM, Jatlow PI: Does melancholia predict response in major depression? J Affect Disord 18:157–165, 1990

Nymgaard K: Studies of the sedation threshold. Arch Gen Psychiatry 1:530–536, 1959

Olsen T, Laurberg P, Weeke J: Low serum triiodothyronine and high serum reverse triiodothyronine in old age: an effect of disease not age. J Clin Endocrinol Metab 47:1111–1115, 1978

Overall JE, Hollister LE, Johnson M, et al: Nosology of depression and differential response to drugs. JAMA 195:946–950, 1966

Pandey GN, Dorus E, Shaughnessy R, et al: Genetic control of platelet monoamine oxidase activity: studies of normal families. Life Sci 25:1173–1178, 1979

Pandey GN, Dorus E, Shaughnessy R, et al: Reduced platelet MAO activity and vulnerability to psychiatric disorders. Psychiatry Res 2:315–321, 1980

Parker G, Tennant C, Blignault I: Predicting improvement in patients with non-endogenous depression. Br J Psychiatry 146:132–139, 1985

Parker G, Hadzi-Pavlovic D, Boyce P: Endogenous depression as a construct: a quantitative analysis of the literature and a study of clinician judgments. Aust N Z J Psychiatry 23:357–368, 1989

Parker G, Hadzi-Pavlovic D, Mitchell P, et al: Psychosocial risk factors distinguishing melancholic and nonmelancholic depression: a comparison of six systems. Psychiatry Res 39:211–226, 1991

Partridge M: Some reflections on the nature of affective disorders, arising from the results of prefrontal leucotomy. J Ment Sci 95:795–825, 1949

Paykel ES: Classification of depressed patients: a cluster analysis derived grouping. Br J Psychiatry 118:275–288, 1971

Paykel ES: Recent life events and clinical depression, in Life Stress and Illness. Edited by Gunderson E, Rahe R. Springfield, IL, Thomas, 1974

Paykel ES: Have multivariate statistics contributed to classification? Br J Psychiatry 139:357–362, 1981

Paykel ES, Prusoff BA, Klerman GL: The endogenous-neurotic continuum in depression: rater independence and factor distributions. J Psychiatr Res 8:73–90, 1971

Paykel ES, Prusoff BA, Tanner J: Temporal stability of symptom patterns in depression. Br J Psychiatry 128:369–374, 1976

Paykel ES, Hollyman JA, Freeling P, et al: Predictors of therapeutic benefit from amitriptyline in mild depression: a general practice placebo-controlled trial. J Affect Disord 14:83–95, 1988

Perris H: Life events and depression, part I: effect of sex, age and civil status. J Affect Disord 7:11–24, 1984a

Perris H: Life events and depression, part II: results in diagnostic subgroups and in relation to the recurrence of depression. J Affect Disord 7:25–36, 1984b

Perris H, Eisemann M, Ericsson U, et al: Attempts to validate a classification of unipolar depression based on family data: symptomatological aspects Neuropsychobiology 9:103–107, 1983

Peselow ED, Goldring N, Fieve RR, et al: The dexamethasone suppression test in depressed outpatients and normal control subjects. Am J Psychiatry 140:245–247, 1983

Peselow ED, Baxter N, Fieve RR, et al: The dexamethasone suppression test as a monitor of clinical recovery. Am J Psychiatry 144:30–35, 1987

Pfohl B, Stangl D, Zimmerman M: The implications of DSM-III personality disorders for patients with major depression. J Affect Disord 7:309–318, 1984

Pollitt JD: Suggestions for a physiological classification of depression. Br J Psychiatry 3:489–495, 1965

Price LH, Nelson JC, Charney DS, et al: The clinical utility of family history diagnosis for the diagnosis of melancholia. J Nerv Ment Dis 172:5–11, 1984

Prusoff BA, Paykel ES: Typological prediction of response to amitriptyline: a replication study. Int Pharmacopsychiatry 12:153–159, 1977

Prusoff BA, Weissman MM, Klerman GL, et al: Research diagnostic criteria subtypes of depression. Arch Gen Psychiatry 37:796–801, 1980

Puchall LB, Coursey RD, Buchsbaum MS, et al: Parents of high-risk subjects defined by levels of monoamine oxidase activity. Schizophr Bull 6:338–346, 1980

Puig-Antich J, Dahl R, Ryan N, et al: Cortisol secretion in prepubertal children with major depressive disorder: episode and recovery. Arch Gen Psychiatry 46:801–809, 1989a

Puig-Antich J, Goetz D, Davies M, et al: A controlled family history study of prepubertal major depressive disorder. Arch Gen Psychiatry 46:406–418, 1989b

Rabkin JG, Quitkin FM, Stewart JR, et al: The dexamethasone suppression test with mildly to moderately depressed outpatients. Am J Psychiatry 140:926–927, 1983

Rao VAR, Coppen A: Classification of depression and response to amitriptyline therapy. Psychol Med 9:321–325, 1979

Reynolds CF III, Kupfer DJ: Sleep research in affective illness: state of the art circa 1987. Sleep 10:199–215, 1987

Reynolds CF III, Shipley JE: Sleep in depressive disorders, in Psychiatry Update: American Psychiatric Association Annual Review, Vol 4. Edited by Hales RE, Frances AJ. Washington, DC, American Psychiatric Press, 1985

Rice J, McGuffin P, Goldin LR, et al: Platelet monoamine oxidase activity: evidence for a single major locus. Psychiatry Res 7:325–335, 1982

Rickels K, Feighner JP, Smith WT: Alprazolam, amitriptyline, doxepin and placebo in the treatment of depression. Arch Gen Psychiatry 42:134–141, 1985

Riesby N, Gram LF, Bech P, et al: Imipramine: clinical effects and pharmacokinetic variability. Psychopharmacology 54:263–272, 1977

Ritti A: Folie a double-forme, in Dictionaire Encyclopédique des Sciences Medicales, Vol 3, 4th Series. Edited by Dechambre A. Paris, Asselin et Houzeau, 1876, pp 321–339

Roberts JM: Prognostic factors in the electro-shock treatment of depressive states, I: clinical features from history and examination. J Ment Sci 105:693–702, 1959a

Roberts JM: Prognostic factors in the electro-shock treatment of depressive states II: the application of specific tests. J Ment Sci 105:703–713, 1959b

Rose JT: Reactive and endogenous depressions: response to ECT. Br J Psychiatry 109:213–217, 1963

Rosenthal SH, Klerman GL: Content and consistency in the endogenous depressive pattern. Br J Psychiatry 112:471–484, 1966

Roth M: The phenomenology of depressive states. Can Psychiatr Assoc J 4 (suppl):32–52, 1959

Roth M, Gurney MWP, Mountjoy CQ: The Newcastle rating scales. Acta Psychiatr Scand Suppl 310:42–54, 1983

Roy A, Breier A, Doran AR, et al: Life events in depression: relationship to subtypes. J Affect Disord 9:143–148, 1985

Rubin RT, Poland RE, Lesser IM, et al: Neuroendocrine aspects of primary endogenous depression, IV: pituitary-thyroid axis activity in patients and matched control subjects. Psychoneuroendocrinology 12:333–347, 1987

Rush AJ, Giles DE, Roffwarg HP, et al: Sleep EEG and dexamethasone suppression test findings in outpatients with unipolar major depressive disorders. Biol Psychiatry 17:327–341, 1982

Rush AJ, Schlesser MA, Roffwarg HP, et al: Relationships among the TRH, REM latency and dexamethasone suppression tests: preliminary findings. J Clin Psychiatry 44:23–29, 1983

Rush AJ, Erman MK, Schlesser MA, et al: Alprazolam vs amitriptyline in depressions with reduced REM latencies. Arch Gen Psychiatry 42:1154–1159, 1985

Rush AJ, Jarrett RB, Gullion CM, et al: Are biological abnormalities related to prior course of depressive illness (abstract)? Biol Psychiatry 25:56A, 1989a

Rush AJ, Giles DE, Jarrett RB, et al: Reduced REM latency predicts response to tricyclic medication in depressed outpatients. Biol Psychiatry 26:61–72, 1989b

Rush AJ, Giles DE, Schlesser MA, et al: Dexamethasone response, TRH stimulation, REM latency, and subtypes of depression. Unpublished data, 1994a

Rush AJ, Giles DE, Schlesser MA, et al: The dexamethasone suppression test in patients with affective disorders. Unpublished data, 1994b

Ryan ND, Puig-Antich J, Rabinovich H, et al: The clinical picture of major depression in children and adolescents. Arch Gen Psychiatry 44:854–861, 1987

Sands SE: Electro-convulsive therapy in 301 patients in a general hospital. BMJ 2:289–293, 1946

Sargent W: The physical treatments of depression: their indications and proper use. J Neuropsychiatry 2 (suppl):1–7, 1961

Sargent W, Slater E: An Introduction to Physical Methods of Treatment in Psychiatry. Edinburgh, E & S Livingstone, 1946

Schatzberg AF, Rothschild AJ: Psychotic (delusional) major depression: should it be included as a distinct syndrome in DSM-IV? Am J Psychiatry 149:733–745, 1992

Schlesser MA, Rush AJ, Witschy JK, et al: TRH stimulation test in depressive illness subtypes. Paper presented at the 7th World Congress of Psychiatry. Vienna, Austria, July 1983

Shagass C, Jones AL: A neurophysiological test for psychiatric diagnosis: results in 750 patients. Am J Psychiatry 114:1002–1010, 1958

Simpson GM, Pi EH, Gross L, et al: Plasma levels and therapeutic response with trimipramine treatment of endogenous depression. J Clin Psychiatry 49:113–116, 1988

Snyder PJ, Utiger RD: Response to thyrotropin-releasing hormone (TRH) in normal man. J Clin Endocrinol 34:380–385, 1972

Spitzer RL, Endicott J, Robins E: Research Diagnostic Criteria: rationale and reliability. Arch Gen Psychiatry 36:773–782, 1978

Stokes PE, Stoll PM, Koslow SH, et al: Pretreatment DST and hypothalamic-pituitary-adrenocortical function in depressed patients and comparison groups: a multicenter study. Arch Gen Psychiatry 41:257–267, 1984

Strauss EB: Discussion on the diagnosis and treatment of the milder forms of the manic-depressive psychosis. Proc R Acad Med 23:894–895, 1930

Strober M: Follow-up of affective disorder patients. Paper presented at the American Psychiatric Association, New York, May 1983

Strober M, Carlson GA: Bipolar illness in adolescents with major depression. Arch Gen Psychiatry 39:549–558, 1982

Strongin EI, Hinsie LE: A method for differentiating manic-depressive depressions from other depression by means of parotic secretions. Psychiatr Q 13:697–704, 1939

Taylor MA, Redfield J, Abrams R: Neuropsychological dysfunction in schizophrenia and affective disease. Biol Psychiatry 16:467–479, 1981

Thase ME, Hersen M, Bellack AS, et al: Validation of a Hamilton subscale for endogenomorphic depression. J Affect Disord 5:267–278, 1983

Thompson K, Hendrie H: Environmental stress in primary depressive illness. Arch Gen Psychiatry 26:130–132, 1972

van Praag HM, Uleman AM, Spitz JC: The vital syndrome interview. Psychiatr Neurol Neurochir 68:329–349, 1965

von Knorring L: Morbidity risk for psychiatric disorders in relatives of patients with neurotic-reactive depression, in Anxious Depression: Assessment and Treatment. Edited by Racagni G, Smeraldi E. New York, Raven, 1987

von Knorring L, Oreland L: Visual averaged evoked responses and platelet monoamine oxidase activity as an aid to identify a risk group for alcoholic abuse: a preliminary report. Prog Neuropsychopharmacol Biol Psychiatry 2:385–392, 1978

von Knorring L, Perris C, Oreland L, et al: Morbidity risk for psychiatric disorders in families of probands with affective disorders divided according to levels of platelet MAO activity. Psychiatry Res 15:271–279, 1985

Waldman H: Die Tageschwankung in der Depression als rhythmisches Phanomenon. Fortschritte der Neurologie-Psychiatrie 40:83–104, 1982

Wenzel KW, Meinhold H, Herpich M: TRH-Simulationstest mit Alters-und-geschlechtsabhangingem: TSH-Anstieg bei Normalpersonen. Klin Wochenschr 52:722–727, 1974

Wieberg A, Gottfries C-G, Oreland L: Low platelet monoamine oxidase activity in human alcoholics. Med Biol 55:181–186, 1977

Wing JK, Cooper JE, Sartorius N: The Measurement and Classification of Psychiatric Symptoms. London, Cambridge University Press, 1974

Winokur G: Controversies in depression, or do clinicians know something after all? in Treatment of Depression: Old Controversies and New Approaches. Edited by Clayton PC, Barrett JE. New York: Raven, 1983

Winokur G: The validity of neurotic-reactive depression: new data and reappraisal. Arch Gen Psychiatry 42:1116–1122, 1985

Winokur G: Family (genetic) studies in neurotic depression. J Psychiatr Res 21:357–363, 1987

Winokur G, Pitts FN: Affective disorder, I: is reactive depression an entity? J Nerv Ment Dis 138:541–547, 1964

Winokur G, Black DW, Nasrallah A: Depressions secondary to other psychiatric disorders and medical illnesses. Am J Psychiatry 145:233–237, 1988

Winter H, Herschel M, Propping P, et al: A twin study of three enzymes (DBH, COMT, MAO) of catecholamine metabolism: correlations with MMPI. Psychopharmacology 57:63–69, 1978

World Health Organization: Mental Disorders: Glossary and Guide to Their Classification in Accordance with the Ninth Revision of the International Classification of Diseases. Geneva, World Health Organization, 1978

Young MA, Scheftner WA, Klerman GL, et al: The endogenous subtype of depression: a study of its internal construct validity. Br J Psychiatry 148:257–267, 1986

Young MA, Keller MB, Lavori PW, et al: Lack of stability of the RDC endogenous subtype in consecutive episodes of major depression. J Affect Disord 12:139–143, 1987

Zimmerman M, Spitzer RL: Melancholia: from DSM-III to DSM-III-R. Am J Psychiatry 146:20–28, 1989

Zimmerman M, Coryell W, Pfohl B, et al: Four definitions of endogenous depression and the dexamethasone suppression test. J Affect Disord 8:37–45, 1985a

Zimmerman M, Stangl D, Coryell W: The research diagnostic criteria for endogenous depression and the dexamethasone suppression test: a discriminant function analysis. Psychiatry Res 14:197–208, 1985b

Zimmerman M, Coryell W, Pfohl B, et al: The validity of four definitions of endogenous depression, II: clinical, demographic, familial and psychosocial correlates. Arch Gen Psychiatry 43:234–244, 1986

Zung WWK: Effect of antidepressant drugs on sleeping and dreaming on the depressed patient, III. Biol Psychiatry 1:283–287, 1969

Chapter 10

Should Atypical Depression Be Included in DSM-IV?

Judith G. Rabkin, Ph.D., Jonathan W. Stewart, M.D.,
Frederic M. Quitkin, M.D., Patrick J. McGrath, M.D.,
Wilma M. Harrison, M.D., and Donald F. Klein, M.D.

Statement of the Issue

Although the cluster of affective and vegetative symptoms referred to as atypical depression (AD) has been the object of both research and clinical interest for nearly 20 years, neither DSM-III (American Psychiatric Association 1980) nor DSM-III-R (American Psychiatric Association 1987) provided the necessary criteria for their diagnosis. The issue is whether such provision should be made in DSM-IV and in what manner. In this review, we consider the available research evidence in seven areas: 1) clinical description, 2) treatment response, 3) specificity of response, 4) longitudinal course, 5) family history, 6) laboratory findings, and 7) differential diagnosis. We conclude with recommendations regarding integration of AD in DSM-IV.

Significance of the Issue

Comparison of findings concerning AD between research groups is complicated by the absence of consensually agreed on criteria for AD. No two research groups have used exactly the same definitions, although there are clearly common themes. Our review illustrates the lack of diagnostic consistency in the field today and reveals the need for a common set of criteria for future research.

Method

We included all published studies of patients with unipolar depression who appeared to meet criteria for AD and that provided evidence with respect to the seven issues listed above. Because little has been published in several of these areas, we also cite unpublished data from the Columbia group (defined below).

Results and Discussion: Clinical Description and Criteria for Atypical Depression

The category of AD was first proposed to characterize depressed patients who respond poorly to tricyclic antidepressants and well to monoamine oxidase inhibitors (MAOIs) (Dally and Rohde 1961; Sargant 1960; West and Dally 1959). Nearly 30 years later, it is widely agreed that such depressed patients exist (Quitkin et al. 1988), but the definition of the disorder remains unstandardized. Variations in definition make it difficult to compare findings between research groups. Furthermore, as Aarons (1988) notes, "the question of exactly which 'atypical' clinical characteristics correlate with the putative preferential response of this group to MAOIs has also not been answered" (p. 142). Table 10–1 summarizes the clinical descriptions of AD given by the five groups who have studied characteristics of MAOI responders. The first four groups worked retrospectively, first selecting patients quite broadly defined as depressed, with or without additional diagnostic requirements such as the presence of anxiety. They then sought to characterize MAOI responders. Only the Columbia group has prospectively delineated essential and associated features of AD and then conducted comparative drug trials. We review the work of these groups chronologically.

English Group

The term *atypical depression* was used by West and Dally (1959) and Sargant (1960) to describe patients who were particularly responsive to treatment with iproniazid in contrast to electroconvulsive therapy (ECT) or imipramine. These disorders were characterized by mood reactivity and multiple additional features such as initial insomnia, reversed diurnal variation, fatigue, somatic overreactivity, good premorbid function and personality, and poor response to ECT. These patients tended not to display classical endogenous symptoms such as self-reproach, weight loss, or worse mood in the morning. Overeating and oversleeping were not emphasized, interpersonal sensitivity was not cited.

Table 10–1. Clinical description of atypical depression

Research group	Measure of depression	Vegetative symptoms	Mood reactivity	Anxiety	Other
West and Dally 1959	Associated symptoms (none required)	Associated symptoms (none required) 1. Evening worsening 2. Severe fatigue, lethargy 3. Generalized anxiety, phobias, and panic attacks 4. Somatic preoccupation 5. Premenstrual tension	Not required but considered characteristic	Not required but considered characteristic	1. Endogenous vegetative symptoms said to be absent 2. Good premorbid functioning and personality considered characteristic
Ravaris et al. 1980	RDC major or minor depression	Associated symptoms (none required) 1. Evening worsening 2. Hysterical personality 3. Weight gain 4. Psychic, somatic anxiety 5. Initial insomnia	Not required but considered characteristic	Not required but considered characteristic	
Paykel et al. 1983; Rowan et al. 1982	Moderate depression: score of 7–11 on Raskin 3-area Depression Scale; RDC, ICD-8	Subtype 1: "anxious depression:" psychic anxiety, somatic anxiety, panic attacks Subtype 2: "atypical functional shift": evening worsening, initial insomnia, appetite increase, sleep increase Subtype 3: "nonendogenous depression:" RDC endogenous, Nies-Robinson Diagnostic Index, Newcastle Scale,[a] Klein endogenomorphic, RDC[b] incapacitating			

(continued)

Table 10–1. Clinical description of atypical depression (*continued*)

Research group	Measure of depression	Vegetative symptoms	Mood reactivity	Anxiety	Other
Davidson et al. 1988	RDC major or minor; minimum score of 20 on Hamilton 24-item Depression Scale	Subtype 1: Anxious-vegetative (one required) 1. Hyperphagia 2. Weight gain 3. Evening mood worse Subtype 2: Anxious; no required vegetative features listed above	Required	Required: Minimum score of 8 on Covi Anxiety Scale and significant anxiety, somatic complaints, phobic or panic symptoms	Exclusion: Score on Newcastle Scale signifying endogenous depression
Columbia group (Leibowitz et al. 1984; Quitkin et al. 1989)	RDC major, minor, or intermittent; DSM-III major depression or dysthymia; 10+ on Hamilton 21-item Depression Scale	One of four required 1. Overeating, increased appetite/weight gain 2. Oversleeping 3. Leaden paralysis 4. Pathologic rejection sensitivity	Required	Not required, but history of panic attacks is noted	

[a]Roth et al. 1983.
[b]Spitzer et al. 1978.

Robinson, Ravaris, and Colleagues

In the United States, Robinson and his group were among the first to undertake clinical trials with MAOIs (Ravaris et al. 1976; Robinson et al. 1973). Their basic criterion for study inclusion was that "enough depressive symptoms were present to warrant drug treatment" (Ravaris et al. 1980, p. 1076). In their work, reactivity of mood, anxiety, and the absence of terminal insomnia were the hallmarks of patients who were preferentially responsive to MAOIs.

Paykel, Rowan, and Colleagues

Paykel, Rowan, and colleagues at St. George's Hospital in London conducted a number of studies of nonendogenous depression (Paykel et al. 1983; Rowan et al. 1981, 1982). They identified three clusters of symptoms or features cited in the literature as manifestations of AD: anxiety symptoms with or without depression, reversed vegetative symptoms, and mood reactivity. They focused on outpatients with moderately severe depression. Operational definitions of these formulations of AD are shown in Table 10–1.

Davidson and Colleagues

Davidson and his group have studied AD since the late 1970s, although unlike Robinson, Paykel, and the Columbia group, they have used isocarboxazid rather than phenelzine. For study inclusion, they required an RDC diagnosis of either major or minor depression, as well as the presence of anxiety defined as a minimum score of 8 on the Covi Anxiety Scale (Lipman 1982), including a score of at least 3 on the somatic component. They also required a minimum baseline score of at least 20 on the Hamilton Rating Scale for Depression (24-item version) (Hamilton 1967), depression lasting at least 4 weeks, and presence of significant anxiety, somatic complaints, and phobic or panic symptoms (Davidson et al. 1988).

More specific criteria for AD were later identified for analysis of patient subgroups. These required mood reactivity and nonendogenicity (Newcastle Scale) (Gurney et al. 1972). AD patients were subsequently divided into those with one or more vegetative atypical symptoms (hyperphagia, weight gain, or evening mood worsening), who are referred to as anxious-vegetative AD, and those without any of these vegetative symptoms, referred to as anxious AD.

Columbia Group

The Columbia group designed trials to demonstrate phenelzine superiority over tricyclics in a subset of depressed patients with the essential feature of mood reactivity. In the original study (Liebowitz et al. 1984), patients had to meet RDC criteria (Spitzer et al. 1978) for major, intermittent, or minor depression. Later studies required presence of a DSM-III or DSM-III-R diagnosis of major depression, dysthymia, depression not otherwise specified (NOS), or bipolar disorder NOS. Patients who had a full manic episode were excluded. In addition to the essential criterion of mood reactivity, two or more of four associated features were necessary: oversleeping, overeating, leaden paralysis, and rejection sensitivity. Anxiety and reversed diurnal variation were not included as diagnostic criteria. More recently, this group proposed that the presence of only one associated symptom from the list of four suffices for a diagnosis of AD (Quitkin et al. 1988).

Clinical Picture: Columbia Definition

We present in detail the Columbia operational definition, because no other group has delineated explicit inclusion and exclusion criteria. The time frame is the current episode or past 3 months, except for rejection sensitivity, which refers to any 2-year period since age 18.

The essential criterion of mood reactivity is defined as the capacity to be cheered up, or to respond pleasurably, when presented with positive environmental events. Mood reactivity is rated present if the patient responds with a mood lift of at least 50% toward a hypothetical "100% of normal mood" as experienced at their best, when presented with positive environmental events.

The associated symptom of oversleeping is defined as sleeping at least 10 hours a day, or sleeping at least 2 hours a day more than when not depressed, or spending 2 hours a day in bed, lying down and doing nothing, which is not a consequence of insomnia. Any of these manifestations of hypersomnia must be present at least 3 days a week to meet the criterion.

The symptom of overeating is defined in one of three ways: marked increase in appetite, marked increase in eating (defined as occasional binges, frequent snacks, or other overeating), or weight gain of a least 5 pounds in the past 6 weeks.

The symptom of leaden paralysis is defined as feeling heavy, leaden, or weighted down for at least 1 hour a day at least 3 days a week.

Finally, the symptom of rejection sensitivity requires pathological sensitivity to interpersonal rejection resulting in significant functional impairment. This feature is unique to the Columbia definition and derives from Klein et al.'s (1980) definition of hysteroid dysphoria. It should be emphasized that the majority of Columbia patients manifest this trait. For this feature, the time frame is never the past week but rather the period in adulthood when the person is not depressed, when such a period can be identified. Examples of functional impairment include stormy relationships, frequently failing in important responsibilities, and avoidance of relationships. At least one of three features is required. The first, quality of relationships, refers to how smoothly the patient gets along with others in intimate relationships. The essential ingredient here is the degree of conflict and disruption associated with excessive sensitivity. The second feature is functional impairment in the context of interpersonal sensitivity; this is scored as present if the person reacts to criticism or rebuff by leaving work early, drinking too much, or otherwise displaying substantial maladaptive behavioral responses at least 4 times in a 2-year period. The third feature is avoidance of relationships, defined as avoiding intimate relationships due to rejection sensitivity for at least 2 years. Unlike the other features of AD, rejection sensitivity is regarded as a trait rather than a state, although, as a rule, it is exacerbated during depression. It should be noted that being occasionally touchy or overemotional does not qualify.

Comment

The common element in these descriptions is the reactivity of mood observed or required by all investigators except Paykel. Otherwise, a variety of nonendogenous features are noted that fall into two broad categories: those of anxiety and those of reverse endogenous vegetative symptoms (or what Paykel et al. [1983] refer to as atypical functional shift). Although anxiety is not a defining characteristic for most of the research groups studying AD, their samples generally can be characterized by the presence of some form of anxiety, whether it be "somatic" or "psychic," phobic, or manifested as panic attacks.

It should be noted that, because the Columbia group has found that only one "atypical" symptom appears to be necessary to characterize AD in their conceptualization, and because pathological rejection sensitivity is one of four such symptoms they identify as a qualifying criterion (that is not a vegetative symptom), atypical vegetative behaviors per se may not constitute a necessary characteristic of AD. Nonetheless, as discussed below, AD should not be equated with all nonautonomous depression.

Atypical Depression and Response to MAOIs

Identification of a nosological category by treatment response is an unusual strategy in psychiatry (Klein 1989). When the notion of AD was originally developed, it was generally believed that MAOIs were less effective than tricyclics in the treatment of depression. Consequently, controlled studies of MAOIs in the 1970s concentrated on demonstrating efficacy over placebo in nonendogenous depressed patients, including a subset retrospectively identified as "atypical" who were presumed to exhibit a preferential response. As shown in Table 10–2, three studies independently demonstrated that phenelzine, administered at therapeutic doses, was superior to placebo in treatment of patients with atypical features (Mountjoy et al. 1977; Ravaris et al. 1976; Robinson et al. 1973). More recently, Davidson et al. (1988) showed isocarboxazid to be superior to placebo in patients with major depression accompanied by anxiety and at least one atypical vegetative feature.

Table 10–2. Controlled trials of monoamine oxidase inhibitors (MAOIs) in atypical depression

Investigators	Completers (*n*)	Trial duration	Drug comparisons			Comments	Inclusion criteria
			MAOI PBO	MAOI TCA	TCA PBO		
Robinson et al. 1973	87	6 weeks	PZ > PBO			Special MAOI efficacy noted for "atypical" features such as anxiety, fatigue.	Presence of significant persistent and disabling depressive symptoms required. Age 20+ years. Most referrals from general medical practices.
Ravaris et al. 1976	49	6 weeks	PZ > PBO			PZ 30 mg/day = PBO; PZ 60 mg/day > PBO. Patients had depression and anxiety. Marked improvement: PZ (60 mg) = 67%, PBO = 32%.	Significant depressive symptoms required. Age range 20–80 years.
Mountjoy et al. 1977	83	4 weeks	PZ > PBO			All patients also received a benzodiazepine "for ethical reasons." Maximum PZ dose = 75 mg. Patients had diagnosis of neurotic depression, anxiety neurosis, or agoraphobia.	Mostly inpatients; some day and outpatients. Patients with 2+ symptoms of endogenous depression were excluded. Patients had diagnosis of neurotic depression, anxiety neurosis or agoraphobia.

	N	Duration				Results	Diagnostic criteria
Ravaris et al. 1980	105	6 weeks	PZ > PBO	PZ = AMI	AMI > PBO	Marked improvement: PZ = 56%, AMI = 57%. Maximum dose: PZ = 60 mg, AMI = 150 mg. Both drugs found to have antidepressant and antianxiety effects.	RDC major or minor with significant anxiety. Broad spectrum of symptoms. Patients were included if they had enough depressive symptoms to warrant drug treatment.
Paykel et al. 1983	131	6 weeks	PZ > PBO	PZ = AMI	AMI > PBO	Maximum dose: PZ = 75 mg, AMI = 187.5 mg. No evidence of differential response to AMI and PZ.	RDC major (96%) or minor. Score of 7–11 on Raskin required. Mean illness duration was 11 months (i.e., nonchronic sample).
Davidson et al. 1988	81	6 weeks	ISO > PBO			Maximum dose of ISO = 60 mg/day at week 6. Response rate: ISO = 66%, PBO = 32%. Patients had minimum score of 20 on HAM-D at baseline plus anxiety symptoms. Drug was not superior to PBO for patients who met RDC for minor depression and for those without atypical vegetative symptoms.	RDC major or minor. Covi Anxiety Scale = 8+; Ham-D = 20+; presence of significant anxiety, somatic complaints, and phobic or panic symptoms was required.

Note. PBO = placebo. PZ = phenelzine. AMI = amitriptyline. ISO = isocarboxazid. HAM-D = Hamilton Rating Scale for Depression. RDC = Research Diagnostic Criteria. TCA = tricyclic antidepressant.

The next logical question was whether phenelzine was actually superior to tricyclics in the treatment of AD. Controlled studies conducted in the 1970s reported equal efficacy but did not prospectively develop an atypical depressive sample. Ravaris et al. (1980) found no difference in efficacy between phenelzine and amitriptyline; both were reported to have antianxiety and antidepressant effects. Paykel et al. (1983) also failed to find a difference in clinical response to phenelzine and amitriptyline; both active drugs were superior to placebo.

Over the past 10 years, the Columbia group has conducted four studies of patients with prospectively defined AD comparing phenelzine, imipramine, and placebo. These include the study of 119 AD patients with two or more atypical features (Liebowitz et al. 1988), a replication study of 90 AD patients with two or more associated AD features (Quitkin et al. 1990), Quitkin et al.'s (1988) study of 60 AD patients with only one associated AD feature ("probable" AD study), and a study of 60 depressed mood-reactive patients with no associated features(Quitkin et al. 1989). All patients met DSM-III criteria for major depression and/or dysthymia, or depressive disorder NOS.

These four studies, shown in Table 10–3, together include 269 mood-reactive patients with AD and 60 with mood reactivity but no associated features. Individually and cumulatively, the three studies of AD patients show that these patients more often respond to phenelzine than to imipramine, a difference that is both clinically and statistically significant.

What is noteworthy in all of these studies is not the robust response to phenelzine but a reduced response to imipramine. The fourth study of 60 patients with reactive mood without any associated AD features shows a different pattern of response: imipramine and phenelzine were found to be equal in efficacy, and both were superior to placebo. Only 19 patients received imipramine, however, and the confidence interval limits of 49%–91% preclude firm conclusions that the clinical response to imipramine is higher in this group. Replication is necessary.

During the 1970s and early 1980s, a number of studies with outpatients demonstrated that, at appropriate doses, MAOIs have a considerably broader range of efficacy than initially believed. They may be as effective as tricyclics for the treatment of outpatients with melancholic major depression (e.g., McGrath et al. 1986) and panic disorder (Sheehan 1980–1981) and are effective in social phobia (Liebowitz et al. 1988). Consequently, the finding of MAOI efficacy in AD patients is no longer distinctive (because depressed patients without atypical features also respond).

What *is* extraordinary, in the results available to date, is the finding that mood-reactive patients with at least one associated feature of AD appear to do worse than expected in response to imipramine. This has not been reported by other groups (listed in Table 10–2) or in the clinical literature (e.g., Sovner 1981).

Table 10–3. Columbia group studies of atypical depression (AD)

Investigators	Diagnostic group	Total N (completers)	Percentage improved after 6 weeks (CGI)			Imipramine-phenelzine contrast (CGI)[a]
			Placebo	Imipramine	Phenelzine	
Liebowitz et al. 1988	Reactive mood with 2+ associated features: "original study"	119	28 (13/47)	50 (19/38)	71 (24/34)	$\chi^2 = 3.16$ $P = .08$
Quitkin et al. 1990	Reactive mood with 2+ associated features: "replication" study	90	19 (5/26)	50 (17/34)	83 (25/30)	$\chi^2 = 7.8$ $P = .005$
Quitkin et al. 1988	Reactive mood with only 1 associated feature: "probable" AD	60	29 (7/24)	47 (9/19)	71 (12/17)	$\chi^2 = 1.99$ $P = NS$
Quitkin et al. 1989	Reactive mood with no associated features	60	25 (5/20)	74 (14/19)	75 (15/20)	NS

Note. CGI = Clinical Global Impression.

[a]Combining results for the first 3 studies, 45 of 91 AD patients (49%) responded to imipramine, and 61 of 81 (75%) to phenelzine. $\chi^2 = 12.12$, $P = .001$.

However, the Columbia group has replicated this finding in several ways. First, at the end of these 6-week trials, nonresponders were crossed over to a second treatment in double-blind fashion. Of those who did not respond to placebo ($n = 67$), 63% improved at the end of 6 weeks of treatment with phenelzine, compared to 35% response to imipramine (Quitkin et al. 1991). Imipramine response in phenelzine nonresponders was 39% (7 of 18), whereas phenelzine response among imipramine nonresponders was 68% (26 of 38) (unpublished data).

In the Quitkin et al. (1989) study of 60 patients with reactive mood and no atypical features, among whom the 19 patients treated with imipramine had a 74% response rate, 10 of 11 patients who failed to improve on placebo responded to imipramine, whereas 3 of 4 placebo nonresponders improved on phenelzine. Although small, these numbers show the same trends as those observed in the initial 6-week trial.

Study Differences

The most apparent differences concern sample selection and variations in inclusion and exclusion criteria, including depressive subtype, age, and AD definition. The samples of Paykel et al. and Ravaris et al. appear to include patients with prominent anxious-phobic symptoms in addition to depression, whereas the patients in the Columbia group characteristically manifested vegetative features that Paykel has called "atypical functional shift." These diagnostic differences suggest that the Columbia group may be tapping a different patient population. Their patients are more mildly and more chronically depressed, with earlier age at onset and little evidence of phasic course. Rejection sensitivity is a common feature. It is possible that these characteristics, rather than the specific atypical features often seen, are the central defining features associated with poorer imipramine response and intact phenelzine response. If patients identified by these criteria do indeed have a lower likelihood of responding to tricyclics, this finding has direct relevance for clinical practice. It may also provide a lead in identifying biological differences in subtypes of depression.

Specificity of Treatment Response: Predictive Utility of Symptoms of Atypical Depression

Most investigators working with AD samples have searched for predictors of preferential MAOI treatment response. As shown in Table 10–4, no individual symptom or symptom cluster has been found to be consistently associated with preferential treatment response. No research group has identified and replicated specific AD features associated with superior MAOI response or inferior tricyclic antidepressant treatment response. The available evidence suggests that, for depressed patients with reactive mood, none of the features of AD strongly and consistently predicts clinical response in the individual case. In the aggregate, atypical features appear to be associated with poorer imipramine response and do not predict phenelzine response, which remains high regardless of whether they are present.

Comment: Practical Implications of Identifying the Subtype of AD

Historically, the major practical advantage of identifying AD as a subtype of depressive disorder concerns selection of treatment medication. Because patients with at least one symptom of AD in the presence of reactive mood respond more poorly to imipramine than do other patients, the treating physician may consider another antidepressant class as the first treatment. In the past, this suggested an initial trial with an MAOI, despite the need for dietary compliance, greater risk of side effects, and consequent increased likelihood of drug discontinuation (Agosti et al. 1988).

Newer agents such as fluoxetine might be as effective as MAOIs in treating AD, although no controlled trials have been published to date. In the clinical experience

Table 10–4. Predictors of preferential monoamine oxidase inhibitor response in patients with atypical depression (AD)

Investigators	Predictors	Comment
Ravaris et al. 1980	Reactive mood plus terminal insomnia	Post hoc finding, not tested in new sample
Davidson et al. 1988	Interpersonal sensitivity and phobic avoidance; panic is a negative predictor	No information provided about amount of variance in treatment response accounted for by these variables
Mountjoy et al. 1977	No symptoms or pattern of symptoms found to predict outcome	Specific variables entered into regression equations not specified
Paykel et al. 1983	Concurrent anxiety diagnosis; absence of "characterological" depression; no other symptoms or traits	Unclear how many patients had AD
McGrath et al. 1992	Defining symptoms of overeating, oversleeping, lethargy, and rejection sensitivity only predict poor TCA response if no other symptom present; anxiety and endogenicity not predictive	Only AD studied; large sample, prospective design

Note. TCA = tricyclic antidepressant.

of the Columbia group, the majority of AD patients have responded to fluoxetine. Other preliminary reports on fluoxetine combined with a tricyclic for resistant major depression (Weilburg et al. 1989), bipolar II depression (Simpson and DePaulo 1989), and borderline personality (Cornelius et al. 1989) indirectly suggest possible efficacy for patients with AD.

Evidence Regarding Validity

As Kupfer and Thase (1987) note, "the validity of medical diagnoses traditionally has been tested against several lines of evidence: clinical phenomenology, longitudinal course (natural history), family history, treatment response, and if available, laboratory studies" (p. 35). Clinical phenomenology is described above. The available evidence in the other areas is reviewed here in turn. Because published reports are few; we include analyses of unpublished data from the Columbia group.

Longitudinal Course (Natural History)

Age at onset.   Compared with patients who meet criteria for major depression (including melancholia) or dysthymia but who have no features of AD, the AD patients report sharply earlier age at onset according to the Columbia group, as well as Davidson et al. (1982), Sovner (1981), and Pollitt and Young (1971). The average AD patient reports illness onset starting in high school, compared to the mid-20s or early 30s for the other groups. Although the literature is modest, available evidence points to early age at onset in AD compared with other depression.

Illness course.   Patients with AD tend to have a chronic nonphasic course. Roughly two-thirds of the patients studied at Columbia would meet criteria for DSM-III dysthymia, with or without superimposed major depression, at some time during their illness. Reports of clear-cut episodes interspersed with substantial stretches of well-being are uncommon. In contrast, Thase et al. (1991) found that the majority of their patients selected to have recurrent, phasic major depression also had reversed vegetative symptoms, with or without reactive mood. Chronicity is thus not a necessary characteristic of AD but may characterize patients who seek treatment at a university research clinic, because many melancholic patients at Columbia also describe a chronic illness course.

Davidson et al. (1982) described different patterns of illness for the subtypes of AD they defined. The A type (anxious depression) is considered to be often chronic and persistent over many years. The V type (reversed vegetative symptoms) is said to be intermittent. They noted the problem of describing illness course in patients who may have characterological depression or "subaffective dysthymia" in terms of lack of clarity regarding onset and offset of symptoms. Pollitt and Young

(1971) studied the distribution of typical and atypical depressive symptoms separately in relation to age, for males and females, and for patients with anxiety and with depression. In each of these groups and in the combined sample of 101 anxiety patients and 147 depressed patients, a clear age-related pattern was observed: atypical symptoms were more common in younger adults and typical symptoms appeared more frequently with increasing age and also older age of illness onset. Looked at cross-sectionally, Pollitt and Young's data suggest that atypical symptoms are replaced by typical symptoms. Because this was not a longitudinal analysis, however, their data cannot prove that this occurs, and it is not the experience of the Columbia group.

Another explanation regarding the relation of atypical to typical symptoms over time is that atypical symptoms are manifested during milder phases of illness and convert to typical symptoms as the depression becomes increasingly severe. Some evidence for this idea may be found in Akiskal et al.'s (1978) 4-year prospective study of 100 patients initially diagnosed as having "neurotic depression" according to DSM-II (American Psychiatric Association 1968).

It is generally believed that AD is not as severe as melancholia (Davidson et al. 1982). Even taking into account the fact that atypical symptoms are not given scores on standard ratings scales of severity, the Columbia group found that outpatients with AD have Hamilton scores in the mild to moderate range, and patients with melancholia have higher scores.

In the absence of a well-defined cohort study of patients with AD observed over many years, the hypothesis that AD is a milder variant of melancholia, or that it evolves into endogenous or melancholic depression, cannot be either refuted or demonstrated.

Family History

Only a handful of reports in this area have been published, and none are specific to AD. West and Dally (1959) reported a positive family history of depression in 36% of their MAOI-responsive patients, but type of illness was not reported. Pare and Mack (1971) proposed the existence of two genetically distinct types of depression: one that responds better to MAOIs and the other with a preferential response to tricyclics. As evidence, they cited the observation that first-degree relatives often respond to a given class of antidepressants in the same way that probands do. Whether shared drug response necessarily signifies shared clinical symptoms or an underlying common disorder has not been shown, however.

Stewart et al. (1993) recently analyzed data on familial disorders of depressed patients that he screened over a 7-year period at the Depression Evaluation Service at Columbia. In addition, he also completed a pilot study with blind raters and direct family interviews. These studies are shown in Table 10–5. Cumulatively, the

Table 10–5. Rates of psychiatric disorder in relatives of probands with atypical depression and melancholia as determined by family history interview

Proband diagnosis	N	Relatives	Rate of disorder in relatives (N/100)			
			Major depression	Dysthymic disorder	Atypical depression	Alcohol abuse
Atypical depression	173	736	2.9 (21)[a]	11.8 (87)	3.4 (25)	9.2 (68)
Melancholia	53	297	6.1 (18)	3.4 (10)	1.0 (3)	5.7 (17)
	Statistics		5.99	17.77	4.57	3.46
	$2 \times 2 \, \chi^2$		$P = .01$	$P = .0001$	$P = .03$	$P = .06$

[a]In parentheses are number of relatives with the disorder.
Source. Data from Stewart 1993.

modest available evidence is compatible with the hypothesis that AD tends to show differential familial aggregation.

Laboratory Studies

Sleep studies.   Patients with primary unipolar depressive disorder show a consistent profile of sleep abnormalities. These include shortened initial rapid eye movement (REM) latency, increased REM density, decreased total sleep time, decreased sleep efficiency, and decreased percentage of delta sleep. Patients with bipolar disorder reportedly manifest none of these features except for shortened initial REM latency, which thus appears to be the most consistent sleep abnormality found in affective disorder. The Columbia group (Quitkin et al. 1985) found that the sleep of AD patients was largely equivalent to that of control subjects, but, in contrast, was observed to be clearly and sharply different from the sleep of melancholic patients.

Tyramine excretion.   Sandler et al. (1975) in London noted that severely depressed unipolar patients who would meet current criteria for melancholia excreted significantly lower amounts of sulfate-conjugated tyramine compared with control subjects. The test consists of administering a standardized oral tyramine load and measuring the amount of tyramine excreted in urine over the next 3 hours. Sandler's finding was replicated by Harrison et al. (1984) in a study comparing 38 melancholic patients with 34 control subjects. A group of 51 patients with AD was also included. Overall, the melancholic patients had significantly lower tyramine excretion levels than either the AD patients or the control subjects, who did not differ significantly from each other.

Dichotic listening.   At Columbia, Bruder et al. (1989) compared the dichotic listening performance of 40 atypical patients, compared to 25 melancholic patients and 30 control subjects. Melancholic patients had abnormal perceptual asymmetry on dichotic listening tasks due to poor left-ear performance, which is consistent with hypothesized right-hemispheric dysfunction. In contrast, patients with AD did not differ from control subjects on these tasks.

Comparable findings were not observed for visual tachistoscopic tasks, suggesting either that perceptual asymmetry in melancholia is specific to the auditory modality or that procedural differences or lower reliability of visual tasks may have precluded identification of time differences in this modality as well.

Dextroamphetamine challenge.   The Columbia group gave 0.15 mg/kg i.v. dextroamphetamine to 64 patients, including 24 with AD and 19 with melancholia.

Fifteen of the patients with AD had a dysphoric mood response, compared to 2 of the melancholic patients ($\chi^2 = 11.98$, $P = .001$). Differential mood response to stimulants may distinguish patients with melancholia from those with AD. This dysphoria differs from the clinical history of positive response to oral stimulants reported by many AD patients.

Comment.   Patients with AD generally have results in the normal range on neurophysiological measures, such as the dexamethasone suppression test and polysomnography, that are usually taken in depressed patients, unlike results found in melancholically depressed patients. Patients with AD have usually had normal cerebral asymmetry on testing of cerebral laterality, unlike patients with melancholia, who typically have a reversal of laterality. Cumulatively, these findings suggest that the pathophysiology of AD may be different from that of melancholia.

Relation of Atypical Depression to Other Affective Disorders With Overlapping Features

Seasonal affective disorder.   The symptomatology of seasonal affective disorder (SAD) is similar to that of AD and often includes oversleeping, overeating, and intense lethargy (Terman et al. 1989). Because the associated symptomatology is similar to that of AD, it is reasonable to wonder whether SAD and AD are independent entities. If they are in fact different manifestations of the same disorder, treatment that is effective for one might also benefit the other.

The Columbia group, with Michael Terman, has treated a series of patients with clear-cut SAD in clinical trials. Atypical patients without a seasonal pattern were found unresponsive to light treatment. This differential treatment outcome seems most consistent with SAD and AD representing separate disorders. We are unaware of other data addressing the possible distinction between SAD and AD.

Bipolar disorder.   It is recognized both in the biological and clinical research literature that there is some overlap in sleep profile, clinical symptoms, and medication response between anergic bipolar depressed patients and those with AD. Anergic bipolar depressions are often characterized by oversleeping, low energy, and weight gain, as well as responsivity to MAOIs (e.g., Kupfer et al. 1973). Himmelhoch et al. (1991), in a controlled study of 56 anergic bipolar patients with at least one reversed vegetative symptom of depression, reported preferential response to tranylcypromine compared with imipramine, as previously reported for unipolar patients with AD. In the sleep research literature, bipolar depressed patients have normal sleep efficiency, as do patients with AD, in contrast to other forms of depressive disorder, where sleep is characterized by fragmentation and decreased continuity (Feinberg et al. 1982).

Based on such observations, the question may be asked whether the syndrome described as AD may be a preliminary stage preceding the development of bipolarity or a *forme fruste* of bipolar disorder. There are no longitudinal cohort studies available to address this question directly. Two indirect but related areas of consideration are family history in relatives of patients with AD, and rates of antidepressant-induced mania in atypical versus endogenous patients. If AD were an unrecognized variant of bipolar disorder, increased rates of bipolarity and increased rates of antidepressant-induced mania or hypomania should be seen in the relatives of patients with AD compared with those of unipolar depressed melancholic patients. The available evidence on family history (Stewart, unpublished observations) and rates of tricyclic-induced mania in AD patients (Rabkin et al. 1985) do not support either hypothesis.

Recommendation for Integration of Atypical Depression in DSM-IV

The research literature cumulatively supports the notion that the diagnostic category of AD has clinical utility, as well as preliminary evidence of physiological and biochemical distinctions from other forms of depression. Both for clinical application and to encourage cumulative development of research knowledge across research groups, its inclusion in DSM-IV as a modifier for depressive disorder seems warranted for all DSM-III-R depressive and bipolar categories except mania.

A revised diagnostic system should include the possibility of subcategorization with regard to the presence or absence of associated atypical features, as well as chronicity and severity. This necessarily entails disaggregation of the current DSM-III-R criteria for vegetative symptoms that combine weight loss and weight gain and insomnia and hypersomnia. These need to be listed separately as alternative criteria.

Several concerns have been expressed by the DSM-IV Mood Disorders Work Group about the use of "atypical features" as a modifier. The Work Group notes that its inclusion remains controversial. The treatment response data are limited and need to be replicated across centers and with different comparison medications. Moreover, it is not yet clear how best to define the subtype, and very little has been reported concerning its reliability, prevalence, relationship to other subtypes of depression, and the performance characteristics of various possible defining items.

These cautionary observations notwithstanding, we recommend its inclusion as a modifier for all existing depressive and bipolar categories (excluding mania).

We would define AD subtype in terms of the presence of at least one of four symptoms: overeating/weight gain; oversleeping; severe anergy, defined as leaden paralysis; and dysfunctional rejection sensitivity.

References

Aarons SF: Atypical depression, in Phenomenology of Depressive Illness. Edited by Mann J. New York, Human Sciences Press, 1988, pp 141–157

Agosti V, Stewart J, Quitkin F, et al: Factors associated with premature medication discontinuation among responders to an MAOI or a tricyclic antidepressant. J Clin Psychiatry 49:196–198, 1988

Akiskal HS, Bitar A, Puzantian V, et al: The nosological status of neurotic depression. Arch Gen Psychiatry 35:756–766, 1978

American Psychiatric Association: Diagnostic and Statistical Manual of Mental Disorders, 2nd Edition. Washington, DC, American Psychiatric Association, 1968

American Psychiatric Association: Diagnostic and Statistical Manual Of Mental Disorders, 3rd Edition. Washington, DC, American Psychiatric Association, 1980

American Psychiatric Association: Diagnostic and Statistical Manual Of Mental Disorders, 3rd Edition, Revised. Washington, DC, American Psychiatric Association, 1987

Bruder G, Quitkin F, Stewart J, et al: Cerebral laterality and depression: differences in perceptual asymmetry among diagnostic subtypes. J Abnorm Psychol 98:177–186, 1989

Cornelius J, Soloff P, Perel J, et al: Fluoxetine trial in borderline personality, in New Research Program and Abstracts of the American Psychiatric Association 142nd Annual Meeting, San Francisco, CA, May 1989

Dally PJ, Rohde P: Comparison of antidepressant drugs in depressive illnesses. Lancet 1:18–20, 1961

Davidson J, Miller R, Turnbull C, et al: Atypical depression. Arch Gen Psychiatry 39:527–534, 1982

Davidson J, Giller E, Zisook S, et al: An efficacy study of isocarboxazid and placebo in depression, and its relationship to depressive nosology. Arch Gen Psychiatry 45:120–127, 1988

Feinberg N, Gillin J, Carroll B, et al: EEG studies of sleep and the diagnosis of depression. Biol Psychiatry 17:305–316, 1982

Gurney C, Roth M, Garside R, et al: Studies in the classification of affective disorders. Br J Psychiatry 121:162–166, 1972

Hamilton M: Development of a rating scale for primary depressive illness. British Journal of Social and Clinical Psychology 6:278-296, 1967

Harrison WM, Cooper T, Stewart J, et al: The tyramine challenge test as a trait marker for melancholia. Arch Gen Psychiatry 41:681–685, 1984

Himmelhoch J, Thase M, Mallinger A, et al: Tranylcypromine vs. imipramine in anergic bipolar depression. Am J Psychiatry 148:910–916, 1991

Klein DF: The pharmacological validation of psychiatric diagnosis, in Validity of Psychiatric Diagnosis. Edited by Robins L, Barrett J. New York, Raven, 1989, pp 203–216

Klein DF, Gittelman R, Quitkin F, et al: Diagnosis and Drug Treatment of Psychiatric Disorders, 2nd Edition. Baltimore, MD, Williams & Wilkins, 1980

Kupfer D, Thase M: Validity of major depression: a psychobiological perspective, in Diagnosis and Classification in Psychiatry: A Critical Appraisal of DSM III. Edited by Tischler G. New York, Cambridge University Press, 1987, pp 32–60

Kupfer D, Foster F, Detre T: Sleep continuity changes in depression. J Nerv Ment Dis 34:192–195, 1973

Liebowitz M: Pharmacotherapy of social phobia. J Clin Psychiatry 49:252–257, 1988

Liebowitz M, Quitkin F, Stewart J, et al: Phenelzine v. imipramine in atypical depression. Arch Gen Psychiatry 41:669–677, 1984

Liebowitz M, Quitkin F, Stewart J, et al: Antidepressant specificity in atypical depression. Arch Gen Psychiatry 45:129–137, 1988

Lipman R: Differentiating anxiety and depression in anxiety disorders: use of rating scales. Psychopharmacol Bull 18:69–77, 1982

McGrath PJ, Stewart J, Harrison W: Phenelzine treatment of melancholia. J Clin Psychiatry 47:420–422, 1986

Mountjoy C, Roth M, Garside F, et al: A clinical trial of phenelzine in anxiety depressive and phobic neuroses. Br J Psychiatry 131:486–492, 1977

Pare C, Mack J: Differentiation of two genetically specific types of depression by the response to antidepressant drugs. J Med Genet 8:306–309, 1971

Paykel ES, Rowan PR, Rao B, et al: Atypical depression: nosology and response to antidepressants, in Treatment of Depression: Old Controversies and New Approaches. Edited by Clayton P, Barrett J. New York, Raven, 1983, pp 237–251

Pollitt J, Young J: Anxiety state or masked depression? a study based on the action of monoamine oxidase inhibitors. Br J Psychiatry 119:143–149, 1971

Quitkin F, Rabkin J, Stewart J, et al: Sleep of atypical depressives. J Affect Disord 8:61–67, 1985

Quitkin F, Stewart J, McGrath P, et al: Phenelzine versus imipramine in the treatment of probable atypical depression: defining syndrome boundaries of selective MAOI responders. Am J Psychiatry 145:306–311, 1988

Quitkin F, McGrath P, Stewart J, et al: Phenelzine and imipramine in mood reactive depressives: further delineation of the syndrome of atypical depression. Arch Gen Psychiatry 46:787–793, 1989

Quitkin FM, McGrath PJ, Stewart J, et al: Atypical depression, panic attacks, and response to imipramine and phenelzine. Arch Gen Psychiatry 47:935–941, 1990

Quitkin FM, Harrison W, Stewart J, et al: Response to phenelzine and imipramine in placebo nonresponders with atypical depression: a new application of the crossover design. Arch Gen Psychiatry 48:319–323, 1991

Rabkin J, Quitkin F, McGrath P, et al: Adverse Reactions to monoamine oxidase inhibitors, part II: treatment correlates and clinical management. J Clin Psychopharmacol 5:2–9, 1985

Ravaris C, Nies A, Robinson D, et al: A multiple-dose, controlled study of phenelzine in depression-anxiety states. Arch Gen Psychiatry 33:347–350, 1976

Ravaris C, Robinson D, Ives J, et al: Phenelzine and amitriptyline in the treatment of depression. Arch Gen Psychiatry 37:1075–1080, 1980

Robinson D, Nies A, Ravaris C, et al: The monoamine oxidase inhibitor, phenelzine, in the treatment of depressive-anxiety
states. Arch Gen Psychiatry 29:407–413, 1973

Roth M, Gurney MWP, Mountjoy CQ: The Newcastle rating scales. Acta Psychiatr Scand Suppl 310:42–54, 1983

Rowan P, Paykel E, Parker R, et al: Tricyclic anti-depressant and MAO inhibitor: are there differential effects? in Monoamine Oxidase Inhibitors: The State of the Art. Edited by Youdim M, Paykel E. New York, Wiley, 1981, pp 125–139

Rowan P, Paykel E, Parker R: Phenelzine and amitriptyline: effects on symptoms of neurotic depression. Br J Psychiatry 140:475–483, 1982

Sandler M, Bonham Carter S, Cuthbert M, et al: Is there an increase in monoamine-oxidase activity in depressive illness? Lancet 1:1045–1049, 1975

Sargant W: Some newer drugs in the treatment of depression and their relation to other somatic treatments. Psychosomatics 1:14–17, 1960

Sheehan D, Claycomb J, Kouretas N: Monoamine oxidase inhibitors: prescription and patient management. Int J Psychiatry Med 10:99–121, 1980–1981

Simpson S, DePaulo R: Fluoxetine treatment of bipolar II depression, in New Research Program and Abstracts of the American Psychiatric Association 142nd Annual Meeting, San Francisco, CA, May 1989

Sovner R: The clinical characteristics and treatment of atypical depression. J Clin Psychiatry 42:285–289, 1981

Spitzer RL, Endicott J, Robins E: Research Diagnostic Criteria: rationale and reliability. Arch Gen Psychiatry 35:773–782, 1978

Stewart JW, McGrath P, Rabkin J, et al: Atypical depression: a valid clinical entity? Psychopharmacology 1:479–495, 1993

Terman M, Terman J, Quitkin F, et al: Light therapy for seasonal affective disorder: a review of efficacy. Neuropsychopharmacology 2:1–22, 1989

Thase ME, Carpenter L, Kupfer D, et al: Clinical significance of reversed vegetative subtypes of recurrent major depression. Psychopharmacol Bull 27:17–22, 1991

Weilburg J, Rosenbaum J, Sachs G, et al: New Research Program and Abstracts of the American Psychiatric Association 142nd Annual Meeting, San Francisco, CA, May 1989

West ED, Dally PJ: Effects of iproniazid in depressive syndromes. BMJ 1:1491–1494, 1959

Chapter 11

Should Postpartum Mood Disorders Be Given a More Prominent or Distinct Place in DSM-IV?

Daniel Purnine, M.S., and Ellen Frank, Ph.D.

Statement of the Issues

The aim of this review is to determine whether there is a unique postpartum psychosis and whether nonpsychotic postpartum depression represents a unique diagnostic entity. The milder "maternity blues" are not addressed. The review process involved two steps: 1) a mailed survey requesting opinions from investigators currently working in the area of postpartum disorders and 2) a review of the published literature and some articles in press.

Our examination of the literature on postpartum disorders suggests that a specific syndrome cannot be identified by a unique and consistent constellation of diagnostic validating criteria such as those of Robins and Guze (1970) (age, course, symptoms, family history, etc.). Often, however, enough of these factors in a postpartum patient's presentation (e.g., confusion, lability) are consistent with those observed in other postpartum episodes and discrepant with traditional diagnoses that relying on these diagnoses without modification is problematic.

This work was supported, in part, by NIMH Grant 5-30915 and the John D. and Catherine T. MacArthur Network on the Psychobiology of Depression.

Significance of the Issues

If traditional diagnoses fail to adequately explain one or more presentations of psychiatric disorder that occur puerperally, it may be necessary to consider new diagnostic categories for these presentations. It is important for clinicians to know whether, within traditional diagnostic constructs, some women with postpartum onset demonstrate a unique course, prognosis (McGorry and Connell 1990), or treatment response. The task would then be to identify such patients via symptomatology, personal and family psychiatric history, and/or sociodemographic data.

DSM-III-R (American Psychiatric Association 1987) addresses postpartum disorders only briefly. In the sections on differential diagnosis of both manic and depressive episodes from organic mood syndromes, there is the statement, "because of the difficulty of distinguishing the psychological and physiologic stresses associated with pregnancy and delivery, in this classification such episodes are not considered organic mood syndromes and should be diagnosed as manic (or major depressive) episodes" (pp. 216 and 221). Postpartum disorders go unmentioned in the sections on organic mental syndromes, schizophrenia, delusional disorder, or psychotic disorders not elsewhere classified. Furthermore, the term *postpartum* does not appear in the "Index of DSM-III-R Diagnoses and Selected Diagnostic Terms" (pp. 553–567), making it difficult to locate what little pertinent information is included.

Methods

In general, the Mood Disorders Work Group has been guided by the empirical formulation of Robins and Guze (1970), who argue that a diagnosis is validated by clinical description (symptomatology, course, age at onset, prognosis, and prevalence), as well as by family history data, laboratory findings, and treatment response. In addition, it is important to determine whether there is a specific period of increased risk following parturition or a time at which risk ceases to differ from that in otherwise matched nonchildbearing women.

Letters were mailed to the 21 investigators listed as the first authors of articles discussing postpartum disorders that appeared in the 1986, 1987, and 1988 literature. The letter included a copy of the DSM-III-R criteria for major depressive episode and for manic episode. It asked investigators to comment on the extent to which they felt the DSM-III-R criteria sufficed to describe postpartum disorders and whether, in light of the Robins and Guze criteria, they felt that a case could be made for a separate diagnostic category for postpartum disorders.

For the literature review, sources were limited to English language publications and translated articles or abstracts. Initially, a fairly wide net was cast. This was done by beginning with the volume edited by Brockington and Kumar (1982), *Motherhood and Mental Illness.* Working backward, we reviewed the references included in that volume that appeared to be relevant to the task at hand. Working forward in time, we used the Social Science Citation Index to locate those articles in the post-1982 literature that had referenced the chapters included in the 1982 volume as well as the seminal papers in the pre-1982 literature.

Only articles that included diagnoses made according to a standardized set of criteria (e.g., Research Diagnostic Criteria [RDC; Spitzer et al. 1978], DSM, ICD), as opposed to using a single rating scale, were included, unless the paper provided important information (e.g., sleep or neuroendocrine data) not available in better-characterized samples or was written before the era of specified criteria sets. Those articles describing admissions to psychiatric hospitals (or referral to psychiatric outpatient care in the British system) within 4 weeks of parturition were also included, on the assumption that hospitalization was an indicator of sufficient severity of illness to warrant inclusion. Some large epidemiological studies were based on chart notes or diagnoses not made by the author(s). Further consideration was given to the generalizability of the findings, with studies involving consecutive admissions being given the greater weight. Studies were included only if the same size approximated a minimum of 50 subjects, unless the study provided specific information that was directly relevant to the Robins and Guze validators and was considered to be of particularly high quality.

Results

Survey Results

Twelve responses were received from the investigator survey. Most were brief and indicated that the DSM-III-R criteria were satisfactory as written; however, several noteworthy suggestions were made. Some supported more explicit recognition for postpartum mood disorders, citing the heuristic value and likely improvements in identification and treatment. One investigator suggested providing for a special designation of postpartum mental disorders on Axis III. Another advocated the identification of "disorders of the mother-infant relationship," which are milder than those that might be classified under sections on child abuse and neglect.

There was support for our decision to consider depressive episodes in the postpartum period as more akin to major depressive disorder than to "organic" mood syndromes. However, it was pointed out that weight loss is a normal aspect of postpartum adjustment, as is appetite increase, especially in women who are breast-feeding, and that sleep difficulties and fatigue need to be placed in context. Thus, vegetative symptoms may be less clearly indicative of depression during this period than cognitive and affective changes.

Results of the Literature Review

Historical background. It has been recognized for centuries that the puerperal period may be associated with mental illness. Although today puerperal disorders are typically divided into three categories that reflect severity (puerperal psychosis, postpartum depression, and maternity blues), the two less severe categories are of fairly recent interest and have received attention mainly in the last two decades (Kendell 1985).

The seminal 19th century works of Esquirol and Marcé provide an often-quoted background for current struggles over the distinction of puerperal psychosis/depression as diseases or syndromes. Esquirol (as quoted in Herzog and Detre 1976) described an illness with delirium as the usual presenting feature, and today "disturbances of the consciousness" and confusion remain prominent in the literature.

In Marcé's (1858) *Insanity in Pregnant, Puerperal and Lactating Women,* 29 of 44 cases were diagnosed with mania, 10 with melancholia. "Puerperal mania has neither in its psychotic manifestations nor its physical symptoms anything specific to itself" (Marcé 1858, p. 204, as quoted in Brockington et al. 1982). However, a unique constellation of symptoms was thought to define a syndrome that was different from nonpuerperal affective disorders and contained bizarre behavior and what Brockington calls "transitory intellectual enfeeblement."

As a result of Kraepelin's influence, puerperal psychoses have long been described as falling into one of three categories: toxic, schizophrenic, or affective (Berrios and Hauser 1988; Kendler 1986). Many of the early descriptions resembled toxic/infectious states. Over the years, the introduction of antibiotics and more sterile hospital settings have accompanied the decline of these "organic" psychoses (Thomas and Gordon 1959). Seager (1960) reviewed early studies in which one-third to one-half of cases were found to be suffering from toxic confusional psychosis, with a sharp drop in the 1950s to as low as 1.5 per 1,000 cases. Protheroe's (1969) early group, 1927–1941, had notably more "clouding of consciousness" than did the 1942–1961 group, also suggesting a reduction in the organic nature of psychoses in the puerperium.

Reviewing 12 studies from 1911 to 1958, Thomas and Gordon (1959) found that, early in the century, most puerperal psychosis involved patients with manic depression, with few patients with schizophrenia observed. The trend reversed by mid-century. Brockington et al. (1982) extended the list of studies to 1978, at which point the distribution looked widely varied and inconclusive. The dominance of one diagnostic group over the other seems to depend on geography as well as history. Herzog and Detre (1976) pointed out two decades ago that affective diagnoses dominated in England, whereas diagnoses of schizophrenia were more common in the United States. They suggested, as did Brockington et al. (1982), that Americans overdiagnosed schizophrenia at that time; this was probably due to "broader criteria for the concept of schizophrenia . . . in the American literature" (Jansson 1964, p. 14) before DSM-III. In a long-term study of puerperal psychosis, Protheroe (1969) found 6 organic, 37 schizophrenic, and 91 affective cases. Schizophrenia comprised 11% of Arentsen's (1968) diagnoses, the remainder being mostly affective.

A study by Davidson and Robertson (1985) supported the present rarity of organic psychosis among puerperals, but found an equal distribution of schizophrenia and bipolar disorder. More common now, however, schizophrenia represents a small minority among puerperal diagnoses in both the United States and Britain. Dean and Kendell (1981) found that 82% of patients with postpartum psychiatric disorders had depression, mania, or hypomania, and less than 2% had schizophrenia, a distribution often replicated (Meltzer and Kumar 1985; Platz and Kendell 1988). Today, the severe puerperal mental disorders are largely characterized as affective illnesses (Brockington et al. 1982; Kendell 1985; McNeil 1988; Schopf et al. 1984). Whether this should be attributed to actual changes in the nature of the disorder (perhaps a function of the cohort effect for depressions in general, observed in the Epidemiologic Catchment Area (ECA) study and its offshoots), to changes in diagnostic fashions, or to a combination of the two is difficult to say. A preponderance of affective illness makes sense if, in fact, the puerperium is merely a period of increased risk for that which is already latent.

Problems of defining puerperal mental illness. Unfortunately, the literature has largely "failed to distinguish among the maternity blues, postpartum affective psychoses, and mild to moderate postpartum depression" (Hopkins et al., 1984, p. 498). The psychotic/neurotic division is sometimes used as a continuum-like measure as opposed to a sampling criterion (e.g., Dean and Kendell's [1981] finding that patients with puerperal depression were more psychotic than nonpuerperal patients).

Despite the vague diagnostic focus of many of the articles we reviewed, most of them identified with one of the following terms: *postpartum psychosis, postpartum depression (nonpsychotic),* or the more generic *puerperal mental illness.* Articles in the latter category are sometimes represented in our analysis of puerperal psychosis, because criteria and descriptions were often very similar to descriptions of postpartum psychosis (Davidson and Robertson 1985; Dean and Kendell 1981; Grundy and Roberts 1975; Meltzer and Kumar 1985; Nott 1982; Paffenbarger 1964; Paffenbarger and McCabe 1966; Pugh et al. 1963; Seager 1960; Wilson et al. 1972). It turns out that it is actually easier to identify studies that included *non*psychotic major or minor depression (e.g., O'Hara et al. 1984) than to ascertain what is included in the studies of more severe disorders. This may be because interest in less severe postpartum disorders is a more recent phenomenon and thus coincides with a general requirement for greater diagnostic specificity in the psychiatric literature.

Authors frequently use the term *postpartum psychosis* synonymously with *severe psychiatric postpartum disorders* (Schopf et al. 1985, p. 164). This is the broad conceptualization applied to postpartum psychosis in most of the literature. Hospital admission or diagnosis of schizophrenia, mania, major depression, and even milder conditions often suffice as an inclusion criterion (Kendell et al. 1981; McNeil 1987, 1988; Platz and Kendell 1988; Schopf et al. 1984, 1985; Thuwe 1974; Whalley et al. 1982), without separate attention to the psychotic process itself. This issue is rarely addressed, the most explicit instance being in a study by Brockington et al. (1981), which had an inclusion stipulation that one of two psychiatrists considered the patient "psychotic." Unfortunately, in a later article regarding "puerperal psychosis," 89 of 104 subjects were listed as depressive (major, major-probable, minor), without specific mention of psychotic process (Brockington et al. 1988). Meltzer and Kumar (1985) caution against overapplying the psychotic label, because only 7 of 31 of their patients with puerperal major depression showed firm evidence of "alienation from reality." Using this more rigid criterion, their estimated incidence of puerperal "psychosis" fell from 1.6 to 0.6 per 1,000 births (Meltzer and Kumar 1985).

Temporal criteria either for onset or for psychiatric admission do not define a puerperal illness per se but, as an independent variable, restrict the subject sample to the investigator's idea of the postpartum risk period (or sometimes a portion thereof) for the purpose of sample purity. This has been as stringent as 2 weeks after parturition (Brockington et al. 1981; Dean et al. 1989) or as late as 12 months postpartum (Meltzer and Kumar 1985). More common criteria are 6 months, 3 months, or 6 weeks.

Symptom picture of postpartum psychosis.   Separating the puerperal diagnoses into depressed and manic, Dean and Kendell (1981) found that patients with puerperal depression were more psychotic, disoriented, agitated, and emotionally labile and showed more symptoms of slowness than did nonpuerperal matched control subjects. Interestingly, almost all of the difference was accounted for by a small minority of patients who had organic signs. Among manic patients, there were no significant symptom differences between puerperal patients and control subjects (Dean and Kendell 1981).

One of the most common clusters of possibly distinctive symptoms of postpartum psychoses is the "confusion" mentioned earlier. Widely defined, this refers to symptoms akin to delirium. Despite evidence that such symptoms have declined over the years, Brockington et al. (1981) found that confusion was a dominant feature in 24% of patients and tended to accompany the more abrupt onsets. Similar figures are the 23% found by Protheroe (1969) and the 25% found by Reich and Winokur (1970), although the latter was coincident with the rate of confusion in patients with nonpuerperal psychosis as well.

In addition to confusion, Brockington et al. (1981) found more "incompetence" and fewer schizophrenic symptoms in patients with puerperal psychosis. A20preponderance of manic symptoms was found (elation, lability of mood, increased activity and sociability), suggesting a link to bipolar disorder, a relationship addressed later in this review.

Symptom picture of nonpsychotic puerperal depression.   As with postpartum psychoses, there is a "paucity of empirical data on the features of postpartum depression" (Hopkins et al. 1984, p. 502). Research has centered on prevalence and predisposing agents, rather than the symptom picture. Several studies (e.g., O'Hara et al. 1984) have concentrated on the proportion of prospectively followed pregnant women who meet one or another set of criteria for depressive disorder. Thus, these investigators focus on the presence or absence of conventional depressive symptoms with no mention of whether unique symptoms might also be present in the postpartum period.

In the opinion of Hemphill (1952), puerperal depression does form a distinct entity, one that "in many ways resembles involutional melancholia" (p. 1234). Common features are said to be a lack of concentration, ideas of guilt and unworthiness, motor agitation, and great anxiety regarding suicide and compulsions of violence to the child. One wonders whether Hemphill's description may not include a fair proportion of psychotic women and/or women in the process of developing psychotic features.

Pitt's (1968) assertion of an "atypical depression" following childbirth has set the modern stage for debate over whether there is a unique depression in the puerperium. Of his patients with puerperal depression, almost all had anxiety, which sometimes overshadowed the depression. Common symptoms were hypochondriasis, fatigue, and anorexia. On the Maudsley Personality Inventory (Eysenck 1958), they were more neurotic and less extroverted than control subjects. Sleep disturbance was manifest as difficulty getting to sleep rather than early-morning awakening. Pitt states that only 1 of 33 cases showed "classical depression."

Cooper et al. (1988) generally do not support Pitt's view of a unique symptom picture but did find that patients with depression at 6 months postpartum had greater loss of interest and loss of concentration than patients with nonpuerperal depression ($P < .001$). Pitt also found that "a few patients complained of impaired concentration" (Pitt 1968, p. 1327).

Course and prognosis.   Little specific research attention has focused on the course of postpartum disorders. With respect to psychoses and other severe puerperal mental illnesses, the distinguishing feature is rapid onset of symptoms, with many women developing florid symptomatology over the course of 24–48 hours, typically beginning 2 or 3 days after birth (Sneddon et al. 1981). Women exhibiting the most extreme symptomatology (e.g., catatonia) also appear to show rapid recovery (Steiner 1979). Otherwise, the course of puerperal psychoses does not appear to differ from psychoses appearing at other times. Women with nonpsychotic puerperal depressions appear to experience a course of illness no different from that observed at other times, although no systematic comparisons have yet been made.

Although the question of prognosis is rarely addressed directly, several investigators observed that the prognosis for postpartum psychotic episodes may be somewhat better than for episodes of similar symptomatic configuration appearing at other times. Steiner (1979) suggests that short-term prognosis is related to symptom onset within 3 weeks of delivery, response to treatment within 10 days of hospitalization, and the presence of physical problems before, during, and after delivery rather than to specific diagnostic factors.

Sneddon et al. (1981) describe their experience with 48 cases admitted to a mother and baby unit. For the 32 women with acute puerperal psychosis, prognosis was good, with 29 women returning to essentially normal function and confidence in themselves as parents and marital partners. Outcome was considerably worse for women with chronic schizophrenia and severe personality disorder diagnoses.

Period of risk after birth.   The onset of various mental disturbances just after parturition is the key to their distinction and the core of their definition. "The time relation of the condition, a peak of cases shortly after delivery, is too striking to reconcile with a view that pregnancy has no place as a factor in causation, despite the nonspecific reaction" (Thomas and Gordon 1959, p. 371). Paffenbarger (1964) studied the records of women who were psychiatric inpatients within 6 months of parturition and found that 34% of admissions were within 1 week and 68% within 1 month of delivery. Reviewing admissions during pregnancy and in the 9 months after parturition, Pugh et al. (1963) discovered a large excess of admissions for psychoses in the first 3 months postpartum. A smaller but significant trend was found for other diagnoses collectively. In studies of similar design, Nott (1982) also found an increased rate of psychosis, but not of other diagnoses, after childbirth; Kendell et al.

(1976) found a rise in both functional psychoses and depressive illnesses in the 3 months after parturition.

The studies of generic puerperal mental illness support this temporal relationship (Dean and Kendell 1981; Kendell et al. 1976, 1981, 1987), as do those specifically of postpartum psychoses (Arentsen 1968; Paffenbarger et al. 1961; Schopf et al. 1985). For nonpsychotic depression, however, the puerperium is not even clearly a time of measurable increased risk, as is discussed in the following section.

Prevalence of nonpsychotic depression. Looking at the first 3 months after childbirth, Kumar and Robson (1984) found 14% of mothers with "affective disorder." Watson et al. (1984) identified affective disorder in 12% of a prospective sample at 6 weeks after birth. O'Hara et al. (1984) originally found 12% with major or minor depression (RDC) in the first 9 weeks after delivery, a 3% increase over the antenatal rate. In a more recent study (O'Hara et al. 1990), these investigators found a rate of 10.4% in the first 9 weeks postpartum, compared to 7.7% in the second trimester. Troutman and Cutrona (1990), Cooper et al. (1988), and Cutrona (1983) also found no significant increase after childbirth. The findings of Cox et al. (1982) resemble most current figures (13% at 3–5 months), but the antenatal rate of 4% offers rare support that pregnancy may confer some protection. The rates of nonpsychotic puerperal depression tend to fall between 10% and 15%, not significantly different from rates in nonchildbearing matched control subjects (O'Hara et al. 1990).

Prevalence of psychotic episodes. Estimates of the incidence of severe or psychotic episodes of puerperal mental illness are quite low. In 1961, Paffenberger et al. cited a range from 0.5 to 3.5 per 1,000 pregnancies. This agrees with the work of Hemphill (1952), in which 37 of 37,000 (1/1,000) maternity hospital admissions resulted in psychiatric admission. Note that these included a wide array of diagnoses. Paffenberger (1964) and Paffenberger and McCabe (1966) report incidence in the 6 months after birth as 1.9 per 1,000. This approximated the rate in nonchildbearing women, but of note was the pronounced peak in the first month postpartum. Incidence of *puerperal mental illness,* defined as any mental disorder referred to a psychiatrist, in the first month after birth was 1.9 per 1,000 (Grundy and Roberts 1975). Kendell et al. (1976) found 9 cases of functional psychoses over the 90 days postpartum in a survey of 2,257 pregnancies, or about 4 per 1,000. Nott (1982) reported 1.15 per 1,000 psychoses over 90 days postpartum. In 1981, Kendell et al. found that 2.0 per 1,000 births lead to psychiatric admission. An extension of that study later yielded 2.2 per 1,000 (Kendell et al. 1987). In a review of the case notes, about half of these admissions suggested psychotic symptoms. Nott's and Kendell's groups, respectively, found 12 and 14.5 times the prenatal incidence in the postpartum period, defined as 3 months after parturition. Using hospital records, Meltzer and Kumar (1985) report incidence of 1.6 per 1,000. This stands in agreement with the bulk of the literature, but with stricter temporal and clinical criteria for "puerperal psychosis," this rate dropped to 0.6 per 1,000.

Recurrence. The risk of puerperal mental illness increases greatly for women who have had episodes with previous births. However, if the risk of nonpuerperal episodes also rises, it may be that these individuals simply have a higher susceptibility to mental illness in general. Protheroe (1969) determined that 41% of women who had further pregnancies had recurrences. In 1961, Paffenbarger et al. studied the chart histories of 41 patients who each had at least one subsequent pregnancy; 51% had further episodes. The recurrence rate per birth was 35%. In a study by Davidson and Robertson (1985), the risk of psychosis with further pregnancies was 33% in general. It varied with the diagnosis, as would be expected in the recurrence rates of nonpuerperal disorders.

Family history data. Family history data in women with severe puerperal disorders have shown only weak and conflicting trends. Thuwe (1974) studied the descendants of women who had experienced puerperal psychosis during the period 1872–1926 in Goteborg, Sweden. She found significantly more psychiatric disorder in the offspring of these women than in control subjects. Kadrmas et al. (1979) found fewer affective disorders in first-degree relatives of patients with puerperal bipolar disorder than in those of patients with nonpuerperal bipolar disorder, although the trend was not significant. Schopf et al. (1985) found a lack of family history of affective psychoses in women with puerperal episodes. Dean et al. (1989), using family study methods, found that women with only puerperal episodes had higher psychiatric morbidity in their families than did control bipolar patients when general practitioner treatment was taken into account.

Laboratory findings. Given the many hormonal theories concerning the etiology of postpartum psychoses and depression, surprisingly few laboratory studies have been conducted in women experiencing these illnesses. Most address the more prevalent maternity blues. According to one theory, the sudden fall of progesterone occurring between the first and second stages of labor is responsible for the increased number of depressions. Only Nott et al. (1976) have attempted to explore this relationship. Because no case of mood disturbance in their sample was severe, their findings, although suggestive of a relationship, are of questionable generalizability to the more severe syndromes (Campbell and Winokur 1985).

Other physiological theories have focused on the catecholamine hypothesis of mood disorders. Treadway et al. (1969) found a significant correlation between decreased urinary norepinephrine and severity of postpartum depression. This and other research suggesting a role for free tryptophan and cortisol levels (Handley et al. 1980) are also of constrained generalizability, because it is questionable whether any of the women studied had a severe or major depression.

Using the dexamethasone suppression test (DST), Singh et al. (1986) found that positive DST was more common in psychoses and depression occurring postpartum than at other times. However, an 80% rate of positive DST in normal women 5 days postpartum suggests that the escape from dexamethasone suppression was related to general postpartum hormonal changes as opposed to anything specific to puerperal mental illness.

In a larger study of endorphins in cerebrospinal fluid, Lindstrom et al. (1978) examined fraction I and II endorphins in four patients with puerperal psychosis. Three of the four showed elevated levels of both fractions in the acute drug-free stage. Treatment with electroconvulsive therapy (ECT) or neuroleptics resulted in normal endorphin levels in all of these women. These findings were not different, however, for the acutely ill schizophrenic or manic patients studied.

Treatment response data.   Surprisingly, we located no studies comparing treatment response in puerperal women with treatment response in women with comparable diagnoses appearing at other times in the life cycle. It has been recommended that prophylactic lithium be given as soon as possible after delivery as a preventive measure in women with a history of bipolar disorder. This would seem to be especially indicated for women with a history of bipolar episodes with postpartum onsets (Robinson and Stewart 1986; Stewart 1988).

Controlled studies may be indicated on the effectiveness of estrogen treatment. It may not only prevent "the blues" (Hamilton 1982), but in 50 patients with previous postpartum illnesses, its use was accompanied by *no* recurrences, whereas the literature suggests a 30%–50% recurrence per pregnancy in patients with previous postpartum psychiatric illness (J. A. Hamilton, personal communication, 1989).

Risk factors for postpartum psychoses.   It appears that primiparous women are at greater risk for puerperal psychoses. In general population studies by Kendell et al. (1981), 62% of postpartum psychoses were primiparae, whereas 47% of all births were primiparae. Most other percentage estimates of primiparity among postpartum psychoses fall in the same range (Arentsen 1968; Bratfos and Haug 1966; Meltzer and Kumar 1985; Protheroe 1969).

Evidence for this relationship has not been found by all investigators, however (Grundy and Roberts 1975; Seager 1960). Hemphill (1952) found a relationship to parity only for puerperal schizophrenia but not for postpartum psychoses in general. McNeil reported that primiparity did not seem to be related to generic postpartum psychoses but was tied to a subgroup with onset before 3 weeks postpartum (McNeil 1987) and a subgroup with exclusively puerperal episodes (McNeil 1988). The proportion of puerperally ill women who are primiparous may not represent the true nature of the disorder, however, because many women who experience a severe postpartum illness after the birth of a first child may then elect to have no more children.

Social stressors have been investigated as catalysts for puerperal disorders. Whereas social class has repeatedly failed to show a connection, single-mother status continues to receive attention for puerperal psychoses, and marital conflict for nonpsychotic depressions. The proportion of single mothers in Kendell et al.'s (1981) investigation was 14% for puerperal psychiatric patients, double that of the control group ($P < .10$). Meltzer and Kumar (1985) also found a rate of 14%, although they did not cite a rate for single motherhood in their general population.

Single mothers may be more prone to puerperal illness as a result of the stressful anticipation of single parenting and, perhaps, the stigma of having an illegitimate child. The high proportion of single mothers among the puerperally mentally ill may, however, simply reveal a greater likelihood for these women to be admitted to the hospital, because they are without the support of a husband at home (Kendell et al. 1981). Single motherhood was not found to be related to puerperal disorders by Davidson and Robertson (1985), McNeil (1987), Paffenbarger (1964), Paffenbarger et al. (1961), or Protheroe (1969).

The role of obstetric factors is no clearer. Paffenbarger (1964) and Paffenbarger and McCabe (1966) claimed that a lighter birth weight and a shorter gestation period resulted in puerperal mental illness. Neither claim was confirmed by Grundy and Roberts (1975). Kendell et al. (1981) also failed to support the link with length of gestation but did find a significant relationship between postpartum psychoses and cesarean section, a trend supported by Nott (1982) but with numbers too small to establish significance.

Risk factors for nonpsychotic depression in the puerperium. As with the more severe puerperal disorders, risk of nonpsychotic depression after childbirth is higher in those with a psychiatric history (Ballinger et al. 1979; O'Hara et al. 1983; Paykel et al. 1980; Tod 1964; Watson et al. 1984). A higher level of depressive symptoms (measured by Beck Inventory [Beck 1978]) during pregnancy has been associated with postpartum depression (O'Hara et al. 1982, 1983, 1984). Yet O'Hara (1986) found "women with depression during pregnancy were not the ones who were depressed after delivery, so that prepartum and postpartum depression appeared to be independent" (p. 572). Kumar and Robson (1984) had similar conclusions, although Frank et al. (1987) found patients with lifetime histories of both prepartum and postpartum episodes.

Symptoms of anxiety during pregnancy have been thought to correlate positively with puerperal depression (Dalton 1971). Hayworth et al. (1980) measured anxiety and hostility at 36 weeks gestation and found that high levels of both related to depression at 6 weeks postpartum (subjects were not assessed for depression antenatally, however). Tod (1964) found that pathological anxiety during pregnancy occurred in all cases of puerperal depression. An absence of this relationship was found by Pitt (1968), Cox et al. (1982), and Kumar and Robson (1984).

More stressful life events occurred before and after delivery in women who became depressed (O'Hara et al. 1983). The association with social stress and life events has been supported (O'Hara 1986; O'Hara et al. 1982; Paykel et al. 1980) but not by all studies (Hopkins et al. 1987; Pitt 1968). A biological link to puerperal depressions was suggested in one study by the lesser presence of stressful events in the 38 weeks before postpartum onsets compared with prepartum onsets (Martin et al. 1989). A preventative role for social support has been both supported (O'Hara et al. 1983; Paykel et al. 1980) and contested (Hopkins et al. 1987).

Evidence regarding obstetric risk factors and complications (Cox et al. 1982; Hopkins et al. 1987; O'Hara et al. 1983, 1984; Pitt 1968) has been conflicting and inconclusive. No relationship with prolonged labor has been found (Cox et al. 1982; Pitt 1968). O'Hara et al. (1984) and Hopkins et al. (1987) found that child care stressors were related to depression; however, Hopkins et al. measured maternal perception of infant temperament, a source of possible bias.

Dissatisfaction with the marital relationship or a poor marriage probably increases risk of depression in the puerperium (Ballinger et al. 1979; Kumar and Robson 1984; O'Hara 1986; Paykel et al. 1980; Watson et al. 1984), as it does at other times. As with the more severe puerperal disorders, postpartum depression is apparently not associated with social class (Ballinger et al. 1979; Hayworth et al. 1980; Pitt 1968; Tod 1964; Watson et al. 1984), marital status (Hayworth et al. 1980; Watson et al. 1984), or primiparity (Ballinger et al. 1979; Cox et al. 1982; Hayworth et al 1980; O'Hara et al. 1982; Tod 1964; Watson et al. 1984).

Alignment of puerperal psychoses with existing diagnoses and distinguishing purely puerperal patients.   We noted earlier that postpartum disorders were once aligned more strongly with schizophrenia and even toxic psychoses. In a cluster analysis of schizophrenic patients, Hays (1978) suggested that puerperal patients represented a unique subgroup, characterized by thought disorder, catatonic symptoms, and lability of mood; however, a connection with affective disorders, particularly bipolar disorder, has lately received the most attention, because investigators have begun distinguishing women who have had only postpartum episodes ("pure puerperals") from those having onset at other times as well ("mixed" cases).

Perhaps pure cases are the victims of a true puerperal illness, their identification and description typically confounded by the inclusion of patients with other disorders, the onsets of which are *provoked* by childbirth/parturition or simply happen to *coincide* with childbirth.

In a follow-up of women who had been hospitalized for puerperal psychiatric disorders (mostly affective), Schopf et al. (1984) found that 65% had at least one nonpuerperal relapse. Although the course of these patients' illnesses did not differ from that of their diagnostic category in general, those with exclusively puerperal episodes did "seem to be nosologically independent from the traditionally recognized endogenous psychoses" (Schopf et al. 1984, p. 54). Considering the rarity of having just one lifetime episode and the lack of a family history of affective psychosis in these women, Schopf considered their disorder a separate clinical entity.

Whalley (1982) confined his puerperally ill group to those without prior psychiatric history and notes that 10% of Protheroe's (1969) subjects had an earlier, nonpuerperal episode, so that "these puerperal episodes might have been relapses of established (manic-depressive) disorder" (Whalley et al. 1982, p. 180). McNeil (1988) also distinguished between pure and mixed cases, adding a group who had never had puerperal illness. The first two groups more commonly had affective disorders, the latter, schizophrenia.

The symptom picture in postpartum manic depression is similar to that of manic-depressive episodes occurring at other times (Bratfos and Haug 1966; Dean and Kendell 1981; Reich and Winokur 1970). Kadrmas et al. (1979) considered that perhaps puerperal bipolar patients "have the same illness (as nonpuerperal bipolar patients), but that some people need a stronger stimulus (parturition) to bring about the illness" (p. 554). The fact that puerperal bipolar patients had fewer recurrences and tended to have fewer affectively ill relatives than nonpuerperal bipolar patients points to "heterogeneity within the bipolar system" (p. 553), a sentiment echoed by Dean et al. (1989). It also suggests a "lesser vulnerability" model of severe puerperal mental illness. The findings of a study by Platz and Kendell (1988) support this idea, because there were more psychiatric admissions, subsequent to the index case, for nonpuerperal psychotic patients than for puerperal psychotic patients. Dean et al. (1989) studied the family history, symptom picture, and prognosis for manic-depressive patients, also distinguishing between patients with a mixed history of puerperal and nonpuerperal episodes, patients with nonpuerperal episodes only, and pure puerperal patients. The pure group had a better prognosis with fewer relapses than the other groups, implying less vulnerability for the former. However, the puerperal-only group actually showed *increased* psychiatric morbidity in relatives. In the study by Kadrmas et al. (1979), puerperal bipolar patients also had Schneiderian symptoms, reflecting alienation from reality, more often than bipolar control subjects.

Discussion

Considering the dearth of evidence for symptom specificity, unique family history, biological correlates, or treatment response, it is questionable whether mild to moderate depression that occurs postpartum represents a distinct clinical entity that should be afforded a separate diagnostic label in DSM-IV. Postpartum psychoses and bipolar episodes that appear in the first few weeks after delivery may represent a somewhat different case. It does appear that at least a subset of women with severe puerperal mental illness present with a symptom picture that includes features not ordinarily observed in other affective psychoses. Of particular note are the confusion and disorientation apparent in approximately one-quarter of puerperal psychotic patients. Because Dean et al. (1989) have identified some differences between women with puerperal disorders only and those with a mixed history of puerperal and nonpuerperal episodes, it would be important to know how the symptomatic picture, including confusion, relates to the distinction between puerperal-only versus mixed cases and to the family history of psychiatric disorder. Studies examining the stronger temporal link to parturition among bipolar presentations should also employ the "mixed versus pure" distinction, as should laboratory studies. Perhaps there is a distinct group of severe postpartum mental illnesses that have a unique pathophysiology but have yet to be isolated.

It is possible that severe postpartum disorders are actually of two origins, with concomitant differences in the presentation of illness. One yields a manic or mixed presentation and is seen in women with a vulnerability to bipolar illness. This syndrome, which appears quite precipitously, may represent a "pure subgroup which has features different from nonpuerperal manic depressives" (C. Dean, personal communication, 1988) and may be triggered by the *specific* physiological/endocrinological changes associated with parturition. A second form, which may present as a purely depressive disorder or as a schizophrenic disorder, has a more variable time to onset (up to a few months in some studies) and may be triggered by the more *general* stress of giving birth and new motherhood.

Recommendations

The current research evidence does not justify inclusion of separate diagnostic categories for either nonpsychotic or psychotic postpartum mental disorders; however, specific aspects of these illnesses may be relevant in deciding whether these disorders should be given a more prominent place in DSM-IV. At the very least, the "Index of Diagnostic Terms" should lead the user of DSM-IV to information concerning postpartum disorders.

We suggest the inclusion of qualifiers under the description of the following: 1) major depressive disorder, 2) bipolar disorder, manic and depressed, 3) schizoaffective disorder, and 4) psychotic disorder not otherwise specified. A qualifier such as "with postpartum onset of psychotic features" should be followed by a description of the confusion that often accompanies these disorders. This qualifier statement (like modifiers for seasonal, atypical, melancholic) should allow for a discussion of specific treatment and prevention recommendations. This is particularly relevant because 1) there is a strikingly high rate of recurrence of postpartum episodes in women who have subsequent deliveries, 2) there is a risk for inadequate development of the mother-infant relationship in women whose postpartum disorders are of extended duration or in women who are separated from their infant as a result of their psychiatric disorder, and, most important, 3) it would allow DSM-IV to note the small but devastating risk of infanticide in women who experience severe postpartum mental illness.

References

American Psychiatric Association: Diagnostic and Statistical Manual of Mental Disorders, Third Edition, Revised. Washington, DC, American Psychiatric Association, 1987

Arentsen K: Postpartum psychosis: with particular reference to the prognosis. Danish Medical Bulletin 15:97–100, 1968

Ballinger CB, Buckley DE, Naylor GJ, et al: Emotional disturbance following childbirth: clinical findings and urinary excretion of cyclic AMP. Psychol Med 9:293–300, 1979

Beck AT: Depression Inventory. Philadelphia, PA, Philadelphia Center for Cognitive Therapy, 1978

Berrios GE, Hauser R: The early development of Kraepelin's ideas on classification: a conceptual history. Psychol Med 18:813–821, 1988

Bratfos O, Haug JO: Puerperal mental disorders in manic-depressive females. Acta Psychiatr Scand 42:285–294, 1966

Brockington IF, Kumar R (eds): Motherhood and Mental Illness. New York, Academic Press, 1982

Brockington IF, Cernik KF, Schofield EM, et al: Puerperal psychosis, phenomena and diagnosis. Arch Gen Psychiatry 38:829–833, 1981

Brockington IF, Winokur G, Dean C: Puerperal psychosis, in Motherhood and Mental Illness. Edited by Brockington IF, Kumar R. New York: Academic Press, 1982, pp 37–70

Brockington IF, Margison FR, Schofield E, et al: The clinical picture of the depressed form of puerperal psychosis. J Affect Disord 15:29–37, 1988

Campbell S, Winokur G: Postpartum affective disorders: selected biological aspects, in Postpartum Psychiatric Disorders. Edited by Inwood DG. Washington, DC, American Psychiatric Press, 1985, pp 20–35

Cooper PJ, Campbell EA, Day A, et al: Non-psychotic psychiatric disorder after childbirth: a prospective study of prevalence, incidence, course and nature. Br J Psychiatry 152:799–806, 1988

Cox JL, Connor Y, Kendell RE: Prospective study of the psychiatric disorders of childbirth. Br J Psychiatry 140:111–117, 1982

Cutrona CE: Causal attributions of perinatal depression. J Abnorm Psychol 92:161–172, 1983

Dalton K: Prospective study into puerperal depression. Br J Psychiatry 118:689–692, 1971

Davidson J, Robertson E: A follow-up study of postpartum illness, 1946–1978. Acta Psychiatr Scand 71:451–457, 1985

Dean C, Kendell RE: The symptomatology of puerperal illness. Br J Psychiatry 139:128–133, 1981

Dean C, Williams RJ, Brockington IF: Is puerperal psychosis the same as bipolar manic-depressive disorder? A family study. Psychol Med 19:637–647, 1989

Eysenck H: A short questionnaire for the measurement of two dimensions of personality. J Appl Psychol 42:14–17, 1958

Frank E, Kupfer DJ, Jacob M, et al: Pregnancy-related affective episodes among women with recurrent depression. Am J Psychiatry 144:288–293, 1987

Grundy PF, Roberts CJ: Observations on the epidemiology of post partum mental illness. Psychol Med 5:286–290, 1975

Hamilton JA: The identity of postpartum psychosis, in Motherhood and Mental Illness. Edited by Brockington IF, Kumar R. New York, Academic Press, 1982, pp 1–16

Handley SL, Dunn TL, Waldron G, et al: Tryptophan, cortisol, and puerperal mood. Br J Psychiatry 146:498–508, 1980

Hays P: Taxonomic map of the schizophrenias with special reference to puerperal psychosis. BMJ 2:755–757, 1978

Hayworth J, Little BC, Carter SB, et al: A predictive study of postpartum depression: some predisposing characteristics. Br J Med Psychol 53:161–167, 1980

Hemphill RE: Incidence and nature of puerperal psychiatric illness. BMJ 2:1232–1235, 1952

Herzog A, Detre T: Psychotic reactions associated with childbirth. Diseases of the Nervous System 37:229–235, 1976

Hopkins J, Marcus M, Campbell SB: Postpartum depression: a critical review. Psychol Bull 95:498–515, 1984

Hopkins J, Campbell SB, Marcus M: Role of infant-related stressors in postpartum depression. J Abnorm Psychol 96:237–241, 1987

Jansson B: Psychic insufficiencies associated with childbearing. Acta Psychiatr Scand Suppl 172:7–26, 156–163, 1964

Kadrmas A, Winokur G, Crowe R: Post partum mania. Br J Psychiatry 135:551–554, 1979

Kendell RE: Invited review: emotional and physical factors in the genesis of puerperal mental disorders. J Psychosom Res 29:3–11, 1985

Kendell RE, Wainwright S, Hailey A, et al: The influence of childbirth on psychiatric morbidity. Psychol Med 6:297–302, 1976

Kendell RE, Rennie D, Clarke JA, et al: The social and obstetric correlates of psychiatric admission in the puerperium. Psychol Med 11:341–350, 1981

Kendell RE, Chalmers JC, Platz C: Epidemiology of puerperal psychosis. Br J Psychiatry 150:662–673, 1987

Kendler K: Kraepelin and the differential diagnosis of dementia praecox and manic-depressive insanity. Compr Psychiatry 27:549–558, 1986

Kumar R, Robson KM: A prospective study of emotional disorders in childbearing women. Br J Psychiatry 144:35–47, 1984

Lindstrom LH, Widerlov E, Gunne LM, et al: Endorphins in human cerebrospinal fluid: clinical correlations to some psychotic states. Acta Psychiatr Scand 57:153–164, 1978

Martin CJ, Brown GW, Goldberg DP, et al: Psycho-social stress and puerperal depression. J Affect Disord 16:283–293, 1989

McGorry PM, Connell S: The nosology and prognosis of puerperal psychosis: a review. Compr Psychiatry 31:519–534, 1990

McNeil TF: A prospective study of postpartum psychoses in a high risk group. Acta Psychiatr Scand 75:35–43, 1987

McNeil TF: Women with nonorganic psychosis: psychiatric and demographic characteristics of cases with versus without postpartum psychotic episodes. Acta Psychiatr Scand 78:603–609, 1988

Meltzer ES, Kumar R: Puerperal mental illness, clinical features and classification: a study of 142 mother-and-baby admissions. Br J Psychiatry 147:647–654, 1985

Nott PN: Psychiatric illness following childbirth in Southampton: a case register study. Psychol Med 12:557–561, 1982

Nott PN, Franklin M, Armitage C, et al: Hormonal changes and mood in the puerperium. Br J Psychiatry 128:379–383, 1976

O'Hara MW: Social support, life events, and depression during pregnancy and the puerperium. Arch Gen Psychiatry 43:569–573, 1986

O'Hara MW, Rehm LP, Campbell SA: Predicting depressive symptomatology: cognitive-behavioral models and postpartum depression. J Abnorm Psychol 91:457–461, 1982

O'Hara MW, Rehm LP, Campbell SA: Postpartum depression: a role for social network and life stress variables. J Nerv Ment Dis 171:336–341, 1983

O'Hara MW, Neunaber DJ, Zekoski EM: Prospective study of postpartum depression: prevalence, course, and predictive factors. J Abnorm Psychol 93:158–171, 1984

O'Hara MW, Zekoski EM, Philipps LH, et al: Controlled prospective study of postpartum mood disorders: comparison of childbearing and nonchildbearing women. J Abnorm Psychol 99:3–15, 1990

Paffenbarger RS: Epidemiological aspects of parapartum mental illness. Br J Prevent Soc Med 18:189–195, 1964

Paffenbarger RS, McCabe LJ: The effect of obstetric and perinatal events on risk of mental illness in women of childbearing age. Am J Public Health 56:400–407, 1966

Paffenbarger RS, Steinmetz CH, Pooler BG, et al: The picture puzzle of the postpartum psychoses. J Chronic Dis 13:161–173, 1961

Paykel ES, Emms EM, Fletcher J, et al: Life events and social support in puerperal depression. Br J Psychiatry 136:339–346, 1980

Pitt B: "Atypical" depression following childbirth. Br J Psychiatry 114:1325–1335, 1968

Platz C, Kendell RE: A matched control follow-up and family study of "puerperal psychoses." Br J Psychiatry 153:90–94, 1988

Protheroe C: Puerperal psychosis: a long-term study, 1927–1961. Br J Psychiatry 115:9–30, 1969

Pugh TF, Jerath BK, Schmidt WM, et al: Rates of mental disease related to childbearing. N Engl J Med 268:1224–1228, 1963

Reich T, Winokur G: Postpartum psychoses in patients with manic depressive disease. J Nerv Ment Dis 151:60–68, 1970

Robins E, Guze S: Establishment of diagnostic validity in psychiatric illness: its application to schizophrenia. Am J Psychiatry 126:107–111, 1970

Robinson GE, Stewart DE: Postpartum psychiatric disorders. Can Med Assoc J 134:31–37, 1986

Schopf J, Bryois C, Jonquiere M, et al: On the nosology of severe psychiatric post-partum disorders. Eur Arch Psychiatr Neurol Sci 234:54–63, 1984

Schopf J, Bryois C, Jonquiere M, et al: A family heredity study of postpartum "psychoses." Eur Arch Psychiatr Neurol Sci 235:164–170, 1985

Seager CP: A controlled study of postpartum mental illness. J Ment Sci 106:214–230, 1960

Singh B, Gilhotra M, Smith R, et al: Postpartum psychoses and the dexamethasone suppression test. J Affect Disord 11:173–177, 1986

Sneddon J, Kerry RJ, Bant WP: The psychiatric mother and baby unit: a three-year study. The Practitioner 225:1295–1299, 1981

Spitzer RL, Endicott J, Robins E: Research Diagnostic Criteria: rationale and reliability. Arch Gen Psychiatry 35:773–782, 1978

Steiner M: Psychobiology of mental disorders associated with childbearing. Acta Psychiatr Scand 60:449–464, 1979

Stewart DE: Prophylactic lithium in postpartum affective psychosis. J Nerv Ment Dis 176:485–489, 1988

Thomas CL, Gordon JE: Psychosis after childbirth: ecological aspects of a single impact stress. Am J Med Sci 238:363–388, 1959

Thuwe I: Genetic factors in puerperal psychosis. Br J Psychiatry 125:378–385, 1974

Tod EDM: Puerperal depression: a prospective epidemiological study. Lancet 2:1264–1266, 1964

Treadway CR, Kane FJ, Jarrahi-Zadeh A, et al: A psychoendocrine study of pregnancy and puerperium. Am J Psychiatry 125:1380–1385, 1969

Troutman BR, Cutrona CE: Nonpsychotic postpartum depression among adolescent mothers. J Abnorm Psychol 99:69–78, 1990

Watson JP, Elliot SA, Rugg AJ, et al: Psychiatric disorder in pregnancy and the first postnatal year. Br J Psychiatry 144:453–462, 1984

Whalley LJ, Roberts DF, Wentzel J, et al: Genetic factors in puerperal affective psychoses. Acta Psychiatr Scand 65:180–193, 1982

Wilson JE, Barglow P, Shipman W: The prognosis of postpartum mental illness. Compr Psychiatry 13:305–316, 1972

Chapter 12

Validity of Seasonal Pattern as a Modifier for Recurrent Mood Disorders in DSM-IV

Mark S. Bauer, M.D., and David L. Dunner, M.D.

Statement of the Issues

Seasonal pattern (SP) was adopted in DSM-III-R (American Psychiatric Association 1987) as a modifier for recurrent major depressive disorder, bipolar disorder, and bipolar and depressive disorders not otherwise specified (NOS). The purpose of this chapter is to delineate options for revision of SP as a modifier for recurrent mood disorders in DSM-IV in light of more recent empirical evidence.

Significance of the Issues

Historical background regarding the development of SP criteria for DSM-III-R has recently been summarized (Spitzer and Williams 1989). Briefly, evidence for inclusion of seasonal affective disorder (SAD) came to the attention of the DSM-III Mood Disorders Work Group relatively late in the process of developing the Mood Disorders section. However, the Work Group felt that the evidence was strong enough to consider inclusion of SAD as a disorder or SP as a modifier. Consultation with Drs. Norman Rosenthal and Michael Terman and discussions among the Work Group members led to the current form of the criteria.

Before publication of DSM-III-R, most researchers in SAD used the criteria for winter depression proposed by the National Institute of Mental Health (NIMH)

Preparation of this manuscript was supported in part by a Physician Scientist Award (K11-MH00720) and a Young Investigator Award from the National Alliance for Research in Schizophrenia and Depression (NARSAD) to M.S.B.

Table 12–1.   Comparison of diagnostic schemata for winter depression/seasonal pattern

Rosenthal criteria for winter depression[a]	DSM-III-R criteria for seasonal pattern modifier
1. Recurrent fall/winter depressions	Regular onset within a 60-day period
2. No seasonally varying psychosocial	Same stressor
3. Regularly occurring nondepressed periods in spring and summer	Regular remission or switch to (hypo)mania within a 60-day period
4. At least two of the depressions occurred during consecutive years	At least 3 episodes, 2 in consecutive years; ratio of 3:1 seasonal:nonseasonal
5. At least one of the depressions has met RDC for major depression	Modifies bipolar disorder, recurrent major depressive disorder, depressive disorder not otherwise specified
6. No other Axis I pathology	Other diagnoses do not exclude application of the modifier

Note. RDC = Research Diagnostic Criteria.
[a]Rosenthal et al. 1989.

group led by Rosenthal (Rosenthal et al. 1984). Because of some concerns about the final form of the DSM-III-R modifier, the majority of researchers have continued to use the Rosenthal criteria. The most recent version of those criteria for SAD (Rosenthal et al. 1989) is compared to the DSM-III-R SP modifier criteria in Table 12–1. Note that SP was written to be applied to either winter or summer seasonal depressions. Because the prevalence of the latter syndrome appears to be much lower than winter depression (Rosen et al. 1990) and because only a few dozen patients of the summer type have been studied to date, mainly at one center (Wehr et al. 1989), the term *SAD* is used here to refer only to winter-type SP. All but one study reviewed in this chapter used one of the two criteria sets described in Table 12–1 for winter depression; the remaining study (Garvey et al. 1988) used similar criteria, requiring full major depressive episodes for at least two consecutive winters. Use of the terms *SAD* and *SP* here is dictated by context.

Methods

Review Methods

We solicited data from researchers in the field on several occasions, including annual meetings of the Society for Light Treatment and Biological Rhythms. In addition, all available literature on SAD published in the English language was reviewed. The search was conducted by reviewing journals since 1985 that had published articles on affective disorders or biological rhythms. Whenever a relevant article was found, the reference list was inspected, and additional references were located by title. The search was considered exhaustive when no further titles were revealed that had not already been found. Abstract books for each annual meeting for the Society of Light Treatment and Biological Rhythms and the Society for Research in Biological Rhythms were also reviewed. No computerized National Library of Medicine (NLM) search was conducted because of lack of key-word-based search strategies relevant to the topic.

Criteria for Validity

Several methods for assessing the validity of a putative neuropsychiatric syndrome are in current use. The literature on SP has been reviewed in light of three such approaches. First, Robins and Guze (1970) suggested that if a group of clinical features comprises a valid and separate disorder, five criteria should be fulfilled. These criteria have served as the basis for the Mood Disorders Work Group's evaluation of disorders and modifiers for inclusion or revision: 1) clinical characteristics form a consistent pattern in patients with the disorder; 2) laboratory studies reveal abnormalities that can identify patients with that syndrome; 3) exclusion criteria are available to eliminate borderline or doubtful cases, leaving as homogeneous a group as possible; 4) follow-up studies reveal a relatively homogeneous outcome for patients with the disorder; and 5) family studies show higher rates of that disorder in relatives of patients with the disorder than in relatives of patients with other disorders. A sixth criterion, treatment response as assessed in formal treatment studies, may also help to distinguish distinct clinical entities.

Second, Kendell (1982) emphasized diagnostic reliability and separability of a syndrome from similar syndromes. Specifically, he suggested that 1) a disorder should have explicit criteria that can be reliably applied in relevant settings, and 2) groups of characteristics that distinguish a disorder should separate it from similar disorders. Distribution frequencies for such characteristics should manifest "points of rarity" or "nonlinearities" that separate similar disorders (see Bauer and Whybrow, Chapter 13, this volume).

Finally, Spitzer and Williams (1989) suggested at a conference on SAD research that four types of diagnostic validity are necessary for SAD or SP to be considered a distinct neuropsychiatric syndrome: face validity, descriptive validity, predictive validity, and construct validity.

Results

SP/SAD and the Robins-Guze Criteria

Consistent symptom pattern. Clinical characteristics of patients with SAD are summarized in Table 12–2. Most studies reveal a preponderance of females among

SAD patients in excess of that usually expected in recurrent major depressive disorder. Age at onset is usually mid-20s, with SAD appearing to be extremely rare in children in the two metropolitan areas studied thus far (reviewed in Sonis 1989). The proportion of SAD with bipolar spectrum versus unipolar spectrum disorders is inconsistent across studies.

No information is available regarding the proportion of patients exhibiting SP for major affective episodes versus for recurrent dysphoric periods. Neither the Rosenthal criteria nor DSM-III-R is specific in this regard. The former require only one major depressive episode retrospectively, whereas the latter can be applied to depressive disorder NOS, which would include Research Diagnostic Criteria (Spitzer et al. 1978) minor depressive episodes. There is no information regarding differences in demographics, clinical features, or outcome between those who qualify for major mood disorder and those who fit into the residual depressive disorder NOS category.

Patients with SAD have been described as having "atypical" or "reverse vegetative" symptoms (Table 12–2). Most studies indicate that SAD patients have prominent lethargy, increased sleep, increased appetite and weight, and "carbohydrate" craving. However, two caveats are in order. First, these characteristics may not represent the only, or even most common, clinical pattern for those who fulfill criteria for SAD/SP. The method of recruitment for the first seven studies listed was media or referral based (M/R). Symptom patterns are invariably described in this sort of recruitment, which includes word of mouth, interviews, newspaper articles, and sometimes advertisements. Thus, the recruitment of patients with that particular symptom pattern may become a self-fulfilling prophecy. This sort of referral method leads to what is denoted in Table 12–2 as a "SAD-weighted population base." In addition, one study screened patients for clinic entry based on the presence of such a symptom pattern ("SAD-weighted screening"). Whereas this sort of recruitment and screening may be very appropriate for certain sorts of studies, it limits the use of such data for purposes of validating the syndrome. To our knowledge only one data set exists that reports symptom frequency in SP patients garnered from a nonenriched referral base (Garvey et al. 1988). The percentage endorsing each symptom in that study was roughly comparable to that reported in other SAD studies, but only hypersomnia and "carbohydrate" craving were significantly greater in the SAD than in the nonseasonal sample.

The second problem is one of specificity. The reverse vegetative symptom pattern is also common in nonseasonal patients (e.g., with bipolar disorder) (Thase 1989). The two studies from nonenriched patient bases provide only weak support for the hypothesis that the "reverse vegetative" symptom pattern distinguishes SP from nonseasonal depressions. Specifically, Garvey et al. (1988) found that only increased sleep and "carbohydrate" craving were significantly more common in SP

Table 12–2.   Clinical characteristics of seasonal affective disorder

Study site	NIMH	SW	UK-S	UK-M	NY	AK	PH	IA	PT
Study characteristics									
Year reported	1984/9	1986/9	1989	1989	1989	1989	1991	1988	1989
Number of subjects	29/156	22/63	51	45	163	17	23	18	18
Method of recruitment	M/R	M/R	M/R	M/R	M/R	M/R	M/R	Practice	Clinic
SAD-weighted population base?	Yes	Yes	Yes	–	Yes	Yes	Yes	No	No
SAD-weighted screening?	No	Yes	No	No	No	–	No	No	No
Demographics									
% Female	89	78	90	71	83	94	57	61	–
Age at presentation (years)	40	44	42	47	39	38	36	–	–
Clinical characteristics									
Met criteria for current MDE	–	–	100	100	<73	–	100	–	–
Unipolar	7[a]	90	29	–[d]	47	18	74	45	83
Bipolar w/hypomania	76[a]	8	51	46[d]	23	82	26	33	–
Bipolar w/mania	17[a]	–	20	–	3	0	0	22	–
Age at onset of affective symptoms	27	32	24	28	21	25	25	22[e]	–
Prior pharmacological prescription	69	66	49	71	42	57	39	–	100
Symptom profile (% with symptom present)									
Depressed mood	100	91[b]	96	100	95	–	96	–	–
Anxiety	72	86	86	91	76	–	30	89	–
Decreased physical activity	100	100	100	100	97	–	83	94	–
Decreased sleep	–	–	–	–	–	–	9	–	–
Increased sleep	97	82	2 hr[c]	60	71	–	78	72[e]	NS[f]
Decreased appetite	28	45	16	49	2	–	4	–	Less[f]
Increased appetite	66	45	74	40	77	–	52	50	NS
Decreased weight	17	23	6	38	5	–	0	–	–
Increased weight	76	55	84	40	78	–	48	–	NS
"Carbohydrate" craving	79	77	82	47	88	–	43	67[e]	–

(continued)

Table 12–2. Clinical characteristics of seasonal affective disorder (*continued*)

Study site	NIMH	SW	UK-S	UK-M	NY	AK	PH	IA	PT
Family history (% probands with positive family history)									
Affective illness	69	64	–	47	51	57	35	55	–
SAD	37	14	–	7	23	15	9	–	–
Suicide	–	20	–	11	–	–	9	–	–
Alcoholism	19	18	–	13	20	42	22	33	–

NIMH = Washington, DC (Rosenthal et al. 1984), and other data (Thompson 1989).

SW = Switzerland: Wirz–Justice et al. (1986, 1989) statistics corroborated in an enlarged sample (*n* = 112; A. Wirz–Justice, personal communication, 1991).

UK-S = Southampton (Thompson 1989).

UK-M = Maudsley (Winton and Checkley 1989).

NY = New York (Terman et al. 1989b).

AK = Anchorage (Hellekson 1989).

PH = Philadelphia (Bauer et al. 1991).

IA = Iowa City (Garvey et al. 1988).

PT = Pittsburgh (Thase 1989).

M/R = media/referral source. Practice = private practice. MDE = major depressive episode. Clinic = mood disorders research clinic. – = no information.

SAD = seasonal affective disorder.

[a]Data from 1989 (enlarged) sample.

[b]All symptom profile data from earlier study; remainder from 1989.

[c]Mean increase.

[d]Bipolar by Research Diagnostic Criteria.

[e]Significantly greater in SAD than in nonseasonal recurrent unipolar depressive patients; see text for details.

[f]Significantly less in SAD than in nonseasonal depressive patients; see text for details.

than in nonseasonal depression. Thase (1989) found that decreased appetite, but not increased sleep, increased appetite, or increased weight, occurred more frequently in SP patients.

Laboratory abnormalities.   As with other neuropsychiatric syndromes, clinically useful diagnostic tests are not available. Phase, or timing with respect to the light-dark cycle, of the nocturnal peak of circadian rhythm of serum melatonin has been reported to be abnormal in patients with SAD (Lewy et al. 1987). However, subsequent studies have provided only partial replication (Dahl et al. 1990), and extension to other circadian rhythms (Dahl et al. 1990; Levandosky et al. 1991) has not been consistent with the original melatonin findings.

Distinct boundaries.   The delineation of SP involves particularly its separation from 1) subsyndromal seasonal mood and behavior changes and 2) nonseasonal forms of affective illness. The ability to differentiate SAD from subsyndromal seasonal changes in mood and behavior is made particularly difficult by the application of SP to depressive disorder NOS (and diagnosis of SAD by Rosenthal criteria in patients with recurrent minor depressive episodes), because the difficulties inherent in diagnosing minor mood disorders, such as dysthymic disorder and cyclothymic disorder (see Keller and Russell, Chapter 1, and Howland and Thase, Chapter 2, this volume), compound the difficulties inherent in diagnosing a mood disorder based on its temporal characteristics (see Bauer and Whybrow, Chapter 13, this volume).

To complicate matters further, mood, energy, sleep, and appetite disturbances characteristic of SAD may represent a continuously distributed general population characteristic. For example, Kasper et al. (1988, 1989a, 1989c) have proposed that persons who do not meet criteria for SAD but score high on Seasonal Pattern Assessment Questionnaire (SPAQ) indices of seasonality comprise a separate syndrome ("subsyndromal SAD" or "S-SAD"). The most recent summary of criteria for S-SAD (Kasper 1991) indicates that it differs from SAD in that persons with S-SAD have never experienced a major affective episode in winter, and neither they nor anyone else suggested that they seek treatment for winter symptoms. However, as with SAD, these criteria have not been investigated from the perspective of validity. For example, in the Philadelphia sample, 52% of patients with SP had never sought treatment prior to evaluation (Bauer et al. 1991), yet they met criteria for current major depressive episode and recurrent major depressive disorder or bipolar disorder.

Furthermore, three random-sample survey studies of the general population (Kasper et al. 1989c; Rosen et al. 1990; Terman et al. 1989a, 1989b) have identified prominent "seasonality" in a large proportion of nonclinical samples using a self-report instrument, the SPAQ (Rosenthal et al. 1989). Up to 10%–20% of the samples were found to have prominent difficulties with decreased energy, increased sleep, increased appetite, and weight gain during the winter. The distribution of such seasonality scores was unimodal and skewed to the right. In these studies, the most severe (far right) tail of these general population samples score in the range of diagnosed SAD patients and are thought to represent undiagnosed SAD cases. Prevalence of SPAQ-defined SAD in these studies is as high as 10% at the latitude of New England. Although the SPAQ is a relatively new instrument, existing data do support its reliability (Thompson et al. 1988) and validity (Bartko and Kasper 1989; Rosenthal et al. 1987; Thompson et al. 1988). Thus, there is support for the construct validity of seasonality as a traitlike characteristic, although its precise relationship with clinically defined SAD remains to be elucidated.

There is some evidence from other studies of nonclinical samples that depressed mood may become more prominent in the winter (Eastwood et al. 1985). Furthermore, Terman et al. (1989a) suggested that symptoms consistent with SAD or S-SAD, but not other psychopathological symptoms or traits, show seasonal variation with winter peaks (Terman et al. 1989a). However, the variance explained by a seasonal component in that general population study was quite small, on the order of 5%. At present, our knowledge of seasonality of mood must be regarded as quite rudimentary (Lacoste and Wirz-Justice 1989).

Separation of patients with SP from patients with nonseasonal depressive episodes that occur in winter further complicates delineation of boundaries. Nonseasonal forms of affective illness are not distinguished from SAD on the basis of clinical and demographic characteristics, as summarized above. Furthermore, although early studies indicated that affective episodes peak primarily in spring and early fall (Goodwin and Jamison 1990), more recent prospectively gathered data indicate that episodes of affective illness in a nonseasonal population may also peak in winter (Thase 1989). This suggests that most winter major depressive episodes may not be part of an SP mood disorder. Furthermore, prominent seasonality has been described in other indices of psychiatric morbidity in general, including suicide, hospital admissions for depression, initial visits to psychiatrists for treatment, initial prescriptions of antidepressant medication, and administration of antidepressant treatment (Wehr and Rosenthal 1989).

Similarly, patients with nonseasonal mood disorders may show high levels of seasonality, as measured by the SPAQ. Pande et al. (1991) administered the SPAQ to 28 patients with "mood-reactive atypical depression" that did not meet criteria for SP because of chronicity of mood episode and found SPAQ scores in the S-SAD or SAD range in 57%. The items reported reflect winter worsening of mood, energy, sleep, and appetite typical of SAD. SPAQ scores characteristic of patients with SAD have also been described in 11.4% of inpatients with major depressive disorder, although the proportion who actually had diagnosable SAD was not reported

(Kasper and Kamo 1990). A similar degree of seasonality has also been described in approximately 65% of a sample of bulimic patients, only 14% of whom concurrently met criteria for a mood disorder with SP (R. Levitan, A. Kaplan, R. Joffe, A. Levitt, personal communication, May 27, 1991). Bulimic patients in this sample also often described a dramatic increase in binge frequency during the winter.

Homogeneous outcome.   Most studies indicate an age at onset of affective symptoms in the mid-20s and presentation in the late 30s to early 40s. There is little published information on long-term outcome. However, in a series of five patients followed for 3–9 years, the seasonal pattern of depressive symptoms appeared stable (A. Wirz-Justice, personal communication, 1991). On the other hand, in a small sample from Pittsburgh, 33% (6 of 18) no longer qualified for the diagnosis of SAD (by Rosenthal criteria) after 1 year (Thase 1989). Three had experienced different onset or offset, two had not recovered in summer, and one developed a summer depressive episode. Thase suggested that these changes may have been due to treatment with, and maintenance on, tricyclic antidepressants. Alternatively, the syndrome may not be as stable over time as commonly assumed, or the criteria for diagnosis, based on retrospective recollection of pattern of symptoms over time, may not have high specificity.

By definition, the hallmark of SP is homogeneous short-term outcome (i.e., regular remission in spring or summer and regular recurrence in fall or winter). Controversy has surrounded the DSM-III-R adoption of the 60-day window criteria for onset and offset (Criteria 1 and 3 in Table 12–1). There has been little reported research, none of it prospective, regarding these criteria. One abstract reported that in 46 patients diagnosed with SAD, 41% had episode onset within a 60-day window, 67% within 90 days, and 89% within 120 days (Takahashi 1990). On the other hand, none of 23 patients in the Philadelphia study who met Rosenthal criteria for SAD were excluded by the DSM-III-R 60-day window criteria for SP (Bauer et al. 1991). In further support of the similarity of these two criteria sets, Elster and Wirz-Justice found no difference in rate of response to light treatment in patients who fulfilled all SP criteria, some SP criteria, or only Rosenthal criteria (A. Wirz, personal communication, 1991).

As noted above, both Rosenthal and DSM-III-R criteria include patients who experience winter recurrence of both major and minor affective episodes. There is no information as to whether episode severity in patients with SP "breeds true," or whether short- or long-term outcome differs between those who have a recurrent major affective disorder and those with recurrent dysphoria.

Familial aggregation.   Studies of family history (Table 12–2) indicate that 35%–69% of probands with SAD have first-degree relatives with some form of affective illness; 7%–37% of probands have a family history of SAD, with 9%–20% having a family history of suicide. Alcoholism has been found in a sizable minority (13%–42%). No studies are available comparing SP and nonseasonal depressive patients.

Treatment response. Response to treatment with bright white light, perhaps at specific times of the day, has been another hallmark of SAD (Rosenthal et al. 1984; Terman et al. 1989b). Most of the reported studies describe clinically relevant decreases in depression rating scale scores of more than 50% or remission of episode by categorical criteria after 1–2 weeks of treatment in 50%–60% of patients, although maximal response may not be reached until the third week of treatment (Bauer et al. 1991). Interestingly, mild symptoms present in persons with S-SAD may respond to light treatment identical to that used to treat SAD (Kasper et al. 1989a, 1989b). Those studies and one other (Rosenthal et al. 1987) have, in contrast, found no effect of light treatment on behavior and mood in normal subjects over a similar period (7 days), although recent data from a controlled study of 4 weeks of bright light treatment in control subjects indicates that bright light may induce manic symptoms detectable by clinician rating (Bauer et al. 1991).

In contrast to the studies in patients with SP, studies of the effects of light in patients with nonseasonal depression have shown much more modest effects, albeit in very short-term (1-week) paradigms. Interestingly, the first report of light treatment of nonseasonal depressive patients is actually contemporaneous with the first SAD studies (Kripke et al. 1983). Open and controlled trials of bright light alone or in combination with antidepressants substantiated the original findings, which were shown to be independent of season of occurrence of episode (Deltito et al. 1991; Dietzel et al. 1986; Kripke et al. 1983, 1989, 1992; Peter 1986; Prasko and Prasnova 1988; Volz et al. 1990). However, not all controlled trials have demonstrated statistically significant effects (Kripke et al. 1987; Mackert et al. 1991; Yerevanian et al. 1986), although the overall effect size in these studies appears to be similar to that of 1 week's treatment with chemical antidepressants in nonseasonal depressive episodes (Kripke et al. 1992). Thus, light responsivity does not appear to be unique to SAD, although the dramatic 1- to 2-week response time may be.

Although most of the studies of the clinical characteristics of SAD note that at least 40% of patients have been treated with pharmacotherapy, no formal retrospective studies of response to such treatments have been reported. To our knowledge, only two controlled prospective treatment studies of potential antidepressant compounds have been reported in SP. Whereas d-fenfluramine was superior to placebo in treating 18 patients with SAD in a crossover paradigm (O'Rourke et al. 1989), melatonin suppression using atenolol was not efficacious (Rosenthal et al.

1988). A structured open trial of the monoamine oxidase inhibitor tranyl-cypromine reported marked effects in patients with winter depression (Dilsaver and Jaeckle 1990).

SP/SAD and the Kendell Guidelines

Explicit and reliable criteria. DSM-III-R criteria for SP and Rosenthal criteria for SAD are, for the most part, explicit. Both criteria sets have the disadvantage of depending, in an unspecified percentage of cases, on the poorly operationalized syndromes of minor depressive disorder and depressive disorder NOS. Furthermore, neither criteria set has been studied with regard to diagnostic reliability.

Separability from similar disorders. Population studies indicate that seasonality, defined on the basis of SPAQ score, has a unimodal, right-skewed distribution. Therefore, seasonality itself does not categorically differentiate patients with SP from normal subjects. Similarly, as summarized above, prominent seasonality and seasonal worsening of symptoms in mood and other psychiatric disorders suggest that such characteristics will also not be useful in discriminating SP from nonseasonal syndromes.

On the other hand, clinical response to short-term (less than 14-day) light treatment may differentiate SP from nonseasonal depressive patients. However, this hypothesis has not yet been directly tested. Furthermore, it is not clear whether depressive episodes during the winter in nonseasonal depressive illness respond to light, which would suggest that the season of occurrence of the depressive episode is the distinguishing characteristic rather than the pattern of episodes in a particular patient over time.

SP/SAD and Diagnostic Validity

Face validity. According to Spitzer and Williams (1989), face validity, the most impressionistic type of validity, is the degree to which people who are expert in the field think the concept is an important distinction. SP without doubt has struck a chord in clinicians and researchers in the area of mood disorders. Interestingly, support for face validity comes from another quarter as well. As noted above, 52% of patients in the Philadelphia sample meeting criteria for SP had never seen a mental health professional for any purpose before evaluation in our program. Such "lay experts" did not characterize their problems as mental health related, but a newspaper query regarding depression in the winter that went away in spring clearly made sense to them.

Descriptive validity.   Descriptive validity represents the extent to which the defining features of an illness are unique to that illness. As reviewed above, the clinical
characteristics of SP are not unique to those depressive episodes. Demographics
and family history are thus far noncontributory as well. However, the one clinical
feature that may, ironically, provide the most support for descriptive validity is the
fact that symptoms reliably disappear in spring or summer.

Predictive validity.   Data concerning predictive validity, the degree to which a
syndrome is characterized by a unique natural history or a unique response to
treatment, provide perhaps the strongest support for SP as a distinct diagnostic
entity. Both spring-summer remissions and response to short-term treatment with
bright light therapy may be uniquely characteristic of SP. However, despite the
promise that light treatment appears to hold for many individuals with SP, there
are still no data from comparative studies of SP and nonseasonal depression that
could substantiate the apparent distinctiveness of treatment response in SP. Similarly, strong support would be lent to the validity of SP as a separate diagnostic
category if antidepressants effective in nonseasonal depression were less efficacious
in SP depressive episodes.

In addition, it is not clear to what degree SP is stable throughout the course of
a recurrent mood disorder. Of interest is the often-quoted study of prevalence of
SAD along the eastern seaboard of the United States (Rosen et al. 1990). The
strongest predictor of SAD in that study was not actually latitude but age, with
younger age associated with SAD in logistic regression modeling. The next strongest
predictor was an age-by-latitude interaction, indicating that younger persons were
vulnerable for SAD and that living at higher latitudes increased the risk of expression of the syndrome. In contrast, older individuals were relatively protected
wherever they lived. One possible interpretation, among several, is that one may
"outgrow" SAD. Obviously this has not yet been directly tested, since the syndrome
was first described only in 1984.

Construct validity.   Finally, construct validity refers to the degree to which the
core characteristics and boundaries of an entity are known. In biomedical settings
this usually refers to the degree to which the etiology or pathophysiological processes involved in an illness are understood. Evidence regarding the underlying
processes again derives from natural history and treatment response. Fall-winter
onset, spring-summer remission, and response to light administration all support
the conceptualization of light being involved in the pathogenesis of, and/or recovery
from, depressive episodes in SP. Beyond that, however, knowledge is minimal.
Whereas hypotheses concerning circadian rhythm abnormalities have been investigated most intensively and provide the most powerful heuristic models for

understanding SAD, the simple phase-shift hypothesis appears to need revision (Levandosky et al. 1991; Terman et al. 1989b). Exploration of noncircadian hypotheses regarding the efficacy of bright light is in a very rudimentary stage.

Discussion

Options: Modifier? Disorder? Trait?

The Mood Disorders Work Group is considering several options regarding whether and how to define seasonality in DSM-IV. One option is to delete the modifier because, like the concept of "neurotic depression," its boundaries are too ill defined and its definition relies too heavily on theoretical constructs. However, evidence reviewed above, particularly natural history and treatment response data, was felt to be sufficient to merit retention of SP in some form in DSM-IV. On the other end of the spectrum, making SP into a separate mood disorder, SAD, was considered but was found to be without sufficient supporting evidence.

Review of the evidence regarding seasonality in normal subjects and in patients without mood disorders led to evaluation of several additional options. A case can be made, in view of the traitlike aspects of seasonality, that it may more properly belong on Axis II for diagnosis in persons with or without other psychiatric symptoms who have dysfunction due to wintertime changes in mood, weight, energy, and sleep. A related option is that SP may be an appropriate modifier for *any* psychiatric disorder that worsens in winter. However, data at this time are too scant for these options to be viable, although characterization of seasonality of mood and other symptoms in patients with nonaffective psychiatric disorders and in normal subjects is clearly an important area for further study. In summary, then, current evidence indicates that SP is appropriate as a modifier for mood disorders.

Options: Review of Current Criteria

Two of the criteria for SP are relatively uncontroversial. First, exclusion on the basis of a seasonally varying psychosocial stressor (e.g., final examinations for students; seasonally determined unemployment) appears relatively straightforward and is found as well in the Rosenthal criteria. Second, although the Rosenthal criteria exclude other Axis I psychopathology, there is precedent in the DSM system for allowing multiple diagnoses; there is no reason not to adopt this additional exclusionary criterion as needed for specific research studies.

The 60-day windows for onset and offset have sparked perhaps the most heated discussions among investigators and clinicians. Despite widespread research concerning SAD, data on the onset window are limited to two abstracts that discuss a total of 69 patients, as summarized above. The Japanese series (Takahashi et al. 1990) strongly support widening of the onset window beyond 60 days. Widening the window to 90 days would permit fairly wide intra-individual variation of onset times (e.g., September 1 to December 1). The advantage is that this would accommodate variability both due to random distribution of onset around an ideal mean and to nonrandom factors that may hasten or delay onset for a particular year (e.g., environmental stressors). However, widening the window any further could compromise face and construct validity. For example, a 120-day window would allow onset to vary from August 1 to December 1 in the same individual from year to year, corresponding to a difference in day length at the time of onset of 4.67 hours at the latitude of Philadelphia and 5.15 hours at the latitude of Seattle.

No data exist concerning the offset window. Overall, there is little consensus concerning the operationalization of remission of any mood episode. DSM-III-R currently defines *full remission* as having "no significant signs or symptoms of the disturbance for at least 6 months" (p. 218). Adoption of a requirement for full remission (or a switch to a hypomanic or manic episode) would make an offset criterion unnecessary, because it would preclude spring-summer depressive pathology.

No information is available regarding the appropriateness of the 3:1 ratio for seasonal:nonseasonal episodes; the same is true for the Rosenthal criterion of 2 consecutive years with winter episodes. If the diagnosis is stable over long periods, the 3:1 requirement would provide for a relatively homogeneous group descriptively, while not erroneously excluding many patients who truly have SP. On the other hand, if SP is a valid diagnosis, but one that may change over several years as the Pittsburgh data indicate (Thase 1989), then the 3:1 ratio would exclude a large proportion of patients who would be diagnosed with SP (e.g., four nonseasonal episodes followed by 4 years of winter-only episodes). A concern regarding the Rosenthal criteria, which simply require two consecutive winters with depressive symptoms, is that they allow an unspecified number of additional nonwinter episodes. A decision regarding optimal episode-counting rules will have to rely on formal studies of natural history or discovery of diagnostically relevant biological markers or other external validators.

There has been little discussion of the application of SP to non-major mood disorders. This may be because the Rosenthal criteria, used by most SAD researchers to date, allow the diagnosis of SAD in the context of recurrent minor depressions as long as there is one retrospectively documented major depressive episode. Perhaps because of this vagueness, it is common practice in SAD research not to document the proportion of subjects with recurrent major mood disorders or to report treatment, neuroendocrine, or other results stratified on the basis of current major versus minor mood episodes. With the growing awareness of subsyndromal variants of SAD, the boundaries of the syndrome become murkier as the basic disorder that is modified by SP becomes less pronounced. Thus, differentiating episodes on the basis of severity may be necessary if the validity of SP/SAD is to be well tested. However, limiting application of SP to major mood disorders would doubtless exclude a large proportion of the patients who provided the basis for the validity evidence reviewed above.

Recommendations

Regarding the most controversial aspects of SP, the window and the number of seasonal versus nonseasonal episodes, several options are recommended for consideration. First, no change could be made in the window criteria, with a disclaimer in the text indicating that the window criteria are not precise and that clinical judgment must be used in the presence of strong evidence for SP. Alternatively, the window may be explicitly widened, although to a maximum of 90 days.

Regarding episode pattern over time, criteria may remain unchanged, with another text disclaimer for clinical judgment. Similarly, 2 or 3 years of SP may be required with "substantially" more seasonal than nonseasonal episodes as a criterion.

We favor a more explicitly operationalized criteria set, achieved by requiring 2 consecutive years with SP with no intervening nonseasonal depressive episodes. In this case, a person would need only a relatively short course to qualify for SP; however, sample homogeneity would be at least as great as that of groups defined by the Rosenthal criteria, which require 2 consecutive years of stable onset and offset of symptoms but are not explicit regarding intercurrent episodes (Table 12–1). On the other hand, this definition may formally exclude those with, for example, a winter depressive episode in each of the past 3 years with one summer episode last year. However, such patients could clearly be included in research studies if desired. More important, this approach minimizes the pseudoprecision of episode ratios determined retrospectively and defines the syndrome in a relatively simple manner that will allow for the study of its stability over time.

References

American Psychiatric Association: Diagnostic and Statistical Manual of Mental Disorders, 3rd Edition, Revised. Washington, DC, American Psychiatric Association, 1987

Bartko J, Kasper S: Seasonal changes in mood and behavior: a cluster analytic approach. Psychiatry Res 28:227–239, 1989

Bauer M, Kurtz J, Batt L, et al: Mood and behavioral effects of four-week light treatment in winter depressives and controls. Proceedings of the Third Annual Meeting of the Society for Light Treatment and Biological Rhythms. Toronto, Ontario, Canada, June 1991

Dahl K, Avery D, Savage M, et al: Endocrine rhythms in seasonal affective disorder during a constant routine. Soc Neurosci Abstr 16:603, 1990

Deltito J, Moline M, Pollak C, et al: The effect of bright light treatment on non-SAD bipolar spectrum depressed patients. Soc Light Treatment Biol Rhythms Abstr 3:17, 1991

Dietzel M, Saletu B, Lesch O, et al: Light treatment in depressive illness: polysomnographic, psychometric, and neuroendocrinologic findings. Eur Neurol Del 25 (suppl):93–103, 1986

Dilsaver S, Jaeckle R: Winter depression responds to an open trial of tranylcypromine. J Clin Psychiatry 51:326–329, 1990

Eastwood M, Whitton J, Kramer P, et al: Infradian rhythms: a comparison of affective disorders and normal persons. Arch Gen Psychiatry 42:295–299, 1985

Garvey M, Wesner R, Godes M: Comparison of seasonal and nonseasonal affective disorders. Am J Psychiatry 145:100–102, 1988

Goodwin F, Jamison K: Manic-Depressive Illness. New York, Oxford University Press, 1990, pp 183–184

Hellekson C: Phenomenology of seasonal affect disorder, in Seasonal Affective Disorders and Phototherapy. Edited by Rosenthal N, Blehar M. New York, Guilford, 1989, pp 33–45

Kasper S, Rogers A, Yancey A, et al: Phototherapy in subsyndromal seasonal affective disorder and "diagnosed" controls. Pharmacopsychiatry 21:428–429, 1988

Kasper S: Quo vadis S-SAD? Newsletter of the Society for Light Treatment and Biological Rhythms 3:16–18, 1991

Kasper S, Kamo T: Seasonality in major depressed inpatients. J Affect Disord 19:243–248, 1990

Kasper S, Rogers S, Yancey A, et al: Phototherapy in individuals with and without subsyndromal seasonal affective disorder. Arch Gen Psychiatry 46:837–844, 1989a

Kasper S, Rogers S, Yancey A, et al: Psychological effects of light therapy in normals, in Seasonal Affective Disorders and Phototherapy. Edited by Rosenthal N, Blehar M. New York, Guilford, 1989b, pp 260–270

Kasper S, Wehr T, Bartko J, et al: Epidemiological findings of seasonal changes in mood and behavior. Arch Gen Psychiatry 46:823–831, 1989c

Kendell R: The choice of diagnostic criteria for biological research. Arch Gen Psychiatry 39:1334–1339, 1982

Kripke D, Risch S, Janowsky D: Bright white light alleviates depression. Psychiatry Res 10:105–112, 1983

Kripke D, Gillin J, Mullaney D, et al: Treatment of major depressive disorders with bright white light for five days, in Chronobiology and Psychiatric Disorders. Edited by Halaris A. New York, Elsevier, 1987, pp 207–218

Kripke D, Mullaney D, Savides T, et al: Phototherapy for nonseasonal major depressive disorders, in Seasonal Affective Disorders and Phototherapy. Edited by Rosenthal N, Blehar M. New York, Guilford, 1989, pp 342–346

Kripke D, Mullaney D, Klauber M, et al: Controlled trial of bright light for nonseasonal major depressive disorders. Biol Psychiatry 31:119–134, 1992

Lacoste V, Wirz-Justice A: Seasonal variation in normal subjects: an update of variables current in depression research, in Seasonal Affective Disorders and Phototherapy. Edited by Rosenthal N, Blehar M. New York, Guilford, 1989, pp 167–229

Levandosky A, Joseph-Vanderpool J, Hardin T, et al.: Core body temperature in patients with seasonal affective disorder and normal controls in summer and winter. Biol Psychiatry 29:524–534, 1991

Lewy A, Sack R, Miller L, et al: Antidepressant and circadian phase-shifting effects of light. Science 235:352–354, 1987

Mackert A, Volz H-P, Stieglitz R-D, et al: Phototherapy in nonseasonal depression. Biol Psychiatry 30:257–268, 1991

O'Rourke D, Wurtman J, Wurtmann R, et al: Treatment of seasonal depression with d-fenfluramine. J Clin Psychiatry 50:343–347, 1989

Pande A, Haskett R, Greden J: Seasonality in mood-reactive atypical depression. Soc Biol Psychiatry Abstr 29:127A, 1991

Peter K: First results with bright light in affective psychosis. Psychiatr Neurol Med Psychol 38:384–390, 1986

Prasko J, Prasnova H: The acceleration of antidepressants' effects by using phototherapy in endogenous depression. Annual Meeting, CINP, Munich, 1988

Robins E, Guze S: Establishment of diagnostic validity in psychiatric illness: its application to schizophrenia. Am J Psychiatry 126:107–111, 1970

Rosen L, Targum S, Terman M, et al: Prevalence of seasonal affective disorder at four latitudes. J Psychiatr Res 31:131–144, 1990

Rosenthal NE, Sack DA, Gillin JC, et al: Seasonal affective disorder: a description of the syndrome and preliminary findings with light-therapy. Arch Gen Psychiatry 41:72–80, 1984

Rosenthal N, Rotter A, Jacobsen F, et al: No mood-altering effects found after treatment of normal subjects with bright light in the morning. Psychiatry Res 22:1–9, 1987

Rosenthal N, Jacobsen F, Sack D, et al: Atenolol in seasonal affective disorder: a test of the melatonin hypothesis. Am J Psychiatry 145:52–55, 1988

Rosenthal N, Kasper S, Schulz P, et al: New concepts and developments in seasonal affective disorder, in Seasonal Affective Disorder. Edited by Thompson C, Silverstone T. London, Clinical Neuroscience Publishers, 1989, pp 97–132

Sonis W: Seasonal affective disorder of childhood and adolescence, in Seasonal Affective Disorders and Phototherapy. Edited by Rosenthal N, Blehar M. New York, Guilford, 1989, pp 46–54

Spitzer R, Williams J: The validity of seasonal affective disorder, in Seasonal Affective Disorders and Phototherapy. Edited by Rosenthal N, Blehar M. New York, Guilford, 1989, pp 79–84

Spitzer RL, Endicott J, Robins E: Research Diagnostic Criteria: rationale and reliability. Arch Gen Psychiatry 35:773–782, 1978

Takahashi K: Multicenter study of SAD in Japan: a preliminary report. Abstracts of the Annual Meeting, Society for Light Treatment and Biological Rhythms. New York, May 1990, p 12

Terman M, Botticelli S, Link B, et al: Seasonal symptom patterns in New York: patients and population, in Seasonal Affective Disorder. Edited by Thompson C, Silverstone T. London, Clinical Neuroscience Publishers, 1989a, pp 77–96

Terman M, Terman J-S, Quitkin F, et al: Light therapy for seasonal affective disorder: a review of efficacy. Neuropsychopharmacology 2:1–22, 1989b

Thase M: Comparison between seasonal affective disorder and other forms of recurrent depression, in Seasonal Affective Disorders and Phototherapy. Edited by Rosenthal N, Blehar M. New York, Guilford, 1989, pp 64–78

Thompson C: The syndrome of seasonal affective disorder, in Seasonal Affective Disorder. Edited by Thompson C, Silverstone T. London, Clinical Neuroscience Publishers, 1989, pp 37–58

Thompson C, Stinson D, Fernandez M, et al: A comparison of normal, bipolar, and seasonal affective disorder subjects using the Seasonal Pattern Assessment Questionnaire. J Affect Disord 14:257–264, 1988

Volz HP, Mackert A, Steiglitz RD, et al: The effect of bright white light therapy on nonseasonal depressive disorder: preliminary results. J Affect Disord 19:15–21, 1990

Wehr T, Rosenthal N: Seasonality and affective illness. Am J Psychiatry 146:829–839, 1989

Wehr T, Giesen H, Schulz P, et al: Summer depression: description of the syndrome and comparison with winter depression, in Seasonal Affective Disorders and Phototherapy. Edited by Rosenthal N, Blehar M. New York, Guilford, 1989, pp 55–68

Winton F, Checkley S: Clinical characteristics of patients with seasonal affective disorder, in Seasonal Affective Disorder. Edited by Thompson C, Silverstone T. London, Clinical Neuroscience Publishers, 1989, pp 59–68

Wirz-Justice A, Bucheli C, Graw P, et al: Light treatment of seasonal affective disorder in Switzerland. Acta Psychiatr Scand 74:193–204, 1986

Wirz-Justice A, Graw P, Bucheli C, et al: Seasonal affective disorder in Switzerland: a clinical perspective, in Seasonal Affective Disorder. Edited by Thompson C, Silverstone T. London, Clinical Neuroscience Publishers, 1989, pp 69–76

Yerevanian B, Anderson J, Grota L, et al: Effects of bright incandescent light on seasonal and nonseasonal major depressive disorder. Psychiatry Res 18:355–364, 1986

Chapter 13

Validity of Rapid Cycling as a Modifier for Bipolar Disorder in DSM-IV

Mark S. Bauer, M.D., and Peter C. Whybrow, M.D.

Statement of the Issues

Dunner and Fieve (1974) provided the first definition of rapid cycling, based on data from a study of treatment outcome in bipolar disorder. They found that bipolar patients with four or more affective episodes per year failed lithium treatment at a much higher rate than those with fewer episodes and coined the term *rapid cycling* to identify bipolar patients with four or more such episodes per year, emphasizing the poor response of this group to lithium carbonate.

Although this definition became widely accepted in clinical and research usage and served to focus attention on a subset of bipolar patients with a particularly poor prognosis, it is not clear to what extent rapid cycling delineates a distinct subtype of patients with bipolar disorder. This review summarizes the empirical data relevant to the question of whether rapid cycling has sufficient construct validity to become a modifier for bipolar disorder in DSM-IV. Evidence is judged against criteria proposed by Robins and Guze (1970) and by Kendell (1982).

Significance of the Issues

Although the pattern of rapid cycling is noted in the text of DSM-III-R (American Psychiatric Association 1987) as a subtype of the mixed category of bipolar disorder

Preparation of this manuscript was supported by Physician Scientist Award MH00720 and a Young Investigator Award from the National Alliance for Research in Schizophrenia and Depression (NARSAD) to M.S.B. and a NARSAD Established Investigator Award to P.C.W.

or as a subtype of bipolar disorder not otherwise specified (NOS), the practical importance to clinicians and researchers of having a distinct modifier has never been reviewed. Such a putatively refractory form of affective illness deserves review, because refractory affective illness must become an important focus for research in the coming decades (Prien and Gelenberg 1989) and because persons with refractory illness take up a disproportionate amount of health care effort. Characterization of specific subtypes of affective illness that have particular treatment implications may benefit research and clinical care.

Methods

Review Strategies

A comprehensive review of the literature on bipolar disorder was carried out with two strategies. First, computer-assisted searches on bipolar disorder were conducted via Medline of the National Library of Medicine from 1970 to 1991. Second, reference lists of relevant articles were reviewed for additional articles. The search was considered comprehensive when no references were found by one method that had not already been found by the other. Case reports were excluded from review because it was judged that they would be of limited value in assessing the validity of rapid cycling as a syndrome. The interested reader is directed to earlier extensive reviews of rapid cycling for more such information (Alarcon 1985; Roy-Byrne et al. 1984). Manuscripts that were under review or in press were also solicited from workers in related fields.

The Definition of Rapid Cycling

The definition of rapid cycling as originally proposed by Dunner and Fieve (1974) identifies a distinct group of patients who 1) have bipolar disorder and 2) experience four or more affective episodes in 12 months. Although the specific cutpoint of four episodes per year may at some point be replaced, it has provided the working definition of rapid cycling for the last 15 years. It is therefore appropriate for this definition to be the starting point for the "self-rectification and increasing refinement" (Robins and Guze 1970) of the diagnosis.

Criteria for Validity

Evidence for validity of rapid cycling as a modifier was evaluated against two complementary sets of criteria to determine whether a collection of characteristics delineates a distinct neuropsychiatric syndrome. Those proposed by Robins and Guze (1970) outline explicit criteria for the identification of a set of clinical characteristics as a psychiatric disorder. Kendell (1982) emphasized the need for developing explicit criteria based on empirical data for psychiatric syndromes and outlined strategies for establishing the reliability and validity of such "operational" definitions.

Results

Rapid Cycling and the Robins-Guze Criteria

In their review of schizophrenia, Robins and Guze (1970) proposed that a group of symptoms in psychiatric patients represents a distinct disorder if five criteria are fulfilled: 1) clinical characteristics form a consistent pattern in patients with the disorder; 2) laboratory studies reveal abnormalities that can identify patients with that syndrome; 3) exclusion criteria are available to eliminate borderline or doubtful cases, leaving as homogeneous a group as possible; 4) follow-up studies reveal a relatively homogeneous outcome for patients with the disorder; and 5) family studies show higher rates of that disorder in relatives of patients with the disorder than in relatives of patients with other disorders. A sixth criterion, treatment response as assessed in formal treatment studies, may also help to distinguish distinct clinical entities.

Clinical characteristics.   Rapid cycling, defined as four or more affective episodes in 12 months, has thus far been applied only to bipolar affective disorder. In an early report, Dunner et al. (1977) reported that 40 of 390 patients with bipolar disorder exhibited a rapid cycling course, compared to none of 84 patients with unipolar depression. Prien et al. (1984) found a rapid cycling course in bipolar but not unipolar subjects. Similarly, Coryell et al. (1991) found rapid cycling in only 0.4% of patients with recurrent unipolar depression. Note that, although patients with rapid cycling have bipolar disorder, they may exhibit only depressive episodes during a period of prospective observation (Bauer et al. 1990). On the other hand, Angst et al. (1990) have recently described a sample of persons with unipolar depression in Switzerland who have frequent brief depressive episodes, without evidence of manic symptoms. This syndrome of "recurrent brief depression" also appears to be similar to major depressive disorder in terms of age at onset, family history, and level of impairment. Interestingly, the syndrome is approximately evenly distributed across sexes, unlike either rapid cycling bipolar disorder (see below) or major depressive disorder. Thus, a second affective syndrome characterized by brief but severe episodes has been described.

Dunner's original study reported a prevalence of 13% (Dunner and Fieve

1974), with more recent data from the Collaborative Program on the Psychobiology of Depression indicating a prevalence of 18.5% (Coryell et al. 1991). Estimates have ranged from 4.2%, with the criterion of at least four affective episodes per year over 2 years (Prien et al. 1984), to 27% (Tondo et al. 1981). Although prevalence estimates derived from such studies depend on referral patterns to those centers, it is clear that rapid cycling is not a rare phenomenon in secondary or tertiary care centers. Prior or current use of antidepressants (see below) may also affect prevalence figures.

Patients with rapid cycling are equally divided between bipolar I and II subtypes (Bauer et al. 1990; Dunner 1979). Clinical characteristics do not distinguish rapid cycling from non–rapid cycling bipolar patients during depressive episodes (Dunner et al. 1977) or manic or hypomanic episodes (Bauer et al. 1990), although rapid cycling patients may exhibit a dysphoric manic profile less frequently than non–rapid cycling bipolar patients (Post et al. 1989).

Rapid cycling occurs predominantly in women, with 75%–95% of rapid cycling patients being female in most (Bauer et al. 1990; Coryell et al. 1991; Dunner and Fieve 1974; Tondo et al. 1981; Wehr et al. 1988) but not all (Joffe et al. 1987) studies. This is in contrast to the even gender distribution in bipolar disorder in general (Weissman and Boyd 1983). No other patient characteristics distinguish patients with rapid cycling from those with non–rapid cycling bipolar disorder, including age, age at onset of affective symptoms, and duration of affective symptoms (Coryell et al. 1991; Roy-Byrne et al. 1984).

Laboratory studies. As is currently true for all the other forms of affective disorder, there are no laboratory studies by which one can validly and reliably identify rapid cycling, at least not with sufficient predictive validity for clinical or research use. However, the presence of specific risk factors for a disorder may provide clues to its pathophysiology and therefore indicate fruitful directions for investigation of laboratory abnormalities. Three risk factors have been associated with rapid cycling across several studies: gender, antidepressant use, and hypothyroidism.

As noted above, the vast majority of rapid cycling patients in most studies are women. However, despite descriptions of menstrually linked mood cycles in some rapid cycling patients (Bauer et al. 1990; Price and DiMarzio 1986), most affective episodes occur without temporal relationship to the menstrual cycle (Bauer et al. 1990). Furthermore, rapid cycling occurs in both pre- and postmenopausal women and can continue through menopause (Wehr et al. 1988). Thus, although the association between gender and rapid cycling is strong, there does not appear to be a strong link with fluctuations of gonadal axis function.

Antidepressants have been well documented to induce or exacerbate rapid cycling in prospective studies (Tondo et al. 1981; Wehr and Goodwin 1979a, 1979b,

1979c; Wehr et al. 1988) and may contribute to frequency of episodes in 33%–51% of rapid cycling patients (Wehr et al. 1988). However, Coryell et al. (1991) have suggested that it is the presence of depression rather than antidepressant use per se that is associated with rapid cycling. Patients with antidepressant-associated rapid cycling are not distinguishable from spontaneously rapid cycling patients in terms of clinical characteristics, thyroid status, or outcome (Bauer et al. 1990), suggesting that patients with spontaneous and antidepressant-induced rapid cycling do not represent distinct clinical groups.

The most common thyroid axis abnormality in unselected bipolar patients is a blunted TSH response to TRH infusion (e.g., Amsterdam et al. 1983). In contrast, the most common finding in rapid cycling bipolar patients is hypothyroidism or evidence that may reflect a milder degree of thyroid hypofunction. Rapid cycling patients have been shown to have an increased incidence of hypothyroidism during treatment with lithium carbonate (Cho et al. 1979), a higher prevalence of hypothyroidism from various causes (Bauer et al. 1990; Cowdry et al. 1983), and a greater increase in TSH in response to treatment with lithium carbonate (Cowdry et al. 1983) than non–rapid cycling bipolar patients. Hypothyroidism occurs more frequently in women than men, as does rapid cycling. Some evidence indicates that the association of rapid cycling with hypothyroidism may be stronger than its association with female gender; this finding has led to the hypothesis that hypothyroidism may be the mechanism responsible for the female preponderance in rapid cycling (Bauer et al. 1990). Negative studies include that by Wehr et al. (1988), who found an extraordinarily high rate of hypothyroidism in non–rapid cycling bipolar patients (37%) and a prevalence rate of 47% among rapid cycling patients, well above that usually reported. Joffe et al. (1987) also reported no association. However, their study was atypical in reporting a non–rapid cycling sample that was 83% female, far higher than the proportion of women in most studies of bipolar disorder in general (Weissman and Boyd 1983). Coryell et al. (1991) also reported no difference between rapid cycling and non–rapid cycling bipolar patients in response to general queries about history of thyroid problems.

Boundaries of rapid cycling.   The boundaries of rapid cycling are defined by the occurrence of a given number of affective episodes over a period of time. Thus, delineation of the putative syndrome depends on severity and duration of pathological mood states and number of mood states per unit time. The criteria defined by Dunner and Fieve (1974) of four or more affective episodes per 12 months are explicit and should be easily applied. However, classic observations of patients with rapid cycling focused on those with brief but severe episodes who are not easily accommodated by the Dunner-Fieve definition, because their episodes would have been counted as a single mixed episode according to DSM-III-R or Research

Diagnostic Criteria (RDC; Spitzer et al. 1978). However, most investigators employ severity criteria that separate rapid cycling from cyclothymic disorder by requiring mood states in rapid cycling to meet severity criteria for major affective episodes according to the diagnostic system used for at least a full day (see Coryell et al. 1991).

The effect of including persons with brief but severe episodes, as in recurrent brief depression (Angst et al. 1990), is that episode frequency may, not unexpectedly, be much higher than four episodes per 12 months (e.g., Bauer et al. 1990; Kukopolis et al. 1980; Roy-Byrne et al. 1984, 1985; Wehr and Goodwin 1979a, 1979b, 1979c; Wehr et al. 1982). In fact, there is evidence that the optimal cut-point for rapid cycling may be greater than four episodes per year (see below, "Rapid Cycling and Kendell Strategies" section).

Course and outcome.   Rapid cycling can occur at any time during the course of bipolar disorder, from the onset of bipolar disorder to several decades after the initiation of symptoms. Rapid cycling can also begin as early as the late teens or as late as the ninth decade of life. There are no apparent clinical differences between rapid cycling of early versus late onset in terms of course or severity of illness (Bauer and Whybrow 1991).

Rapid cycling has often been considered explicitly or implicitly to be a cyclic disorder (Roy-Byrne et al. 1984; Wehr and Goodwin 1979a, 1979b, 1979c; Wehr et al. 1982). However, evidence for true periodicity in the disorder is scant beyond descriptions of patients with classic 48-hour cycling, which appears to be quite rare (Wehr 1989). Furthermore, a cyclic pattern may not be specific to those with four or more episodes per 12 months (Stancer et al. 1970).

Most empirical evidence indicates that rapid cycling has a complex temporal pattern, as was initially described by Kraepelin (1921, pp. 139 and 188). More recently, Dunner et al. (1977) noted that affective episodes tend to come in doublets or triplets, whereas Kukopolis et al. (1980) reported prognostic differences depending on the sequence of mood states. Recently presented data indicate that chaotic, rather than cyclic, behavior may characterize the mood pattern over time in rapid cycling bipolar patients but not in control subjects (Bauer and Whybrow 1991; Gottschalk et al. 1990).

Most studies indicate that poor prognosis is a hallmark of rapid cycling. Rapid cycling patients experience many more episodes over the course of their illness than do non–rapid cycling bipolar patients. The magnitude of the difference is striking: rapid cycling patients at the National Institute of Mental Health (NIMH) had experienced 56.7 episodes since the onset of their disorder, compared to 8.2 for non–rapid cycling bipolar patients (Roy-Byrne et al. 1985). In both early (Dunner and Fieve 1974) and more recent (Wehr et al. 1988) reports, fewer than one-third of rapid cycling patients responded to pharmacotherapy, despite development of several alternatives to lithium during the intervening 14 years. The latter study found that only 14% of rapid cycling patients entered remission when their antidepressants were discontinued, despite continued lithium therapy.

On the other hand, the Collaborative Program reported the analysis of their data relevant to rapid cycling and concluded that "the prognosis of rapid cycling patient is more benign than is generally assumed" (Coryell et al. 1991) based on decreasing prevalence of rapid cycling in those identified with rapid cycling during the index year of the study. However, although data presented indicate that rapid cycling may not be an "end-stage" form of bipolar disorder in the majority of cases, there is no evidence that patients who met criteria for rapid cycling in the first, but not subsequent, years were symptom free during those later years or that those patients were less impaired than during periods of rapid cycling. Thus, although it is not clear to what degree rapid cycling "breeds true," available evidence indicates that its natural history is that of a chronic and severe affective disorder, the course of which may be modulated by antidepressants and other pharmacological agents.

Family studies.   Several studies indicate that families of rapid cycling probands differ from those of other affectively ill patients. Dunner et al. (1977) found a positive family history of bipolar disorder in 45.5% of bipolar II rapid cycling patients versus 25% of non–rapid cycling bipolar II patients. There was no difference, however, in family history of rapid cycling versus non–rapid cycling bipolar I patients. Similarly, 81.8% of rapid cycling bipolar II patients had a family history of affective disorder compared to 58.8% of non–rapid cycling bipolar II patients, again with no difference between these bipolar I subgroups. Wehr et al. (1988) found that first-degree relatives of rapid cycling bipolar patients had somewhat higher rates of unipolar disorder (40% versus 26%) and somewhat lower rates of bipolar disorder (26% versus 37%) than did those of non–rapid cycling bipolar patients. However, rapid cycling occurred only in families of rapid cycling probands (13% versus 0%). Interestingly, that sample of rapid cycling families had nearly double the rate of alcoholism found in non–rapid cycling families (30% versus 16%).

In contrast, Nurnberger et al. (1988) reported no difference in rates of rapid cycling or affective disorder in relatives of rapid cycling versus non–rapid cycling affective (primarily schizoaffective) patients, although they did not differentiate between bipolar I and II and schizoaffective probands. Coryell et al. (1991) found no difference between the families of rapid cycling and non–rapid cycling probands in terms of proportion of relatives with a lifetime history of mania (4.1% versus 4.2%) or depression (20.1% versus 19.6%) by proband report and no difference in either mania (2.2% versus 4.2%) or depression (27.2% versus 33.0%) when direct interviews were done. Similarly, no differences in incidence of mania and depression were found when a smaller number of relatives were interviewed 6 years after the initial evaluation.

Treatment response.   Dunner and Fieve's initial study of rapid cycling (1974) found that 59% of non–rapid cycling bipolar patients responded to lithium treatment, compared to only 18% of rapid cycling patients. This poor response rate has been replicated in several more recent studies of lithium alone (Prien et al. 1984; Wehr et al. 1988) or in combination with other therapies (Kukopolis et al. 1980). Thus, the diagnosis has clear predictive validity: patients with rapid cycling do not respond as well as non–rapid cycling patients to lithium treatment. Interestingly, two early studies indicate that bipolar patients with a cyclic course whose episode frequency is less than four per 12 months also respond poorly to lithium (Dunner and Fieve 1974; Stancer et al. 1970), raising the question of whether lack of response to lithium may relate to the temporal pattern of affective episodes rather than being a function of number of episodes.

Alternative treatment strategies have been suggested in numerous case reports (reviewed in Alarcon 1985; Roy-Byrne et al. 1984). Most of the agents mentioned were investigated more extensively at NIMH (Wehr et al. 1988), usually with dismal results. However, promising treatment results using high doses of the thyroid hormones thyroxine or triiodothyronine in addition to other psychotropic medications have been reported in two small series of rapid cycling patients (Bauer and Whybrow 1990; Stancer and Persad 1982), although placebo-controlled trials have been conducted in only a small number of patients thus far (Bauer and Whybrow 1990).

A number of studies have supported a role for the anticonvulsants, particularly carbamazepine, in the treatment of various aspects of bipolar disorder (Kishimoto et al. 1983; Okuma et al. 1981; Post 1988). Most of those studies primarily included patients who were not responsive to lithium, suggesting that there was a high proportion of rapid cycling patients in the patient samples. Thus it is reasonable to suppose that carbamazepine may be effective in prophylaxis of lithium-resistant rapid cycling. However, only two studies have reported results specifically in rapid cycling patients. Data from both Kishimoto et al. (1983) and Post et al. (1986) indicate that patients with a rapid cycling course may respond better to carbamazepine than patients with a non–rapid cycling course. Calabrese and Delucchi (1990) also reported successful results using the anticonvulsant valproic acid in an open treatment protocol for a large sample of rapid cycling bipolar patients.

In summary, the hallmark of rapid cycling remains nonresponsiveness to lithium. Furthermore, two studies suggest that rapid cycling patients may respond better to carbamazepine than non–rapid cycling patients. Although cautious optimism is warranted regarding treatment modalities besides lithium, the most striking finding in reviewing treatment studies is the paucity of controlled data specifically concerning treatment response in rapid cycling patients.

Rapid Cycling and Kendell Strategies

Kendell (1982) emphasized the importance of using specific, explicit criteria to develop reliable definitions of distinct psychiatric syndromes. He further suggested that a useful definition should validly identify a homogeneous group of patients and suggested that validity of a definition must ultimately be based on identifying a group of patients who share a common etiology or a common biological predisposition. He proposed that the first practical steps in identifying homogeneous groups on empirical grounds should focus on identifying boundaries between similar psychiatric syndromes on the basis of clinical and other characteristics. Accordingly, to be considered valid, the diagnosis of rapid cycling should be made reliably and should provide evidence of boundaries that exclude similar syndromes.

Reliability.   The identification of rapid cycling is built on 1) the diagnosis of individual affective episodes as currently defined and 2) their frequency. We are aware of no evidence regarding reliability of diagnosis of rapid cycling comparing independent raters, as appears to be the case for modifiers currently in DSM-III-R such as seasonal pattern. Regarding frequency of episodes, most rapid cycling patients have far more than four episodes per year (Bauer et al. 1990; Roy-Byrne et al. 1985), suggesting that number of episodes should present diagnostic problems in few patients.

Evidence for boundaries.   Kendell proposed that psychiatric syndromes X and Y that have overlapping symptomatic profiles are separate entities if there exist "points of rarity" in the frequency distribution of some laboratory or a clinical characteristic that appears in the two syndromes in varying degrees. Similarly, if the relationship between some clinically relevant variable and a spectrum of diagnostic categories or characteristics shows evidence of "nonlinearity" (e.g., graphical discontinuity; discussed in greater detail with regard to rapid cycling in Bauer and Whybrow 1991), then there is support for separating the spectrum into two clinical syndromes at the point of nonlinearity. He pointed out, however, that he knew of no empirical data to confirm the existence of such nonlinearities.

Interestingly, the relationship between gender and episode frequency in bipolar disorder appears to provide an example of such a nonlinearity. Most studies of unselected bipolar patients indicate that approximately 50% are women (reviewed in Weissmann and Boyd 1983), in contrast to the female preponderance among rapid cycling patients (see above). Utilizing data on gender distribution versus episode frequency in rapid cycling that has been previously reported (Bauer et al. 1991), evidence of nonlinearity emerges (Figure 13–1). The even gender distribution found in bipolar patients in general is seen in rapid cycling patients with 4–11 episodes per year. However, the proportion of women increases dramatically as episode frequency increases beyond 11 episodes per year. Whether the optimal cutoff for episode frequency in rapid cycling is closer to 12 than 4 episodes per year remains to be determined by subsequent studies using multiple research strategies.

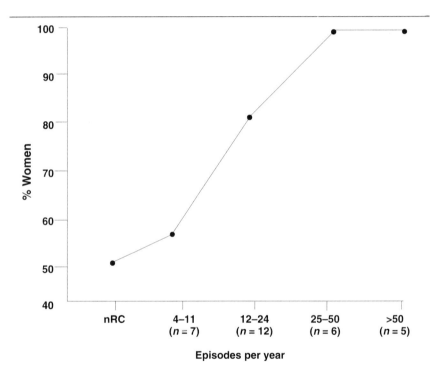

Figure 13–1. Data from Bauer et al. (1990) have been reanalyzed to illustrate the relationship between gender and episode frequency. Most studies of unselected bipolar populations indicate that approximately 50% of bipolar patients are women (Weissmann and Boyd 1983). This is similar to the 58% proportion in rapid cycling patients with 4–11 episodes per year. However, the proportion of women increases markedly at 12 episodes per year. This may reflect a "nonlinearity" (Kendell 1982) in the relationship between gender and episode frequency in bipolar illness, providing support for the delineation of rapid cycling as a distinct form of bipolar illness.
Source.   Bauer MS, Whybrow PC: "Rapid Cycling Bipolar Disorder: Clinical Features, Treatment, and Etiology," in *Advances in Neuropsychiatry and Psychopharmacology, Volume 2: Refractory Depression.* Edited by Amsterdam JD. New York, Raven, 1991, p. 198. Used with permission.

Nonetheless, the existence of this break in linearity supports the separation of rapid cycling as a distinct clinical entity.

Discussion

Overview of Evidence Regarding Construct Validity of Rapid Cycling

The inclusion of rapid cycling as a modifier for bipolar disorder is supported by several sorts of evidence. Among clinical characteristics, female preponderance among rapid cycling patients is in marked contrast to the even gender distribution in bipolar disorder in general; furthermore, the high proportion of women among rapid cycling patients cannot be explained simply by occurrence of menstrually linked affective episodes. No other clinical characteristics appear to distinguish rapid cycling patients.

Although no diagnostic laboratory studies are available, as in most neuropsychiatric disorders, risk factors may delineate specific pathophysiological factors that may distinguish patients with rapid cycling bipolar disorder from those with non-rapid cycling bipolar disorder. Risk factors that have been associated with rapid cycling across several studies include gender, antidepressant use, and hypothyroidism. However, studies are not unanimous in endorsing any of these factors.

The boundary of four or more affective episodes per year, provided in the Dunner-Fieve definition, is explicit but may not be the optimal cutpoint for defining a homogeneous group. Furthermore, the issue of defining individual episodes for rapid cycling patients with brief but severe episodes has not yet been resolved.

Although some investigators have viewed rapid cycling as an end-stage form of bipolar disorder, other evidence indicates that the phenomenon may be time limited. However, evidence from both early general clinic studies and more recent research center studies indicate that patients with rapid cycling comprise a group with chronic affective illness. Note that other time-limited clinical syndromes may delineate distinct groups of patients with mood disorders. The most prominent example of this is the occurrence of a manic episode in patients with a history of major depressive episodes, which changes the diagnosis from major depressive to bipolar disorder, with its associated prognostic, genetic, and treatment-response implications.

Most but not all family history studies comparing rapid cycling with non–rapid cycling bipolar disorder indicate that rapid cycling patients may have families that are particularly highly loaded for affective illness and perhaps for alcoholism. There are few data concerning whether rapid cycling per se runs in families or what genetic model might explain the occurrence of rapid cycling.

Most treatment studies indicate that patients with a rapid cycling course do not respond well to lithium. There is some evidence that they may respond better to carbamazepine than non–rapid cycling patients.

The diagnosis of rapid cycling is easily operationalized. Evidence of "non-linearity" in the relationship of number of episodes per year and gender support the differentiation of patients with bipolar disorder according to episode frequency and suggests that the optimal cutpoint may be closer to 12 than 4 episodes per year.

Options for the Rapid Cycling Modifier

Evidence reviewed above is based on the original definition proposed by Dunner and Fieve (1974) of four or more affective episodes in 12 months, with additional explicit requirements for episode delineation in the case of brief but severe episodes (Bauer et al. 1990; Coryell et al. 1991). Two implications follow from this simple phenomenological definition. First, no reference to episode cyclicity per se is included. The evidence reviewed above indicates that this is appropriate. Second, the definition is based on descriptive criteria alone and therefore does not distinguish between spontaneous and antidepressant-induced rapid cycling. This also appears to be appropriate because these groups do not differ on clinical characteristics and both share a poor prognosis. Several specific options for rapid cycling were considered by the DSM-IV Mood Disorders Work Group.

1. *Keep classification as in DSM-III-R (i.e., split patients with rapid cycling between bipolar disorder mixed and bipolar disorder NOS.* Two lines of reasoning support this option: a) the clinical data summarized above are not sufficient to justify inclusion or b) although the evidence above supports inclusion of the modifier in some form, formal acceptance should await clear data regarding rules for episode counting. The disadvantage to this option is that these issues would be more difficult to resolve while rapid cycling remains split between two already heterogeneous categories. As noted above, it is not surprising, in light of the lack of recognition of rapid cycling in standard psychiatric nosologies, that no placebo-controlled trials have been reported that were undertaken specifically in rapid cycling patients; data relevant to treatment response in such trials have been without exception from post hoc analyses.

2. *Include rapid cycling as a modifier, defined as four or more episodes per 12 months, counting only full-duration manic, hypomanic, or major depressive episodes.* The advantage to this option is its simplicity in application, based on the counting of episodes for which diagnostic reliability is well established. The requirement of at least four episodes in 12 months is more simple than the requirements for certain other modifiers in DSM-III-R, such as the 3:1 episode ratio over at least 3 years

required for seasonal pattern. The major disadvantage is that this definition would exclude a large proportion of patients currently considered to have rapid cycling who have brief but severe episodes.

3. *Include rapid cycling, defined as four or more episodes per 12 months, counting both full duration and truncated episodes (i.e., those that meet severity but not duration criteria for an episode of mania, hypomania, or major depression).* This option incorporates the general approach used by most researchers in the field and therefore reflects the database for the evidence outlined in this chapter. The reasoning is that the length criteria for affective episodes that are currently required by DSM-III-R and the RDC (Spitzer et al. 1978) are designed to separate more from less severely ill patients and lose their utility when applied to such a severely and consistently ill group of patients. The symptom severity dimension is necessary to differentiate patients with rapid cycling from those with cyclothymic disorder. The disadvantage to this approach is that current nosological systems are not yet well equipped to characterize brief mood episodes; similar difficulties exist in the definition of symptom resolution. Switches from an episode of one polarity to the other provide little problem in definition. This would ensure the counting of only discrete affective episodes and would differentiate rapid cycling patients from patients with "double depression" (Keller and Shapiro 1982; Kocsis and Frances 1987), who exhibit "cycling below the line" (Wehr et al. 1988), and would further exclude patients with chronic mixed manic and depressive symptoms. However, criteria for remission duration are at this point arbitrary and not standardized among workers in the field. Thus, as for other episodic mood disorders, optimal definition awaits consensus in the field regarding resolution of symptoms.

4. *Adopt options 2 or 3 but change the cutpoint for episodes per year.* With the exception of the results summarized above that are consistent with an optimal cutpoint for rapid cycling of 12–24 episodes per year, little evidence supports a specific boundary other than 4 episodes per 12 months. However, results from the MacArthur/DSM-IV Rapid Cycling Data Reanalysis Study currently under way may provide more information on this issue. (Results will appear in a subsequent volume of the *DSM-IV Sourcebook.*)

Recommendations

Based on the evidence discussed above, the recommendation of the Mood Disorders Work Group is to include rapid cycling as a modifier for bipolar disorder as described under Option 3. However, there are several outstanding issues that await input from the results of the MacArthur/DSM-IV Rapid Cycling Data Reanalysis Study and from feedback based on the experience of the mental health profession at large. First, the optimal number of episodes per year to identify rapid cycling needs to be determined in view of the best currently available data. Second, the effect of allowing truncated episodes to count as individual episodes, rather than counting them as a single mixed episode, needs to be considered in more detail. Specifically, the minimum length of each mood state and the demarcation of episode boundaries in rapid cycling must be clarified (e.g., is a switch to a mood episode of the "opposite polarity" sufficient to separate episodes? How long should remission be between mood episodes of the same polarity to count mood episodes as separate?). The approach of the Data Reanalysis Study is to address these issues by investigating the effect of differing definitions of rapid cycling on both diagnostic reliability and validity according to the criteria discussed above.

References

Alarcon R: Rapid cycling affective disorders: a clinical review. Compr Psychiatry 26:522–540, 1985

American Psychiatric Association: Diagnostic and Statistical Manual of Mental Disorders, 3rd Edition, Revised. Washington, DC, American Psychiatric Association, 1987

Amsterdam J, Winokur A, Lucki I, et al: A neuroendocrine test battery in bipolar patients and healthy subjects. Arch Gen Psychiatry 40:515–521, 1983

Angst J, Merikangas K, Scheidegger P, et al: Recurrent brief depression: a new subtype of affective disorder. J Affect Disord 19:87–98, 1990

Bauer M, Whybrow P: Rapid cycling bipolar affective disorder, II: treatment of refractory rapid cycling with high dose thyroxine, a preliminary study. Arch Gen Psychiatry 47:435–440, 1990

Bauer M, Whybrow P: Rapid cycling bipolar disorder: clinical features, treatment, and etiology, in Advances in Neuropsychiatry and Psychopharmacology, Vol 2: Refractory Depression. Edited by Amsterdam J. New York, Raven, 1991

Bauer M, Whybrow P, Winokur A: Rapid cycling bipolar affective disorder, I: association with grade I hypothyroidism. Arch Gen Psychiatry 47:427–432, 1990

Calabrese J, Delucchi G: Spectrum of efficacy of valproate in 55 patients with rapid cycling bipolar disorder. Am J Psychiatry 147:431–444, 1990

Cho J, Bone S, Dunner D, et al: The effect of lithium treatment on thyroid function in patients with primary affective disorder. Am J Psychiatry 136:115–116, 1979

Coryell W, Endicott J, Keller M: Rapidly cycling affective disorder: demographics, diagnosis, family history, and course. Arch Gen Psychiatry 49:126–131, 1991

Cowdry R, Wehr T, Zis A, et al: Thyroid abnormalities associated with rapid cycling bipolar illness. Arch Gen Psychiatry 40:414–420, 1983

Dunner D: Rapid cycling bipolar manic depressive illness. Psychiatr Clin North Am 2:461–467, 1979

Dunner D, Fieve R: Clinical factors in lithium carbonate prophylaxis failure. Arch Gen Psychiatry 30:229–233, 1974

Dunner D, Patrick V, Fieve R: Rapid cycling manic depressive patients. Compr Psychiatry 18:561–565, 1977

Gottschalk A, Bauer M, Whybrow P: A chaotic form of affective illness. Biol Psychiatry 27:99A, 1990

Joffe R, Kutcher S, MacDonald C: Thyroid function and bipolar affective disorder. Psychiatry Res 25:117–121, 1987

Keller M, Shapiro R: "Double depression": superimposition of acute depressive episodes on chronic depressive disorders. Am J Psychiatry 139:438–442, 1982

Kendell R: The choice of diagnostic criteria for biological research. Arch Gen Psychiatry 39:1334–1339, 1982

Kishimoto A, Ogura C, Hazama H, et al: Long-term prophylactic effects of carbamazepine in affective disorders. Br J Psychiatry 43:327–332, 1983

Kocsis J, Frances A: A critical discussion of DSM-III dysthymic disorder. Am J Psychiatry 144:1534–1542, 1987

Kraepelin E: Manic-Depressive Insanity and Paranoia, 1921 Edition. Translated by Barclay R. Birmingham, AL, Classics of Psychiatry & Behavioral Science, 1989

Kukopulos A, Reginaldi D, Laddomada P, et al: Course of the manic-depressive cycle and changes caused by treatments. Pharmacopsychiatry 13:156–167, 1980

Nurnberger J, Guroff J, Hamovit J, et al: A family study of rapid-cycling bipolar illness. J Affect Disord 15:87–91, 1988

Okuma T, Inanaga K, Otsuki S, et al: A preliminary double-blind study of the efficacy of carbamazepine in prophylaxis of manic-depressive illness. Psychopharmacology 73:95–96, 1981

Post R: Approaches to treatment-resistant bipolar affectively ill patients. Clinical Neuropharmacology 11:93–104, 1988

Post R, Rubinow D, Ballenger J: Conditioning, sensitization, and the longitudinal course of affective illness. Br J Psychiatry 149:191–201, 1986

Post R, Rubinow D, Uhde T, et al: Dysphoric mania: clinical and biological correlates. Arch Gen Psychiatry 46:353–358, 1989

Price W, DiMarzio L: Premenstrual tension syndrome in rapid-cycling bipolar affective disorder. J Clin Psychiatry 47:415–417, 1986

Prien R, Gelenberg A: Alternative to lithium for preventive treatment of bipolar disorder. Am J Psychiatry 146:840–848, 1989

Prien R, Kupfer D, Mansky P, et al: Drug therapy in the prevention of recurrences in unipolar and bipolar affective disorders: report of the NIMH Collaborative Study group comparing lithium carbonate, imipramine, and a lithium carbonate-imipramine combination. Arch Gen Psychiatry 41:1096–1104, 1984

Robins E, Guze S: Establishment of diagnostic validity in psychiatric illness: its application to schizophrenia. Am J Psychiatry 126:107–111, 1970

Roy-Byrne P, Joffe R, Uhde T, et al: Approaches to the evaluation and treatment of rapid-cycling affective illness. Br J Psychiatry 145:543–550, 1984

Roy-Byrne P, Post R, Uhde T, et al: The longitudinal course of recurrent affective illness: life chart data from research patients at the NIMH. Acta Psychiatr Scand Suppl 317:3–34, 1985

Spitzer R, Endicott J, Robins E: Research Diagnostic Criteria: rationale and reliability. Arch Gen Psychiatry 35:773–782, 1978

Stancer H, Persad E: Treatment of intractable rapid-cycling manic-depressive disorder with levothyroxine: clinical observations. Arch Gen Psychiatry 39:311–312, 1982

Stancer H, Furlong W, Godse D: A longitudinal investigation of lithium as a prophylactic agent for recurrent depressions. Can Psychiatr Assoc J 15:29–40, 1970

Tondo L, Laddomada P, Serra G, et al: Rapid cyclers and antidepressants. Int Pharmacop-
    sychiatry 16:119–123, 1981
Wehr T: Causes and treatments of rapid cycling affective disorder, in Antidepressant
    Therapies: Applications for the Outpatient Practitioner. Edited by Amsterdam J. New
    York, Marcel Dekker, 1989
Wehr T, Goodwin F: Rapid cycling between mania and depression caused by maintenance
    tricyclics. Psychopharmacol Bull 15:17–19, 1979a
Wehr T, Goodwin F: Rapid cycling in manic-depressives induced by tricyclic antidepressants.
    Arch Gen Psychiatry 36:555–559, 1979b
Wehr T, Goodwin F: Tricyclics modulate frequency of mood cycles. Chronobiologia
    6:377–385, 1979c
Wehr T, Goodwin F, Wirz-Justice A, et al: 48-hour sleep-wake cycles in manic-depressive
    illness: naturalistic observations and sleep deprivation experiments. Arch Gen Psychia-
    try 39:559–565, 1982
Wehr T, Sack D, Rosenthal N, et al: Rapid cycling affective disorder: contributing factors and
    treatment responses in 51 patients. Am J Psychiatry 145:179–184, 1988
Weissmann M, Boyd J: The epidemiology of affective disorders, in Neurobiology of Mood
    Disorders. Edited by Post R, Ballenger J. Baltimore, MD, Williams & Wilkins, 1983,
    pp 60–75

Section II

Late Luteal Phase Dysphoric Disorder

Chapter 14

Late Luteal Phase Dysphoric Disorder

Judith H. Gold, M.D., F.R.C.P.C., Jean Endicott, Ph.D.,
Barbara L. Parry, M.D., Sally K. Severino, M.D.,
Nada Stotland, M.D., and Ellen Frank, Ph.D.

Introduction

Late luteal phase dysphoric disorder (LLPDD) was first proposed as a new diagnostic category to be included in DSM-III-R (American Psychiatric Association 1987). Because research data were felt to be preliminary, however, the diagnosis was not included as an official category in DSM-III-R and was instead placed in Appendix A of the manual as a "proposed diagnostic category needing further study." After much discussion, the diagnosis was called late luteal phase dysphoric disorder to distinguish it from premenstrual syndrome (PMS), a condition that gives equal emphasis to physical symptoms. The diagnostic criteria suggested for LLPDD in the DSM-III-R appendix are as follows:

A. In most menstrual cycles during the past year, symptoms in B occurred during the last week of the luteal phase and remitted within a few days after onset of the follicular phase. In menstruating females, these phases correspond to the week before, and a few days after, the onset of menses. (In nonmenstruating females who have had a hysterectomy, the timing of luteal and follicular phases may require measurement of circulating reproductive hormones.)

B. At least five of the following symptoms have been present for most of the time during each symptomatic late luteal phase, at least one of the symptoms being either (1), (2), (3), or (4):

(1) marked affective lability, e.g., feeling suddenly sad, tearful, irritable, or angry
(2) persistent and marked anger or irritability
(3) marked anxiety, tension, feelings of being "keyed up," or "on edge"

(4) markedly depressed mood, feelings of hopelessness, or self-deprecating thoughts

(5) decreased interest in usual activities, e.g., work, friends, hobbies

(6) easy fatigability or marked lack of energy

(7) subjective sense of difficulty in concentrating

(8) marked change in appetite, overeating, or specific food cravings

(9) hypersomnia or insomnia

(10) other physical symptoms, such as breast tenderness or swelling, head-aches, joint or muscle pain, a sensation of "bloating," weight gain

C. The disturbance seriously interferes with work or with usual social activities and relationships with others.

D. The disturbance is not merely an exacerbation of the symptoms of another disorder, such as major depression, panic disorder, dysthymia, or a personality disorder (although it may be superimposed on any of these disorders).

E. Criteria A, B, C, and D are confirmed by prospective daily self-ratings during at least two symptomatic cycles. (The diagnosis may be made provisionally prior to this confirmation.)

Note: For coding purposes, record 300.90 Unspecified Mental Disorder (Late Luteal Phase Dysphoric Disorder). (p. 369)

The suggestion to include LLPDD in DSM-III-R aroused a great deal of controversy. Many critics felt that the diagnosis would be stigmatizing or would become a wastebasket term used when a more specific diagnosis was difficult. It was also feared that the term might be used inappropriately in forensic situations or in child custody disputes. Furthermore (especially in view of the controversy about possible misuse), the research literature was viewed as inadequate in sup-porting the clinical utility of the proposed diagnosis, in suggesting how it might best be defined, and in indicating its prevalence in the overall population of women. There was also concern that the late luteal phase symptoms might be so common that it would be inappropriate to call them pathological (Stotland 1991). Ultimately, it was hoped that research as well as clinical discourse would be encouraged by the decision to include LLPDD in the appendix of DSM-III-R (Spitzer et al. 1989).

Statement of the Issues

The LLPDD Work Group set out to determine whether there are sufficient data to justify including such a diagnosis in DSM-IV or, alternatively, whether it should remain in an appendix to facilitate further research on the validity and clinical utility of LLPDD. The basic issues are the validity and clinical utility of the proposed diagnosis of LLPDD. Is there a clinically significant mental disorder associated with the menstrual cycle that can be demarcated from other mental disorders?

Issues that bear on this question include

1. What is the likely prevalence of such a diagnosis in various clinical settings and in community samples? Are these symptoms so ubiquitous as to be considered "normal" (and thus inappropriate to be categorized as a mental disorder) or so rare as to be clinically insignificant?

2. Does the research literature indicate that the proposed diagnosis occurs as a primary condition or only as an exacerbation of other disorders? What is the degree and nature of comorbidity with other disorders? What, if any, is its association with psychosis?

3. What is the course and the stability of the disorder?

4. What are the familial factors associated with it?

5. What are the biological findings associated with the proposed disorder?

6. Do data exist to support effective and specific treatment for LLPDD?

7. What are the potential social, forensic, and occupational risks of including the LLPDD diagnosis in DSM-IV? How would the existence of these risks be assessed? Do these risks differ from those associated with other physical and mental disorders?

8. What would be the optimal criteria for this disorder? How reliably can the diagnosis be made? Are prospective ratings necessary? What are the performance characteristics of the proposed items in DSM-III-R and other items tested in clinical research studies?

9. If LLPDD appears to be a useful diagnosis, where is it best placed in the classification?

10. What is the best name for this disorder?

Literature Review Methodology

Methods

Because the criteria for LLPDD were proposed in 1987, the time lag between their introduction and the publication of the results of studies has limited the number of reports relevant to the issues just outlined. However, one measure of the utility of the LLPDD criteria is the considerable extent to which they have been accepted by both preclinical (e.g., Schmidt et al. 1991) and clinical (e.g., Harrison et al. 1989a; Stone et al. 1990) research groups. By mid-1991, at least one paper per month that made use of the LLPDD criteria was appearing in the literature.

The LLPDD Work Group has conducted a critical, comprehensive, and systematic review of the literature on premenstrual disorders, including unpublished articles obtained from a number of researchers in this area. Special attention has been given to studies performed since 1983. Extensive literature searches have been made using a number of databases such as Medline, Psychological Abstracts, Index Medicus, Biological Retrieval Service, and Medlars.

Over 400 articles have been reviewed. Emphasis has been given to studies using prospective daily ratings for at least one menstrual cycle and involving control groups or double-blind crossovers. Studies that did not meet these criteria but that have been quoted extensively or have been influential in guiding research inquiries or treatment methods have also been reviewed.

As mentioned above, because the term *LLPDD* was newly introduced in 1987, there are a limited number of published studies that use this name or the DSM-III-R criteria. Most researchers refer to PMS, and some do not define how that diagnosis was made. The definitions most commonly used, when noted, are based on the 1983 National Institute of Mental Health (NIMH) consensus that subjects meet the following: 1) a marked change of 30% in intensity of symptoms 6 days prior to menses and 2) 2 months of daily ratings of these symptoms.

The Work Group examined the literature for data validating the existence of the LLPDD diagnosis or the symptoms of PMS. The symptoms of PMS have often not been defined exactly but generally must occur between ovulation and menses and disappear after the onset of menses. LLPDD is distinguished from PMS by a clear emphasis on mood and behavioral changes as opposed to somatic changes, more stringent criteria regarding the severity of the complaints and their interference with functioning, the need for confirmation over two cycles rated prospectively, and the number and type of symptoms required for the diagnosis.

Methodological Problems in the Literature

It is important to detail a number of methodological problems in the literature that have been encountered during this analysis.

1. There are a number of different definitions used for the diagnosis of PMS and many variations in how the diagnosis is made. Investigators often do not specify how the diagnosis was made other than by a phrase such as "prospectively confirmed PMS." Severity of symptoms and degree of impairment are rarely specified. It is difficult to compare studies because subjects are likely to be heterogeneous with respect to severity, functional impairment, and symptom profile. This highlights the need for well-defined criteria. It is not known

if data from these studies are comparable to what would be obtained if the DSM-III-R criteria for LLPDD had been used.

2. Sample sizes are small in many studies.

3. Many studies do not use control groups.

4. Many studies do not use prospective daily ratings. It has been demonstrated that retrospective ratings often overdiagnose premenstrual conditions. On the other hand, prospective ratings have been criticized as possibly biased if the subject is aware of the purpose of the study. Prospective ratings also have not always been confirmed by observers, by clinical interviews, or by psychological testing. This area remains controversial (Severino and Moline 1989).

5. Sample selection may result in bias. There have been no published population surveys. Subjects in most studies have been volunteers who knew the nature of the study, so that the results may reflect biases (Severino et al. 1989).

6. The duration of symptoms and their timing in the cycle is often not delineated, and the degree of change in the severity of symptoms during the cycle and the resultant amount of incapacity needed to make the diagnosis are unclear.

7. Multiple hormone samples are needed throughout the cycle to establish cyclical variation and menstrual cycle phase. Optimally, because of circadian rhythms and the pulsatile secretion of some hormones, samples should be collected throughout the day. Very few studies have done this (Parry et al. 1989).

Results

Prevalence

It is reported that 20%–40% of women say they have some premenstrual symptoms (Severino and Moline 1989), and approximately 5% say that these symptoms have a significant impact on their lives. However, there are no published studies of the prevalence of LLPDD or PMS in the general population based on prospective daily ratings. Data from Rivera-Tovar and Frank's (1990) study of university women, who were unaware of the focus of the study and who prospectively rated LLPDD symptoms over 90 days, give a point prevalence rate of 4.6% over two cycles. This finding is consistent with the 3.4% prevalence for severe PMS found by R. F. Haskett (unpublished data, 1987) in a general population survey. A report from the Duke site of the Epidemiologic Catchment Area study, using an expanded questionnaire (Stout and Steege, ASPOG Annual Meeting, 1990), noted an overall prevalence of 6.8%, using seven questions included in the criteria for LLPDD retrospectively.

Differential Diagnosis and Lifetime and Concurrent Comorbidity

Once diagnostic criteria are proposed for a new disorder, the first questions addressed should be: Can clinicians identify individuals who meet the proposed criteria, and What are the major differential diagnostic issues encountered? The concurrent and lifetime comorbidity with other disorders is of related importance.

As is the case with most mental disorders, the clinical features included in the criteria for LLPDD are shared by other disorders. Furthermore, the clinical features may also be present in conditions that do not reach a level of severity and associated impairment that would warrant being considered a disorder (e.g., mild premenstrual changes or syndromes).

Three components are of major importance for the differential diagnosis of LLPDD: 1) the timing of the appearance (late luteal phase) and disappearance (follicular phase) of a constellation of clinical symptoms, 2) evidence that the symptoms are associated with serious interference with work or usual social activities or relationships with others, and 3) evidence that the disturbance is not merely an exacerbation of the symptoms of another disorder. As is the case with most disorders in DSM-III-R, there are no explicit guidelines regarding how these clinical decisions are to be made.

Results of literature review. The articles listed in Table 14–1 indicate that it is possible for clinicians to identify groups of women who meet criteria for LLPDD and do not have any (other) current DSM-III-R Axis I or Axis II disorders (Harrison et al. 1989a, 1989c, 1990; Parry et al. 1989; Pearlstein et al. 1990; Rausch et al. 1988). In several of the studies, the authors identified women with other relatively mild conditions who met criteria for superimposed LLPDD as well (i.e., they had a distinct and severe syndrome of additional clinical features that were present during the late luteal phase of the cycle and absent during the follicular phase) (Harrison et al. 1989b; Stone et al. 1990).

Although, as noted above, it is possible to identify women who clearly meet the LLPDD criteria, women who seek treatment for premenstrual problems are often found to have current mental or other medical conditions that may account for many, if not all, of their "premenstrual" complaints. The most frequent conditions requiring differential diagnostic attention are indicated in Tables 14–2, 14–3, and 14–4. The studies noted in the tables indicate that the following mental disorders are found with sufficient frequency to warrant careful efforts to determine differential diagnoses in all women who seek treatment for LLPDD: major mood disorders, dysthymia, anxiety disorders, somatoform disorders, bulimia, substance use disorders, and personality disorders (Harrison et al. 1989b; Hart and Russell

1986; McMillan and Pihl 1987; R. C. Reid et al., unpublished data; Severino et al. 1989; Stout and Steege 1985). Clinicians should also be alert to the possibility that other, nonmental medical disorders may be present. Frequently mentioned examples include seizure and thyroid disorders, cancer, lupus, anemia, and various infections (Keye et al. 1986).

For the most part, studies that report on the rates of current disorders other than LLPDD have not addressed the problems in differentiating LLPDD superimposed as an additional diagnosis on an ongoing condition from exacerbation of that condition. One frequently finds that a woman with another ongoing condition has some worsening of the ongoing symptoms or the appearance of new problems during the late luteal phase of the cycle (Bäckström et al. 1984; Breier et al. 1986; Endicott and Halbreich 1988; Friedman et al. 1982; Gladis and Walsh 1987; Price et al. 1987; Slen 1984) (see Table 14–3). In such instances, it is often not possible

Table 14–1. Clinical application of DSM-III-R criteria for late luteal phase dysphoric disorder (LLPDD)

Reference	*N* subjects	Comments
Rausch et al. 1988	16	Met DSM-III-R criteria for LLPDD
Harrison et al. 1989a	11	Met DSM-III-R criteria for LLPDD
Harrison et al. 1989b	86	Met criteria for LLPDD with no other Axis I or II disorder
	54	Met criteria for LLPDD and also had a relatively mild current anxiety or affective disorder, substance abuse disorder, or personality disorder
Harrison et al. 1989c	14	Sought treatment for severe premenstrual dysphoric changes; diagnosed as meeting criteria for LLPDD with no current Axis I or II disorder
Parry et al. 1989	6	Selected with LLPDD
Harrison et al. 1990	30	Met criteria for LLPDD with no other Axis I or II disorder
Pearlstein et al. 1990	78	Met criteria for LLPDD with no Axis I diagnosis
Stone et al. 1990	50	Met criteria for LLPDD with no Axis I disorder
	20	Met criteria for LLPDD but also had an Axis I disorder

Source. Reprinted from Endicott J: "Differential Diagnoses and Comorbidity," in *Premenstrual Dysphorias: Myths and Realities.* Edited by Gold JH, Severino SK. Washington, DC, American Psychiatric Press, 1994, p. 5. Used with permission.

Table 14–2. Evidence of current mental or other medical disorders in women with self-identified premenstrual problems

Reference	N subjects	Comments	Findings based on data from follicular phase
McMillan and Pihl 1987	28	Met criteria for premenstrual from major depressive syndrome	10 (37%) were found to have intermittent depression throughout the menstrual cycle.
Stout and Steege 1985	100	Sought evaluation for PMS after passing telephone screening	64% showed evidence of problems during the follicular phase according to the Minnesota Multiphasic Personality Inventory (31% neurotic, 11% characterologic, 5% psychotic, 17% unclassified); 25% had clinically significant depression during the follicular phase according to the Beck Depression Inventory.
Hart and Russell 1986	31 12	Reported PMS Reported no problems	There were significant follicular phase differences in depression, anxiety, tension, and irritability, indicating that many of the women with PMS had problems throughout the cycle. No breakdown of numbers of women who accounted for the higher scores was provided.
Keye et al. 1986	68 34	Responded to a newspaper article about premenstrual problems No complaints	Many medical conditions were identified: hypertension (2), systemic lupus erythematosus (1), galactorrhea (5), breast mass (1), endometriosis (2), meningioma (1). 50% were currently under the care of a psychologist, but the number with current mental disorders was not noted.
Harrison et al. 1989b	195	Sought treatment for premenstrual anxiety, depression, or irritability; completed at least one cycle of daily ratings; and passed an initial telephone interview	87 (45%) had a current mental disorder.

Reid et al.[a]	122	Referred to tertiary care PMS clinic	30 women who had high high follicular as well as luteal phase problems (12 had premenstrual exacerbation, 11 were high without exacerbation, 7 had drop in symptoms in late follicular phase only).
Severino et al. 1989	58	Self-referred for premenstrual difficulties	12 (21%) had a current anxiety or depressive disorder, 1 had another psychiatric disorder.

Note. PMS = premenstrual syndrome.
Source. Reprinted from Endicott J: "Differential Diagnoses and Comorbidity," in *Premenstrual Dysphorias: Myths and Realities.* Edited by Gold JH, Severino SK. Washington, DC, American Psychiatric Press, 1994, pp. 7–8. Used with permission.
[a]Reid RL, Hahn PM, VanVugt DA: "Characteristics of the Menstrual Cycle in Women Attending a Premenstrual Clinic, I: Implications for Diagnosis," unpublished data, 1993.

Table 14–3.   Evidence of premenstrual exacerbation of other mental disorders

Reference	Condition	Sample	Measures	Findings
Gladis and Walsh 1987	Bulimia	15 women who did not respond to placebo	Eating diaries	The mean scores for binges per day were compared for 5-day cycle segments; the segment just before menses was significantly higher than all other segments except the one just preceding it (days −10 to −5).
Bäckström et al. 1984	Epilepsy	Unknown	Seizure records	Cases were used to demonstrate that some women show a pattern of increased seizure frequency during the luteal phase, but the frequency with which this occurs was not noted.
Price et al. 1987	Bulimia	10 women with normal menstrual cycles	Weekly record of no. of binges for 2 months	All 10 increased binge eating; 5 showed marked increases (2 moderate and 3 small). The phase effect was significant for the total group.
Breier et al. 1986	Agoraphobia and panic attacks	43 with agoraphobia and panic attacks	Reports	51% of the women with agoraphobia had premenstrual exacerbation of symptoms.
Endicott and Halbreich 1988	Major depression	24 at depression clinic	Premenstrual Assessment Form[a]	83% reported worsening of depression and/or addition of symptoms premenstrually.
Slen 1984	Alcoholism	33 with regular cycles	Time of hospital admission	Significantly more subjects were admitted when they were menstruating, perhaps due to less control premenstrually.
Friedman et al. 1982	Mixed diagnosis	45 inpatients	Interview	28 (62%) met criteria for a premenstrual syndrome that differed from their usual symptoms.

Source. Reprinted from Endicott J: "Differential Diagnoses and Comorbidity," in *Premenstrual Dysphorias: Myths and Realities.* Edited by Gold JH, Severino SK. Washington, DC, American Psychiatric Press, 1994, p. 9. Used with permission.
[a]Halbreich U, Endicott J, Schacht S, et al.: "The Diversity of Premenstrual Changes as Reflected in the Premenstrual Assessment Form (PAF)." *Acta Psychiatr Scand* 65:46–65, 1982.

to determine whether she would meet all of the criteria for LLPDD if the other medical condition were not present. No systematic studies were found that have focused on this issue; therefore, the frequency with which women would be found to have superimposed LLPDD is unclear.

Studies that have focused on lifetime comorbidity of mental disorders in women with LLPDD and no other current medical disorder usually indicate that these women have a higher rate of past mood and anxiety disorders than do women without severe premenstrual problems (Harrison et al. 1989b; Ling and Brown 1990; Pearlstein et al. 1990; Severino et al. 1989) (see Table 14–4). Unfortunately, most of the studies that have reported on lifetime comorbid conditions have failed to clearly differentiate women with LLPDD alone from those with exacerbations of ongoing mental disorders or concurrent comorbid mental disorders. As indicated in Table 14–4, few articles were found that made this distinction. The studies noted in this table indicate that comorbidity of

Table 14–4. Evidence of prior lifetime comorbidity of other mental disorders with late luteal phase dysphoric disorder (LLPDD)

Reference	Subjects	Lifetime diagnosis
Harrison et al. 1989b	86 women who met criteria for LLPDD with no other Axis I or II disorders	70% prior major depressive disorder of 4 weeks or more 16% prior panic disorder 7% prior alcohol abuse 7% prior drug abuse
	61 control subjects with no premenstrual problems	41% prior major depressive disorder of 4 weeks or more 5% prior panic disorder 8% prior alcohol abuse 3% prior drug abuse
Pearlstein et al. 1990	78 women with no current Axis I or II disorders	46% prior major depressive disorder 69% prior major or minor depressive disorder 14% prior anxiety disorder
Ling and Brown 1990	83 women	48% history of depression
Severino et al. 1989	58 women	40% prior episode of anxiety or depressive disorder 4% prior substance abuse

Source. Reprinted from Endicott J: "Differential Diagnoses and Comorbidity," in *Premenstrual Dysphorias: Myths and Realities.* Edited by Gold JH, Severino SK. Washington, DC, American Psychiatric Press, 1994, p. 11. Used with permission.

prior disorders is relatively high, particularly with the major mood disorders.

There are many anecdotal reports that women with severe mood problems limited to the late luteal phase of the menstrual cycle are at high risk for subsequently developing episodes of other disorders, particularly depression. Information on premenstrual relapse or recurrence of mental disorders or other conditions is shown in Table 14–5. In the absence of prospective studies of women who meet the proposed criteria for LLPDD in the absence of a concurrent Axis I or Axis II disorders, however, the degree of risk cannot be estimated.

The degree of functional impairment experienced by women with prospectively confirmed LLPDD has been examined in 78 women presenting for treatment (E. Frank, A. D. Rivera-Tovar, and T. B. Pearlstein, unpublished data). On the Social Adjustment Scale-Self Report (SAS-SR), subjects had luteal phase scores comparable to those observed by Weissman et al. (1978) in clinically depressed women. In the follicular phase, these subjects had social adjustment scores in the good to excellent range. Although the mean Global Assessment Score (GAS) (Endicott et al. 1976) for these subjects was 84.9 in the follicular phase, it dropped to an average of 69.7 in the luteal phase ($P < .0001$).

Summary and conclusions.   Clinicians and investigators have demonstrated that it is possible to identify women who meet the criteria for LLPDD in the absence of other current medical disorders. These studies also indicate that the criteria as proposed can be applied in a relatively stringent manner. Many women who seek treatment are found not to have documented late luteal phase problems of sufficient severity to meet the criteria. Thus, the proposed criteria appear to have achieved the aim of differentiating milder premenstrual syndromes from premenstrual disorders. The differential diagnosis of LLPDD superimposed on another ongoing disorder, however, has been less well studied. The criteria as proposed in DSM-III-R do not offer sufficient guidelines for determining whether clinical worsening during the late luteal phase of the menstrual cycle reflects an exacerbation of another condition or superimposed LLPDD.

The studies reviewed indicate that many women who seek treatment for premenstrual problems will not be found to have a clear-cut and distinct condition that meets the proposed LLPDD criteria because the symptoms are not present, are not severe enough, or cannot be differentiated from some chronic mental or other medical condition. Daily ratings are essential to establish the timing and patterns of changes in clinical features. If cycle changes in the specified clinical features are documented, the differential diagnosis of LLPDD from premenstrual changes or syndromes is primarily dependent on evidence of associated severe interference with social and occupational functioning.

As is the case with other disorders in DSM-III-R, better guidelines for deter-

Table 14–5. Evidence of premenstrual relapse or recurrence of mental disorder or other conditions

Reference	Condition	Sample	Measures	Findings
Brockington et al. 1988	Puerperal psychosis	8 patients	Relapse	10–17 relapses occurred during days −1 to −4 before menses.
Abramowitz et al. 1982	Depressive and schizophrenic disorder	39 depressed, 76 schizophrenic	Hospital admission	41% of the depressed women, but no schizophrenic women, had increased likelihood of having been admitted the day before or the day after menses started.
Hatotani et al. 1979	Periodic psychoses	47 with more than three episodes	Onsets	23 women had onsets regularly during the middle or later half of the menstrual cycle, none during the follicular period after menses, 3 during menses; 21 were irregular.
d'Orban and Dalton 1980	Violent criminal acts	50 with regular cycles	Criminal behavior	44% committed their offenses during the paramenstruum. Timing of offenses was unrelated to symptoms of premenstrual tension.
Luggin et al. 1984	Various conditions	121 acute admissions	Admission date	More admissions than expected took place during the menstrual period and fewer intermenstrual.

Source. Reprinted from Endicott J: "Differential Diagnoses and Comorbidity," in *Premenstrual Dysphorias: Myths and Realities.* Edited by Gold JH, Severino SK. Washington, DC, American Psychiatric Press, 1994, p. 10. Used with permission.

mining the necessary degree of "interference" or impairment are needed for this distinction to be made more reliably. If cyclic changes in clinical features are documented in an individual with another ongoing disorder, the diagnosis of superimposed LLPDD is more difficult to make, because the rules for attribution of impairment to the cyclic features are not given in the proposed criteria. To date, a definitive study that attempts to differentiate between a premenstrual diagnosis that is superimposed on a preexisting mental disorder versus an exacerbation of an existing disorder has not been carried out. For the most part, the clinicians who have applied the proposed criteria for LLPDD have not complained about problems of judging "how much change is clinically significant change." This issue has been primarily one of great interest for research investigators, who want to have more explicit guidelines for sample selection.

The levels of comorbidity with other mental disorders, both current and lifetime, are quite high. Some have proposed that the dysphoric mood changes seen premenstrually be considered as simply prodromal or residual manifestations of major mood disorders. Such a proposal is likely to obscure differences among groups of women with lifetime major mood disorders, some of whom also meet the criteria for LLPDD and some of whom do not. Certainly it would be premature to assume that every woman who meets the criteria for LLPDD will eventually have a major mood disorder. That the two conditions frequently exist together does not necessarily mean they are manifestations of the same condition. The levels of comorbidity reported here are not dissimilar to those reported for panic disorder or alcohol abuse and major mood disorders in women. It is unlikely that a proposal would be made to subsume such comorbidity under the single diagnosis of major mood disorder.

Psychotic Symptoms and LLPDD

Because of anecdotal reports of recurring psychosis associated with the menstrual cycle (Leetz et al. 1988), the question has arisen as to whether psychotic features are an important component of LLPDD.

Table 14–6 summarizes studies of psychotic disorders that may be related to the menstrual cycle. The attempts to differentiate periodic psychoses from schizophrenic or affective psychoses is not new (Gjessing 1938; Vaillant 1964) (see Table 14–7).

Early in the twentieth century, Kraepelin (1903/1971) made the link between periodic psychoses and the menstrual cycle:

> We still have to mention a small group which runs a pronounced periodic course either in the introductory stages of the disease or during its whole duration. . . .
> In the female sex they are frequently connected with the menstrual periods in this

way, that the attack begins with the commencement of the menses or even a short time before, and then lasts about one or two weeks till it makes way for a clear interval lasting usually somewhat longer. (pp. 129–131)

Hatotani et al. began publishing reports in the 1950s on atypical psychoses in women, characterized by 1) acute onset of illness that tended to recur at intervals; 2) clinical symptoms of emotional disturbances, clouding of consciousness, and psychomotor disturbances; and 3) premorbid immature character with poor self-control (Hatotani et al. 1962). Because these studies were based on retrospective histories and included some women with menstrual cycle abnormalities, their value is solely to document the observation of a link between the menstrual cycle and the occurrence of psychotic symptoms.

Leonhard (1961) classified the endogenous psychoses as diagnoses to be distinguished from either schizophrenic illness or manic-depressive illness. Leonhard's cycloid psychosis was considered a distinct entity that was more prevalent in women.

Cutting et al. (1978) investigated patients with cycloid psychosis (73 patients) in comparison to patients diagnosed with schizophrenia (73 patients), depressive

Table 14–6. Psychotic diagnoses in the literature

Diagnosis	Reference(s)
Premenstrual psychosis	Verghese 1963; Williams and Weekes 1952
Hyperestrogenic cyclic psychosis	Lingjaerde and Bredland 1954
Periodic psychosis (atypical endogenous psychosis)	Takagi 1959; Wakoh et al. 1960; Hatotani et al. 1962, 1979; Endo et al. 1978; Berlin et al. 1982
Periodic insanity	Evans 1893
Cycloid psychosis[a]	Leonhard 1961; Perris 1973, 1974; Cutting et al. 1978
Atypical psychosis[a]	Perris 1973, 1974
Periodische (rekurrente)[a] schizophrenia	Perris 1973, 1974
Periodic catatonia[a]	Perris 1973, 1974
Periodic psychosis of puberty	Wenzel 1960; Altschule and Brem 1963; Teja 1976; Berlin et al. 1982
Recurrent menstrual psychosis	Felthous et al. 1980
Puerperal psychosis-premenstrual relapse	Dennerstein et al. 1983; Brockington et al. 1987
Remitting schizophrenia	Vaillant 1964
Schizophreniform psychosis	Gerada and Reveley 1988

[a]Leonhard's classification.

Table 14-7. Common features of the schizophrenia-like psychoses

Date	Author	Eponym	Recovery	Acute picture resembles schizophrenia	Good premorbid adjustment	Psychologically understandable symptoms	Precipitating cause	Symptoms of psychotic depression	Heredity-positive psychotic depression	Acute onset	Con-fusion	Concern with dying
1849	Bell	Bell's mania	Yes	Yes	Yes					Yes	Yes	
1861	Griesinger	Melancholia with stupor	Yes	Yes				Yes		Yes	Yes	Yes
1862	Bucknill and Tuke	Acute dementia	Yes	Yes				Yes		Yes		
1903	Kraepelin	Mixed conditions of manic-depressive insanity	Yes	Yes		Yes		Yes		Yes	Yes	Yes
1913	Kirby	Catatonic syndrome allied to manic-depressive insanity	Yes	Yes	Yes	Yes	Yes	Yes		Yes		Yes
1920	Kempf	Homosexual panic	Yes?	Yes				Yes		Yes	Yes	Yes
1921	Hoch	Benign stupor	Yes	Yes		Yes	Yes	Yes	Yes?	Yes	Yes	Yes
1924	Bleuler	Hysterical twilight state	Yes	Yes		Yes		Yes			Yes	Yes
1933	Kasanin	Schizoaffective psychosis	Yes	Yes	Yes	Yes	Yes	Yes	Yes?	Yes		
1937	Langfeldt	Schizophreniform state	Yes	Yes	Yes	Yes	Yes	Yes	Yes	Yes	Yes	
1938	Gjessing	Gjessing's syndrome	Yes	Yes	Yes					Yes	Yes	
1944	Keiser	Reactive state of adolescence	Yes	Yes		Yes	Yes	Yes		Yes		Yes
1947	Adland	Acute exhaustive psychosis	Yes	Yes	Yes	Yes	Yes	Yes		Yes	Yes	Yes
1950	Meduna	Oneirophrenia	Yes	Yes			Yes			Yes	Yes	
1961	Leonhard	Cycloid psychoses	Yes	Yes	Yes	Yes		Yes		Yes	Yes	Yes
Present		Adolescent turmoil	Yes	Yes		Yes	Yes			Yes	Yes	Yes

Source. Reprinted from Vaillant GE: "An Historical Review of the Remitting Schizophrenia." *Journal of Nervous and Mental Disease* 138:48–56, 1964. Used with permission. Copyright by Williams & Wilkins, 1964.

psychosis (73 patients), mania (73 patients), and schizoaffective illness (49 patients). To meet criteria for the diagnosis of cycloid psychosis, the following had to apply: 1) a psychotic episode in which hallucinations, delusions, or marked thought disorder were present; 2) at least one episode of depression (or elation) alternating with either normal mood, elation, or depression present during the psychotic episode; 3) at least two of the following five were present—paranoia-like symptoms, perplexity, pananxiety, ecstasy, and motility disturbances. Two features distinguished cycloid psychosis from the other groups: the high proportion of women and the particular outcome (Table 14–8, from Cutting et al. 1978, pp. 641–642).

There are also reports in the literature of women with other psychiatric diagnoses who have premenstrual exacerbations of their symptoms. Ota et al. (1954) described women with both schizophrenic and manic illness whose relapses occurred during the premenstrual and menstrual phases of their cycles. Swanson et al. (1964) reported 21 psychotic women with premenstrual worsening of symptoms and 5 psychotic women without premenstrual worsening of symptoms. All but 4 patients improved when treated with Enovid 5 mg bid, 20 days each month. They did not specify which women did not respond to treatment. Simpson et al. (1962, 1964) reported very similar findings.

Eight articles on this topic have appeared in the literature since 1980: a theoretical paper (Felthous and Robinson 1981), six case reports, and one paper describing eight women. Subjects ranged in age from 15 to 34 years. One subject was diagnosed with schizophreniform psychosis, nine had a premenstrual relapse of puerperal psychosis, one had periodic psychosis of puberty, and three had the diagnosis of recurrent menstrual psychosis. A summary of the articles reporting findings about specific women appears in Table 14–9.

Summary.   The question of a link between menstrual cycle hormones and psychotic symptoms is not new. It has arisen historically in the context of symptomatology (i.e., periodic psychoses in women) and in the context of treatment response (i.e., the use of progesterone and estrogen to maintain remission of symptoms in periodic psychoses). No prospective studies have been reported that address the question of psychotic symptoms and PMS or LLPDD. There seems to be very little support within the literature for the addition of symptoms of psychosis to the diagnostic criteria for LLPDD. Instead, psychotic symptoms should be described as a possible associated feature of the disorder. This would encourage clinicians and researchers to inquire routinely about these symptoms.

Course of the Disorder

There has been very little systematic study of the course and stability of LLPDD. It is stated that premenstrual symptoms can begin at any age after menarche. Those

Table 14–8. Distinguishing features of cycloid psychosis

	Cycloid	Manic	Depressive	Schizophrenic	Schizoaffective
Sex (% female)	90	53**	55**	51**	47**
Immediate outcome (%)					
Recovery	50	40	39	15**	39
Good outcome	40	34*	48	36**	41
Poor outcome	10	26*	13	49**	20
Follow-up success (%)	92	90	89	93	96
Follow-up period (years)	10	6.5*	7	7.5	8
Subsequent outcome (% of traced patients)					
Well throughout	21	44**	60**	26	36
Further admissions	72	53*	24**	68	62
Other psychiatric attention	7	3	16	6	2
Annual rate/patient					
New admissions	0.28	0.18**	0.06**	0.20*	0.20*
New episodes	0.30	0.19**	0.09**	0.21*	0.21*
Time in hospital (months)	0.86	0.46*	0.24**	2.52**	1.32

Note. Significance between "cycloid" and another group (t test or χ^2), * $P < .05$; ** $P < .01$.
Source. Reprinted from Cutting JC, Clare AW, Mann AH: "Cycloid Psychosis: An Investigation of the Diagnostic Concept." *Psychological Medicine* 8:637–648, 1978. Used with permission.

Table 14–9. Studies concerning premenstrual exacerbation of psychotic symptoms, 1980–1991

Study	Subject	Age (years)	Symptoms	Diagnosis	Family history	Episode	Days before menses	Unsuccessful treatments	Successful treatments
Labbate et al. 1991	1	35	Anxiety Irritability Emotional lability Paranoid delusions Auditory hallucinations	Recurrent premenstrual psychosis	Unknown	1	10	Antipsychotics Antidepressants Birth control pills Pyridoxine	Carbamazepine Level of 8–10 µg/ml
Gerada and Reveley 1988	1	34	Perplexity Anxiety Paranoid delusions Mute, restless Depressed Auditory hallucinations	Schizophreniform psychosis	Paternal uncle (schizophrenia) Cousin (schizophrenia)	1 2 3 4 5 6	6 4–6 4–6 4–6 6 Premenses	Haloperidol Lithium	Dydrogesterone 10 mg Days 12–26
Leetz et al. 1988	1	34	Manic excitement Delusions Hallucinations Disorientation	Periodic menstrual psychosis	Unknown	1	Several days before	Neuroleptics Lithium	Medroxyprogesterone acetate 100 mg im once a month
Brockington et al. 1987	1	24	Talked excitedly Punning She felt she was a computer Delusions	Premenstrual relapse of puerperal psychosis	At age 16, patient had 2 brief premenstrual psychotic episodes lasting 2 weeks: Semistuporous Decreased movement Strange statements about God and Devil Decreased eating Decreased sleep Perplexed Delusions	1 2 3 4 5	"Shortly" "A few days" 8 10 2		Progesterone and estrogen

(continued)

Table 14–9. Studies concerning premenstrual exacerbation of psychotic symptoms, 1980–1991 (*continued*)

Study	Subject	Age (years)	Symptoms	Diagnosis	Family history	Episode	Days before menses	Unsuccessful treatments	Successful treatments
	2	18	Increased activity Decreased sleep Telepathic powers	"	Trifluoperazine 10 mg daily	1 2	2 1	ECT Chlorpromazine	
	3	25	Disruptive Disheveled Overactive Irritable Distractible Delusions	"	At age 23, she was treated for premenstrual tension Cannabis abuse for 5 years	1 2	4 2		
	4			"		1	2		
	5			"		1 2 3	0–4 3 (–)		
	6			"		1	4		
	7			"		1 2	0 2		
	8			"		1	1		
Dennerstein et al. 1983	1	26	Disheveled Perplexed Loose associations Delusions Visual and tactile hallucinations Emotional lability Paranoid IQ = 63	Premenstrual relapse of puerperal psychosis	Since age 13, menarche, had depression 2–3 days before each menses Father: paranoid, schizophrenia Sister: schizophrenia Paternal uncle: paranoid, schizophrenia	1 2 3 4 5 6	? (~38 days post-partum) ? (~79 days post-partum) ? (~100 days post-partum) Premenstrual Premenstrual Premenstrual	Chlorpromazine ECT Norinyl-1	Danazol 600 mg daily Fluphenazine decanoate 25 mg every 2 weeks

Study	N	Age	Symptoms	Diagnosis	History			Treatment	Contraceptive
Berlin et al. 1982	1	15	Incoherent speech Insomnia Hallucinations Agitation Emotional lability Aimless wandering Public disrobing Staring into space Neglect of hygiene Strike out at others	Periodic psychosis of puberty	Premenstrual episodes present since age 12			Chlorpromazine Thioridazine Haloperidol Tricyclic anti-depressants Lithium Psychotherapy	21-day oral progesterone agent
Felthous et al. 1980	1	21	Argumentative Agitated Insomniac Dissociated thought Delusions Self-destructive thoughts Anuretic	Recurrent menstrual psychosis	Psychotic episodes began at age 14	1 2 4	0 0 0	Lithium Chlorpromazine	Ortho-Novum 1/50–21

who seek treatment are usually in their 30s. The average age at onset is unknown for LLPDD. Symptoms usually remit with menopause. However, much greater attention to collection of longitudinal data is needed (S. K. Severino, unpublished presentation, NIMH Workshop, 1989).

In a highly sophisticated recent study of the timing of premenstrual mood changes, Schmidt et al. (1991) examined three groups of women with prospectively confirmed PMS. By manipulating hormone levels through exogenous administration of the progesterone antagonist mifepristone and human chorionic gonadotropin or placebo, they were able to create one group in which menses occurred at midcycle, and the hormonal milieu at what ordinarily would have been the luteal phase was altered; a second group in which the hormonal milieu was also altered, but bleeding occurred at the expected time; and a third group in which the hormonal milieu was not altered. All three groups nonetheless experienced the symptoms of PMS at the time that would have been the luteal phase. Neither the blockade of the action of progesterone nor truncation of the luteal phase altered the course or severity of the symptoms of PMS. They speculate that LLPDD may be a cyclical mood disorder that becomes entrained to the menstrual cycle in much the same way that seasonal affective disorder appears to be entrained to the circannual cycle. To test this hypothesis, it would be necessary to manipulate hormone levels through several cycles, a procedure that is unlikely to ever be carried out. Alternatively, PMS may be triggered by hormonal events occurring earlier in the cycle. Regardless of the interpretation of the results of Schmidt et al., the study does call into question the appropriateness of referring to this syndrome as late luteal phase dysphoric disorder because it appears that its expression is not dependent on the late luteal phase hormonal environment.

Familial Factors

Familial studies of premenstrual symptoms are inconclusive in their findings. Finnish investigators reported that 70% of daughters of mothers with "premenstrual tension" also had symptoms, compared to only 37% of daughters of unaffected mothers (Kantero and Widholm 1971b). Dalton et al. (1987) reported that symptoms of PMS are likely to occur in both monozygotic twins if they occur in one. Concordance rates were significantly higher in monozygotic twins (93%) than in dizygotic twins (44%) or in sibling control subjects (31%). The difference between dizygotic twins and sibling control subjects was not significant. Another survey of twins also suggests that symptoms are hereditary (Van den Akker et al. 1987).

Biological Studies

Gonadal steroids/gonadotropins.   Rubinow et al. (1988) examined estradiol (E_2), progesterone (P), follicle-stimulating hormone (FSH), luteinizing hormone (LH), testosterone-estradiol-binding globulin (TBG), dihydroepiandrosterone sulfate (DHEA), dehydrotestosterone (DHT), prolactin, and cortisol in 17 women with prospectively confirmed PMS and 9 control subjects, diagnosed using daily ratings for two cycles with 30% change criteria and Schedule for Affective Disorders and Schizophrenia (SADS) interviews. Blood samples were drawn at 8 A.M. during the early, mid-, and late follicular and the early, mid-, and late luteal menstrual cycle phases. There were no diagnosis-related changes in any of the hormones. The authors suggest the need for dynamic rather than baseline measures to examine biological differences in PMS patients.

Hammarbäck et al. (1989) examined 18 PMS patients (no control subjects) who had been diagnosed using daily ratings for two cycles. Blood samples for E_2, P, FSH, and LH were taken daily in the luteal phase. Increased E_2 and P levels were associated with increased symptomatology. Increased FSH levels were inversely related to symptoms of breast swelling and tenderness. The authors suggested that the relationship between E_2, P, and FSH may be important in the production of PMS symptoms.

Watts et al. (1985) measured E_2, P, FSH, LH, cortisol, prolactin, thyroid-stimulating hormone (TSH), and testosterone in control subjects and in 35 PMS patients who had been diagnosed by daily prospective ratings recorded for 2 months. Blood samples were taken between 8:30 A.M. and 5:00 P.M. (the study did not control for possible circadian variation) during weeks 1–4 of the menstrual cycle. Ovulation was determined by ultrasound. PMS patients were found to have earlier ovulation, possibly a longer luteal phase, and increased cortisol levels. Although there was some suggestion of a phase-advance of the E_2 peak in PMS patients versus control subjects, the levels of these and other measured hormones did not differ significantly between the two groups. In contrast, Ying et al. (1987) examined a group of 83 infertile patients undergoing timed endometrial biopsy for the assessment of luteal phase adequacy. Their data suggest that the hormonal milieu associated with luteal phase defects do not correlate with premenstrual symptoms.

Halbreich et al. (1986) examined the rate of change of gonadal hormones in relation to PMS symptomatology. Seventeen women with PMS that had been prospectively confirmed using daily ratings, the Premenstrual Assessment Form (PAF) (Endicott et al. 1986) and the SADS (Endicott and Spitzer 1978) and who showed varying degrees of premenstrual changes and three control subjects had blood drawn between 8:00 A.M. and 10:00 A.M. three times per week to determine E_2 and P levels. Clinical assessment was used to determine the severity of premenstrual changes. A faster rate of change of progesterone levels was associated with more severe symptomatology with a time lag of 4–7 days between the hormonal increase or decrease and the presentation of symptoms.

Bäckström et al. (1985) studied seven PMS patients diagnosed using 1 month of prospective ratings and seven control subjects who had undergone hysterectomy. Their methods included enucleation of the corpus luteum. The luteal phase of PMS patients was associated with decreased progesterone and FSH levels and increased E_2 levels. The authors suggested that these findings may implicate increased inhibin levels in PMS. Many of the women had uterine fibroids and other medical reasons for hysterectomy. Because of the difficulty of performing the techniques involved, the study has not been replicated.

Summary: Although the studies are variable, the majority of well-controlled studies do not support consistent changes in E_2, P, FSH, or LH in PMS patients compared to asymptomatic control subjects. Because Hammarback's work suggests that spontaneous anovulatory cycles cause disappearance of cyclical symptoms in women with premenstrual syndrome, it may be that it is the indirect effect of ovarian steroids in relation to other neurotransmitter, neuroendocrine, or circadian systems that precipitates premenstrual mood changes rather than simply direct effects of the increased or decreased levels of these steroid hormones.

Neurovegetative signs (sleep, appetite) and psychophysiological responses.   Both-Orthman et al. (1988) examined appetite changes in 21 PMS patients diagnosed by 3 months of daily self-ratings and 13 control subjects confirmed as not having PMS by 2 months of daily ratings. Based on the PAF (Endicott et al. 1986), increased appetite correlated with depressed mood in PMS patients. These findings led the authors to suggest links between PMS and atypical depressions and to implicate the possible role of the serotonin system.

Mauri et al. (1988) examined self-reports of sleep during the premenstrual phase for 14 PMS patients who had been diagnosed via prospective assessments and for 26 control subjects. Their methods included use of two retrospective questionnaires, the Post-Sleep Inventory (Webb et al. 1976) and the Premenstrual Tension Syndrome Form (a yes/no questionnaire) (Steiner et al. 1980). PMS patients reported increased sleep disturbances during the luteal phase. Sleep disturbances discriminated between PMS patients and control subjects with 82% accuracy. The questionnaires, however, were based on subjective, retrospective reports.

Parry et al. (1989) measured sleep EEG, temperature, and wrist movement activity during the menstrual cycle in eight PMS patients and eight control subjects who had been screened with 2 months of daily ratings and weekly ratings using the Hamilton Rating Scale for Depression (Hamilton 1960) and the Beck Depression Inventory (Beck et al. 1979). Sleep EEG recordings were made twice weekly for one menstrual cycle. Activity was measured daily with a wrist actogram, and temperature was measured by means of a nocturnal indwelling rectal probe. PMS patients had more stage II sleep and less rapid eye movement (REM) sleep than control subjects. There were no significant differences between the groups with regard to daily wrist activity measurements. PMS patients had an earlier minimum nocturnal temperature than the control subjects at all phases of the menstrual cycle, but the differences were not statistically significant. Both groups had increased awakenings during the late luteal phase. The sleep changes in the PMS patients, although different from those in control subjects, did not parallel sleep changes characteristic of patients with major depressive disorders.

More recently, Lee et al. (1990) examined sleep changes in healthy women during the follicular and luteal phases. In women reporting more negative symptoms premenstrually on the Profile of Mood States (McNair et al. 1971) (subjects were not evaluated for LLPDD a priori), there was an associated decrease in delta-wave sleep.

Van den Akker and Steptoe (1989) examined psychophysiological responses (heart rate, skin conductance, and electromyography results) in 16 women reporting severe premenstrual symptoms and in 8 control women but found no marked differences in resting autonomic activity.

Summary: Although the findings need to be replicated in larger samples, the studies support differences between PMS patients and control subjects in neurovegetative signs and symptoms (sleep and appetite) during the menstrual cycle. Differences in neurovegetative signs may suggest underlying biological differences in the regulation of these systems, the anatomic and physiological bases of which currently remain unknown.

Neuroendocrine: thyroid.   Brayshaw and Brayshaw (1987), in a very controversial study using retrospective questionnaires, identified 20 women with PMS and 12 without PMS. The authors performed thyroid-releasing hormone (TRH) infusions and then treated symptomatic women with levothyroxine (T_4/Synthroid). They claimed that the women with PMS showed increased TSH responses to TRH and that 100% of the women with PMS responded to levothyroxine. The main criticisms of the study are that the women with PMS were not diagnosed using prospective ratings and that the subject population included patients with thyroid disorder, affective disorder, or anorexia but not PMS, and there were no outcome measures.

In contrast, Roy-Byrne et al. (1987) found no differences between patient and control groups or between the follicular and luteal menstrual cycle phase when they measured TSH and prolactin levels after TRH infusion. The sample included 14 women with prospectively confirmed PMS and control subjects (documented by daily ratings and 30% change criteria). The investigators did report increased variability of TSH responses to TRH (blunted and augmented responses) in symptomatic patients compared with control subjects.

Casper et al. (1989) also found no differences in TSH or prolactin response to TRH during either the follicular or luteal phases in 15 PMS patients and 19 control subjects. Subjects for this study were selected via ratings of visual analogue scales recorded every third day for one cycle for control subjects and two cycles for PMS patients.

More recently, Nikolai et al. (1990) studied baseline thyroid function (thyroxine [T$_4$], triiodothyronine [T$_3$] uptake, T$_3$, TSH, and TSH response to TRH) in 15 control subjects and 44 women with PMS diagnosed by daily diaries using the scoring system of Abraham (1983). The results showed that there was no significant thyroid disease in PMS patients and that levothyroxine was no better than placebo in the treatment of PMS.

Neuroendocrine: prolactin.   Parry et al. (1991) found that, in eight PMS patients who completed daily ratings for several cycles, there were normal TSH responses but enhanced prolactin responses to TRH administered during the follicular and luteal menstrual cycle phases. In addition, in this study, cerebrospinal fluid (CSF) samples for 3-methoxy-4-hydroxyphenylglycol (MHPG), homovanillic acid (HVA), 5-hydroxyindoleacetic acid (5-HIAA), β-endorphin, γ-aminobutyric acid (GABA), and prostaglandins were obtained from PMS patients during an asymptomatic follicular and a symptomatic luteal menstrual cycle phase. MHPG levels in CSF were significantly higher during the premenstrual phase than during the follicular phase. Follicular and luteal phase dexamethasone suppression tests (DSTs) were performed in subsequent months after initial circadian hormone profiles of cortisol were obtained. Baseline cortisol levels showed significant increases during the late follicular phase, which was probably an effect of estrogen. Of these patients, 62% showed nonsuppression to dexamethasone; however, this abnormality occurred during both the follicular and luteal menstrual cycle phases.

Neuroendocrine: cortisol.   Other groups have examined differences in cortisol levels in PMS patients and normal control subjects. Haskett et al. (1984) examined urinary free cortisol (UFC) and DST in 42 PMS patients who were selected on the basis of self-report scales and clinical interviews during the follicular and luteal phases (no daily ratings; no control subjects). A 1-mg DST was administered, and levels of UFC (24 hours) were obtained on cycle days 9 and 26. There was no cortisol hypersecretion, and there was normal 4:00 P.M. suppression of cortisol after DST. No changes were found in UFC levels between follicular and luteal phases. The authors suggest that PMS is not a model for endogenous depression.

Roy-Byrne et al. (1986) also examined the DST in 11 women with prospectively confirmed PMS (daily ratings for 2 months). No follicular-luteal differences in DST results were found in either PMS patients or control subjects.

Steiner et al. (1984) examined the circadian profile of prolactin, growth hormone (GH), and cortisol in two women with PMS and in two control subjects assessed by Moos's (1968) Menstrual Distress Questionnaire—Today version (MDQ-T). Blood samples were obtained every 30 minutes for 24 hours during the follicular and luteal phases. There were increased prolactin levels during the luteal phase in both PMS patients and control subjects (normal GH and cortisol). The small sample size limits the generalizability of the findings, however.

Neuroendocrine: glucose.   Reid et al. (1986) examined oral glucose tolerance by administering a 5-hour glucose tolerance test to six women with PMS (assessed by Steiner et al.'s [1980] Premenstrual Tension Questionnaire, not daily ratings) and five normal control subjects. Glucose tolerance did not differ between the follicular and luteal phases or between control subjects and PMS patients. There were no differences in glucose, insulin, or glucagon responses to naloxone. Denicoff et al. (1990) also examined glucose tolerance tests during the follicular and luteal phases in 11 women with prospectively confirmed PMS. Although the women experienced hypoglycemic symptoms, these were not specific to the luteal phase and did not resemble the women's PMS symptoms.

Diamond et al. (1989) performed hyperglycemic clamp studies in control women during midfollicular and midluteal menstrual cycle phases and found that glucose metabolism is impaired in the luteal phase of the menstrual cycle, an effect that could not be explained by differences in the plasma insulin response. However, these subjects were not selected or screened for menstrually related mood disorders.

Neuroendocrine: melatonin.   Parry et al. (1990) examined the melatonin circadian profile in eight PMS patients (documented by 2 months of daily ratings) and eight age-matched control subjects during the early follicular, late follicular, midluteal, and late luteal menstrual cycle phases. The PMS patients showed significantly lower levels of melatonin than the control subjects and a significant phase-advance of the melatonin offset at all menstrual cycle phases. These findings suggest chronobiological disturbances in PMS patients.

Summary: Although a variety of differences in neuroendocrine systems are reported, there are no consistent findings with respect to thyroid, cortisol, prolactin, or glucose abnormalities in PMS patients compared with control subjects. The differences in melatonin secretion between PMS patients and control subjects hold promise, but remain to be replicated.

Serotonin and other neurotransmitter systems.   Ashby et al. (1988) examined alterations of serotonergic mechanisms and monoamine oxidase in PMS patients who had been diagnosed using daily visual analogue scales for anxiety for two menstrual cycles and by the Minnesota Multiphasic Personality Inventory (MMPI) (Hathaway and McKinley 1970). The criteria used in this study required a 30% increase in the mean ratings recorded during the follicular phase compared with the luteal phase. Blood samples were obtained premenstrually (days −9 to −1) and postmenstrually (days 5–9) for platelet uptake and content of 5-hydroxytryptophan, monoamine oxidase, and tryptophan. The V_{max} (concentration) of 5-hydroxytryptophan uptake and content was lower premenstrually in PMS patients than in control subjects. Monoamine oxidase concentrations were lower postmenstrually than premenstrually. There were no significant changes in tryptophan concentrations. This study focused only on women with PMS anxiety, and sample size is not described. However, as the authors discuss, their findings suggest that changes in serotonergic circadian rhythms play a role in PMS. A follow-up report by Ashby et al. (1990) suggests that plasma obtained from PMS patients caused less stimulation of 5-hydroxytryptophan uptake than did plasma from the control group.

Taylor et al. (1984) also examined serotonin levels and platelet uptake in 16 PMS patients assessed by the MDQ (Moos 1968). Blood levels were drawn during the premenstrual and postmenstrual phases. The V_{max} of serotonin was significantly lower during the premenstrual phase. There were no differences in K_m (affinity) values. The study used no control subjects, the screening of subjects was not described, and the cycle phase was not documented. However, the findings are consistent with those of Ashby et al. (1988).

Rapkin et al. (1987) examined serotonin levels in whole blood in 14 women with PMS and 13 age-matched control subjects selected according to symptom diaries kept for 1 month, results of the Profile of Mood States (McNair et al. 1971), and the 30% criteria described earlier in this section. Blood samples were obtained during the late luteal and premenstrual phases. Serotonin levels in PMS patients were lower during the last 10 days of the cycle. Although the time of day at which samples were collected was not specified and diaries were obtained for only 1 month, this was otherwise a methodologically sound study.

Malmgren et al. (1987) examined platelet serotonin uptake and vitamin B_6 treatment in 19 women with PMS and 19 age-matched control subjects who completed the MDQ (Moos 1968) and Spielberger et al. (1970) anxiety questionnaires on cycle days 5–7 and 25–27. Blood samples were obtained during the premenstrual and postmenstrual phases. There were stable V_{max} and K_m values at both menstrual cycle phases. There were no group differences: lower V_{max} values occurred in spring. There was no effect of vitamin B_6. A limitation of this study was that daily ratings were not obtained.

U. Halbreich (personal communication, December 1988) reported that in women seeking treatment for dysphoric premenstrual changes (prospectively evaluated), the pharmacokinetic disposition of tryptophan was not changed during the menstrual cycle. They did observe a premenstrual blunting of prolactin and cortisol responses to an 8-g tryptophan loading dose, which suggests a role for the serotonergic system in symptom formation.

Rojansky et al. (1991) report that imipramine receptor binding was lower in prospectively evaluated women with dysphoric premenstrual changes than in control subjects during the early luteal phase. Although there was no consistent change from the asymptomatic early luteal phase to the symptomatic late luteal phase, the authors suggest that a preexisting vulnerability to the development of premenstrual dysphoric changes might be related to impaired gonadal hormone modulation of the serotonergic system.

In addition to the CSF studies of dopamine, serotonin, and norepinephrine reported by Parry et al. (1990, 1991) (see "Neuroendocrine" section), in which an increase in MHPG levels in CSF was found premenstrually in PMS patients, Halbreich et al. (personal communication, December 1991) reported an increase in the numbers of α_2-adrenergic receptors in women with dysphoric PMS during the follicular phase and even more so during the late luteal phase compared with normal control subjects.

In previous studies, Schrijver et al. (1987) reported increased urinary MHPG excretion in PMS patients, and DeLeon-Jones et al. (1982) reported downregulation of premenstrual urinary MHPG with therapeutic lithium treatment.

Summary: With the exception of Malmgren et al.'s (1987) study in which daily ratings were not obtained, the other studies of serotonin levels in PMS patients compared with control subjects show a consistent decrease in the V_{max} or levels of serotonin premenstrually. Studies with larger sample sizes in well-diagnosed PMS patients and control subjects are needed to replicate these findings, but the results to date show a consistent trend. Given that melatonin is synthesized from serotonin, these data are consistent with the previously reported data on melatonin (see "Neuroendocrine" section).

Some preliminary data from Parry et al.'s (1991) CSF studies and from the urinary and plasma studies of DeLeon-Jones et al. (1982), U. Halbreich (unpublished data, December 1991), and Schrijver et al. (1987) suggest a role for the noradrenergic system.

β-**Endorphin.** Chuong et al. (1985) examined neuropeptide levels in 20 PMS patients and 20 control subjects. Patients completed the MDQ (Moos 1968) and daily diaries for 3 months. Control subjects completed diaries for 1 month. Blood samples were collected every 2–3 days for 1 month for *β*-endorphin. *β*-Endorphin levels were lower in PMS patients than in control subjects. In PMS patients, levels during the luteal phase were lower than during the follicular phase. There were no changes in neurotensin, human pancreatic peptide, vasointestinal peptide, gastrin, or bombesin levels. Although the study was limited by the fact that only peripheral, not central, levels were measured, the authors suggest that β-endorphin levels may be a state marker for PMS (circadian effects were not taken into account).

Facchinetti et al. (1987) also examined plasma β-endorphin in 11 PMS patients and 8 control subjects who completed MDQ every 2 days. Blood samples were collected every 2–3 days for 1 month to determine levels of β-endorphin and β-lipotropin. PMS patients showed a decrease in β-endorphin levels premenstrually and during menses but normal values during the follicular phase. No changes were found in control subjects, and no changes in β-lipotropin levels were found during the menstrual cycle. Although there were no daily ratings, the investigators did do prospective assessments using the Menstrual Distress Questionnaire every other day. The authors implicate the failure of central opioid tonus premenstrually.

Tulenheimo et al. (1987) examined plasma β-endorphin immunoreactivity in 12 PMS patients who had been diagnosed using daily records (0–3 severity) and 14 control subjects. Morning blood samples were collected during the mid- and late follicular phases, the early and late luteal phases, and the premenstrual cycle phase. No differences in estradiol, progesterone, LH, or cortisol were found between groups. β-Endorphin levels were lower in PMS patients than in control subjects during the luteal phase. There were no menstrual cycle phase differences. The results of this study, showing lowered β-endorphin levels in PMS patients compared with control subjects in the luteal phase, agree with similar trends found in other studies.

Giannini et al. (1989) reported that 21 of 53 women with LLPDD had significant declines in serum β-endorphin levels on the 20th day of the cycle that were associated with increased anxiety, physical discomfort, decreased concentration, and increased calorie consumption. However, there were no control patients, serum levels of β-endorphin were less well substantiated than plasma levels, the sampling was infrequent, and 32 women had no decline in β-endorphin levels.

Summary: Although differences in assay sensitivity and circadian variability need to be accounted for, the studies consistently show a trend of decreased β-endorphin levels in PMS patients compared with control subjects during the luteal phase. The major limitation of these studies is that plasma β-endorphin is a peripheral measure. Measures of β-endorphin in CSF of PMS patients do not decline premenstrually (Parry et al. 1991).

Other potential substrates (prostaglandins, vitamins, electrolytes, CO_2 inhalation). Jakubowicz et al. (1984) examined prostaglandins in 80 PMS patients treated with mefenamic acid. Prostaglandin levels were measured for three cycles in 19 of the 80 patients, who were selected using a daily symptom checklist for one cycle. Blood samples were obtained every 3 days. Although 86% of patients improved when administered 500 mg of mefenamic acid three times daily versus placebo, there were no changes in prostaglandin levels during the menstrual cycle, and prostaglandin levels were lower in patients than in control subjects.

Mira et al. (1988) examined vitamins and trace elements in women with PMS. Thirty-eight patients with PMS and 23 control subjects completed prospective symptom reports for three cycles. Samples were collected during the midfollicular and premenstrual cycle phases for magnesium, zinc, and vitamins A, E, and B_6. No differences between groups were found during the cycle for any of the nutritional parameters.

Chuong et al. (1990) examined vitamin A levels at 2- to 3-day intervals throughout three menstrual cycles in 10 PMS patients and 10 control subjects diagnosed using daily diaries. No significant changes were noted between the control subjects and the patients during either the luteal or the follicular phase.

Varma (1984) examined hormones and electrolytes in 25 PMS patients and 10 control subjects selected using daily visual analogue scales. Blood samples were obtained on days 3, 7, 11, 15, 19, 24, and 27 of each cycle. No differences in sodium or potassium levels were found between the women with PMS and control subjects, and there were no menstrual cycle phase differences. Although there was a slight increase in cortisol levels during the luteal phase in the women with the most severe PMS, levels were still in the normal range. No differences between groups were found for estradiol, progesterone (slight increase in estrogen-to-progesterone ratio in PMS patients in luteal phase), prolactin, FSH, or LH.

Rojansky and Halbreich (1991) examined the severity of symptoms and hormonal correlates in 78 sterilized (tubal ligation) and nonsterilized women with prospectively confirmed PMS. No significant differences could be demonstrated between groups. The authors concluded that premenstrual symptoms are not associated with tubal sterilization.

Harrison et al. (1989) found that women with LLPDD were more sensitive to the anxiety-provoking properties of CO_2 inhalation (double breath or rebreathing) and lactate infusion than were asymptomatic control subjects. In this study, none of the control subjects developed intense anxiety or panic attacks, whereas more than half of the women with LLPDD did so. These findings suggest that patients with LLPDD and anxiety disorders may have a shared vulnerability.

Summary: The studies do not support prostaglandin, nutritional (vitamin), or electrolyte disturbances in PMS patients. The work on CO_2 inhalation suggests biological differences between patients with LLPDD and control subjects and perhaps a shared vulnerability of patients with LLPDD and those with anxiety or panic disorders.

Overview summary. A review of the current literature clearly indicates that a precise understanding of the biological differences between patients suffering from premenstrual affective, cognitive, and behavioral symptomatology cannot be obtained without close attention to the diagnostic criteria used in the different studies. The absence of standardized criteria is the rate-limiting factor in furthering the search for biological differences in these individuals. Studies that examine similar systems cannot be compared if research groups use variable selection criteria. Thus, the first step in exploring the biological vulnerabilities that predispose women to severe premenstrual mood disturbances is to develop standardized diagnostic criteria to enhance sample homogeneity.

The most consistent data appear to lie in the realm of the neurotransmitter system, serotonin (which includes melatonin, as the latter is synthesized from the former), and some suggestions for the adrenergic (which regulates the timing of melatonin release) and β-endorphin systems, although the case for these systems is much less strong.

Several methodologically sound studies suggest that biological differences in PMS patients versus control subjects may be more a trait than a state marker. These findings further emphasize the necessity for distinguishing patient from control groups using rigorous diagnostic criteria (as is needed for genetic linkage studies, for example). Such diagnostic specificity will then allow for comparison of biological differences in other psychiatric diagnostic categories (e.g., affective disorder, panic disorder). The studies on biological differences in patients with premenstrual mood disorders versus normal control subjects suggest that PMS patients may have a biological vulnerability, manifested most readily in the serotonergic and melatonin systems (with possible contributions from the noradrenergic system) that is unmasked premenstrually. Like the postpartum period for affective illness, the threshold for presentation or the protective factor may be lowered during the premenstrual phase because of the interaction of the altered hormonal milieus with neurotransmitter, neuroendocrine, and circadian systems. There may also be an altered response to steroid effects on the brain at this time because of altered receptor substrate sensitivity.

Treatment Studies

This section provides an overview of the most stringent PMS treatment efficacy studies to date. Second, it discusses treatments that, by mode of administration or suppression of ovulation, might be considered to validate the diagnosis of LLPDD. For this review, studies were grouped into seven categories: 1) ovulation suppression, 2) progesterone and dydrogesterone, 3) nutritional supplements, 4) diuretics, 5) psychopharmacological agents, 6) melatonin suppressors, and 7) miscellaneous treatments. It is important to note that treatments are grouped according to their use in particular studies, and many treatments have a greater number of effects than are mentioned in this review.

In reviewing PMS treatment studies, one must bear in mind certain methodological limitations that are inherent in research on this disorder:

1. Because of the cyclical nature of PMS and LLPDD, researchers are limited in the amount of time they may spend observing the phenomenon, and symptoms may not always appear reliably or with the same intensity in each cycle. To assess these cyclical changes adequately, long baseline periods are needed, along with extended follow-up periods, so that symptom improvement or deterioration can be observed. The problem with these long observation periods is twofold. First, the most severe cases may drop out of studies during the no-treatment baseline period, and second, those who respond quickly to treatment may lose their motivation to continue in follow-up once they are well.

2. In contrast to LLPDD, PMS is a heterogeneous disorder, having varied manifestations that can include any of over 150 symptoms. Typological categories of PMS have been suggested as a means of making subjects more homogeneous in clinical trials, but no single typology has demonstrated its validity or usefulness. In fact, most women meet criteria for more than one typological subgroup, making comparisons between subgroups difficult, if not impossible.

Ovulation suppression.   Many treatments that are effective at reducing or eliminating PMS symptoms seem to do so by suppressing ovulation. Table 14–10 lists the treatments, such as danazol, luteinizing hormone–releasing hormone (LHRH) agonists, estradiol plus norethisterone, and oophorectomy.

Danazol is a gonadotropin-releasing hormone agonist that most likely exerts its effects by suppressing the gonadotropin surge at ovulation (Watts et al. 1987). Of the four studies reviewed here, two were designed in a double-blind, crossover manner. In the first, Gilmore et al. (1985) found that danazol (400 mg daily) was superior to placebo, but side effects were a problem for many of the 36 women completing the study. Sarno et al. (1987) studied a lower dose of danazol (200 mg/day), which was given only in the presence of premenstrual symptoms. This lower, cyclical dose of danazol was also superior to placebo for symptom relief but without the side effects noted in the study by Gilmore et al. (1985). In two single-blind, randomized studies, Watts et al. (1985, 1987) looked at the efficacy of danazol in subjects receiving doses of 100, 200, and 400 mg compared with a control group receiving placebo. Once again, danazol was superior to placebo, with side effects becoming problematic at the high dose. The results of these four studies suggest that a relatively low, cyclical dose of danazol has effects comparable to those of higher doses but is better tolerated. In addition, cyclical administration of danazol seems to keep estradiol and gonadotropin levels normal throughout the menstrual cycle.

Table 14–10 summarizes the results of two studies of estradiol plus norethisterone. One study, by Watson et al. (1989), was performed in a double-blind, crossover manner, using implants of placebo or 200 mg of estradiol. Magos et al. (1986) used a 100-mg estradiol implant or placebo in a double-blind, longitudinal study. In both studies, daily scores from the MDQ (Moos 1968) provided a measure of treatment outcome. Also common to both studies was the use of oral norethisterone (5 mg daily), taken by subjects premenstrually to promote normal menstruation. In both studies, estradiol plus norethisterone was superior to placebo for relief of premenstrual symptoms. Watson et al. (1989) found that some women experienced skin irritation and discoloration at the site of the estradiol patch. Whereas Magos et al. (1986) noted no side effects with the estradiol implants, they warned of the possibility of hyperestrogenemia with this form of treatment.

The efficacy of buserelin, an LHRH agonist, was tested in three studies, with mixed results. Hammarbäck and Bäckström (1988) performed the only double-blind, crossover trial, in which buserelin (400 μg daily) or placebo was administered by nasal spray, and symptoms were rated daily on a visual analogue scale. They found that buserelin was superior to placebo for all symptoms studied. At the 400-μg daily dose, women became anovulatory while continuing to menstruate regularly, with no development of postmenopausal symptoms. Bancroft et al. (1987) also used nasal-spray administration in their placebo-controlled trial of buserelin (600 μg daily). Active treatment was given for long-term ($n = 10$) and short-term ($n = 10$) periods. Five women from the long-term group received placebo after their symptoms had stabilized after receiving buserelin. The results of this study were mixed, with buserelin superior for mood symptoms, bloating, and breast tenderness but not for irritability and low energy. In addition, many side effects were seen, including hot flushes, labile mood, hypomania, and loss of libido.

Muse et al. (1984) used a daily injection of 50 μg of an LHRH agonist or placebo in a single-blind, crossover study in which the efficacy of buserelin was demonstrated only for physical symptoms. Hot flushes were a side effect of treatment in this study, and the authors also cautioned that osteoporosis may develop if this treatment is given over an extended period. Despite mixed results, the use of buserelin as a treatment for PMS symptoms remains promising.

The final method of ovulation suppression reviewed here is accomplished by surgical rather than pharmacological means. Studies of oophorectomy and hysterectomy followed by a regimen of estrogen replacement indicated that this form of treatment eliminated mood and physical symptoms associated with PMS. Summaries of two such studies are found in Table 14–10. In studies by Casper and Hearn

Table 14–10. Ovulation suppression

Reference	Treatment	Measures	Methods	Results
Gilmore et al. 1985	Danazol	MDQ	36 women; 400 mg danazol or placebo daily for 3 mo; MDQ daily	Danazol superior to placebo
Sarno et al. 1987	Danazol	MSQ	14 women; 200 mg danazol or placebo daily, from onset of symptoms until menses, for 2 mo	Danazol superior to placebo
Watts et al. 1985	Danazol	Total wk 4 score of each symptom; cyclical change scores (wk 4/wk 2)	100 ($n = 10$), 200 ($n = 10$), or 400 ($n = 10$) mg danazol or placebo ($n = 10$) daily for 3 mo	Danazol superior to placebo for 5 of the 7 symptoms studied
Watts et al. 1987	Danazol	Total wk 4 score of each symptom; cyclical change scores (wk 4/wk 2)	100 ($n = 10$), 200 ($n = 10$), or 400 ($n = 10$) mg danazol or placebo ($n = 10$) daily for 3 mo	200- and 400-mg doses best for cyclical irritability; 400-mg dose best for weekly irritability; breast pain lower on all danazol doses
Muse et al. 1984	LHRH agonist	Premenstrual assessment calendar; plasma LH, FSH, estradiol, and progesterone	8 women; 50 µg LHRH agonist or placebo daily for 3 mo	Active treatment superior to placebo for reducing only physical symptoms and abolishing cyclical hormone fluctuations
Bancroft et al. 1987	LHRH agonist (buserelin)	VAS; urinary estrogen and pregnanediol	600 µg nasal buserelin daily for 18–65 wk ($n = 10$) or 3–11 wk ($n = 10$); 5 long-term placebo once symptoms were under control	No change in hormones; improvement in mood, bloating, and breast tenderness for long-term treatment; no differences for short-term treatment
Hammarbäck and Bäckström 1988	LHRH agonist (buserelin)	Plasma estrogen and progesterone; VAS	23 women; 400 µg nasal buserelin or placebo daily for 3 mo; blood samples weekly	No changes in hormones; buserelin superior to placebo for all symptoms

(continued)

Table 14–10. Ovulation suppression *(continued)*

Reference	Treatment	Measures	Methods	Results
Magos et al. 1986	Estradiol + norethisterone	MDQ; retrospective VAS; General Health Questionnaire	68 women; 100 mg estradiol sc + 5 mg norethisterone po for 7 days, 9 days before menses; physician review every 3 mo; MDQs daily	Based on MDQ active Tx superior to placebo; no differences on any other measures
Watson et al. 1989	Estradiol + norethisterone	MDQ; PDQ	40 women; 200 µg estradiol sc + 5 mg norethisterone or placebo for 3 mo; questionnaires daily	Active treatment superior to placebo
Casper and Hearn 1990	Oophorectomy and hysterectomy + estrogen	PRISM; Campbell's Overall Life Satisfaction (Campbell et al. 1976); Index of General Affect (Campbell et al. 1976); POMS; Quality of Life Questionnaire (Evans et al. 1985)	14 women with treatment-resistant PMS; oophorectomy and hysterectomy performed on all women but one, who had already had hysterectomy; 6-week follow-up and PRISM calendar completed at 6 mo	Surgical intervention eliminated premenstrual symptoms
Casson et al. 1990	Oophorectomy and hysterectomy + estrogen	PRISM	14 women with treatment-resistant PMS; oophorectomy and hysterectomy performed; PRISM calendar completed at two points during a follow-up year	Surgical intervention eliminated premenstrual symptoms

Note. FSH = follicle-stimulating hormone. LH = luteinizing hormone. LHRH = luteinizing hormone–releasing hormone. MDQ = Menstrual Distress Questionnaire (Moos 1968). MSQ = Menstrual Symptom Questionnaire (Abraham 1980). PDQ = Personality Diagnostic Questionnaire (Magos et al. 1986). PMS = premenstrual syndrome. POMS = Profile of Mood States (McNair et al. 1971). PRISM = Prospective Record of the Impact and Severity of Menstrual Symptomatology (Reid 1985). VAS = visual analog scale.

Source. Reprinted from Rivera-Tovar A, Rhodes R, Pearlstein TB, et al.: "Treatment Efficacy," in *Premenstrual Dysphorias: Myths and Realities.* Edited by Gold JH, Severino SK. Washington, DC, American Psychiatric Press, 1994, pp. 101–102. Used with permission.

(1990) and Casson et al. (1990), women were selected on the basis of their unresponsiveness to previous medical therapy. In both studies, symptoms were recorded using Reid's Prospective Record of the Impact and Severity of Menstrual Symptomatology (PRISM) calendar (Reid 1985) for 2 months before and up to 1 year following surgery.

Overall, suppression of ovulation seems promising as a treatment for severe physical and affective symptoms of PMS. Whereas both pharmacological and surgical treatments are effective, pharmacological treatments are more desirable, because they allow for ovulation suppression through less radical means with essentially the same effect as surgery and with the reversibility not afforded by a surgical procedure.

Progesterone and dydrogesterone.   Several studies have tested the efficacy of progesterone, as well as that of its optical isomer dydrogesterone, for the treatment of PMS symptoms. The details of these studies can be found in Table 14–11.

Eight progesterone studies are reviewed here, all of which were designed in a double-blind, crossover manner. In all but two studies, treatment was administered by vaginal suppository. The doses in these six studies ranged from 200 to 800 mg daily, whereas doses in the two oral-treatment studies were either unreported (Dennerstein et al. 1985) or less than 10 mg daily (Jordheim 1972).

Of the eight studies reviewed, the most recent, by Freeman et al. (1990), also had the strongest study design. Subject selection was based on 2 months of prospective symptom rating followed by 2 months of placebo treatment, during which subjects continued to rate symptoms on a daily symptom record. Subjects were then randomly assigned to groups receiving either placebo or active treatment with progesterone (400 or 800 mg/day), with subjects receiving 2 months of each treatment, for a total of 6 months of double-blind, crossover treatment. Daily symptom records and patients' global improvement ratings showed no efficacy of progesterone at either dose level. This result is in agreement with those of all other studies except Dennerstein et al. (1985), who found progesterone superior to placebo. The Dennerstein study, however, had a much smaller sample size ($N = 23$) than did that by Freeman et al. (1990) ($N = 121$), and it failed to report the progesterone dose tested. Based on this information and the negative results of the other six studies, progesterone cannot be recommended as a treatment for the symptoms of PMS.

Dydrogesterone, the optical isomer of progesterone, has also been studied as a possible treatment for PMS, and Table 14–11 reports the results of three such studies. Dennerstein et al. (1986) and Sampson et al. (1988) performed double-blind, crossover studies, in which dydrogesterone (20 mg daily) was given during the luteal phase only. In addition, these two studies based diagnosis and treatment

Table 14–11. Progesterone and dydrogesterone

Reference	Treatment	Measures	Methods	Results
Andersch and Hahn 1985	Progesterone	Modified CPRS scale	15 women; after 1-mo baseline, 100 mg vaginal progesterone or placebo twice daily, from 10 days before menses or at first symptoms until menses onset, for 1 mo	No differences
Dennerstein et al. 1985	Progesterone	MDQ; BDI; STAI; MACL; daily symptom reports	23 women; oral active treatment or placebo (no doses given) for 2 mo	Progesterone clinically and statistically superior to placebo
Freeman et al. 1990	Progesterone	Daily symptom reports; patient global improvement ratings	121 women; 4-mo washout period, then randomized to groups receiving 400- and 800-mg progesterone suppositories daily for 2 mo; treatment on days 16–28 of each mo	No significant differences
Jordheim 1972	Progesterone (2.5 mg) + diuretic (2 mg)	Subjects' daily record	21 women; active treatment or placebo 3 times daily, from 10 days before menses, for 4 mo	No differences
Maddocks et al. 1986	Progesterone	BDI; Irritability Scale; STAI; MDQ, Form-T; PMTS self-rating scale	20 women, 1-mo symptom rating; 400 mg vaginal progesterone or placebo daily from day 12 of cycle, for 3 mo	No differences
Richter et al. 1984	Progesterone	Subjects' rankings of best cycles; authors' daily symptom rating scale	22 women assigned to treatment sequence consisting of 800 mg vaginal progesterone or placebo daily from day 15 to menses onset, 4 treatment cycles	No differences
Sampson 1979	Progesterone	MDQ; retrospective self-assessment	1-mo MDQ ratings; part 1: subjects ($n = 35$) received 400 mg progesterone or placebo daily for 1 mo; part 2: subjects ($n = 26$) received 800 mg progesterone or placebo daily for 1 mo	No preferences for either treatment

van der Meer et al. 1983	Progesterone	4-point symptom scale	13 women; 400 mg rectal progesterone or placebo daily, midcycle to menses onset, for 2 mo; gynecologist visit monthly	No differences
Dennerstein et al. 1986	Dydrogesterone	MDQ; STAI; MACL; daily symptom rating	24 women; 1-mo daily ratings, then 200 mg dydrogesterone or placebo daily on days 12–26 of each mo, for 2 mo; women interviewed in menstrual period of each cycle	No differences, but treatment effect was noted
Kerr et al. 1980	Dydrogesterone	Gynecologist's assessment; plasma progesterone levels; symptom diaries	67 women; 20 mg active treatment or placebo daily on days 12–26 each mo in a single-blind trial, for 6 mo	Subjects' diaries showed active treatment superior to placebo for 3 of 13 symptoms studied
Sampson et al. 1988	Dydrogesterone	MDQ	69 women; after 1-mo symptom rating, 20 mg dydrogesterone or placebo daily, balanced, for 2 mo	No overall efficacy of dydrogesterone

Note. BDI = Beck Depression Inventory (Beck et al. 1979). CPRS = Comprehensive Psychopathological Rating Scale (Asberg et al. 1978). Irritability Scale (Buss and Durkee 1957). MACL = Mood Adjective Checklist (Mackay et al. 1978). MDQ = Menstrual Distress Questionnaire (Moos 1968). PMTS = Premenstrual Tension Syndrome (Haskett and Abplanalp 1983). STAI = State Trait Anxiety Inventory (Spielberger et al. 1970).

Source. Reprinted from Rivera-Tovar A, Rhodes R, Pearlstein TB, et al.: "Treatment Efficacy," in *Premenstrual Dysphorias: Myths and Realities.* Edited by Gold JH, Severino SK. Washington, DC, American Psychiatric Press, 1994, pp. 106–107. Used with permission.

outcome on the MDQ (Moos 1968), which was completed by subjects daily. Neither study found dydrogesterone beneficial in the treatment of PMS.

In a single-blind, placebo-controlled study, Kerr et al. (1980) also administered dydrogesterone at a dose of 20 mg/day on a cyclical basis. This study, however, lacked prospective symptom rating to confirm the PMS diagnosis, although patients did keep daily symptom diaries during the treatment phase of the study. Results of this study were somewhat cloudy, because gynecologists' assessments showed no clear efficacy of active treatment, and individuals' diaries showed dydrogesterone to be superior to placebo for very few symptoms.

Based on the group means for the hormonal studies discussed here, the use of progesterone and dydrogesterone in the treatment of PMS does not appear to be beneficial.

Nutritional supplements.   A third group of studies, shown in Table 14–12, concentrated on the efficacies of various nutritional supplements for the alleviation of PMS symptoms. Seven of the 14 studies were concerned with vitamin B_6 (pyridoxine), but other nutrients, such as vitamin E, calcium, and evening primrose oil, as well as a nutrient combination called Optivite, were also studied.

Of the various nutrient supplements mentioned, only two have been demonstrated to be superior to placebo for relief of the symptoms of PMS. The first such treatment, studied by London et al. (1987), was vitamin E (α-tocopherol). In this randomized, double-blind study, 22 subjects received active treatment (400 IU daily), and 19 subjects received placebo for 3 months. Treatment outcome for the study was based on a questionnaire that included symptoms classified by Steiner et al. (1980a) and those in Abraham's (1980) four symptom categories.

Results of the vitamin E study showed this treatment to be superior to placebo clinically, although not statistically, for the relief of PMS. No side effects were reported for vitamin E, but one woman taking placebo did complain of headache, chest pain, anxiety, and paranoid ideation.

A double-blind, crossover study by Thys-Jacobs et al. (1989) demonstrated the efficacy of calcium (1,000 mg daily) for the treatment of PMS. Documentation of symptoms before, during, and 1 month after treatment was facilitated by daily symptom questionnaires. Subjects ($N = 33$) also rated treatment preference retrospectively, and once again, calcium was superior to placebo. Side effects such as nausea, constipation, flatulence, and gastrointestinal discomfort were noted with the active treatment.

Another nutritional supplement studied was evening primrose oil (Efamol), which contains γ-linolenic acid, a derivative of cis-linoleic acid and a critical precursor of prostaglandin E_1. Levels of cis-linoleic acid have been found to be higher in PMS patients than in control subjects, but with reduced metabolites,

Table 14–12. Nutritional supplements

Reference	Treatment	Measures	Methods	Results
London et al. 1987	α-Tocopherol	Questionnaire based on symptom classification of Steiner et al. (1980a) and Abraham (1984)	400 IU ($n = 22$) or placebo ($n = 19$) given for 3 mo; symptoms in follicular and luteal phases rated in all cycles	Active treatment superior to placebo in 3 of 4 Abraham categories and Steiner symptoms but not at $P < .05$
Thys-Jacobs et al. 1989	Calcium	Daily symptom scores; retrospective global assessment	33 women; 1,000 mg calcium carbonate or placebo daily for 3 mo, then a 4th mo of symptom scoring	Calcium superior to placebo
Callender et al. 1988	Evening primrose oil + vitamin supplement	Daily symptom diary; BDI; Salkind Inventory; subjective report	10 women; 3,000 mg Efamol + Efavit (750 mg ascorbic acid, 30 mg zinc sulfate, and 150 mg each niacin and vitamin B_6) or placebo, from day 7 to day 1 of menses, for 2 mo, with washout between	Subjective improvement in 70% of active treatment and 30% of placebo cycles; no differences in Beck or Salkind scores
Khoo et al. 1990	Evening primrose oil	4-point rating scale of symptoms	38 women met authors' criteria for PMS based on 1-mo symptom rating; Efamol or placebo given for 3 mo	No significant differences between treatments
Stephenson et al. 1988	Evening primrose oil + vitamin E	MDQ	70 women; 2-mo symptom rating; 8 capsules daily, active treatment or placebo, for 3 mo; monthly visit to nurse; MDQs completed 3 days/wk	No differences between treatments
Chakmakjian et al. 1985	Optivite	MSQ; self-rating of symptoms	Subjects (n = 31) took 6 tablets of Optivite or placebo daily for 3 cycles; MSQ completed in wk 2 and 4 of all cycles	16 subjects preferred Optivite, 7 preferred placebo, 8 had no preference; MSQ scores lower for PMT-A and PMT-C on Optivite

(continued)

Table 14–12. Nutritional supplements (*continued*)

Reference	Treatment	Measures	Methods	Results
Stewart 1987	Optivite	Self-rating of symptoms	3 mo of Optivite or placebo; 4 tablets/day in 1st 2 wk, then 8 tablets/day ($n = 119$); or 2 tablets/day in 1st 2 wk, then 4 tablets/day ($n = 104$)	Optivite superior to placebo only in high-dose trial
Abraham and Hargrove 1980	Pyridoxine	MSQ; daily weight records	25 women; 500 mg pyridoxine or placebo daily for 3 mo; daily weight and MSQ ratings	Pyridoxine superior in 22 subjects, as shown by MSQ score
Barr 1984	Pyridoxine	Daily symptom records	48 women; 200 mg pyridoxine or placebo daily, from cycle day 10 to day 3 of menses, for 2 mo	Pyridoxine superior to placebo
Hagen et al. 1985	Pyridoxine	Global VAS; self-rating of symptoms; plasma magnesium	Subjects ($n = 34$) received 100 mg pyridoxine or placebo daily for 2 mo; VAS completed at end of each 2-mo period	Treatments equivalent; order effect observed
Harrison et al. 1984	Pyridoxine	Physician's CGI; PAF; daily self-rating scale	Placebo nonresponders ($n = 20$) given 50–150 mg pyridoxine + 1.5–6.0 g L-tryptophan daily for 3 mo	No differences between treatments
Kendall and Schnurr 1987	Pyridoxine	Daily symptom records; PAF; MDQ; Form-T	55 women; 150 mg pyridoxine or placebo daily for 2 mo; daily MDQ and symptom records	Pyridoxine superior to placebo for autonomic and behavioral symptoms only
Malmgren et al. 1987	Pyridoxine	Platelet serotonin uptake	300 mg pyridoxine or placebo daily, from cycle day 15 to day 1 of menses, for 2 mo	No differences between treatments

| Williams et al. 1985 | Pyridoxine | Investigator's final assessment; daily record of tablets taken and symptom severity | 50–200 mg pyridoxine (n = 204) or placebo (n = 230) for 3 cycles | No difference in individual symptoms, but overall results showed pyridoxine to be superior to placebo |

Note. BDI = Beck Depression Inventory (Beck et al. 1979). CGI = Clinical Global Impressions Scale. MDQ = Menstrual Distress Questionnaire (Moos 1968). MSQ = Menstrual Symptom Questionnaire (Abraham 1980). PAF = Premenstrual Assessment Form (Endicott et al. 1986). PMT-A and PMT-C = Premenstrual Tension Syndrome—Subtype A and Premenstrual Tension Syndrome—Subtype C (Abraham 1980). VAS = visual analog scale.
Source. Reprinted from Rivera-Tovar A, Rhodes R, Pearlstein TB, et al.: "Treatment Efficacy," in *Premenstrual Dysphorias: Myths and Realities.* Edited by Gold JH, Severino SK. Washington, DC, American Psychiatric Press, 1994, pp. 109–111. Used with permission.

suggesting a low conversion rate of *cis*-linoleic acid to γ-linolenic acid (Brush 1984). γ-Linolenic acid, administered by means of evening primrose oil, was thought to be capable of overcoming any block in prostaglandin E_1 production. Although Callender et al. (1988) reported subjective improvement during 70% of cycles in which active treatment was given and only 30% of cycles in which placebo was given, they found no differences in other outcome measures. This lack of treatment efficacy was more clearly demonstrated in studies by Khoo et al. (1990) and Stephenson et al. (1988). The weight of evidence from these three double-blind, crossover studies suggests that evening primrose oil is not an effective treatment for PMS symptoms.

Two efficacy studies of Optivite, a multivitamin multimineral supplement, have provided mixed results for PMS treatment. Chakmakjian et al. (1985) performed a double-blind, crossover study of Optivite (six tablets daily) and placebo therapy. Table 14–12 shows the results of this study, which indicated no clear efficacy of the active treatment. Stewart (1987), in a random, double-blind study, suggested that Optivite is efficacious at a relatively high dose (8 tablets daily) but not at a lower one (4 tablets daily). The results of both of these studies would suggest that perhaps a third study, in which patients are given at least 8 tablets daily, would help to answer the question of the efficacy of Optivite for the treatment of PMS.

As mentioned previously, vitamin B_6 accounted for 7 of the 14 nutritional supplement studies reviewed here. Overall, the studies, shown in Table 14–12, suggest that B_6 is not clearly any more efficacious than placebo and is therefore not an effective treatment for PMS. In fact, all but three studies found no efficacy whatsoever of vitamin B_6. Abraham and Hargrove (1980) performed a double-blind, crossover study using a 500-mg/day vitamin B_6 dose. They used their Menstrual Symptom Questionnaire as an outcome measure. In this study, active treatment was superior to placebo for 22 of 25 women.

Barr (1984) found a cyclical (i.e., administered from cycle day 10 to day 3 of menses), 200-mg daily dose of vitamin B_6 to be superior to placebo, based on subjects' daily symptom records. This study, however, did not require prospective confirmation of premenstrual symptoms before subject selection. The third study supporting vitamin B_6 use was performed by Williams et al. (1985) in a placebo-controlled, double-blind manner. Results of this study were based on subjects' diary cards, which provided a record of the number of tablets taken and the severity of symptoms experienced. Subjects' compliance in completing these cards was low, with only half of all cards turned in, many of which were incomplete. Another complicating factor in the study was that a dose effect was evident, with improvement more likely as the number of tablets taken increased, regardless of the treatment given.

To sum up, evidence from studies of nutritional supplements suggests that only vitamin E and calcium hold any promise as treatments for premenstrual syndrome. There is, however, a need for replication of results in both cases, because each of these treatments was tested in only one study.

Diuretics. The use of diuretics in the treatment of PMS has been extensively studied. Table 14–13 lists the various diuretics included in this review. Although bromocriptine has been the focus of the majority of this research, its efficacy remains unclear. Bromocriptine is a dopamine agonist that has been proposed to exert its effects by inhibiting the release of prolactin and stimulating the excretion of electrolytes, causing diuresis (Kullander and Svanberg 1979). All but two of the eight bromocriptine studies described here were performed in a double-blind, crossover manner; the other two (Steiner et al. 1983; Ylostalo et al. 1982) were designed as placebo-controlled trials. In every study but that by Steiner et al. (1983), the medication dose ranged from 2.5 to 5.0 mg/day, and administration was limited to the luteal phase of each cycle. Results of studies by Andersen et al. (1977), Ghose and Coppen (1977), Kullander and Svanberg (1979), and Steiner et al. (1983) revealed no differences between bromocriptine and placebo. Studies by Andersch and Hahn (1982), Benedek-Jaszmann and Sturtevant (1976), Graham et al. (1978), and Ylostalo et al. (1982) produced mixed results, with only a few symptoms alleviated by the active treatment. Based on this information, it seems that, at best, bromocriptine is only partially effective at reducing the symptoms of PMS, most often exerting relief only for breast symptoms. This particular diuretic, then, holds little promise as a treatment for the full premenstrual syndrome.

Hoffman (1979) reported on the efficacy of ammonium chloride (1,950 mg/day) plus caffeine (600 mg/day), tested in a double-blind, crossover study. This study concentrated on weight gain as the primary symptom of interest. Diuretic was superior to placebo for reduction of premenstrual weight gain, but no mention was made regarding the relief of any mood or other physical symptoms. For the time being, then, this treatment may be considered effective for only a small part of the overall PMS symptomatology.

A double-blind, crossover study comparing chlorthalidone (25–50 mg/day), lithium carbonate (24 mg/day), and placebo was performed by Mattson and von Schoultz (1974). Prospective daily rating was not a part of this study; rather, women and their physicians made independent ratings of symptoms once during the luteal phase of each cycle. According to these ratings, all treatments improved all symptoms. In fact, more women preferred placebo than lithium or chlorthalidone. Another finding of interest was that the diuretic effect of lithium observed in this study was not seen when women took chlorthalidone, a well-known diuretic.

Metolazone in various doses was studied by Werch and Kane (1976). In this double-blind, crossover study, body weight was the primary outcome measure, but

Table 14–13. Diuretics

Reference	Treatment	Measures	Methods	Results
Hoffman 1979	Ammonium chloride + caffeine	Weight records, days 14–17, 18–23, and 24	22 women; 1,950 mg ammonium chloride + 600 mg caffeine or placebo daily on cycle days 18–24	Diuretic superior to placebo
Andersch and Hahn 1982	Bromocriptine	Plasma progesterone, prolactin; self-rating, physical symptoms	35 women; 2.5 mg bromocriptine daily for 3 mo or placebo daily for 1 mo, from symptom onset; blood samples in luteal phase of each cycle	Bromocriptine superior for reducing finger and leg swelling; no other differences
Andersen et al. 1977	Bromocriptine	Self-rating of symptoms; plasma progesterone, pro-lactin, and estradiol	21 women; 5.0 mg bromocriptine or placebo daily, from day of expected ovulation to menses onset; symptoms rated on cycle days 7–26	No difference between treatments
Benedek-Jaszmann and Sturte-vant 1976	Bromocriptine	Plasma prolactin, FSH, LH estradiol, and progesterone; urinary potassium, sodium, and creatinine	10 women; 5.0 mg bromocriptine or placebo daily for 1 cycle, from day 10 until menstruation	Bromocriptine superior for physical and mood symptoms; no effect on creatinine; increased sodium and potassium excretion
Ghose and Coppen 1977	Bromocriptine	MSQ	13 women; 1.5 mg bromocriptine or placebo daily, from 10 days before menses onset	No difference between treatments
Graham et al. 1978	Bromocriptine	Daily record of body weight, breast size, and basal body temperature; daily symptom rating	8 women; 2.5 mg bromocriptine daily, days 14–16, and 5.0 mg/day until menstruation, or placebo daily, for 2 mo	Bromocriptine improved bloating and psychiatric symptoms; no changes in other physical symptoms

Study	Drug	Measures	Design/dose	Results
Kullander and Svanberg 1979	Bromocriptine	Self-rating of symptoms; plasma estradiol, FSH, LH, progesterone, and prolactin	10 women; 5 mg bromocriptine or placebo daily, from day 14 until menstruation, for 2 mo	No treatment differences for symptom relief; bromocriptine reduced prolactin levels and increased FSH and LH
Steiner et al. 1983	Bromocriptine	VAS; MDQ; MAACL; STAI; HRSD Carroll Depression Scale	2.5 ($n = 8$), 5.0 ($n = 8$), or 7.5 ($n = 8$) mg bromocriptine or placebo ($n = 6$) daily for 3 consecutive mo; physician visits on days 9 and 26 of each mo	No difference between treatments
Ylostalo et al. 1982	Bromocriptine	Daily weight records; subject symptom ratings	2.5–5 mg bromocriptine or placebo ($n = 18$), or 5–10 mg norethisterone daily from day 12 to menses onset; placebo in cycles 1 and 4, active treatment in cycles 2 and 3	Bromocriptine superior to placebo and norethisterone, but norethisterone better tolerated
Mattsson and von Schoultz 1974	Lithium or chlorthalidone	Physician's symptom ratings; subject symptom ratings	18 women; 25 mg chlorthalidone daily in wk 1, then 50 mg daily, or placebo; 24 mEq/day in 2 premenstrual wk	No difference between treatments
Werch and Kane 1976	Metolazone	Body weight; self-rating of symptoms	1.0 ($n = 13$), 2.5 ($n = 15$), and 5.0 ($n = 5$) mg metolazone daily; excessive diuresis at 5-mg dose, so switched to a lower dose	Less weight gain in diuretic cycles; less water retention and negative affect as well
O'Brien et al. 1979	Spironolactone	PMI (luteal VAS–follicular VAS score)	18 women; 100 mg spironolactone or placebo daily on days 18–26 for at least 1 mo	Spironolactone superior to placebo on PMI

(continued)

Table 14–13. Diuretics (*continued*)

Reference	Treatment	Measures	Methods	Results
Vellacott et al. 1987	Spironolactone	Daily weight records; daily symptom records; plasma hormone levels; urinary aldosterone	100 mg spironolactone ($n = 31$) or placebo ($n = 32$) daily, from day 12 to menses onset, for 2 mo; blood sample on day 21 of each cycle	Spironolactone superior to placebo on many symptoms, but none reached significance; no other differences between treatments

Note. FSH = follicle-stimulating hormone. HRSD = Hamilton Rating Scale for Depression (Hamilton 1960). LH = luteinizing hormone. MAACL = Multiple Affect Adjective Check List (Zuckerman and Lubin 1965). MDQ = Menstrual Distress Questionnaire (Moos 1968). MSQ = Menstrual Symptom Questionnaire (Abraham 1980). PMI = Premenstrual Mood Index. STAI = State Trait Anxiety Inventory (Spielberger et al. 1970). VAS = visual analog scale. Carroll Depression Scale (Carroll et al. 1981).

Source. Reprinted from Rivera-Tovar A, Rhodes R, Pearlstein TB, et al.: "Treatment Efficacy," in *Premenstrual Dysphorias: Myths and Realities.* Edited by Gold JH, Severino SK. Washington, DC, American Psychiatric Press, 1994, pp. 114–116. Used with permission.

subjects ($N = 46$) also rated several other symptoms, both physical and affective. Once again, prospective ratings were not made on a daily basis; rather, symptoms were rated during bimonthly physician visits. At the end of treatment, subjects receiving metolazone at all doses showed significant improvement of symptoms when compared with placebo. In addition, the lower doses of metolazone seemed just as effective as the higher doses, but without side effects such as excessive diuresis and weakness.

The final diuretic discussed here is spironolactone, and the results of two studies of this drug are shown in Table 14–13. Both studies were conducted in a double-blind manner, with spironolactone (100 mg/day) or placebo administered during the luteal phase of each cycle. O'Brien et al. (1979) found spironolactone to be superior to placebo, based on a premenstrual mood index, calculated from daily visual analogue scales of symptom severity. Vellacott et al. (1987) found that, although spironolactone was generally better than placebo for relief of PMS symptoms, this relief failed to reach statistical significance for all symptoms but bloating.

It thus appears that diuretics in general should be considered as possible treatments for premenstrual bloating or weight gain, but there is little evidence of their efficacy for other PMS symptoms.

Psychopharmacological agents.   In recent years, several studies have examined the efficacy of psychopharmacological agents as treatments for PMS. Table 14–14 shows the various anxiolytics and antidepressants included in this review.

The anxiolytic alprazolam has been the focus of three recent studies in which treatment was administered only during the luteal phase of each cycle. Harrison et al. (1987, 1990) performed two double-blind, crossover studies of alprazolam at doses ranging from 0.25 to 4 mg/day. Smith et al. (1987) used a 0.75-mg/day alprazolam dose, also in a double-blind, crossover study. In all three studies, subject selection was based on at least 1 month of prospective symptom rating to confirm the diagnosis of PMS, and symptom rating was continued throughout the treatment phase. The results of these studies confirm the superiority of alprazolam over placebo for relief of PMS symptoms. Treatment in all cases was tapered off at the end of each month to avoid withdrawal symptoms.

Another anxiolytic found efficacious as a PMS treatment is buspirone. Treatment in a study by Rickels et al. (1989) was given only during the luteal phase of each menstrual cycle, as was done in the alprazolam studies. The medication dose in this placebo-controlled, double-blind study was 20 mg/day. Although buspirone seems promising for the treatment of PMS, more efficacy studies are necessary to support the findings discussed here.

Clomipramine is among the antidepressants that have been studied as a treatment for PMS. Details of a study by Eriksson et al. (1990) are shown in Table

Table 14–14. Psychopharmacologic agents

Reference	Treatment	Measures	Methods	Results
Harrison et al. 1987	Alprazolam	CGI; GAS	34 women; 0.25–4 mg alprazolam or placebo daily, from symptom onset to menses onset, for 3 mo, with tapering of drug	Alprazolam superior to placebo
Harrison et al. 1990	Alprazolam	CGI; GAS; DRF; PAF	30 women; 0.5–4 mg alprazolam or placebo daily from symptom onset to menses onset, for 3 mo, with tapering of drug; PAF completed at end of each cycle	Alprazolam superior to placebo
Smith et al. 1987	Alprazolam	Daily symptom diary	14 women; 0.75 mg alprazolam or placebo daily, from cycle day 20 through day 2 of menses, for 2 mo, with tapering of drug	Alprazolam superior to placebo
Rickels et al. 1989	Buspirone	Daily symptom diary	Placebo nonresponders assigned to 20 mg buspirone ($n = 17$) or placebo ($n = 17$) daily during last 12 days of cycle for 3 mo	Buspirone superior to placebo
Eriksson et al. 1990	Clomipramine	VAS; subject ratings	Placebo nonresponders ($n = 5$) given 25–50 mg clomipramine daily for 5 cycles; symptoms rated daily	Clomipramine superior to placebo
Rickels et al. 1990	Fluoxetine	Daily Symptom Rating Scale; HRSD	10 women; 1-mo rating, then 1 mo on placebo, and 20 mg fluoxetine daily for at least 2 mo; 10 women in placebo control group	Fluoxetine superior to placebo
Stone et al. 1991	Fluoxetine	DRF; GAS	20 mg fluoxetine ($n = 9$) or placebo ($n = 6$) daily for 2 mo; clinic visit in each luteal phase for GAS	Fluoxetine superior to placebo

Singer et al. 1974	Lithium	Global Clinical Scale; Target Symptoms Scale; self-rating scale	14 women; 750–1,000 mg lithium carbonate or placebo daily, with target blood level of drug of 0.8–1.3 mEq/L	No differences between treatments
Steiner et al. 1980b	Lithium	VAS; MDQ; MACL; STAI; CDS	15 women; 600–900 mg lithium carbonate daily, after a no-treatment baseline cycle	Efficacy of lithium not shown
Harrison et al. 1989	Nortriptyline	DRF; PAF; CGI	11 women; 50–125 mg nortriptyline daily, given to placebo nonresponders	Nortriptyline superior to placebo in 8 of 11 subjects

Note. CDS = Carroll Depression Scale (Carroll et al. 1981). CGI = Clinical Global Impressions Scale. DRF = Daily Rating Form (Endicott et al. 1986). GAS = Global Assessment Scale (Endicott et al 1976). HRSD = Hamilton Rating Scale for Depression (Hamilton 1960). MACL = Mood Adjective Checklist (Mackay et al. 1978). MDQ = Menstrual Distress Questionnaire (Moos 1968). PAF = Premenstrual Assessment Form (Endicott et al. 1986). STAI = State Trait Anxiety Inventory (Spielberger et al. 1970). VAS = visual analog scale.

Source. Reprinted from Rivera-Tovar A, Rhodes R, Pearlstein TB, et al.: "Treatment Efficacy," in *Premenstrual Dysphorias: Myths and Realities.* Edited by Gold JH, Severino SK. Washington, DC, American Psychiatric Press, 1994, pp. 119–120. Used with permission.

14–14. In this study, placebo responders were screened out, and nonresponders were treated with 25–50 mg clomipramine daily. Visual analogue scales of symptoms showed clomipramine to be superior to placebo for this dose range, which is lower than the dose generally used in the treatment of depression. Still, this study had only five subjects, making replication with a larger sample desirable. Side effects such as sedation, constipation, and dry mouth were reported, even at this relatively low clomipramine dose.

The results of two studies of fluoxetine, another antidepressant, are shown in Table 14–14. Both Rickels et al. (1990) and Stone et al. (1991) found a 20-mg/day dose of fluoxetine superior to placebo for PMS relief. Prospective ratings for at least 1 month were used in both studies as a means of selecting subjects who met DSM-III-R criteria for LLPDD. Although fluoxetine was found to be a beneficial treatment for PMS, some side effects (nausea, insomnia, headache, dizziness, nervousness, increased appetite, decreased libido) were noted.

Nortriptyline was the subject of one study by Harrison et al. (1989). Only subjects who showed no previous response to placebo and whose symptoms met DSM-III-R criteria for LLPDD for 2 months prior to treatment ($N = 11$) were selected for the study. Doses of 50–125 mg/day nortriptyline were found superior to placebo in 8 of the 11 women participating in the study. As is the case with other promising treatments, replication with a larger sample, possibly in a double-blind, crossover manner, is desirable.

Of all the psychopharmacological agents discussed here, only lithium has been shown to be ineffective as a treatment for PMS. Singer et al. (1974) and Steiner et al. (1980b) failed to show any benefit of lithium at doses ranging from 600 to 1,000 mg daily. Based on these findings and on the high frequency of side effects (nausea, tremor, dizziness), lithium is not recommended for the treatment of PMS.

In summary, it is evident that most of the anxiolytic and antidepressant agents discussed here have been beneficial as treatments for PMS. Only lithium has been shown ineffective for this purpose. There remains, however, a need for study replication for treatments such as buspirone, clomipramine, and nortriptyline.

Melatonin inhibition.   Table 14–15 lists studies of treatments intended to suppress melatonin secretion. Included in this group are bright light, atenolol, and propranolol.

Bright light has a tendency to suppress melatonin secretion in early evening, with a rebound later in the night, whereas atenolol and propranolol are β-adrenergic agonists that suppress melatonin secretion throughout the night. Parry et al. (1987) studied a 24-year-old woman who had a history of LLPDD only in fall and winter. As shown in Table 14–15, the subject underwent four different treatment trials: 1) phototherapy presented daily from 6:00 P.M. to 11:00 P.M. during luteal

Table 14–15. Melatonin inhibition

Reference	Treatment	Measures	Methods	Results
Rausch et al. 1988	Atenolol	MDQ; BDI; Steiner rating scale; HRSD; POMS	16 women; 2-mo symptom rating before treatment, with DSM-III-R criteria met; 50 mg atenolol or placebo daily from 10 days before menses, for 1 mo	Trend toward lower symptom scores on atenolol but not significant on most measures
Parry et al. 1987	Light, propranolol, or atenolol	HRSD; blood melatonin	1 woman; LLPDD in fall and winter; 4 trials: 1) 2,500 lux daily from symptom onset; 2) light plus placebo or melatonin (1.6 mg), or placebo alone; 3) propranolol (40 mg) or placebo, then 1 mo at half dose; 4) atenolol or placebo 1 mo each	All 3 forms of treatment superior to placebo
Parry et al. 1989	Light	HRSD; BDI; VAS	6 women; 2,500 lux, 2 h daily in morning and evening from 7 days before to menses onset, for 1 mo	Only evening light significantly improved symptoms

Note. BDI = Beck Depression Inventory (Beck et al. 1979). HRSD = Hamilton Rating Scale for Depression (Hamilton 1960). LLPDD = late luteal phase dysphoric disorder. MDQ = Menstrual Distress Questionnaire (Moos 1968). POMS = Profile of Mood States (McNair et al. 1971). VAS = visual analog scale. Steiner rating scale (Steiner et al. 1980a).

Source. Reprinted from Rivera-Tovar A, Rhodes R, Pearlstein TB, et al.: "Treatment Efficacy," in *Premenstrual Dysphorias: Myths and Realities.* Edited by Gold JH, Severino SK. Washington, DC, American Psychiatric Press, 1994, p. 123. Used with permission.

phase; 2) light plus placebo and then light plus melatonin, to determine whether melatonin would reverse the therapeutic effect of light; 3) propranolol (40 mg) or placebo nightly during the luteal phase, with a subsequent cycle of treatment at half the original dose; and 4) atenolol (50 mg/day) for 1 month followed by 1 month of placebo. All three active treatments were found beneficial in the relief of depressive symptoms occurring during the luteal phase.

A double-blind, crossover study of atenolol (50 mg/day) was performed by Rausch et al. (1988). The 16 women in the study were accepted only after meeting DSM-III-R criteria for LLPDD. Based on outcome measures including the MDQ (Moos 1968), the Profile of Mood States (McNair et al. 1971), the Beck Depression Inventory (Beck et al. 1979), and the Hamilton Rating Scale for Depression (Hamilton 1960), atenolol was beneficial for reduction of premenstrual symptomatology, although not all symptom improvement reached significance.

Finally, Parry et al. (1989) reported results of a randomized, crossover trial of morning versus evening light (2,500 lux). Six women met DSM-III-R criteria for LLPDD and entered the study. Light therapy was presented in 2-hour sessions during luteal phases, with Hamilton (1960) and Beck (1979) measures taken at the end of each luteal phase. Results of this study showed that, although there were no significant differences between morning and evening light therapy, the evening treatment was more promising, significantly improving Hamilton scores and nearly doing so for Beck scores.

The treatment of premenstrual syndrome by melatonin inhibition has shown some promise, as demonstrated in the three studies discussed here. One problem presented by the light studies is the lack of a placebo-control condition.

Miscellaneous treatments.   Several PMS treatments in this review were not appropriate for inclusion within the various categories discussed thus far. Many of these treatments have been supported by research and the details of these studies can be found in Table 14–16.

Clonidine, which decreases the amount of norepinephrine released at presynaptic sites, was studied by Giannini et al. (1988). This 4-month, double-blind, crossover study demonstrated the efficacy of a 17 mg/kg daily clonidine dose, based on luteal phase scores on the Brief Psychiatric Rating Scale (Overall and Gorham 1962). Although results were encouraging, the outcome measure tracked only psychiatric symptoms, and no mention was made of any physical symptom measure. Another complicating factor was selection of women with PMS symptoms, but no mention of any particular selection criteria. Further study, using more extensive outcome measures and appropriate selection criteria, is recommended if clonidine is to be considered a valid treatment for PMS.

Toth et al. (1988) studied the effects of an antibiotic, doxycycline, on symptoms

Table 14–16. Miscellaneous treatments

Reference	Treatment	Measures	Methods	Results
Giannini et al. 1988	Clonidine	Brief Psychiatric Rating Scale	24 women; 17 mg clonidine or placebo daily for 2 mo	Clonidine superior to placebo
Toth et al. 1988	Doxycycline	VAS; Menstrual Flow Questionnaire	1-mo baseline; 200 mg doxycycline ($n = 15$) or placebo ($n = 15$) daily for 2 mo; 6-mo follow-up visit	Doxycycline superior to placebo at 6-mo follow-up
Prior and Vigna 1987	Exercise	Menstrual Cycle Questionnaire	8 women in conditioning group, 6 women in sedentary control group. Studied normal menstrual symptoms	Exercise improved only physical symptoms
Gunston 1986	Mefenamic acid	Daily symptom checklist; subjective assessment	42 women; 1-mo baseline then 750 mg mefenamic acid or placebo daily, days 11–26, for 4 mo	Mefenamic acid superior to placebo according to subjective assessment
Jakubowicz et al. 1984	Mefenamic acid	Daily symptom checklist	80 women in open trial, 19 in double-blind, crossover study; 1,500–2,000 mg mefenamic acid or placebo daily	Mefenamic acid superior to placebo
Mira et al. 1986	Mefenamic acid	VAS (mood); questionnaire (physical)	15 women; 3-mo rating, then 1,000–2,000 mg mefenamic acid or placebo daily	Mefenamic acid superior for most symptoms
Wood and Jakubowicz 1980	Mefenamic acid	Daily symptom checklist; subjective performance	37 women; 1-mo baseline, then 1,500 mg mefenamic acid or placebo daily, from symptom onset for 1 mo	Mefenamic acid superior to placebo according to subjective reports
Chuong et al. 1988	Naltrexone	MDQ; basal body temperature; daily diary	20 women; 2 no-treatment cycles, then 50 mg naltrexone or placebo daily for 3 mo, followed by 1 mo of no treatment and 3 mo of alternative treatment	Naltrexone superior to placebo
Nikolai et al. 1990	L-Thyroxine	MSD	15 no-treatment control subjects and 44 PMS subjects; 2-mo rating, then PMS subjects given 1.6 μg/kg L-thyroxine or placebo for 2 mo	No differences between treatments

Note. MDQ = Menstrual Distress Questionnaire (Moos 1968). MSD = Menstrual Symptom Diary (Abraham 1980). VAS = visual analog scale. Brief Psychiatric Rating Scale (Overall and Gorham 1962). Menstrual Flow Questionnaire (Macleod Laboratory, New York Hospital–Cornell Medical Center).
Source. Reprinted from Rivera-Tovar A, Rhodes R, Pearlstein TB, et al.: "Treatment Efficacy," in *Premenstrual Dysphorias: Myths and Realities.* Edited by Gold JH, Severino SK. Washington, DC, American Psychiatric Press, 1994, p. 127. Used with permission.

of PMS. An infectious etiology was proposed for some PMS cases (subclinical endometrial or ovarian infection), and it was deemed possible that doxycycline could clear up such infections and relieve PMS symptoms. Women received 200 mg/day doxycycline (n = 15) or placebo (n = 15) for 2 months in this double-blind study. Based on visual analogue scale scores, doxycycline was significantly better than placebo at relieving PMS symptoms, even up to 6 months after treatment had ceased. Treatment of PMS with doxycycline, then, appears promising; but, once again, study replication is necessary.

Prior and Vigna (1987) have suggested that exercise may be an effective treatment for premenstrual syndrome, based on a prospective controlled study of the effect of conditioning exercise on normal menstrual symptomatology. Conditioning exercise consisted of running 3 or 4 days a week, with gradual increases of about 10% per week in mileage and intensity. Based on menstrual cycle questionnaire scores from days 2 to 5 of three cycles, exercise appeared efficacious for reduction of normal menstrual symptoms. In order for a study of this nature to be conducted with women having PMS, it is important that appropriate selection criteria and outcome measures be used. Unlike pharmaceutical studies, exercise trials cannot be performed in a double-blind manner, so environmental and other variables must be considered. Prior and Vigna stressed the need for documentation of the menstrual cycle, energy output of the exercise, and the nutritional changes and social interactions involved in both training and non-training groups in studies of this type.

Results of three double-blind, crossover studies and one double-blind, placebo-controlled trial of mefenamic acid are found in Table 14–16. This agent appears to act as a prostaglandin inhibitor in the relief of PMS. All four of the mefenamic acid studies agreed that this treatment was superior to placebo for relief of most PMS symptoms. Treatment in all cases was given in the luteal phase of each cycle, generally at symptom onset. Medication doses in the studies ranged from 750 mg/day (Gunston 1986) to 2,000 mg/day (Jakubowicz et al. 1984; Mira et al. 1986). In the two higher-dose studies, side effects such as nausea, skin rash, and diarrhea were reported. To sum up, mefenamic acid appears effective as a cyclically administered PMS treatment, even at half the 2,000-mg/day maximum dose used here.

In 1988, Chuong et al. reported the results of a double-blind, crossover study of naltrexone, a narcotic agonist that does not appear to have any addiction or withdrawal risks. Daily diaries and MDQ (Moos 1968) demonstrated the superiority of cyclic administration of naltrexone (50 mg/day) over placebo for symptom relief. Some side effects reported at this naltrexone dose were nausea, decreased appetite, and dizziness, which the authors have suggested may be reduced by decreasing or dividing the medication dose. Study replication, perhaps with a lower medication dose, is recommended in the case of this treatment.

Nikolai et al. (1990) performed a double-blind, placebo-controlled study of L-thyroxine as a possible treatment for PMS, following a suggestion that some form of thyroid hypofunction may be at least partly responsible for the appearance of PMS symptoms. After 2 months of treatment with either 1.6 µg/kg L-thyroxine (n = 22) or placebo (n = 22), Nikolai et al. found no benefit of L-thyroxine, as shown by Abraham's (1980) Menstrual Symptom Diary.

Overview summary.   Treatment efficacy studies could be used as validators for LLPDD in one of three ways: 1) treatments administered premenstrually, aimed at relieving only luteal phase symptoms; 2) continuous treatment with ovulation suppressors, eliminating the menstrual cycle; or 3) continuous treatment, often at a dose considered subtherapeutic for other disorders such as depression and anxiety. With these criteria, 21 of the 31 different PMS treatments could be considered to provide some evidence of the validity of the PMS diagnosis.

When administered in a cyclic fashion, treatments such as alprazolam, bromocriptine, buspirone, dydrogesterone and progesterone, light therapy, mefenamic acid, metolazone, naltrexone, and spironolactone were superior to placebo for relief of at least some premenstrual symptoms. Like other mood and anxiety disorders, PMS has been found to be responsive to a variety of interventions affecting multiple biological systems. The studies of alprazolam are of particular interest because this is a drug with high potential for the development of dependence and dose escalation, neither of which were observed in the studies discussed in this review. Furthermore, alprazolam appeared to provide relief from the full syndrome.

The most obvious group of validating studies concerned ovulation suppressors such as danazol, estradiol, buserelin, and oophorectomy. These treatments, by effectively halting the cyclic fluctuations in reproductive hormone levels, served to decrease or abolish severe premenstrual complaints.

One treatment that was effective at a relatively low dose was clomipramine, normally used in the treatment of depression. When used for premenstrual complaints, a low dose of clomipramine was significantly better than placebo. In addition, irritability, and *not* dysphoria, as might be expected, was the symptom most improved by clomipramine. Other continuous treatments that were effective were atenolol, calcium, clonidine, doxycycline, fluoxetine, and propranolol.

It should be noted that although nonpharmacological methods of PMS management have been reported, no published study has used a placebo control or suitable comparison condition. For this reason, nonpharmacological treatment studies have not generally been included in this review, with the exception of oophorectomy, exercise, and light therapy. There is also considerable discussion in the literature of oral contraceptives as a means of ameliorating both premenstrual and menstrual complaints. Again, no published studies could be found that in-cluded appropriate subject selection criteria, random assignment, or placebo controls.

Social, Forensic, and Occupational Issues

Psychiatric and other medical diagnostic entities are conceptualizations that arise out of social beliefs, needs, and contexts and have social implications ranging from access to care and insurance reimbursement to exemption from work, culpability, and exclusion from positions of responsibility (Kutchins and Kirk 1989). The LLPDD diagnosis would, by definition, be limited to one gender, and would be directly related to women's menstrual/reproductive function (Parlee 1980). These facts are, in themselves, neither positive nor negative. Most illnesses related to reproductive organs and functions are limited to one gender. Elucidation of a gender-related illness results in social advantages and disadvantages for diagnosed sufferers: legitimization and stigma.

The social context of the origin of premenstrual complaints consists of per-sonal and societal beliefs about gender and menstrually-related impairment (Loth-stein 1985), and its implications include all potentially positive and negative effects of official medical recognition of menstrually related impairment on the self-image, medical/psychiatric care, and social roles of women (Parlee 1980). This section addresses the issues raised at the beginning of this chapter from the social perspec-tive. Both the positive and negative potential social implications are considered in each case.

Data and criteria for the diagnosis.   The psychosocial meanings of menstruation and of female gender may cause serious methodological problems for studies of a late luteal phase disorder of mood. In many cultures (including ours), menstrual taboos are widely practiced and are associated with externally imposed limitations on women's activities, either at the time of each menstrual period or throughout the reproductive years. Taboos range from proscriptions on sexual intercourse to banishment to a "menstrual hut" outside regular living quarters for the duration of menses. Orthodox Judaism, traditionally and in modern America, requires that women attend a ritual communal bath, the "mikvah," after each period, to cleanse themselves of menstrual impurity before resuming sexual and even physical contact with their husbands (Reik 1964). Such practices raise a question: what is the effect of the monthly expectation of "pollution" and exclusion on women's subjective state and behavior? Are they causally associated with the resentment/anger, lability, dysphoria, and other symptoms reported premenstrually by some women?

Studies performed in the United States clearly indicate that both women and men expect women to experience negative changes in mood and behavior associated with the menstrual cycle, and during the premenstrual phase in particular. The attention accorded the putative syndrome was and continues to be associated with the appearance of a large number of articles in the popular press focusing on and reifying "premenstrual syndrome." New over-the-counter medications for this condition have been developed and marketed extensively. These social realities may demonstrate popular awareness of a real psychiatric problem, but they also complicate any attempt to gather data about psychiatric symptoms related to the menstrual cycle.

Socially defined gender roles and behaviors expected of men and women have also received considerable attention by scholars concerned with the social etiology and effects of premenstrual complaints (Parlee 1974). For example, women are expected to exhibit affect and change affect more easily than men. The distinction between affective responsiveness and "emotional lability," a DSM-III-R criterion for the LLPDD disorder, cannot be made with validity or reliability (Verbrugge 1979).

One exception to the expectation of emotional expression in women is anger. Displays of anger by men tend to be regarded as normative, even as evidence of strength and assertion, whereas women's anger is considered "masculine," pathological, and/or negative and is actively discouraged and suppressed by society. This view is held by women as well as men. Anger is a component of at least two of the criteria for LLPDD as published in the appendix of DSM-III-R. Should there be some cyclic variation of mood and response to events, and should that variability include anger, the anger will be perceived as symptomatic, which is to say negative and abnormal, by both men and women. The perception might hold regardless of the circumstances provoking the anger (Phillips 1989). Some writers have suggested that, given the circumstances (domestic violence, poverty, unsupported parenthood) of many women in our society, it is absence of anger that should be posited as abnormal and maladaptive rather than the reverse. Insofar as mood variability is perceived, it will also tend to be attributed to the menstrual cycle (Heilbrun 1989).

The attribution of symptoms or perceived impairment to the menstrual cycle is so pervasive in our society that the criteria for the diagnosis have had to undergo successive refinements (Abplanalp et al. 1980). Retrospective reports of premenstrual symptoms could not be confirmed by prospective data gathering. There are still only a small number of reports in the published literature using DSM-III-R criteria that include 2 months of prospective symptoms ratings (Christiansen 1986). Criteria for other DSM disorders do not require such lengthy symptom documentation. Few clinical and/or research subjects will comply with requirements for more than 2 months of ratings. The rigor of this requirement could be seen as discriminatory against those who suffer from the disorder (Spitzer et al. 1989). At the same time, however, this requirement is dictated by both the empirical findings of discrepancies between retrospective and prospective ratings and the attribution issues just discussed, and there is little evidence that even 2 months is sufficient to establish a menstrual-cycle–related disease. We have not examined studies, if any exist, that address the compliance of sufferers from more established disorders who are required to rate symptoms daily. It is not clear whether the difficulty is universal or whether it is particular to premenstrual complaints.

The tendency to attribute problems to, or even to perceive them as being related to, the menstrual cycle also complicates prospective rating systems, whether the ratings are done by the patient or by an outside observer. Both men and women in our society believe that women suffer from some degree of dysphoria and decreased function during the premenstruum and/or menses. Almost all studies have been performed on volunteers who believed themselves to suffer from PMS. In almost all studies, women have recorded their menstrual cycles and their physical and psychological symptoms on the same instruments. The research or clinical investigation serves strongly to reinforce the belief that symptoms and the menstrual cycle are related (Metcalf et al. 1989).

Studies of variations in mood and functioning over time that do not include explicit or implicit links to the menstrual cycle reveal very different patterns (Hamilton et al. 1989). Some studies demonstrate that men experience changes in state or mood that are as intense as those experienced by women, even if not in the same chronological pattern. Although attempts have been made, it is impossible to blind women to their menstrual cycle without eliminating it. For one thing, it is clear that there are cyclic physical changes and symptoms (Eckholm 1985). Women may become extremely sensitive to subtle manifestations as they progress through their reproductive years (Fisher et al. 1989; Wilson and Keye 1989).

If religious and cultural beliefs and taboos concerning menstruation occasioned so much psychological distress for women that they were disabled during the premenstrual phase, official professional recognition of this psychological disability might acknowledge suffering, focus attention on its social etiology, and facilitate the development of strategies to address the causes of the syndrome. However, imputation of the symptoms to a physiological, rather than a cultural, etiology might reinforce the taboos and stigma and undermine current efforts to foster cultural openness about menstruation and its acceptance as a natural and healthy process (Stewart 1989).

Prevalence and differentiation from other disorders.   The stipulation of prospective confirmation may disqualify many women who are convinced that they have the disorder. This raises two concerns. First, there are few psychiatric disorders that more people believe they have than can be confirmed. Many of the patients who present with the complaint of PMS, but are diagnosed with another psychiatric disorder, actively and forcefully refuse the appropriate diagnosis, even when there is specific, effective, and available treatment for it (Rapkin et al. 1989). This raises questions about the validity of the diagnosis, its differentiation from other psychiatric disorders, and the clinical implications of formalizing the more "desirable" diagnosis with a place in the official nomenclature. The second and related concern is the effect of exclusion from the diagnosis on subjectively symptomatic women.

Patients who have undergone hysterectomy without oophorectomy, and who therefore experience no menstrual bleeding, have been studied in an attempt to factor out subjects' knowledge of menstrual cycle phase, but a number of physical changes alert women to menstrual cycle phase (McEwen 1988). Hysterectomy could heighten their attention to these changes. When the hysterectomy is performed because of uterine pathology, the end of menstruation may be experienced as a loss of a valued feminine function, so that evidence of continued ovarian function assumes more importance.

Researchers in the field have struggled with the severity of change criteria for the symptoms comprising the defined disorder. Percentage change, absolute severity plotted on a scale, or any criterion is a more or less arbitrary imposition of a differentiation between normal and abnormal. This may be true for any disease. It is a particular issue for LLPDD because there are inconsistencies in the rating criteria used in different studies. It is contradictory to posit that symptoms must be limited to the late luteal phase and then to use a percentage change criterion. Patients with significant and persistent symptoms throughout the cycle would thus be included.

Placement of the disorder within the nomenclature.   Although some medical and psychiatric conditions are, by their nature, confined to one gender or the other, identifying a menstrually related psychiatric disorder as a free-standing entity or a special kind of affective disorder raises conceptual problems as well as related social problems (McCurdy-Myers and Caplan, unpublished observations). LLPDD, by definition, would be an illness related to a hormonal cycle (Youngs and Reame 1985). Because derangements of other hormones result in behavioral and affective symptoms as well, one may question the rationale for establishing as a psychiatric disease entity one hormonally related set of symptoms characteristic only of women. Male hormones have not been specifically singled out as etiological in disorders in which they may be implicated, such as those characterized by aggression.

There are other alternatives. Hormonally caused disorders could be classified as medical, rather than psychiatric, disorders. This would, however, contribute to the old notion that psychiatric disorders are limited to those without identifiable physical etiologies rather than being disorders whose signs and symptoms are those of cognition, mood, and behavior. A category of hormone-related psychiatric disorders could be established. Or hormonal and other physical contributors to psychiatric illnesses could be indicated by numbers after the decimal points in the diagnostic codes. This approach would be consistent with the finding that many patients who complain of PMS actually have mood disorders that may be worse premenstrually (Hamilton et al. 1989).

Social, forensic, and occupational risks of the diagnosis for women. Although the question concerning social, forensic, and occupational risks is framed in terms of negative implications of the diagnosis, positive implications for women might also exist. It is reassuring when a name and etiology for one's symptoms is identified. Specific treatments may be developed as research is facilitated by consensually accepted disease criteria.

Risks for women fall into two categories. The first is the risk that the establishment of a menstrually related psychiatric disorder poses for all women. It might confirm the cultural belief that menstruation causes disability and makes women less fit for positions of responsibility (although women, and even PMS sufferers, are generally considered fit for the demands of motherhood, accusations of "PMS" can be a factor in child-custody cases) (Dalton 1979; Mullen 1980). In the event that PMS as an official psychiatric diagnosis is used as a defense in criminal trials (it has been used but mostly unsuccessfully in recent years), the negative impact would be even more potent, with the menstrual cycle seen to dispose women to acts of violence and abuse (Chait 1986; Holtzman 1988).

A more subtle problem, but one that is perhaps more problematic for the field, is the impact of a narrowly defined LLPDD diagnosis on the majority of women who now present for treatment of PMS and who would be excluded (Reid 1987). A possible benefit is that the accurate etiologies of their complaints might be identified and specific treatment offered (Klerman 1990). However, it has already been demonstrated that many such women refuse and are offended by the diagnoses for which they qualify and, therefore, do not receive effective treatment for them. The inclusion of LLPDD in the psychiatric nomenclature would tempt treating clinicians to give patients this label they so desire. This misdiagnosis might compound the cultural belief that many women are psychiatrically disabled by the menstrual cycle and distort the gathering of information about the incidence of psychiatric illnesses.

Discussion

One of the more heated controversies during the preparation of DSM-III-R was whether to include LLPDD in the classification. Arguments for this diagnosis included the contention that LLPDD is a clinically significant condition supported by research and clinical literature and that its omission from DSM-III-R might result in underdiagnosis or misdiagnosis with failure to give appropriate treatment. Arguments against the inclusion of LLPDD in DSM-III-R included the relative paucity of the clinical and research literature, the possibility that it might encourage inappropriate diagnosis and treatment, and the potential for stigmatizing women. Additional questions were raised about whether this condition is best conceptualized as a mental disorder (as opposed to an endocrinological or gynecological disorder) and whether consideration should also be given to including disorders that may be related to male hormones (e.g., aggressiveness). After much discussion, the compromise solution for DSM-III-R was to include LLPDD in an appendix for categories needing further study, in the hope that this would encourage additional research. Indeed, this has clearly been the case, and the DSM-IV Work Group on LLPDD has benefited from an accumulating literature on this condition. Current discussions rely more heavily on the interpretation of empirical data than was previously possible.

The criteria for this proposed disorder, and the examination they are undergoing, are far more strict than those applied to the other DSM-IV diagnoses. Perhaps eventually a similarly rigorous procedure will be adopted for all mental disorders with resultant far-reaching scientific and treatment benefits.

Studies of signs and symptoms related to the menstrual cycle are complicated by methodological difficulties and social attributions, and these must be taken into account in evaluating the extent to which the existing literature provides evidence of a clinically useful and valid diagnosis. Studies using the DSM-III-R criteria for LLPDD have begun to appear in the psychiatric literature; however, a larger number of methodologically sound studies using these criteria would increase our confidence in both the utility and validity of the diagnosis. A data reanalysis of several large data sets on LLPDD has been conducted by this Work Group and will be reported in a later volume of the *DSM-IV Sourcebook*. The results suggest that optimal criteria for LLPDD differ only slightly from those proposed in the appendix of DSM-III-R (Hurt et al. 1992).

If research is to validate LLPDD, then many different questions must be addressed. Does LLPDD have a prevalence small enough not to be commonplace but not so small as to be trivial? Furthermore, if such a disorder exists, it must be found to have symptoms that are predominantly emotional and behavioral rather than physical. Other important validators must include course of the disorder, genetic factors, treatment response, and biological test results. Finally, it would be important to determine whether criteria can be developed that will not be misunderstood and misused.

The initial findings of the literature review and data reanalysis suggest the following about LLPDD: 1) unlike PMS, which has been reported in 20%–40% of menstruating women, approximately 5% of menstruating women might meet the criteria for LLPDD; 2) LLPDD is associated with clinically significant distress and functional impairment; 3) although the symptoms of LLPDD are not infrequently superimposed on other mental disorders, some women with no history of other mental disorders meet the criteria for LLPDD; 4) the items included in the DSM-III-R definition of LLPDD perform well with respect to sensitivity and specificity; 5) abnormalities in several biological systems (e.g., serotonin, melatonin, noradrenergic) have been associated with clinically significant premenstrual dysphoria; and 6) several different types of somatic treatment (e.g., ovulation suppressants, antidepressants, anxiolytics) show some promise of efficacy.

Stigma is associated with most mental disorders, and the ramifications of this stigma must be weighed against the consequences of failing to include the diagnosis, which would imply that the condition does not merit medical attention. Risks of undertreatment, overtreatment, and inappropriate treatment exist. There is concern for the effect that a diagnosis such as the proposed LLPDD might have on the general perception of women as being capable members of society. Discussion of this issue remains speculative and is based on women's treatment experiences with other complaints and on the myths and prejudices that surround menstruation. The potential occupational, social, and forensic risks of including such a diagnosis in the nomenclature are unknown.

Another issue is the choice of name. In DSM-III-R, the term *late luteal phase dysphoric disorder* was chosen in preference to the original term considered by the DSM-III-R committee *(premenstrual dysphoric disorder)* for two reasons: 1) to emphasize the distinction between this disorder and premenstrual syndrome (PMS), with its less severe and less specific premenstrual symptomatology; and 2) to include women with the disorder who no longer menstruate because of hysterectomy. The problems with the term *late luteal phase dysphoric disorder* are that it is cumbersome and is potentially misleading because the symptoms may not be exclusively related to the endocrine state of the late luteal phase. It has been suggested that the term *premenstrual dysphoric disorder* be substituted for *late luteal phase dysphoric disorder* in DSM-IV.

The Work Group continues to review and interpret the evidence on which it must base its recommendation about LLPDD in DSM-IV. There is accumulating, but preliminary, evidence that a disorder meeting the criteria for LLPDD as proposed in the DSM-III-R appendix does exist in a small number of women and is associated with significant functional impairment. However, there are many methodological problems in the research to date. Well-designed studies using the LLPDD criteria are just beginning to appear in the literature. There are several etiological leads in biological and treatment research but no consensus on the biological origins of the symptoms.

Recommendations

Several options have been proposed. Option 1 would be to continue to place the criteria set in an appendix and not to include this disorder in the official part of the classification. Option 2 is inclusion in the nomenclature. Option 3 reflects a view that, although this condition may be clinically significant, it is best not conceptualized as a mental disorder and would be included in the section for Other Clinically Significant Conditions That May Be a Focus of Diagnosis or Treatment. Option 4 is to omit this category from DSM-IV. Finally, if LLPDD is not included as a separate diagnosis in DSM-IV, it could be listed as an example in the mood disorder not otherwise specified and/or anxiety disorder not otherwise specified categories. At this point in the process, the Work Group has not completed its review of the full range of evidence to determine its recommendations.

References and Further Reading

General

American Psychiatric Association: Diagnostic and Statistical Manual of Mental Disorders, Third Edition, Revised. Washington, DC, American Psychiatric Association, 1987

Anderson M, Severino S, Hurt SW, et al: Premenstrual syndrome research: using the NIMH guidelines. J Clin Psychiatry 49:484–486, 1988

Asberg M, Perris C, Schalling D, et al: The CPRS: development and applications of a psychiatric rating scale. Acta Psychiatr Scand Suppl 271:1–69, 1978

Buss AH, Durkee A: An inventory for assessing different kinds of hostility. J Consult Clin Psychol 21:343–349, 1957

Campbell A, Converse PE, Rodgers WL: The Quality of American Life: Perceptions, Evaluations, and Satisfactions. New York, Russell Sage, 1976

Carroll BJ, Feinberg M, Smouse PE, et al: The Carroll Rating Scale for Depression, I: development, reliability and validation. Br J Psychiatry 138:194–200, 1981

Dalton K, Dalton M, Guthrie K: Incidence of the premenstrual syndrome in twins. BMJ 295:1027–1028, 1987

Endicott J: Current mental or other disorders found in women seeking treatment for "premenstrual problems." Paper submitted to the LLPDD Work Group, DSM-IV Task Force, 1989

Endicott J, Halbreich U: Retrospective report of premenstrual depressive changes: factors affecting confirmation by daily ratings. Psychopharmacol Bull 18:109–112, 1982

Evans DR, Burns JE, Robinson WE, et al: The Quality of Life Questionnaire: a multidimensional measure. Am J Community Psychol 13:305–310, 1985

Gallant SJ, Hamilton JA: On a premenstrual psychiatric diagnosis: what's in a name? Professional Psychol 19:271–278, 1988

Gallant SJ, Hamilton JA: Problematic aspects of diagnosing premenstrual phase dysphoria. Professional Psychol 20:60–68, 1990

Gallant SJ, Popiel DA, Hoffman DM: Using daily ratings to confirm PMS/LLPDD, I: effects of demand characteristics and expectations. Part II: what makes a real difference? Psychosom Med 54:149–166, 1992a

Gallant SJ, Popiel DA, Hoffman DM: Using daily ratings to confirm PMS/LLPDD, II: what makes a real difference? Psychosom Med 54:149–166, 1992b

Gise LH, Lebovits AH, Paddison PL, et al: Issues in the identification of premenstrual syndromes. J Nerv Ment Dis 178:228–234, 1990

Hamilton JA, Gallant SJ: Debate on late luteal phase dysphoric disorder (letter). Am J Psychiatry 147:1106, 1990

Haskett RF, Abplanalp JM: Premenstrual Tension Syndrome: diagnostic criteria and selection of research subjects. Psychiatry Res 9:125–138, 1983

Hurt SW, Schnoor PP, Severino FK, et al: LLPDD and six hundred seventy women evaluated for premenstrual complaints. Am J Psychiatry 149:525–530, 1992

Kantero RL, Widholm O: Gynecological findings in adolescence, II: the age of menarche in Finnish girls in 1969. Acta Obstet Gynecol Scand Suppl 14:7–18, 1971a

Kantero RL, Widholm O: A statistical analysis of the menstrual patterns of 8,000 Finnish girls and their mothers, IV: correlations of menstrual traits between adolescent girls and their mothers. Acta Obstet Gynecol Scand Suppl 14:30–36, 1971b

Mackay C, Cox T, Burrows G, et al: An inventory for the measurement of self-reported stress and arousal. Br J Soc Clin Psychol 17:282–284, 1978

McCurdy-Myers J, Caplan P: Is late luteal phase dysphoric disorder a legitimate diagnostic category, unpublished paper, 1990

Paddison PL, Gise LH, Lebovits AH, et al: Sexual abuse and premenstrual syndrome: comparison between a lower and higher socioeconomic group. Psychosomatics 31:265–272, 1990

Parlee MB: The premenstrual syndrome. Psychol Bull 80:454–465, 1973

Parry B: Biological differences in LLPDD research studies. Paper submitted to the LLPDD Work Group, DSM-IV Task Force, 1991

Rivera-Tovar AD, Frank E: Late luteal phase dysphoric disorder in young women. Am J Psychiatry 147:1634–1636, 1990

Rubinow DR, Schmidt PJ: Models for the development and expression of symptoms in premenstrual syndrome. Psychiatr Clin North Am 12:53–65, 1989

Schmidt PJ, Nieman LK, Grover GN, et al: Lack of effect of induced menses on symptoms in women with premenstrual syndrome. N Engl J Med 324:1174–1179, 1991

Severino SK, Moline ML: Premenstrual Syndrome: A Clinician's Guide. New York, Guilford, 1989

Severino SK, Hurt S, Schnurr P: Database Study Proposal for the LLPDD Work Group, DSM-IV Task Force, 1989

Severino SK, Wagner DR, Moline ML, et al: High nocturnal body temperature in premenstrual syndrome and late luteal phase dysphoric disorder. Am J Psychiatry 148:1329–1335, 1991

Spielberger CD, Gorsush RL, Lushene RE: State Trait Anxiety Inventory (STAI) Manual. Palo Alto, CA, Consulting Psychologists Press, 1970

Spitzer R, Severino S, Williams JBW, et al: Late luteal phase dysphoric disorder and DSM-III-R. Am J Psychiatry 146:892–897, 1989

Stotland N: Social, Psychoanalytic and Legal Implications of LLPDD, paper submitted to the LLPDD Work Group, DSM-IV Task Force, 1991

Van den Akker OB, Stern GS, Neale MC, et al: Genetic and environmental variations in menstrual cycle: histories of two British twin samples. Acta Genet Med Gemellol (Roma) 36:541–548, 1987

Zuckerman M, Lubin B: Manual for Multiple Affect Adjective Check List. San Diego, CA, Education and Industrial Testing Services, 1965

Differential Diagnosis and Comorbidity

Abramowitz ES, Baker AH, Fleiscler SF: Onset of depressive psychiatric crisis and the menstrual cycle. Am J Psychiatry 139:475–478, 1982

Bäckström T, Landgren S, Zetterland B, et al: Effects of ovarian steroid hormones on brain excitability and their relation to epilepsy seizure variation during the menstrual cycle, in Advances in Epileptology, Vol 15. Edited by Porter RJ, Mattson RH, Ward AA Jr, et al. New York, Raven, 1984, pp 269–277

Breier A, Charney DS, Henniger GR: Agoraphobia with panic attacks. Arch Gen Psychiatry 43:1029–1036, 1986

Brockington IF, Kelly A, Hall P, et al: Premenstrual relapse of puerperal psychosis. J Affect Disord 14:287–292, 1988

Endicott J, Spitzer RL, Fleiss JL, et al: The Global Assessment Scale: a procedure for measuring overall severity of psychiatric disturbance. Arch Gen Psychiatry 33:766–771, 1976

Endicott J, Halbreich U: Clinical significance of premenstrual dysphoric changes. J Clin Psychiatry 49:486–489, 1988

Friedman RC, Hurt SW, Charkin J, et al: Sexual histories and premenstrual affective syndrome in psychiatric inpatients. Am J Psychiatry 139:1484–1486, 1982

Gladis MM, Walsh BT: Premenstrual exacerbation of binge eating in bulimia. Psychiatry 144:1592–1595, 1987

Harrison WM, Endicott J, Nee J: Treatment of premenstrual depression with nortriptyline: a pilot study. J Clin Psychiatry 50:136–139, 1989a

Harrison WM, Endicott J, Nee J, et al: Characteristics of women seeking treatment for premenstrual syndrome. Psychosomatics 30:405–411, 1989b

Harrison WM, Sandberg D, Gorman J, et al: Provocation of panic with CO_2 inhalation in patients with premenstrual dysphoria. J Psychiatr Res 27:183–192, 1989c

Harrison WM, Endicott J, Nee J: Treatment of premenstrual dysphoria with alprazolam: a pilot study. Arch Gen Psychiatry 47:270–276, 1990

Hart WG, Russell JW: A prospective comparison study of premenstrual syndrome. Med J Aust 68:634–637, 1986

Hatotani N, Nishikubo M, Litayama I: Periodic psychosis in the female and the reproductive process, in Psychoneuroendocrinology in Reproduction. Edited by Zichella L, Pancheri P. New York, Elsevier/North-Holland, 1979, pp 55–68

Keye WR Jr, Hammend DC, Strong T: Medical and psychological characteristics of women presenting with premenstrual problems. Obstet Gynecol 68:634–637, 1986

Ling FW, Brown CS: Clinical phenomenology of PMS: implications for the physician in a nonpsychiatric specialty area (abstract book #40). Paper presented at the Fourth National Institute of Mental Health International Research Conference on the Classification and Treatment of Mental Disorders in General Medical Settings, Bethesda, MD, June 1990

Luggin R, Bernsted L, Peterson B, et al: Acute psychiatric admission related to the menstrual cycle. Acta Psychiatr Scand 69:461–465, 1984

Margus AL, Brincat M, Studd JWW: Trend analysis of the symptoms of 150 women with a history of premenstrual syndrome. Am J Obstet Gynecol 155:277–282, 1986

McMillan MJ, Pihl RO: Premenstrual depression: a distinct entity. J Abnorm Psychol 92:149–154, 1987

d'Orban PT, Dalton J: Violent crime and the menstrual cycle. Psychol Med 10:353–359, 1980

Parry BL, Berga SL, Mostofi N, et al: Morning versus evening bright light treatment of late luteal phase dysphoric disorder. Am J Psychiatry 146:1215–1217, 1989

Pearlstein TB, Frank E, Rivera-Tovar A, et al: Prevalence of Axis I and Axis II disorders in women with late luteal phase dysphoric disorder. J Affect Disord 20:129–134, 1990

Price MA, Torem MS, DiMarzio LR: Premenstrual exacerbation of bulimia. Psychosomatics 28:378–379, 1987

Rausch JL, Janowsky DS, Golshan S, et al: Antenol treatment of late luteal phase dysphoric disorder. J Affect Disord 15:141–147, 1988

Schnurr PP: Measuring amount of symptom change in the diagnosis of premenstrual syndrome psychological assessment. J Consult Clin Psychol 1:277–283, 1989

Severino SK, Hurt SW, Shindledecker RD: Late luteal phase dysphoric disorder: spectral analysis of cyclic symptoms. Am J Psychiatry 146:1155–1160, 1989

Slen WW: A note on menstruation and hospital admission date of intoxicated women. Biol Psychiatry 19:1133–1136, 1984

Stone AB, Pearlstein TB, Brown WA: Fluoxetine in the treatment of premenstrual syndrome. Psychopharmacol Bull 26:331–335, 1990

Stout AL, Steege JF: Psychological assessment of women seeking treatment for premenstrual assessment. J Psychosom Res 29:621–629, 1985

Watkins PC, Williamson DA, Falhowski C: Prospective assessment of late luteal phase dysphoric disorder. J Psychopathol Behav Assess 11:249–259, 1989

Weissman MM, Prusoff BA, Thompson WD, et al: Social adjustment by self-report in a community sample and in psychiatric outpatients. J Nerv Ment Dis 166:317–326, 1978

Psychotic Symptoms and LLPDD

Adland ML: Review, case studies, therapy, and interpretation of the acute exhaustive psychoses. Psychiatr Q 21:38–69, 1947

Altschule MD, Brem J: Periodic psychosis of puberty. Am J Psychiatry 119:1176–1178, 1963

Bell LV: On a new form of disease. Am J Insanity 6:97–127, 1849

Berlin FS, Bergey GK, Money J: Periodic psychosis of puberty: a case report. Am J Psychiatry 139:119–120, 1982

Billig O, Bradley JD: Combined shock and corpus luteum hormone therapy. Am J Psychiatry 102:783–787, 1945

Bleuler E: Textbook of Psychiatry (4th German ed.). Translated by Brill AA. New York, Macmillan, 1924

Blumberg MA, Billig O: Hormonal influence upon "puerperal psychosis" and "neurotic conditions." Psychiatr Q 16:454–462, 1942

Bower WH, Altschule MD: Use of progesterone in the treatment of post-partum psychosis. N Engl J Med 254:157–160, 1956

Brockington IF, Kelly A, Hall P, et al: Premenstrual relapse of puerperal psychosis. J Affect Disord 14:287–292, 1987

Bucknill JC, Tuke DH: Psychological Medicine. London, John Churchill, 1862

Cutting JC, Clare AW, Mann AH: Cycloid psychosis: an investigation of the diagnostic concept. Psychol Med 8:637–648, 1978

Dennerstein L, Judd F, Davies B: Psychosis and the menstrual cycle. Med J Aust 1:524–526, 1983

Endo M, Diaguji M, Asano Y, et al: Periodic psychosis recurring in association with menstrual cycle. J Clin Psychiatry 39:456–461, 465–466, 1978

Evans BD: Periodic insanity, in which the existing cause appears to be the menstrual function: report of a typical case. Med News 538, 1893

Felthous AR, Robinson DB: Oral contraceptive medication in prevention of psychotic exacerbations associated with phases of the menstrual cycle. J Preventive Psychiatry 1:5–15, 1981

Felthous AR, Robinson DB, Conroy RW: Prevention of recurrent menstrual psychosis by oral contraceptive. Am J Psychiatry 137:245–246, 1980

Gerada C, Reveley A: Schizophreniform psychosis associated with the menstrual cycle. Br J Psychiatry 152:700–702, 1988

Gjessing R: Disturbances of somatic functions in catatonia with a periodic course, and their compensation. Mental Science 84:608–621, 1938

Griesinger W: Mental Pathology and Therapeutics (2nd German ed.). London, New Sydenham Society, 1867

Hatotani N, Ishida C, Yura R, et al: Psychophysiological studies of typical psychosis: endocrinological aspects of periodic psychoses. Folia Psychiatrica et Neurologica Japonica 16:248–292, 1962

Hatotani N, Nishikubo M, Kitayama I: Periodic psychoses in the female and the reproductive process in psychoneuro-endocrinology, in Reproduction. Edited by Zichella L, Pancheri P. New York, Elsevier/North-Holland, 1979, pp 55–67

Hoch A: Benign Stupors: A Study of a New Manic-Depressive Reaction Type. New York, Macmillan, 1921

Janowsky DS, Gorney R, Kelley B: "The Curse": vicissitudes and variations of the female fertility cycle. Psychosomatics 7:242–247, 1966

Janowsky DS, Gorney R, Mandell AJ: The menstrual cycle. Arch Gen Psychiatry 17:459–469, 1967

Kasanin J: The acute schizoaffective psychoses. Am J Psychiatry 13:97–126, 1933

Keiser S: Severe reactive states and schizophrenia in adolescent girls. Nerv Child 4:17–25, 1944

Kempf EJ: Psychopathology. St. Louis, MO, Mosby, 1920

Kirby GH: The catatonic syndrome and its relation to manic-depressive insanity. J Nerv Ment Dis 40:694–704, 1913

Kraepelin E: Dementia Praecox and Paraphrenia (1903). Translated by Barclay RM. New York, Robert E Kreiger, 1971

Labbate LA, Shearer G, Waldrep DA: A case of recurrent premenstrual psychosis (letter). Am J Psychiatry 148:147, 1991

Langfeldt G: The prognosis in schizophrenia and the factors influencing the course of the disease. Acta Psychiatr Scand Suppl 13, 1937

Leetz KL, Rodenhauser P, Wheelock J: Medroxyprogesterone in the treatment of periodic menstrual psychosis. J Clin Psychiatry 49:372–373, 1988

Leonhard K: Cycloid psychoses: endogenous psychoses which are neither schizophrenic nor manic-depressive. J Ment Sci 107:633–648, 1961

Lingjaerde P, Bredland R: Hyperestrogenic cyclic psychosis. Acta Psychiatr Scand 29:355–364, 1954

Meduna LJ: Oneiroophrenia. Urbana, University of Illinois Press, 1950

Ota Y, Mukai T, Gotoda K: Study on the relationship between psychotic symptoms and sexual cycle. Folia Psychiatria et Neurologica Japonica 8:207–217, 1954

Perris C: Cycloid psychoses: historical background and nosology. Nord Psykiatr Tidsskr 27:369–378, 1973

Perris C: A study of cycloid psychosis. Acta Psychiatr Scand Suppl 253:1–77, 1974

Schmidt HJ: The use of progesterone in the treatment of postpartum psychosis. JAMA 121:190–192, 1943

Simpson GM, Radinger N, Rochlin D, et al: Enovid in the treatment of psychic disturbances associated with menstruation. Dis Nerv Syst 23:589–590, 1962

Simpson GM, Rochlin D, Kline NS: Further studies of enovid in the treatment of psychiatric patients. Dis Nerv Syst 25:484–486, 1964

Swanson DW, Barron A, Floren A, et al: The use of norethynodrel in psychotic females. Am J Psychiatry 1120:1101–1103, 1964

Takagi H: Periodic psychosis in preadolescence. Psychiatr Neurol Jpn 61:1194–1208, 1959

Teja JS: Periodic psychosis of puberty. J Nerv Ment Dis 162:52–57, 1976

Vaillant GE: An historical review of the remitting schizophrenia. J Nerv Ment Dis 138:48–56, 1964

Verghese A: The syndrome of premenstrual psychosis. Indian J Psychiatry 5:160–163, 1963

Wakoh T, Takekoshi A, Yoshimoto S, et al: Patho-physiological study of the periodic psychosis (atypical endogenous psychosis) with special reference to the comparison with chronic schizophrenia. Mie Medical Journal 10:317–340, 1960

Wenzel U: Periodishce Umdammerungen in der Pubertat. Arch fur Psychiatrie und Zeit-schrift f.d. ges Neurologie 201:133–150, 1960

Williams EY, Weekes LR: Premenstrual tension associated with psychotic episodes. J Nerv Ment Dis 116:321–329, 1952

Biological Studies

Abraham GE: Nutritional factors in the etiology of the premenstrual tension syndrome. J Reprod Med 28:446–464, 1983

Ashby CR, Carr LA, Cook CL, et al: Alteration of platelet serotonergic mechanisms and monoamine oxidase activity in premenstrual syndrome. Biol Psychiatry 24:225–233, 1988

Ashby CR, Carr LA, Cook CL, et al: Alteration of 5-HT uptake by plasma fractions in the premenstrual syndrome. J Neural Transm Gen Sect 79:41–50, 1990

Bäckström T, Smith S, Lothian H, et al: Prolonged follicular phase and depressed gonado-tropins following hysterectomy and corpus luteectomy in women with premenstrual tension syndrome. Clin Endocrinol (Oxf) 22:723–732, 1985

Beck AT, Rush AJ, Shaw ES, et al: Cognitive Therapy of Depression. New York, Guilford, 1979

Both-Orthman B, Rubinow DR, Hoban C, et al: Menstrual cycle phase-related changes in appetite in patients with premenstrual syndrome and in control subjects. Am J Psychiatry 145:628–631, 1988

Brayshaw ND, Brayshaw DD: Premenstrual syndrome and thyroid dysfunction. Integrative Psychiatry 5:179–193, 1987

Casper RF, Patel-Christopher A, Powell AM: Thyrotropin and prolactin response to thyrotropin-releasing hormone in premenstrual syndrome. J Clin Endocrinol Metab 68:608–612, 1989

Chuong CJ, Coulam CB, Kao PC, et al: Neuropeptide levels in premenstrual syndrome. Fertil Steril 44:760–765, 1985

Chuong CJ, Dawson EB, Smith ER: Vitamin A levels in premenstrual syndrome. Fertil Steril 54:643–647, 1990

DeLeon-Jones FA, Val E, Herts C: MHPG excretion and lithium treatment during premenstrual tension syndrome: a case report. Am J Psychiatry 139:950–952, 1982

Denicoff KD, Hoban C, Grover GW, et al: Glucose tolerance testing in women with premenstrual syndrome. Am J Psychiatry 147:477–480, 1990

Diamond MP, Simonson DC, De Fronzo RA: Menstrual cyclicity has a profound effect on glucose homeostasis. Fertil Steril 52:204–208, 1989

Endicott J, Spitzer RL: A diagnostic interview: the Schedule for Affective Disorders and Schizophrenia. Arch Gen Psychiatry 35:837–844, 1978

Endicott J, Nee J, Cohen J, et al: Premenstrual changes: patterns and correlates of daily ratings. J Affect Disord 10:127–135, 1986

Facchinetti F, Martignoni E, Petraglia F, et al: Premenstrual fall of plasma β-endorphin in patients with premenstrual syndrome. Fertil Steril 47:570–573, 1987

Giannini et al: B-endorphin related symptoms in late luteal disorder. APA Abstract, New Research 227, May 1989

Halbreich U, Endicott J, Goldstein S, et al: Premenstrual changes and changes in gonadal hormones. Acta Psychiatr Scand 74:576–586, 1986

Hamilton M: A rating scale for depression. J Neurol Neurosurg Psychiatry 23:56–62, 1960

Hammarbäck S, Damber JE, Bäckström T, et al: Relationship between symptom severity and hormone changes in women with premenstrual syndrome. J Clin Endocrinol Metab 68:125–130, 1989

Harrison WM, Sandberg D, Gorman JM, et al: Provocation of panic with carbon dioxide inhalation in patients with premenstrual dysphoria. Psychiatry Res 27:183–192, 1989

Haskett RF, Steiner M, Carroll BJ: A psychoendocrine study of premenstrual tension syndrome. J Affect Disord 6:191–199, 1984

Hathaway SR, McKinley JC: Minnesota Multiphasic Personality Inventory. Minneapolis, University of Minnesota, 1970

Jakubowicz DL, Godard E, Dewhurst J: The treatment of premenstrual tension with mefenamic acid: analysis of prostaglandin concentrations. Br J Obstet Gynaecol 91:78–84, 1984

Lee KA, Shaver JF, Giblin EC, et al: Sleep patterns related to menstrual cycle phase and premenstrual affective symptoms. Sleep 13:403–409, 1990

Malmgren R, Collins A, Milsson CG: Platelet serotonin uptake and effects of vitamin B_6 treatment in premenstrual tension. Neuropsychobiology 18:83–88, 1987

Mauri M, Reid RL, MacLean AW: Sleep in the premenstrual phase: a self-report study of PMS patients and normal controls. Acta Psychiatr Scand 78:82–86, 1988

McNair DM, Lorr M, Pruppleman LF: Profile of Mood States. San Diego, CA, Educational and Industrial Testing Service, 1971

Mira M, Steward PM, Abraham SF: Vitamin and trace element status in premenstrual syndrome. Am J Clin Nutr 47:636–641, 1988

Moos RH: The development of a menstrual distress questionnaire. Psychosom Med 30:853–867, 1968

Nikolai TF, Mulligan GM, Gribble RK, et al: Thyroid function and treatment in premenstrual syndrome. J Clin Endocrinol Metab 70:1108–1113, 1990

Parry BL, Mendelson WB, Duncan WC, et al: Longitudinal sleep EEG temperature and activity measurements across the menstrual cycle in patients with premenstrual depression and in age-matched controls. Psychiatry Res 30:285–303, 1989

Parry BL, Berga SL, Kripke DF, et al: Altered waveform of plasma nocturnal melatonin secretion in premenstrual depression. Arch Gen Psychiatry 47:1139–1146, 1990

Parry BL, Gerner RH, Wilkins JN, et al: CSF and neuroendocrine studies of premenstrual syndrome. Neuropsychopharmacology 5:127–137, 1991

Rapkin AJ, Edelmuth E, Chang LC, et al: Whole-blood serotonin in premenstrual syndrome. Obstet Gynecol 70:533–537, 1987

Reid RL, Greenaway-Coates A, Hahn PM, et al: Oral glucose tolerance during the menstrual cycle in normal women and women with alleged premenstrual "hypoglycemic" attacks: effects of naloxone. J Clin Endocrinol Metab 62:1167–1172, 1986

Rojansky N, Halbreich U: Prevalence and severity of premenstrual changes after tubal sterilization. J Reprod Med 36:551–555, 1991

Rojansky N, Halbreich U, Zander K, et al: Imipramine receptor binding and serotonin uptake in platelets of women with premenstrual changes. Gynecol Obstet Invest 31:146–152, 1991

Roy-Byrne PP, Rubinow DR, Qwirtsman H, et al: Cortisol response to dexamethasone in women with premenstrual syndrome. Neuropsychobiology 16:61–63, 1986

Roy-Byrne PP, Rubinow DR, Hoban C, et al: TSH and prolactin responses to TRH in patients with premenstrual syndrome. Am J Psychiatry 144:480–484, 1987

Rubinow DR, Hoban G, Grover GN, et al: Changes in plasma hormones across the menstrual cycle in patients with menstrually related mood disorders and in control subjects. Am J Obstet Gynecol 158:5–11, 1988

Schrijver J, Louwerse ES, Bruinse HW, et al: Increased urinary MHPG excretion in premenstrual syndrome (PMS): the effect of vitamin B_6. Journal of Psychosomatic Obstetrics and Gynaecology 6:179–186, 1987

Spielberger CD, Gorsuch RL, Lushene RE: STAI Manual. Palo Alto, CA, Consulting Psychologists Press, 1970

Steiner M, Haskett RF, Carroll BJ: Premenstrual tension syndrome: the development of research diagnostic criteria and new rating scales. Acta Psychiatr Scand 62:177–190, 1980

Steiner M, Haskett RF, Carroll BJ: Circadian hormone secretory profiles in women with severe premenstrual tension syndrome. Br J Obstet Gynaecol 91:466–471, 1984

Taylor DL, Matthew RJ, Ho BT, et al: Serotonin levels and platelet uptake during premenstrual tension. Neuropsychobiology 12:16–18, 1984

Tulenheimo A, Laatkainen T, Salminen K: Plasma β-endorphin immunoreactivity in premenstrual tension. Br J Obstet Gynaecol 94:26–29, 1987

Van den Akker D, Steptoe D: Psychophysiological responses in women reporting severe premenstrual symptoms. Psychosom Med 51:319–328, 1989

Varma TR: Hormones and electrolytes in premenstrual syndrome. Int J Gynaecol Obstet 22:51–58, 1984

Watts JFF, Butt WR, Edwards LR, et al: Hormonal studies on women with premenstrual tension. Br J Obstet Gynaecol 92:247–255, 1985

Webb WB, Bonnet M, Blume G: A post-sleep inventory. Percept Mot Skills 43:987–993, 1976

Ying YK, Soto-Albors CE, Randolph JS, et al: Luteal phase defect and premenstrual syndrome in an infertile population. Obstet Gynecol 69:96–98, 1987

Treatment Efficacy

Abraham GE: Premenstrual tension. Current Problems in Obstetrics and Gynecology 3:3–39, 1980

Abraham GE, Hargrove JT: Effect of vitamin B_6 on premenstrual symptomatology in women with premenstrual tension syndromes: a double blind crossover study. Infertility 3:155–165, 1980

Andersch B, Hahn L: Bromocriptine and premenstrual tension: a clinical and hormonal study. Pharmatherapeutica 3:107–113, 1982

Andersch B, Hahn L: Progesterone treatment of premenstrual tension: a double-blind study. J Psychosom Res 29:489–493, 1985

Andersen AN, Larsen JF, Steenstrup OR, et al: Effect of bromocriptine on the premenstrual syndrome: a double-blind clinical trial. Br J Obstet Gynecol 84:370–374, 1977

Bancroft J, Boyle H, Warner P, et al: The use of an LHRH agonist, buserelin, in the long-term management of premenstrual syndromes. Clin Endocrinol 27:171–182, 1987

Barr W: Pyridoxine supplements in the premenstrual syndrome. Practitioner 228:425–427, 1984

Beck AT, Rush AJ, Shaw ES, et al: Cognitive Therapy of Depression. New York, Guilford, 1979

Benedek-Jaszmann LJ, Sturtevant H: Premenstrual tension and functional infertility: etiology and treatment. Lancet 1:1095–1098, 1976

Brush MSG: Abnormal essential fatty acid levels in plasma in women with PMS. Am J Obstet Gynecol 150:363–364, 1984

Callender K, McGregor M, Kirk P, et al: A double-blind trial of evening primrose oil in the premenstrual syndrome: nervous symptom subgroup. Human Psychopharmacology Clinical and Experimental 3:57–61, 1988

Casper RF, Hearn MT: The effect of hysterectomy and bilateral oophorectomy in women with severe premenstrual syndrome. Am J Obstet Gynecol 162:105–109, 1990

Casson P, Hahn PM, Van Vugt DA, et al: Lasting response to ovariectomy in severe intractable premenstrual syndrome. Am J Obstet Gynecol 162:99–105, 1990

Chakmakjian ZH, Higgins CE, Abraham GE: The effect of a nutritional supplement, Optivite for Women, on premenstrual tension syndromes, II: effect on symptomatology, using a double blind cross-over design. J Appl Nutr 37:12–17, 1985

Chuong C, Coulam C, Bergstralh E, et al: Clinical trial of naltrexone in premenstrual syndrome. Obstet Gynecol 72:332–336, 1988

Dennerstein L, Spencer-Gardner C, Gotts G, et al: Progesterone and the premenstrual syndrome: a double-blind crossover trial. BMJ 290:1617–1621, 1985

Dennerstein L, Morse C, Gotts G, et al: Treatment of premenstrual syndrome: a double-blind trial of dydrogesterone. J Affect Disord 11:199–205, 1986

Eriksson E, Lisjo P, Sundblad C, et al: Effect of clomipramine on premenstrual syndrome. Acta Psychiatr Scand 81:87–88, 1990

Freeman E, Rickels K, Sondheimer S, et al: Ineffectiveness of progesterone suppository treatment for premenstrual syndrome. JAMA 264:349–353, 1990

Ghose K, Coppen A: Bromocriptine and premenstrual syndrome: controlled study. BMJ 1:147–148, 1977

Giannini AJ, Sullivan B, Sarachene J, et al: Clonidine in the treatment of premenstrual syndrome: a subgroup study. J Clin Psychiatry 49:62–63, 1988

Gilmore DH, Hawthorn RJS, Hart D: Danol for premenstrual syndrome: a preliminary report of a placebo-controlled double-blind study. J Int Med Res 13:129–130, 1985

Graham JJ, Harding PE, Wise PH, et al: Prolactin suppression in the treatment of premenstrual syndrome. Med J Aust 2:18–20, 1978

Gunston KD: Premenstrual syndrome in Cape Town, II: a double-blind placebo-controlled study of the efficacy of mefenamic acid. S Afr Med J 70:159–160, 1986

Hagen I, Nesheim B, Tuntland T: No effect of vitamin B6 against premenstrual tension: a controlled clinical study. Acta Obstet Gynecol Scand 64:667–670, 1985

Hamilton M: A rating scale for depression. J Neurol Neurosurg Psychiatry 23:56–62, 1960

Hammarbäck S, Bäckström T: Induced anovulation as treatment of premenstrual tension syndrome: a double-blind crossover study with GnRH-agonist versus placebo. Acta Obstet Gynecol Scand 67:159–166, 1988

Harrison WM, Endicott J, Rabkin JG, et al: Treatment of premenstrual dysphoric changes: clinical outcome and methodological implications. Psychopharmacol Bull 20:118–122, 1984

Harrison WM, Endicott J, Rabkin JG, et al: Treatment of premenstrual dysphoria with alprazolam and placebo. Psychopharmacol Bull 23:150–153, 1987

Harrison WM, Endicott J, Nee JC: Treatment of premenstrual depression with nortriptyline: a pilot study. J Clin Psychiatry 50:136–139, 1989

Harrison WM, Endicott J, Nee JC: Treatment of premenstrual dysphoria with alprazolam: a controlled study. Arch Gen Psychiatry 47:270–275, 1990

Hoffman JJ: A double-blind crossover clinical trial of an OTC diuretic in the treatment of premenstrual tension and weight gain. Current Therapeutic Research 26:575–580, 1979

Jakubowicz D, Godard E, Dewhurst J: The treatment of premenstrual tension with mefenamic acid: analysis of prostaglandin concentrations. Br J Obstet Gynecol 91:78–84, 1984

Jordheim O: The premenstrual syndrome. Acta Obstet Gynecol Scand 51:77–80, 1972

Kendall KE, Schnurr PP: The effects of vitamin B6 supplementation on premenstrual symptoms. Obstet Gynecol 70:145–149, 1987

Kerr G, Day J, Munday M, et al: Dydrogesterone in the treatment of the premenstrual syndrome. Practitioner 224:852–855, 1980

Khoo SK, Munro C, Battistutta D: Evening primrose oil and treatment of premenstrual syndrome. Med J Aust 153:189–192, 1990

Kullander S, Svanberg L: Bromocriptine treatment of the premenstrual syndrome. Acta Obstet Gynecol Scand 58:375–378, 1979

London RS, Murphy L, Kitlowski KE, et al: Efficacy of alpha-tocopherol in the treatment of the premenstrual syndrome. J Reprod Med 32:400–404, 1987

Maddocks S, Hahn P, Moller F, et al: A double-blind placebo-controlled trial of progesterone vaginal suppositories in the treatment of premenstrual syndrome. Am J Obstet Gynecol 154:573–581, 1986

Magos L, Brincat M, Studd JW: Treatment of the premenstrual syndrome by subcutaneous estradiol implants and cyclical oral norethisterone: placebo controlled study. BMJ 292:1629–1633, 1986

Malmgren R, Collins A, Nilsson C: Platelet serotonin uptake and effects of vitamin B6 treatment in premenstrual tension. Neuropsychobiology 18:83–88, 1987

Mattsson B, von Schoultz B: A comparison between lithium, placebo, and a diuretic in premenstrual tension. Acta Psychiatr Scand Suppl 255:75–84, 1974

McNair DM, Lorr M, Droppleman LF: EDITs Manual for the Profile of Mood States. San Diego, CA, Educational and Industrial Testing Service, 1971

Mira M, McNeil D, Fraser I, et al: Mefenamic acid in the treatment of premenstrual syndrome. Obstet Gynecol 68:395–398, 1986

Moos RH: The development of a menstrual distress questionnaire. Psychosom Med 30:853–867, 1968

Muse K, Cetel N, Futterman L, et al: The premenstrual syndrome: effects of "medical ovariectomy." N Engl J Med 311:1345–1349, 1984

Nikolai TF, Mulligan GM, Gribble RK, et al: Thyroid function and treatment in premenstrual syndrome. J Clin Endocrinol Metab 70:1108–1113, 1990

O'Brien PMS, Craven D, Selby C, Symonds EM: Treatment of premenstrual syndrome by spironolactone. Br J Obstet Gynecol 86:142–147, 1979

Overall JE, Gorham DR: The Brief Psychiatric Rating Scale. Psychol Rep 10:799–812, 1962

Parry B, Rosenthal N, Tamarkin L, et al: Treatment of a patient with seasonal premenstrual syndrome. Am J Psychiatry 144:762–766, 1987

Parry BL, Berga SL, Mostofi N, et al: Morning versus evening bright light treatment of late luteal phase dysphoric disorder. Am J Psychiatry 146:1215–1217, 1989

Prior J, Vigna Y: Conditioning exercise and premenstrual symptoms. J Reprod Med 32:423–428, 1987

Rausch JL, Janowsky DS, Golshan S, et al: Antenolol treatment of late luteal phase dysphoric disorder. J Affect Disord 15:141–147, 1988

Reid RL: Premenstrual syndrome, in Current Problems in Obstetrics and Gynecology. Edited by Leventhal JM, Hoffman JJ, Keith LG, et al. Chicago, IL, Year Book Medical, 1985, pp 1–57

Richter M, Haltvick R, Shapiro S: Progesterone treatment of premenstrual syndrome. Current Therapeutic Research 36:840–850, 1984

Rickels K, Freeman E, Sondheimer S: Buspirone in treatment of premenstrual syndrome (letter). Lancet 1:777, 1989

Rickels K, Freeman E, Sondheimer S, et al: Fluoxetine in the treatment of premenstrual syndrome. Current Therapeutic Research 48:161–166, 1990

Sampson G: Premenstrual syndrome: a double-blind controlled trial of progesterone and placebo. Br J Psychiatry 135:209–215, 1979

Sampson GA, Heathcote PR, Wordsworth J, et al: Premenstrual syndrome: a double-blind cross-over study of treatment with dydrogesterone and placebo. Br J Psychiatry 153:232–235, 1988

Sarno AP, Miller EJ, Lundblad EG: Premenstrual syndrome: beneficial effects of periodic, low-dose danazol. Obstet Gynecol 70:33–36, 1987

Singer K, Cheng R, Schou M: A controlled evaluation of lithium in the premenstrual tension syndrome. Br J Psychiatry 124:50–51, 1974

Smith S, Rinehart JS, Ruddock VE, et al: Treatment of premenstrual syndrome with alprazolam: results of a double-blind, placebo-controlled, randomized crossover clinical trial. Obstet Gynecol 70:37–43, 1987

Steiner M, Haskett RF, Carroll B: Premenstrual tension syndrome: the development of research diagnostic criteria and new rating scales. Acta Psychiatrica Academica 62:117–190, 1980a

Steiner M, Haskett R, Osmun J, et al: Treatment of premenstrual tension with lithium carbonate. Acta Psychiatr Scand 61:96–102, 1980b

Steiner M, Haskett RF, Osmun JN, et al: The treatment of severe premenstrual dysphoria with bromocriptine. Journal of Psychosomatic Obstetrics and Gynecology 2:223–227, 1983

Stephenson MJ, Milner R, Lamont J, et al: Treatment of premenstrual syndrome with oil of evening primrose: a randomized controlled trial. Proceedings of the 16th Annual Meeting of the North American Primary Care Research Group, Ottawa, Ontario, Canada, 1988

Stewart A: Clinical and biochemical effects of nutritional supplementation on the premenstrual syndrome. J Reprod Med 32:435–441, 1987

Stone AB, Pearlstein TB, Brown WA: Fluoxetine in the treatment of premenstrual syndrome. Psychopharmacology Bull 26:331–335, 1990

Stone AB, Pearlstein TB, Brown WA: Fluoxetine in the treatment of late luteal phase dysphoric disorder. J Clin Psychiatry 152:290–293 , 1991

Thys-Jacobs S, Ceccarelli S, Bierman A, et al: Calcium supplementation in premenstrual syndrome: a randomized crossover trial. J Gen Intern Med 4:183–189, 1989

Toth A, Lesser M, Naus G, et al: Effect of doxycycline on premenstrual syndrome: a double-blind randomized clinical trial. J Int Med Res 16:270–279, 1988

van der Meer YG, Benedek-Jaszmann LJ, van Loenen AC: Effect of high-dose progesterone on the premenstrual syndrome: a double-blind cross-over trial. Journal of Psychosomatic Obstetrics and Gynecology 2–4:220–222, 1983

Vellacott ID, Shroff NE, Pearce MY, et al: A double-blind, placebo-controlled evaluation of spironolactone in the premenstrual syndrome. Curr Med Res Opin 10:450–456, 1987

Watson NR, Savas M, Studd JWW, et al: Treatment of severe premenstrual syndrome with oestradiol patches and cyclical oral norethisterone. Lancet 2:730–732, 1989

Watts JF, Edwards RL, Butt WR: Treatment of premenstrual syndrome using danazol: preliminary report of a placebo-controlled, double-blind, dose ranging study. J Int Med Res 13:127–128, 1985

Watts JF, Butt WR, Edwards RL: A clinical trial using danazol for the treatment of premenstrual tension. Br J Obstet Gynecol 94:30–34, 1987

Werch A, Kane R: Treatment of premenstrual tension with metolazone: a double-blind evaluation of a new diuretic. Current Therapeutic Research 19:565–572, 1976

Williams MJ, Harris R, Dean B: Controlled trial of pyridoxine in the premenstrual syndrome. J Int Med Res 13:174–179, 1985

Wood C, Jakubowicz D: The treatment of premenstrual syndromes with mefenamic acid. Br J Obstet Gynecol 87:627–630, 1980

Ylostalo P, Kauppila A, Poulakka J, et al: Bromocriptine and norethisterone in the treatment of premenstrual syndrome. Obstet Gynecol 59:292–297, 1982

Social, Forensic, and Occupational Findings

Abplanalp J, Haskett RF, Rose RM: The premenstrual syndrome. Advances in Psychoneuroendocrinology 3:327–347, 1980

American Psychiatric Association: Diagnostic and Statistical Manual of Mental Disorders, 3rd Edition, Revised. Washington, DC, American Psychiatric Association, 1987

Brooks J, Ruble D, Clark A: College women's attitudes and expectations concerning menstrual-related changes. Psychosom Med 98:288–298, 1977

Chait LR: Premenstrual syndrome and our sisters in crime: a feminist dilemma. Women's Rights Law Reporter 9:267–293, 1986

Christiansen D: Correlates of confirmed premenstrual dysphoria. J Psychosom Res 33:307–313, 1986

Dalton K: Once a Month. Pomona, CA, Hunter House, 1979

Eckholm E: Premenstrual problems seem to beset baboons. The New York Times, June 4, 1985, p C2

Fisher M, Trieller K, Napolitano B: Premenstrual symptoms in adolescents. Journal of Adolescent Health Care 10:369–375, 1989

Hamilton JA, Gallant SA: On a premenstrual psychiatric diagnosis: what's in a name? Prof Psychol 198:271–278, 1988

Hamilton JA, Gallant SA, Lloyd C: Evidence for a menstrual-linked artifact in determining rates of depression. J Nerv Ment Dis 177:359–365, 1989

Harrison W, Endicott J: Characteristics of women seeking treatment for PMS. Psychosomatics 30:405–411, 1989

Heilbrun AB Jr, Frank ME: Self-preoccupation and general stress level as sensitizing factors in premenstrual and menstrual distress. J Psychosom Res 33:571–577, 1989

Holtzman E: Premenstrual syndrome as a legal defense, in The Premenstrual Syndromes. Edited by Gise LH, Kase NG, Berkowitz RL. New York, Churchill Livingstone, 1988, pp 137–143

Klerman GL: The psychiatric patient's right to effective treatment: implications of Osheroff v. Chestnut Lodge. Am J Psychiatry 147:409–427, 1990

Koeske RK, Koeske GF: An attributional approach to moods and the menstrual cycle. J Pers Soc Psychol 31:473–478, 1975

Kutchins J, Kirk SA: DSM-III-R: the conflict over new psychiatric diagnoses. Health Soc Work 14:91–101, 1989

Lothstein LM: Female sexuality and feminine development: Freud and his legacy. Adv Psychosom Med 12:57–70, 1985

McCurdy-Myers J, Caplan P: Is late luteal phase dysphoric disorder a legitimate diagnostic category? (unpublished paper)

McEwen BS: Basic research perspective: ovarian hormone influence on brain neurochemical functions, in The Premenstrual Syndromes. Edited by Gise LH, Kase NG, Berkowitz RL. New York, Churchill Livingston, 1988, pp 21–33

Metcalf MG, Livesey JH, Wells JE, et al: Mood cyclicity in women with and without the premenstrual syndrome. J Psychosom Res 33:407–418, 1989

Mullen PD: Once a month. Women Health 5:84–85, 1980

Norden MJ: Fluoxetine in borderline personality disorder. Prog Neuro-Psychopharmacol Biol Psychiatr 13:885–893, 1989

Osofsky HJ, Blumenthal S (eds): Premenstrual Syndrome: Current Findings and Future Directions. Washington, DC, American Psychiatric Press, 1985

Parlee MB: The premenstrual syndrome. Psychol Bull 30:454–465, 1973

Parlee MB: Stereotypic beliefs about menstruation: a methodological note on the Moos Menstrual Distress Questionnaire and some new data. Psychosom Med 36:229–240, 1974

Parlee MB: Social and emotional aspects of menstruation, birth, and menopause, in Psychosomatic Obstetrics and Gynecology. Edited by Youngs DD, Ehrhardt AA. New York, Appleton-Century-Crofts, 1980, pp 67–79

Phillips JW: Caffeine and premenstrual syndrome (letter to editor). American Journal of Public Health 79:1680, 1989

Rapkin AJ, Chang LC, Reading AE: Mood and cognitive style in premenstrual syndrome. Obstet Gynecol 74:644–649, 1989

Reid RL: Premenstrual syndrome. AACC ENDO 5:1–12, 1987

Reik T: Pagan Rites in Judaism. New York, Farrar Strauss, 1964

Ruble DN: Premenstrual symptoms: a reinterpretation. Science 197:291–292, 1977

Scully D, Bart P: A funny thing happened on the way to the orifice: women in gynecology textbooks, in Changing Women in a Changing Society. Edited by Huber J. Chicago, IL, University of Chicago Press, 1973, pp 283–288

Smith S, Schiff I: The premenstrual syndrome: diagnosis and management. Fertil Steril 52:527–543, 1989

Spitzer RL, Severino SK, Williams JBW, et al: Late luteal dysphoric disorder and DSM-III-R. Am J Psychiatry 146:892–897, 1989

Stewart DE: Positive changes in the premenstrual period. Acta Psychiatr Scand 79:400–405, 1989

Verbrugge LM: Female illness rates and Illness behavior. Women Health 4:61–79, 1979

Wilson CA, Keye WR: A survey of adolescent dysmenorrhea and premenstrual symptom frequency: a model program for prevention, detection and treatment. Journal of Adolescent Health Care 10:317–322, 1989

Youngs DD, Reame N: Psychoendocrinology and the menstrual cycle, psychosomatic obstetrics and gynecology. Adv Psychosom Med 12:25–34, 1985

Section III

Anxiety Disorders

Introduction to Section III

Anxiety Disorders

Michael R. Liebowitz, M.D.

This chapter is an introduction to the work of the Anxiety Disorders Work Group. The Work Group consisted of Michael R. Liebowitz, M.D. (chairperson of the Work Group and head of the Social Phobia sub-Work Group); David H. Barlow, Ph.D. (vice-chairperson and head of the Specific Phobia, Generalized Anxiety Disorder, and Mixed Anxiety and Depression sub-Work Groups); James C. Ballenger, M.D. (cohead of the Panic Disorder/Agoraphobia sub-Work Group); Jonathan Davidson, M.D. (cohead of the Posttraumatic Stress Disorder sub-Work Group); Edna B. Foa, Ph.D. (head of the Obsessive-Compulsive Disorder and cohead of the Posttraumatic Stress Disorder sub-Work Groups); and Abby J. Fyer, M.D. (cohead of the Panic Disorder/Agoraphobia sub-Work Group).

The Work Group, in conjunction with an internationally renowned group of collaborators who functioned as members of sub-Work Groups or advisers, was responsible for considering issues and criteria for panic disorder with and without agoraphobia, agoraphobia without a history of panic disorder, social phobia, simple phobia, obsessive-compulsive disorder (OCD), posttraumatic stress disorder (PTSD), generalized anxiety disorder (GAD), and mixed anxiety and depression. We followed the standard format for DSM-IV, which involved a conservative attitude toward change, seeking compatibility with ICD-10 (World Health Organization 1990) wherever possible and basing revisions on empirical data from literature reviews, reanalyses of existing databases, and field trials. Inconsistencies, gaps, and illogicalities in DSM-III-R (American Psychiatric Association 1987) were also clarified wherever possible. Data from reanalyses of existing studies and field trials are not yet available and will be considered in later volumes of the *Sourcebook*. The comments in this introductory chapter are based on the deliberations of the Anxiety Disorders Work Group and the DSM-IV Task Force to date and especially on information gathered in the very extensive and numerous literature reviews conducted by members of the sub-Work Groups, which are presented in integrated form by disorder in the chapters that follow in this section.

General Issues for the Anxiety Disorders Section

In DSM-III-R, panic attacks were described in the section on panic disorder, despite the implicit assumption that they could occur with other anxiety disorders as well, and that only unexpected panic attacks were specific to panic disorder. For purposes of clarity, it is proposed to state this explicitly in DSM-IV, and to define panic attacks separately at the beginning of the Anxiety Disorders section before describing any of the specific disorders.

With regard to the definition of a panic attack, DSM-III-R specified that panic attack symptoms develop suddenly and increase in intensity within 10 minutes of the first C symptom noticed in the attack. As a clarification, DSM-IV proposes that panic attack symptoms develop abruptly and reach a crescendo within 1020minutes. It is thought that this better captures the crescendo-like nature of panic attacks.

In addition, review of the literature suggested that subtypes of panic attacks (unexpected, situationally bound, and situationally predisposed) could be defined on the basis of when the attacks occur in relation to entering feared situations. Unexpected panic attacks are not associated with situational triggers, and are prototypical of panic disorder. Situationally bound panic attacks are exclusively associated with situational triggers and predictably occur almost immediately on exposure to those situations or objects; they are prototypical of social and specific phobias. Situationally predisposed panic attacks are more likely to occur on exposure to certain situational triggers but are variable in the frequency and timing with which they occur. They tend to be associated with panic disorder with agoraphobia but not exclusively.

Panic Disorder Without Agoraphobia, Panic Disorder With Agoraphobia, Agoraphobia Without a History of Panic Disorder

The principal areas focused on for DSM-IV were threshold, cognitive, and boundary issues (see Ballenger and Fyer, Chapter 15, this volume).

A major issue for panic disorder in DSM-IV was to find empirical support for the minimum number of symptoms required for a panic attack and for the minimum number of attacks (and/or type of associated cognitions) needed to define panic disorder. In DSM-III (American Psychiatric Association 1980) and DSM-III-R, these were arrived at principally by expert consensus. Review of the literature suggested that a minimum threshold of four symptoms probably most reliably and validly defines a panic attack but that the existing database was too sparse to firmly support this conclusion. In particular, some patients describe limited symptom attacks characterized by fewer than four symptoms that are otherwise similar to unexpected panic attacks in nature and sequelae.

The second threshold issue involved the number of panic attacks and associated features necessary to meet criteria for panic disorder. DSM-III-R required four attacks (one of which must be unexpected) in 4 weeks, or one or more attacks followed by at least a month of persistent worry about having another attack. Review of the existing literature revealed that requiring four panic attacks in 4 weeks might be overly restrictive because of clinical and community reports of suffering and disability on the part of those with "infrequent panic" (i.e., individuals who have panic attacks, some of which are unexpected, who fail to meet this frequency criteria). However, the literature did not suggest an alternative fixed number of panic attacks that could better serve as a minimum threshold. Therefore, the alternative option of recurrent unexpected panic attacks is being considered, subject to evaluation in a field trial.

With regard to the other threshold (i.e., one panic attack plus a month of worry), it was felt that the worry criterion could possibly be expanded to more accurately reflect the full range of fears experienced by individuals who have a panic attack. Specifically, review of the literature suggested that three cognitions are typically present in panic attacks and between attacks in panic disorder. These are of physical catastrophe, loss of control, and social embarrassment. However, it was felt that such cognitions might not always be identifiable in routine clinical practice. Thus, the proposed alternative to worry about having another panic attack is a month or more of persistent concern about having additional panic attacks *or* worry about the implications of the attack or its consequences (e.g., losing control, having a heart attack, "going crazy"). To heighten diagnostic precision and facilitate the differential diagnosis from other anxiety disorders, it is proposed that this worry criterion must be met in addition to the criterion requiring recurrent unexpected panic attacks.

With regard to the boundaries between panic disorder and agoraphobia and social and simple phobias, the literature reviews and Work Group deliberations revealed that, whereas prototypical cases were easy to distinguish, it was very difficult to define criteria that clearly demarcated the boundaries. In the end, it seemed most realistic to leave the differential diagnosis to clinical judgment. In the criteria for panic disorder, it is proposed to add "The anxiety or phobic avoidance is not better accounted for by another mental disorder such as . . . social phobia." As a guide, the criteria would also contain "Consider the diagnosis of specific phobia when the avoidance is limited to a few specific situations or social phobia when the avoidance is limited to social situations."

To promote adoption of a single international set of criteria, the ICD-10 definition of agoraphobia is considered for DSM-IV as an alternative to a modified DSM-III-R definition. This would read "an interrelated and overlapping cluster of phobias involving fears of characteristic situations." However, no data from the existing literature were found to evaluate this alternative.

Other issues evaluated in the panic disorder/agoraphobia literature reviews included the relationship of panic disorder to cardiac complaints, irritable bowel symptoms, and alcohol abuse; the potential role of laboratory provocations of panic in routine clinical practice; and the relationship of agoraphobia to panic attacks. It was concluded that the extensive overlap between cardiac complaints and panic disorder makes it very important to educate primary care physicians about panic disorder. With regard to irritable bowel syndrome, greater attention to its possible overlap with panic disorder is needed. The same is true for alcohol abuse and panic disorder, with recognition that alcohol withdrawal can be confused with panic disorder unless the patient is reevaluated after a suitable time for acute withdrawal has elapsed.

Review of the literature suggested that laboratory provocations of panic attacks with such agents as sodium lactate or carbon dioxide have been important research tools but are not yet considered to have demonstrated sufficient sensitivity and specificity to be employed clinically.

Finally, although it is proposed that agoraphobia without a history of panic attacks continues to be included in DSM-IV because community studies continue to record such cases, it is rarely seen in studies of clinical samples. As discussed in the Panic Disorder chapter, the reasons for this discrepancy are not yet clear. What does seem clear is that among patients with panic disorder and agoraphobia, the agoraphobia usually follows the panic attacks and is subsequently mediated by the expectation of panicking in particular situations.

Specific Phobias

The principal issues for the specific phobias (see Craske et al., Chapter 16, this volume) were the boundaries with panic disorder/agoraphobia and the possible existence of subtypes. The recommendation was also made to change the diagnostic label from simple to specific phobias to improve definitional clarity and achieve conformity with ICD-10.

The literature review revealed that it was difficult to define a clear boundary between specific phobias and panic disorder/agoraphobia. Overall, the reviews found that cued fear, anxiety, or panic is the essence of a specific phobia, as opposed to unexpected (uncued) panics and fear of such panic attacks in panic disorder. Some controversy arose, however, in applying this principle to certain specific situational phobias (driving, flying, heights, bridges, enclosed spaces, tunnels). One review done by the Specific Phobia group concluded that the mode of onset should determine the boundary between specific phobia and agoraphobia. The recommendation was that any situational phobia for which the onset of fear and avoidance was due to an unexpected panic attack in a situation about which the person had not previously been anxious (this was modified to additionally include one or more unexpected panic attacks outside the phobic situation on the basis of Epidemiologic Catchment Area [ECA] reanalyses) should be viewed as a mild form of agoraphobia, whereas situational phobias with other modes of onset would be classified as specific phobias. This view was not adopted for DSM-IV, however, because it conflicted with the findings of the agoraphobia reviews, which recommended that either the DSM-III-R or the ICD-10 (or both) definitions of agoraphobia be used. Both of these definitions of agoraphobia exclude fears of single situations no matter what their origin.

To incorporate these findings, the criteria for specific phobia are reworded to emphasize the immediate and predictable relationship between the phobic stimulus and the anxiety response, in contrast to unexpected panic attacks, which do not always occur immediately on being exposed to a feared situation or even with every exposure to that situation. However, the criteria also include the feature "The anxiety or phobic avoidance is not better accounted for by another mental disorder, such as . . . Panic Disorder With Agoraphobia (e.g., fear of having unexpected panic attacks) or Agoraphobia Without History of Panic Disorder" to emphasize that clinical judgment must also play a role in the differential diagnosis.

The literature review also supported the subdivision of specific phobia into several subtypes, including natural environment type (e.g., animals, insects, storms, and water); blood, injection, injury type; situational type (e.g., cars, planes, heights, elevators, and tunnels/bridges); and other type (e.g., phobic avoidance of situations that may lead to choking, vomiting, or contracting an illness). Blood injection phobias were found to differ from other types of specific phobias in several ways, including age at onset, family concordance, and frequent association with fainting. Individuals with situational phobias differed from those with animal phobias in having a later age at onset, greater probability of an unexpected panic attack as the trigger, and a greater likelihood of a familial history of situational than animal phobia (and the reverse for probands with animal phobias). Choking phobia also seemed to have clearly identifiable features, although it was unclear whether it was prevalent enough to warrant classification as a distinct subtype.

Another issue reviewed by the Work Group was the relationship of illness phobia to hypochondriasis. The review of the literature suggested that disease conviction (fear or belief of having a disease) was more consistent with hypochondriasis, whereas exaggerated illness fears without disease conviction (fear of getting a disease) were consistent with a diagnosis of specific phobia. Some patients with OCD also have exaggerated fears of getting diseases, but compulsive rituals are present as well.

The Work Group also reviewed the literature on the relationship of phobias induced by traumatic events to PTSD. They recommend that phobia of a circumscribed object or situation that develops following a traumatic stressor (sufficient to meet criterion A of PTSD) should be considered a specific phobia unless full PTSD criteria are met. A PTSD type of syndrome that develops after exposure to a subtraumatic stressor (insufficient to meet criterion A of PTSD) would not meet the DSM-III-R definition of PTSD.

Social Phobia

The principal issues regarding social phobia were subtypes, relationship to avoidant personality disorder and to avoidant disorder of childhood or adolescence, boundaries with panic disorder and agoraphobia, and whether social anxiety and/or avoidance secondary to an Axis III condition should automatically be excluded from social phobia.

Social phobia was originally conceptualized by Marks (1970) as encompassing excessive anxiety and/or avoidance of a broad range of social, interactional, and performance situations, all linked by the common theme of excessive concern with scrutiny and evaluation by others. DSM-III established criteria for social phobia but defined it narrowly to approximate performance anxiety, relegating more generalized social fears to avoidant personality disorder. DSM-III-R defined social phobia more broadly and established the subtype of generalized social phobia to designate individuals who feared most social situations. As discussed in the chapter on social phobia (Schneier et al., Chapter 17, this volume), review of the literature revealed some empirical support for this dichotomy in terms of pharmacological responsivity, responses during laboratory challenge, and so on; however, it was felt that it might be possible to portray nongeneralized social phobia with greater precision if two subtypes in addition to generalized social phobia were delineated: performance type for pure performance anxiety and limited interactional type for difficulties in one or two but not most social situations. These subclassification systems are being compared for validity and reliability via reanalyses of existing data sets.

In DSM-III, avoidant personality disorder was an exclusion for social phobia. This was dropped in DSM-III-R, at the same time that avoidant personality disorder criteria were changed to become more interpersonally focused. The result, as revealed by the literature review, is that there is now substantial overlap between social phobia, particularly its generalized form, and avoidant personality disorder. However, although we believe that demonstrations of the efficacy of pharmacological and cognitive behavioral treatment argue for social phobia being the more useful designation in cases of overlap, sufficiently convincing data to validate narrowing the definition of, or eliminating, avoidant personality disorder to do away with the overlap with social phobia are lacking.

Social phobia may also overlap extensively with avoidant disorder of childhood or adolescence. Child researchers and clinicians report that avoidant disorder is used in lieu of social phobia to diagnose children and adolescents, because in DSM-III-R it is an exclusion for social phobia. An overall principle of DSM-IV is that continuity between child and adult diagnoses is desirable whenever possible. To this end, an option for DSM-IV is to drop avoidant disorder of childhood and adolescence and to amplify the criteria and text for social phobia to make them fully suitable for children and adolescents.

With regard to the boundary of social phobia and panic disorder, DSM-III-R excluded social or performance anxiety/avoidance secondary to fear of having a panic attack from social phobia. Individuals with social phobia can have panic attacks; what DSM-III-R meant to exclude from social phobia, but did not explicitly say, was fear of an *unexpected* panic attack. In addition, some patients can have unexpected panic attacks that lead to performance or social avoidance, at which time they would not be called social phobic. However, the unexpected panic attacks may subside, but the social or performance anxiety/avoidance persist. At this time, taking a cross-sectional rather than historical perspective, social phobia might be the most clinically appropriate diagnosis. Overall, it was thought best to leave the differential diagnosis to clinical judgment by including the following statement in the criteria for social phobia: "The fear and avoidance is not better accounted for by Panic Disorder With Agoraphobia." The reasons social phobia should be differentiated from panic disorder are covered in detail in the literature review summary (see Schneier et al., Chapter 17). In essence, not to differentiate them would blur the boundaries between two disorders that seem pathophysiologically distinct.

An important issue that remains to be fully resolved is whether social anxiety/avoidance secondary to medical conditions such as tremors, stuttering, and burns or scars should continue to be completely excluded from social phobia, as it is now in DSM-III-R. No empirical basis for this exclusion was found in the literature review. Three options are therefore being considered for DSM-IV. The first is to drop the exclusion entirely, which would include in social phobia seriously disfigured or medically impaired individuals whose level of social anxiety or avoidance, although extensive, may not be excessive for their condition. This might greatly inflate the prevalence of social phobia. We may also currently lack the data to fully evaluate this as an option. The second option is to continue the blanket exclusion, which carries the liability that individuals with secondary social phobia who would benefit from recognition and treatment as social phobic patients will not receive them. The third option is to expand social phobia to include individuals with medical disabilities whose social anxiety or avoidance exceeds what is generally expected with that level of medical disability, reasoning that such individuals have some tendency toward excessive concerns with evaluation or scrutiny by others. The difficulty with this option is the possible unreliability involved in determining when social anxiety is excessive for a given medical disability or problem. These options are being studied as far as possible through data reanalyses. If the data suggest that some change from DSM-III-R is indicated but are insufficient to delineate which option to choose, it may be advisable to maintain the DSM-III-R exclusion in DSM-IV but include social phobia secondary to medical conditions as an example of an anxiety disorder not otherwise specified and as a candidate diagnosis in need of further study in the appendix. This will serve to raise clinical awareness and stimulate further research.

Other issues examined in the literature reviews for social phobia include delineation of the boundaries of social phobia with substance use disorders, shyness, and test anxiety; determination of whether physiological and biochemical characteristics could help define social phobia; and consideration of cross-cultural aspects in the definition of the disorder.

Given the frequent co-occurrence of substance abuse and social phobia, the literature review concluded that the importance of making the differential diagnosis should be mentioned in the text or criteria. It is proposed that the statement that the fear and avoidance (of social phobia) is not due to a substance-induced anxiety disorder (e.g., alcohol withdrawal) be included in DSM-IV. The data also suggest that some patients with substance abuse require additional treatment for comorbid social phobia.

The literature review found that *shyness* overlaps with social phobia but is a larger, more inclusive, and less well-defined term. Test anxiety also appears on review to bear many similarities to social phobia, and it was recommended that it be included as an example of social phobia in the text or the criteria.

Review of the physiological and biochemical literature on social phobia found that current data are insufficient to be incorporated meaningfully into DSM-IV criteria. However, physiological data do support the existence of social phobic subtypes, and biochemical findings do support the differentiation of social phobia from panic disorder.

Cross-cultural studies reveal that social phobia is not a culture-bound syndrome, although cultural conditions can affect its prevalence. Studies in Japan and Korea suggest that social phobia may have a delusional variant there, but this needs further study before DSM criteria are amended.

Obsessive-Compulsive Disorder

The principal issues concerning OCD included the definition and relationship of obsessions and compulsions; the issue of senselessness; the boundaries with worry, hypochondriasis, and body dysmorphic disorder; and the possibility of OCD subtypes (see Foa et al., Chapter 18, this volume).

After close study of the DSM-III-R criteria for OCD, the Work Group found a certain contradiction in the definition of obsessions and compulsions. Obsessions were defined as 1) "recurrent and persistent ideas, thoughts, impulses, or images that are experienced, at least initially, as intrusive and senseless;" and 2) "the person attempts to ignore or suppress such thoughts or impulses or to neutralize them with some other thought or action" (p. 247). The acts listed under 2 are generally thought to be compulsions performed in response to the obsession. However, the DSM-III-R definition of compulsions states that they are behaviors, leaving in limbo the classification of mental acts carried out in response to obsessions. Are they mental compulsions, or further obsessions? The DSM-IV Work Group felt that such mental acts (counting, magical thinking, etc.) function as compulsions and are handled in behavior therapy in a manner similar to how behavioral compulsions such as hand washing or checking are handled. The DSM-IV definition of compulsions was therefore amended to include such mental acts that function to reduce the distress from obsessions.

The DSM-III-R criteria required that obsessions be experienced, at least initially, as senseless. The review of the literature revealed that OCD patients seem to fall on a continuum with regard to how senseless they consider their obsessions and that requiring all obsessions to meet a standard of senselessness would exclude some otherwise appropriate patients from the OCD category. For this reason, for DSM-IV, the Work Group is considering substituting the term *ego-dystonic*. This would have a broader connotation (i.e., that the obsessions were not experienced as voluntarily produced but rather as thoughts that invaded consciousness and were experienced as senseless or repugnant).

The Work Group reviewed the literature comparing worry and obsessions to see whether there was any blurring of the boundary between GAD and OCD. They concluded that obsessions tended to focus on different themes than worry (dirt/contamination, religion, sex, and aggression rather than the more real-life problems of family, money, and work) and that worry was less intrusive or ego-dystonic. Therefore, to sharpen the boundary between OCD and GAD, it is proposed that the OCD criteria include the feature "the thoughts, impulses, or images are not simply excessive worries about real-life problems."

The boundary between OCD and hypochondriasis was also reviewed. A potential for overlap was discerned; some OCD patients present with primarily somatic obsessions, which might meet criteria for hypochondriasis, whereas some hypochondriacal patients also have checking compulsions related to their illness fears and might meet criteria for OCD. However, no study has actually focused on how many patients meet criteria for both disorders. This area was felt to need further study, and no immediate suggestions were made for the DSM-IV OCD criteria.

The similarities of body dysmorphic disorder (BDD) and OCD were also highlighted by the literature review. Although the evidence was considered insufficient to warrant reclassifying BDD as a subtype of OCD, it was felt that the similarities should be mentioned in the text for OCD.

Two proposals for subtyping OCD are included in the *DSM-IV Options Book* (American Psychiatric Association 1991). The first has three levels based on degree of insight: with insight, if a person recognizes that the obsessions and compulsions are excessive and unreasonable; with overvalued ideas, if the person maintains that the obsessions and compulsions are not unreasonable or excessive but acknowledges the validity of contrary evidence; and with delusions, if delusions about the content of the obsessions or compulsions are a prominent feature. The literature review found that these distinctions were comprehensible but expressed concern that they were not sufficiently clear to be of diagnostic utility. The review noted that senselessness of obsessions and compulsions was most appropriately conceptualized as a continuum ranging from full recognition of the unreasonableness of the obsessions and compulsions to delusional conviction about them. This subtyping schema was included in the *Options Book* as one way to reflect the range of senselessness with which OCD can be associated.

The second subtyping option for OCD is the ICD-10 schema of predominantly obsessions, predominantly compulsions, and mixed type. It was felt that clinical observation offered some validation for these subtypes, but no systematic studies were found that have examined the issue. It was included as an option to be tested in the DSM-IV OCD field trial.

Posttraumatic Stress Disorder

Literature reviews of PTSD covered a variety of issues, including definition of the stressor, cohesiveness of symptomatology across victim groups, where PTSD should be placed in DSM-IV, the diagnostic implications of biological findings, variations in course and duration and their implications as regards subtyping, epidemiology, and the effects of chronic and repeated trauma (see Davidson et al., Chapter 19, this volume).

With regard to the stressor criterion, the literature review found that the risk of developing PTSD tended to be proportional to the magnitude of the stressor; that particular stressor characteristics such as threat to life, physical harm, exposure to grotesque death or atrocity, and loss of or injury to a loved one modestly correlated with the development of PTSD development; and that subjective experiences of helplessness, fear, or perceived threat to life or of violence were possibly related to PTSD development. The review recommended a stressor definition that emphasized the characteristics of the event, retained some restrictiveness, and eliminated DSM-III-R's seemingly less reliable references to the unusualness of the experience and universality of the distress. This was incorporated as option A1 in the *DSM-IV Options Book*. The literature review also recommended considering the performance characteristics of definitions, which include an aspect of subjective appraisal (option A2) or the ICD-10 stressor criterion (option A3).

The literature reviews examining PTSD symptom patterns in children, disaster victims, combat veterans, and crime victims concurred in recommending against any major change in the DSM-III-R format for intrusive, avoidant, or hyperarousal features. In some samples, however, avoidant symptoms were less frequent, and the recommendation was made to consider lowering the minimum required number of avoidant symptoms from three to two so that the diagnosis would not be unreasonably restrictive. This will be tested in the field trial.

The literature review also weighed the evidence for reclassifying PTSD as a dissociative disorder, placing it in a new category of stress response disorders (or a more narrow category of disorders of extreme stress not elsewhere classified), or maintaining it as an anxiety disorder. The review recommended that PTSD be assigned to a separate category for disorders of extreme stress, to better reflect etiology and to achieve compatibility with ICD-10. It noted, however, that the rest of DSM-IV, like its predecessors, is descriptive rather than etiological and that more than trauma is required to induce PTSD in most cases. If that reclassification did not occur, the review concluded that available data supported retaining PTSD among the anxiety disorders, which is the position taken in the *Options Book*.

Biological findings of tonic and phasic autonomic hyperactivity in PTSD were considered consistent with the traumatic origin of the disorder. The review concluded that more prominence should be given to physiological hyperactivity in response to reminders of the trauma. The recommendation was made to move this feature from the hyperarousal to the intrusive symptom category. The impact of this will be tested in the field trial.

With regard to variations in course and duration and their implications for subtyping PTSD, the reviews suggested that

1. The 1-month minimum duration of symptoms be dropped as a requirement, and no minimum duration be required.
2. A 1-month lapse following the initial trauma should be required before the diagnosis can be made.
3. Less than 3 months of symptoms would be called the acute form and 3 months or more the chronic form. PTSD symptoms beginning more than 6 months (or 3 months) after the trauma would be called the delayed form.

These recommendations were incorporated into option E3 in the *Options Book,* to be considered along with DSM-III-R's 1-month minimum duration (option E1) and a 3-month minimum duration (option E2).

The review examined epidemiological data and concluded that they support separate classification of PTSD in a Stress Disorder section in DSM-IV (see above) but no evidence for changing the criteria.

The literature review was felt to offer "extensive but unsystematized support for the concept of a complex post-traumatic syndrome (DESNOS) in survivors of prolonged, repeated victimization." It was felt that the syndrome was distinct from PTSD and in need of further empirical study.

Although not covered in the literature reviews, for clinical accuracy, depiction of trauma reminders was broadened from "events" to "internal or external cues" in several of the intrusive criteria.

Generalized Anxiety Disorder

Issues of concern with regard to GAD included its differential diagnosis from affective, somatoform, and obsessive-compulsive disorders and from normal worry; the reliability and utility of the somatic symptom list; and whether pathological worry should continue to be a necessary criterion (see Moras et al., Chapter 20, this volume).

The literature review found some overlap with dysthymia and major depression, but no recommendations for changes in criteria were made. It was found that there is the potential to overdiagnose GAD in the presence of hypochondriasis; therefore, the caveat that, if hypochondriasis is present, the focus of anxiety and worry is not about having a serious illness, was added to the criteria for GAD.

Literature reviews pertaining to the differences in cognitive symptoms in GAD versus OCD are discussed in the section on OCD. The term *unrealistic* has been removed from the descriptors of worry in GAD to emphasize that GAD worries tend to be about real-life issues. This is consonant with adding to the definition of obsessions that they are not just excessive worries about real-life problems.

The literature also suggests that uncontrollability and disruptiveness might be dimensions that distinguish pathological from normal worry. This led to the recommendation to include the following feature of pathological worry in the criteria for GAD: "The person finds it difficult to control the worry and to focus attention on the tasks at hand." To further differentiate GAD from normal worry, it is proposed that several other features be added to the DSM-IV criteria: the worry has to be pervasive (focused on many life circumstances) rather than be about two or more life circumstances, as in DSM-III-R; and the worry or associated somatic symptoms have to cause significant impairment in social or occupational functioning or marked distress.

The literature review also revealed that the reliability of the DSM-III-R GAD definition was below that of other anxiety disorders in several systematic studies with structured interviews and trained raters. The changes outlined above were designed to reduce several sources of unreliability. The 18-item somatic symptom list in DSM-III-R's criterion D also contributed to GAD's unreliability, although the literature was not consistent in suggesting which symptoms could be most reliably rated. Pilot studies were then carried out to determine which somatic symptoms could be most reliably rated and were most predictive of GAD. This led to option E3 of the DSM-IV GAD proposal, which emphasizes somatic symptoms such as restlessness, being easily fatigued, feeling keyed up or on edge, difficulty concentrating or mind going blank, or irritability.

Many patients in primary care and cross-cultural samples report distressing and/or disabling anxiety and depressive symptoms that do not meet DSM-III-R syndromal criteria. This has given rise to consideration of a mixed anxiety and depression category for DSM-IV (see below), which is being explored through a field trial. It is expected, however, that the field trial will also be informative with regard to GAD, especially on the issue of whether there is a substantial subset of patients who meet the somatic but not the cognitive (worry) criteria for the disorder and, if so, whether GAD should be modified so that worry is not a necessary criterion.

Mixed Anxiety and Depression

ICD-10 proposes to include a new category of mixed anxiety and depression that is meant to designate patients with symptoms of anxiety and depression that are sufficiently distressing and/or impairing to warrant a psychiatric diagnosis but are lacking the features to meet one of the existing anxiety or affective diagnoses. Although the ICD-10 category has no operational criteria or validating data, it was decided that the Anxiety Disorders Work Group would conduct a literature review as a first step toward considering the category for DSM-IV (see Moras et al., Chapter 21, this volume).

The literature review found reports of the existence of such patients, particularly in primary care settings, where practitioners felt that they were numerous but not adequately diagnosed because they did not fit an existing DSM-III-R category. However, it remains to be seen whether such findings are confirmed when subjects are interviewed by trained raters using structured interviews. It was therefore recommended that a DSM-IV field trial be undertaken to further study the issue of a "subsyndromal" (by DSM-III-R standards) mixed anxiety-depression category.

The literature reviews also examined the issue of whether some patients with both anxiety and depressive features that currently meet DSM-III-R thresholds for an anxiety or affective disorder might be better conceptualized as having a mixed anxiety-depressive disorder. Available comorbidity data on DSM-III and DSM-III-R anxiety and mood disorders did not argue for the existence of such a disorder, although psychometric studies did suggest that some symptoms were common to both anxiety and affective disorders. Given that a syndromal level mixed anxiety-depressive disorder would represent a radical departure from the DSM-III and DSM-III-R principle of separating the anxiety and affective disorders, it was recommended that this not be pursued for DSM-IV.

References

American Psychiatric Association: Diagnostic and Statistical Manual of Mental Disorders, 3rd Edition. Washington, DC, American Psychiatric Association, 1980

American Psychiatric Association: Diagnostic and Statistical Manual of Mental Disorders, 3rd Edition, Revised. Washington, DC, American Psychiatric Association, 1987

American Psychiatric Association: DSM-IV Options Book: Work in Progress. Washington, DC, American Psychiatric Association, 1991

Marks IM: The classification of phobic disorders. Br J Psychiatry 116:377–386, 1970

World Health Organization: ICD-10 Chapter V: Mental and Behavioral Disorders: Diagnostic Criteria for Research. Geneva, Switzerland, World Health Organization, 1990

Chapter 15

Panic Disorder and Agoraphobia

James C. Ballenger, M.D., and Abby J. Fyer, M.D.

Statement of the Issues

Panic Disorder Without Agoraphobia

1. Should DSM-IV retain the same criterion for frequency of panic attacks (PA) used in DSM-III-R (American Psychiatric Association 1987)?
2. Should DSM-IV retain the requirement of four symptoms to qualify for a PA?
3. Should DSM-IV use the cognitive features of PAs in panic disorder (PD) more extensively?
4. Should DSM-IV retain the requirement for spontaneous PAs?
5. Can the criteria better describe the typical PD patient?
6. Should some subclassifications of PD be used (e.g. cardiac, neurological, gastrointestinal)?
7. How can the boundary with social phobia be defined?
8. Can biological tests be used in the diagnosis?

Panic Disorder With Agoraphobia

1. Should the DSM-IV criteria be more compatible with the ICD-10 criteria?
   a. Should the postulated etiologic link between PD and agoraphobia that is included in DSM-III-R be retained, removed, or deemphasized?
   b. Should the typical agoraphobic situations be described more fully?
   c. Should the DSM-IV utilize the ICD-10 idea that the agoraphobic phobias are "interrelated and overlapping"?
2. What is the boundary of agoraphobia and simple/specific phobias?

Significance of the Issues

The DSM-III-R PD and agoraphobia criteria have been the subject of considerable discussion and controversy over the past few years (Aronson 1987; Buller 1990; Jablensky 1985; Liebowitz and Fyer 1990; Margraf et al. 1986, 1987; Skodol 1989). The argument has been made that the use of the specific frequency chosen for PAs in previous criteria sets, either one in each of 3 weeks (DSM-III, American Psychiatric Association 1980) or one in each of the preceding 4 weeks (DSM-III-R), is arbitrary. Also, most experts and clinicians feel these numbers are not representative of typical patients whose PA frequency varies greatly over time and among individuals. Clinicians and researchers have argued that these arbitrary numerical criteria lead to situations in which patients with different and/or "subclinical" frequency configurations are not diagnosed with PD despite significant symptomatology and morbidity (Weissman et al. 1989). Previous criteria also describe the most severe end of the PD spectrum and may miss patients with less frequent PAs who do have significant morbidity and who would benefit from treatment.

It is also unclear how the PA frequency criterion relates to or works with the other arm of the diagnostic criteria in DSM-III-R (i.e., one PA plus a month of worry about the recurrence of a PA). Little is known about how these two significantly different criteria diagnose patients—whether they diagnose the same groups of patients or whether they even generate different prevalence rates for PD. Perhaps the frequency criterion diagnoses the severe end of the spectrum and the "one plus a month" criterion diagnoses a group of individuals with less severe symptoms.

There is considerable controversy, especially among psychologists (Barlow 1986, 1988a; Clark 1986; Moras et al. 1990), regarding whether the catastrophic cognitions of PD are characteristic of the disorder and should be used in the diagnosis. Perhaps even more critical is the theoretical argument that the tendency to employ a catastrophic cognitive style may be central to the development of PD and therefore to the efficacy of the new cognitive treatments.

There has been considerable theoretical controversy concerning whether a "spontaneous" PA is essential to the diagnosis of PD. This primarily arises because many PD patients with or without agoraphobia may initially have spontaneous attacks, but later in the course of their illness, the spontaneous attacks may become less frequent or disappear entirely and be replaced by situational PAs. Others argue that the requirement for at least one spontaneous attack is primarily utilized because of a specific biological theory of PD that is not proved and that theory-driven criteria should be removed from DSM-IV. However, arguments for retention of the spontaneous attacks center on their utility in defining boundaries with other disorders that also include PAs, although few if any spontaneous PAs (e.g., obsessive-compulsive disorder, social phobia).

There are several subclassifications that some clinicians and researchers feel could be usefully introduced in DSM-IV to allow patients with these disorders to be more frequently and accurately diagnosed. The most prominent proposed subclassifications are for patients with primary cardiovascular presentations, including those who do not have fear or panic as a symptom and those with gastrointestinal or irritable bowel presentations. Ideally, subclassification would draw attention to the different presentations of these patients that often lead to failure to recognize the syndrome as PD.

The field of biological study of PD, especially provocative-challenge tests, is well developed relative to other psychiatric syndromes. An external objective test would be extremely useful in increasing the validity (and credibility) of diagnosis and should be considered for inclusion in DSM-IV.

There has been controversy since the publication of DSM-III-R over the required linkage of PD and agoraphobia, both on theoretical and empirical grounds. Some argue that there are no valid data supporting the theory that PAs are required for the subsequent development of agoraphobia. This argument is most frequently made by European psychiatrists, who also feel that agoraphobia is a much more important syndrome than PD and that its importance was reduced in DSM-III-R when it was made a subset of PD. Empirically, there are also a few clinical data sets that suggest that there is a substantial group of agoraphobic patients (as high as 25%) who do not report a history of PD or even PAs before the development of agoraphobia (Fava et al. 1988). These data sets describe patients who had agoraphobia first and then developed PAs, obviously arguing against the required sequence of PAs first, followed by secondary development of agoraphobia. This issue has practical significance because the European view was adopted in ICD-10, making it difficult in this instance to meet one of the major goals of DSM-IV, i.e., to make DSM-IV compatible with ICD-10.

In DSM-III-R, a similar precedence was given to PD over social phobia, which led to some confusion when individuals with presumed social phobia had prominent unexpected PAs. The DSM-IV should attempt to more definitively define the boundary between social phobia and PD, presumably by use of the distinction between unexpected PAs and social- or performance-related anxiety episodes.

Defining the boundary between agoraphobia and simple or specific phobias is important because it has implications for the prevalence and treatment of the various disorders. Many clinicians feel the treatments for agoraphobia and simple or specific phobias are different. Whether a person who is phobic of flying because he or she has PAs in airplanes is considered to have a simple or specific phobia or agoraphobia might influence choice of treatment (i.e., behavioral and pharmacological). The boundary issues for agoraphobia and social phobia would have similar implications because the treatments for these conditions are also not identical.

Method and Results

Frequency and Symptom Thresholds for Panic Disorder[1]

This review summarizes data relevant to two threshold (i.e., case-identification) issues in the diagnosis of PD: 1) the required number of PAs and the time period over which these are counted and 2) the minimum number of symptoms needed to define a PA.

The articles included were collected by 1) computerized literature search using Medlars II (1980–1989) and Medline (1980–1989) services under topics of diagnosis, assessment, monitoring, prevalence, and epidemiology with anxiety disorders, PD, and agoraphobia; 2) telephone requests to 11 investigators working in this area for either manuscripts in press or preparation or names of colleagues engaged in related work; 3) systematic review of references cited by all relevant articles in the computer search and from telephoned investigators. Only articles published, in press, or submitted for publication are included. Studies that did not report sampling method or definition of PAs or disorder were excluded.

PA Frequency

Prevalence.   Data from epidemiological, analog, and patient samples suggest that there is a significant population of individuals who report PAs but at a frequency less than is required to meet either the DSM-III (three in 3 weeks) or DSM-III-R (four in 4 weeks) diagnostic criteria.

Epidemiologic studies: Three direct-interview studies of stratified general-population samples (Angst et al. 1989; Eaton et al. 1988; Von Korff and Eaton 1989; Wittchen 1986) found lifetime and/or current rates of infrequent panic between 2% and 3%. In two studies, the rate of infrequent panic was about twice that of PD (Angst et al. 1989; Eaton et al. 1988; Von Korff and Eaton 1989). In the third, it was about equal to that of PD (Wittchen 1986). Two additional general-population studies using either telephone (Salge et al. 1988) or postal (Katerndahl 1987) surveys found somewhat higher rates of infrequent panic (14% and 18%, respectively).

Analog studies: The 1985 study of college students reported by Norton et al. was the first to focus attention on subthreshold infrequent panic. These earlier findings have now been replicated and amplified by both Norton et al. (1986) and

[1]Abby J. Fyer, M.D., and Hilary Rassnick, M.A.

Telch et al. (1989b). Both groups administered a self-report panic- and anxiety-focused questionnaire to large numbers of college psychology students. The earlier Norton et al. study (1985) found that 22% of students reported at least one PA but fewer than three in the past 3 weeks. The subsequent study (Norton et al. 1986) replicated the 22% rate for any PA, but found that in only 5% of subjects was at least one attack *unexpected.*

Telch et al. (1989b) found a similar proportion (4.4%) of individuals who reported lifetime occurrence of at least one unexpected DSM-III-R panic attack who did not meet criteria for PD. However, individuals who met the low-threshold DSM-III-R criteria (one attack plus 1 month of apprehension about the next attack) would be excluded from Telch et al.'s but not Norton et al.'s infrequent panic group. The Telch et al. report does not distinguish between subjects meeting either one or both of the two DSM-III-R entry criteria.

Two additional studies reported high rates of PAs among nonpatient populations but did not distinguish between subjects who did and did not meet disorder criteria. Of 151 psychology students surveyed by Rapee et al. (1988) with a self-report anxiety questionnaire, 14% reported lifetime occurrence of at least one unexpected PA. Brown and Cash (1989) found a 26% 1-year prevalence of at least one DSM-III PA among the 509 responding university staff and faculty surveyed with a similar instrument but omitting explicit mention of unexpectedness.

Clinical studies: Katon et al. (1987b) reported that 9% of 195 sequentially assessed family practice outpatients met current and 19% met past criteria for *simple panic,* defined as having had at least one but never three DSM-III PAs in 3 weeks. However, 75% of these individuals with infrequent panic had had at least six attacks. Beitman et al. (1988) found that 24% of 33 cardiology outpatients with normal angiography met similar criteria for the *past 3 weeks.* However, past PD was not ruled out. In contrast, Von Korff et al. (1987), using similar methodology, reported only a 1.4% prevalence of PD among an unselected series of primary care patients.

A fourth study by Stirton and Brandon (1988) used a self-report questionnaire to survey the registry of a British general practice. Responders who reported any panic symptoms were followed up with a semistructured clinical interview. Of the respondents in this study, 8% reported infrequent panic.

Lepine et al. (1989) recruited volunteers from a random sample of French psychiatrists in private practice. Of the 1,271 patients evaluated, 43% had had at least one DSM-III PA (four symptoms) in their life. However, only about one-half (21% of the sample) met the four in 4 weeks frequency criterion. An additional 13% met the less restrictive DSM-III-R threshold (one plus a month of apprehension about the next attack).

Methodological Issues in Measurement of Panic

There appear to be no negative studies concerning the existence of infrequent panic. The convergence of findings using a variety of sampling and assessment methods seems to provide substantial evidence that this syndrome is as prevalent as, or more prevalent than, DSM-III PD. However, the methodology of a number of the cited investigations has been significantly criticized. Most investigators either did not use state-of-the-art assessment methods (i.e., a highly trained clinician using a semi-structured interview of known reliability) or were incomplete or ambiguous in their application of PA criteria. Inexperienced or insufficiently trained interviewers or subjects (in self-report studies) and imprecise use of diagnostic requirements could result in an overestimate of the prevalence of subthreshold panic syndromes. This might occur through mistaken inclusion of other types of anxiety (e.g., anticipatory surges before entering a phobic situation, intense or dramatically reported response to interpersonal conflict) or nonanxious episodic disturbances (e.g., seizures) in the panic category. There is not enough information to allow for fact-based conclusions concerning the impact of different assessment methods (self-report, clinician, nonclinician) and PA definition on prevalence rates. However, the available data, we review, provide some initial guidelines and directions for further work.

An additional interpretive difficulty has been the failure to acknowledge or accommodate limitations inherent in cross-sectional assessment of a transient and often untreated phenomenon (Rice et al. 1986). However, this is not discussed, because loss of recall most likely results in either underestimation of subdisorder rates or misclassification of full-disorder subjects in the subthreshold group.

Studies comparing clinician, nonclinician, and self-report assessment of panic: Several clinical series indicate good to excellent reliability for diagnosis of PAs and PD by clinicians using semistructured diagnostic interviews (Barlow 1985; Di-Nardo et al. 1983; Fyer et al. 1989; Mannuzza et al. 1989). One study reported excellent reliability for "ever having had a spontaneous PA" (Fyer et al. 1989). Results concerning retrospective assessment of frequency of unexpected or other PAs within a specific time period are mixed (Barlow 1988a; Margraf et al. 1987). Four available comparisons of self-report and interviewer diagnosis in nonclinical samples indicate that the former method yields higher panic rates.

Comparison of clinician assessment to lay interviewer administration of the Diagnostic Interview Schedule (DIS) (Robins et al. 1981) has been the focus of considerable discussion. The data suggest disagreement but no clear directional trend. The largest reported sample (Markowitz et al. 1989; Weissman et al. 1989) includes 14 Epidemiologic Catchment Area (ECA) subjects diagnosed by lay interviewer DIS as PD and reinterviewed using the Schedule for Affective Disorders and

Schizophrenia, Lifetime Version (Modified for the Study of Anxiety Disorders) (SADS-LA) (Fyer et al. 1985; Mannuzza et al. 1986). On reinterview, 11 met DSM-III PD criteria, whereas 3 had no panic but had other anxiety or affective disorders.

PA definitions: In this context, the critical DSM-III PA criteria are those hypothesized to reflect a qualitative distinction between panic and other severe anxiety (Klein and Klein, 1989a, 1989b, 1989c). These include unexpected, sudden onset, crescendo course, multiple, simultaneously associated symptoms and exclusion of association with simple or social phobias (i.e., stimulus-bound attacks). In clinical settings, these qualities have been found to distinguish many social phobic and most generalized anxiety and simple phobic patients from PD patients (Barlow et al. 1985; Liebowitz et al. 1985b; Mannuzza et al. 1989).

Only two studies have directly addressed this issue in subdisorder populations. Both reported that more rigorous application of the particular criterion studied (unexpectedness, unexpectedness plus crescendo) decreased supposed prevalence. Norton et al. (1986) rated panic occurrence (sudden intense anxiety accompanied by four symptoms) and unpredictability (out of the blue) in two separate sequential questions. Only about one-quarter of those with current panic reported "unexpected" panic as required by the DSM-III/DSM-III-R criteria (22% versus 6%). The most common panic situations reported by those with predictable panic were social encounters.

Brown and Cash (1989) found that introducing additional distinctions between panic and other anxiety into the standard Anxiety Questionnaire (Norton et al. 1985) panic screening question considerably reduced frequency of self-reported current panic (4 weeks) in a nonclinical population (22% to 12%). The modification included an additional description of panic as a "sudden rush" of anxiety and explicit exclusion of intense anxiety associated with "life worries."

Summary: Effects of Interviewer Versus Self-Report Assessment, Panic Definition, and Sample Procedures on Prevalence of Infrequent Panic

Very few studies unequivocally fulfill state-of-the-art assessment standards. Two (Beitman et al. 1988; Stirton and Brandon 1988) appear exempt from these criticisms and provide strong support for the existence of infrequent panic and the prevalence of the syndrome in nonpsychiatric medical settings. Clinician assessment and established interview schedules were used in one clinical (Katon et al. 1987a, 1987b) and two epidemiological (Angst et al. 1989; Wittchen 1986) investigations. Unfortunately, all three are unclear about certain aspects of their criteria for PA definition. The remaining epidemiological studies and all of the analog data are dependent on self-report or lay interviewer assessments. Most also suffer from unclear or incomplete panic definitions.

However, the central question with respect to thresholds for panic frequency and symptom criteria is whether false-positive assessments could account for the majority of identified subthreshold cases. Although further investigation is needed, available data suggest that methodological improvements would significantly decrease the number of, but probably not eliminate, those with infrequent panic. However, at present, only rough estimates of the number of affected individuals involved (i.e., infrequent panic and consequent illness behavior) can be made.

The multiple between-study methodological differences make it difficult to disentangle the specific effects of any one procedure. However, some information can be gained by comparing rates across studies. The direct-interview epidemiological studies that achieved high completion rates found prevalences of 2%–3% regardless of whether a clinical (Angst et al. 1989; Wittchen 1986) or lay (Eaton et al. 1988; Von Korff and Eaton 1989) interview was used. All report some attempt to exclude individuals who had *not* had at least one unexpected attack.

The DIS, on which the Eaton et al. and Von Korff et al. reports are based, is structured so that only individuals who meet criteria for a phobic disorder are asked whether they have ever had an attack that was not in a phobic situation. Angst et al. (1989) reported difficulties in making this distinction in a number of instances. The term *crescendo* was not explicitly used in the panic definitions of these studies. However, Angst et al. did require *terror* in addition to the DSM-III/DSM-III-R *anxiety, fear,* or *discomfort.*

To carry the exercise further, these limitations can be taken into account by assuming a 50% false-positive rate (the highest found in the comparative clinician/self-report). This reduces the estimated number of those with infrequent panic to 1%–1.5% of the population. On the basis of Angst et al.'s and the ECA's data, treatment seeking or impairment would be found in from one-fourth to one-half of these individuals.

Are Individuals With "Infrequent Panic" Ill?

The relatively sparse data available concerning the association of infrequent panic with impairment, treatment seeking, or subject distress often make it difficult to assess the existence (if any) of a relationship between "illness" behavior and infrequent panic. However, even within these limitations, the data suggest that a subset of those with infrequent panic are ill. Moreover, although the proportion of ill individuals is lower among those with infrequent panic than those with disorder-level panic, there is some indication that degree of disability among affected individuals in both groups is similar.

Help seeking/medication use/impairment.   In four of five available studies, 25% of those with infrequent panic compared to 50% of PD subjects reported seeking professional help for anxiety symptoms (Angst et al. 1989; Katon et al. 1987b; Salge et al. 1988; Telch et al. 1989b). In the fifth, none of the subjects had sought help for panic (Norton et al. 1986). Telch et al. study observed a progressively downward gradient for the percentage seeking professional help for anxiety symptoms (48% disorder versus 23% infrequent versus 10% nonpanic) with significant between-group differences ($P < .01$). Significance statistics are not reported in the remaining studies due to the small number of cases. Telch found a similar proportional relationship between panic frequency and report of medication use for anxiety (18% versus 13% versus 5%; $P < .01$).

In the study by Angst et al. (1989), 3 of 14 of those with infrequent panic reported severe work impairment, 1 subject had moderate impairment, and the remaining 10 had none. Interestingly, although the proportion of those who were severely impaired was greater, a similar bimodal distribution of this variable was seen in the PD group (severe 4 of 9 impairment, 5 of 9 no impairment).

Subjective distress. Angst et al. (1989) also asked subjects to rate "subjective suffering" on a scale of 1–100. Mean scores for infrequent and PD groups were 73 and 97 ($P < .003$). Another aspect of subjective distress is "anticipatory anxiety" or "worry about panic." Lepine et al. (1989) found that "persistent fear of having another attack for at least 1 month" was reported by more than 90% of psychiatric outpatients who had at least one full PA but did not meet the four in 4-week criterion. In the study by Telch et al. (1989b), only 10% of those with infrequent panic but 73% of those with disorder-level panic (DSM-III-R) reported significant fear of their next attack. However, because the disorder group includes individuals who met either of the two DSM-III-R threshold criteria (four in 4 weeks or one plus 1 month of anxiety), these data do not directly address the degree of association between attack frequency and apprehension.

Other illness variables. In their analyses of the ECA data, Eaton et al. (1988) found that of the 3.8% of the subjects who reported lifetime occurrence of PAs that had "interfered a lot with their lives," one-half (1.9% of the study population) denied ever having had at least three PAs in 3 weeks. In the same data set, Weissman et al. (1989) found a significantly increased risk for suicide attempts and ideation among those with both frequent and infrequent panic compared with control subjects without panic symptoms.

Are Individuals With Infrequent Panic Similar to More Restrictively Defined PD Subjects With Respect to Standard Validity Measures?

Cross-sectional variables: demographic characteristics. Data from epidemiological, analog, and clinical settings indicate that those with infrequent and DSM-III disorder-level panic are similar with respect to sex ratio and *mean* age at onset (Angst et al. 1989; Beitman et al. 1988; Katon et al. 1987b; Telch et al. 1989b; Von Korff and Eaton 1989).

The ECA studies have also reported similar distribution of subthreshold PA syndromes (simple PAs, severe and recurrent panic) and PD across educational, marital, and ethnic variables. Higher risks for all three panic syndromes were found among women compared with men, individuals with less than high school education, and widowed, separated, or divorced persons compared with those currently or never married (Von Korff and Eaton 1989; Von Korff et al. 1985).

Although similarities appear to outweigh differences, two studies have also noted areas of partial demographic divergence. In the ECA data set, simple panic (nonsevere, fewer than three in 3 weeks) has its peak number of onsets (35%) between ages 15 and 19 years. Only about 20% of the onsets of severe and recurrent panic and PD occur between these ages. However, PD has a second peak in age at onset (25–30 years) which is not seen for the subthreshold syndromes (Von Korff and Eaton 1989). About 15% of PD, 10% of severe and recurrent panic, and 5% of simple panic onsets are reported in these years. Interestingly, a similar bimodal age-at-onset distribution for the disorder has been previously reported in clinical samples and attributed to physiological and medical disturbances in the older patients (Klein 1964). Angst et al. (1989) reported a significant difference in female-male ratio only among the subthreshold group (2:1 versus 6:1, $P < .01$).

Panic symptomatology.   There is some disagreement as to the extent to which PAs reported by those with infrequent panic resemble those of individuals meeting DSM-III PD criteria. However, the overall similarities seem greater than the differences. The number and type of "associated symptoms" are the only factors that have been systematically studied. On the average, those with infrequent panic report slightly fewer symptoms per attack than subjects meeting disorder criteria. In the three studies reporting this comparison for those with infrequent versus disorder-level panic, the respective figures were 4 versus 6 (median, Von Korff et al. 1985), 4 versus 7 (mean, Telch et al. 1989b), and 7 versus 10 (mean, Rapee et al. 1988).

Findings of the four reports comparing relative frequency of the different DSM-III/DSM-III-R "associated symptoms" are inconsistent. Three found no significant between-group differences (Katerndahl 1990; Lepine et al. 1989; Von Korff et al. 1985), two found significantly decreased frequency of trembling among infrequent panic subjects in both Angst et al's (1989) small epidemiological sample (5/14 versus 8/9, $P < .05$) and Telch et al.'s (1989b) college students (50% versus 77%, $P < .01$). Telch et al. also found that subdisorder subjects were significantly less likely to report another 7 of the 14 symptoms, including fear of dying (18%

versus 52%) or going crazy (26% versus 64%), derealization (30% versus 60%), nausea (26% versus 50%), dizziness (31 versus 50%), numbness/tingling (18% versus 41%), and chest pain (16% versus 36%). In contrast, Angst et al. (1989) found no other significant differences, although fear of losing control was less likely among those with sporadic panic (7/14 versus 8/9).

Psychiatric comorbidity. Both epidemiological and clinical data suggest similar and highly elevated risks for lifetime major depression (MDD) among both PD and infrequent panic subjects. Angst et al. 1989 reported rates of lifetime MDD of 36% and 44%, respectively, in the two groups across three primary care outpatient groups: PD (95%), simple (infrequent) panic (72%), and nonpanicking control subjects (29%). Differences between controls and both panic groups reached significance in 2-day comparisons ($P < .01$).

Although infrequent panic can be associated with avoidance, there are insufficient data to assess whether phobias are as common among this population as in disorder-level subjects (Weissman et al. 1986). For example, recent epidemiological and clinical data on agoraphobia with panic indicate that infrequent panic occurred in one-half to one-third of these subjects (Barlow et al., Chapter 16 in this volume; Weissman et al. 1986). Both Salge et al. (1988) and Norton et al. (1985) reported panic-attributed avoidance among a substantial minority of those with infrequent panic (35% [20 of 58] and 18% [4 of 22], respectively).

However, only two small between-group comparisons are available. Katon et al. (1987a) found an upward gradient in mean number of phobias in nonpanic control subjects, in those with subthreshold panic, and in those with disorder level panic, respectively. Both panic groups differed significantly from control subjects (1.2 versus 3.3, and 1.2 versus 4.8, $P < .001$). This relationship was maintained even when the analysis was limited to individuals with panic who reported no panics during the 3 months prior to assessment (3.3 versus 2.5 versus 1.4, $P < .05$ for both two-way comparisons) (Katon et al. 1987a). Angst et al. (1989) found that 2 of 9 with PD compared to 0 of 14 with sporadic panic in the Zurich epidemiological study were also given a diagnosis of agoraphobia.

Family and twin studies. A number of studies indicate that PD is familial (Crowe 1985). If restrictively defined PD and infrequent panic reflect variable clinical presentations of the same underlying heritable diathesis, then it would be expected that 1) PD and infrequent panic will each be familial, and 2) both PD probands and probands who have infrequent panic but not PD will transmit separately increased risks for *both* PD and infrequent panic to their relatives compared with relatives of not ill or general population relatives. Similarly, shared genetic diathesis would be indicated by increased monozygotic (MZ) compared to dizygotic (DZ) concordance for each (and therefore both) among co-twins of probands with each syndrome.

Although these studies have not been done, partial data support the hypothesis of commonality. Torgerson (1983), in a small sample of DSM-III anxiety disorder patients, found only a slight excess of MZ versus DZ concordance for PD. However, if generalized anxiety disorder (GAD) patients with infrequent panic were included in the PD group, MZ twins had five times as great a concordance for anxiety disorders with PAs as DZ twins. Crowe et al. (1983) reported an increased risk for "probable" PD among first-degree relatives of PD probands compared with relatives of not-ill control subjects. "Probable" PD included individuals with *either* fewer than the DSM-III three attacks in 3 weeks *or* less than four associated symptoms per PA. Family history data from those with nonclinical panic (of whom 22 of 24 had fewer than three attacks in the past 3 weeks) also indicate increased risk for PAs among first-degree relatives of these subjects compared with relatives of nonpanicking control subjects (Norton et al. 1986).

Biological assessment/treatment outcome.   Cowley et al. (1987) reported similar and significantly elevated panic and anxiety symptom response to intravenous sodium lactate in patients with DSM-III PD and DSM-III GAD plus a history of subdisorder panic frequency compared with GAD patients who did not have a history of panic and normal control subjects. Similar increased panicogenic response to sodium lactate has been reported among patients with MDD and bulimia who also report "infrequent" unexpected panic compared with patients with these disorders but no panic history and/or control subjects who are not ill (Gorman et al. 1985; Liebowitz et al. 1985a; McGrath et al. 1985).

Although clinical experience and case reports suggest similar treatment response among groups with frequent and infrequent panic, neither open clinical series nor comparative controlled trials have been published.

Longitudinal studies.   One hypothesis concerning infrequent panic is that it represents an early or "between" phase of the full disorder. Patients in retrospective studies often report isolated or "infrequent" attacks that occurred months or years before the onset of the disorder. Lifetime histories of waxing and waning panic frequency as well as a recurrent episodic course are also common (Breier et al. 1986; Uhde et al. 1985b).

Von Korff and Eaton (1989), working with the ECA data, reported that approximately half of subjects classified as having infrequent panic at initial interview met criteria for panic disorder at the 1-year follow-up. Furthermore, the follow-up interview indicated that the 1-year incidence rate of PD (i.e., the number of new cases during that year) among individuals with a history of PAs but *not* PD was considerably higher than among subjects who had never had either attacks or disorder.

Is There Evidence for an "Inherent" Threshold (i.e., a Cumulative Level of PA Frequency Beyond Which Either the Association With "Illness" or Similarity to Disorder-Level Subjects With Respect to Validity Measures Rises Significantly)?

Most studies do not address this issue because all those with infrequent panic were included in one group regardless of specific attack frequency. An exception is the ECA data, which created two levels: "simple" and "severe and recurrent" panic.

Direct comparisons of rates of "illness" among those with simple, severe, and disorder-level panic have not been reported. With respect to age at onset and symptom count, those with severe panic were more similar to those with simple panic on the former but closer to disorder-level subjects on the latter.

A previous ECA report (Von Korff et al. 1985) suggests a higher rate of limited-symptom attacks among those with infrequent compared with frequent panic. Twenty-nine percent of simple panic subjects reported fewer than three symptoms per attack, compared to 8% of those with recurrent panic and 6% of disorder level subjects.

Are Those With Limited-Symptom Panic Ill? Do They Resemble the More Restrictively Defined Group With Respect to Standard Validity Measures?

There are few data directly addressing these questions. The ECA findings indicate that 1.7% of the United States adult population have had "severe" limited-symptom attacks (i.e., attacks with three or fewer symptoms that subjects told a doctor about, that subjects took medication for more than once, or that interfered "a lot" in the subject's life). An additional 2.1% have had "nonsevere" attacks and/or attacks limited to phobic situations (these three groups are not reported separately).

The study of agoraphobia without a history of PD has provided examples in which limited-symptom attacks are associated with avoidance (Barlow et al., Chapter 16 in this volume; Klein and Klein 1989a; Weissman and Merikangas 1986). However, the proportion of those with limited-symptom panic who develop this complication is not known.

Results of the two direct comparisons of symptoms occurring during full and limited-symptom attacks are incomplete and contradictory. Katerndahl (1990) reported no systematic differences in symptom frequency between limited-symptom (three symptoms or fewer) and full panics among a general-population sample assessed by self-report. The most frequently reported symptoms in the latter group were fears of dying, going crazy, or losing control (41%) and palpitations (37%).

In contrast, in an ambulatory cardiac monitoring of DSM-III PD patients, palpitations (64%), chest pain (31%), and nausea (26%) were the symptoms most commonly reported during limited-symptom attacks. Fears of dying (0%) and going crazy or losing control (5%) were rare (Margraf et al. 1987; Taylor et al. 1986).

Is There Evidence for an "Inherent" Threshold (i.e., Critical Number of Associated Symptoms Above Which Either Illness Behavior Is More Common and/or Standard Validity Measures Reflect Similarity to the More Restrictively Defined Disorder Group)?

Studies assessing different rates of illness behavior among subjects with different numbers of panic symptoms (e.g., two, three, four, or more) have not been reported. In addition, sparse data are available addressing the possible qualitative distinction between attacks characterized by two, three, four, or more symptoms.

Several studies indicate significant rates of limited-symptom attacks among clinical panic/anxiety samples (Barlow 1988a; Fyer et al. 1989; Taylor et al. 1986). One ambulatory monitoring study reported that PAs with fewer than three symptoms were briefer and less intense than those with four or more symptoms. Fewer of the limited-symptom attacks met the cardiac monitoring criteria for panic (38% versus 64%) (Taylor et al. 1986). However, neither type of symptoms nor quality of onset distinguished these groups.

Summary and Implications for DSM-IV PD Criteria

Panic Frequency

Review of the currently available literature suggests that previous PA frequency requirements (four in 4 weeks, three in 3 weeks) might be inappropriately restrictive and therefore consideration should be given to changing the PA threshold in DSM-IV:

1. Convergent data from epidemiological, analog, and clinical studies indicate the existence of a significant number of individuals with "infrequent panic," (i.e., individuals who have DSM-III-R PAs but are excluded from the diagnostic category only because of failure to meet the frequency criterion).

2. A substantial number of those with "infrequent panic" report panic associated with treatment seeking, functional impairment, or subjective distress. In at least some cases, the degree of morbidity does not differ from that seen in disorder-level subjects.

3. Those with "infrequent panic" closely resemble disorder-level subjects with respect to traditional measures of diagnostic validity. The clinical phenomenology and demography of the two groups are similar. Preliminary twin study, family history, and biological challenge data are also consistent with commonality between these two groups. However, prospective longitudinal, family, and treatment studies have not been reported.

Although significant methodological limitations exist in some studies, the extent of the limitations does not appear sufficient to contradict these conclusions. However, further studies using more rigorous definitions of PAs and more careful assessment of the relationship between attacks and morbidity are needed.

The literature suggests two strategies for ascertaining a more appropriate panic frequency threshold. Both require further empirical assessment (i.e., reanalysis of existing data sets and/or field trials). One option for DSM-IV is to continue to use the less restrictive part of the DSM-III-R threshold criterion (at least one PA followed by persistent fear of another attack for at least 1 month) while eliminating its more restrictive (four in 4 weeks) arm. This has the advantage of preserving some degree of continuity. In addition, the study by Lepine et al. (1989) suggests that in a clinical psychiatric population, this less restrictive DSM-III-R alternative encompasses many of those who meet other PD criteria but do not fulfill the frequency requirement. The Lepine et al. study is the only one to address this issue, however, and is confined to a clinical psychiatric population. Moreover, because the majority of panic sufferers still do not reach psychiatric settings, additional field trials in psychiatric, other medical, and nonclinical settings would be needed to assess the reliability and validity of this definition as well as its impact on prevalence. The potential contribution of alternative and/or additional "cognitive" criteria (e.g., excessive worries about health that develop in conjunction with panic symptoms) could also be investigated as part of this process.

If the frequency requirement is eliminated, establishment of a *standardized* set of optional subcategories (e.g., lifetime history of four attacks in 4 weeks; lifetime history of only one attack, 1 month of worry about the next attack; and possibly for treatment studies, four attacks in the past 4 weeks) could be used to maintain clarity of communication in further studies of possible importance of panic frequency for course, treatment outcome, etc. One logical strategy would be to reanalyze existing epidemiological data sets to see whether the pattern of association between different levels of subthreshold panic frequency (e.g., one attack per lifetime, six attacks per lifetime) and rates of "illness" behaviors suggest any inherent "disorder" thresholds. These would then be further evaluated in field trials.

Several available studies (Katon 1986; Von Korff and Eaton 1989; Von Korff et al. 1985) suggest the possibility of a continuum of severity between those with subthreshold and disorder-level panic with respect to number of symptoms, illness behavior, and comorbidity. However, sample sizes are small, and/or the roles of potentially contributing dependent variables (attack frequency, intensity, symptoms pattern, etc.) are not clearly delineated.

Limited-Symptom Panic

Based on the literature review, individuals who have *only* limited-symptom attacks (fewer than four symptoms) appear to constitute a small percentage of the panic population (less than one-quarter of those with nonclinical and infrequent panic and about 5%–10% of disorder-level subjects). Descriptive data are very limited, and data concerning family history, demographic, biological, and treatment characteristics have not yet been developed. There are no clear indications from the available data as to whether this group should be included or excluded from the diagnostic category.

Ongoing research of existing epidemiological data sets may soon provide further information. However, given the small number of individuals reporting attacks with three but not four symptoms, the most conservative course at present seems to be to maintain the four-symptom threshold in DSM-IV. By limiting application of the term *panic* to the most severe, and therefore most salient, events (Rubin 1986), the requirement for four simultaneous symptoms also improves reliability and probably facilitates assessment of such qualities as crescendo and sudden onset.

Role of Negative Cognitions in Panic Disorder With or Without Agoraphobia[2]

The issues reviewed concerning negative cognitions include 1) whether there are specific negative cognitions that distinguish PD patients from other psychiatric patients and individuals who are not ill and 2) the content and prevalence of these catastrophic cognitions in PD patients. Relevant literature was identified and abstracted from computer searches of the Medline and Psychological Abstracts databases for the past 5 years, and relevant earlier references were obtained from these papers and abstracted. Twenty-two studies were included on the basis of satisfactory methodology and contribution to one of the following aspects of PD: 1) the nature of cognitive abnormalities in PD/agoraphobia, 2) whether these cognitions differ between PD and other groups, and 3) the relationship between abnormal cognitions and avoidance behavior. Additionally, the baseline measurements of 100 patients with PD and agoraphobia and 61 PD patients in two controlled treatment trials were examined for the presence or absence of negative cognitions beyond the level displayed by nonanxious normal subjects. This substudy addressed the question: Do all PD patients have disordered cognitions?

---

[2]W. Stewart Agras, M.D.

What are the fears evoked in PD/agoraphobia by experience of panic?   In the first systematic study of the ideational components associated with anxiety, Hibbert (1984) compared patients with GAD or PD using a carefully structured interview. Patients with PD had significantly more thoughts of illness, death, and loss of self-control than GAD patients. There was no difference between groups on thoughts of social embarrassment. In a similar but uncontrolled study, Ottaviani and Beck (1987) examined the cognitions in a group of 30 PD patients using a semistructured interview. They found that panic arousal was associated with imagery of physical catastrophe (e.g., fainting, death, heart attacks, choking, and psychological catastrophe, such as control or going crazy).

Chambless et al. (1984) developed the Agoraphobic Cognitions Questionnaire, noting two outstanding factors: loss of control and physical consequences of PAs (e.g., illness such as heart attacks). Similarly, Reiss et al. (1986) examined the psychometric properties of the 16-item Anxiety Sensitivity Index (ASI) and concluded that it had unitary properties. The ASI measures the construct of anxious apprehension over the somatic sensations characteristic of fear and anxiety. The perception of the consequences of panic was also assessed using the 20-item Stanford Panic Appraisal Inventory (SPAI) (Telch, unpublished scale, 1987) in a group of 100 agoraphobic patients in our laboratory. The scale was shown to have three factors: fear of medical illness (e.g., heart attack), fear of losing control (e.g., going insane), and fear of social embarrassment. Overall internal consistency of this scale was high (Cronbach alpha = 0.90), with a standard item alpha of 0.89. Overall test-retest reliability was 0.73.

In summary, it appears that PD patients with or without agoraphobia negatively appraise panic symptoms along two dimensions; physical catastrophe and loss of control. There also appears to be a dimension of social embarrassment caused by others' perception of the PA or the feared consequences of a PA, although these data are somewhat less certain.

Is there a particular fear(s) that characterizes this population?   McNally and Foa (1987) found that agoraphobic patients were more likely than normal subjects to interpret bodily sensations associated with anxiety as threatening and that this tendency was reduced following treatment with cognitive-behavior therapy. In a study by Telch et al. (1989a), students meeting DSM-III-R criteria for PD based on questionnaire response had significantly higher ASI scores than normal subjects or those with infrequent panic. Diagnosis in this study may have been inadequate because no direct interviews were held. In another comparison with normal subjects (Zucker et al. 1989), 20 patients with DSM-III-R PD and 10 nonanxious control subjects were interviewed. The interviewers were blind to the diagnosis. The most significant difference found was fear of losing control. Surprisingly, in this study, relatively few patients noted fears of physical catastrophe.

Telch et al. (1989b) compared the cognitions of persons meeting DSM-III-R criteria for PD with those of persons with infrequent panic and found that the PD group had significantly more fears of dying and going insane than those with infrequent panic. In another study (Ganellen et al. 1986), PD patients with and without agoraphobia were compared using an Anxiety Thoughts and Tendencies scale constructed for the study. PD patients had fewer such thoughts than those with agoraphobia. Thus, it appears that there may be a continuum of catastrophic thinking: the least in those with infrequent panic, more in PD patients, and the most in agoraphobic patients.

In a comparison between 11 patients meeting DSM-III criteria for PD and 9 meeting DSM-III criteria for GAD, those with PD had higher somatic concern than the GAD subjects (Barlow et al. 1984). As noted above, Hibbert (1984) made similar findings in his comparison of PD and GAD patients. A comparison demonstrated that PD patients had higher scores on items concerned with fainting, dying, and going crazy than those with simple phobia (Thyer and Himle 1987). In a large study, Chambless and Gracely (1989) compared patients with agoraphobia, PD, GAD, social phobia, obsessive-compulsive disorder, and depression. The agoraphobic patients scored significantly higher than all other groups on fear of bodily sensations associated with anxiety. In addition, the agoraphobic and panic patients scored significantly higher than all other groups on thoughts that their anxiety would cause physical illness. All the clinical groups also scored higher than normal subjects on fears of loss of control and social embarrassment, but they did not differ significantly from one another. Thus, the key factor differentiating agoraphobic and panic patients from patients with other anxiety disorders would seem to be a fear that anxiety will cause physical illness or death. Telch et al. (1989c) compared 35 patients with PD with agoraphobia to 40 patients with PD but no phobic avoidance and found no significant difference on number of PAs, panic symptoms, or panic severity. However, in contrast to the findings described for the previous study, the groups were significantly different on fear of social consequences of panic and of losing control but not on fears of the physical consequences of panic, with the agoraphobic patients showing more fear than the PD patients. A similar but smaller-scale study compared agoraphobic patients with patients with other anxiety disorders and to normal subjects with respect to the ASI (Reiss et al. 1986). Agoraphobic patients scored higher than other anxiety disorder patients on the ASI and the other anxiety disorder patients scored higher than normal subjects.

In a rare physiological study, 10 subjects with PD were compared to 10 subjects with infrequent panic (Beck and Scott 1987). In a visualization of a hospital situation, those with PD demonstrated significantly greater physiological arousal assessed by muscle tension and skin conductance reactivity than those with infrequent panic. This did not occur in other situations. In a second laboratory study where subjects were hyperventilated, 20 PD and 13 GAD subjects were compared (Rapee 1986). The PD subjects reported nearly three times the symptoms compared with the GAD patients. Fears of dying, going insane, and creating a scene were reported by panic but not GAD patients. Fear of losing control was reported by 31.6% of panic and 7.7% of GAD patients.

It can be concluded that agoraphobic patients have a more fearful response to panic than PD patients and that both of these groups have more fears than normal subjects, and more fear than other psychiatric patients, including those with other anxiety disorders. The most consistent difference between PD/agoraphobic patients and other groups is somatic concern.

What percentage of PD and agoraphobic patients have these abnormal cognitions? This question was first addressed in 100 PD patients who met DSM-III criteria for PD with extensive avoidance in a controlled treatment trial. Cognitive response to panic was measured with the SPAI (Telch 1987), a 20-item measure that allows patients to describe the degree to which they have experienced each of the symptoms over the past week. Zucker et al. (1989) demonstrated that a cutoff of 50 on the SPAI was both sensitive and specific in distinguishing between normal subjects and PD patients, and this criterion was utilized. Ninety-three percent of the patients had a score of 50 or higher on this measure. Thus, the vast majority of such patients demonstrate catastrophic thinking in response to panic.

In a second study, the same measure was examined in 61 PD patients with mild or no avoidance. Surprisingly, in this study, 88.5% of this less-disabled group demonstrated catastrophic thinking in response to PAs.

Is there a relationship between cognitions and avoidance?   Emerging data suggest that the cognitive response to anxiety and panic mediates between the two elements cognitions and avoidance in the syndrome of agoraphobia. Ottaviani and Beck (1987) and Hibbert (1984) note that their patients' cognitive misinterpretations of somatic symptoms often triggered PAs. This observation was confirmed by Kenardy et al. (1988b), who used a questionnaire method in a study of 44 agoraphobic patients and found that cognitive factors triggered attacks more than physiological factors.

The first study to monitor cognitions in vivo in conjunction with physiological monitoring (Kenardy et al. 1988b) involved three patients who frequently reported negative cognitions during exposure to feared situations. In two of three PAs, negative cognitions preceded the panic. The authors conclude that physiological change and cognitive interpretation appear to be essential features of a PA. Kenardy et al. (1989) also report on five patients who monitored their cognitions for 1 day while being monitored physiologically. Two PAs were recorded and physiologically confirmed. In both, negative cognitions were associated with panic, but it was not clear if they preceded the attack. In another study, agoraphobic patients with varying degrees of avoidance were assessed prior to exposure to feared situations, and their avoidance was directly determined. It was found that the probability of having a PA accounted for most of the variance in avoidance between subjects (Craske et al. 1988). In addition, predicted intensity, discomfort, and harm from physical symptoms predicted within-subject variation in avoidance.

Chambless and Gracely (1989) studied a large group of patients with agoraphobia and reported that measures of fear predicted level of avoidance behavior, confirming earlier results (Chambless et al. 1984). Similarly, Ganellen et al. (1986) found that their measure of negative cognitions was correlated significantly with global phobia ($r = .59$, $P < .001$), whereas panic frequency and intensity were not. Breier et al. (1986) found, however, that patients who interpreted their first PA as anxiety (i.e., noncatastrophically) took 63 months to develop agoraphobia, whereas those who interpreted the event catastrophically took only 15 months to develop phobic avoidance.

Thus, it appears that PD patients have a variable tendency to interpret bodily sensations associated with anxiety and panic in a catastrophic manner, and that the degree to which this tendency is present predicts the level of agoraphobic avoidance.

What are the implications of all this for diagnostic classification of PD/agoraphobia in DSM-IV?   Both PAs and negative appraisal of the meaning of panic symptoms are essential features of PD with or without agoraphobia. In essence, DSM-III-R recognizes the importance of such cognitions both in the description (although they are described in terms of intense apprehension rather than appraisal of the meaning of panic symptoms) and in the symptom list. A clearer statement regarding the type of cognitions found in PD/agoraphobia might be useful in DSM-IV. Such a requirement might lead to the differentiation of a nonfearful panic group with different prognosis, although further research is needed to make such a differentiation and to establish whether such an addition increases diagnostic reliability and validity.

The literature suggests that three cognitions are typically present in PAs and between attacks in PD:

1. Physical catastrophe (e.g., fear of having a serious illness or of dying during an attack)
2. Loss of control (e.g., fear of going crazy or of doing something uncontrolled)
3. Social embarrassment (e.g., a fear that others will perceive the PA or one of the feared consequences of panic symptoms)

Can Cognitions Be Used to Discriminate Between Panic Disorder and Other Anxiety Disorders?[3]

This part of the review has two sections: 1) studies investigating cognitive disturbance in PD are reviewed to determine whether the cognitions identified by cognitive theorists reliably discriminate PD from other anxiety disorders, and 2) whether the diagnosis of PD could be improved by including cognitive items in the diagnostic criteria is considered.

Interview studies.   Ottaviani and Beck (1987) asked 30 DSM-III PD patients to recall their thoughts during a typical PA. All reported thoughts concerned with either anticipated physical catastrophes (death, heart attack, fainting, loss of breath, illness, and seizure) and/or mental-behavioral catastrophes (loss of control, going crazy). In addition, 12 (40%) feared social humiliation as a result of the physical or mental catastrophe.

   Three interview studies have addressed the question of whether thoughts of the type identified by Ottaviani and Beck (1987) discriminate panic patients from other anxious patients. Each obtained positive results. Hibbert (1984) compared 17 nonphobic patients with PAs to 8 nonphobic patients who did not experience PAs. The two groups differed only in frequency of thoughts concerned with anticipation of death, illness, or loss of control. Rapee (1985) obtained similar results in a larger study that compared the ideation of DSM-III PD patients ($n = 38$) with that of DSM-III GAD patients who had never experienced PAs ($n = 48$). Discriminant function analysis indicated that PD patients were significantly more likely to have thoughts concerned with the anticipation of having a heart attack, fainting, dying, or going mad, whereas GAD patients were more likely to believe that they were unreasonably anxious. Finally, Barlow et al. (1985) investigated the incidence and characteristics of PAs in 108 patients meeting DSM-III criteria for various anxiety disorders or major depression. Only two symptoms, dizziness and the one cognitive item assessed (fear of going crazy, losing control), discriminated PD patients from other patients who had occasional attacks.

Self-monitoring of cognitions during PAs.   In contrast to asking patients to recall thoughts associated with a typical attack, Westling et al. (1989) asked 17 DSM-III-R PD patients to record their cognitions during an attack using a panic diary and then classified the cognitions into mental, physical, or social catastrophes and various noncatastrophic categories. Overall, 79% of PAs were associated with one or more

---

[3]David M. Clark, Ph.D.

types of catastrophic cognition, and *all* patients had at least one PA associated with a catastrophic cognition. Thoughts concerned with physical catastrophes (e.g., dying, heart attack) and mental-behavioral catastrophes (losing control, going mad) were more common than those concerned with social catastrophes (humiliation).

In another self-monitoring study, Rachman et al. (1987) reported that 12 of the 14 patients (86%) who experienced attacks were able to identify catastrophic cognitions similar to those identified by Westling et al. (1989).

Agoraphobic Cognitions Questionnaire (ACQ). The ACQ was developed by Chambless et al. (1984) as a measure of thoughts about the negative consequences of anxiety. Subjects are presented with a list of 14 thoughts and are asked to rate "how often each thought occurs when you are nervous." Factor analyses have revealed that the scale consists of two distinct factors: physical concerns (e.g., heart attack) and social/behavioral concerns (e.g., loss of control). Chambless and Gracely (1989) compared the ACQ responses of 271 outpatients who met DSM-III criteria for PD ($n = 28$), agoraphobia with PAs ($n = 67$), social phobia ($n = 40$), obsessive-compulsive disorder ($n = 33$), GAD ($n = 46$), and dysthymia or MDD ($n = 57$). On the physical concerns factor, PD and agoraphobia with panic patients did not differ from each other but scored significantly higher than all other diagnostic groups.

Fear of bodily sensations. Cognitive theories propose that the panic-related thoughts identified in the above studies are misinterpretations of the bodily sensations experienced in PAs. Consistent with this suggestion, Hibbert (1984), Rachman et al. (1987), and Westling et al. (1989) report that the thoughts that occur in PAs appear to be meaningfully related to the bodily sensations being experienced.

Van den Hout and Griez (1986) administered a 14-item Fear of Autonomic Sensations Questionnaire (FASQ) to DSM-III PD and agoraphobia with PA patients ($n = 29$) and a mixed group of nonpanic neurotic control subjects ($n = 28$). As predicted, panic patients showed significantly greater interoceptive fear.

Foa (1988) administered the Body Sensations Questionnaire (BSQ; Chambless et al. 1984) to five groups of 20 subjects: PD, agoraphobia with PAs, GAD, simple phobia, and normal subjects. Consistent with Van den Hout and Griez's results, both PD groups scored higher than the other anxious patients and normal control subjects.

Finally, Chambless and Gracely (1989) administered the BSQ to patients with DSM-III agoraphobia with PAs, PD, GAD, OCD, and social phobia. The two PD groups obtained the highest scores, but only the agoraphobia with panic patients were significantly different from those with the other anxiety disorders.

Misinterpretation of bodily sensations.   Two sets of investigators have attempted to devise a more direct measure of misinterpretation of bodily sensations. Foa (1988) compared five groups of 20 subjects: PD, agoraphobia with PAs, GAD, simple phobias, and normal. Two types of ambiguous events were presented: descriptions of bodily sensations and ambiguous external events. From the brief report available, it appears that, as predicted, both PD groups differed from the other anxious groups on misinterpretation of bodily sensations but not on misinterpretation of external events.

Clark et al. (1988) compared three groups of 20 subjects: PD with or without agoraphobia, other anxiety disorder (GAD or social phobia), and normal. None of the other anxiety disorder patients had experienced spontaneous PAs. Four types of ambiguous events were presented. Consistent with Foa's study, panic patients were significantly more likely to interpret bodily sensations negatively than other anxious patients ($P < .01$) or normal control subjects ($P < .01$). In addition, this appears to be a highly specific cognitive disturbance because, when equated for current levels of anxiety using analysis of covariance, panic patients did not differ from other anxious patients in their misinterpretation of other ambiguous events (groups 2–4). Comparisons between subgroups indicate that both PD groups (with and without agoraphobia) score higher on misinterpretation of bodily sensations than either GAD ($P < .01$) or social phobia ($P < .05$) patients.

Clark et al. (1988) required both their PD groups (PD and agoraphobia with PAs) to have experienced at least three PAs during a 3-week period in the current episode. To determine whether patients who experience PAs at a lower frequency also misinterpret bodily sensations, an additional group of panic patients ($n = 9$) was recruited. These patients experienced recurrent PAs, some of which were not tied to specific phobic situations, but had never had sufficiently frequent attacks to meet the three attacks in 3 weeks criterion. These individuals with infrequent panic were indistinguishable from the other PD patients and scored higher on misinterpretation of bodily sensations than either GAD patients ($P < .05$) or social phobic patients ($P < .05$).

From the findings described above, it seems that interpretation of bodily sensations as evidence of an *immediately* impending physical or mental disaster distinguishes PD patients from social phobic and GAD patients. Before we can conclude that this interpretive style is specific to PD, we must also consider the relationship between PD and hypochondriasis. However, cognitive theorists (Clark 1988; Salkovskis 1988) have argued that the thinking of panic patients differs from that of hypochondriacal patients in at least two important aspects. First, it is hypothesized that panic patients' interpretations focus on *immediate* catastrophes (e.g., imminent death), whereas hypochondriacal patients' interpretations focus on more long-term threats to health (e.g., gradual development of cardiac disease, cancer). Second, it is hypothesized that hypochondriacal patients misinterpret a wider range of bodily sensations including many stimuli that are not autonomic responses. Salkovskis et al. studied patients meeting DSM-III-R criteria for PD ($n = 24$), hypochondriasis ($n = 19$), or both PD and hypochondriasis ($n = 26$) (Salkovskis, Warwick, and Clark, unpublished data; Warwick and Salkovskis 1990). Compared with hypochondriacal patients, PD patients were significantly more likely ($P < .01$) to interpret group 1 ("panic") bodily sensations as indicative of an immediate catastrophe and were significantly less likely ($P < .05$) to interpret the same sensations as implying a longer-term threat to health. Patients with a joint diagnosis of hypochondriasis and PD made both types of misinterpretation. Hypochondriasis patients scored higher than PD patients on misinterpretation of group 4 ("hypochondriacal") symptoms, but this difference failed to reach significance.

Summary.   The essence of PD is the experience of recurrent PAs, some of which are not the predictable result of exposure to, or anticipation of, a phobic stimulus. At the time DSM-III panic categories were proposed, it was unclear whether patients who fall into these categories have a characteristic set of fears, and ideational content was not included in the diagnostic criteria. However, current data indicate PD is associated with distinctive ideation, and it appears to be reasonable to include this in the diagnostic criteria. By making such a change, the criteria for PD would be brought into line with those of social phobia, GAD, and simple phobia, where ideational content and the specific focus of a patient's fears are important defining features.

DSM-III-R criterion B allows the possibility that an individual could be diagnosed as having PD without the clinician having identified any specific focus of the patient's fears. This is unfortunate because it means that individuals who really have another anxiety disorder (e.g., social phobia or GAD) might be incorrectly diagnosed with PD simply because the clinician has been unable to identify the focus of the patient's fears. By changing the criteria for PD to include what the patient is afraid of, this problem would be avoided.

The studies by Ottaviani and Beck (1987) and Westling et al. (1989) suggest that, with careful interviewing, it is possible to identify feared physical or mental catastrophes in all (or almost all) panic patients. However, in routine clinical practice, it seems unlikely that this will always be the case. For this reason, it might be best to *require* for the diagnosis of PD a fear of PAs and/or thoughts that the sensations experienced in an attack will lead to an immediate physical or mental catastrophe, such as going mad or having a heart attack. Also, the presence of the relevant thoughts could establish the diagnosis of PD even if the patient tends to believe that he/she has a physical problem rather than an anxiety disorder.

"Unexpected" Panic and DSM-IV[4]

The important question reviewed here concerns the necessity of experiencing what has come to be called a "spontaneous" or "unexpected" PA to meet the criteria for PD. In fact, the quality of "expectedness" now forms the core of Criterion A for PD (American Psychiatric Association 1987): "At some time during the disturbance, one or more PAs (discrete periods of intense fear or discomfort) have occurred that were 1) unexpected, i.e., did not occur immediately before or on exposure to a situation that almost always caused anxiety, and 2) not triggered by situations in which the person was the focus of others' attention" (pp. 237–238). This question raises at least two issues on which existing data sets have some bearing. 1) Can investigators from varying persuasions agree on the existence of different "types" of PAs and their definitions? Inherent in this issue is the necessity of distinguishing these attacks from more chronic or background anxiety. 2) Does the evidence support the necessity of one certain type of panic, a "spontaneous" or unexpected panic, occurring at some point during the development of PD?

All data published on definitions and types of panic were reviewed. This included more than 1,300 references accumulated when writing a book on anxiety (Barlow 1988a), abstracting services including the BRS Information Technologies, and PsycSCAN: Clinical Psychology. Unpublished data from the Center for Stress and Anxiety Disorders in Albany, New York, as well as closely related clinics (e.g., The New York State Psychiatric Institute), were also used. The first draft of this paper was sent to Donald Klein for detailed review because of his recent work and extensive experience with definitions and types of panics (e.g., Klein and Klein 1989a, 1989b).

Is there a difference in types of panic?   Some data exist concerning differences between uncued, unexpected, or spontaneous panics and cued panics. Barlow et al. (1985) divided patients into categories based on whether they had ever had an uncued unexpected (spontaneous) PA. Patients with PD with or without agoraphobia comprised one group. Another group was patients who had experienced at least one uncued unexpected panic but did not meet diagnostic criteria for PD with agoraphobia. The third group had never experienced an uncued unexpected panic. The percentage of symptoms endorsed from the 12 DSM-III symptoms was significantly higher in both the PD and the agoraphobic with panic groups. However, differences between those experiencing at least one uncued, unexpected panic and those who had never experienced such a panic occurred for the symptom of

---

[4]David H. Barlow, Ph.D., and Michelle G. Craske, Ph.D.

dizziness (which was associated with the uncued panic).

In Margraf et al.'s (1987) study, situational (cued) attacks were also rated as somewhat more severe but otherwise were phenomenologically similar, although there was a tendency for severely disturbing cognitions (but not somatic symptoms) to be reported more frequently during expected rather than unexpected panics. One study exists comparing PAs occurring within PD with PAs occurring in simple phobic patients during behavioral approach tests. Rachman et al. (1987) administered 69 exposure trials to 20 PD patients of which 30 (43.5%) were associated with a PA. In a corresponding trial with claustrophobic patients, these cued PAs occurred during 36% of 140 trials. Interestingly, claustrophobic subjects tended to report dyspnea, choking, dizziness, and fears of dying and going crazy *more frequently* than PD patients. PD subjects, on the other hand, tended to report palpitations, hot flashes, and trembling more frequently than claustrophobic subjects. Nevertheless, the overall patterns of panic frequency and symptom report were relatively similar.

Clearly, much needs to be done to ascertain the nature of different types of panic. Ideally, this would be carried out with ambulatory monitoring procedures, where both physiological and cognitive measures are collected as well as some indication of the presence of action tendencies such as escape. There is a need for this study not only in patients with PD but also in patients without comorbid PD with a principal diagnosis of simple or social phobia. Examining fear or alarm responses in normal subjects would also be of interest. Data from normal subjects in the study by Taylor et al.. (1986) seem to show differences in normals undergoing emergency reactions compared to PD patients. On the other hand, a later study by Margraf et al. (1987) demonstrated marked similarity in the presenting symptoms of normal subjects with those of patients. These are far too preliminary to draw any conclusions.

Is a "spontaneous" panic necessary for the definition of PD? DSM-III-R definitions clearly state that an individual must experience an unexpected PA (at least initially) to meet the criteria for PD. The individual must then experience a certain number of these attacks in a specified length of time and/or develop anxiety about experiencing another one. Clinical experience would suggest that 100% of patients with PD present with anxiety over the possibility of additional attacks. Evidence has appeared suggesting that anxiety over the possibility of additional PAs is the major distinguishing feature between those with clinical and nonclinical panic, as well as between those who meet definitions for PD and those who do not in a large survey of patients with nonclinical panic (Telch et al. 1989b). This might be the major indication of "caseness."

Furthermore, almost all patients report having experienced an initial unexpected uncued PA that seemed to mark the beginning of their disorder (Barlow 1988a). Occasionally, but rarely, clinicians see patients with agoraphobia who seem not to have experienced a classical PA based on DSM-III-R criteria. For example, of the last 1,455 patients assessed in the Center for Stress and Anxiety Disorders in Albany, New York, 9 patients were seen who received a diagnosis of agoraphobia without panic. Even in these cases, however, at least one marked somatic symptom was present, and the patients reported major fears concerning having these somatic symptoms or limited-symptom attacks while away from home. Therefore, these cases were not diagnosed as having agoraphobia with panic only because of a nosological technicality. In addition, Thyer and Himle (1985) reported 95 of 115 agoraphobic patients met the criteria for agoraphobia with PA, and 20 met the criteria for agoraphobia without panic. However, these investigators also found that all 20 of these patients had some somatic ailment of an unpredictable or sporadic nature such as epilepsy or colitis. It is very possible that those with colitis and related symptoms also met the criteria for limited-symptom attacks. In any case, an unpredictable somatic event (whether functional or organic) seems to serve as a functional equivalent to PAs, in that patients learn to fear the somatic event and avoid situations where it may occur. Because the event is unpredictable, the avoidance can become extensive.

Despite these observations from clinics, epidemiologists report a substantial percentage of people with extensive avoidance who do not present with PAs. Klein and Klein's work (1989a, 1989c) indicates that this may be due to definitional problems, because most of these data were based on retrospective report and collected by lay interviewers. As noted above, these data are subject to distortion, even in the hands of experienced interviewers. In any case, the individuals experiencing somatic symptoms or limited-symptom attacks would seem in every other way to be functionally equivalent to those meeting the criteria for PD, which raises questions about the importance of a retrospective report of four symptoms, a point also made by Klein and Klein (1989c).

It is interesting, however, to consider that a substantial minority (approximately 30%) of patients who present with PD can clearly cite an unfavorable experience with drugs such as anesthesia, cocaine, or marijuana as the setting event for their first panic (e.g., Aronson and Craig 1986; Barlow 1988a; Last et al. 1984). Here the "cause" in terms of a temporally associated event seems clear, and the anesthesia or recreational drug is subsequently avoided. However, a full PD syndrome also develops, including marked sensitivity to a variety of somatic cues and repeated uncued unexpected PAs. It is interesting then to analyze the similarities and differences of this onset with those who have a truly "out of the blue" experience.

Specifically, PD patients with a drug etiology would not seem to be technically classifiable as having an initial uncued panic (Aronson and Logue 1987; Breier et al. 1986; Swinson 1986; Thyer and Himle 1987), although it is clear that they had an unexpected panic. It is also clear that drugs were not a "cue" for them going into the situation, although in many cases drugs subsequently become a cue. It is not initially obvious, however, how a drug-onset PA would differ from a patient who had an initial PA during a public speaking appearance and subsequently develops a discrete social phobia. The major difference seems to be that the PD patient continues to have unexpected and uncued panics, whereas the social phobic patient can always identify the cue and almost always experiences the panic immediately on confronting the situation. Thus, the important point of divergence here would not necessarily be whether the initial (unexpected) PA had a clear precipitant but rather whether *subsequent* PAs were both unexpected and uncued (spontaneous), at least based on the perception of the patient.

However, even this distinction does not entirely work because it is not uncommon for all PAs of chronic PD patients to become cued or "situational." That is, virtually all attacks will occur in situations, such as shopping malls, that the patient has associated with the attacks. Therefore, neither the initial "spontaneity" of the attack or the absence of cues (situations) later on seems to discriminate PD from simple or social phobia.

Data from Barlow's clinic in Albany point to expectancy in terms of the timing of the attack as a discriminating feature. Specifically, when examining the timing of the attack in relation to exposure to the phobic cue or situation, 15% (4 of 27) of simple phobic patients reported that the timing was typically delayed. This compared to 30% (8 of 27) of social phobic patients but 92% (124 of 135) PDs. Thus, although the cue is clear, at least in the mind of the patient, it is not clear when to expect the panic. In other words, it remains unpredictable.

In summary, the initial setting event (cue) for the panic does not seem important. Also, initial panics in most diagnostic categories are unexpected or "out of the blue." What seems important is that at least some of the initial attacks are uncued and some of the attacks probably continue to be either uncued (in the mind of the patient) or, when cues can be identified, the timing of the attacks is typically delayed, thus producing an "unexpected" panic. Whether these attacks represent a basic neurobiological dysregulation or a learned alarm associated with (conditioned to) somatic cues would probably be irrelevant for this classification. All that would be necessary is that the patient, at some time but not necessarily initially, reports an uncued unexpected PA (or temporal discontinuity between the cue and the attack) and develops anxiety focused on the possibility of having another attack or on the consequences of having another attack.

Panic Disorder: Relation to Cardiac and Irritable Bowel Symptoms and Alcohol Abuse[5]

This section of the chapter reviews the existing research and research in progress to answer these questions: 1) Do subgroups of PD patients experience this disorder as frightening cardiac or gastrointestinal symptoms, and should the DSM-IV subcategorize PD with this presentation? 2) Does a subgroup of patients with PD/agoraphobia abuse and/or develop dependence on alcohol, and should DSM-IV subcategorize this overlap? Subcategorization could alert the clinician to atypical presentations of PD, increase diagnostic accuracy, and potentially decrease unnecessary medical testing. There are also increasing data showing that patients with alcohol abuse frequently have one or more associated psychiatric disorders and an emerging awareness that treatment of that disorder may decrease relapse rates.

The research reviewed was gathered from computerized literature searches on the cardiac, irritable bowel, and alcohol abuse overlap with PD. Much of this literature had been included in Dr. Katon's recently published book, *Panic Disorder in the Medical Setting* (Katon 1989), written for the National Institute of Mental Health (NIMH). Research on irritable bowel was also collated for a special article published by the *American Journal of Psychiatry* (Walker et al. 1990a).

In primary care, PD patients often present by selectively focusing on and complaining about the most frightening autonomic somatic symptoms or on a psychophysiological symptom caused by autonomic hyperactivity (e.g., diarrhea, epigastric pain, headache) (Katon 1984).

Several studies have demonstrated that many patients view their symptoms of nervousness and anxiety as appropriate responses to severe physiological sensations (Katerndahl 1988; Ley 1985). These patients are likely to present with concern about one or more autonomic symptoms associated with PD, such as tachycardia, chest pain, or dyspnea, and to answer physician queries about nervousness or anxiety with statements such as "Anyone with the physical symptoms I'm having (chest pain, dyspnea, dizziness . . .) would be frightened" (Katon 1988).

During a study on the prevalence of PD in primary care (Katon et al. 1987b), it was found that a positive response to the one screening question used in the structured psychiatric interview, "Have you ever had a spell or attack when all of a sudden you felt frightened, anxious or very uneasy in situations when most people would not be afraid?" often did not accurately identify a substantial subset of PD patients. These patients were identified by adding several somatic questions, the most sensitive being "Do you ever have sudden episodes of rapid heartbeat or palpitations?"

In a study of 55 primary care patients with PD referred for psychiatric consultation, 89% had initially presented with one or two somatic complaints, and misdiagnosis often continued for months to years (Katon 1984). The three most

---

[5]Wayne J. Katon, M.D.

common complaints were cardiac symptoms (chest pain, tachycardia, irregular heartbeat), gastrointestinal symptoms (especially epigastric distress), and neurological symptoms (headache, dizziness, vertigo, syncope, paresthesias). Clancy and Noyes (1976) have also provided evidence for somatization in PD. They examined the medical records of 71 patients and found that 30 different categories of tests totaling 358 procedures had been carried out (range 0–11, mean 7.5 tests). These patients had 135 specialty consultations, primarily from the cardiology, neurology, and gastroenterology services.

Irritable bowel syndrome (IBS).   IBS is a chronic gastrointestinal syndrome characterized by abdominal discomfort and pain with an alteration in bowel habits (cramping, diarrhea, constipation) in the absence of weight loss or demonstrable gastrointestinal pathology. Drossman et al. (1982) found in an epidemiological study that IBS affects 8%–17% of the general population. Lydiard et al. (1986) described a series of patients who had both IBS and PD. With effective treatment of PD, irritable bowel complaints were also reduced.

In studies that have used structured psychiatric interviews and operational diagnostic criteria, 70%–90% of IBS patients have diagnosable psychiatric problems, most commonly anxiety and depression (Walker et al. 1990a). Fossey et al. (1989) examined 35 consecutive outpatients in a gastroenterology clinic with the Structured Clinical Interview for DSM-III-R (SCID) (Spitzer and Williams 1983). Thirty-eight percent had a lifetime history of PD, and 24% currently had the disorder; 70% had a lifetime history of major depression, and 33% were currently depressed; and 38% were found to have somatization disorder. Walker et al. (1990b) studied 23 patients with IBS and compared them to 10 patients with inflammatory bowel disease. Patients with IBS had a significantly higher lifetime prevalence of PD (30% versus 0%), major depression (65% versus 20%), and somatization disorder (40% versus 0%).

IBS and PD.   The studies on IBS have demonstrated that three psychiatric disorders are associated with this gastrointestinal disorder: PD, major depressive disorder, and somatization disorder. Most of these studies have only examined patients in tertiary care (i.e., referrals to the gastroenterologist). Future studies need to be carried out in community and primary care populations that may have different psychiatric epidemiological patterns. It may be that patients with psychiatric illness are especially likely to be referred due to lack of response to primary care treatments such as bulk and anticholinergic agents. More research is needed to better understand the link between PD and IBS, including family studies, epidemiological studies that do not use exclusion criteria, provocation studies, and treatment studies. It is probably premature, given the lack of research, to subcategorize IBS as a typical presentation of PD. One recommendation might be a notation at the end of the diagnostic criteria (as is already included for mitral valve prolapse) that would read "*Note:* Mitral valve prolapse and IBS may be associated conditions but do not preclude the diagnosis of PD."

Cardiac complaints: association with PD.   The presentation of cardiac complaints by PD patients is likely to lead to expensive and potentially iatrogenic medical testing. Since the middle of the 19th century, cardiologists have described a syndrome of functional cardiac symptoms (chest pain and tachycardia) that was unrelated to organic heart disease (Skerrit 1983). The syndrome was first labeled *DaCosta's syndrome* or *irritable heart* and later *soldier's heart, effort syndrome, neurocirculatory asthenia, hyperdynamic beta-adrenergic circulatory state,* and *hyperventilation syndrome.* Follow-up studies have consistently shown that the risk of subsequent myocardial infarction is low (Kemp et al. 1986), yet 50%–75% have persistent complaints of chest pain and disability after normal coronary arteriograms (Ockene et al. 1980). These patients are frequently described in the medical literature as "cardiac neurotics" or "cardiac cripples" (Caughey 1939).

Past studies documented high anxiety and depression scores on psychological tests of patients who had chest pain and normal coronary angiograms (Costa et al. 1985; Elias et al. 1982) and normal treadmill responses (Channer et al. 1985). Wulsin et al. (1988) screened 49 emergency-room patients with atypical chest pain with a short PD screen and the CES-D and found 43% met criteria for PAs, 16% met criteria for PD, and 39% scored positively for depression.

Three studies have documented that patients with chest pain and negative angiography or treadmill results had a high prevalence of PD (Bass and Wade 1984; Beitman et al. 1987a; Katon et al. 1988). Bass and Wade (1984) studied 99 patients with chest pain undergoing coronary arteriography; 46 had hemodynamically insignificant disease, and 53 had significant coronary adenosis. Twenty-eight (61%) of the 46 with insignificant disease had psychiatric diagnoses, compared to 23% of the 53 with significant obstruction. The most common psychiatric diagnosis in the patients with insignificant disease was anxiety neurosis (in the British nomenclature, the term *PD* is not used), and 52% of this group exhibited polyphobic behavior.

Katon et al. (1988) studied 74 chest pain patients referred to coronary angiography. Using structured interviews, 43% of the 28 patients with chest pain and normal coronary arteries were found to have PD, compared to 5% of 46 patients with chest pain and significant coronary artery stenosis. Patients with chest pain and normal coronary arteries had a significantly higher mean number of autonomic symptoms (tachycardia, dyspnea, dizziness) associated with their chest pain (5.2 versus 3.8, $P < .05$) and were significantly more likely to have atypical chest pain. In a third study, Beitman et al. (1987a) found that 43 (58%) of 74 patients with atypical or nonanginal chest pain and no evidence of coronary artery disease by electrocardiogram, treadmill, or angiography had PD.

Ford (1987) reviewed the association between chest pain and psychiatric illness in the ECA study and found that 2.5% of patients complained of chest pain. Patients with chest pain were four times as likely to have PD, three times as likely to have phobic disorder, and twice as likely to have major depression as control subjects without chest pain.

The above correlations documenting a high association between chest pain and PD have more significant implications for the primary care physician or psychiatrist than for the cardiologist. The cardiologist is more likely to be referred patients with multiple cardiac risk factors and to consequently refer them for cardiac testing. On the other hand, the most common primary care or psychiatric patient is a 20- to 40-year-old woman, a subgroup in which PD has its highest prevalence (Myers et al. 1984), who have a low frequency of coronary artery disease. Moreover, current studies have demonstrated that 40% of primary care patients with PD present with chest pain (Katon 1984). Primary care physicians are the "filter" for cardiac referrals, and thus increased education about the association between chest pain and PD may increase the accuracy of diagnosis and decrease unnecessary medical referrals and testing.

Cardiac symptoms and PD.   There is extensive research linking PD to somatization, especially cardiac complaints. Three recent studies using what is considered to be the cardiac "gold standard" for diagnosis—coronary angiography—have found PD to be associated with chest pain and negative angiography. Moreover, both community, primary care, and emergency-room data support this link. More research is needed to determine causality in this strong association. Thus, family history studies, provocation studies such as lactate infusion or carbon dioxide challenge, and treatment studies are needed to more firmly demonstrate a causal link between PD and chest pain.

The Work Group considered using a subcategorization in DSM-IV that would list a cardiac presentation (chest pain and/or tachycardia), with the patient perceiving the sudden attack of fear or anxiety as secondary to these cardiac symptoms. Thus, the diagnostic criteria might read "at some time during the disturbance, one or more discrete periods of intense fear or discomfort have occurred secondary to chest pain or discomfort. At least some of these periods of fear or discomfort were 1) unexpected and 2) not triggered by situations in which the person was the focus of others' attention." The autonomic symptoms could include all of the same symptoms listed in DSM-III-R except chest pain or discomfort (which are part of Criterion A). However, it was felt that there was insufficient evidence to justify this subcategorization in DSM-IV.

Alcohol abuse.   Ten studies have measured the prevalence of either PD or phobias in patients with alcohol abuse/dependence. The studies of inpatients in alcohol treatment have found prevalence rates for PD that ranged from 5% to 20.8% (excluding the data by Nunes et al. [1988], who studied a small sample of all female patients).

Krystal et al. (1989) reported data from the ECA sample. They found that the presence of alcohol abuse was associated with a large increase in the prevalence of PD. Helzer and Pryzbech (1988) have also shown that patients diagnosed as meeting criteria for alcohol abuse and/or dependence in the ECA were more than twice as likely to have PD. The risk for alcoholism in people with phobias of any type in the ECA project was about 2.5 times higher than in the general population; in persons with PD, the risk was greater than fourfold (Boyd et al. 1984). In the eight studies measuring the prevalence of phobias in patients with alcohol abuse, 3%–52% were found to have phobias, predominantly social phobia and/or agoraphobia. Leaving out the two studies with the most discrepant findings, six studies found prevalence rates of 10%–40%. These prevalence rates suggest that PD and phobic disorders are probably higher in those with alcohol-related disorders than in the general population.

Smail et al. (1984) studied the co-occurrence of these disorders in depth to discern which problem occurred first. The more severely phobic males were also the most alcohol dependent, and those with no phobias were the least alcohol dependent. All phobic alcoholic patients reported that alcohol had helped them to cope in feared situations, and almost all had deliberately used it for this purpose. However, in a subsequent study of 24 hospitalized alcohol abuse patients who also had PD and multiple social phobias, periods of heavy drinking and dependence on alcohol were associated with an exacerbation of agoraphobia and social phobias (Stockwell et al. 1984). Subsequent periods of abstinence were associated with substantial improvements in these anxiety states.

Three of the four other studies that assessed chronology of phobias, PD, and alcohol abuse found that phobias or PD or both preceded alcohol abuse in the majority of patients (Bowen et al. 1984; Mullaney and Trippett 1979; Stockwell et al. 1984). The study by Krystal et al. (1989) of the ECA data found the reverse (i.e., alcohol abuse preceded PD in the majority of cases).

Alcohol abuse/dependence and PD.   Epidemiologically, the research does support an association between PD, phobias (especially social phobias and agoraphobia), and alcohol abuse/dependence. Analogous to major depression, however, care must be taken in diagnosing PD or agoraphobia in the context of alcohol abuse. Alcohol abuse may cause depression, and alcohol withdrawal may precipitate severe anxiety and autonomic nervous system dysfunction. In the section on substance abuse in DSM-IV under "Associated Features," the overlap between PD, social phobia, and agoraphobia should be acknowledged. A caveat should follow stating that alcohol abuse can be secondary to these severe anxiety disorders but may also worsen a preexisting anxiety disorder or perhaps even cause the disorder. Thus, patients must be detoxified for 2–4 weeks (the Substance Abuse Committee suggests 6 weeks) and a reassessment of the anxiety disorder made at that time. If the anxiety disorder is still present, then pharmacological treatment (probably antidepressant but not benzodiazepines) could be initiated. Future treatment studies are needed to determine whether treatment of PD or agoraphobia in abstinent alcohol abuse patients decreases relapse.

In DSM-IV, in the section discussing the differential diagnosis of PD, the overlap with PD and alcohol abuse should also be acknowledged. A statement that the patient must be detoxified from alcohol and then reassessed in 2–4 (6?) weeks before treatment for PD is prescribed will be important to include.

Delineating the Boundaries of Social Phobia: Its Relation to Panic Disorder and Agoraphobia[6]

The purpose of this section of the review is to summarize the literature comparing social phobic disorder to PD and agoraphobia. The following questions were addressed: 1) Is social phobia a distinct clinical syndrome, differing from PD and agoraphobia on a number of variables? 2) What are the principal differential diagnostic features that define the phenomenological boundaries of the syndrome, in particular the boundaries with PD and agoraphobia? (See Schneier et al., Chapter 17, this volume.)

A review of the relevant literature suggests that social phobia is a distinct clinical entity that differs from PD/agoraphobia on a number of variables (Liebowitz 1987; Liebowitz et al. 1985c). Compared with agoraphobia, social phobia is less prevalent (in the community as well as the clinic) (Myers et al. 1984), is about equally represented among males and females who seek treatment for the disturbance (versus a preponderance of females among agoraphobic patients) (Öst 1987; Regier et al. 1984), and has an earlier age at onset. Furthermore, PD and agoraphobia are not found in the families of those with social phobia, nor is social phobia seen in the families of PD/agoraphobic patients (Reich and Yates 1988). Results of biological-challenge studies suggest that social phobia and PD/agoraphobia are characterized by different pathophysiological mechanisms (Liebowitz et al. 1985c). Also, treatment studies show promise in providing some pharmacological dissec-

[6]Salvatore Mannuzza, Ph.D., Abby J. Fyer, M.D., Michael R. Liebowitz, M.D., and Donald F. Klein, M.D.

tion of the syndromes (Liebowitz et al. 1988). Taken together, the above findings underscore the potential significance of further investigations of social phobic disorder to provide additional documentation of its validity and insight into its etiology and treatment.

Perhaps the most significant point of this review is that symptoms must be evaluated within the context of the individual's disturbance. Type of PA (not just "PA"), focus of fear (not just fear of "social" situations), reason for avoidance, etc., must be precisely and thoroughly assessed to formulate an accurate differential diagnosis.

The same logic applies to all symptoms and syndromes in psychiatry. For example, avoidance behavior, a hallmark symptom of the phobic disorders, is diagnostically uninterpretable when viewed out of context. A patient with major depression may avoid people (social withdrawal). A psychotic patient may demonstrate pervasive avoidance (become housebound) because of persecutory delusions. A patient with OCD may avoid public bathrooms because of fears of "giving in" to handwashing compulsions.

The core disturbance in social phobia involves concern about scrutiny, humiliation, and embarrassment, and all other symptoms (e.g., PAs) and behaviors (e.g., avoidance of certain situations) revolve around these concerns. This should probably continue to be a principal part of the diagnostic strategy in DSM-IV for delineating the boundaries of social phobia.

Review of Provocation of Panic Attacks[7]

The principal issue reviewed in this section concerns whether the search for laboratory-based methods of inducing panic have developed to the point where they can be used in the diagnosis of PD.

A comprehensive literature search was performed utilizing key words. The search was then conducted with Medline from 1983 to July 1989 as well as *Excerpta Medica Psychiatr* from 1980 to July 1989. Abstracts were reviewed and important papers studied. We used two papers as key reviews on the subject: "Pharmacological Provocation of Panic Attacks" (Gorman et al. 1987) and "A Neuroanatomical Hypothesis for Panic Disorder" (Gorman et al. 1989). An initial draft of this section was reviewed and edited by Drs. Papp and Gorman. In addition, once the section had been edited several times, a critique was obtained from Dr. Donald Klein, an authority in the field. Every effort was made to reflect the cutting edge of the field and to incorporate current concepts and dilemmas.

PD is unique among psychiatric illnesses because its core symptomatology can

---

[7]Jeremy D. Coplan, M.D., Laszlo A. Papp, M.D., and Jack M. Gorman, M.D.

be provoked in susceptible individuals by pharmacological probes. There has been a recent proliferation of agents reportedly capable of inducing panic symptoms in PD patients, providing psychiatric investigators with an opportunity to address PD at several different levels. First, the investigator is able to establish biochemical, physiological, and neuroimaging concomitants of pharmacologically provoked PAs. Second, agents administered acutely or chronically may block laboratory-induced PAs. This information facilitates the identification of clinically useful therapeutic strategies for treatment of these patients. Third, laboratory-induction of PAs encourages investigators to generate hypotheses designed to uncover the pathophysiology of clinical PD. Generally, hypotheses have attempted to link a specifically known property of a panicogen with its ability to induce panic. The biological system affected by the panicogen is deemed to be dysregulated and is hypothesized to impart a specific vulnerability to the subject that is intimately related to the etiology of PD.

Although this approach has fostered the rapid growth of knowledge concerning PD, it is important to explore the limitations of this line of reasoning. There is a tendency for theories based on the panicogenic effect of a particular agent to inadequately address the panicogenic effects of agents that act on different neurochemical systems. Ideally, a single comprehensive theory concerning the pathogenesis of PD must include an integration of the various mechanisms of the variety of known panicogens. If this task cannot be accomplished, then the disorders could be considered heterogeneous, with different biological subtypes but with a single final common pathway leading to the clinical disorder. Alternatively, there may be several key derangements that occur simultaneously in a given patient. Finally, it is possible, but unlikely, that panicogenic agents do not interact with specific biological abnormalities but rather act to induce panic by the nonspecific induction of subjective stress.

As yet, little emphasis has been placed on the order effect of neurobiological abnormalities in PD. It is conceivable that panicogens may exert their effects at "downstream" sites rendered susceptible via a core defect. Thus, administration of a panicogenic agent may provide valuable information regarding the pathophysiology of PD but may not necessarily address etiological factors of the disorders. Finally, patients with the clinical disorder who fail to respond positively to a particular panicogen need to be considered in the formulation of hypotheses concerning the pathogenesis of PD.

The attributes possessed by the ideal panicogenic agent described by Gorman et al. include

1. The PA should combine physical symptoms of panic with a subjective sense of terror and a desire to flee.

2. The provoked attack should be judged to be symptomatically very similar to the patient's regularly occurring spontaneous PAs.

3. The induction of panic should be specific to patients with a history of spontaneous attacks.

4. The agent, in the panicogenic dose, should be safe for routine administration to human subjects.

5. The effect of the agent provoking panic should be consistent in a given patient. If a desensitization effect to the panicogenic effects of an agent occurs, it should be predictable.

6. Drugs that block spontaneous PAs when given for prolonged periods, such as tricyclic antidepressants, monoamine oxidase inhibitors, and alprazolam, should also block the acute pharmacologically induced attack.

7. Agents that do not block clinical panic acutely or chronically should not block the pharmacologically induced panic.

Despite the stringency of these criteria, a plethora of panicogenic agents have been described that satisfy them to variable degrees. Paradoxically, agents that most fulfill the above criteria, such as sodium lactate, are not necessarily the best understood in terms of their central action. Attempts to create a unifying rubric from which to conceptualize the action of these agents becomes increasingly complex, as new and often discrepant data emerge in the literature.

Conclusions. A detailed review of the relative degree to which the described panicogens fulfill the criteria for panicogenic agents is beyond the scope of this summary, and interested readers are referred to Chapters 10–14 of the *Neurobiology of Panic Disorder* (Ballenger 1990, pp. 158–242). Sodium lactate is probably the most extensively studied and most reliable panicogen, but because of multiple metabolic effects and poorly understood central mechanism of action, research efforts have been directed toward other panicogens. Yohimbine's central action is more clearly understood, but its panicogenic effects have not been as extensively replicated as sodium lactate. The observations that the increases of serum 3-methoxy-4-hydroxyphenylglycol (MHPG) that occur during yohimbine challenge are not seen in lactate-induced panic or natural exposure to phobic stimuli and that imipramine treatment is unable to block yohimbine-induced panic complicate our understanding of yohimbine's effects. CO_2 inhalation appears to closely replicate naturally occurring panic but only causes PAs in a subgroup of PD patients; CO_2 may be of potential use in identifying panic patients with respiratory abnormalities. Isoproterenol has a similar rate of panicogenesis to sodium lactate. Because it crosses the blood-brain barrier poorly, hypotheses concerning its mode of action have been unsatisfying.

The newer serotonergic agents (m-CPP and fenfluramine) are of interest, especially because several effective therapeutic agents appear to work via the serotonergic system. Limitations of these agents include the lack of specificity of their central effects. The similarity of the symptoms induced by these agents to true panic is also questionable.

Models of panic based on biological-challenge studies have contributed greatly to our understanding of the pathophysiology of PD and pathological anxiety states. They have also provided useful tools in evaluating effective interventions in panic. However, it is unclear to what extent they have expanded our knowledge regarding etiological factors in PD.

Questions have been raised regarding the diagnostic utility of panicogens in clinical practice. Even the most reliable panicogens do not have sensitivity that closely approximates a well-conducted clinical interview. Therefore, the pharmacological provocation of panic remains a research tool and cannot be recommended in clinical practice. Future research in the area is warranted to increase the possibility for clinical application of panicogenic agents.

Specific recommendations for DSM-IV.   Despite current clinical and heuristic interest in panic provocation, the Work Group felt that the inclusion of the various laboratory-induced panic responses as specific diagnostic criteria in PD would be premature. A serious limitation to their inclusion is that few centers have conducted consecutive panic provocations on the same subject using different panicogens. It is unclear whether nonresponders to a particular panicogen would respond to alternative panicogens. Strategies of this nature are uncomfortable for investigator and patient alike but may increase levels of diagnostic sensitivity. However, until more data are available, the clinical interview remains the major diagnostic tool.

Is Agoraphobic Avoidance Secondary to Panic Attacks?[8]

To address the extent to which agoraphobic avoidance is secondary to PAs and the resultant diagnostic implications, evidence pertaining to each of the following is reviewed: 1) How frequently is the diagnosis of agoraphobia without panic assigned? Does the clustering of features that characterizes agoraphobia without panic (as currently specified) occur with sufficient frequency to warrant a separate diagnostic category? 2) What is the chronological course between the onset of panic and the onset of agoraphobic avoidance? That is, when both agoraphobic avoidance and PAs are present, is the avoidance preceded by PAs in all cases? 3) Is the maintenance of agoraphobic avoidance strongly related to PAs? 4) To what extent

---

[8]Michelle G. Craske, Ph.D.

do persons with PD differ as a function of their degree of agoraphobic avoidance? That is, is the presence of agoraphobic avoidance associated with features (premorbid and/or comorbid) that are sufficiently distinct to imply a psychopathological process different from the one that is evidenced in persons with PD without agoraphobia? 5) What are the clinical features of persons (if any) who meet the current diagnostic criteria for agoraphobia without a history of PAs? An additional question briefly discussed is whether DSM-IV should expand the number of situations listed as typically avoided in agoraphobia?

Evidence pertaining to each of these issues was gathered by Medlars and Psychological Abstracts computer searches, covering the years 1966 and 1967–1990, respectively. The key words were *panic disorder, agoraphobia,* and *avoidance.* Reference lists from relevant articles were also used.

Prevalence of agoraphobia without a history of panic.   Several community surveys of the prevalence of anxiety disorders have been reported, although the earlier studies (Uhlenhuth et al. 1983; Weissman et al. 1978) did not examine the relationship between panic and agoraphobia in detail. Three subsequent surveys have done so. Angst and Dobler-Mikola (1985) reported results from a subsample of 456 of their large community survey in Zurich. Using a structured interview (structured psychopathological interview and rating of the social consequences of psychic disturbances for epidemiology, SPIKE), they found a "current" and "within the past year" prevalence rate for agoraphobia without PAs in the range of 1.5 per 100, compared to an estimate of 0.7 per 100 for agoraphobia with PAs. However, only agoraphobic patients with concurrent PAs were excluded from the first category. Hence, agoraphobic patients who had panicked in the past might have been included, rendering the group comparison less clear.

Weissman et al. (1986) and Weissman and Merikangas (1986) reported the prevalence of the same two categories, on the basis of data gathered from the ECA study. By using the DIS across five sites with a sample size of more than 15,000, the lifetime rates for agoraphobia without PD or panic symptoms were found to range from 1.4 to 6.6 per 100, whereas the lifetime rates for agoraphobia with PD or panic symptoms ranged from 1.7 to 2.6 per 100 (Weissman et al. 1986). Site variability was marked. In the New Haven site, the rate of agoraphobia without PD was 2.9 per 100, and the rate of agoraphobia with PD was 0.3 per 100. However, closer examination of the New Haven ECA data (Weissman and Merikangas 1986) revealed that many (46.5%) of the subjects categorized as agoraphobia without PD either experienced limited symptom attacks, infrequent PAs, or situational PAs only or attributed the attacks to physical illnesses or other causes. By limiting the category to "pure" agoraphobia without PAs, the rate was reduced to 1.0 per 100.

Finally, Joyce et al. (1989) reported results from the DIS in a New Zealand community sample of 1,498. The estimated lifetime prevalence of agoraphobia (phobic of one or more agoraphobic situations) with PD was 0.8 per 100 and of agoraphobia without PD was 4.3 per 100. Using a more stringent criteria for agoraphobia that required two or more situations that were avoided, the corresponding prevalence estimates were 0.7 and 2.3 per 100. Many of the agoraphobic subjects experienced PAs but did not meet criteria for PD. The rate reduced to 0.6 per 100 for agoraphobia without panic when all subjects who experienced PAs/symptoms were excluded. This figure compares with the rate of 1.0 per 100 obtained by Weissman and Merikangas (1986).

Epidemiological surveys suggest that agoraphobia most often occurs in the absence of PD but most frequently with PA symptoms. The proportions of individuals reporting agoraphobic avoidance without PA symptoms ranges from 0.6 to 1.0 per 100.

A diagnosis of agoraphobia without a history of panic is rarely assigned in clinical practice (Barlow 1988a). Prevalence estimates obtained from research settings, in which the subject pool is comprised of persons seeking treatment, also differ from the ECA estimates. For example, Swinson (1986) reported that agoraphobic avoidance was accompanied by PAs in all of a series of 300 consecutively assessed agoraphobic subjects. It is unclear, however, whether all met criteria for PD. Thyer et al. (1985) examined 115 agoraphobic subjects, of whom 95 (82.6%) experienced PAs (although the number who met criteria for PD is not known). The remaining 20 subjects had a somatic ailment that could be characterized as sporadic or unpredictable, as is characteristic of PAs. Noyes et al. (1986) reported that 80 of 83 agoraphobic subjects experienced a sufficient frequency or severity of PAs to meet criteria for PD, and the remaining 3 subjects experienced infrequent PAs. From a series of 71 consecutively diagnosed agoraphobic subjects at the Center for Stress and Anxiety Disorders in Albany (unpublished data), only 2 (2.8%) met criteria for agoraphobia without a history of PD. In addition, from a total of 1,455 diagnostic evaluations of anxiety disorders, conducted over the course of 6 years at the same center, a diagnosis of agoraphobia without PD was assigned on only 9 (0.06%) occasions. Finally, Pollard et al. (1989) surveyed 93 practitioners with experience in the area of anxiety disorders regarding the number of patients seen in the last 12 months who met DSM-III criteria for agoraphobia with or without PAs. Of 993 subjects, 94% were categorized as with PAs and only 6% as without PAs.

Therefore, community-based surveys yield a much higher prevalence of agoraphobia without PD or PAs than observed in the clinical setting. There are several possible explanations for this discrepancy. First, this may reflect a real difference, as would be consistent with the finding that the presence of PAs tends to increase the likelihood that help will be sought (Barlow 1988a; Boyd 1986). Second, it may reflect an inflation effect in the community survey results, due to the methods by which categories were established. As Weissman et al. (1986) note, "the key DSM-III concept of agoraphobia 'fear of being in a place from which escape might be impossible or difficult in case of incapacitation' is not asked in precisely that way in either the DIS or the SADS. The key concept in the DIS is 'strong fear of something or some situation that is avoided even though there is no real danger'" (p. 790). Such wording might result in the false inclusion of simple phobias such as acrophobia, claustrophobia, air travel phobia, and driving phobias. Furthermore, excessive generalized worry about harm from others or dangers in the environment (e.g., car accidents) might lead to affirmative responses when in fact they are better subsumed under a GAD domain.

Chronology. Examination of chronological course is best conducted through longitudinal research, given the biases and deficiencies of retrospective recall. Unfortunately, all of the studies reviewed entailed retrospective recall.

Breier et al. (1986) examined 55 patients diagnosed with agoraphobia with PAs. Agoraphobic avoidance was recalled as being present prior to the first PA in 1 subject only. The development of agoraphobic avoidance usually occurred within 2 months of the first PA (48.2%). Thirteen (24.1%) recalled that avoidance developed 3–12 months after the first PA, whereas 15 (27.8%) recalled that avoidance developed at least 13 months after the first PA. Garvey and Tuason (1984) found that agoraphobic avoidance followed the initial panic by several weeks in 5 patients (41.7%) and coincided with the initial panic in 7 patients (58.3%). From a series of 65 consecutive diagnoses of PD with agoraphobia from the Center for Stress and Anxiety Disorders in Albany, agoraphobic avoidance was recalled as occurring before the initial PA on only one occasion. The avoidance coincided with or occurred after the initial PA on 40 occasions, whereas the chronological course was not recalled or was not ascertained on 23 occasions. Of the chronological data obtained, the onset of agoraphobia was recalled as occurring after the first panic in 97.6% of the cases. Estimates that correspond to those provided by Breier et al. (1986) are: 45.2% began to avoid within 2 months of the first PA, 19.4% began to avoid between 3 and 12 months after the first PA, and 35.5% began to avoid some time later. These proportions are relatively consistent with those reported by Breier et al. (1986).

In contrast, Fava et al. (1988) examined 20 outpatients who met criteria for agoraphobia and reported that 90% of their subjects experienced phobic symptoms before the onset of panic. Unfortunately, it is difficult to determine the degree to which "phobic symptoms" comprised avoidance of the identifiable cluster of agoraphobic situations. The "prodromal" symptoms that were reported as most often occurring prior to the onset of the first PA included generalized anxiety, phobic anxiety, phobic avoidance, and hypochondriasis. Unfortunately, many of these descriptors were not clearly specified. Phobic anxiety was assessed in reference to agoraphobic situations (measured with the Fear Questionnaire [Marks and Mathews 1979]), and phobic avoidance was apparently present in each of the 18 subjects who feared agoraphobic situations. However, it is not clear how phobic avoidance was assessed.

The most consistent finding, therefore, is that agoraphobic avoidance most often follows the initial PA in persons assigned a diagnosis of PD with agoraphobia.

Maintaining variables. If agoraphobic avoidance is secondary to PAs, then it might be hypothesized that not only the onset but also the maintenance of agoraphobic avoidance is related to dimensions of panic. These dimensions include panic frequency, panic severity, panic typology, and apprehension regarding the occurrence of panic.

Panic Apprehension

Several studies have shown independently that in agoraphobic persons, the degree to which a given situation is avoided depends largely on the degree to which panic is expected to occur in that particular situation. Craske et al. (1988) found that judgments of the likelihood that panic would occur were very predictive of different levels of avoidance exhibited during behavioral approach testing. In addition, such judgments were more predictive than was the length of time since approach to the given situation had been last attempted. Similarly, Telch et al. (1989c) found that concerns about panicking and the perceived resultant negative consequences (social embarrassment and loss of control) in typical agoraphobic situations were more troublesome for individuals with extensive agoraphobic avoidance than for those with minimal avoidance. Mavissakalian (1988) also found, on the basis of self-monitoring and behavioral approach testing, that fear of panic was a mediator of degree of avoidance.

Rachman and colleagues (see Rachman and Bichard 1988, for a review) have conducted a series of studies in which they have microanalytically examined patterns of predicted and actual panic and fear in specific feared situations. Their results have highlighted the way in which unexpectedly high levels of panic and fear serve to increase avoidance behavior, by increasing judgments of the likelihood of panic or the level of fear to be experienced on reexposure to the same phobic situation. Unfortunately, they have specifically measured avoidance only with subjects with snake and spider phobia (Rachman and Lopatka 1986). Replication with persons with PD with agoraphobia is warranted.

Panic Frequency

Another dimension of panic that may relate to the pattern of continued agoraphobic avoidance is the frequency with which PAs occur. However, significant discordance and asynchrony have been observed between measures of the frequency of panic and degree of avoidant behavior. Treatment-outcome studies have demonstrated very significant changes in panic frequency with minimal changes in avoidant behavior and vice versa.

Michelson et al. (1985) reported that approximately 45% of a group of 31 agoraphobic subjects continued to experience "spontaneous" PAs posttreatment, as did approximately 43% at a 3-month follow-up assessment, despite the high degree of improvement in approach behavior exhibited in 67% posttreatment and 61% at follow-up assessment. Klein et al. (1987) concluded, from a path analysis of treatment course data, that improvement in avoidance could occur even while panics continued. It is possible, however, that a reduction in panic frequency (in contrast to an elimination of PAs) accompanied the improvement in avoidance behavior in each of these studies. However, Arnow et al. (1985) noted that panic frequency did not change, on average, as a result of 4 weeks of in vivo exposure, despite improvements in all other measures of phobic avoidance. Similarly, in an analysis of panic and avoidance asynchrony within individuals, Chambless et al. (1986) found that 29% of 35 agoraphobic subjects experienced significant improvements in avoidance without changes in panic frequency. Finally, Clark et al. (1985) observed the converse situation, in which an almost complete elimination of panic was not accompanied by a reduction in avoidance behavior, at least in the short term.

The discordance between panic frequency and avoidance is evident not only with respect to patterns over time but also with respect to group comparisons. Vermilyea (1986) compared the reported frequency of PAs over the 3 weeks prior to assessment between 15 persons with PD and 15 persons with agoraphobia. The frequency of PAs did not differ significantly between groups (11.1 and 9.6, respectively). Craske et al. (1987) found that groups of mild, moderate, and severe avoiders (DSM-III-R nosology) did not differ in terms of panic frequency, despite an increasing trend in mean scores, due to high levels of within-group variability. Furthermore, panic frequency only correlated with reported fear of agoraphobic situations and not with reported avoidance of agoraphobic situations. Rapee and Murrell (1988) observed the same trend and a similar degree of variability. Similarly, Thyer et al. (1985) and Telch et al. (1989c) found that their groups of PD patients with and without agoraphobic avoidance did not differ in terms of panic frequency.

Retrospectively recalled panic frequency and severity have been shown to be exaggerated in comparison with data obtained from continuous self-monitoring (Margraf et al. 1987; Rapee et al. 1990). Therefore, most of the previously mentioned data sets are somewhat questionable. However, self-monitoring of the frequency of panic has yielded rates across groups with different levels of avoidance that are comparable to those obtained from interview data (Vermilyea 1986).

On the other hand, should agoraphobic avoidance successfully reduce the frequency of panic, it is conceivable that very frequent occurrence of panic *initially* accounts for the development of agoraphobic avoidance. Craske et al. (1987) found that the frequency of PAs at the time at which they were recalled as occurring most frequently did not differ between groups with varying levels of avoidance. These data lend support to the hypothesis that panic frequency does not relate strongly to agoraphobic avoidance, although again the findings are susceptible to the inaccuracies of retrospective recall. Longitudinal research is required to fully assess the relationship between panic frequency and the onset of agoraphobic avoidance.

In summary, unlike the degree to which panic is expected to occur in specific situations, the frequency with which panic occurs does not seem to relate to degree of agoraphobic avoidance.

Panic Severity

A third panic dimension that might relate to the maintenance of agoraphobic avoidance is the severity of PAs. Vermilyea (1986) found that groups of subjects with PD and agoraphobia endorsed the same number of symptoms from the DSM-III PA symptom checklist, in reference to the typical recent PAs. The percentages of symptoms endorsed were 80.5% and 81.3%, respectively. In addition, the severity with which each symptom was rated did not differ on average between the groups. In a similar fashion, Sanderson et al. (1987) compared the symptom profiles of typical PAs experienced by 21 subjects with panic with mild agoraphobic avoidance and 30 subjects with panic with moderate to severe agoraphobic avoidance. The percentages of each group reporting the 14 symptoms listed in the DSM-III-R checklist were approximately equal for 10 symptoms, higher in the extensive avoidance group for 2 symptoms, and higher in the mild avoidance group for the other 2 symptoms. That is, the overall percentage of symptoms endorsed did not differ significantly between groups. In addition, the severity ratings for each symptom were comparable between groups. Hence, a close replication of the Vermilyea (1986) data was obtained.

Telch et al. (1989c) reported no differences between the severity of PAs experienced by 40 agoraphobic patients and those experienced by 35 PD subjects. Finally, Oei et al. (personal communication) found that groups of individuals with extensive avoidance and minimal avoidance were not differentiated on the basis of factor scores from the factor analysis of the DSM-III-R checklist. That is, the pattern of symptoms was comparable across groups.

In summary, although agoraphobic avoidance does not seem to be related to variables such as panic frequency, severity, or typology, it does seem to be related to the expectation of panicking in specific agoraphobic situations. However, these findings do not imply that panic expectancy is of causal significance for the development of agoraphobic avoidance.

Features of similarity between groups.   If avoidant behavior can be construed as a feature secondary to panic, as opposed to an independent psychopathological feature, then persons with different levels of agoraphobic avoidance should be relatively similar with respect to measures of other characteristics. If group differences were apparent in terms of age at onset, sex ratio, physiological correlates, and other measures of psychopathology, there might be reason to argue that the addition of agoraphobic avoidance is reflective of a qualitatively different pathological process.

Age at Onset and Duration

The evidence regarding duration and age at onset is contradictory, suggesting either an earlier age at onset for PD with agoraphobia or a comparable age at onset across groups and either a longer average duration for PD with agoraphobia or a comparable duration across groups.

Panic Apprehension

Data reviewed earlier suggest that avoidance of a particular situation is closely related to the degree to which panic is expected to occur in that situation. Another question is the extent to which avoidance relates to generalized apprehension about the recurrence of panic or about the panic-type sensations, regardless of the situational context in which they may occur. Street et al. (1989) found that the average degree to which panic-related sensations were feared, measured using the Body Sensations Questionnaire (Chambless et al. 1984), was very similar across groups who had PD with and without marked agoraphobic avoidance. The ASI (Reiss et al. 1986) similarly measures the construct of anxious apprehension concerning the somatic sensations characteristic of fear and anxiety. In another study, 17 subjects with marked avoidance and 9 subjects with minimal avoidance did not differ on scores from this index (Shadick et al. 1988). McNally and Lorenz (1987) failed to find a significant relationship between ASI scores and avoidance scores from the agoraphobia subscale of the Fear Questionnaire ($r = .20$) (Marks and Mathews 1979). Finally, Adler et al. (1989) asked subjects "How much have you been worrying or how fearful have you been about experiencing a PA over the past month? (0 to 8)." The average rating from 65 subjects with minimal avoidance

(5.1) did not differ significantly from that of 62 subjects with marked avoidance (5.9). In other words, it seems that, in general, the groups are equally apprehensive over the recurrence of panic and panic sensations.

Features of agoraphobia without panic.   The reports from the nine clients who attended the Center for Stress and Anxiety Disorders and were assigned a diagnosis of agoraphobia without panic were examined. They related their avoidance to the following features: limited-symptom attacks (1); fear of incontinence or irritable bowel symptoms (3); fear of physical symptoms resulting from a recent physical trauma, such as stroke and surgery (2); constant symptoms that were never characterized by a "sudden onset" (1); the experience of expected rushes of fear only, without an unexpected rush of fear (1); and missing data (1).

The common feature in all cases was the anticipation of or presence of somatic symptoms. However, the sources for such symptoms were varied. Limited-symptom attacks (i.e., a sudden rush of fear and symptomatology that entailed fewer than four symptoms) were not the primary presentation. Thyer et al. (1985) also noted that their 20 subjects who were diagnosed as agoraphobic without panic experienced somatic symptoms. As described earlier, many of the subjects categorized as agoraphobic without PD in the community surveys experienced PAs or panic symptoms (Joyce et al. 1989; Weissman et al. 1986).

Summary.   The findings can be summarized as follows. First, the diagnosis of agoraphobia without a history of panic is rarely assigned in clinical research settings. The prevalence estimate from a series of 1,455 anxiety diagnoses was .06% (Center for Stress and Anxiety Disorders). The proportion of agoraphobic patients seen clinically who have not experienced panic ranges from 0% to 17.4%, with the mean proportion across studies being 5.1% and the median being 1.4%. Nevertheless, a group of subjects with agoraphobia without a history of PAs or panic symptoms is detected by epidemiological community surveys. The estimates within the nonclinical population range from 0.6 to 1 per 100 for agoraphobia without any type of panic symptoms.

Second, in the group of persons with PD with agoraphobia, agoraphobic avoidance very rarely precedes the first PA. The proportion of persons who recall avoiding prior to panicking ranges from 0% to 2.4%, with the mean proportion across studies being 0.8%.

Third, degree of avoidance at any given time is strongly related to the degree to which panic is anticipated to occur. However, other dimensions of panic, such as the frequency and severity with which PAs occur, and the types of PAs that occur (i.e., expected or unexpected, cued or uncued) are only weakly related to degree of avoidance in general. These findings do not imply that panic expectancy is of causal significance for the development of avoidance but rather that panic expectancy is related to extent of avoidance at any given time once the avoidance has developed as a response.

Fourth, groups of subjects with panic with different levels of avoidance have not been found to differ consistently with respect to age at onset, prevalence of acute versus insidious onset, generalized panic apprehension, premorbid anxious traits, additional anxiety and depressive diagnoses, or physiological measures. Sex ratio does tend to differ between the groups, with the percentage of females increasing as avoidance increases. Also, extensive avoidance has been shown to be associated with higher scores on measures of social sensitivity, neuroticism, and depression. In the absence of longitudinal research, it is not possible to determine whether the latter are a function of agoraphobic avoidance or precede the development of avoidance.

Fifth, examination of patterns of chronicity has yielded contrasting findings. Sixth, familial patterns demonstrate concordance for both agoraphobic avoidance and PAs, but the morbidity for PAs is comparable across groups with different levels of avoidance.

Finally, agoraphobic patients without PD tend to relate their avoidance to the experience of somatic symptoms, some of which comprise limited symptom attacks.

Conclusions.   Together, the evidence suggests that, in the majority of cases, agoraphobic avoidance occurs after the experience of PAs or PA symptoms and is subsequently mediated by the expectation of panicking in particular situations. Despite the evidence suggesting that agoraphobic avoidance is in most cases associated with PAs or PA symptoms, there is no empirical evidence as yet that unequivocally demonstrates that agoraphobic avoidance is primarily a function of the experience of PAs. The evidence does suggest that agoraphobic avoidance is most likely to develop in conjunction with PAs or paniclike symptomatic experiences. However, recognition of the number of persons who experience PA/PD without agoraphobic avoidance lends support to the notion that avoidance emerges for reasons other than or in addition to PAs. Similarly, the number of persons who experience agoraphobic avoidance without panic, which might occur relatively frequently in the general community, suggests that other variables aside from panic play a role in the development of agoraphobic avoidance.

The diagnostic implications from this review rest largely on two issues that need further examination. First, to what extent does the avoidance of individuals who experience PAs or panic symptoms differ from the avoidance that characterizes individuals who do not experience PAs or panic symptoms? This question is difficult to research because so few persons who are avoidant in the absence of

PAs/symptoms seek help, but presumably, community surveys could address the issue of type of avoidance in more detail than has been done to date. Second, to what extent are full PAs functionally different from limited-symptom attacks? The implication from assuming that full and limited-symptom attacks are similar in function is in turn dependent on whether the four symptom criteria for PAs are to be retained. Assuming that full and limited-symptom attacks are functionally similar, then agoraphobic patients who only experience limited-symptom attacks might be included in the current PD with agoraphobia category. However, if the four-symptom criterion is maintained (as currently recommended), then the newly included persons might not meet criteria for PD. Therefore, a discrepancy becomes apparent, because, as is currently specified, individuals must meet criteria for PD to receive a diagnosis of PD with agoraphobia. This is a limitation imposed by retention of the PD symptom criteria.

The extent to which irritable bowel symptoms, vomiting or nausea, and other specific symptoms that are associated with avoidance be considered limited-symptom attacks needs to be further clarified.

A similar set of issues arises for those agoraphobic patients who have not experienced PAs with sufficient frequency to meet the criteria for PD (four in 4 weeks). If the frequency of PA criterion is maintained, a discrepancy will arise. On the other hand, some individuals with infrequent panic would still meet the criteria for PD because they are apprehensive of PAs (for at least a month). Others may report that they are not apprehensive because they are successfully able to prevent the PAs from occurring by avoiding particular situations. In such cases, it would seem logical to assume that their avoidance is a behavioral indicator of apprehension (particularly in light of the previously mentioned research demonstrating the strong association between avoidance and expectancy of panicking). Therefore, those with infrequent panic who avoid would still meet criteria for PD on the basis of apprehension of PAs and are best subsumed under the category of PD with agoraphobia.

A second major diagnostic implication from the review pertains to the current Agoraphobia Without History of PD category. After subsuming agoraphobia with limited-symptom attacks or infrequent attacks under the domain of PD with agoraphobia, very few subjects who present clinically would meet criteria for agoraphobia without history of panic. The prevalence of such persons in the community requires further evaluation to determine whether the estimates obtained are inflated due to methods of questioning or whether a real difference is present between clinical and community samples. However, on the basis of individuals who present in clinical situations, the value of eliminating the category of agoraphobia without history of panic, and diagnosing such persons as anxiety disorder not otherwise specified (NOS) was considered to have some merit, but the Work Group felt the benefits of retaining the category outweighed the disadvantages.

Discussion and Recommendations

PD Without Agoraphobia

Should the PA frequency criterion and options be changed? The issue on which the DSM-IV PD and agoraphobia sub-Work Group has focused the greatest attention has been the previous (DSM-III, DSM-III-R) frequency criterion (e.g., three in 3 weeks or four in 4 weeks). The arguments have been made that these criteria are too restrictive, pseudoscientific, and generate confusion about the typical course of the disorder because they are not representative of the average patient or course of PD. DSM-III-R attempted to deal with this problem in part by adding a second threshold (one PA plus a month's worry about recurrent PAs). The first option would be to retain this two-pronged approach in DSM-IV. This would have the advantage of retaining continuity, and available data justifying a change are not yet overwhelming.

However, several problems with the DSM-III-R threshold criterion have been identified by clinicians and researchers in the field. First, there are no data available at this time about how the "one plus a month of worry" criterion works or how it relates to the "four in 4 weeks" criterion. Also, the requirement of only one PA may be overinclusive and/or unreliable. Some data suggest that the requirement for "one plus a month of worry" specifically about recurrent PAs is too restrictive and does not adequately describe the cognitive worries of as many as 35%–40% of PD patients. Also, the use of only one unexpected PA as a threshold has created boundary problems with simple and social phobias. In some cases, the onset of these phobic disorders is associated with an "unexpected PA" in a particular situation. Although subsequent attacks and anxiety may all be limited to that particular social or specific (simple phobia) situation, the individual might meet the criteria for PD because the first attack was by definition "unexpected."

It is also unclear that two criteria are actually needed. Although data do not currently exist to document that the two diagnostic arms are in fact redundant, most experts believe that the second ("one PA plus a month") would diagnose essentially all patients who would meet the other criterion. The proposed field trial will attempt to empirically uncover a specific frequency of PAs that can better define PD. However, if the trial fails to uncover a specific usable frequency as suspected, one recommended option will be for the primary criterion to essentially utilize the second arm but extend it by including other pertinent cognitive concerns and require recurrent (more than one) PAs; that is, to include worries beyond having another PA to also include worry about other consequences (e.g., losing control, having a heart attack, "going crazy"). This would allow the use and extension of the cognitive aspects of panic as has been recommended in the literature reviews. It appears that this would allow a description of the average patient, most, if not all, of whom have at least a month of anxiety or worry about one or the other of these catastrophic cognitive worries.

From accumulated clinical and epidemiological experience, it is clear that the actual pattern and frequency of PAs is highly variable within and across time in individual patients. We are considering using the phrase "*recurrent* PAs" because it actually seems to be the best descriptor of the frequency that is in fact associated with significant morbidity. The available evidence suggests that isolated or sporadic PAs are not associated with morbidity. It is only when they become "recurrent" that disability results. Because the observed patterns and frequencies are so variable, *recurrent* may be the only truly valid way to describe the pattern that leads to clinical difficulties and disability. The field trial may document this because it appears unlikely that a specific numerical threshold will be defined by the trial.

Given the conservative DSM-IV stance that criteria should not be changed unless there are clear data sets justifying a change, the suggested option 2 could be considered simply a rewording of the DSM-III-R criteria. It is proposed that the "four in 4 weeks" criterion be dropped and that the second criterion arm of "one PA plus a month of worry about having another PA" be used as was allowable in DSM-III-R. This would allow linkage to the remainder of the DSM-III-R criteria, which would be retained but reworded in relatively minor ways: for example, 1) presence of spontaneous PAs, 2) the characteristic symptoms of a PA, 3) four symptoms in each PA, and 4) the characteristic crescendo nature of each PA. These four additional features are very consistent with the DSM-III-R criteria but define the diagnosis without the problematic "four in 4 weeks" criterion, in a manner that most experts agree is more descriptive of the range of typical patients with PD. This would have considerable educational value in that the criteria would educate not only the professional community but also the lay community as to what the typical PD patient "looks like," because one of the primary goals of the DSM-IV is to be educational.

Therefore, the potential new option is to have the first criterion be "recurrent unexpected PAs," retaining the concept that unexpected PAs are the central (and required) feature of the syndrome but that more than one PA is required. Otherwise, the frequency of PAs would not be specified.

It is also proposed that the crescendo idea of the symptoms developing abruptly and reaching maximum intensity (crescendo) within 10 minutes be retained, as well as the criterion of four of the listed symptoms. In summary, the primary options for the PD criteria are to retain the criteria essentially as they were before or to drop the "four in 4 weeks" frequency of PAs and emphasize the second criterion (one plus a month). Available evidence and opinion both support dropping the frequency and placing greater emphasis on the other arm of the DSM-III-R criteria of "one PA plus a month of worry." To support option 2, a field trial will be conducted to determine how this criteria set compares with both arms of the DSM-III-R criteria used together and alone.

The next issue concerns whether a spontaneous PA is, in fact, required for diagnosis. The available evidence strongly suggests continuing the requirement of spontaneity, primarily for its usefulness in defining the boundaries of PD. Some of the other anxiety disorders (e.g., social phobia, obsessive-compulsive disorder) include situational PAs and even spontaneous attacks early in the course, but it appears that only PD continues to have recurrent spontaneous PAs. These recurrent unexpected PAs are, in fact, one of the most characteristic features of PD, and the strategy of using spontaneous PAs to differentiate PD from the other anxiety disorders will probably be heavily utilized in DSM-IV. It remains unclear what percentage of the PAs need to be unexpected. It appears that up to approximately half of the attacks in large clinical populations are spontaneous, but it is unclear how this could be used in the criterion set; therefore, it is proposed that the number (beyond at least one) or percentage of spontaneous attacks not be specified.

Certainly, the evidence strongly supports the continued use of the abrupt/crescendo idea. Continued use of these characteristics attains further importance in the proposals for DSM-IV because of the attempt to better describe the typical PD patient. Certainly, the crescendo idea for PAs is highly descriptive of the typical patient.

The next option was to consider the diagnosis of PAs in patients who only had one, two, or three symptoms, the so-called limited-symptom attacks. Although there is considerable feeling that these limited-symptom attacks are closely related to PAs and lead to similar consequences, the data primarily document that four-symptom attacks should be used to identify patients with PAs. Use of the four-symptom attack criterion defined the individuals in the ECA data set who had significant morbidity when compared with individuals who never had a four-symptom attack, only three-symptom (or fewer) attacks.

The next major issue was whether to employ catastrophic cognitions more extensively in the diagnosis of PD or retain only the DSM-III-R concern of "having another PA." Both of the reviews strongly recommend that the characteristic catastrophic cognitions be used in the diagnosis. Because only 60%–70% of PD patients have the specific catastrophic cognition of fear of recurrence of PAs, it appears that the other common cognitions including worry about "loss of control" or that the anxiety symptoms reflect underlying medical or psychiatric illness should be used. The available data suggest that more than 98% of PD patients have at least one of these characteristic catastrophic cognitions in at least one attack and that it would be helpful in diagnosing PD patients, especially if, as proposed here, either the "one plus" or "recurrent" frequency criteria are used. The proposed options extends the worry after PAs to include "worry about the implications of the attack or its consequences (e.g., losing control, having a heart attack, 'going crazy')."

The option of subclassifying patients into 1) cardiac, 2) gastrointestinal, or 3) alcoholic categories is still an option, but the evidence does not appear to be sufficiently strong to justify subclassification in DSM-IV. Greater emphasis should be placed on the frequent presentation of patients in these particular ways to increase their recognizability and appropriate diagnosis; however, this could probably be emphasized adequately in the text that accompanies the diagnostic criteria.

Not subtyping the so-called nonfearful PD patients may result in some difficulty. It appears that some of these patients do not have enough typical PAs in addition to the nonfearful attacks to meet the proposed PD criteria. Therefore, some of these patients may not be diagnosable using the proposed criteria. However, with our current knowledge base, the extent of this problem is unknown, and the Work Group adopted the conservative stance of not subgrouping these patients until these issues are better understood. However, sufficient emphasis should be placed on this "subgroup" of PD patients in the text, including a full description of their presentation, to improve the extent to which they are recognized and diagnosed appropriately.

The option of including biological tests, particularly the provocative challenge tests, does not appear to be viable at this time because of serious limitations involving the low specificity and sensitivity of the available tests. The boundary with social phobia seems relatively straightforward, and it is proposed that the following be used: 1) that the anxiety be limited to social settings and not occur otherwise, 2) that the fear be specifically of the social consequences of the anxiety (i.e., anxiety symptoms being humiliating or embarrassing), 3) that it be emphasized that spontaneous PAs separate from social situations do not occur, and 4) that the criteria clarify that anxiety in the social situations can take the form of PAs.

PD With Agoraphobia

One issue the group considered early in its deliberations was raised by the European concept that agoraphobia is more important than PD and is not necessarily caused by preexisting PD. This concept was the basis of the ICD-10 decision to give preeminent status to agoraphobia over PD. The Work Group did not conclude available evidence justified a shift to the stance the ICD-10 adopted. However, available evidence suggests that the postulated "tight link" between PD and "subsequent" development of agoraphobic avoidance may not be as clear as previously thought. Although PAs are almost always present at the beginning of the disorder in clinical cases of agoraphobia, there is also strong evidence that continued agoraphobic avoidance is related to continued expectation of PAs but may or may not be correlated with the frequency, severity, or even presence of continued PAs. Therefore, it is concluded that the criteria set should remain the same but that the text should reflect these facts.

A second issue concerns whether the "typical cluster" idea of agoraphobic situations should be described more thoroughly in the criterion set. The characteristic situations derived from study of clinical populations of PD patients are grouped into fears of being in public places, transport vehicles, closed spaces, and meeting/appointments (Johnston et al. 1984). This would have the two additional advantages of making DSM-IV more congruent with ICD-10 and assisting with the difficult boundary issues with simple, nonspecific phobias.

The descriptive term *overlapping and interrelated set of fears* used in ICD-10 seems to have intuitive descriptive value. Use of the concept of "overlapping and interrelated" is perhaps also helpful in the boundary between specific and single phobias. Although this boundary will be specifically studied in the field trial, it would also be possible to utilize this concept to separate agoraphobia from single and specific phobias by having any simple and/or single clinical phobia reclassified in the single and specific phobia category, with multiple or complex phobias being classified as agoraphobia. This would essentially utilize the notion of complexity (as well as "multiple" phobias) as a part of the characteristic definition of agoraphobia. However, the Work Group remains concerned that the phrase "overlapping and interrelated" lacks definitional clarity and may not be useful.

The first option proposed by the Work Group is essentially a rewording of the DSM-III-R criterion A, emphasizing the idea prevalent in the United States that the patient fears incapacitating or embarrassing symptoms. The next option adopts the more European idea of "an overlapping and interrelated cluster of phobias." This option also gives greater emphasis to the fears of the situations themselves rather than fears of places or situations in which symptoms might develop that might be incapacitating or embarrassing.

Certainly the most difficult issue in agoraphobia is the boundary issue with single phobias as represented by the simple phobias and social phobias. There are no currently available data sets that provide a definitive answer concerning where to draw the boundary between agoraphobia and a single phobia. Although this is not particularly difficult in single phobias such as fear of snakes, insects, or thunderstorms, it is most difficult when the single phobia is also characteristically seen in agoraphobic patients with multiple phobias. This is most difficult in situations of single fears such as flying in airplanes, driving, being in elevators. It is proposed that this be studied extensively in a field trial. However, from a conceptual point of view, the principal option appears to tend to diagnose agoraphobia if two or more phobias characteristic of the agoraphobic cluster are present and as a practical matter to tend to leave single phobias in the other categories.

References

Adler CM, Craske MG, Kirschenbaum S, et al: Fear of panic: an investigation of its role in panic occurrence, phobic avoidance and treatment outcome. Behav Res Ther 27:391–396, 1989

American Psychiatric Association: Diagnostic and Statistical Manual of Mental Disorders, 3rd Edition. Washington DC, American Psychiatric Association, 1980

American Psychiatric Association: Diagnostic and Statistical Manual of Mental Disorders, 3rd Edition, Revised. Washington DC, American Psychiatric Association, 1987

Angst J, Dobler-Mikola A: The Zurich study, V: anxiety and phobia in young adults. Eur Arch Psychiatry Neurol Sci 235:171–178, 1985

Angst J, Vollrath M, Merikangas KR, et al: Comorbidity of anxiety and depression in the Zurich cohort study of young adults, in Comorbidity in Anxiety and Mood Disorders. Edited by Maser JD, Cloninger CR. Washington, DC, American Psychiatric Press, 1989, pp 123–137

Arnow BA, Taylor CB, Agras WS, et al: Enhancing agoraphobia treatment outcome by changing couple communication patterns. Behavior Therapy 16:452–467, 1985

Aronson TA: Is panic disorder a distinct diagnostic entity? A critical review of the borders of a syndrome. J Nerv Ment Dis 175:584–594, 1987

Aronson TA, Craig TJ: Cocaine precipitation of panic disorder. Am J Psychiatry 143:643–645, 1986

Aronson TA, Logue CM: On the longitudinal course of panic disorder: developmental history and predictors of phobic complications. Compr Psychiatry 28:244–255, 1987

Ballenger JC (ed): Neurobiology of Panic Disorder. New York, Wiley-Liss, 1990, pp 158–242 (Chapters 10–14)

Barlow DH: The dimensions of anxiety disorders, in Anxiety and the Anxiety Disorders. Edited by Tuma AH, Maser JD. Hillsdale, NJ, Erlbaum, 1985, pp 479–500

Barlow DH: Behavioral conception and treatment of panic. Psychopharmacol Bull 22:802–806, 1986

Barlow DH: Anxiety and Its Disorders: The Nature and Treatment of Anxiety and Panic. New York, Guilford, 1988a

Barlow DH: Current models of panic disorder and a view from emotion theory, in Review of Psychiatry, Vol 7. Edited by Frances AJ, Hales R. Washington, DC, American Psychiatric Press, 1988b

Barlow DH, Cohen AS, Waddell MT, et al: Panic and generalized anxiety disorders: nature and treatment. Behavior Therapy 15:431–449, 1984

Barlow DH, Vermilyea J, Blanchard EB, et al: The phenomenon of panic. J Abnorm Psychol 94:320–328, 1985

Barlow DH, Craske MG, Cerny JA, et al: Behavioral treatment of panic disorder. Behavior Therapy 20:261–282, 1989

Bass C, Wade C: Chest pain with normal coronary arteries: a comparative study of psychiatric and social morbidity. Psychosom Med 14:51–61, 1984

Beck JG, Scott SK: Frequent and infrequent panic: a comparison of cognitive and autonomic reactivity. J Anx Disord 1:47–58, 1987

Beck JG, Taegtmeyer H, Berisford MA, et al: Chest pain without coronary artery disease: an exploratory comparison with panic disorder. J Psychopathol Behav Assess 11:209–229, 1989

Beitman BD, Basha I, Flaker G, et al: Atypical or nonanginal chest pain: panic disorder or coronary artery disease. Arch Intern Med 147:1548–1552, 1987a

Beitman BD, Basha I, Flaker G, et al: Non-fearful panic disorder: panic attacks without fear. Behav Res Ther 25:487–497, 1987b

Beitman BD, Mukerji V, Glaker G, et al: Panic disorder, cardiology patients, and atypical chest pain. Psychiatr Clin North Am 11:387–397, 1988

Bowen RC, Cipywny KD, D'Aray C, et al: Alcoholism, anxiety disorders and agoraphobia. Alcohol: Journal of Clinical and Experimental Research 8:48–50, 1984

Boyd HH: Use of mental health services for the treatment of panic disorder. Am J Psychiatry 143:1569–1574, 1986

Boyd JH, Burke JD, Gruenberg E, et al: Exclusion criteria of DSM-III: a study of co-occurrence of hierarchy-free syndromes. Arch Gen Psychiatry 41:983–989, 1984

Breier A, Charney DS, Heninger GR: Agoraphobia with panic attacks: development, diagnostic stability, and course of illness. Arch Gen Psychiatry 43:1029–1036, 1986

Brown TA, Cash TF: The phenomenon of panic in nonclinical populations: further evidence and methodological considerations. J Anx Disord 3:139–148, 1989

Buller R: Differences in help-seeking for treatment of panic. Presented at Panic Anxiety in Cross-Cultural Perspectives at the 143rd Annual Meeting of the American Psychiatric Association, New York, May 15, 1990

Caughey JL: Cardiovascular neurosis: a review. Psychosom Med 1:311–324, 1939

Chambless DL, Gracely EJ: Fear of fear and the anxiety disorders. Cognitive Therapy and Research 13:9–20, 1989

Chambless DL, Caputo CG, Bright P, et al: Assessment of fear in agoraphobic patients: the body sensations questionnaire and the agoraphobic cognitions questionnaire. J Consult Clin Psychol 52:1090–1097, 1984

Chambless DL, Goldstein AA, Gallagher R, et al: Integrating behavior therapy and psychotherapy in the treatment of agoraphobia. Psychotherapy 23:150–159, 1986

Channer KS, James MA, Papouchado M, et al: Anxiety and depression in patients with chest pain referred for exercise testing. Lancet 11:820–823, 1985

Clancy J, Noyes R: Anxiety neurosis: a disease for the medical model. Psychosomatics 17:90–93, 1976

Clark DM: A cognitive approach to panic. Behav Res Ther 24:461–470, 1986

Clark DM: A cognitive model of panic, in Panic: Psychological Perspectives. Edited by Rachman S, Maser J. Hillsdale, NJ, Erlbaum, 1988

Clark DM, Salkovskis PM, Chalkley AJ: Respiratory control as a treatment for panic attacks. J Behav Ther Exp Psychiatry 16:23–30, 1985

Clark DM, Salkovskis PM, Gelder MG, et al: Tests of a cognitive theory of panic, in Panic and Phobias II. Edited by Hand I, Wittchen HU. New York, Springer-Verlag, 1988

Costa PT, Zonderman AB, Engel BT, et al: The relation of chest pain symptoms to angiographic findings of coronary artery stenosis and neuroticism. Psychosom Med 47:285–295, 1985

Cowley DS, Dager SR, Foster SI, et al: Clinical characteristics and response to sodium lactate of patients with infrequent panic attacks. Am J Psychiatry 144:795–798, 1987

Craske MG, Sanderson WS, Barlow DH: The relationships among panic, fear and avoidance. J Anx Disord 1:153–160, 1987

Craske MG, Rapee RM, Barlow DH: The significance of panic-expectancy for individual patterns of avoidance. Behavior Therapy 19:577–592, 1988

Crowe RR: The genetics of panic disorder and agoraphobia. Psychiatric Developments 2:171–186, 1985

Crowe RR, Noyes R Jr, Pauls DL, et al: A family study of panic disorder. Arch Gen Psychiatry 40:1065–, 1069, 1983

DiNardo PA, O'Brien GT, Barlow DH, et al: Reliability of DSM-III anxiety disorder categories using a new structured interview. Arch Gen Psychiatry 40:1070–1074, 1983

Drossman DA, Sandler RS, McKee DC, et al: Bowel patterns among subjects seeking medical care: use of a questionnaire to identify a population with bowel dysfunction. Gastroenterology 83:529–534, 1982

Eaton WW, Dryman AA, Weissman MW: Panic and phobia, in Psychiatric Disorders in America. Edited by Robins LN, Regier DA. New York, Free Press, 1988

Elias MF, Robbins MA, Blow FC, et al: Symptom reporting, anxiety and depression in arteriographically classified middle-aged chest pain patients. Exper Aging Res 8:45–51, 1982

Fava GA, Grandi S, Canestrari R: Prodromal symptoms in panic disorder with agoraphobia. Am J Psychiatry 145:1564–1567, 1988

Foa EB: What cognitions differentiate panic disorder from other anxiety disorders? in Panic and Phobias II. Edited by Hand I, Wittchen H. New York, Springer-Verlag, 1988

Ford D. The relationship of psychiatric illness to medically unexplained chest pain. Paper presented at Mental Disorders in General Health Care Settings: A Research Conference, Seattle, WA, 1987

Fossey M, Lydiard RB, Marsh WH, et al: Psychiatric morbidity in irritable bowel syndrome. Presented at the 142nd Annual Meeting of the American Psychiatric Association, San Francisco, CA, May 6–11, 1989

Fyer AJ, Endicott J, Mannuzza S, et al: Schedule for Affective Disorders and Schizophrenia: Lifetime Version (Modified for the study of anxiety disorders). New York, Anxiety Disorders Clinic, New York State Psychiatric Institute, 1985

Fyer AJ, Mannuzza S, Martin LY, et al: Reliability of anxiety assessment, II: symptom agreement. Arch Gen Psychiatry 46:1102–1110, 1989

Ganellen RJ, Matuzas W, Uhlenhuth EH, et al: Panic disorder, agoraphobia, and anxiety relevant cognitive style. J Affect Disord 11:219–225, 1986

Garvey MJ, Tuason VB: The relation of panic disorder to agoraphobia. Compr Psychiatry 25:529–531, 1984

Gorman JM, Liebowitz MR, Fyer AJ, et al: Lactate infusions in obsessive-compulsive disorder. Am J Psychiatry 142:864–866, 1985

Gorman JM, Fyer MR, Liebowitz MR, et al: Pharmacological provocation of panic attacks, in Psychopharmacology: The Third Generation of Progress. Edited by Meltzer HY. New York, Raven, 1987, pp 985–993

Gorman JM, Liebowitz MR, Fyer AJ, et al: A neuroanatomical hypothesis for panic disorder. Am J Psychiatry 146:148–161, 1989

Helzer JE, Pryzbech TR: The co-occurrence of alcoholism with other psychiatric disorders in the general population and its impact on treatment. J Stud Alcohol 49:219–224, 1988

Hibbert GA: Ideational components of anxiety: their origin and content. Br J Psychiatry 144:618–624, 1984

Jablensky A: Approaches to the definition and classification of anxiety and related disorders in European Psychiatry, in Anxiety and the Anxiety Disorders. Edited by Tuma AH, Maser J. Hillside, NJ, Lawrence Erlbaum Associates Publishing 1985, pp 735–758

Johnston M, Johnston DW, Wilkes H, et al: Cumulative scales for the measurement of agoraphobia. Br J Clin Psychology 23:133–143, 1984

Joyce PR, Bushnell MA, Oakley-Browne J, et al: The epidemiology of panic symptomatology and agoraphobic avoidance. Compr Psychiatry 30:303–312, 1989

Katerndahl DA: Prevalence of panic attacks. J Fam Pract 24(2):208–209, 1987

Katerndahl DA: The sequence of panic symptoms. J Fam Pract 26:49–52, 1988

Katerndahl DA: Infrequent and limited-symptom panic attacks. J Nerv Ment Dis 178:313–317, 1990

Katon W: Panic disorder and somatization: a review of 55 cases. Am J Med 77:101–106, 1984

Katon W: Panic disorder: epidemiology, diagnosis and treatment in primary care. J Clin Psychiatry 47:21–27, 1986

Katon W: Panic disorder: the importance of phenomenology. J Fam Practice 26:23–24, 1988

Katon W: Panic Disorder in the Medical Setting. Washington, DC, National Institute of Mental Health, Superintendent of Documents, US Government Printing Office, 1989

Katon W, Vitaliano PP, Anderson K, et al: Panic disorder: residual symptoms after the acute attacks abate. Compr Psychiatry 28(2):151–158, 1987a

Katon W, Vitaliano PP, Russo J, et al: Panic disorder: spectrum of severity and somatization. J Nerv Ment Dis 175:12–19, 1987b

Katon W, Hall ML, Russo J, et al: Chest pain: relationship of psychiatric illness to coronary arteriographic results. Am J Med 84:1–9, 1988

Kemp HG, Kronmal RA, Vlietstra RE, et al: Seven year survival of patients with normal or near normal coronary arteriograms: a CASS registry study. J Am Coll Cardiol 7:479–483, 1986

Kenardy J, Oei TPS, Ryan P, et al: Attribution of panic attacks: patient perspective. J Anx Disord 2:243–251, 1988a

Kenardy J, Evans L, Oei TPS: The importance of cognitions in panic attacks. Behavior Therapy 19:471–483, 1988b

Kenardy J, Evans L, Oei TPS: Cognitions and heart rate in panic disorders during everyday activity. J Anx Disord 3:33–43, 1989

Klein DF: Delineation of two drug responsive anxiety syndromes. Psychopharmacol 5:397–408, 1964

Klein DF, Klein HM: The definition and psychopharmacology of spontaneous panic and phobia: a critical review, in Psychopharmacology of Anxiety. Edited by Tyrer PJ. New York, Oxford University Press, 1989a, pp 135–162

Klein DF, Klein HM: The nosology, genetics and theory of spontaneous panic and phobia, in Psychopharmacology of Anxiety. Edited by Tyrer PJ. New York, Oxford University Press, 1989b, pp 163–195

Klein DF, Klein HM: The substantive effect of variations in panic measurement and agoraphobia definition. J Anx Disord 3:45–56, 1989c

Klein DR, Foss DC, Cohen P: Panic and avoidance in agoraphobia: application of path analysis to treatment studies. Arch Gen Psychiatry 44:377–385, 1987

Krystal JH, Leaf P, Bruce M, et al: Aging, alcoholism and panic disorder prevalence. Presented at the 142nd Annual Meeting of the American Psychiatric Association, San Francisco, CA, May 6–11, 1989

Last CG, Barlow DH, O'Brien GT: Precipitants of agoraphobia: role of stressful life events. Psychol Rep 54:567–570, 1984

Lepine JP, Pariente P, Boulenger JP, et al: Anxiety disorders in a French general psychiatric outpatient sample. Soc Psychiatry Psychiatr Epidemiol 24:301–308, 1989

Ley R: Agoraphobia, the panic attack and the hyperventilation syndrome. Behav Res Ther 23:79–81, 1985

Liebowitz MR: Social phobia. Modern Problems of Pharmacopsychiatry 22:141–173, 1987

Liebowitz MR, Fyer AJ: Panic disorder: approaches of DSM-IV. Presented at Panic and Anxiety: A Decade of Progress, Geneva, Switzerland, June 1990

Liebowitz MR, Gorman JM, Fyer AJ, et al: Lactate provocation of panic attacks, II: biochemical and physiological findings. Arch Gen Psychiatry 42:709–719, 1985a

Liebowitz MR, Gorman JM, Fyer AJ, et al: Social phobia: review of a neglected anxiety disorder. Arch Gen Psychiatry 42:729–736, 1985b

Liebowitz MR, Fyer AJ, Gorman JM, et al: Specificity of lactate infusions in social phobia versus panic disorder. Am J Psychiatry 148:947–950, 1985c

Liebowitz MR, Gorman JM, Fyer AJ, et al: Pharmacotherapy of social phobia: an interim report of a placebo-controlled comparison of phenelzine and atenolol. J Clin Psychiatry 49:252–257, 1988

Lydiard RB, Laraia MT, Howell EF, et al: Can panic disorder present as irritable bowel syndrome? J Clin Psychiatry 47:470–473, 1986

Mannuzza S, Fyer AJ, Klein DF, et al: Schedule for Affective Disorders and Schizophrenia: Lifetime Version (Modified for the Study of Anxiety Disorders): rationale and conceptual development. J Psychiatry Res 20:317–325, 1986

Mannuzza S, Fyer AJ, Martin LY, et al: Reliability of anxiety assessment, I: diagnostic agreement. Arch Gen Psychiatry 46:1093–1101, 1989

Margraf J, Ehlers A, Roth WT: Biological models of panic disorder and agoraphobia: a review. Behav Res Ther 24:553–567, 1986

Margraf J, Taylor CB, Ehlers A, et al: Panic attacks in the natural environment. J Nerv Ment Dis 175(9):558–565, 1987

Markowitz JS, Weissman MM, Ouellette R, et al: Quality of life in panic disorder. Arch Gen Psychiatry 46:984–992, 1989

Marks IM, Mathews AM: Brief standard self-rating for phobic patients. Behav Res Ther 17:263–276, 1979

Mavissakalian M: The relationship between panic, phobic and anticipatory anxiety in agoraphobia. Behav Res Ther 26:235–248, 1988

McGrath P, Stewart J, Harrison W, et al: Lactate infusions in patients with depression and anxiety. Psychopharmacol Bull 21(3):555–558, 1985

McNally RJ, Foa EB: Cognition and agoraphobia: bias in the interpretation of threat. Cognitive Therapy and Research 11:567–581, 1987

McNally RJ, Lorenz M: Anxiety sensitivity in agoraphobic patients. J Behav Ther Exp Psychiatry 18:3–11, 1987

Michelson L, Mavissakalian M, Marchione K: Cognitive and behavioral treatments of agoraphobia: clinical, behavioral and psychophysiological outcomes. J Consult Clin Psychol 53:913–925, 1985

Moras K, Craske MG, Barlow DH: Behavioral and cognitive therapies for panic disorder, in Handbook of Anxiety, Vol 4: The Treatments of Anxiety. Edited by Noyes RJ, Roth M, Burrows GD. New York, Elsevier, 1990, pp 311–326

Mullaney JA, Trippett C: Alcohol dependence and phobias: clinical description and relevance. Br J Psychiatry 135:565–573, 1979

Myers JK, Weissman MM, Tischler GL, et al: Six-month prevalence of psychiatric disorders in three communities. Arch Gen Psychiatry 41:959–967, 1984

Norton GR, Barrison B, Hauch J, et al: Characteristics of people with infrequent panic attacks. J Abnorm Psychol 94(2):216–221, 1985

Norton GR, Dorward J, Cox JB: Factors associated with panic attacks in nonclinical subjects. Behavior Therapy 17:239–252, 1986

Noyes R, Crowe RR, Harris EL, et al: Relationship between panic disorder and agoraphobia. Arch Gen Psychiatry 43:227–232, 1986

Nunes E, Quitkin F, Berman C: Panic disorder and depression in female alcoholics. J Clin Psychiatry 49:441–443, 1988

Ockene IS, Shay MJ, Alpert JS, et al: Unexplained chest pain in patients with normal coronary arteriograms: follow-up study of functional status. N Engl J Med 303:1249–1252, 1980

Öst LG: Age of onset in different phobias. J Abnorm Psychol 96:223–229, 1987

Ottaviani R, Beck AT: Cognitive aspects of panic disorders. J Anx Disord 1:15–28, 1987

Pollard CA, Bronson SS, Kenney MR: Prevalence of agoraphobia without panic in clinical settings. Am J Psychiatry 146:559, 1989

Rachman S, Bichard S: The overprediction of fear. Clin Psychol Rev 8:303–312, 1988

Rachman SJ, Lopatka C: Match and mismatch in the prediction of fear, I. Behav Res Ther 24:387–393, 1986

Rachman S, Levitt K, Lopatka C: Panic: the links between cognitions and bodily symptoms, I. Behav Res Ther 25:411–423, 1987

Rainey JM, Pohl RB, Williams M, et al: A comparison of lactate and isoproterenol anxiety states. Psychopathology 17:74–82, 1984

Rapee RM: Distinction between panic disorder and generalized anxiety disorder: clinical presentation. Aust N Z J Psychiatry 19:227–232, 1985

Rapee R: Differential response to hyperventilation in panic disorder and generalized anxiety disorder. J Abnorm Psychol 95:24–28, 1986

Rapee RM, Murrell E: Predictors of agoraphobic avoidance. J Anx Disord 2:203–217, 1988

Rapee RM, Ancis JR, Barlow DH: Emotional reactions to physiological sensations: panic disorder patients and non-clinical symptoms. Behav Res Ther 26(3):265–269, 1988

Rapee RM, Craske MG, Barlow DH: Subject-described features of panic attacks using self-monitoring. J Anx Disord 4:171–181, 1990

Regier DA, Myers JK, Kramer M, et al: The NIMH epidemiological catchment area program: historical context, major objectives, and study population characteristics. Arch Gen Psychiatry 41:934–941, 1984

Reich J, Yates W: Family history of psychiatric disorders in social phobia. Compr Psychiatry 29:72–75, 1988

Reiss S, Peterson RA, Gursky DM, et al: Anxiety sensitivity, anxiety frequency and the prediction of fearfulness. Behav Res Ther 24:1–8, 1986

Rice JP, McDonald-Scott P, Endicott J, et al: The stability of diagnosis with an application to bipolar II disorder. Psychiatry Res 19:285–296, 1986

Robins LN, Helzer JE, Croughan J, et al: The National Institute of Mental Health Diagnostic Interview Schedule: its history, characteristics, and validity. Arch Gen Psychiatry 38:381–389, 1981

Rubin DC (ed): Autobiographical Memory. New York, Cambridge University Press, 1986

Salge RA, Beck JG, Logan AC: A community survey of panic. J Anx Disord 2:157–167, 1988

Salkovskis PM: Phenomenology, assessment and the cognitive model of panic, in Panic: Psychological Perspectives. Edited by Rachman S, Maser J. Hillsdale, NJ, Erlbaum, 1988

Sanderson WS, Rapee RM, Barlow DH: The DSM-III-Revised anxiety disorder categories: description and patterns of comorbidity. Poster presented at Association for Advancement of Behavior Therapy Annual Meeting, Boston, MA, 1987

Shadick R, Craske MG, Barlow DH: Courage and avoidance behavior. Poster presented at Association for Advancement of Behavior Therapy Annual Meeting, New York, 1988

Skerrit PW: Anxiety and the heart: a historical review. Psychol Med 13:17–25, 1983

Skodol AE: Problems in Differential Diagnosis: From DSM-III to DSM-III-R in Clinical Practice. Washington, DC, American Psychiatric Press, 1989

Smail P, Stockwell T, Canter S, et al: Alcohol dependence and phobic anxiety states, I: a prevalence study. Br J Psychiatry 144:53–57, 1984

Spitzer RL, Williams JRB: Structured Clinical Interview for DSM-III. New York, New York State Psychiatric Institute, 1983

Stirton RF, Brandon S: Preliminary report of a community survey of panic attacks and panic disorder. J R Soc Med 81(6):392–393, 1988

Stockwell T, Smail S, Hodgson R, et al: Alcohol dependence and phobic anxiety states, II: a retrospective study. Br J Psychiatry 144:58–63, 1984

Street LL, Craske MG, Barlow DH: Sensations, cognitions and the perceptions of cues associated with expected and unexpected panic attacks. Behav Res Ther 27:189–198, 1989

Swinson RP: Reply to Klein. Behavior Therapist 9:110–128, 1986

Taylor CB, Shiekh J, Agras WS, et al: Ambulatory heart rate changes in patients with panic attacks. Am J Psychiatry 143:478–482, 1986

Telch MJ: The Panic Appraisal Inventory. Unpublished scale, University of Texas, 1987

Telch MJ, Shermis MD, Lucas JA: Anxiety sensitivity: unitary personality trait or domain-specific appraisals? J Anx Disord 3:25–32, 1989a

Telch MJ, Lucas JA, Nelson P: Nonclinical panic in college students: an investigation of prevalence and symptomatology. J Abnorm Psychol 98(3):1–7, 1989b

Telch MJ, Brouillard M, Telch CF, et al: Role of cognitive appraisal in panic-related avoidance. Behav Res Ther 27:373–383, 1989c

Thyer BA, Himle J: Temporal relationship between panic attack onset and phobic avoidance in agoraphobia. Behav Res Ther 23:607–608, 1985

Thyer BA, Himle J: Phobic anxiety and panic anxiety: how do they differ? J Anx Disord 1:59–67, 1987

Thyer BA, Himle J, Curtis GC, et al: Comparison of panic disorder and agoraphobia with panic attacks. Compr Psychiatry 26:208–214, 1985

Torgerson S: Genetic factors in anxiety disorders. Arch Gen Psychiatry 40:1085–1089, 1983

Uhde TW, Boulenger DP, Vittone B, et al: Human anxiety and nonadrenergic function: preliminary studies with caffeine, clonidine and yohimbine, in Proceedings of the Seventh World Congress of Psychiatry. New York, Plenum, 1985a

Uhde TW, Boulenger JP, Roy-Byrne PP, et al: Longitudinal course of panic disorder. Prog Neuropsychopharmacol Biol Psychiatry 9:39–51, 1985b

Uhde TW, Roy-Byrne PP, Vittone BJ, et al: Phenomenology and neurobiology of panic disorder, in Anxiety and the Anxiety Disorders. Edited by Tuma AH, Maser JD. Hillsdale, NJ, Erlbaum, 1985c

Uhlenhuth EH, Balter MB, Mellinger GD, et al: Symptom checklist syndromes in the general population. Arch Gen Psychiatry 40:1167–1173, 1983

van den Hout MA, Griez E: Experimental panic: biobehavioral notes on empirical findings, in Panic and Phobias. Edited by Hand I, Wittchen HU. New York, Springer-Verlag, 1986

Vermilyea JA: A comparison of anxiety in "normal" and anxiety disordered populations. Unpublished doctoral dissertation, The University of Albany, State University of New York, 1986

Von Korff M, Eaton WW: Epidemiologic findings on panic, in Panic Disorder: Theory, Research and Therapy. Edited by Baker R. New York, Wiley, 1989

Von Korff MR, Eaton WW, Keyl PM: The epidemiology of panic attacks and panic disorder: results of three community surveys. Am J Epidemiol 122(6):970–981, 1985

Von Korff M, Shapiro S, Burke JD, et al: Anxiety and depression in a primary care clinic. Arch Gen Psychiatry 44(2):152–156, 1987

Walker EA, Roy-Byrne PP, Katon WJ: Irritable bowel syndrome and psychiatric illness. Am J Psychiatry 147:565–572, 1990a

Walker EA, Roy-Byrne PP, Katon WJ, et al: Psychiatric illness and irritable bowel syndrome: a comparison with inflammatory bowel disease. Am J Psychiatry 147:1656–1661, 1990b

Warwick HMC, Salkovskis PM: Hypochondriasis. Behav Res Ther 28:105–117, 1990

Weissman MM, Merikangas KR: The epidemiology of anxiety and panic disorders: an update. J Clin Psychiatry 47:11–17, 1986

Weissman MM, Myers JK, Harding PS: Psychiatric disorders in a US urban community. Am J Psychiatry 135:459–462, 1978

Weissman MM, Leaf PJ, Blazer DG, et al: The relationship between panic d and agoraphobia: an epidemiological perspective. Psychopharmacol Bull 22:787–791, 1986

Weissman MM, Leckman JF, Merikangas KR, et al: Depression and anxiety disorders in parents and children: results from the Yale family study. Arch Gen Psychiatry 41:845–852, 1984

Weissman MM, Klerman GL, Markowitz JS, et al: Suicidal ideation and suicide attempts in panic disorder and attacks. N Engl J Med 321:1209–1214, 1989

Westling BE, Stjernlof K, Öst LG: Self-monitoring of cognitions during panic attacks. Presented at Annual Conference of Association for Advancement of Behaviour Therapy, 1989

Wittchen HU: Epidemiology of panic attacks and panic disorders, in Panic and Phobias I. Edited by Hand I, Wittchen HU. New York, Springer, 1986, pp 18–27

Wulsin LR, Hillard JR, Geier P, et al: Int J Psychiatry Med 18:315–323, 1988

Zucker D, Taylor CB, Brouillard M, et al: Cognitive aspects of panic attacks: content, course and relationship to laboratory stressors. Br J Psychiatry 155:86–91, 1989

Chapter 16

Specific (Simple) Phobia

Michelle G. Craske, Ph.D., David H. Barlow, Ph.D.,
David M. Clark, Ph.D., George C. Curtis, M.D.,
Elizabeth M. Hill, Ph.D., Joseph A. Himle, M.S.W.,
Yue-Joe Lee, M.D., Julie A. Lewis, B.A., Richard J. McNally, Ph.D.,
Lars-Goran Öst, Ph.D., Paul M. Salkovskis, Ph.D., and
Hilary M. C. Warwick, B.M., M.R.C.Psych.

Statement of the Issues

This report represents an integrative review of six different review papers that were requested by the Simple Phobia Subcommittee. As an initial step, the subcommittee recommended changing the diagnostic label from simple phobia to specific phobia. The recommendation was based on recognition of the value of consistency between DSM-IV and ICD-10 (World Health Organization 1990) nosology, especially because the term *specific phobia* more aptly describes the disorder. Hereafter in the review, the term *specific phobia* is used.

The subcommittee identified two major areas for consideration. The first area concerned clarification of the boundary between specific phobias and panic disorder with agoraphobia (PDA) or agoraphobia without a history of panic (A). Differential diagnosis between PDA/A and specific phobias is difficult in many cases, because several situations are listed as being commonly feared and/or avoided in both categories of disorder. The second major area of consideration concerned the feasibility of specifying distinct subtypes within the specific phobia category. It was believed that evidence for distinctiveness in terms of age at onset, sex ratio, response to treatment, and the like would support the notion of distinguishing among subtypes of specific phobias.

In addition, the subcommittee raised questions concerning the differentiation between specific phobias of illness and hypochondriasis and between traumatic-etiology phobias and posttraumatic stress disorder (PTSD). Specifically, the following questions were addressed by the six review papers:

1. To what extent are "situational" phobias of driving, enclosed places, heights, and public transportation distinct from agoraphobia, and distinct from other types of specific phobias, such as animal phobias? In other words, is there evidence to suggest that "situational" phobias be classified as either a subtype within the specific phobia category or as part of PDA/A?

2. What is the role of panic attacks in specific phobias, and is the fear experienced in a specific phobic reaction distinct from panic attacks experienced in PDA? In other words, are there features of phobic fear that are sufficiently distinct from panic attacks for the purposes of clarifying the boundaries between specific phobias and PDA?

3. Is there evidence to suggest that blood/injury phobia is a distinct subtype within the diagnosis of specific phobia?

4. Is there evidence to suggest that choking phobia is a distinct subtype within the diagnosis of specific phobia?

5. How are illness phobias differentiated from a diagnosis of hypochondriasis, or should illness phobias be subsumed under the diagnosis of hypochondriasis?

6. Is there evidence to suggest that specific phobias that develop following a trauma of posttraumatic stress proportions should be considered specific phobias or symptoms of PTSD?

Significance of the Issues

As stated above, the main issues covered by the review papers pertained to providing better guidelines for distinguishing between specific phobias and PDA or A, and to the validity of distinguishing among subtypes of specific phobias. In both cases, the ramifications for research methodology and clinical practice are clear. Basic agreement about the defining features of the population under study is necessary before attempting to examine the effectiveness of different treatments for different anxiety disorders. The treatment issue extends to the effectiveness of different treatments for different types of specific phobias.

The difficulty differentiating between specific phobias and PDA has been highlighted by diagnostic reliability studies and clinical anecdotal reports. The diagnosis of specific phobia tends to be less reliable than the diagnoses of the majority of other anxiety disorders (DiNardo et al. 1983; Manuzza et al. 1989). The difficulty differentiating between specific phobias and PDA is due largely to the overlap in the types of situations that are commonly feared and/or avoided in both disorders. Driving, flying, traveling by bus or train, heights, and enclosed places are common circumscribed phobic situations, and they belong to the cluster of agoraphobic situations from which it is difficult to escape in the event of a panic attack or some other physical ailment. Furthermore, fears of circumscribed objects or situations are sometimes associated with "panicky" feelings. However, little explicit guidance is provided in DSM-III-R (American Psychiatric Association 1987) for determining the diagnostic assignment of someone, for example, who is very anxious about and who panics while driving but who is neither anxious about nor panics with respect to any other situation. In this case, the particular situation (i.e., driving) and the report of panicking resembles PDA, but the circumscribed nature of the phobia resembles specific phobia. Diagnoses for PDA are usually more reliable than for specific phobias, because the *number* of situations anticipated or avoided is usually sufficient to provide enough evidence to the diagnostician for a PDA diagnosis. However, the issue of diagnostic assignment is less clear in the case of fear/avoidance of a single, circumscribed situation.

Traditionally, research studies have grouped the various specific phobias (e.g., animal phobias, height phobias, driving phobias) together. In parallel with this research trend has been a tendency to assume that the same type of treatment approach is equally appropriate for all specific phobias. However, several more recent studies have suggested that marked differences exist across the various phobic objects or situations (Himle et al. 1989; Öst 1987). The differences have included age at onset, sex distribution, and familial patterns, in addition to response to treatment intervention. The extent to which these differences are suggestive of varying psychopathologies, courses, and prognoses was considered important to evaluate, because such variation would support the notion of specifying subtypes within the diagnosis of specific phobia.

Method

Because each review paper used slightly different methods of review, the specific methods used for each review are described just prior to presenting the results of that review. In each case, the reviews were conducted in a systematic and comprehensive fashion while maintaining an objective perspective for the presentation of results. The assignment of topics to certain reviewers was based on consideration of accessibility to relevant databases and expertise in the area being reviewed.

Results

Specific "Situational" Phobias: A Variant of Agoraphobia[1]

The major issue addressed by this review is the extent to which fear and avoidance of certain situations (driving, flying, heights, and enclosed places) are distinct from agoraphobia and from animal phobias. It was reasoned that if the situational phobias were not distinct from agoraphobia but were distinct from animal phobias, then their inclusion under the diagnosis of PDA/A might be considered. If situational phobias were distinct from agoraphobia and animal phobias, then subtyping within the specific phobia diagnosis might be considered.

No explicit boundary was drawn between mild agoraphobia and agoraphobia-like specific phobias in DSM-III-R, other than by offering examples of each. In DSM-III-R, heights and enclosed places consistently appear as examples of specific phobias, whereas bridges, tunnels, and travel by bus or train consistently appear as examples of agoraphobia. The same strategy was incorporated into the methodology of the recent Epidemiologic Catchment Area (ECA) study, where all phobias of heights and enclosed places were coded as simple phobias regardless of what other symptoms were present or absent. Similarly, all phobias of bridges, tunnels, and public transportation, including airplanes, buses or trains, were coded as agoraphobia regardless of what other symptoms were present. A reanalysis of the ECA data is presented at the end of this summary of the Curtis et al. review.

Method. Original research reports that met the following criteria were included in the review: the report included groups or subgroups of subjects diagnosed as having simple phobia using DSM-III, DSM-III-R, or RDC (Spitzer et al. 1978) criteria or contained enough information to permit the reviewers to assign this diagnosis; the report permitted further classification of subjects with circumscribed phobias as phobias of animals or of specific situational stimuli (heights, enclosures, driving, flying, elevators, buses, trains, bridges, tunnels, etc.); the report contained information on age at onset, sex ratio, comorbidity, family history, response to treatment, or any other potentially useful information about subjects with animal or specific situational fears. If these three criteria were not present, an alternative strategy was to include studies that reported factor analyses and permitted examination of factor loadings of animal fears/phobias or specific situational fears/phobias.

To initiate the literature search, the titles of all documents containing a word that included *phobia* were retrieved from Medline and Psychological Abstracts databases. To retrieve the desired factor analytic studies, the same search procedures were followed using the search terms *fear and factor* and *phobia and factor*. Computer searches were augmented by examining bibliographic citations in rele-

---

[1]Curtis GC, Himle JA, Lewis JA, Lee Y-J: "Specific Situational Phobias: Variant of Agoraphobia?" Paper requested by the Simple Phobia Subcommittee of the DSM-IV Anxiety Disorders Work Group, 1989.

vant chapters of several recent books reviewing the construct of anxiety. In total, 93 articles were examined.

Results. The authors noted that difficulties with interpretation of the results were encountered given the lack of controlled studies comparing different types of phobias and the variability across studies in methods of classification. Three main groups of phobias were compared: 1) situational phobias (driving, flying, enclosed places, tunnels, bridges, and heights), 2) animal phobias, and 3) agoraphobia.

Sex ratio: The ratios indicated a similarity between groups with situational phobias and agoraphobia, in which the percentage of males was slightly higher than was the case for groups with animal phobias. The figures reported most frequently for agoraphobia and situational phobias were 10%–13% males, in contrast to 9% males for animal phobias (Table 16–1). However, the trends were not marked and were not replicated in community samples. It is possible that sex ratios in clinical samples are affected by sex differences in treatment seeking behavior. Sex ratio data were obtained from the following sources: Bourdon et al. 1988; Fava et al. 1988; Himle et al. 1989, 1991; Lautch 1971; Liddell and Lyons 1978; Marks 1970, 1981; Marks and Gelder 1966; Martin et al. 1969; Öst 1987; Philips 1985; Raguram and Bhide 1985; Snaith 1968; Takeya et al. 1978; Thorpe and Burns 1983; Whitehead et al. 1978.

Age at onset: With the exception of height phobia, the age at onset of the situational phobias was very similar to that of agoraphobia (early to mid-20s), and contrasted with the early-childhood onset for animal phobias (Table 16–2). Height phobias tended to develop in late childhood/early adolescence. The authors noted that age at onset is influenced by mode of acquisition, because traumatic etiology is less likely to be related to a typical age at onset. Therefore, interpretation of age at onset should take etiology into consideration. Age at onset data were obtained from the following sources: Barlow 1988; Craske et al., unpublished; Himle et al. 1989; Himle et al. unpublished; Jerremalm et al. 1986; Liddell and Lyons 1978; Marks 1970; Marks and Gelder 1966; Mendel and Klein 1969; Öst 1987; Philips 1985; Sheehan et al. 1981; Takeya et al. 1978; Thyer and Curtis 1983.

Panic attack etiology: Although panic attacks were rarely recalled as being the trigger for the development of animal phobias, a substantial minority (estimates ranging from 4% to 50%) of patients with situational phobias experienced panic attacks (e.g., Himle et al. 1991), as did the majority of agoraphobic patients (Barlow 1988). However, variability was noted among the various situational phobias with respect to the occurrence of panic attacks. Etiology data were obtained from the following sources: Barlow 1988; Craske et al., unpublished; DiNardo et al. 1988; Himle et al. unpublished; Kleinknecht 1982; Liddell and Lyons 1978; Marks 1970; McNally and Steketee 1985; Munjack 1984; Murray and Foote 1979; Öst 1985, 1987.

Table 16–1.   Sex ratios

Study	N	% Male
Animal phobias		
Marks and Gelder 1966	18	6
Martin et al. 1969	19	0
Whitehead 1978	12	17
Whitehead et al. 1978	14	7
Ladouceur 1983	36	3
McNally and Steketee 1985	22	9
Watts and Sharrock 1985	35	6
Raguram and Bhide 1985	2	0
Öst 1987	50	4
Himle et al. 1989	25	0
Situational phobias		
Marks and Gelder 1966	12	25
Himle et al. 1989	46	43
Takeya et al. 1978	16	88
Bourque and Ladouceur 1980	50	30
Williams et al. 1985	38	42
Marshall 1988	20	55
Öst 1987	40	10
Matthew et al. 1982	48	19
Munjack 1984	30	17
Solyom et al. 1973	40	30
Howard et al. 1983	56	20
Marks 1981	13	15
Agoraphobia		
Thorpe and Burns 1983		
1956–1980	625	10–37
Clinical projects	40	12
National survey	963	11
Lader et al. 1967	11	0
Martin et al. 1969	28	39
Munjack and Moss 1981	68	15
Neiger et al. 1981	97	14
Sheehan et al. 1981	100	15
Raguram and Bhide 1985	26	85
Thyer et al. 1985	34	15
Öst 1987	100	13
Fava et al. 1988	20	35

Source. Curtis GC, Himle JA, Lewis JA, Lee Y-J: "Specific Situational Phobias: Variant of Agoraphobia?" Paper requested by the Simple Phobia Subcommittee of the DSM-IV Anxiety Disorders Work Group, 1989.

Comorbidity: The authors concluded that the issue of comorbidity between various types of phobias, panic attacks, and depression requires further evaluation. To some extent, this evaluation was achieved by the reanalysis of the ECA data set (see below). Comorbidity data were obtained from the following sources: Alfin 1987; Barlow 1988; Bowen and Hohout 1979; Howard et al. 1983; Lader et al. 1967; Liddell and Lyons 1978; Marks 1970, 1981; Matthew et al. 1982; Munjack and Moss 1981; Norton et al. 1985, 1986; Philips 1985; Solyom et al. 1973.

Familial aggregation: There was some evidence to suggest an aggregation within families by class of phobia. In other words, probands with phobias of animals were

Table 16–2.   Age at onset

Study	N	Mean age at onset (years)
Animal phobias		
Marks and Gelder 1966	18	4.4
Martin et al. 1969	19	4.8
Marks 1970	30	4.0
Öst 1987	50	6.9
Himle et al. 1989	25	14.9
Craske et al., unpublished, 1993	28	17.4[a]
Situational phobias		
Marks and Gelder 1966	12	23
Himle et al. 1989	46	27
Takeya et al. 1978	16	32
Bourque and Ladouceur 1980	50	9
Williams et al. 1985	38	12
Öst 1987	40	21
Munjack 1984	30	33
Solyom et al. 1973	40	28
Marks 1981	13	55
Agoraphobia		
Thorpe and Burns 1983		
1956–1980		20–31
Clinical projects	40	27
National survey	963	28
Martin et al. 1969	28	24
Sheehan et al. 1981	100	24
Munjack and Moss 1981	68	27
Öst 1987	100	28
Fava et al. 1988	20	31

[a]Omitting 28.6% who reported having the phobia "all my life."

Source.   Curtis GC, Himle JA, Lewis JA, Lee Y-J: "Specific Situational Phobias: Variant of Agoraphobia?" Paper requested by the Simple Phobia Subcommittee of the DSM-IV Anxiety Disorders Work Group, 1989.

likely to have first-degree relatives with phobias of animals also (although not usually of the same animal). Similarly, probands with situational phobias tended to have relatives with phobias of other types of situations. However, the data were limited within this area, and further investigation is needed. Familial data were obtained from the following sources: Fyer et al. unpublished; Himle et al. 1989; Liddell and Lyons 1978.

Treatment response: The authors noted that the evidence pertaining to response to treatment is not currently sufficient for the determination of differential patterns according to type of phobia. Treatment response data were obtained from the following sources: Cameron et al. 1987; Marks 1970, 1981; Thyer and Curtis 1984.

Factor analyses: Unfortunately, the factor analytic studies rarely met the conventional minimal standards for ensuring factor stability. Therefore, considerable variability was noted in factor loadings, although there was a consistent trend for fears of animals and insects to load on the same factor. Factor analysis data were obtained from the following sources: Arrindell 1980; Bates 1971; Beck and Emery 1985; Hallam and Hafner 1978; Landy and Gaupp 1971; Lawlis 1971; Meikle and Mitchell 1974; Ollendick 1989; Rothstein et al. 1972; Rubin and Lawlis 1969; Rubin et al. 1968; Scherer and Nakamura 1968; Torgersen 1979; Wilson and Priest 1968.

In summary, the strongest evidence for commonality between situational phobias and agoraphobia and for a separation between situational phobias and animal phobias was age at onset (with the exception of height phobia). The same trends were partially supported by panic attack etiology and familial aggregation patterns.

Discussion.   The authors recommended that, in light of the similarities between situational phobias and agoraphobia, and the contrasts with animal phobias, the "mild" avoidance category of the agoraphobia diagnosis be broadened to include any situational phobias (driving, flying, heights, bridges, enclosed places, tunnels) for which the onset of fear and avoidance is due to an unexpected panic attack in a situation about which the person had not previously been anxious. Situational phobias with other modes of onset should be classified as specific phobias.

Heterogeneity of DSM-III-R Simple Phobia and the Simple Phobia/Agoraphobia Boundary: Evidence From the ECA Study[2]

The authors reanalyzed the ECA data set (Reiger et al. 1984) for phobias to further assess the viability of situational phobias as a variant of agoraphobia. Their reanal-

---

[2]Curtis GC, Hill EM, Lewis JA: "Heterogeneity of DSM-III-R Simple Phobia and the Simple Phobia/Agoraphobia Boundary: Evidence From the ECA Study." Preliminary report to the Simple Phobia Subcommittee of the DSM-IV Anxiety Disorders Work Group, 1990.

ysis is presented in detail in another report but is summarized in the current review because the results are pertinent to the final consensus recommendations.

Method.   Copies of the ECA data tape, the Diagnostic Interview Schedule (DIS; Robins et al. 1981), and the ECA diagnostic algorithm for generating DSM-III (American Psychiatric Association 1980) diagnoses from the interview data were obtained. The diagnostic algorithms were ignored, so that each of the 12 phobia items were examined in their own right. The phobia items were tunnels or bridges, being in a crowd, public transportation, going out of the house alone, being alone, heights, being in a closed place, storms, water, spiders/mice/bugs/snakes/bats, being near other harmless animals or dangerous animals that cannot get at you, and any other fear. Of the total of 13,538 interviews from four different sites (Baltimore, MD, St. Louis, MO, Durham, NC, and Los Angeles, CA), 1,123 reported one and only one of the phobia items, and 2,265 subjects reported more than one phobia. Various forms of statistical clustering followed by stepwise logistic regressions were conducted.

Results.   Three main clusters were identified. The first was an "agoraphobia" cluster, consisting of being alone, going out of the house alone, and crowds. Fear of enclosed places was added to the agoraphobia cluster, given 1) similarities in terms of comorbidity rates with other variables (i.e., panic attacks, social phobia, alcoholism, depression, and schizophrenia), and 2) items in the agoraphobia cluster were predictive of claustrophobia, and vice versa. The second was a "childhood" cluster, consisting of animals, storms, and being in water. The third was a group of inconsistently or weakly clustering items, including tunnels or bridges, public transportation, and any other fear. Height phobia was considered to be separate from the three clusters, given its uniquely high proportion of males (57.7% of subjects with only height phobias and 40.2% of all subjects with height phobias versus 36% in the agoraphobia cluster and 31% in the childhood cluster).

The most powerful discriminator among the clusters was age at onset, which was considerably older in the agoraphobia cluster (24 years) than in the childhood cluster (8.8 years). The age at onset for claustrophobia peaked in childhood (2–7 years), but a secondary peak seemed to occur in the 20s, yielding an overall mean age at onset of 15.5 years. A similar, almost bimodal distribution was found for age at onset for tunnels/bridges and public transportation. The peak age at onset for height phobias was young (2–7 years), but the spread of onset did not extend as high as for the phobias of enclosed places, tunnels/bridges, and public transporta-tion, yielding a slightly lower average age at onset of 14.7 years.

Comorbidity patterns also discriminated among the two strongest clusters. Although the childhood cluster items were more prevalent, the fears were associated less strongly with other phobias and psychiatric conditions than were the agoraphobia cluster items.

The third group of inconsistently clustering items was difficult to interpret because of the lack of specification inherent in the items themselves (i.e., tunnels or bridges, various forms of public transportation, and any other fear). However, their ages at onset tended to follow a similar trend of peaking in childhood, with many new cases developing through the early adult years. Fears of heights and enclosed places overlapped with this third cluster in two ways: first, in terms of age at onset distributions (as described above), and second, because heights and enclosures typically form part of public transportation and tunnels/bridges situations.

Discussion.   The ECA data revealed some trends that were at variance with the review of available literature regarding the commonality between situational phobias and agoraphobia (summarized earlier). That is, many of the situational phobias did not clearly cluster with agoraphobic situations, particularly in terms of comorbidity patterns and co-occurrence rates. Fear of enclosed places was associated most strongly with agoraphobic situations.

The authors recommended that situational phobias that begin with an unexpected panic attack in the subsequently phobic situation, and in which there is a history of one or more panic attacks or two or more limited symptom attacks outside the phobic situation, be classified as mild agoraphobia. Situational phobias that do not meet the aforesaid criteria should be diagnosed in a separate category, perhaps called specific phobia not otherwise specified (NOS). The cluster of phobias that includes fear of animals, storms, and water might be considered another separate category. Also, the authors recommended that blood/injury phobias be assigned to a separate diagnostic category of blood/injury phobia. Any remaining fears of circumscribed objects or situations should be classified as specific phobia NOS.

Boundary Between Simple Phobia and Panic Disorder[3]

This review addressed the issue of differentiation between specific phobias and PDA using a different set of variables for comparison. In particular, features of the fear response itself, as it is experienced in response to circumscribed phobic situations, were contrasted with panic attacks. The features that were examined included

---

[3]Craske MG: "The Boundary Between Simple Phobia and Panic Disorder With Agoraphobia." Paper requested by the Simple Phobia Subcommittee of the DSM-IV Anxiety Disorders Work Group, 1989.

symptom profile, physiological patterns, expectancy/predictability, and focus of apprehension.

Two questions were asked. First, are the features of PDA cued panic attacks (i.e., panic in response to an anticipated situation) different from phobic fear? Second, are the features of PDA uncued panic attacks (i.e., "out of the blue" or spontaneous attacks) different from phobic fear? It was reasoned that if the features of panic attacks (cued and uncued) are clearly different from phobic reactions, then descriptive features exclusive to phobic fear might be elucidated for the purpose of enhancing differential diagnoses. On the other hand, if the features of panic attacks are indistinguishable from phobic fear, then the difference between PDA and specific phobia is more likely to reside in either the nature of the object or situation that is feared or in the occurrence (versus features) of uncued panic attacks.

Method.   Original research reports were obtained from Medlars and Psychological Abstracts databases covering the years 1966–1989, using the key words *simple phobia, agoraphobia,* and *panic.* The search was augmented by use of citations from recent books concerning the construct of anxiety. The author noted that the review was impeded by lack of controlled studies comparing PDA with different types of specific phobias. In addition, difficulties were encountered when comparing across studies, due to inconsistent use of the terms *fear* and *anticipatory anxiety.*

Results.   Comparisons were made in terms of symptom profile, physiology of fear, predictability of fear, and focus of apprehension.

Symptom profile: Symptom data were gathered from retrospective interviewing, concurrent self-monitoring under naturally occurring conditions (for PDA panic attacks only), and experimental induction conditions. A majority of individuals with specific phobias (from 75% to 100%) report the presence of four or more symptoms (from the DSM-III-R panic attack checklist) when anxious or fearful about their phobic object or situation (e.g., Barlow et al. 1985; Rachman et al. 1987). On average, groups of individuals with PDA tend to endorse a higher percentage of the symptoms from the checklist, but severity and rank ordering of symptoms differed very little from the ratings provided by groups of individuals with various specific phobias. In addition, several studies of PDA subjects who self-monitored their panic attacks in the natural environment have shown that situational (or cued) attacks and spontaneous (or uncued) attacks are very similar in terms of symptom profiles and endorsement ratios (e.g., Krystal et al. 1988; Margraf et al. 1987).

On the other hand, there was preliminary evidence to suggest different symptom profiles across the various types of specific phobias. For example, the rank ordering of symptoms tended to differ for those with blood/injury phobias (L. G. Öst, personal communication) in comparison with a group of those with mixed simple phobias and in comparison with those with PDA panic attacks (Table 16–3). Furthermore, those with animal phobias may endorse fewer symptoms than those with other types of specific phobias (Craske et al. 1993; Craske et al., unpublished data). In addition, those with claustrophobia tended to report particularly strong symptom patterns when forced to confront enclosed places, according to experimental work conducted by Rachman et al. (1988b). In fact, individuals with claustrophobia endorsed a higher percentage of symptoms than did those with PDA during their behavioral testing procedures (Rachman et al. 1988a, 1988b). Symptom profile data were obtained from the following sources: Barlow et al. 1985;

Table 16–3.   Mean severity and frequency of report of panic attack symptoms

	Mixed					
	Panic disorder[a] (N = 190)		Simple phobia[a] (N = 35)		Injection phobia[b] (N = 50)	
Panic attack symptoms	Mean (1–4)	%	Mean (1–4)	%	Mean (1–4)	%
Dyspnea	2.0	61.5	2.4	48.6	1.8	42.0
Choking	2.0	40.1	2.4	14.3	2.4	34.0
Tachycardia	2.5	83.4	2.5	77.1	2.9	78.0
Chest pain/ discomfort	2.0	41.2	1.4	22.9	2.0	22.0
Sweating	2.0	65.1	2.2	77.1	3.3	96.0
Dizziness/ unsteadiness/faintness	2.3	86.1	2.0	51.4	3.3	83.0
Nausea/abdominal distress	1.9	51.9	2.3	20.6	2.8	78.0
Derealization/ depersonalization	2.3	58.3	2.3	25.7	2.1	42.0
Paresthesias	2.0	57.2	1.3	20.0	2.0	20.0
Hot/cold flashes	2.1	65.2	1.7	51.4	3.1	72.0
Trembling/shaking	2.2	77.5	1.9	65.7	2.9	66.0
Fear of dying	2.6	53.5	2.0	25.7	2.0	8.0
Fear of going crazy/ losing control	2.7	70.1	2.5	57.1	2.9	32.0

[a]Center for Stress and Anxiety Disorders, Albany, New York.
[b]L. G. Öst, personal communication, 1989.
Source.   Craske MG: "The Boundary Between Simple Phobia and Panic Disorder With Agoraphobia." Paper requested by the Simple Phobia Subcommittee of the DSM-IV Anxiety Disorders Work Group, 1989.

Craske et al., unpublished; Krystal et al. 1988; Margraf et al. 1987; Rachman and Levitt 1985; Rachman et al. 1987, 1988b; Rapee et al. 1990; Street et al. 1989.

Physiological patterns: There was a paucity of studies suitable for the purpose of comparing phobic reactions and panic attacks in this area. In addition, many of the studies were flawed by inadequate controls and the discordance between subjective reports of fear. Also, the degree of physiological arousal that is apparent in both disorders complicates the issue. To date, there is no available evidence to suggest that the peripheral physiology (e.g., heart rate, blood pressure, respiration) of specific phobic reactions differs from the physiology of PDA cued panic attacks (e.g., Cook et al. 1988; Nesse et al. 1980; Taylor 1977), with the exception of one specific phobia.

Blood/injury phobia has a distinct diphasic physiological basis, characterized by an occasional, although inconsistent, initial acceleration, followed by a consistently observed deceleration in heart rate and blood pressure. The deceleration phase seems to account for the frequent fainting behavior in individuals with this group of phobias (e.g., Johansson and Öst 1982). Physiological data were obtained from the following sources: Abelson and Curtis 1989; Cook et al. 1988; Curtis et al. 1976, 1979; Graham et al. 1961; Johansson and Öst 1982; Ko et al. 1983; McGlynn et al. 1973; Nesse et al. 1980, 1985; Öst 1987; Öst et al. 1982, 1984a, 1984b; Prigatano and Johnson 1974; Sartory et al. 1977; Taylor 1977; Taylor et al. 1986; Woods et al. 1987.

Expectancy/predictability: Predictability is an important variable to assess because a hallmark feature of PDA is the unexpected nature of the panic attacks. However, for the current review, expectancy was examined in relation to cued attacks only. (The unpredictability inherent in uncued or 'spontaneous' panic attacks clearly differentiates between the two disorders.) The question addressed was whether PDA situational/cued attacks are any more or less expected/predictable than the fear experienced by those with specific phobias when confronting their phobic stimuli.

Frequently, PDAs report that although certain situations are anticipated for fear of experiencing a panic attack, the likelihood that panic will occur and the precise point in time when panic will occur during exposure to the situation are not fully predictable. This contrasts with the general assumption that individuals with phobias become predictably more fearful as the phobic stimulus is approached.

In a series of studies conducted by Rachman et al. (1988a, 1988b), individuals with claustrophobia reportedly experienced unexpected episodes of fear (i.e., panic) in claustrophobic situations. That is, their prediction that a rush of fear or panic was unlikely to happen was not accurate. In fact, individuals with claustrophobia were found to have an equivalent number of occasions during which they

panicked unexpectedly to those with PDA (during behavioral approach to anticipated situations) (e.g., Rachman et al. 1988a, 1988b). However, the extent to which
the reactions of those with claustrophobia were unexpected is unclear. It is possible
that individuals with claustrophobia are sometimes unsure about being fearful on
any given occasion of exposure to a claustrophobic situation, but rarely are they
truly surprised by the occurrence of a fearful reaction. Furthermore, the degree to
which individuals with other types of specific phobias (e.g., animal phobias)
experience unexpected rushes of fear or panic is in need of investigation.

The issue of the precise time at which fear is experienced in anticipated
situations has not been fully examined. During retrospective reporting, the majority of individuals with specific phobias report that they typically feel anxious or
fearful immediately on encountering the phobic situation, although variations
across type of specific phobia are marked (Craske et al. 1993; Craske et al.,
unpublished data). In contrast, individuals with PDA report that their fear is more
typically delayed when they encounter anticipated situations. Further investigation
is needed, however, because onset of fear may have been confused with onset of
anticipatory anxiety. Expectancy data were obtained from the following sources:
Craske et al. 1993; Craske et al., unpublished data; Margraf et al. 1987; Rachman
and Levitt 1985; Rachman and Lopatka 1986a, 1986b; Rachman et al. 1988b;
Somerville et al. 1983; Street et al. 1989; Teghtsoonian and Frost 1982.

Focus of apprehension: The cognitive component in anxiety is featured in the
DSM-III-R diagnostic criteria for PD/PDA, social phobia, and generalized anxiety
disorder. The focus of apprehension in PD/PDA is clearly on experiencing another
panic attack or its perceived consequences (e.g., losing control, going crazy, or
dying). In the criteria for simple phobia, the focus of apprehension is specified as
a rule-out only: "other than fear of having a panic attack (as in Panic Disorder) or
of humiliation or embarrassment in certain social situations (as in Social Phobia)"
(p. 244).

Traditionally, it has been assumed that the focus of apprehension in specific
phobias is tied directly to perceived harm from aspects of the phobic situation (e.g.,
being bitten by a dog, a plane crashing, or an elevator getting stuck). However,
several investigations have shown otherwise. For example, it has been found that
individuals with animal phobias are frequently concerned about panicking or losing
control (McNally and Steketee 1985), as are those with driving phobias (Munjack
1984), claustrophobia (e.g., Rachman et al. 1987), and needle phobias (e.g., Kaver
et al. 1989). Consistent with these reports are the two factors found to account for
up to 90% of the variance in fear ratings for specific phobic situations. These factors
are labeled danger expectancy (or concerns about the dangerous nature of the
situation, such as concerns about a plane crashing) and anxiety expectancy (or
concerns about the consequences from anxiety reactions in the situation, such as

concerns about losing control within the confines of an enclosed place) (Gursky and Reiss 1987; Reiss et al. 1988). Anxiety expectancy closely resembles the "panic-apprehension" experienced by those with PD/PDA.

The extent to which an anxiety expectancy predominates may vary across the different types of phobias. Preliminary data suggest that individuals with claustrophobia in particular are concerned with losing control and panicking (Craske et al. 1993).

The high prevalence of fears of panicking and losing control in response to circumscribed objects or situations makes the issue of differential diagnosis between PD/PDA and specific phobias more difficult. However, clinical wisdom would suggest that, in the case of specific phobias, anxiety expectancy is limited to the presence of the phobic stimulus. In contrast, a hallmark feature of PDA is persistent apprehension about the recurrence of panic even when an identifiable situational trigger is neither anticipated nor present. Data pertaining to focus of apprehension were obtained from the following sources: Chambless et al. 1984; Clark et al. 1988; Craske et al. 1993; Ehlers and Margraf 1989; Foa 1988; Gursky and Reiss 1987; Hugdahl and Öst 1985; Kaver et al. 1989; Kleinknecht and Lenz 1989; McNally and Steketee 1985; Munjack 1984; Rachman et al. 1987; Reiss 1987; Reiss et al. 1986; van den Hout et al. 1987.

Discussion.   The author of this section (Craske) concluded that much more research is needed because the boundary between specific phobias and PDA seems to depend to a large extent on the particular type of phobia in question. A MacArthur-funded project is being conducted by Craske to address these issues. However, it is suggested that differential diagnosis might be enhanced by giving consideration to the content of apprehension, pervasiveness of panic-apprehension, and presence of uncued panic attacks.

It is suggested that the criteria for specific phobias allow for worry about experiencing panic in the phobic situation. However, if panic-apprehension pervades beyond the actual or anticipated presence of the phobic stimulus and/or if uncued panic attacks exist, then a diagnosis of PDA should be considered. Furthermore, it is suggested that when a PDA diagnosis is assigned, an additional diagnosis of specific phobia may be assigned if fear of a circumscribed stimulus is associated with definite worry about danger or harm from the stimulus itself. For example, an individual may experience uncued panic attacks, worry persistently about the recurrence of panic, and be phobic of driving for fear of being hit by other vehicles on the road. In this case, a codiagnosis of PD/PDA and specific phobia would be warranted. Finally, it is suggested that the criteria for specific phobias recognize that panic attacks occur and may sometimes be unexpected, although anxiety is usually aroused immediately on encountering the phobic stimulus.

Blood Phobia: A Specific Phobia Subtype in DSM-IV[4]

The primary issue addressed in this review was the validity or feasibility of considering blood phobia as a distinct subtype within the specific phobia diagnostic category. Blood phobia can be defined as the fear and avoidance of situations involving exposure (direct or indirect) to blood, injury, wounds, etc. If escape from the situation is not possible, there is a high probability of fainting due to a marked drop in blood pressure and/or heart rate. Obviously, including blood phobia as a subtype would suggest particular treatment implications.

Method. A computer search was conducted using Medline and Psychological Abstracts databases covering the period 1972–1989. The key words were *blood phobia, injury phobia,* and *vaso-vagal syncope.* This search yielded 17 papers describing 1–15 case studies and only 2 controlled studies. Data from Öst's own sample of 81 subjects with blood phobias were also included for the purposes of review (Öst 1991). The case studies were: Babcock and Powell 1982; Cohn et al. 1976; Curtis and Thyer 1983; Elmore et al. 1980; Gudjonsson and Sartory 1983; Kozak and Miller 1985; Kozak and Montgomery 1981; Lloyd and Deakin 1975; McGrady and Bernal 1986; Orwin 1972; Öst et al. 1989; Richards 1988; Thyer and Curtis 1985; Wardle and Jarvis 1981; and Yule and Fernando 1980.

Results. The review provided a full description of the features of blood phobia for purposes of comparison with the available data regarding features of other specific phobias.

Prevalence: The prevalence of blood phobia is in the range of 3%-4.5% (Agras et al. 1969; Costello 1982; Lapouse and Monk 1959; Miller et al. 1974). However, it should be cautioned that estimates of prevalence were gathered prior to implementation of the DSM-III criteria and are therefore tentative.

Sex ratio: In the published series of studies, 63% of blood phobic samples were males (e.g., Thyer et al. 1985), although only 35% of Öst's (1991) 81 blood phobics were males.

Age: The mean age at onset was 8.5 years (range 2–20 years) (e.g., Öst 1991; Thyer et al. 1985). The mean age at which treatment was sought was approximately 30 (range 16–55 years).

Etiology: The mode of acquisition was ascertained by Öst (1991) through questioning and recall, and the findings are therefore of questionable accuracy. However, the majority of those with blood phobias associated the onset of their

---

[4]Öst L-G: "Blood Phobia: A Specific Phobia Subtype in DSM-IV." Paper requested by the Simple Phobia Subcommittee of the DSM-IV Anxiety Disorders Work Group, 1989.

phobia with traumatic conditioning experiences, including unexpected panic attacks (45% of the females and 57% of the males). The second most frequent mode of acquisition was modeling or observing another person reacting with anxiety in response to blood/injury (26% of females and 25% of males). Information was cited as the mode of acquisition by 8% of the females and 7% of the males. Finally, 21% of females and 11% of males were unable to recall any specific instance or mode of acquisition.

Course: According to the case study reports, blood phobia tends to be chronic, usually with a gradual worsening of the phobia over time. However, data were restricted to phobic patients seeking treatment, so that no information was available concerning rates of spontaneous remission.

Familial patterns: A very high incidence of blood phobia is evident in family members. Interviewing of first-degree relatives of 25 blood phobic patients at Öst's center resulted in 64% of the patients having at least one relative with blood phobia.

Comorbidity: Approximately half of the group of blood phobic patients have at least one other phobia, although it is not usually as severe or as impairing as the blood phobia. The degree of impairment from blood phobia can be quite severe, including inability to obtain necessary medical treatment, fearing future pregnancy, or dropping out of medical school (Öst, unpublished; Thyer et al. 1985).

Physiology: A distinct physiological response characterizes blood phobia (Öst et al. 1984b). This response sometimes includes initial acceleration (i.e., increased heart rate and blood pressure) and usually includes deceleration (i.e., decreased heart rate and blood pressure). Consequently, approximately 75% of those with blood phobias report a history of fainting in the phobic situation.

Treatment response: Blood phobias have been shown to respond well to a procedure designed to counteract deceleration of heart rate and blood pressure (Öst et al. 1984a). The procedure is called applied tension and contrasts with the method of applied relaxation usually used to control anxiety reactions.

Blood phobia versus injection phobia: According to the data set collected by Öst (unpublished), blood and injection phobias share many features, including the particularly salient features of fainting history and physiological response to the phobic situation. On the other hand, fewer individuals with injection phobias (approximately 22%) report that family relatives have the same phobia. Features of blood and injection phobias are compared in Table 16–4.

In summary, blood (and injection) phobias differ from other types of specific phobias in several ways. First, mean age at onset is significantly later than for animal phobias but significantly earlier than for dental phobia and claustrophobia. Second, a significantly higher proportion of those with blood phobias report family members with blood phobias comparison with the concordance ratios for family relatives of those with animal phobias, dental phobias, and claustrophobia. In addition,

Table 16–4.   Blood phobia versus injection phobia

	Blood phobia	Injection phobia
Sex (%)		
Female	65.4	74.6
Male	34.6	25.4
Age at onset (years)	8.6 ± 177 3.9	8.1 ± 177 5.0
Fainting history (%)	70.4	58.2
Number of fainting episodes	10.8 ± 177 3.9	7.8 ± 177 11.4
Relative with same phobia (%)	60.5	22.2
Mutilation Questionnaire	19.9 ± 177 4.2	17.3 ± 177 5.8

Note. Values are means ± SD, except for percentages.
Source. Öst L-G: "Blood Phobia: A Specific Phobia Subtype in DSM-IV." Paper requested by the Simple Phobia Subcommittee of the DSM-IV Anxiety Disorders Work Group, 1989.

fainting is very rarely reported by individuals with other types of phobias, who tend to show a pattern of physiological acceleration as opposed to deceleration when confronted with their phobic stimuli.

In conclusion, blood phobia is distinct from other phobias (excluding injection phobia) in terms of fainting history and physiological response. Blood phobia is distinct from all other phobias, including injection phobia, in terms of the number of first-degree relatives reporting the same type of phobia.

Discussion.   The author suggests that a blood/injection phobia be identified as a subtype of specific phobia.

Fear of Choking: A Simple Phobia Subtype?[5]

The purpose of this review was to examine the validity of identifying choking phobia as a distinct subtype of specific phobia. Choking phobia is characterized by fear and avoidance of swallowing pills, food, or fluids. Fear of choking often produces significant weight loss, as well as having additional social implications, such as inability to eat when alone.

---

[5]McNally RM: "Fear of Choking: A Simple Phobia Subtype?" Paper requested by the Simple Phobia Subcommittee of the DSM-IV Anxiety Disorders Work Group, 1989.

Method.   Articles on this topic were located via the Medline database, using the key words *choking phobia, hypersensitive gag reflex, globus hystericus, dysphasia, airway obstruction,* and *vomiting phobia.* In addition, reference lists of the Medline-located articles were used to locate other potentially relevant papers. Cases involving fears of vomiting rather than choking per se, cases involving swallowing difficulties without associated fear, and cases involving nonfearful dysphagia stemming from organic disease were not included in the review. The search yielded 23 case reports and no controlled investigations (Bradley and Narula 1987; Brown et al. 1986; Chatoor et al. 1988; Greenberg et al. 1986, 1988; Kaplan and Evans 1978; Kaplan 1987; Landy 1988; Liebowitz 1987; Lukach and Bruce 1988; McNally 1986; McNally et al. 1990; Philips 1985; Puhakka and Kirveskari 1988; Solyom and Sookman 1980; Wilks and Marks 1983; Wilson et al. 1988).

Results.   On the basis of the case reports, the following descriptive features were found to characterize choking phobia.

Prevalence and sex ratio: Evidence regarding prevalence and sex distribution for choking phobia was not available. However, no obvious sex differences were noted.

Age at onset and etiology: The onset of choking phobia seems to be traumatic in the majority of cases (e.g., after an incident of choking or nearly choking on food) (e.g., Greenberg et al. 1988; McNally 1986). Consequently, there appears to be no characteristic age at onset; age at onset has been recorded from early childhood to old age.

Comorbidity: Choking phobia has been reported to occur separately and in conjunction with panic disorder, oppositional defiant disorder, and depression.

Response to treatment: Case studies have shown that choking phobia responds consistently to graduated exposure in vivo and to medications that attenuate panic attacks (e.g., imipramine and alprazolam) (e.g., Chatoor et al. 1988; Greenberg et al. 1988; Solyom and Sookman 1980).

Differential diagnoses: Differentiation from other disorders was suggested using the following guidelines: 1) If the fear of choking occurs only during panic attacks, a diagnosis of panic disorder is suggested. 2) If the individual is afraid of swallowing inedible objects versus choking, a diagnosis of obsessive-compulsive disorder is suggested. 3) If the individual is afraid of embarrassment rather than choking, a diagnosis of social phobia is suggested. 4) If the individual is afraid of becoming fat, a diagnosis of anorexia nervosa is suggested. 5) If the individual experiences a "lump in the throat" sensation and is not afraid of choking, a diagnosis of globus is suggested. 6) If the individual is intolerant of objects in the mouth rather than being fearful of choking and dying, a diagnosis of hypersensitive gag reflex is suggested. 7) If the individual suffered a choking incident and continues to experience intrusive memories of the event, a diagnosis of PTSD is suggested.

Discussion.   Although choking phobia seems to have clearly identifiable features, it is unclear whether it occurs with sufficient prevalence to warrant a distinct subtype classification.

Hypochondriasis, Illness Phobia, and Other Anxiety Disorders[6]

Several issues relating to hypochondriasis were addressed in this review paper. The basis for defining the boundaries between hypochondriasis and specific phobias is the most relevant issue here. A related issue concerned whether disease conviction and illness phobia represent two distinct components of hypochondriasis, as suggested by Kellner (1985) and Pilowsky (1967).

Method.   The review of available literature was complemented by results from an investigation conducted by the authors in which several diagnostic groups were compared with regard to their behaviors, attitudes, and fears of unexpected physiological changes. Of main interest to the current review was the group of patients with a diagnosis of hypochondriasis, who were subdivided according to degree of disease phobia. Subjects completed a series of questionnaires, including a questionnaire designed to examine interpretations of ambiguous situations concerning external and internal events. Examples of the items included "your heart is beating fast and pounding," "a member of your family is late arriving home," and "you notice lumps under the skin of your neck." In addition, subjects rated the frequency with which they carried out a number of health-related behaviors, such as seeking reassurance from relatives or medical services and checking their bodies for signs of illness. Various standardized questionnaires were also employed, including the Agoraphobia Cognitions Questionnaire (Chambless et al. 1984), the Fear Questionnaire (Marks and Mathews 1979), and a measure of hypochondriacal-related symptoms and behaviors called the Illness Questionnaire (Warwick and Salkovskis 1989).

Results.   Results from the literature review are followed by a summary of the relevant findings from the authors' empirical investigation.

   Literature review: The presence of two separate components of hypochondriasis, called disease conviction and disease phobia, has been supported through factor analytic studies and control group comparisons (Kellner et al. 1987; Pilowsky

---

[6]Salkovskis PM, Warwick HMC, Clark DM: "Hypochondriasis, Illness Phobia, and Other Anxiety Disorders." Paper requested by the Simple Phobia and Panic Disorder Subcommittees of the DSM-IV Anxiety Disorders Work Group, 1990.

1967). In addition, there is some preliminary evidence to suggest that exposure-based treatments may be more effective in patients who show the phobic pattern of behavior (Salkovskis and Warwick 1986; Warwick and Marks 1988).

In some cases of hypochondriasis, the main feature seems to be a fear of contracting an illness rather than the belief that one has a disease. That is, the illness phobia component seems to be stronger than the disease conviction component. In this case, the main behavioral feature is avoidance of anxiety-triggering stimuli. It has been proposed that illness phobia may be best classified as a specific phobia. However, diagnosis is difficult because more general fears of illness are not tied to specific phobic stimuli. A recent example of the confusion that is possible concerns patients with worries over AIDS. As expected, the emergence of AIDS and the attendant publicity have been associated with anxieties in persons at little risk for contracting the illness. Many of these cases could have been classified as either hypochondriasis or illness phobia given the lack of clear definitions. In other words, the overlap with illness phobia arises because the definition of hypochondriasis includes the *fear* of having or, *belief* that one has, a disease persists despite medical reassurance.

Empirical investigation: Hypochondriacal patients almost all showed high degrees of disease conviction, although small subgroups of low disease conviction and high disease phobia, and vice versa, existed. A median split procedure was used to compare subjects with high and low disease conviction and disease phobia. In contrast to those who scored high on disease phobia, high levels of disease conviction were associated with higher scores on the core aspects of hypochondriasis, such as misinterpretations of bodily symptoms and checking behaviors. Frequency of anxiety symptom was associated with disease conviction also.

The authors conclude that the definition of hypochondriasis probably incorporates two phenomenologically distinct entities of illness phobia and disease conviction. However, it is unclear at this point to what extent the illness phobia component of hypochondriasis is the same as a specific phobia.

Discussion. It is recommended that fear of developing or being exposed to illnesses such as AIDS or cancer, and avoidance of stimuli associated with such illnesses, be considered a specific phobia as long as the person does not believe that he or she has the illness. On the other hand, it is suggested that the diagnostic criteria for hypochondriasis specify the need for a disease conviction component.

Distinction Between Traumatic Simple Phobia and PTSD[7]

Given that some specific phobias develop after harmless but frightening experiences in the to-be-phobic situation, whereas others develop after traumatic, life-threatening events, the distinction between pathological fears and PTSD at times becomes questionable. The distinction can become blurred in two ways. First, the individual can be exposed to a traumatic stressor meeting the criterion for a full PTSD type of event but only exhibit signs and symptoms of a specific phobia. Second, an individual may be exposed to a subtraumatic stressor that does not qualify for criterion A of PTSD and yet exhibit signs and symptoms of PTSD. For example, Thyer and Curtis (1983) described a woman who accidentally killed a group of frogs while mowing her lawn. Although diagnosed as a having a phobia, she evidently exhibited other symptoms suggestive of PTSD.

Method.   Articles were collected from Medline and Psychological Abstracts databases, with the key words *traumatic phobia, posttraumatic phobia, posttraumatic fears, etiology of phobias,* and *intersection of posttraumatic stress and simple phobia.* The search yielded 27 citations, several of which were considered pertinent (Burstein 1984; Chatoor et al. 1988; Fairbank et al. 1981; Gislason and Call 1982; Goorney and O'Connor 1971; Horowitz et al. 1979; McCaffrey and Fairbank 1985; McNally and Steketee 1985; Munjack 1984; Öst 1987; Thyer and Curtis 1983).

Results and discussion.   The review summarized a number of published cases involving specific phobias following a traumatic event. The conclusions from the review were that individuals who experienced a trauma of PTSD proportions but who display features of specific phobias (e.g., Fairbank et al. 1981; Goorney and O'Connor 1971) should be diagnosed as having specific phobias. The case of subtraumatic events followed by PTSD-type reactions is more difficult (e.g., Thyer and Curtis 1983), because inclusion of such cases under the PTSD diagnosis depends on revisions to the PTSD criterion in which the nature of the trauma is specified.

Discussion and Recommendations

In this section of the integrative review, the issues considered to reach consensus and the specific diagnostic recommendations made by the Work Group for the diagnosis of specific phobia are covered.

---

[7]McNally RM: "On the Distinction Between Traumatic Simple Phobia and Posttraumatic Stress Disorder." Paper requested by the Simple Phobia Subcommittee of the DSM-IV Anxiety Disorders Work Group, 1989.

Differential Diagnosis Between Specific Phobia and PD/PDA

The reviews by Curtis et al. and by Craske highlighted the need to give further consideration to the differentiation between specific phobias and panic disorder with agoraphobia or agoraphobia without a history of panic. In particular, these reviews pointed out that 1) the situational phobias of public transportation, heights, and enclosed places overlap the two diagnostic categories of specific phobias and agoraphobia; 2) similarities exist between some situational phobias (particularly claustrophobia) and agoraphobia in terms of age at onset, and occurrence of panic attacks; and 3) in contrast to earlier assumptions, individuals with specific phobias can be most concerned with the possibility of panicking when confronted with their phobic situations. However, not enough similarities were noted to warrant assigning all phobias of public transportation, enclosed places, and heights to the agoraphobia category. Claustrophobia seemed to associate most closely with agoraphobia, but even in this case, there was sufficient variability within the domain of claustrophobia to discount the notion that all cases of claustrophobia represent a variant of agoraphobia.

Curtis et al. recommended two provisos to the inclusion of situational phobias under the domain of agoraphobia. First, they suggested that the onset of the situational phobia must be characterized by an unexpected panic attack in a situation about which the person had not previously been anxious. Second, the situational phobia must be accompanied by panic attacks in other situations. According to their recommendations, fear/avoidance of elevators that developed after an unexpected panic attack in an elevator, and that co-occurred with panic attacks in other situations, would meet criteria for agoraphobia. If panics were not experienced elsewhere, then an agoraphobia diagnosis would not be considered.

Alternatively, Craske emphasized the importance of focus of apprehension and, possibly, the extent to which anxiety is experienced immediately on exposure to the phobic stimulus, for differentiating specific phobias from PDA. It was suggested that worry about dangerous aspects of the situation (as opposed to panicking, losing control, and so on) was not necessary for a diagnosis of specific phobia, but predominance of danger expectancy was a useful aid for differentiating specific phobias from agoraphobic avoidance. For example, a fear of driving that was associated mostly with worrying about being hit by other cars would be considered a specific phobia, even if a diagnosis of PDA was coexistent. In contrast, a fear of driving associated mostly with the possibility of panicking and losing control would be considered agoraphobic, assuming the presence of other essential features of PDA (e.g., the experience of uncued panic attacks or pervasive worrying about panic in the absence of identifiable triggers).

Further consideration was given to each set of recommendations. It was pointed out that reliance on the subjective report of focus of apprehension is problematic, because phobic individuals are not able to specify what it is they are most worried about on every occasion. On the other hand, focus of apprehension is integrated into the criteria for several other anxiety disorders, such as social phobia and generalized anxiety disorder.

Reliance on mode of acquisition (initial unexpected panic attack) for diagnostic decision making was also questioned. Features of phobic disorders may not cluster according to their mode of acquisition. For example, there is no evidence to date to suggest that driving phobias that begin after an unexpected panic attack differ significantly from driving phobias that begin after a car accident. Further empirical investigation is needed to evaluate the significance of an unexpected panic attack etiology.

The combination of an unexpected panic attack etiology plus panic attacks in other situations seems a more compelling basis for an agoraphobia diagnosis. However, the Work Group questioned potential departures from the "gist" of agoraphobia. For example, it is conceivable that an individual with a flying phobia, whose phobia developed after an unexpected panic attack during a flight, and who experiences panic attacks while driving and waiting in lines, is currently phobic of flying due to the threat of crashing in poor weather conditions. In this case, the flying phobia itself is related to concerns about dangerous aspects of the situation as opposed to concerns about panicking or inability to escape in the event of a panic attack. Under these conditions, the flying phobia may be best considered as a specific phobia despite the mode of onset and the possible coexisting PDA diagnosis. If, on the other hand, the flying phobia was related to concerns about losing control in the trapped situation of a flight, then assignment to the PDA category would be more appropriate. As stated earlier, the extent to which an unexpected panic attack etiology (even in the presence of panic attacks in other situations) is predictive of presenting phobic features is not known. Future investigation may reveal a consistent relationship between unexpected panic attack onset and phobic features, which are distinct from the phobic features associated with other modes of onset. If so, then the recommendations made by Curtis et al. would be preferred to relying on subjective reports about focus of apprehension. However, the Work Group agreed that the recommendations by Curtis et al. may be premature at this point.

It was recommended that a specific phobia diagnosis is appropriate under most conditions for the description of fear of a circumscribed object or situation, regardless of the mode of onset. The notion of fear of a 'circumscribed object or situation' was given predominance, even if the situation is one that appears in the cluster of agoraphobia situations. If the phobic situation is feared because of a concern about dangerous, harmful, or aversive aspects of the situation (e.g., crashing in a plane, being bitten by a dog, or the "slimy" skin of a snake), a specific phobia diagnosis is clearly appropriate. If the phobic situation is feared because of a concern about panicking (or its consequences, such as losing control), a specific phobia diagnosis is appropriate, as long as panic is not pervasively anticipated. On the other hand, if panic is pervasively anticipated (i.e., in the absence of the specific phobic stimulus), then a diagnosis of PDA should be considered. Finally, experiencing anxiety immediately on exposure to the phobic stimulus was considered another possible way of differentiating specific phobias from agoraphobia.

More information will be gathered with respect to the situational phobias from a MacArthur project that is under way. However, the ECA findings presented by Curtis et al. suggest that special attention should be given to claustrophobia, because it clusters most reliably with agoraphobia.

Subtypes Within the Diagnosis of Specific Phobia

Literature reviews by Curtis et al., McNally, and Öst all highlight features specific to different types of phobias. Curtis et al. suggest that fears of animals, storms, and water cluster strongly. A weaker cluster was comprised of tunnels/bridges, public transportation, and other fears. Height phobia and claustrophobia were inconsistently associated with the second cluster. However, they had similar age-at-onset distributions. Also, heights and enclosures are components of the situations of tunnels/bridges and public transportation. On the other hand, fear of heights was quite distinct from other phobias in terms of the high percentage of males, and claustrophobia was closer to an agoraphobia cluster in terms of patterns of comorbidity.

Öst presented evidence to show that blood and injection phobias are similar to each other and distinct from other phobias, particularly in terms of fainting history and physiological fear profile. Öst suggested that because injury phobia is almost always related to seeing blood, the term *injury* be dropped. Other members of the Work Group questioned this recommendation, because tissue injury was considered to be a better statement of the common denominator than was blood. Consequently, the term *blood/injury/injection* was recommended by the Work Group.

McNally reviewed a number of studies showing that choking phobia was a fairly distinct type of phobia, particularly because the onset is almost invariably linked to trauma (usually choking on food). However, the Work Group agreed that it is premature to propose a separate subtype for choking phobia, because the prevalence of this phobia is unknown.

Overall, the Work Group recommended that certain subtypes be specified within the diagnosis of specific phobia. These included "natural environment" phobias (animals, water, and storms) and blood/injury/injection phobias. The possibility of a broad cluster of "situational" phobias (heights, enclosed places, public transportation) was also recommended, in addition to an "other" subtype.

Differentiation Between Specific Phobias and Hypochondriasis

The Work Group agreed with the suggestions by Salkovskis et al. that disease conviction was more consistent with a hypochondriasis diagnosis, whereas illness phobia without disease conviction was consistent with a specific phobia diagnosis. The importance of further specification of the criteria for hypochondriasis was recognized.

Differentiation Between Specific Phobias and PTSD

Finally, the Work Group agreed that a phobia of a circumscribed object or situation that follows a traumatic event should be considered a specific phobia. However, diagnosis of a posttraumatic syndrome following a subtraumatic event is dependent on the criterion defining the events that precipitate PTSD.

Specific Diagnostic Recommendations

On the basis of the Work Group consensus and comments from other members of the DSM-IV Task Force, the following recommendations were made for the diagnostic criteria for specific phobias:

1. Fear cued by the presence of, or anticipation of the presence of, a specific object or situation (e.g., flying, heights, animals, getting an injection, seeing blood).
2. Exposure to the phobic stimulus predictably provokes an immediate anxiety response or immediate panic attack.
3. The phobic stimulus is avoided or endured with anxious anticipation.
4. The person recognizes that the fear is excessive or unreasonable.
5. The avoidance and/or anxious anticipation interferes significantly with the person's normal routine, with usual social activities or relationships with others, or with appropriate health or dental care, or there is marked distress about having the phobia.
6. The anxiety or phobic avoidance is not otherwise accounted for by another mental disorder, such as obsessive-compulsive disorder (e.g., fear of contamination), PTSD (e.g., avoidance of stimuli associated with a severe stressor), social phobia (e.g., avoidance of social situations because of fear of embarrassment), or agoraphobia without history of panic disorder (e.g., fear of having a panic attack in different situations).

Subtypes:
  Natural environment (e.g., animals, storms, and water)
  Blood, injury, injection
  Situational (e.g., public transportation, tunnels, bridges, elevators, flying, and driving)
  Other

It was recommended that a description of ways of differentiating specific phobias (particularly situational phobias) from panic disorder with agoraphobia, or agoraphobia without a history of panic disorder, hypochondriasis, and PTSD be provided in the text section.

References

Abelson JL, Curtis GC: Cardiac and neuroendocrine responses to exposure therapy in height phobics: disynchrony within the "physiological response system." Behav Res Ther 27:561–567, 1989

Agras S, Sylvester D, Oliveau D: The epidemiology of common fears and phobias. Compr Psychiatry 10:151–156, 1969

Alfin PL: Agoraphobia: a study of family of origin characteristics and relationship patterns. Smith College Students Social Work 57:134–154, 1987

American Psychiatric Association: Diagnostic and Statistical Manual of Mental Disorders, 3rd Edition. Washington, DC, American Psychiatric Association, 1980

American Psychiatric Association: Diagnostic and Statistical Manual of Mental Disorders, 3rd Edition, Revised. Washington, DC, American Psychiatric Association, 1987

Arrindell W: Dimensional structure and psychopathology correlates of the fear survey schedule (FSS-III) in a phobic population: a factorial definition of agoraphobia. Behav Res Ther 18:229–242, 1980

Babcock HH, Powell DH: Vasovagal fainting: deconditioning an autonomic syndrome. Psychosomatics 23:969–973, 1982

Barlow DH: Anxiety and Its Disorders: The Nature and Treatment of Anxiety and Panic. New York, Guilford, 1988

Barlow DH, Vermilyea J, Blanchard EB, et al: The phenomenon of panic. J Abnorm Psychol 94:320–328, 1985

Bates HD: Factoral structure and MMPI correlates of a fear survey schedule in a clinical population. Behav Res Ther 9:355–360, 1971

Beck AT, Emery G: Anxiety Disorders and Phobias: A Cognitive Perspective. New York, Basic Books, 1985

Bourdon KH, Boyd JH, Rae DS, et al: Gender differences in phobias: results of the ECA community survey. J Anx Disord 2:227–241, 1988

Bourque P, Ladouceur R: An investigation of various performance-based treatments with agoraphobics. Behav Res Ther 18:161–170, 1980

Bowen RC, Hohout J: The relationship between agoraphobia and primary affective disorders. Can J Psychiatry 24:317–322, 1979

Bradley PJ, Narula A: Clinical aspects of pseudodysphagia. J Laryngol Otol 101:689–694, 1987

Brown SR, Schwartz JM, Summergrad P, et al: Globus hystericus syndrome responsive to antidepressants. Am J Psychiatry 143:917–918, 1986

Burstein A: Treatment of post-traumatic stress disorder with imipramine. Psychosomatics 25:681–687, 1984

Cameron OG, Liepman MR, Curtis GC, et al: Ethanol retards desensitisation of phobias in non-alcoholics. Br J Psychiatry 150:845–849, 1987

Chambless DM, Caputo GC, Bright P, et al: Assessment of fear in agoraphobics: the Body Sensations Questionnaire and the Agoraphobia Cognitions Questionnaire. J Consult Clin Psychol 52:1090–1097, 1984

Chatoor I, Conley C, Dickson L: Food refusal after an incident of choking: a post-traumatic eating disorder. J Am Acad Child Adolesc Psychiatry 27:105–110, 1988

Clark DM, Salkovskis PM, Gelder M, et al: Tests of a cognitive theory of panic, in Panic and Phobias II. Edited by Hand I, Wittchen HU. Berlin, Springer-Verlag, 1988

Cohn CK, Kron RE, Brady JP: A case of blood-illness-injury phobia treated behaviorally. J Nerv Ment Dis 162:65–68, 1976

Cook EW III, Melamed BG, Cuthbert BN, et al: Emotional imagery and the differential diagnosis of anxiety. J Consult Clin Psychol 56:734–740, 1988

Costello CG: Fears and phobias in women: a community study. J Abnorm Psychol 91:280–286, 1982

Craske MG, Zarate R, Burton T, et al: Specific fears and panic attacks: a survey of clinical and nonclinical samples. J Anx Disord 7:1–19, 1993

Craske MG, Burton TM, Rapee RM, et al: Simple phobics presenting for treatment: what are their fears? Unpublished data, 1993

Curtis GC, Thyer B: Fainting on exposure to phobic stimuli. Am J Psychiatry 140:771–774, 1983

Curtis G, Buxton M, Lippman D, et al: "Flooding in vivo" during the circadian phase of minimal cortisol secretion: anxiety and therapeutic success without adrenal cortical activation. Biol Psychiatry 11:101–107, 1976

Curtis GC, Nesse R, Buxton M, et al: Plasma growth hormone: effect of anxiety during flooding in vivo. Am J Psychiatry 136:410–414, 1979

DiNardo PA, O'Brien GT, Barlow DH, et al: Reliability of DSM-III anxiety disorder categories using a new structured interview. Arch Gen Psychiatry 40:1070–1074, 1983

DiNardo PA, Guzy LT, Jenkins JA, et al: Ecology and maintenance of dog fears. Behav Res Ther 26:241–244, 1988

Ehlers A, Margraf J: The psychophysiological model of panic attacks, Anxiety Disorders Annual Series of European Research in Behavior Therapy. Edited by Emmelkamp PMG, 1989

Elmore RT Jr, Wildman EW, Westefeld JS: The use of systematic desensitization in the treatment of blood phobia. J Behav Ther Exp Psychiatry 11:277–279, 1980

Fairbank JA, DeGood DE, Jenkins CW: Behavioral treatment of a persistent post-traumatic startle response. J Behav Ther Exp Psychiatry 12:321–324, 1981

Fava GA, Grandi S, Canestrari R: Prodromal symptoms in panic disorder with agoraphobia. Am J Psychiatry 145:1564–1567, 1988

Foa EB: What cognitions differentiate panic disorder from other anxiety disorders? in Panic and Phobias II. Edited by Hand I, Wittchen HU. Berlin, Springer-Verlag, 1988

Fyer AJ, Manuzza S, Gallops MS, et al: Familial transmission of simple phobias and fears: a preliminary report. Arch Gen Psychiatry 47:252–256, 1990

Gislason IL, Call JD: Dog bite in infancy: trauma and personality development. Journal of the American Academy of Child Psychiatry 21:203–207, 1982

Goorney B, O'Connor PJ: Anxiety associated with flying: a retrospective survey of military aircrew psychiatric casualties. Br J Psychiatry 119:156–166, 1971

Graham DT, Kabler D, Lunsford L: Vasovagal fainting: a diphasic response. Psychosom Med 23:493–507, 1961

Greenberg DB, Stern TA, Weilburg JB: Fear of choking. J Fam Pract 22:547–548, 1986

Greenberg DB, Stern TA, Weilburg JB: The fear of choking: three successfully treated cases. Psychosomatics 29:126–129, 1988

Gudjonsson GH, Sartory G: Blood-injury phobia: a "reasonable excuse" for failing to give a specimen in a case of suspected drunken driving. J Forensic Science Society 23:197–201, 1983

Gursky DM, Reiss S: Identifying danger and anxiety expectancies as components of common fears. J Behav Ther Exp Psychiatry 18:3–8, 1987

Hallam RS, Hafner RJ: Fears of phobic patients: factor analyses of self-report data. Behav Res Ther 16:1–6, 1978

Himle JA, McPhee K, Cameron OG, et al: Simple phobia: evidence for heterogeneity. Psychiatry Res 28:25–30, 1989

Himle JA, Crystal D, Curtis GC, et al: Mode of onset of simple phobia subtypes: further evidence for heterogeneity. Psychiatry Res 36:37–43, 1991

Horowitz MJ, Wilner N, Alvarez W: Impact of events scale: measure of subjective stress. Psychosom Med 41:209–218, 1979

Howard WA, Murphy SM, Clarke JC: The nature and treatment of fear of flying: a controlled investigation. Behavior Therapy 14:557–567, 1983

Hugdahl K, Öst LG: Subjectively rated physiological and cognitive symptoms in six different clinical phobias. Personality and Individual Differences 6:175–188, 1985

Jerremalm A, Jansson L, Öst L: Individual response patterns and the effects of different behavioral methods in the treatment of dental phobia. Behav Res Ther 24:587–596, 1986

Johansson J, Öst LG: Perception of autonomic reactions and actual heart rate in phobic patients. J Behav Assess 4(2):133–143, 1982

Kaplan PR, Evans IM: A case of functional dysphagia treated on the model of fear of fear. J Behav Ther Exp Psychiatry 9:71–72, 1978

Kaplan RM: More on the globus hystericus syndrome. Am J Psychiatry 144:528–529, 1987

Kaver A, Hellstrom K, Öst LG: Cognitions in needle phobia. Poster presented at World Congress of Cognitive Therapy, Oxford, England, June 1989

Kellner R: Functional somatic symptoms and hypochondriasis. Arch Gen Psychiatry 42:821–833, 1985

Kellner R, Abbott P, Winslow WW, et al: Fear, beliefs and attitudes in DSM-III hypochondriasis. J Nerv Ment Dis 175:20–25, 1987

Kleinknecht RA: The origins and remission of fear in a group of tarantula enthusiasts. Behav Res Ther 20:437–443, 1982

Kleinknecht RA, Lenz J: Blood/injury fear, fainting, and avoidance of medically related situations: a family correspondence study. Behav Res Ther 27:537–547, 1989

Ko GN, Elsworth JD, Roth RH, et al: Panic induced elevation of plasma MHPG levels in phobic-anxious patients: effects of clonidine and imipramine. Arch Gen Psychiatry 40:424–430, 1983

Kozak MJ, Miller GA: The psychophysiological process of therapy in a case of injury-scene-elicited fainting. J Behav Ther Exp Psychiatry 16:139–145, 1985

Kozak MJ, Montgomery GK: Multimodal behavioral treatment of recurrent injury-scene-elicited fainting (vasodepressor syncope). Behavioral Psychotherapy 9:316–321, 1981

Krystal J, Woods S, Hill C: Characteristics of self-defined panic attacks. New research presentation at 141st Annual Meeting of American Psychiatric Association, Montreal, Canada, May 1988

Lader MH, Gleder MG, Marks IM: Palmar skin conductance measures as predictors of response of desensitization. Psychosom Res 11:283–290, 1967

Ladouceur R: Participant modelling with or without cognitive treatment for phobias. J Consult Clin Psychol 51:942–944, 1983

Landy FJ, Gaupp LA: A factor analysis of the FSS-III. Behav Res Ther 9:89–93, 1971

Landy G: Fear of choking and food refusal. J Am Acad Child Adolesc Psychiatry 27:514–515, 1988

Lapouse R, Monk MA: Fears and worries in a representative sample of children. Am J Orthopsychiatry 29:803–818, 1959

Lautch H: Dental phobia. Br J Psychiatry 119:151–158, 1971

Lawlis GF: Response styles of a patient population on the fear survey schedule. Behav Res Ther 9:95–102, 1971

Liddell A, Lyons M: Thunderstorm phobias. Behav Res Ther 16:306–308, 1978

Liebowitz MR: Globus hystericus and panic attacks. Am J Psychiatry 144:390–391, 1987

Lloyd GG, Deakin HG: Phobias complicating treatment of uterine carcinoma. BMJ 5:440, 1975

Lukach B, Bruce BK: Behavioral treatment of an oral liquid medication phobia in a liver transplant candidate. Paper presented at the meeting of the Association for Advancement of Behavior Therapy, New York, November 1988

Manuzza S, Fyer AJ, Martin LY, et al: Reliability of anxiety assessment, I: diagnostic agreement. Arch Gen Psychiatry 46:1093–1101, 1989

Margraf J, Taylor CB, Ehlers A: Panic attacks in the natural environment. J Nerv Ment Dis 175:558–565, 1987

Marks IM: The classification of phobic disorders. Br J Psychiatry 116:377–378, 1970

Marks IM: Space "phobia": a pseudo-agoraphobic syndrome. J Neurol Neurosurg Psychiatry 44:387–391, 1981

Marks IM, Gelder MG: Different ages of onset in varieties of phobia. Am J Psychiatry 123:218–221, 1966

Marks IM, Mathews AM: Brief standard self-rating for phobic patients. Behav Res Ther 17:263–267, 1979

Marshall WL: Behavioral indices of habituation and sensitization during exposure to phobic stimuli. Behav Res Ther 26:67–77, 1988

Martin I, Marks IM, Gelder M: Conditioned eyelid responses in phobic patients. Behav Res Ther 7:115–124, 1969

Matthew RJ, Weinman ML, Semchuk KM, et al: Driving phobia in the city of Houston. Am J Psychiatry 139:1049–1051, 1982

McCaffrey RJ, Fairbank JA: Behavioral assessment and treatment of accident-related post-traumatic stress disorder: two case studies. Behavior Therapy 16:406–416, 1985

McGlynn FD, Puhr JJ, Gaynor R, et al: Skin conductance responses to real and imagined snakes among avoidant and non-avoidant college students. Behav Res Ther 11:417–426, 1973

McGrady AV, Bernal GAA: Relaxation based treatment of stress induced syncope. J Behav Ther Exp Psychiatry 17:23–27, 1986

McNally RJ: Behavioral treatment of a choking phobia. J Behav Ther Exp Psychiatr 17:185–188, 1986

McNally RJ, Steketee GS: The etiology and maintenance of severe animal phobias. Behav Res Ther 23:431–435, 1985

McNally RJ, Cassiday KL, Calamari JE: Taijin-kyofu-sho in a black American woman: behavioral treatment of a "culture-bound" anxiety disorder. J Anx Dis 4:83–87, 1990

Meikle S, Mitchell MC: Factor analysis of the fear survey schedule with phobics. J Clin Psychol 30:44–46, 1974

Mendel JGC, Klein DF: Anxiety attacks with subsequent agoraphobia. Compr Psychiatry 10:190–195, 1969

Miller LC, Barret CL, Hampe E: Phobias of childhood, in Child Personality and Psychopathology: Current Topics, Vol 1. Edited by Davids A. New York, Wiley, 1974, pp 89–134

Munjack DJ: The onset of driving phobia. J Behav Ther Exp Psychiatry 15:305–308, 1984

Munjack DJ, Moss HB: Affective disorders and alcoholism in families of agoraphobics. Arch Gen Psychiatry 38:869–871, 1981

Murray EJ, Foote F: The origins of fear of snakes. Behav Res Ther 17:489–493, 1979

Neiger S, Atkinson L, Quarrington B: A factor analysis of personality and fear variables in phobic disorders. Can J Behav Med 13:336–348, 1981

Nesse RM, Curtis GC, Brown GM, et al: Anxiety induced by flooding therapy for phobias does not elicit prolactin secretory response. Psychosom Med 42(1):25–31, 1980

Nesse RM, Curtis GC, Thyer BA, et al: Endocrine and cardiovascular responses during phobic anxiety. Psychosom Med 47(1):320–332, 1985

Norton GR, Harrison B, Hauch J, et al: Characteristics of people with infrequent panic attacks. J Abnorm Psychol 94:216–221, 1985

Norton GR, Dorward J, Cox BJ: Factors associated with panic attacks in non-clinical subjects. Behavior Therapy 17:239–252, 1986

Ollendick TH: Fears in children and adolescents: reliability and generalizability across gender, age and nationality. Behav Res Ther 27:19–26, 1989

Orwin A: Breathe less, fear less: a method used to treat blood phobia. Nursing Mirror 16:25–26, 1972

Öst LG: Ways of acquiring phobias and outcome of behavioral treatment. Behav Res Ther 23:683–689, 1985

Öst LG: Age at onset of different phobias. J Abnorm Psychol 96:223–229, 1987

Öst LG: Acquisition of blood and injection phobia and anxiety response patterns in clinical patients. Behav Res Ther 29:323–332, 1991

Öst LG, Johansson J, Jerremalm A: Individual response patterns and the effects of different behavioral methods in the treatment of claustrophobia. Behav Res Ther 20:445–460, 1982

Öst LG, Lindahl IL, Sterner U, et al: Exposure in-vivo vs. applied relaxation in the treatment of blood phobia. Behav Res Ther 22:205–216, 1984a

Öst LG, Sterner US, Lindahl IL: Physiological responses in blood phobics. Behav Res Ther 22:109–117, 1984b

Öst LG, Sterner US, Fellenius J: Applied tension, applied relaxation, and the combination in the treatment of blood phobia. Behav Res Ther 27:109–121, 1989

Philips HC: Return of fear in the treatment of a fear of vomiting. Behav Res Ther 23:45–52, 1985

Pilowsky I: Dimensions of hypochondriasis. Br J Psychiatry 113:89–93, 1967

Prigatano GP, Johnson HJ: Autonomic nervous system changes associated with a spider phobic reaction. J Abnorm Psychol 83(2):169–177, 1974

Puhakka HJ, Kirveskari P: Globus hystericus: globus syndrome? J Laryngol Otol 102:231–234, 1988

Rachman SJ, Levitt K: Panics and their consequences. Behav Res Ther 23:585–600, 1985

Rachman S, Lopatka C: Match and mismatch in the prediction of fear, I. Behav Res Ther 24:387–393, 1986a

Rachman S, Lopatka C: Match and mismatch of fear in Gray's theory, II. Behav Res Ther 24:395–601, 1986b

Rachman S, Lopatka C, Levitt K: Panic: the links between cognitions and bodily symptoms, I. Behav Res Ther 25(5): 411–423, 1987

Rachman S, Lopatka C, Levitt K: Experimental analyses of panic, II: panic patients. Behav Res Ther 26(1):33–40, 1988a

Rachman S, Levitt K, Lopatka C: Experimental analyses of panic, III claustrophobic subjects. Behav Res Ther 26(1):41–52, 1988b

Raguram R, Bhide AV: Patterns of phobic neurosis: a retrospective study. Br J Psychiatry 147:557–560, 1985

Rapee RM, Craske MG, Barlow DH: Subject described features of panic attacks using a new self-monitoring form. J Anx Disord 4:171–181, 1990

Reiger DA, Myers JK, Kramer M, et al: The NIMH Epidemiologic Catchment Area (ECA) program: historical context, major objectives, and study population characteristics. Arch Gen Psychiatry 41:934–941, 1984

Reiss S: Theoretical perspectives on the fear of anxiety. Clin Psychol Rev 7:585–596, 1987

Reiss S, Peterson RA, Gursky DM, et al: Anxiety sensitivity, anxiety frequency and the prediction of fearfulness. Behav Res Ther 24:1–8, 1986

Reiss S, Peterson RA, Gursky DM: Anxiety sensitivity, injury sensitivity, and individual differences in fearfulness. Behav Res Ther 26:341–345, 1988

Richards D: Blood phobia. Nursing Times 84:49–51, 1988

Robins LN, Helzer JE, Croughan J, et al: National Institute of Mental Health Diagnostic Interview Schedule, Version III. St. Louis, MO, Washington University School of Medicine, 1981

Rothstein W, Holmes GR, Boblitt WE: A factor analysis of the fear survey schedule with a psychiatric population. J Clin Psychol 28:78–80, 1972

Rubin BM, Katlin ES, Weiss BW, et al: Factor analysis of a fear survey schedule. Behav Res Ther 6:65–75, 1968

Rubin SE, Lawlis GF: Factor analysis of the 122 item fear survey schedule. Behav Res Ther 7:381–386, 1969

Salkovskis PM, Warwick HMC: Morbid preoccupations, health anxiety and reassurance: a cognitive behavioural approach to hypochondriasis. Behav Res Ther 24:597–602, 1986

Sartory G, Rachman SJ, Grey S: An investigation of the relationship between reported fear and heart rate. Behav Res Ther 15:435–438, 1977

Scherer MW, Nakamura CY: A fear survey schedule for children (FSS-FCC): a factor analytic comparison with manifest anxiety (CMAS). Behav Res Ther 6:173–182, 1968

Sheehan DV, Sheehan KE, Minichiello WE: Age at onset of phobic disorders: a re-evaluation. Compr Psychiatry 22:544–553, 1981

Snaith RP: A clinical investigation of phobias. Br J Psychiatry 114:673–697, 1968

Solyom L, Sookman D: Fear of choking and its treatment: a behavioural approach. Can J Psychiatry 25:30–34, 1980

Solyom L, Shugar R, Bryntwick S, et al: Treatment of fear of flying. Am J Psychiatry 130:423–427, 1973

Somerville JW, Barrios FX, Merritt BR, et al: Misattribution in a fearful situation following different modes of arousal. Perceptual and Motor Skills 56:45–46, 1983

Spitzer RL, Endicott J, Robins E: Research Diagnostic Criteria: rationale and reliability. Arch Gen Psychiatry 35:773–782, 1978

Street LL, Craske MG, Barlow DH: Sensations, cognitions and the perception of cues associated with expected and unexpected panic attacks. Behav Res Ther 27:189–198, 1989

Takeya T, Baron JB, Ohno Y, et al: Comparative study of post-traumatic and psychogenic acrophobia (fear of height). Agressologie 19:91–92, 1978

Taylor CB: Heart-rate changes in improved spider-phobic patients. Psychological Reports 41:667–671, 1977

Taylor CB, Sheikh J, Agras WS, et al: Ambulatory heart rate changes in patients with panic attacks. Am J Psychiatry 143:478–482, 1986

Teghtsoonian R, Frost RO: The effects of viewing distance on fear of snakes. J Behav Ther Exp Psychiatry 13(3):181–190, 1982

Thorpe GL, Burns LE: The Agoraphobic Syndrome. New York, Wiley, 1983

Thyer BA, Curtis GC: The repeated pretest-posttest single-subject experiment: a new design for empirical clinical practice. J Behav Ther Exp Psychiatry 14:311–315, 1983

Thyer BA, Curtis GC: The effects of ethanol intoxication on phobic anxiety. Behav Res Ther 22:556–610, 1984

Thyer BA, Curtis GC: On the diphasic nature of vasovagal fainting associated with blood-injury-illness phobia. Pavlovian Journal of Biological Science 20:84–87, 1985

Thyer BA, Himle J, Curtis GC: Blood-injury-illness phobia: a review. J Clin Psychol 41:451–459, 1985

Torgersen S: Nature and origin of common phobic fears. Br J Psychiatry 134:343–351, 1979

van den Hout MA, van der Molen M, Griez E, et al: Specificity of interoceptive fears to panic disorders. J Psychopathol Behav Assess 9:99–106, 1987

Wardle J, Jarvis M: The paradoxical fear response to blood, injury and illness: a treatment report. Behavioral Psychotherapy 9:13–24, 1981

Warwick HMC, Marks IM: Behavioural treatment of illness phobia. Br J Psychiatry 152:239–241, 1988

Warwick HMC, Salkovskis PM: Cognitive therapy of hypochondriasis, in Cognitive Therapy in Clinical Practice. Edited by Scott J, Williams JMG, Beck AT. London, Croom Helm, 1989

Watts F, Sharrock R: Relationships between spider constructs in phobics. Br J Med Psychol 58:149–153, 1985

Whitehead WE: Flooding treatment of phobias: does chronic diazepam increase effectiveness? J Behav Ther Exp Psychiatry 9:219–225, 1978

Whitehead WE, Robinson A, Blackwell B, et al: Effects of diazepam on phobic avoidance behavior and phobic anxiety. Biol Psychiatry 13:59–64, 1978

Wilks CGW, Marks IM: Reducing hypersensitive gagging. British Dental Journal 155:263–265, 1983

Williams SL, Turner SM, Peer DF: Guided mastery and performance desensitization treatments for severe agoraphobia. J Consult Clin Psychol 53:237–247, 1985

Wilson GD, Priest HF: The principal components of phobic stimuli. J Clin Psychol 24:191, 1968

Wilson JA, Deary IJ, Maran AGD: Is globus hystericus? Br J Psychiatry 153:335–339, 1988

Woods SW, Charney DS, McPherson AH, et al: Situational panic attacks: behavioral, physiological, and biochemical characterization. Arch Gen Psychiatry 44:365–375, 1987

World Health Organization: ICD-10 Chapter V: Mental and Behavioral Disorders: Diagnostic Criteria for Research. Geneva, Switzerland, World Health Organization, 1990

Yule W, Fernando P: Blood phobia—beware. Behav Res Ther 18:587–590, 1980

Chapter 17

Social Phobia

Franklin R. Schneier, M.D., Michael R. Liebowitz, M.D.,
Deborah C. Beidel, Ph.D., Abby J. Fyer, M.D.,
Mark S. George, M.D., Richard G. Heimberg, Ph.D.,
Craig S. Holt, Ph.D., Donald F. Klein, M.D.,
Andrew P. Levin, M.D., R. Bruce Lydiard, M.D., Ph.D.,
Salvatore Mannuzza, Ph.D., Lynn Y. Martin, R.N., M.S., C.S.,
A. Egido Nardi, M.D., Diana Roscow Terrill, M.A.,
Robert L. Spitzer, M.D., Samuel M. Turner, Ph.D.,
Thomas W. Uhde, M.D., Ivan Vasconcelos Figueira, M.D., and
Marcio Versiani, M.D.

Statement of the Issues

The Social Phobia sub-Work Group identified the following issues for review: delineation of boundaries of social phobia with panic disorder, with avoidant personality disorder, with substance use disorders, with shyness, with test anxiety, with generalized anxiety disorder, and with physical disabilities that cause social anxiety; definition of subtypes within social phobia; determination of whether physiological and biochemical characteristics may help define social phobia; and consideration of cross-cultural aspects in the definition of the disorder.

Significance of the Issues

The lack of clear definition of several boundaries of social phobia has been problematic for clinicians and researchers. At the diagnostic threshold level, social phobia has appeared contiguous with other forms of social or performance anxiety, such as shyness, test anxiety, and anxiety secondary to a physical disability. It is unclear whether these related problems should be classified as social phobia.

Shyness is a lay term for the common subclinical condition characterized by fear of negative evaluation, avoidance of certain social settings, and heightened somatic response when in fearful situations. It is unclear whether shyness and social phobia represent parallel, overlapping, or completely different syndromes.

Test anxiety has been described in psychology literature as the occurrence of somatic sensations and worries prior to and during scholastic examinations. It shares with social phobia the core fear of negative evaluation and embarrassment.

Certain physical disabilities or medical conditions may lead to social anxiety and phobic avoidance. When social phobia occurs secondary to a medical condition, such as Parkinson's disease, it is unclear whether it should be considered a separate disorder. It might be considered unrelated to social phobia, related to social phobia but different from primary social phobia (e.g., a subtype of social phobia), or the same as social phobia.

Certain other psychiatric disorders have been observed to commonly co-occur with social phobia, but it is uncertain whether they are functionally related. Clarification of the relationships of social phobia to other psychiatric disorders may be useful in treatment selection and in defining research subject groups.

One such group of disorders is the substance use disorders and alcohol abuse and dependence in particular. Social phobia and substance abuse often appear to co-occur, and the issue of whether both disorders should be considered separately, or whether they should be considered parts of a single process, may be important in guiding treatment.

The extent to which the anxiety features of social phobia overlap with those of other anxiety disorders is another common clinical and research problem. Panic disorder and agoraphobia especially have been noted to overlap with social phobia, and it has been reported that differentiating them from DSM-III-R (American Psychiatric Association 1987) social phobia is difficult. When the fears present in generalized anxiety disorder include social anxieties, the relationship of generalized anxiety disorder to social phobia may also be difficult to define.

The relationship of social phobia to avoidant personality disorder has been unclear. DSM-III-R apparently broadened the definition of social phobia to include many persons with avoidant personality disorder by removing the hierarchical decision rule that had prohibited the dual diagnosis of social phobia and avoidant personality disorder. Empirical data might validate an appropriate border for social phobia in this area.

Linked to the broader definition of social phobia in DSM-III-R was the introduction of the generalized subtype, defined by fear of most social situations. The reliability and validity of this subtyping approach remain to be established, and alternative subtyping approaches might be considered. If the generalized subtype is retained, a complementary "nongeneralized" subtype should be named and defined.

Expansion of research into physiological and biochemical aspects of social phobia has raised the issue of whether biological measures might help validate the social phobia diagnosis or the subtypes within social phobia. Are there physiological or biochemical measures that distinguish individuals with social phobia from normal subjects or from those with other anxiety disorders or that distinguish subtypes within social phobia?

DSM-III-R definitions of social phobia were largely based on American and western European psychiatric research and experience. A consideration of the manifestations of social phobia in other cultures, however, may help distinguish its most universal and fundamental attributes from those that are culture specific.

Overall Methods

Systematic and comprehensive reviews of the existing literature pertaining to each issue were assigned to Social Phobia sub-Workgroup advisers and their associates as follows: shyness—D. Beidel, S. Turner; test anxiety—D. Beidel; relationship to physical disorders associated with social anxiety—R. B. Lydiard, M. George, D. Roscow, and T. Uhde; panic disorder and agoraphobia—S. Mannuzza, A. Fyer, M. Liebowitz, D. Klein; generalized anxiety disorder—M. Verisiani, A. Nardi, I. Vasconcelos; substance abuse—F. Schneier and R. B. Lydiard; avoidant personality disorder—F. Schneier, R. Spitzer; subtypes—R. Heimberg, C. Holt; physiological and biochemical findings—A. Levin; cross-cultural issues—M. Liebowitz. Methods of each review are detailed below.

Individual Issues: Methods, Results, and Discussion

Relationship of Shyness and Social Phobia

Methods.   Literature searches in psychological and psychiatric journals were conducted with computer and manual search procedures. Population samples included children and adults and patients described as either socially phobic or shy. There is a difference in subject selection procedures for the two conditions, because studies of shyness used or parental self-reports, whereas social phobic subjects were usually selected on the basis of clinician interviews. Furthermore, a wide variety of definitions of shyness have been employed by different investigators. Shy and socially phobic individuals were compared on demographic and familial factors, component characteristics, and life consequences.

Results.   The prevalence of shyness has been reported to be 20%–40% among college students (Spielberger et al. 1984; Zimbardo 1977), 38%–46% among fifth-grade students (Lazarus 1982), and 28% of boys and 32% of girls (ages 8–10 years) in the Berkeley Guidance Study (Caspi et al. 1988). In contrast, the Epidemiologic Catchment Area (ECA) study indicated that only 2%–3% of the population has Diagnostic Interview Schedule (DIS)/DSM-III (American Psychiatric Association 1980) social phobia (Robins et al. 1984).

Somatic arousal symptoms such as blushing, muscle twitching, palpitations, trembling, and sweating appear to be similar in both social phobia and shyness (Amies et al. 1983; Turner et al. 1989). Similarly, laboratory evaluations have demonstrated that both groups show some differences from normal subjects in regard to heart rate/blood pressure response to social stressors (Kagan et al. 1988; Turner et al. 1986b). There have been no empirical comparisons, however, of symptom profiles or autonomic reactivity between the two groups.

There is great consistency between descriptions of cognitions reported by shy and social phobic groups. Social phobic individuals engaged in social interaction report fewer positive and more negative thoughts than normal control subjects (Nyman and Heimberg 1985; Turner et al. 1986b). Fear of negative evaluation has been demonstrated to be a problem in shy subjects (Ludwig and Lazarus 1983; Pilkonis 1977). Again, there have been no empirical comparisons of cognitions between the two groups. In regard to behavior, social skills deficits and avoidance of social situations have been reported in some social phobic individuals (Emmel-kamp et al. 1985; Marks 1985; Turner et al. 1986a) and some shy subjects (Harris 1984; Pilkonis 1977).

In regard to functioning, impairment in occupational, social, and vocational spheres has been documented in social phobia (Amies et al. 1983; Liebowitz et al. 1985b; Turner et al. 1986a). Shy boys have been reported on follow-up (Caspi et al. 1988) to be older than nonshy boys at age of marriage, fatherhood, and entering a stable career. Shy girls were more likely than nonshy girls to follow a life pattern that included marriage, childbearing, and homemaking. Impairment in function has not been demonstrated for shy individuals to the same extent that has been demonstrated for social phobic individuals.

Discussion.   In summary, based on existing data, there is no unambiguous way to differentiate shyness from social phobia in DSM-IV criteria. It appears that the two syndromes are similar with respect to behavioral, cognitive, and somatic parameters. The groups differ in respect to prevalence, with shyness reported in 20%–50% of subjects studied and social phobia present in only 2%–3% of the general population. Shyness appears to be a much larger and more heterogeneous category that overlaps social phobia to a substantial but unmeasured degree. Shyness, unlike social phobia, does not require distress or impairment, yet shyness does not represent only the less severe end of a social phobia continuum. If a boundary between social phobia and shyness is to be delineated in diagnostic criteria, the term *shyness* as it is now used will need to be more clearly defined.

Relationship of Test Anxiety and Social Phobia

Methods. Literature searches in psychology and psychiatry journals were conducted with computer and manual search procedures. For test anxiety, population samples consisted almost exclusively of high school and college students. The literature review was confined to English language articles and research conducted with human subjects. There is a large literature on test anxiety, but this review focuses on a few classic papers describing its dimensions and investigations examining the relationship of test anxiety to other social-evaluative fears or trait anxiety. Additionally, studies that directly assessed cognitive or somatic aspects of test anxiety and that could be related to the same parameters found in social phobia are reviewed.

Results. Test anxiety has been hypothesized to consist of cognitive and somatic components (Liebert and Morris 1967). The cognitive component includes fears of failure and negative evaluation. The somatic component denotes the autonomic arousal that occurs before and during the examination. Symptoms of test anxiety could result in inability to attend to relevant aspects of an examination (Meichenbaum 1972), thus impairing academic performance.

It has been suggested that a subgroup of test-anxious young adults also report worries about social relationships (Sarason 1975). In an empirical study (Pilkonis 1977) of 154 undergraduates, test anxiety was positively correlated with public self-consciousness, private self-consciousness, social anxiety, and fear of negative evaluation. Another study of 36 test-anxious individuals (Goldfried et al. 1978) reported elevated measures of social anxiety and fear of negative evaluation. Test-anxious individuals tended to also fear job interviews, public speaking, and attending a party. Additionally, test anxiety has been documented in public-speaking social phobic patients seeking treatment at an anxiety disorders clinic (Turner et al. 1986b). Of the sample interviewed concerning anxiety in social situations, 19% endorsed testing as a situation that created significant distress.

Another study examined psychophysiological responses of test-anxious children (Beidel 1988). Of 25 children with test anxiety, 15 (60%) met criteria for an anxiety disorder, with 6 (24%) meeting criteria for social phobia and 6 (24%) meeting criteria for overanxious disorder. During both test-taking and public-speaking tasks, test-anxious children had significantly higher heart rates than non-test-anxious peers. The pattern of response was similar to that previously reported for adults with social anxiety (Turner et al. 1986b).

Discussion. Studies of test-anxious populations find elevated levels of social-evaluative anxiety, and one study of social phobic subjects found a 19% rate of test anxiety. Additionally, physiological response in test-anxious subjects appeared similar to that reported for social phobia. There appears to be overlap between test anxiety and social phobia, which is not surprising, given that testing requires the evaluation of one's work by others with the possibility of embarrassment or humiliation. Fears of social phobic situations such as public speaking or performing on stage similarly involve potential evaluation by others. Therefore, although test anxiety is not an overtly social fear it may be similar enough to be included within the definition of social phobia. One option for DSM-IV would be to include test anxiety as an example of social phobia. Another option would be to mention the association in the text of DSM-IV but to avoid including it in the criteria for social phobia until the relationship undergoes further empirical study.

Social Phobia Secondary to Physical Disability

Methods. Four conditions associated with secondary social anxiety—stuttering, benign essential tremor (BET), Parkinson's disease, and breast modification—were assessed. Literature on stuttering was reviewed by conducting both Medline and Psychological Abstracts searches back to 1965, confined to articles published in English and studies conducted in humans. Additionally, reference lists of 11 journals from 1985 to 1989 were reviewed for relevant articles. Five textbooks were also reviewed. For BET, a Medline search extending back to 1974 was limited to articles published in English and using human subjects. Reference lists of six journals for the past 5 years were reviewed, in addition to four standard textbooks on movement disorders. For Parkinson's disease, Medline was searched back to 1965 and Psychological Abstracts back to 1983. Six textbooks were also reviewed. For breast modification, Medline was searched back to 1965 with articles published in English and human studies only. Psychological Abstracts were reviewed back to 1983, and three textbooks were also reviewed.

Results. No data were found regarding the prevalence of DSM-III or DSM-III-R social phobia in those who stutter. DSM-III and DSM-III-R criteria exclude the diagnosis of social phobia if it is only related to concerns about stuttering. Nevertheless, social avoidance and anxiety have been reported to occur commonly among those who stutter. Among stutterers, anxiety may be an impediment to speaking fluently (Bloodstein 1987), and fluency may be worse when speaking to superiors (Sheehan et al. 1967) or larger audiences (Porter 1939) but better when speaking to children (Ramig et al. 1982) or when speaking alone. Personality inventory testing of stuttering patients suggests that they are less assertive (Cohen et al. 1975), and have more interpersonal sensitivity (Sermas and Cox 1982) and social anxiety (Greiner et al. 1985) than control groups. Pharmacological studies using anxiolytic drugs (DiNardo et al. 1983; Holliday 1959; Kent and Williams 1959; Leanderson and Levi 1967; Maxwell and Paterson 1958; Rustin et al. 1981) have suggested that anxiety reduction was an important therapeutic component when improvement occurred.

No data were found regarding the prevalence of social phobia in patients with BET. It is clear, however, that the underlying essential/familial tremor may be exaggerated during times of stress. This worsening of the tremor with stress can be blocked by beta-blockers and benzodiazepines (Gengo et al. 1986; Thompson et al. 1984), drugs that have also been suggested to be useful for social anxiety (Koller et al. 1986). Whereas clinical experience suggests that patients with BET develop avoidance behaviors resembling social phobia, data regarding a true comorbidity between social phobia and BET are lacking. Psychogenic tremor has been reported in some anxious patients but without diagnostic details (Koller et al. 1986).

In a study of 24 patients with Parkinson's disease, 9 (38%) were diagnosed as having a DSM-III-R anxiety disorder, and 4 of these 9 received a diagnosis of social phobia (Stein et al. 1990). Three other patients exhibited symptoms of social anxiety, but due to the exclusion criterion concerning anxiety that is limited to self-consciousness and embarrassment about Parkinsonian symptoms being apparent to others, these patients did not receive a DSM-III-R diagnosis. In another study of 12 patients with anxiety disorders and Parkinson's disease, the clinical onset of the anxiety disorder occurred with or after the onset and treatment of neurological symptoms in 9 (75%). Psychiatric illness in such cases may be a psychological response to chronic disease, a function of the medical treatment of the disease, and/or a function of some common pathophysiological process.

No studies directly investigated the association between social anxiety (or phobia) and mastectomy, breast reconstruction, or augmentation mammoplasty. Anecdotal evidence suggests that women undergoing these procedures often experience marked social anxiety or avoidance either before or after breast modification. One study found that 81% of women seeking augmentation mammoplasty believed that other people constantly looked at them, particularly noticing their bust size (Bale et al. 1980). In childhood, this concern resulted in shyness and avoidance of sports due to avoidance of showering with others (Sihm et al. 1978). Similarly, another study of adults found that 95% of subjects seeking breast augmentation refused to appear naked in front of partners or in front of other women, compared to 5% of control subjects (Schlebusch and Levin 1983). Augmentation mammoplasty has been reported to increase participation in physical exercise, sexual contact, self-confidence, and social interaction (Jonsson et al. 1984; Sihm et al. 1978).

Discussion.   Although there is clinical evidence for the association of considerable secondary social anxiety and avoidance in each of the physical disorders assessed, systematic data on their relationship with social phobia exist only for Parkinson's disease. In one study, social phobic symptoms were present in 7 of 24 patients with Parkinson's disease. DSM-III-R criteria exclude diagnosis of social phobia if the fear is only related to another disorder.

Several options exist for defining this boundary in DSM-IV. The exclusion for social phobia secondary to a physical disorder could be left essentially intact. This would retain the most homogeneous definition of social phobia, because secondary social phobia might differ from primary social phobia in certain features (e.g., later age at onset). It would, however, fail to alert clinicians to secondary social anxiety that is causing impairment and may be treatable independent of the underlying physical disorder. An alternate option would be to drop the exclusion completely, permitting the diagnosis of social phobia even if it is focused only on a particular physical abnormality. An intermediate option would allow the diagnosis of social phobia if the fear of embarrassment about the social ramifications of the primary disorder is clearly in excess of that usually associated with the disorder. The last option requires that diagnosticians have familiarity with levels of social anxiety "usually" associated with physical conditions.

Boundary With Substance Use Disorders

Methods.   A computer search was conducted with Medline from 1980 to 1989 and with Psychological Abstracts from 1980 to 1989. It was confined to journals published in English and research conducted with human subjects. The reference lists of four journals from 1985 to 1989 were also reviewed.

Results.   Studies that examined the prevalence of substance abuse in social phobia or the prevalence of social phobia among those with substance abuse are listed in Tables 17–1 and 17–2, respectively. Studies that examined mixed phobic populations without specifying a social phobic diagnosis were excluded.

Four studies examined the rate of alcohol abuse/dependence in social phobic populations. Schneier et al. (1989) found a 16% rate of history of Research Diagnostic Criteria (RDC) alcoholism in an anxiety clinic population of 98 DSM-III-R social phobic patients who had previously been screened to exclude current alcoholism. Another study (Barlow et al. 1986a) found only a 5% prevalence of comorbid DSM-III alcohol abuse among 19 DSM-III social phobic patients presenting to an anxiety clinic. Of 11 DSM-III social phobic patients presenting to another anxiety clinic, 4 (36%) had problematic drinking, as measured by the Michigan Alcoholism Screening Test (Thyer et al. 1986). Finally, in another study

(Amies et al. 1983), 20% of DSM-III social phobic patients reported alcohol "taken in excess."

Three of the above studies (Amies et al. 1983; Barlow et al. 1986a; Thyer et al. 1986) also examined the rate of alcohol abuse/dependence in anxiety disorders other than social phobia. In each of these studies, the rate was highest among those with social phobia, although the difference was not always significant. No reports were found on the prevalence of abuse/dependence of substances other than alcohol.

Five studies have examined the rate of social phobia in those with substance abuse or, more specifically, in those with alcohol abuse. Among 75 inpatients with RDC alcoholism, 21% were given lifetime RDC diagnoses of probable or definite social phobia (Chambless et al. 1987). In another sample of abstinent individuals who had been diagnosed with DSM-III alcohol abuse, 8% met DSM-III criteria for social phobia (Stravynski et al. 1986). Among 60 alcoholic individuals who were either in an inpatient unit ($n = 52$) or attending Alcoholics Anonymous ($n = 8$), 39% were diagnosed by a clinical rating scale as social phobic during their last period of drinking (Smail et al. 1984). In a group of 48 alcoholic inpatients, 12.5% met lifetime RDC for social phobia (Bowen et al. 1984). Finally, of 102 alcoholic inpatients, 56% were diagnosed by a clinical rating scale as experiencing subjective distress and/or disabling avoidance in regard to social situations (Mullaney and Trippett 1979).

In respect to clinical characteristics associated with these dual diagnoses, one

Table 17–1.   Substance/alcohol abuse in social phobia populations

Study	N	Social phobia diagnostic criteria	Setting	% with substance abuse	Substance abuse diagnosis and criteria
Schneier et al. 1989	98	DSM-III-R	Outpatient	16	RDC alcoholism[a]
Barlow et al. 1986a	19	DSM-III	Outpatient	5	DSM-III alcohol abuse
Thyer et al. 1986	11	DSM-III	Outpatient	36	MAST alcoholism
Amies et al. 1983		DSM-III	Outpatient	20	Alcohol taken in excess

Note.   RDC = Research Diagnostic Criteria. MAST = Michigan Alcohol Screening Test.
[a]Past history of.

study found that social phobic subjects with a history of alcoholism had more severe social phobia, were more likely to have the generalized subtype of social phobia, and were less likely to be married than those without a history of alcoholism (Schneier et al. 1989). There were no other differences in demographics. Another study reported that in a comparison of alcoholic inpatients with social phobia to nonalcoholic social phobic patients in an anxiety clinic, there were no significant differences in demographic variables, Fear Questionnaire (Marks and Mathews 1979) scores, or depression.

Age at onset of social phobia preceded that of alcohol abuse in 15 of 16 dual-diagnosis patients in one study (Schneier et al. 1989). In another study, the mean age at onset of social phobia preceded that of alcoholism (14.6 versus 23.6 years), and for 80% of patients with an anxiety disorder and alcoholism, the anxiety disorder had an earlier onset (Chambless et al. 1987). In a third study, social phobia preceded alcoholism in 70% of dual-diagnosis patients. Several studies have reported that at least 40% of individuals with alcoholism and social phobia claim to have used alcohol to self-medicate anxiety (Schneier et al. 1989; Smail et al. 1984; Stravynski et al. 1986). Another study of 15 individuals with DSM-III social phobia who used any alcohol or anxiolytic drugs found that 46% reported using alcohol to feel more sociable at a party and 50% reported intentional use of alcohol prior to attending a social event (Turner et al. 1986a).

Table 17–2. Social phobia in substance/alcohol abuse populations

Study	N	Substance abuse diagnosis and criteria	Setting	% with social phobia	Social phobia diagnostic criteria
Chambless et al. 1987	75	RDC alcoholism	Inpatient	21	RDC
Stravynski et al. 1986	96	Clinical alcoholism	Inpatient	8	DSM-III
Smail et al. 1984	60	Clinical alcoholism	Inpatient	39[a]	Other
Bowen et al. 1984	48	RDC alcoholism	Inpatient	12.5	RDC
Mullaney and Trippett 1979	102	Clinical alcoholism	Inpatient	56[b]	Other

Note. RDC = Research Diagnostic Criteria.
[a]During last drinking period.
[b]"Fully or borderline social phobia."

Discussion. Three of four studies of the rate of comorbid alcohol abuse/dependence in those with social phobia found a higher rate of alcoholism than the reported lifetime prevalence in the general population of 8%–10% in men and 3%–5% in women (Schuckit 1986). In each of three studies that also measured the rate of alcoholism in patients with other anxiety disorders, the rate of alcoholism was highest in social phobia, despite several factors that may have led to underestimation of alcoholism in those with clinical social phobia. One study (Schneier et al. 1989) excluded patients with current alcohol abuse, and the other three studies used DSM-III criteria for social phobia, which excluded those more severe cases that might be given a DSM-III diagnosis of avoidant personality disorder instead. This group of patients may be at highest risk for alcoholism.

Five studies of social phobia among alcoholic inpatients found rates of 8%–56%, substantially higher than the reported 0.9%–2.6% prevalence of DSM-III social phobia in the general U.S. population (Myers et al. 1984). The two studies with the highest rates (Mullaney and Trippett 1979; Smail et al. 1984) took place in England and did not use standardized diagnostic criteria. The study with the lowest rate of social phobia among alcoholic patients used DSM-III criteria but also found a 35% rate of avoidant personality disorder, and many of these patients might have been considered social phobic by DSM-III-R criteria. Overall, the findings suggest an elevated prevalence of social phobia among alcoholic inpatients.

Clinical characteristics of these dual-diagnosis patients were examined mainly in two studies, the results of which did not completely agree. Patients with alcoholism and social phobia were similar to nonalcoholic social phobic patients in most respects. One study found that social phobia tended to be more severe in patients with comorbid alcoholism. Three studies that examined age at onset in dual-diagnosis patients found that social phobia generally preceded alcoholism.

Additionally, four studies found high rates of self-reported self-medication of social phobia with alcohol. This finding must be interpreted cautiously in light of the retrospective nature of these reports and the absence of a normal control group. Nevertheless, it raises the possibility that alcoholism may sometimes occur as a direct complication of social phobia. It is also possible that social phobia may sometimes occur as a complication of alcoholism, given the high rates of social phobia reported during periods of drinking.

Given that social phobia and substance abuse disorders often co-occur, yet neither disorder is an essential feature of the other, it seems that substance use disorders specifically should be mentioned in the DSM-IV social phobia text or in the social phobia criteria. The principle that patients with acute substance abuse should not be given other psychiatric diagnoses on more than a provisional basis until detoxified appears to be supported here and could be included in social phobia criteria. However, the data also suggest that some patients with substance abuse will require additional treatment for comorbid social phobia.

Border With Panic Disorder and Agoraphobia

Method. The literature comparing social phobia with panic disorder and agoraphobia was reviewed using Medline and Psychlit searches and manual review of 11 journals and recent textbooks on anxiety.

Results. Social phobic subjects have been shown to differ from subjects with panic disorder and agoraphobia in several respects. Both general population and clinic sample data suggest that agoraphobia is more prevalent than social phobia and that the rates of social phobia and panic disorder are roughly comparable (Table 17–3). Social phobia appears to be equally common across genders among clinic patients in contrast to agoraphobia, which is much more common in females, both in the general population and among clinic attendees (Table 17–4). Studies reporting age at onset have consistently shown earlier onsets for social phobia than for agoraphobia (Table 17–5).

Studies suggest that the relatives of panic and agoraphobic patients are not at an increased risk for social phobia, nor are relatives of social phobic patients at an increased risk for panic disorder or agoraphobia (Noyes et al. 1986; Reich and Yates 1988a). Biological challenge comparisons of the disorders are discussed below in the section on physiological and biochemical aspects of social phobia. In regard to response to pharmacotherapy, tricyclics, monoamine oxidase inhibitors (MAOIs), and alprazolam are effective in the treatment of panic disorder (reviewed by Gorman 1987), but beta-blockers do not reduce clinical spontaneous panic attacks (Noyes et al. 1984), nor does pretreatment with beta-blockers prevent lactate-induced panic attacks (Gorman et al. 1983) in panic disorder patients. The few systematic pharmacological studies of the treatment of social phobia (Deltito and Perugi 1986; Falloon et al. 1981; Liebowitz 1987; Pecknold et al. 1982) suggest that beta-blockers are successful only in the acute (prn) reduction of certain aspects of performance anxiety; MAOIs are effective in reducing social anxiety; tricyclics do not appear to be efficacious in treating social discomfort in general, or social phobia in particular (Liebowitz 1987); and high-potency benzodiazepines such as alprazolam are effective in symptom reduction (Lydiard et al. 1988; Reich and Yates 1988b). If the pharmacological findings for social phobia are confirmed in subsequent studies, beta blocker efficacy (for performance anxiety) and tricyclic efficacy for panic may distinguish social phobia from panic disorder/agoraphobia.

Several investigators have reported substantial comorbidity between social phobia, agoraphobia, and panic disorder (Table 17–6). However, the use of various

Table 17–3. Prevalence of social phobia, agoraphobia, and panic disorder in community samples of the general population and clinical samples of anxiety disorder patients

Nature of sample/ investigator	N	% with diagnosis of:		
		Social phobia	Agoraphobia	Panic disorder
Community samples				
Myers et al. 1984[a]				
New Haven, CT	3,058	NA	2.8	0.6
Baltimore, MD	3,481	2.2	5.8	1.0
St. Louis, MO	3,004	1.2	2.7	0.9
Pollard and Henderson, 1987, 1988				
Full DSM-III criteria	500	2.0	2.8	NA
Minus distress criterion	500	20.6	—	NA
Clinical samples				
Barlow 1985	102[b]	19	40	17
DiNardo et al. 1983	51[b]	16	45	16
Marks 1970	800[c]	8	60	NR

Note. NA = not assessed. NR = not reported.
[a]6-month prevalence rates.
[b]Consecutive referrals to an anxiety clinic who were given a primary anxiety disorder diagnosis.
[c]Total phobic patients seen at Maudsley Hospital "in the last decade."

diagnostic criteria and the resulting rates, which vary widely make the extent of comorbidity virtually indeterminate.

The type of anxiety attack a patient experiences may differ between social phobia and panic disorder. The Schedule for Affective Disorders and Schizophrenia—Lifetime Anxiety version (SADS-LA; Fyer et al. 1985; Mannuzza et al. 1986) distinguishes three types of panic attacks: spontaneous, which are unexpected or "out of the blue"; situationally predisposed, for which the probability of having an attack is increased in certain situations; and stimulus bound, which are almost invariably experienced when anticipating, or being exposed to, the phobic stimulus. Panic disorder in DSM-III-R is by definition associated with spontaneous panic attacks. Stimulus-bound attacks are often observed in those with social phobia (e.g., almost invariably panicking when signing a check in the presence of a bank teller). Situationally predisposed attacks are observed in panic disorder patients (e.g., panic risk is increased, but panics are not inevitable, when entering a crowded subway) and social phobic patients (e.g., panic risk is increased, but panics are not inevitable, when attending a social affair).

According to DSM-III-R, in social phobia, "exposure to the specific phobic stimulus (or stimuli) almost invariably provokes an immediate anxiety response." This anxiety reaction may be experienced as subjective (e.g., distress, apprehensiveness, or discomfort), somatic (e.g., trembling, sweating, or palpitations), some combination of these (as in a limited symptom attack), or a full-blown panic attack (with sudden terror plus multiple accompanying symptoms). There are, however, no available data on whether those with social phobia typically experience an "immediate" phobic response to phobic stimuli or a more gradual response.

Barlow et al. (1985) studied the frequency of panic attacks across DSM-III anxiety disorders and found that 16 of 19 social phobic patients (84%) and 6 of 7 simple phobic patients (86%) reported experiencing a panic attack, which was defined as "a sudden rush of intense fear or anxiety or feelings of impending doom" accompanied by at least 4 (of 12) associated symptoms. These rates dropped to 50% of social phobic patients and 33% of simple phobic patients when the DSM-III frequency criterion (at least three attacks in 3 weeks) was applied. Only a minority of the panic attacks experienced by the simple and social phobic patients were spontaneous.

The specificity of social situations as precipitants of panic attacks occurring in

Table 17–4.   Sex ratio of social phobia, agoraphobia, and panic disorder

Nature of sample/investigator	Social phobia		Agoraphobia		Panic disorder	
	N	% Female	N	% Female	N	% Female
Nonclinical samples						
Myers et al. 1984						
New Haven, CT	NA	—	88	84	20	80
Baltimore, MD	78	72	213	79	37	70
St. Louis, MO	38	71	88	87	26	69
Pollard and Henderson 1987, 1988						
Full DSM-III criteria	10	40	14	57	NA	—
Minus distress criterion	103	67	—	—	NA	—
Clinical samples						
Amies et al. 1983	87	40	57	86	NA	—
Marks 1970	64	50	480	75	NR	—
Solyom et al. 1986	47	47	80	86	NR	—
Thyer et al. 1985	42	52	95	80	62	57

Note. N = number of subjects with the indicated diagnosis. NA = not assessed. NR = not reported.

social phobia has been reported to be a distinguishing feature of social phobia. It has been suggested, however, that differentiating social from nonsocial situations is not always clear. In a study of the test-retest reliability of anxiety diagnoses (Mannuzza et al. 1989), 27% of all diagnostic disagreements for social phobia resulted from inadequate clarification of the patient's primary disturbance. Many of these discrepancies concerned the social-nonsocial distinction. In one case, both raters diagnosed social phobia. However, one rater made the additional diagnosis of simple phobia of airplanes. The other rater clarified, by obtaining additional information, that the patient's avoidance of airplanes was related to his social phobia. When asked, hypothetically, whether he would fly if the plane were empty, the patient responded, "No problem. It's the people, not the plane." In another case, both raters diagnosed panic disorder. However, one rater made the additional diagnosis of social phobia, because the patient (presumably) feared and avoided public speaking, eating in public, and asking directions. The other rater clarified that these situations, although "social," were essentially no different from other situations that the patient avoided (cars, trains, buses, etc.). The major concern in all involved a fear of having a panic attack.

Table 17–5.   Ages at onset (years) of social phobia and agoraphobia

Investigator	Social phobia		Agoraphobia	
	N	Mean age at onset	N	Mean age at onset
Amies et al. 1983	87	19.0	57	24.0
Burns and Thorpe 1977	NA	—	963	28.0
Cameron et al. 1986	37	14.3	NR	—
Doctor 1982	NA	—	404	28.1
Marks and Gelder 1966	25	18.9	84	23.9
Marks and Herst 1970	NA	—	1,200	29.0
Öst 1987	80	16.3	100	27.7
Shafar 1976	20	20.0	68	32.0
Sheehan et al. 1981	NA	—	100	24.1
Solyom et al. 1986	47		80	
First symptoms		16.6		24.5
Disorder		23.5		26.0
Thyer et al. 1985	42	15.7	95	26.3
Turner et al. 1986b	21	16.5	NA	—

Note.   N = number of subjects with the indicated diagnosis. NA = not assessed. NR = not reported.

Liebowitz et al. (1985b) described a developmental sequence observed in some panic/agoraphobic patients that they refer to as "secondary social phobia":

> Also problematic is how to classify patients who develop spontaneous panic attacks leading to panic disorder or agoraphobia and then, as aspects of a larger syndrome, begin to avoid certain performance or social situations . . . such patients . . . do fear embarrassment or humiliation were they to have a panic attack in front of others, and thus avoid giving speeches, giving parties, etc. (p. 729)

Munjack et al. (1987) compared 20 panic disorder patients, some of whom had social fearfulness ("secondary social phobics") to 20 social phobic patients with no spontaneous panic attacks ("primary social phobics") on self-ratings of the SCL-90R (Derogatis 1983). Panic patients scored significantly higher than social phobic patients on the somatization factor. Social phobic patients scored significantly higher than panic patients on the interpersonal sensitivity factor. The authors concluded that primary and secondary social phobias are distinct. In addition, they indicated, "it is our impression that there is virtually no overlap between these two groups in circumstances that invoke their social discomfort" (p. 50).

Conversely, panic disorder and social phobia may coexist and may be difficult

Table 17–6. Comorbidity among social phobia (SP), agoraphobia (AGP), and panic disorder (PD)

	Primary diagnosis						
	Social phobia			Agoraphobia		Panic disorder	
Investigator	N	% AGP	% PD	N	% SP	N	% SP
Barlow et al. 1986a	19	0	0	41	17	17	35
de Ruiter et al. 1989							
Interference procedure[a]	3	0	33	56	11	17	6
Temporal procedure[b]	5	60	0	27	0	10	0
Sanderson et al. 1987[c]	?	?	?	?	28	?	?
Solyom et al. 1986	47	30[d]	NR	80	55[e]	NR	—
Stein et al. 1989	NA	—	—	—	—	35[f]	46

Note. N = number of subjects with the primary diagnosis. NA = not assessed. NR = not reported.
[a]Primary diagnosis based on degree of functional impairment.
[b]Primary diagnosis based on first syndrome to develop.
[c]Summarized in Turner and Beidel 1989.
[d]"Clinically significant agoraphobia."
[e]"Clinically significant social phobia."
[f]66% met criteria for agoraphobia.

to differentiate. Stein et al. (1989) reported that 16 (46%) of patients with DSM-III-R panic disorder also had social phobia. They found that, in many cases, it was difficult, if not impossible, to distinguish whether the patient's social anxiety or phobias were unrelated to the fear of having a panic attack.

There is some evidence that the anxiety symptoms of social phobic and panic/agoraphobic patients differ. Blushing and muscle twitching were reported to be more common in those with social phobia, whereas limb weakness, difficulty breathing, dizziness and faintness, buzzing or ringing in the ears, and fainting were more common among those with agoraphobia (Amies et al. 1983). In another study (Reich et al. 1988), significantly fewer social phobic than panic disorder patients reported palpitations, chest pains, tinnitus, blurred vision, headaches, and fear of dying. Significantly fewer panic disorder than social phobic patients reported dry mouth. A third study (Cameron et al. 1986) reported similar findings.

Liebowitz et al. (1985a) observed that, whereas social phobic patients often report feeling more comfortable when alone, panic disorder patients are comforted by the presence of significant others. There is some empirical support for the clinical observation that panic/agoraphobic patients experience less anxiety when accompanied by a familiar companion. Sinnott et al. (1981) had agoraphobic patients rate a questionnaire with respect to the severity of the anxiety-provoking effect of several situations. Items that specified being unaccompanied showed significantly higher fear ratings than items that specified being accompanied ("by someone sympathetic and supportive").

Discussion.   Review of the literature suggests that social phobia and panic disorder/agoraphobia differ on a variety of characteristics. Compared with agoraphobia, social phobia is less prevalent (in the community as well as the clinic), is about equally represented among males and females who seek treatment for the disturbance (versus a preponderance of females among agoraphobic patients), and has an earlier age at onset. Furthermore, panic disorder and agoraphobia are not overrepresented in the families of social phobic patients, nor is social phobia in the families of panic/agoraphobic patients. Anxiety symptoms differ between the two disorders. Results of biological challenge studies suggest that social phobia and panic disorder/agoraphobia are characterized by different pathophysiological mechanisms, and treatment studies show promise in providing pharmacological dissection of the syndromes. Although these statistical differences support the distinction between the disorders, they are not definitive enough to be considered diagnostic criteria.

In general, the two disorders may best be distinguished by the focus of the patient's fear and reasons for avoidance. The core disturbance in social phobia involves concerns about scrutiny, humiliation, and embarrassment; all other symptoms (e.g., panic attacks) and behaviors (e.g., avoidance of certain situations) revolve around these concerns. However, when significant social anxiety is present in an individual with panic disorder, it may be difficult to determine whether the focus of such social anxiety is (secondary) fear of being observed during a panic attack or is primary. The significance of "secondary" (versus "primary") social phobia is largely unexplored (e.g., with respect to treatment, familial psychiatric history, prognosis, and other factors). Until this issue is clarified, researchers should distinguish panic patients who avoid social situations due to fear of having a panic attack in front of others, from those with a full social phobic syndrome with intrinsic fear of social situations. The social phobia criteria might therefore exclude social phobia secondary to panic disorder, as did the DSM-III-R criteria. The terminology is further complicated because a social anxiety episode in pure social phobia may take the form of a panic attack, and this could be acknowledged in the social phobia criteria.

The situation of social phobia secondary to panic is analogous to that in which an embarrassing physical disorder (e.g., Parkinson's disease) precedes the onset of social phobia, and in regard to DSM-IV, it would be most concise for a single criterion to address both forms of "secondary" social phobia. Because differentiating panic disorder and agoraphobia has the special difficulties discussed above, however, it is desirable in the DSM-IV social phobia criteria to separately exclude social phobia secondary to panic disorder, apart from the criteria options for other "secondary" social phobia. The panic disorder/social phobia distinction could be discussed further in the text.

Another possibility considered was the potentially more reliable approach of omitting any panic disorder exclusion criterion and permitting the diagnosis of social phobia, even when apparently caused by primary panic disorder. This would have the disadvantage of increasing prevalence of social phobia and ignoring the partially validated distinctions between panic disorder and social phobia, which are reviewed above. The other extreme would exclude any social phobia if panic disorder is present, but this would negate social phobia that appears independent of preexisting panic disorder.

Boundary With Generalized Anxiety Disorder

Method. A Medline search was conducted for the years 1980–1989. Three journals were also searched for relevant papers from 1985 to 1989.

Results. Three studies have reported the prevalence of generalized anxiety disorder in social phobia to be 55%, 21%, and 17%, respectively (Barlow et al. 1986a; Versiani et al. 1988, 1989). The last study was the largest, including 250 patients diagnosed by DSM-III-R criteria using the Structured Clinical Interview for DSM-III-R (SCID; Spitzer et al. 1987). No studies were found reporting the prevalence of social phobia in generalized anxiety disorder.

Barlow et al. (1986b) compared generalized anxiety disorder to social phobia and concluded that generalized anxiety disorder may be distinguished as an independent category on the basis of "apprehensive expectation or chronic worry focused on multiple life situations." They state that generalized anxiety disorder symptomatology can be distinguished from phobic disorders on the basis of chronicity, early onset, and lack of relationship to specific stimuli.

Versiani et al. (1988,1989) reported that most social phobic patients did not experience high levels of anxiety related to nonsocial situations. In a comparison of 250 primary social phobic patients and 72 patients with generalized anxiety disorder, generalized anxiety disorder patients scored higher on the Hamilton Anxiety and Depression scales (Hamilton 1967) and on the SCL-90 (Derogatis 1983), except for the subscale rating "interpersonal sensitivity." Insomnia was more common in generalized anxiety disorder.

Two other studies have examined differences in symptomatology between these groups. Reich et al. (1988) found that social phobic patients have a lower frequency of headaches and fear of dying and a higher frequency of sweating, flushing, and dyspnea in comparison with generalized anxiety disorder patients. Cameron et al. (1986) reported similar findings.

Discussion. The small amount of data available suggest that current distinctions between generalized anxiety disorder and social phobia may be partially validated by differences in rates of particular characteristic symptoms. Insufficient data exist to suggest any recommendations for changes in criteria for DSM-IV.

Boundary With Avoidant Personality Disorder

Method. A search was conducted of the psychiatric and psychological literature for empirical studies of comorbid social phobia and avoidant personality disorder. Included were computer searches with Medline from 1980 to 1989 and with Psychological Abstracts from 1980 to 1989. The computer search was confined to journal articles published in English and research conducted with human subjects. The indexes of four journals from 1985 to 1989 were also reviewed for relevant papers. Recent studies and review articles were examined.

Results. Evaluation of the overlap of these diagnoses is complicated by the substantial changes in the criteria for social phobia and avoidant personality disorder from DSM-III to DSM-III-R. According to the hierarchical schema of DSM-III, a diagnosis of social phobia was not given if the marked anxiety and avoidance of certain social situations was due to avoidant personality disorder. In DSM-III-R, the hierarchical schema was dropped, so that some patients previously diagnosed as having only avoidant personality disorder might now be given the additional diagnosis of social phobia. It seems likely that many of these patients now dually diagnosed would be in the "generalized" subtype of DSM-III-R social phobia, with fear of most social situations.

The criteria for avoidant personality disorder also changed substantially from DSM-III to DSM-III-R. Criteria of "desire for affection and acceptance" and "low self-esteem" were deleted in DSM-III-R. New criteria of "has no close friends or confidants (or only one) other than first-degree relatives," "is reticent in social situations because of a fear of saying something inappropriate or foolish, or of being unable to answer a question," "fears being embarrassed by blushing, crying, or showing signs of anxiety in front of other people," and "exaggerates the potential difficulties, physical dangers, or risks involved in doing something ordinary but outside his or her usual routine, e.g., may cancel social plans because she anticipates being exhausted by the effort of getting there" were added for DSM-III-R (p. 353). Additionally, whereas DSM-III required the presence of all five criteria to make the diagnosis, DSM-III-R requires only four of seven criteria to be present.

Several studies have examined these disorders using DSM-III criteria. In a study of 289 outpatients in Norway (Alnaes and Torgersen 1988), DSM-III diagnoses were made for Axis I using the SCID (Spitzer et al. 1987) and for Axis II using the Structured Interview for DSM-III Personality Disorders (SIDP; Pfohl et al. 1983), with suspension of the hierarchical rule excluding social phobia in the presence of avoidant personality disorder. Avoidant personality disorder was present in 9 of 10 patients with social phobia.

Only two papers were found that empirically compared subjects with DSM-III social phobia and avoidant personality disorder. Turner et al. (1986a) noted that the distinction between these disorders is clinically difficult to assess. They compared 10 patients with DSM-III social phobia with 8 subjects with DSM-III avoidant personality disorder on a battery of self-report instruments and in a series of structured social interactions, during which physiological reactivity, type of cognitions, and behavioral manifestations of skill and anxiety were monitored. Individuals diagnosed as avoidant personality disorder reported distress in more social situations, more somatic anxiety symptoms, more hypersensitivity in social interactions, more depression, and more tendency to ruminate than subjects with social phobia. During the structured social interactions, there were no differences between the disorders in psychophysiological and cognitive variables; however, subjects with avoidant personality disorder were less socially skilled.

Stravynski et al. (1986) examined clinical characteristics of patients with

DSM-III social phobia ($n = 7$), avoidant personality disorder ($n = 34$), or agoraphobia ($n = 8$) who were attending an alcoholism rehabilitation program. Diagnosis was made by two independent evaluators. Half of the diagnostic disagreement between raters (13 of 26) was over the social phobia versus avoidant personality disorder distinction, which apparently was difficult to assess. The groups did not differ significantly in sex, mean age, rate of unemployment, education, or rate of living alone, but yearly income was lowest in the social phobia group. Measures of alcoholism did not differ between groups. Scores on the Fear Questionnaire (Marks and Mathews 1979), Beck Depression Inventory (Beck et al. 1961), and the State-Trait Anxiety Inventory (Spielberger 1983) did not differ between social phobia and avoidant personality disorder. Patients with avoidant personality disorder were less likely than patients with social phobia to report their most difficult situation as "being observed in groups" (36% versus 80%).

In regard to treatment response, Turner (1987) reported that seven DSM-III social phobic patients with a personality disorder were less responsive to cognitive-behavior therapy than were six social phobic patients without any personality disorder. The relevance of these results to the social phobia/avoidant personality disorder distinction is unclear, however, since only two of the seven personality disorder patients had avoidant personality disorder. Additionally, the method used for making the personality disorder diagnosis, pretreatment Minnesota Multiphasic Personality Disorder (MMPI) combined with posttreatment DSM-III criteria, is questionable.

Deltito and Perugi (1986) reported a case of DSM-III avoidant personality disorder responding to a monoamine oxidase inhibitor, a treatment that has been shown to be efficacious in social phobia (Liebowitz et al. 1988).

Greenberg and Stravynski (1983) have suggested that the therapeutic implication of the DSM-III division between social phobia and avoidant personality disorder could be that social phobia responds to exposure therapy, whereas avoidant personality disorder requires social skills training in addition to exposure. Although this hypothesis has not been tested directly, it is not supported by evidence indicating that exposure therapy alone may be insufficient for many social phobic patients (Butler 1985) and that social skills training may be effective in social phobia (Falloon et al. 1981). Heimberg et al. (1987) have suggested that the two groups may differ in desire to confront avoided situations, which may be absent in the avoidant personality disorder patient who has adopted avoidance as a comfortable lifestyle.

Among studies using DSM-III-R criteria, Reich et al. (1989) reported rates of DSM-III-R avoidant personality disorder among 14 social phobic patients of 21.4% and 35.7%, as diagnosed by the Personality Disorder Questionnaire (Hyler et al. 1983) and Millon Clinical Multiaxial Inventory (Millon 1983), respectively.

DSM-III-R avoidant personality disorder criteria (from a preliminary version of the SCID-II [Spitzer and Williams 1986]) were rated weekly for 8 weeks during treatment of social phobic patients with alprazolam. Scores for six of the nine avoidant personality disorder criteria decreased significantly in frequency during treatment. The three criteria that did not show significant improvement involved "no close friends or confidants," "feelings easily hurt by criticism or disapproval," and "exaggerates the potential dangers or risks of everyday situations."

Deltito and Stam (1989) reported two additional cases of avoidant personality disorder responding to pharmacotherapy with MAOIs.

Discussion.   The few existing studies comparing social phobia and avoidant personality disorder, whether by DSM-III or DSM-III-R criteria, have found that the disorders share most characteristics and frequently coexist (when the DSM-III exclusion criterion for avoidant personality disorder is dropped). Several studies suggest that the DSM-III distinction between the two disorders is difficult to assess clinically, and there is some evidence for similarities in treatment response. Data on populations diagnosed by DSM-III-R criteria are meager but suggest substantial overlap in diagnosis and treatment response for the two groups. It is possible that social phobia and avoidant personality disorder criteria describe overlapping subpopulations of the same disorder, with avoidant personality disorder representing the more severe end of a continuum. Research in progress may help clarify this relationship.

Subtypes of Social Phobia

Method.   A search of the psychological and psychiatric literatures was conducted to locate studies of relevance to the subtype issue that were published from 1985 to 1989. Both empirical articles and review articles were examined, and unpublished works, papers presented at scientific meetings, and works in press familiar to the authors were included. Nine journals were specifically searched.

Results.   Several previous attempts have been made to derive subtypes in studies of socially anxious college students. Pilkonis (1977) derived two clusters: those with public shyness focused on behavioral deficits that may be scrutinized by others, and those with private shyness focused more on internal sensations. Other studies (Fremouw et al. 1982; Gross and Fremouw 1982) clustered subjects into groups described as high in self-reported perception of physiological arousal but low in actual arousal or high in cognitive distortion but low in physiological arousal. Turner and Beidel (1985) clustered socially anxious subjects into one group that experienced both high frequency of negative thinking and high physiological arousal and another that experienced only high frequency of negative thinking but not physiological arousal.

Other investigators (Lewin et al. 1986; McNeil and Lewin 1986) divided socially anxious undergraduates into four groups comprised of all possible combinations of high or low speech anxiety and high or low general social anxiety. Generally, socially anxious subjects were more impaired on questionnaire measures of social distress, but performance in a behavioral challenge (speech task) was unrelated to questionnaire scores (McNeil and Lewin 1986). In contrast, on the speech task, high speech anxious subjects were significantly more impaired than low speech anxious subjects. The only significant contributor to speech performance was speech anxiety, although the performance of the low speech anxious/high generally socially anxious group approached that of the speech anxious groups.

In a second study (Lewin et al. 1986), all four groups completed measures of positive and negative self-statements and participated in two behavioral tests, one speech and one social interaction. Of the screening sample, 2% ($n = 1,080$) reported high speech anxiety in the absence of general social anxiety, whereas 3.2% reported high anxiety in both domains. In response to the speech task, high speech anxious groups reported more negative self-statements and fewer positive self-statements and showed more behavioral disruption than low speech anxious subjects. In the social interaction task, however, the high speech anxious/low general socially anxious group performed well and reported a preponderance of positive self-statements. The authors conclude that a subset of socially anxious subjects is fearful of public speaking but not of general social interaction and may be discriminated from other socially anxious subjects on the basis of both self-report and behavioral performance.

Only three studies have directly studied the subtype issue with patients who have been diagnosed according to DSM-III or DSM-III-R criteria, but the data from some others may also be relevant. Pollard and Henderson (1988) reported results of an epidemiological study of 500 subjects. Their structured interview was constructed according to DSM-III criteria. It did not, therefore, include information about generalized social phobia, but it did include a detailed study of limited/discrete social phobias. Of the 500 subjects interviewed, 10 (2%) met DSM-III criteria for the diagnosis of social phobia. However, if the criterion of significant distress was suspended, fully 22.6% of their sample reported at least one social phobia. This broke down into 20.6% reporting public-speaking/performance fears, 2.8% fears of writing in the presence of others, 1.2% fears of eating in public restaurants, and 0.2% fears of using public restrooms. No other situations were sampled.

Heimberg et al. (1989) reported the first direct comparison of generalized social phobic patients (as defined by DSM-III-R) and limited/discrete social phobic patients. They compared 35 generalized social phobic patients with a group of 22 social phobic patients with fears of public speaking on demographic characteristics, response to a series of questionnaire measures, and subjective, behavioral, and physiological responses to an individualized behavioral challenge. Those with generalized social phobia were found to be younger, less educated, and less likely to be employed than those with public-speaking phobia. Clinical assessors rated those with generalized social phobia as having more severe phobias and more functional impairment. They appeared more anxious, more depressed, and more concerned about negative social evaluation, and they endorsed more negative and fewer positive self-statements about social interaction. It should be noted that the two groups did not differ in their self-report of social phobic anxiety or specific fears of public speaking.

Generalized and public-speaking phobic patients also did not differ in the subjective anxiety they reported in response to behavioral challenge. However, observer ratings of anxiety and performance suggested poorer performance and greater overt anxiety on the part of those with generalized social phobia. Of special importance to this review are the findings from the assessment of physiological arousal (heart rate reactivity) because the two groups showed very different patterns: although the two groups were similar at baseline, those with generalized social phobia showed a modest increase of 4–5 beats per minute (bpm) over baseline during the behavioral challenge, whereas those with public-speaking phobia showed a dramatic increase in heart rate (19–20 bpm) in the first minute of the behavioral challenge, which then gradually decreased (to approximately 9 bpm) over the course of the challenge. The investigators summarized these data to suggest that those with generalized social phobia may show their greatest impairment in the cognitive and behavioral realms, whereas those with public-speaking phobia may be most vulnerable in the cognitive and physiological realms. The findings have some similarity to data with socially anxious students reported by Turner and Beidel (1985), described above.

Levin et al. (1993) reported a similar study comparing 28 individuals with generalized social phobia and 9 individuals with limited/discrete phobias to a group of 14 normal control subjects. Of the 9 individuals with limited/discrete phobias, 8 feared public speaking and 1 was phobic of public restrooms, so the results of Levin et al. (1989) are generally comparable to those of Heimberg et al. (1989). It is important to note that all subjects participated in the same standardized behavioral challenge (a speech task). Those with generalized social phobia were younger than either limited/discrete or control subjects. Similar to Heimberg et al.'s findings, those with generalized social phobia showed greater observer-rated behavioral disruption during the challenge, although this was only evident at the beginning and middle of the challenge and not at the end. Both limited/discrete and control subjects showed greater cardiac arousal than those with generalized social phobia during the challenge, but there were few differences in arousal between limited/discrete phobic and control subjects. A series of biochemical measures (plasma epinephrine, norepinephrine, cortisol) failed to differentiate the groups.

The third study that used DSM-III-R to define groups of generalized and limited/discrete social phobic patients examined differences in their familial and social background (Bruch and Heimberg, in press). Preliminary results from that study suggest that, relative to those with limited/discrete phobias, individuals with generalized social phobia were more likely to label themselves as shy and to believe that other people also saw them that way, to report fewer dates in the time period from the beginning of junior high school until age 21, and to see their mothers as shy or social phobic. They also reported that their families were less inclined to socialize with other families in a group, although there were no differences in how much stress their parents placed on the opinions of others.

Scant data exist on differential treatment response by social phobia subtype. In the realm of psychosocial treatment, three studies have attempted to divide social phobic patients into subgroups other than by the generalized versus discrete distinction and to determine whether this strategy led to differences in treatment outcome. Trower et al. (1978) described two groups as "social phobic" and "socially inadequate." Both groups were treated with either social skills training or systematic desensitization. The former group showed benefit with either approach, whereas the latter appeared to benefit only from social skills training. Öst et al. (1981) took a similar approach and designated patients as either "behavioral reactors" (failing to demonstrate adequate social skills in a behavioral test) or "physiological reactors" (showing a high level of cardiac arousal in the behavioral test). Subjects were treated with social skills training or applied relaxation. In this study, there did appear to be a treatment matching effect. Behavioral reactors fared better with social skills training, and physiological reactors fared better with applied relaxation. Jerremalm et al. (1986) divided social phobic subjects into "cognitive reactors" (showing a high degree of cognitive distortion in response to a questionnaire) or physiological reactors but failed to find a difference in response to self-instructional training or applied relaxation.

Heimberg (1986) reported a study on the prediction of response to cognitive-behavioral group treatment of social phobia. The DSM-III-R social phobic subtype was the first predictor to enter the regression equation, accounting for 21% of the variance in outcome. Limited/discrete social phobic subjects showed the most positive treatment response, although those with generalized social phobia also improved.

Data on differential response to pharmacological intervention are also scanty.

Liebowitz et al. (1985b) review data suggesting the efficacy of beta-blockade in the treatment of performance anxiety among normal musicians, public speakers, and other people vulnerable to stage fright. However, no study yet completed has examined the social phobic subtype as a prospectively determined variable affecting treatment outcome. Liebowitz et al. (1988) have done so in their controlled trial of the effectiveness of phenelzine, atenolol, and placebo, but published data do not include subtype-by-treatment data. Levin et al. (1993), in their review of pharmacological treatments, suggest that there may be a differential response to atenolol versus phenelzine by subtype. Specifically, phenelzine may be more effective for those with generalized social phobia, whereas atenolol may be more effective for those with limited/discrete social phobias. Evaluations of this assertion awaits the analysis of data for the full cohort of subjects in that study.

Discussion.   Two general conclusions can be drawn. First, there do appear to be a variety of meaningful differences between social phobic patients who have been categorized into the DSM-III-R generalized versus limited/discrete subtypes. These appear in analyses of their demographic characteristics, social and family background, degree of overall impairment, behavioral and physiological response to behavioral challenge, and possibly their response to psychosocial and pharmacological intervention. Second, there are a multitude of conceptual issues that remain unresolved and a great deal of research that needs to be conducted before we are on solid ground in evaluating the subtypes issue.

One possible problem with the DSM-III-R approach is in its definition of subtypes. It gives only a brief definition of the generalized subtype: "specify generalized type if the phobic situation includes most social situations." All other (limited/discrete) social phobic presentations were lumped together simply by their exclusion from the generalized category. Although this crude subdivision has some validity as discussed above, alternative definitions should be considered.

Anecdotal reports suggest that the generalized subtype distinction can be difficult to make in many cases, partly due to difficulty in defining "most" social situations. If a patient shows significant anxiety and/or impairment in heterosexual relationships but copes without anxiety on the job and in same-sex social interactions, what is the appropriate subtype designation? The patient does not fit the generalized category because *most* situations are not feared, yet he or she fears many more situations than the individual with prototypical public speaking phobia in the nongeneralized (limited/discrete) subtype.

An alternative to subtypes based on quantity of social situations feared would be based on quality of social situations. One approach would divide social phobia into two subtypes: one involving situations with qualities of performance, the other involving fear of social interactions. The distinction appears to have greater face validity than the current one based on "most" situations, but its true validity remains to be demonstrated. A similar possibility would create a third intermediate category for subjects with fear of social interactions that is not generalized to most social situations. This would provide a separate subtype for individuals such as those who fear dating but do not fear most social situations.

Yet another proposed model was considered but is not being included as an option. It would have divided social phobia into two disorders: circumscribed social phobia, limited to discrete, performance-like fears; and social anxiety disorder, encompassing all social interactive fears and the current generalized social phobia. Creating two disorders would have several advantages. It would restrict the term *social phobia* to its traditional meaning relating to circumscribed situations. It would ease the integration of avoidant disorder of childhood into social anxiety disorder, because children may manifest social avoidance without being aware of a feared phobic object. It would ease integration of avoidant personality disorder, which may share many features of generalized, but not discrete, social phobia. Disadvantages of the two-disorder model include it being a more major nosological shift, lack of empirical evidence to support its proposed advantages, and difficulties in coding an additional diagnosis while maintaining compatibility with ICD-10 (World Health Organization 1990).

The proposed subtypes are

- *Performance type:* if the phobic stimulus involves public performance of activities that can be engaged in comfortably if the individual is doing them while alone (e.g., playing a musical instrument, giving a speech, urinating, writing, eating) and does not meet the definition of generalized type.
- *Limited interactional type:* if the phobic stimulus is restricted to one or two socially interactive situations, such as going out on dates or speaking to authority figures.
- *Generalized type:* if the phobic situation includes most social situations (also consider the diagnosis of avoidant personality disorder).

Reanalysis of existing data, using this three-subtype model, will allow examination of the reliability and validity of this option. If the data show that the three subtypes lack reliability or validity, the subtypes could either be collapsed into a two-subtype definition or eliminated.

Physiological and Biochemical Aspects of Social Phobia

Method. Studies using DSM-III and DSM-III-R social phobic subjects as well as analogue groups (e.g., students selected by elevated scores on self-report) and subjects presenting with social phobic complaints but no formal diagnosis are included in this review. An effort was made to include all relevant physiological and biochemical studies that used DSM-III or DSM-III-R criteria to diagnose social phobia. Several studies reporting physiology have been omitted because they focus on predicting response to behavioral treatment and not diagnostic validity.

Results.   The search for trait markers in social phobia has been limited to a few reports. An early study of autonomic reactivity by Lader (1967) found that socially anxious patients had more resting spontaneous galvanic skin resistance fluctuations and habituated more slowly to tones than normal subjects. Increased reactivity was also noted in agoraphobic patients. These interesting results have not been reproduced in DSM-III–defined groups.

As to neuroendocrine markers, Tancer et al. (1990) reported normal 24-hour urinary free cortisol, dexamethasone suppression test, and growth hormone responses to clonidine in DSM-III–defined social phobic patients. In contrast to this negative finding, mitral valve prolapse has been reported to be more frequent in social phobic patients (8 of 30) compared with normal subjects (2 of 30), although panic disorder was not clearly excluded in this report (Chaleby and Ziady 1988). Another group (Benca et al. 1986) reported two patients with social phobia and mitral valve prolapse but concluded that these patients may have had panic disorder as well.

The most prevalent research strategy in social anxiety and social phobia has been observation of physiological and biochemical response patterns during exposure to phobic situations. Studies in unscreened normal subjects have documented significant increases in pulse, blood pressure, and plasma catecholamines during public speaking (Dimsdale and Moss 1980; Taggart et al. 1973) and musical performance (Neftel et al. 1982). Increases observed were up to 50 bpm (Taggart et al. 1973) for pulse and 2%–300% for plasma epinephrine (Dimsdale and Moss 1980). These studies were unique because they involved observations during maximally stressful real-life circumstances such as grand round presentations. In contrast, observations of analogue and clinically defined social phobic subjects have never utilized such potent stimuli, making it difficult to compare the results in normal subjects to those in anxiety subjects.

Analogue studies, usually of college students, have evaluated physiological responses during role-played socialization or performance challenge. Borkovec et al. (1974) and Twentyman and McFall (1975) found that anxious subjects had approximately 10 bpm greater increases in heart rate during socialization with opposite-sex confederates compared with nonanxious subjects. Results during public speaking in analogue groups are weaker, with at least one group (Knight and Borden 1979) finding similar heart rate responses in anxious and nonanxious groups.

Other studies have evaluated the responses of clinically defined socially anxious subjects. Although investigators did not use DSM-III, subjects were usually defined by having sufficient social phobic complaints to seek treatment. Two of these studies documented increases in autonomic measures during or in anticipation of challenge (Kanter and Goldfried 1979; Öst et al. 1981). A third report also included a normal control group (Beidel et al. 1985) and found small but significantly greater increases in heart rate and systolic blood pressure in clinically anxious subjects during public speaking and social interaction. In addition, they found that heart rate and systolic blood pressure returned to baseline more slowly over the course of interaction or impromptu speech in the anxious subjects compared with normal subjects.

Like the non-DSM-III studies, the DSM-III literature is varied in its use of control subjects and testing of validity. Heimberg et al. (1985) describe heart rate and behavioral and subjective responses in seven social phobic patients during individualized phobic challenges. On average, subjects showed significant 4- to 6-bpm increases in heart rate during performance, but the authors noted a wide variability in response patterns. In addition, there was great variability in heart rate response when the challenges were repeated over a 14-week course of cognitive-behavioral therapy. Behavioral and subjective variables improved more consistently over the course of the treatment. This study did not employ control subjects, but it does suggest variability in heart rate responses across similar exposures.

A later study by Heimberg et al. (1987a) found heart rate responses up to 8 bpm increases in social phobic patients during 4-minute personally relevant behavioral simulations. They were weakly correlated ($r = .35-.40$) to somatic but not to cognitive self-report, suggesting that autonomic responsiveness is not directly related to subjective responses. In a similar repeated-challenge design, Emmelkamp et al. (1985) also found inconsistent heart rate responses during socialization challenge in 34 DSM-III social phobic patients over the course of six cognitive-behavioral treatments.

In a study more relevant to issues of diagnostic validity, Turner et al. (1986b) compared DSM-III–defined social phobic patients, socially anxious nonclinical subjects, and normal control subjects during two socialization challenges and a speech. Heart rate reactivity, although significant, varied only 3 bpm between tasks and was not significantly different between groups. Systolic blood pressure, in contrast, was higher in a speaking task than in a same-sex interaction for both the anxious groups and was higher in the anxious groups than in normal subjects. Only the DSM-III clinical subjects showed greater increases in heart rate in the opposite-sex interaction over the same-sex interaction. The results indicate that analogue groups may share some of the characteristics of clinical samples and do differ from normal subjects.

The only study of biochemical response during behavioral challenge involved 37 DSM-III-R–defined social phobic patients and 14 control subjects observed during a 10-minute simulated speech (Levin et al. 1993). Although patients demonstrated significantly more behavioral and subjective responses during a 10-minute speech, control subjects showed greater heart rate increases (17% versus 11%) during the speech compared with patients. In contrast, patients and control subjects had similar biochemical responses: 60%–70% increases in plasma epinephrine, 30%–35% increases in norepinephrine, and no significant changes in cortisol. A more stressful challenge might have revealed biochemical differences between the groups.

Investigations comparing social phobic patients with other anxiety subjects are limited but provocative. Lader's (1967) pre-DSM-III measurements of skin conductivity suggested that socially anxious subjects share increased reactivity with agoraphobic patients compared with normal subjects and simple phobic patients, who did not differ. Johansson and Öst (1982), comparing poorly defined social phobic patients and claustrophobic patients, reported significantly higher heart rates during resting baseline in the social phobic patients (78 versus 73 bpm). During challenge (with a speech for the social phobic patients and confinement for the claustrophobic patients), the social phobic patients again had higher heart rates (94 versus 78 bpm).

Lang et al. (1983) employed a repeated-challenge design to compare socially anxious college students (an analogue group) and subjects with snake phobias. During exposure to snakes, the snake phobic group had significantly greater increases in heart rate than the socially anxious groups, but both groups had similar heart rate responses to public-speaking simulation.

Similar results were reported by Cook et al. (1988) in a comparison of DSM-III social phobic, simple phobic, and agoraphobic patients responding to personalized phobic scripts. Simple phobic patients showed significantly greater increases in heart rate and skin conductivity compared with agoraphobic patients, with social phobic patients falling between the two groups. In contrast to the earlier study (Lang et al. 1983), social phobic patients also developed greater heart rate increases during a standardized speech script performed by all three groups.

Limited biochemical challenge data are available concerning DSM-III social phobic patients. Liebowitz et al. (1985a) infused social phobic patients with 0.5 M racemic sodium lactate. Although panic patients have experienced panic attacks at a 50%–70% rate during infusion (Liebowitz et al. 1984), only 1 of 15 social phobic patients experienced an anxiety episode during lactate infusion. Papp et al. (1988) found that infusion of epinephrine produced social anxiety symptoms in only 1 of 11 social phobic patients, despite significant increases in heart rate and blood pressure. This challenge took place in a laboratory devoid of social or evaluative cues. In contrast, 38 of 62 panic patients panicked during infusion of the beta-adrenergic agonist isoproterenol, versus only 1 of 29 control subjects (Pohl et al. 1985). The results suggest that response to adrenergic stimulation differs between panic patients and social phobic patients.

Results from carbon dioxide inhalation are less clear in distinguishing panic and social phobic patients. Gorman et al. (1988) reported that 12 of 31 panic patients and 0 of 8 social phobic patients experienced anxiety during inhalation of 5% carbon dioxide. When the concentration was increased to 7%, 6 of 9 panic patients and 3 of 3 social phobic patients had anxiety attacks. Rapee et al. (1986) reported that single-breath inhalation of 50% carbon dioxide produced less anxiety in social phobic patients compared with panic patients. In contrast, A. J. Fyer (personal communication, 1988) found equal effects in both groups with 35% single-breath challenges. Overall, sensitivity to carbon dioxide appears to be shared between panic and social phobic patients, but factors such as threshold may modulate response.

Reports of physiological differences between subtypes are discussed above in the section on subtypes.

Discussion. The data on physiological and biochemical aspects of social phobia suggest several conclusions. First, virtually every study demonstrates increases in heart rate during performance or socialization in patients with social phobia. It is unclear, however, whether those with social phobia experience more arousal than normal subjects under similar circumstances. In regard to trait markers, none have been established in rigorously defined samples. Physiological measures have not been shown to reliably differentiate social phobia from other anxiety disorders. The biochemical challenge literature does suggest that panic disorder and social phobia are distinct, although it requires more investigation with a range of anxiogenic compounds under differing sets of environmental cues. Preliminary evidence suggests physiological differences between subtypes in social phobia, which should be taken into consideration in future comparisons of social phobic subjects to other groups. In summary, current physiological and biochemical data are insufficient to be incorporated meaningfully into DSM-IV criteria.

Cross-Cultural Issues

Methods. English language literature searches of Medline from 1983 to 1989 and of Psychlit from 1974 to 1989 were conducted for references to social phobia in societies outside of the United States and Europe. In addition, reference lists of all major articles on social phobia were scanned for citations relevant to cross-cultural issues. Of the 15 references found, 9 were useful and are discussed below.

Results. Data on Mexican Americans come from the Los Angeles site of the National Institute of Mental Health (NIMH) ECA study (Karno et al. 1989). Mexican Americans born in Mexico, Mexican Americans born in the United States, and non-Hispanic whites born in the United States were compared in terms of lifetime prevalence rates of anxiety disorders. There were no significant differences for social phobia. Mexican Americans born in Mexico and non-Hispanic whites born in the United States both had prevalences of 2.3%, whereas Mexican Americans born in the United States had a prevalence of 3.4%.

Phobic disorders in India and Great Britain were studied by reviewing outpatient records of an Indian and a British research hospital and comparing subsamples matched for age and sex (Chambers et al. 1986). Sudden death and illness phobias were more common in India, whereas agoraphobia and social phobia were more common in Great Britain. It is unclear, however, whether the findings can be generalized beyond these two institutions.

Chaleby (1987) believes that social phobia is a "notably common disorder among Saudis." This conclusion is based on the finding that social phobia was diagnosable in 13% of the patients with "neurotic disorders" seeking help at King Faisal Specialist Hospital in Riyadh. It is not clear from the paper, however, how that figure was ascertained.

Between October 1983 and May 1985, 35 patients who met DSM-III criteria for social phobia were compared to a 3-month sample of 270 general psychiatry patients. The social phobic patients differed in several ways. They had a higher male-to-female ratio (80% versus 44%), were younger (mainly in their 20s), were more highly educated, and had a higher occupational status. These are all probably highly correlated, however, because males and younger people have more educational and occupational opportunities in Saudi Arabia.

As in American social phobic patients, other psychiatric features were common: 21 patients were also depressed, 10 had somatization, 5 had psychotic symptoms, 7 had simple phobia, 13 had agoraphobia, 9 had panic attacks, 4 had obsessive-compulsive disorder, 2 were alcoholic, and 2 had sexual dysfunction. Only 22 of the 35 (63%) presented for the treatment of social phobia, but Chaleby gives the impression that all 35 met criteria using DSM-III hierarchical exclusions.

In a separate publication (Chaleby and Ziady 1988), 8 of 30 social phobic patients had echocardiographic evidence for mitral valve prolapse, as opposed to a 7% incidence in the normal population. They fail to specify, however, how many of those social phobic patients also had panic disorder, which has already been associated with mitral valve prolapse.

Japanese psychiatrists have long been interested in interpersonal fears and phobias, beginning with Morita's work in the 1920s. Japanese psychiatrists use the term *taijin kyofu* to describe a spectrum of conditions involving a "phobia of interpersonal relations" (Kasahara 1987; Lee 1987).

Kasahara (1987) divides the spectrum into four levels of increasing severity. The first is transient excessive self-consciousness that often occurs in adolescence. The second approximates American notions of social phobia. The third is associated with certain delusional beliefs, such as believing one has a bad smell that causes discomfort to others whenever one is in public, despite reassurance to the contrary. These are accompanied by ideas of reference, because actions of others such as touching their noses are interpreted as confirming evidence. The term *quasi delusional* is used because the beliefs tend to fluctuate in conviction from obsession to overvalued idea to delusion and are usually not accompanied by other delusional ideas (Kasahara 1987; Lee 1987; Takahashi 1989). Japanese psychiatrists themselves are unsure whether to include this form of interpersonal fear with social phobia or with psychoses. The fourth form occurs in association with schizophrenia, either before or after psychotic decompensation.

A feature that seems far more common to social phobia in Japan than in the United States is the fear of making others uncomfortable. For example, erythrophobia or fear of blushing troubles Japanese patients because blushing may be discomforting to others, whereas in the United States, blushing is embarrassing because it reveals one's own unease. Similarly, a fear of staring leads to interpersonal avoidance in Japan because staring makes others uncomfortable (Kasahara 1970). These differences are probably due to cultural influences, because Japan and Korea place great emphasis on relating harmoniously to others.

Discussion.   The data suggest that social phobia is not a culture-bound syndrome, although cultural conditions can affect its prevalence. Thus, cultures that place a great emphasis on external appearance or behavior appear likely to be associated with a higher prevalence of social phobia. This is a testable hypothesis using the anthropological literature.

This survey raises questions as to the boundary of social phobia with psychosis. Based on the attention it has received from psychiatric investigators, the delusional belief of making others uncomfortable because of some imagined bodily malfunction appears more common in Japan and Korea than in Western societies. This may be a pathophysiologically different condition from what we in the West think of as social phobia and might be better classified with the psychoses. Alternatively, it could be a culturally shaped alternative expression of social phobia that is pathophysiologically similar, or it could be a more severe, delusional form of social phobia analogous to delusional depression or obsessive-compulsive disorder with overvalued or delusional ideation. The most sensible approach is to acknowledge the uncertainty, leaving open the possibility that delusional states can be forms of social phobia. Definitive answers await clinical and epidemiological studies of both traditional and delusional social phobia in Western and Asian societies.

Recommendations

1. Shyness is currently too heterogeneous and ambiguous a category to be either included or excluded in DSM-IV social phobia criteria.
2. Test anxiety clearly overlaps with social phobia, but it is unclear whether its association is close enough for test anxiety to be included explicitly in social phobia criteria. It is suggested that in reanalysis of existing data sets, the rate of test anxiety in social phobic populations be examined to clarify this issue.
3. In regard to social phobia secondary to physical disability or secondary to other psychiatric disorders, the following options have been proposed for consideration and validation by reanalysis of existing data at five research centers. See the "Physical Disability" section above for discussion of their rationale.

   a. If another disorder is present, the fear in criterion A is not limited to embarrassment about the social ramifications of having the disorder (e.g., stuttering, trembling in Parkinson's disease, or exhibiting abnormal eating behavior in anorexia nervosa).

   b. If another disorder is present, the fear of embarrassment about the social ramifications of having the disorder is clearly in excess of that usually associated with the disorder, e.g., severe social isolation in a person with stuttering, trembling (in Parkinson's disease), or abnormal eating behavior (in anorexia nervosa).

   c. No exclusion criterion for fear limited to embarrassment about another disorder.

4. Criteria should exclude substance-induced anxiety disorders, and the relationship of social phobia to substance use disorders should be addressed in the DSM-IV social phobia text.
5. With respect to the border with generalized anxiety disorder, insufficient data exist to suggest that any changes should be made from DSM-III-R criteria. Future studies should assess the extent of comorbidity between these disorders and determine whether patients with comorbidity are more similar to either of the pure diagnostic groups.
6. With respect to the border with avoidant personality disorder, insufficient data exist to suggest that any changes should be made from DSM-III-R criteria. Further empirical studies are required to determine the extent to which

avoidant personality disorder and social phobia overlap or differ in clinical characteristics (including social skills and avoidance behavior), course of illness, treatment response, and family history. These studies should include subtyping of social phobia as generalized and nongeneralized to determine overlap for both subgroups of social phobia. The current criteria, which permit codiagnosis of social phobia and avoidant personality disorder should facilitate comparison of these diagnostic groups.

7. In regard to subtypes, a three-category option has been proposed for consideration and validation by reanalysis of existing data at five research centers. The reanalysis will examine the reliability of resubtyping subjects in existing data sets and it will examine validity by comparing the coherence of resulting subtypes with respect to a variety of validators. Based on the results of the reanalysis, the subtype definitions may be modified further.

8. Current physiological and biochemical data are insufficient to be meaningfully incorporated into DSM-IV criteria. Future studies should examine biological markers with attention to subtypes within social phobia.

9. Studies of social phobia in non-Western cultures have raised the issue of whether delusional forms of social anxiety should be included within social phobia. Because this is unclear, criteria should neither include nor exclude delusional states.

References

Alnaes R, Torgersen S: The relationship between DSM-III symptom disorders (Axis I) and personality disorders (Axis II) in an outpatient population. Acta Psychiatr Scand 78:485–492, 1988

American Psychiatric Association: Diagnostic and Statistical Manual of Mental Disorders, 3rd Edition. Washington, DC, American Psychiatric Association, 1980

American Psychiatric Association: Diagnostic and Statistical Manual of Mental Disorders, 3rd Edition, Revised. Washington, DC, American Psychiatric Association, 1987

Amies PL, Gelder MG, Shaw PM: Social phobia: a comparative clinical study. Br J Psychiatry 142:174–179, 1983

Bale S, Lisper H, Palm B: A psychological study of patients seeking augmentation mammoplasty. Br J Psychiatry 136:133–138, 1980

Barlow DH: The dimensions of anxiety disorders, in Anxiety and the Anxiety Disorders. Edited by Tuma AH, Maser JD. Hillsdale, NJ, Lawrence Erlbaum, 1985, pp 479–500

Barlow DH, Vermilyea J, Blanchard EB, et al: The phenomenon of panic. J Abnorm Psychol 94:320–328, 1985

Barlow DH, DiNardo PA, Vermilyea BB, et al: Co-morbidity and depression among the anxiety disorders: issues in diagnosis and classification. J Nerv Ment Dis 174:63–72, 1986a

Barlow DH, Blanchard EB, Vermilyea JA, et al: Generalized anxiety and generalized anxiety disorder: description and reconceptualization. Am J Psychiatry 143:40–44, 1986b

Beck AT, Ward CH, Mendelson M, et al: An inventory for measuring depression. Arch Gen Psychiatry 4:561–571, 1961

Beidel DC: Psychophysiological assessment of anxious emotional states in children. J Abnorm Psychol 97:80–82, 1988

Beidel DC, Turner SM, Dancu CV: Physiological, cognitive, and behavioral aspects of social anxiety. Behav Res Ther 23:109–117, 1985

Benca R, Matuzas W, Al-Sadir F: Social phobia, MVP, and response to imipramine. J Clin Psychopharmacol 6:50–51, 1986

Bloodstein A: A Handbook on Stuttering. The National Easter Seal Society, Chicago, 1987

Borkovec TD, Stone NM, O'Brien GT, et al: Evaluation of a clinically relevant target behavior for analogue outcome research. Behav Ther 5:503–513, 1974

Bowen RC, Cipywnyk D, D'Arcy C, et al: Alcoholism, anxiety disorders, and agoraphobia. Alcoholism (NY) 8:48–50, 1984

Bruch MA, Heimberg RC: Differences in perceptions of parental and personal characteristics between generalized and nongeneralized social phobics. J Anx Disord (in press)

Burns LE, Thorpe GL: The epidemiology of fears and phobias (with particular reference to the National Survey of Agoraphobics). J Int Med Res 5:1–7, 1977

Butler G: Exposure as a treatment for social phobia: some instructive difficulties. Behav Res Ther 23:651–657, 1985

Cameron OG, Thyer BA, Nesse RM, et al: Symptom profiles of patients with DSM-III anxiety disorders. Am J Psychiatry 143:1132–1137, 1986

Caspi A, Elder GH Jr, Bem DJ: Moving away from the world: life course patterns in shy children. Dev Psychol 24:824–831, 1988

Chaleby K: Social phobia in Saudis. Soc Psychiatry 22:167–170, 1987

Chaleby K, Ziady G: Mitral valve prolapse and social phobia. Br J Psychiatry 152:280–281, 1988

Chambers J, Yeragani VK, Keshavan MS: Phobias in India and the United Kingdom. Acta Psychiatr Scand 74:388–391, 1986

Chambless DL, Cherney J, Caputo GC, et al: Anxiety disorders and alcoholism: a study with inpatient alcoholics. J Anx Disord 1:9–40, 1987

Cohen LR, Thompson PF, Ruppel RW, et al: Assertive training: an adjunct to fluency shaping. Journal of Fluency Disorders 1:10–25, 1975

Cook EW, Melamed BG, Cuthbert BN, et al: Emotional imagery and the differential diagnosis of anxiety. J Consult Clin Psychol 56:734–740, 1988

Deltito JA, Perugi G: A case of social phobia with avoidant personality disorder treated with MAOI. Compr Psychiatry 2:255–258, 1986

Deltito JA, Stam A: Psychopharmacological treatment of avoidant personality disorder. Compr Psychiatry 30:498–504, 1989

Derogatis LR: SCL-90-R Administration, Scoring, and Procedures: Manual II. Towson, MD, Clinical Psychometric Research, 1983

de Ruiter C, Rijken H, Garssen B, et al: Comorbidity among the anxiety disorders. J Anx Disord 3:57–68, 1989

DiCarlo LM, Katz J, Batkin S: An exploratory investigation of the effect of DSM-III anxiety disorder categories using a new structured interview. Arch Gen Psychiatry 40:1070–1074, 1983

Dimsdale JE, Moss J: Plasma catecholamines in stress and exercise. JAMA 243:340–342, 1980

DiNardo PA, O'Brien GT, Barlow DH, et al: Reliability of meprobamate on stuttering behavior. J Nerv Ment Dis 128:558–561, 1983

Doctor RM: Major results of a large-scale pretreatment survey of agoraphobics, in Phobia: A Comprehensive Summary of Modern Treatments. Edited by Dupont RL. New York, Brunner/Mazel, 1982, pp 203–214

Emmelkamp PMG, Mersch PP, Vissia E, et al: Social phobia: a comparative evaluation of cognitive and behavioral interventions. Behav Res Ther 23:365–369, 1985

Falloon IRH, Lloyd GG, Harpin RE: Real-life rehearsal with nonprofessional therapists. J Nerv Ment Dis 169:180–184, 1981

Fremouw WJ, Gross R, Monroe J, et al: Empirical subtypes of performance anxiety. Behav Assess 4:179–193, 1982

Fyer AJ, Endicott J, Mannuzza S, et al: Schedule for Affective Disorders and Schizophrenia—Lifetime Version (modified for the study of anxiety disorders). New York: Anxiety Disorders Clinic, New York State Psychiatric Institute, 1985

Gengo FM, Kalonaros GC, McHugh WB: Attenuation of response to mental stress in patients with essential tremor treated with metoprolol. Arch Neurol 43:687–689, 1986

Goldfried MR, Linehan MM, Smith JL: Reduction of test anxiety through cognitive restructuring. J Consult Clin Psychol 46:32–39, 1978

Gorman JM: Panic disorders. Mod Prob Pharmacopsychiatry 22:36–90, 1987

Gorman JM, Levy GF, Liebowitz MR, et al: Effect of acute B-adrenergic blockade on lactate-induced panic. Arch Gen Psychiatry 40:1079–1082, 1983

Gorman JM, Fyer AJ, Goetz R, et al: Ventilatory physiology of patients with panic disorder. Arch Gen Psychiatry 45:31–39, 1988

Greenberg D, Stravynski A: Social phobia (letter). Br J Psychiatry 143:526, 1983

Greiner JR, Fitzgerald HE, Cooke PA, et al: Assessment of sensitivity to interpersonal stress in stutterers and non-stutterers. Journal of Communication Disorders 18:215–225, 1985

Gross RT, Fremouw WJ: Cognitive restructuring and progressive relaxation for treatment of empirical subtypes of speech-anxious subjects. Cognitive Therapy and Research 6:429–436, 1982

Hamilton M: Development of a rating scale for primary depressive illness. Br J Soc Clin Psychol 6:278–296, 1967

Harris PR: Shyness and psychological imperialism: on the dangers of ignoring the ordinary language roots of the terms we deal with. Eur J Social Psychol 14:169–181, 1984

Heimberg RG: Predicting the outcome of cognitive-behavioral treatment of social phobia. Paper presented at the annual meeting of the Society for Psychotherapy Research, Wellesley, MA, June 1986

Heimberg RG, Beckler RE, Goldfinger K, et al: Treatment of social phobia by exposure, cognitive restructuring, and homework assignments. J Nerv Ment Dis 173:236–245, 1985

Heimberg RG, Gansler D, Dodge CS: Convergent and discriminate validity of the cognitive-somatic anxiety questionnaire in a social phobic population. Behav Assess 9:379–388, 1987a

Heimberg RG, Dodge CS, Becker RE: Social phobia, in Anxiety and Stress Disorders. Edited by Michelson L, Ascher ML. New York, Guilford, 1987b, pp 280–309

Heimberg RG, Hope DA, Dodge CS, et al: DSM-III-R subtypes of social phobia: comparison of generalized social phobic patients and public speaking phobics. J Nerv Ment Dis 178:172–179, 1989

Heimberg RG, Dodge CS, Hope DA, et al: Cognitive behavioral group treatment for social phobia: comparison to a credible placebo control. Cognitive Therapy and Research 14:1–23, 1990

Holliday AR: Effect of meprobamate on stuttering. Northwest Medicine 58:837–841, 1959

Hyler SE, Rieder RD, Spitzer RL, et al: Personality Diagnostic Questionnaire (PDQ). New York, New York State Psychiatric Institute, 1983

Jerremalm A, Jansson L, Öst LG: Cognitive and physiological reactivity and the effects of different behavioral methods in the treatment of social phobia. Behav Res Ther 24:171–180, 1986

Johansson J, Öst LG: Perception of autonomic reactions and actual heart rate in phobic patients. J Behav Assess 4:133–143, 1982

Jonsson C, Engman K, Asplund O: Psychological aspects of breast reconstruction following mastectomy. Scand J Plast Reconstr Hand Surg 18:317–325, 1984

Kagan J, Reznick JS, Snidman N: Biological bases of childhood shyness. Science 240:167–171, 1988

Kanter NJ, Goldfried MR: Relative effectiveness of rational restructuring and self-control desensitization in the reduction of interpersonal anxiety. Behav Ther 10:472–490, 1979

Karno M, Golding JM, Bunam A, et al: Anxiety disorders among Mexican Americans and non-Hispanic whites in Los Angeles. J Nerv Ment Dis 177:202–209, 1989

Kasahara Y: Fear of eye-to-eye confrontation among neurotic patients in Japan, in Japanese Culture and Behavior. Edited by Lebra TS, Lebra WT. University of Hawaii Press, 1970, pp 289–387

Kasahara Y: Social phobia in Japan and Korea. East Asia Academy of Cultural Psychiatry, Department of Psychiatry, College of Medicine, Seoul National University, 1987, pp 3–14

Kent LR, Williams DE: Use of meprobamate as an adjunct to stuttering therapy. Journal of Speech and Hearing Disorders 24:64–69, 1959

Knight ML, Borden RJ: Autonomic and affective reactions of high and low socially-anxious individuals awaiting public performance. Psychophysiology 16:209–213, 1979

Koller W, Biary M, Cone S: Disability in essential tremor: effective treatment. Neurology 36:1001–1004, 1986

Lader MH: Palmar skin conductance measures in anxiety and phobia states. J Psychosom Res 11:271–281, 1967

Lang PJ, Levin DN, Miller GA, et al: Fear behavior, fear imagery, and the psychophysiology of emotion: the problem of affective response integration. J Abnorm Psychol 92:276–306, 1983

Lazarus PJ: Incidence of shyness in elementary-school age children. Psychol Rep 51:904–906, 1982

Leanderson R, Levi L: A new approach to the experimental study of stuttering and stress. Acta Oto-Laryngol Suppl 224:311–316, 1967

Lee SH: Social phobia in Korea, in Social Phobia in Japan and Korea. East Asia Academy of Cultural Psychiatry, Department of Psychiatry, College of Medicine, Seoul National University, 1987, pp 24–53

Levin AP, Schneier FM, Liebowitz MR: Social phobia: biology and pharmacology. Clin Psychol Rev 9:129–140, 1989

Levin AP, Saoud JB, Strauman T, et al: Responses of "generalized" and "discrete" social phobics during public speaking. J Anx Disord 7:207–222, 1993

Lewin MR, Guilfoyle E, McNeil DW: Distinctions between public speaking anxiety and generalized social anxiety. Paper presented at the annual meeting of Southwestern Psychological Association, Fort Worth, TX, April 1986

Liebert RM, Morris LW: Cognitive and emotional components of test anxiety: a distinction and some initial data. Psychol Rep 20:975–978, 1967

Liebowitz MR: Social phobia. Mod Probl Pharmacopsychiatry 22:141–173, 1987

Liebowitz MR, Fyer AJ, Gorman JM, et al: Lactate provocation of panic attacks, I: clinical and behavioral findings. Arch Gen Psychiatry 41:764–770, 1984

Liebowitz MR, Fyer AJ, Gorman JM, et al: Specificity of lactate infusions on social phobia versus panic disorders. Am J Psychiatry 142:947–950, 1985a

Liebowitz MR, Gorman JM, Fyer AJ, et al: Social phobia: review of a neglected anxiety disorder. Arch Gen Psychiatry 42:729–736, 1985b

Liebowitz MR, Gorman JM, Fyer AJ, et al: Pharmacotherapy of social phobia: an interim report of a placebo-controlled comparison of phenelzine and atenolol. J Clin Psychiatry 49:252–257, 1988

Ludwig RP, Lazarus PJ: Relationship between shyness in children and constricted cognitive control as measured by the Stroop Color-Word Test. J Consult Clin Psychol 51:386–389, 1983

Lydiard RB, Laraia MT, Howell EF, et al: Alprazolam in social phobia. J Clin Psychiatry 49:17–19, 1988

Mannuzza S, Fyer AJ, Klein DF, et al: Schedule for Affective Disorders and Schizophrenia—Lifetime Version (modified for the study of anxiety disorders): rationale and conceptual development. J Psychiatr Res 20:317–325, 1986

Mannuzza S, Fyer AJ, Martin LY, et al: Reliability of anxiety assessment, I: diagnostic agreement. Arch Gen Psychiatry 46:1093–1101, 1989

Marks IM: The classification of phobic disorders. Br J Psychiatry 116:377–386, 1970

Marks IM: Behavioral treatment of social phobia. Psychopharmacol Bull 21:615–618, 1985

Marks IM, Gelder MG: Different ages of onset in varieties of phobia. Am J Psychiatry 123:218–221, 1966

Marks IM, Herst ER: A survey of 1,200 agoraphobics in Britain. Soc Psychiatry 5:16–24, 1970

Marks IM, Mathews AM: Brief standard self-rating for phobic patients. Behav Res Ther 17:263–267, 1979

Maxwell RDH, Paterson JW: Meprobamate in the treatment of stuttering. BMJ #5075, April 1958, pp 873–874

McNeil DW, Lewin MR: Public speaking anxiety: a meaningful subtype of social phobia? Paper presented at the annual meeting of the Association for Advancement of Behavior Therapy, Chicago, IL, November 1986

Meichenbaum DH: Cognitive modification of test anxious college students. J Consult Clin Psychol 39:370–380, 1972

Millon T: Millon Clinical Multiaxial Inventory, 3rd Edition. Minneapolis, MN, National Computer Services, 1983

Mullaney JA, Trippett CJ: Alcohol dependence and phobias: clinical description and relevance. Br J Psychiatry 135:565–573, 1979

Munjack DJ, Brown RA, McDowell DE: Comparison of social anxiety in patients with social phobia and panic disorder. J Nerv Ment Dis 175:49–51, 1987

Myers JK, Weissman MM, Tischler GL, et al: Six-month prevalence of psychiatric disorders in three communities. Arch Gen Psychiatry 41:959–967, 1984

Neftel K, Adler R, Kappell K, et al: Stage fright in musicians: a model illustrating the effect of beta blockers. Psychosom Med 44:461–469, 1982

Noyes R, Anderson DJ, Clancey J, et al: Diazepam and propranolol in panic disorder and agoraphobia. Arch Gen Psychiatry 41:287–292, 1984

Noyes R, Crowe RR, Harris EL, et al: Relationship between panic disorder and agoraphobia: a family study. Arch Gen Psychiatry 43:227–232, 1986

Nyman D, Heimberg RG: Heterosocial anxiety among college students: a reasonable analogue to social phobia? Paper presented at the Association for Advancement of Behavior Therapy, Houston, TX, 1985

Öst LG: Age of onset in different phobias. J Abnorm Psychol 96:223–229, 1987

Öst LG, Jerremalm A, Johansson J: Individual response patterns and the effects of different behavioral methods in the treatment of social phobia. Behav Res Ther 19:1–16, 1981

Papp LA, Gorman JM, Liebowitz MR, et al: Epinephrine infusions in patients with social phobia. Am J Psychiatry 145:733–736, 1988

Pecknold J, McClure D, Appeltauer L, et al: Does tryptophan potentiate clomipramine in the treatment of agoraphobic and social phobic patients? Br J Psychiatry 140:484–490, 1982

Pfohl B, Stangl D, Zimmerman M: Structured Interview for DSM-III Personality Disorders (SIDP), 2nd Edition. Iowa City, University of Iowa College of Medicine, 1983

Pilkonis PA: Shyness, public and private, and its relationship to other measures of social behavior. Journal of Personality 45:585–595, 1977

Pohl R, Rainey J, Ortiz A, et al: Isoproterenol-induced anxiety states. Psychopharmacol Bull 21:424–427, 1985

Pollard CA, Henderson JG: Prevalence of agoraphobia: some confirmatory data. Psychol Rev 60:1305, 1987

Pollard CA, Henderson JG: Four types of social phobia in a community sample. J Nerv Ment Dis 176:440–445, 1988

Porter AK: Studies in the psychology of stuttering, XIV: stuttering phenomena in relation to size and personnel of audience. J Speech Dis 4:323–333, 1939

Ramig PR, Krieger SM, Adams MR: Vocal changes in stutterers and non-stutterers when speaking to children. Journal of Fluency Disorders 7:369–384, 1982

Rapee R, Mattick R, Murrell E: Cognitive mediation in the affective component of spontaneous panic attacks. J Behav Ther Exp Psychiatry 17:245–253, 1986

Reich J, Yates W: Family history of psychiatric disorders in social phobia. Compr Psychiatry 29:72–75, 1988a

Reich J, Yates W: A pilot study of treatment of social phobia with alprazolam. Am J Psychiatry 145:590–594, 1988b

Reich J, Noyes R, Yates W: Anxiety symptoms distinguishing social phobia from panic and generalized anxiety disorders. J Nerv Ment Dis 176:510–513, 1988

Reich J, Noyes R, Yates W: Alprazolam treatment of avoidant personality traits in social phobic patients. J Clin Psychiatry 50:91–95, 1989

Robins LN, Helzer JE, Weissman MM, et al: Lifetime prevalence of specific psychiatric disorders at three sites. Arch Gen Psychiatry 41:949–958, 1984

Rustin L, Cuhr A, Cook PJ, et al: Controlled trial of speech therapy versus oxprenolol for stammering. BMJ 283:517–518, 1981

Sanderson WC, Rapee RM, Barlow DH: The DSM-III-R revised anxiety disorder categories: descriptions and patterns of comorbidity. Paper presented at the annual meeting of the Association for Advancement of Behavior Therapy, Boston, MA, November 1987

Sarason IG: Test anxiety, attention, and the general problem of anxiety, in Stress and Anxiety, Vol 1. Edited by Spielberger CD, Sarason IG. Washington, DC, Hemisphere/Wiley, 1975, pp 165–188

Schlebusch L, Levin A: A psychological profile of women selected for augmentation mammoplasty. S Afr Med J 64:481–483, 1983

Schneier FR, Martin LY, Liebowitz MR, et al: Alcohol abuse in social phobia. J Anx Disord 3:15–23, 1989

Schuckit MA: Genetic and clinical implications of alcoholism and affective disorder. Am J Psychiatry 143:140–147, 1986

Sermas CE, Cox MD: The stutterer and stuttering: personality correlates. Journal of Fluency Disorders 7:141–158, 1982

Shafar S: Aspects of phobic illness: a study of 90 personal cases. Br J Med Psychol 49:221–236, 1976

Sheehan DV, Sheehan KE, Minichiello WE: Age of onset of phobic disorders: a reevaluation. Compr Psychiatry 22:544–553, 1981

Sheehan J, Hadley R, Gould E: Impact of authority on stuttering. J Abnorm Psychol 72(3):290–293, 1967

Sihm F, Jagd M, Pers M: Psychological assessment before and after augmentation mammoplasty. Scand J Plast Reconstr Surg Hand Surg 12:295–298, 1978

Sinnott A, Jones B, Fordham AS: Agoraphobia: a situational analysis. J Clin Psychol 37:123–127, 1981

Smail P, Stockwell T, Canter S, et al: Alcohol dependence and phobic anxiety states, I: a prevalence study. Br J Psychiatry 144:53–57, 1984

Solyom L, Ledwidge B, Solyom C: Delineating social phobia. Br J Psychiatry 149:464–470, 1986

Spielberger CD: Manual for the State-Trait Anxiety Inventory, Revised. Palo Alto, CA, Consulting Psychologists Press, 1983

Spielberger CD, Pollans CH, Worden TJ: Anxiety disorders, in Adult Psychopathology and Diagnosis. Edited by Turner SM, Hersen M. New York, Wiley, 1984, pp 263–303

Spitzer R, Williams JBW: The Structured Clinical Interview for DSM-III-R Personality Disorders. New York, Biometrics Research Department, New York State Psychiatric Institute, 1986

Spitzer R, Williams JB, Gibbon M: Structured Clinical Interview for DSM-III-R. New York, Biometrics Research Department, New York State Psychiatric Institute, 1987

Stein MB, Shea CA, Uhde TW: Social phobic symptoms in patients with panic disorder: practical and theoretical implications. Am J Psychiatry 146:235–238, 1989

Stein MB, Heuser IJ, Juncos JL, et al: Anxiety disorders in patients with Parkinson's disease. Am J Psychiatry, 147:147–220, 1990

Stravynski A, Lamontagne Y, Lavallee YJ: Clinical phobias and avoidant personality disorder among alcoholics admitted to an alcoholism rehabilitation setting. Can J Psychiatry 31:714–719, 1986

Taggart P, Carruthers M, Somerville W: Electrocardiogram, plasma catecholamines and lipids, and their modification by oxprenolol when speaking before an audience. Lancet 2:341–346, 1973

Takahashi T: Social phobia syndrome in Japan. Compr Psychiatry 30:45–52, 1989

Tancer ME, Stein MB, Gelernter CS, et al: The hypothalamic-pituitary-thyroid axis in social phobia. Am J Psychiatry 147:929–933, 1990

Thompson C, Lang A, Parkes JD, et al: A double-blind trial of clonazepam in benign essential tremor. Clin Neuropharmacol 7:83–88, 1984

Thyer BA, Parrish RT, Curtis GC, et al: Ages of onset of DSM-III anxiety disorders. Compr Psychiatry 26:113–121, 1985

Thyer BA, Parrish RT, Himle J, et al: Alcohol abuse among clinically anxious patients. Behav Res Ther 24:357–359, 1986

Trower P, Yardley K, Bryant B, et al: The treatment of social failure: a comparison of anxiety-reduction and skills acquisition procedures on two social problems. Behav Modif 2:41–60, 1978

Turner SM: The effects of personality disorder diagnosis on the outcome of social anxiety symptom reduction. Journal of Personality Disorders 1:136–143, 1987

Turner SM, Beidel DC: Empirically derived subtypes of social anxiety. Behav Ther 16:384–392, 1985

Turner SM, Beidel DC: Social phobia: clinical syndrome, diagnosis, and comorbidity. Clin Psychol Rev 9:3–18, 1989

Turner SM, Beidel DC, Dancu CV, et al: Psychopathology of social phobia and comparison to avoidant personality disorder. J Abnorm Psychol 95:389–394, 1986a

Turner SM, Beidel DC, Larkin KT: Situational determinants of social anxiety in clinic and non-clinic samples: physiological and cognitive correlates. J Consult Clin Psychol 54:523–527, 1986b

Turner SM, Beidel DC, Dancu CV, et al: An empirically derived inventory to measure social fears and anxiety: the social phobia and anxiety inventory. J Consult Clin Psychol 1:35–40, 1989

Twentyman CT, McFall RM: Behavioral training of social skills in shy males. J Consult Clin Psychol 43:384–395, 1975

Versiani M, Mundim FD, Nardi AE, et al: Tranylcypromine in social phobia. J Clin Psychopharmacol 8:279–283, 1988

Versiani M, Nardi AE, Mundim FD: Fobia social. J Bras Psiq 38:251–263, 1989

World Health Organization: ICD-10 Chapter V: Mental and Behavioral Disorders: Diagnostic Criteria for Research. Geneva, Switzerland, World Health Organization, 1990

Zimbardo PG: Shyness: What It Is, What To Do About It. Boston, MA, Addison-Wesley, 1977

Chapter 18

Obsessive-Compulsive Disorder

Edna B. Foa, Ph.D., Michael Jenike, M.D.,
Michael J. Kozak, Ph.D., Russell Joffe, M.D., Lee Baer, Ph.D.,
David Pauls, Ph.D., Deborah C. Beidel, Ph.D.,
Steven A. Rasmussen, M.D., Wayne Goodman, M.D.,
Richard P. Swinson, M.D., F.R.C.P., Eric Hollander, M.D., and
Samuel M. Turner, Ph.D.

Statement of the Issues

The changes proposed for the obsessive-compulsive disorder (OCD) criteria in DSM-IV reflect the following issues:

1. The DSM-III-R (American Psychiatric Association 1987) criteria for OCD imply that obsessions are distressing. It is proposed to make this criterion explicit.
2. The DSM-III-R OCD criteria do not distinguish between obsessions and worries, hypochondriacal concerns, and body dysmorphic preoccupations.
3. The DSM-III-R criteria for OCD emphasize that individuals with OCD recognize their obsessions and compulsions as senseless, unreasonable, or excessive. This emphasis seems to contradict empirical data and clinical observations.
4. The DSM-III-R criteria for obsessions imply that some compulsions are mental acts (e.g., silent praying, repeating phrases). However, in the criteria for compulsions, only behavioral acts are mentioned.
5. ICD-10 (World Health Organization 1990) subdivides OCD into three categories: mostly obsessions, mostly compulsions, both obsessions and compulsions. Is this division useful? Should DSM-IV adopt it?

Three literature reviews were prepared to address issue 2, and one review was done on issue 3. Issues 4 and 5 were considered in a paper analyzing problems with current criteria and will be addressed as part of a field study. The issues discussed in these reviews are summarized below. Three additional reviews addressed issues more relevant to descriptive text than to criteria (Gilles de la Tourette's Syndrome and Obsessive-Compulsive Disorder [Pauls, unpublished]; Biological Aspects of Obsessive-Compulsive Disorder [Joffe and Swinson, unpublished]; The Relationship Between Obsessive-Compulsive Personality and Obsessive-Compulsive Disorder [Jenike and Baer, unpublished]) and therefore are not summarized here.

Significance of the Issues

1. Defining Obsessions as Distressing and Unwanted

DSM-III-R implies but does not explicitly state that the content of obsessions is aversive. Therefore, preoccupation with positive events, as in daydreaming about a sex partner, might be diagnosed as an obsession. To disallow this, it is proposed that DSM-IV explicitly state that the content of obsessions is unpleasant for the patient. This is important because successful behavioral and pharmacotherapies for OCD seem to operate in part by reducing distress associated with obsessions.

2. Distinction Between Obsessions and Worries, Hypochondriacal Concerns, and Body Dysmorphic Preoccupations

Dwelling on unpleasant thoughts is common to several disorders, notably generalized anxiety disorder (GAD), hypochondriasis, and body dysmorphic disorder. To obviate misdiagnoses, the features that distinguish obsessions from worries and preoccupations should be clearly stated in the criteria for obsessions. This is particularly important for patients with obsessions but no compulsions.

3. Should the Criteria for OCD Retain the Requirements That Obsessions and Compulsions Be Viewed by the Patient as Senseless or Excessive?

Early descriptions of OCD noted that patients' thinking is characterized by irrationality and insanity (Westphal 1878). However, the influence of Janet (1908) and Schneider (1925), who argued that obsessions are recognized by patients as absurd and ego-alien, strongly contributed to the various DSM versions. The lack of such recognition that is sometimes observed in OCD received little attention. More recently, there has been renewed acknowledgment in the literature that at least some individuals with OCD do not recognize their obsessions or compulsions as senseless. If patients are broadly distributed on the recognition continuum, then the idea that obsessions and compulsions are viewed as senseless should be de-emphasized in DSM-IV; otherwise, patients who fall on the far end of the continuum may be erroneously excluded.

4. Are There Mental Compulsions?

The DSM-IV seems simultaneously to maintain the traditional view that obsessions are mental events and compulsions are behavioral events and to endorse the view that thoughts can be compulsions (i.e., can reduce obsessional distress). This leads to confusion because mental compulsions ("neutralizing thoughts") are considered under the rubric of obsessions. In accordance with the traditional view, DSM-III-R describes compulsions as "repetitive, purposeful, and intentional behaviors which are designed to neutralize or prevent discomfort." The idea that thoughts can also neutralize or prevent discomfort is absent from the definition of compulsions. This ambiguity can lead to diagnosing a patient as pure obsessional when obsessions and only mental compulsions are present. Because there is evidence that different behavioral treatments are effective for obsessions and for compulsions, it is important to diagnose these accurately.

5. Should DSM-IV Adopt the ICD-10 Subcategories of a) Obsessions b) Compulsions, and c) Obsessions and Compulsions?

This issue is related to the question mentioned above concerning mental versus behavioral rituals, in that the ICD-10 subcategories are based on a distinction between obsessions and compulsions. One justification for a categorization is the extent to which "natural" groupings of symptoms occur. Another justification is different responses to treatment. As mentioned above, patients with pure obsessions respond differently to behavioral treatment than patients with obsessions and compulsions.

Methods and Results

1. Are Obsessions Distressing?

DSM-III-R reflects the view about OCD that emphasizes the dynamic functional relationship between obsessions and compulsions. Accordingly, obsessions are events that elicit distress, such as thoughts of being contaminated, thoughts of being responsible for a catastrophe, impulses to kill one's child, or blasphemous images.

In DSM-III-R, however, the view that obsessions are distressing is expressed only indirectly in the definition of obsessions and by implication in the definition of compulsions. Accordingly, although obsessions are not explicitly defined as aversive, the individual is said to attempt to "ignore, suppress, or neutralize" them. It is explicitly stated that compulsive behavior is designed to reduce discomfort. It has been proposed to correct this ambiguity in DSM-IV by specifying that obsessions "are experienced as intrusive and unwanted and cause marked anxiety or distress." No paper was commissioned on this question. However, below is a summary of evidence for the view that obsessions are distressing.

Evidence that obsessions increase anxiety comes from findings indicating that ruminative thoughts give rise to greater elevation of heart rate and increased skin conductance response than do neutral thoughts (Boulougouris et al. 1977; Rabavilas and Boulougouris 1974). In addition, both actual and imaginary confrontation with contamination has been found to result in increases in heart rate, subjective anxiety (Hodgson and Rachman 1972; Kozak et al. 1988) and skin conductance response (Hornsveld et al. 1979). Such physiological changes have been repeatedly found to be associated with anxiety.

2. Distinction Between Obsessions and Worries, Hypochondriacal Concerns, and Preoccupations

On the Nature of Obsessional Thoughts and Worry:
Similarities and Dissimilarities[1]

A computer search of the Medline and Psychological Abstracts databases was used to identify articles addressing the issue of obsessional thought, worry, and the relationship between the two constructs. Key words included *obsessional thoughts, rumination, obsessive ideation, obsessionality, intrusive thoughts, worry, anxiety,* and *depression.* The search was conducted on literature published from 1970 to 1989. In addition, the reference sections of articles identified in this search were screened, as were major research articles and books in the area of OCD that were published from 1980 to 1989.

The terms *obsession* and *worry* are commonly used by the lay public and mental health professionals alike to refer to thinking of a perseverative nature. Similarly, the term *rumination* is used to describe both obsessional thought processes and worry. Throughout the psychological and psychiatric literature, all three terms have been used interchangeably to describe cognitive processes that are part of the obsessive-compulsive syndrome. The focus of this review was the relationship between worry and obsessions. Unfortunately, little empirical research exists directly exploring the relationship between obsessions and worry. There is a consid-

---

[1]Turner and Beidel.

erable descriptive literature on the phenomenology of obsessional behavior and conceptual and theoretical speculation on the nature of obsessive ideation. Also, there is an emerging literature on worry as it is manifested in both normal and psychopathological states. These literatures were considered in an effort to compare and contrast these two types of cognitive phenomena.

Phenomenology of obsessional thinking.   Obsessions are repetitive and intrusive thoughts, images, and impulses that are considered unacceptable by the individual, lead to subjective distress, and are accompanied by some form of resistance. The presence of these unwanted and uncontrollable mental events is typically viewed as "ego-alien" and may be considered senseless, repugnant, blasphemous, obscene, or some combination of these. In approximately 70%–75% of cases, the obsessions are accompanied by one or more compulsions (Akhtar et al. 1975). The requirement that patients resist the unwanted obsessions has been seen as an important characteristic of the disorder and is incorporated into the DSM-III-R definition of obsession: "the person attempts to ignore or suppress such thoughts or impulses or to neutralize them with some other thought or action" (p. 245). Furthermore, the individual "recognizes that the obsessions are the product of his or her own mind, and are not imposed from without" (p. 245). The latter point is particularly important because it allows clear differentiation of obsessions from ideation of control and thought insertion associated with psychotic states. Although the internally derived quality of obsessive ideation is central to the definition, it should be noted that obsessions can be instigated by the external environment (Likierman and Rachman 1980). For example, following the onset of OCD, various stimuli in the environment such as sharp objects, words, or individuals can cue the onset of obsessive ideation. The triggering of obsessions by environmental factors is consistent with the observation that episodes of obsessions and compulsions often wax and wane with environmental stress (Rasmussen and Tsuang 1984) and is certainly consistent with our own clinical experience with OCD patients.

Recently, there have been a number of efforts directed at classifying obsessional phenomena. The most common method of classification is based on form and content. Akhtar et al. (1975) identified six forms of obsessions: obsessive doubt, obsessive thinking, obsessive impulse, obsessive fear, obsessive image, and a miscellaneous form. The latter relates to phenomena that appear obsessional in nature but cannot be classified in any of the five other categories. An example of the miscellaneous type, presented by Akhtar et al. (1975), was the repeated and unwanted intrusion into consciousness of a musical tune.

In addition to the six forms, Akhtar et al. (1975) delineated six categories of content: dirt and contamination, aggression, inanimate-interpersonal (e.g., locks, bolts, and other safety devices, orderliness in arrangement), sex, religion, and miscellaneous. The miscellaneous category included such obsessions as those related to the human anatomy, historical facts, and musical hits. The most common obsessional form was doubting, which was experienced by 74% of the sample, whereas dirt and contamination was the most prominent obsessional content (46%). Akhtar et al. cogently pointed out that both the form and content of obsessions are likely to be influenced by cultural patterns and that cross-cultural studies are necessary to fully address this issue.

Khanna and Channabasavanna (1988) also generated six forms that seem to essentially describe the same behaviors but with slightly different terminology. Their categories included obsessional thought, obsessional doubts, obsessional fears, obsessional urges, obsessional images, and obsessive convictions. These authors found that the single most common form was obsessional doubt (12.33%). Six content areas of obsessions were delineated (dirt and contamination, religion, sex, death, illness, aggression), with dirt and contamination the most prominent theme (14.25%), confirming Akhtar et al.'s (1975) findings. As in the case of form, there were few differences in the classification of obsessional content. Whereas Akhtar et al. (1975) included illness in the dirt and contamination category, Khanna and Channabasavanna (1988) classified illness as a separate category. Also, these authors did not include a miscellaneous category and placed death in an entirely separate category.

Employing a somewhat different strategy, Mavissakalian (1979) attempted to forge a unitary view of obsessional and compulsive phenomena by proposing a functional classification system. In this conceptualization, obsessions were defined as anxiety producing and compulsions as anxiety reducing. External and internal obsessive-compulsive behavior was considered to be functionally equivalent. Four forms were proposed: obsessions, obsessions plus successful compulsions (anxiety reducing), obsessions plus obsessionalized compulsions (anxiety increasing), and rituals consisting mainly of stereotyped overt or covert behaviors (autonomous of anxiety and/or obsessions). A very similar characterization was made by Foa and Tillmanns (1980). These are interesting attempts at classification that have potential theoretical as well as treatment implications. However, because in these classification systems obsessions are intimately intertwined with compulsions, they are not discussed further here.

Controllability, uncontrollability, and obsessional ideation. Although issues of controllability are most often studied in relation to depression, they are emerging as an important area of inquiry for the anxiety disorders as well (cf. Barlow 1988). The inability to control unwanted, intrusive, and often abhorrent thoughts, images, or impulses is central to our current concept of obsessional thinking, and it seems clear that the uncontrollability of obsessions is a source of distress for OCD patients.

Generally, it has been assumed that much of the uncontrollability was related to the unpleasant and frequently unacceptable themes of obsessions and to their ability to instigate arousal (e.g., Rachman and Hodgson 1980). Indeed, survey data have shown that the uncontrollability of intrusive thoughts is associated with the subjective perception of the thought in a negative light and with accompanying arousal (e.g., Salkovskis 1985). However, Edwards and Dickerson (1987) reported that intrusive thoughts of a pleasant nature were perceived as equally difficult to control as unpleasant intrusive thoughts. In a study designed to directly assess the relationship of unpleasantness and uncontrollability, England and Dickerson (1988) concluded that unpleasantness of the theme had little relationship to uncontrollability. This is an interesting finding, and should it be replicated with a patient population, additional consideration of this issue will be required.

In a series of three studies, Rachman and de Silva (1978) reported that normal and abnormal obsessions were similar in form and meaning and somewhat similar in content. Abnormal obsessions tended to last longer and were more discomforting, more intense, and more frequent. They were also more strongly resisted and harder to dismiss. Salkovskis and Harrison (1984) replicated part of the Rachman and de Silva study and reported similar results.

Some characteristics of worry and its relationship to obsessions.   Until recently, there was little empirical research on worry, a phenomenon that is ubiquitous, easily understood by the lay population, and associated with many daily experiences. Like obsessions, worry can be found in normal and abnormal populations (Borkovec et al. 1991). In an early definition of worry, Borkovec et al. (1983) defined it as "a chain of thoughts and images, negatively affect-laden and relatively uncontrollable. The worry process represents an attempt to engage in mental problem-solving on an issue whose outcome is uncertain but contains the possibility of one or more negative outcomes. Consequently, worry relates closely to fear process" (p. 10). Borkovec et al. (1983) further noted that worry can at times be spontaneous and at other times be cued by fear-producing stimuli. Defined in this fashion, the similarity to obsessional thinking is readily apparent. Studies of intrusive thinking in normal subjects have been applied when discussing the parameters of worry. Similarly, the relationship of worry to characteristics such as uncontrollability, unpleasantness, and mood have been discussed. However, it is unclear if this literature applies to the concept of worry, because its content seems to differ from that of obsessionality.

Although frequently used interchangeably in the literature (and interchangeably with the term *worry* as well), a number of authors have pointed to differences between obsessions and ruminations. For example, Beech (1974) defined ruminations as prolonged and often fruitless attempts to solve a self-set problem to which there is no real or apparent solution. Similarly, Woodruff et al. (1974) described obsessive ideas as thoughts that repeatedly intrude into consciousness, whereas ruminations were defined as prolonged inconclusive thinking about a subject. Considering these definitions, worry appears to most approximate rumination. Also, implied in these definitions is the notion that ruminations are self-initiated, a major difference from the intrusive nature of obsessions. The tendency to worry or ruminate about issues of concern is pervasive and seems to be related to an endless number of encounters associated with the normal course of daily living. Thus, one is likely to be concerned about issues of health, finances, academic performance, and the like. In making the differentiation from what was termed *morbid preoccupation,* Hoogduin (1986) noted that "the content of the thought is usually connected with real problems or experiences that cause unhappiness. It is more often than not consistent with the patient's personality and/or previous history. Obsessional thoughts by contrast, usually conflict with the personality norms, and previous history" (p. 40). There is a considerable literature on the worry associated with test anxiety, a highly prevalent condition among young school-children and to some extent among students in higher education. Although intense worry is associated with the anticipation of test-taking and may be uncontrollable at that time, such individuals do not tend to be worried about test-taking to a great degree in the absence of needing to take a test (Liebert and Morris 1967). The implication of this is clear: worry seems to be largely self-initiated and to be in response to a specific circumstance.

Worry or apprehensive expectation is considered to be the core feature of GAD (Barlow 1988) and is a major feature of the DSM-III-R criteria. In examining the domains of worry in GAD patients, Sanderson and Barlow (1986) reported that the most common sphere of worry related to life circumstances (e.g., family, money, work, and illness). In a later study from the same laboratory, Craske et al. (1988) used these categories in addition to a miscellaneous category to examine the worries of normal subjects and GAD patients. The worries of GAD patients and normal subjects did fit into these categories, but as might be expected, the worries of the patient group were more intense. Also, 64% of the GAD patients compared to 88% of the normals identified a specific precipitant to their worries. Finally, GAD patients considered their worries to be less controllable than did the normal subjects. Similarly, Borkovec et al. (1991) reported that the most frequent worries reported by GAD patients in their clinic were family/interpersonal issues and the miscellaneous category, whereas illness/health/injury was the least reported. To reiterate, worry appears to be more self-induced and appears to be related to current ongoing difficulties more than obsessions. Much of what we know about worry is derived from the study of GAD, which in DSM-III-R is defined primarily by maladaptive worrying.

Clearly, the content of worries seen in GAD patients is rather different from the content of obsessions in OCD patients. Thus, GAD patients do not often report the concern with dirt and contamination, aggressive impulses, or horrific images so characteristic of OCD. In many instances, it appears that the onset is more often self-initiated, even if there is some perception of uncontrollability, but worries also seem to be associated with mood. It is unclear just how intrusive are the worries associated with GAD. A second major difference appears to be the form of the obsessions when compared to worries. Thus, images and impulses do not appear to be part of the GAD picture. Worries typically appear in the form of a thought. Consistent with this view, Borkovec et al. (1991) redefined worry as involving "predominantly conceptual, verbal linguistic, as opposed to imaginal, activity in both normals and GAD clients" (p. 22).

Attempts by GAD patients to resist worrying were not different from attempts by normal control subjects, 64.9% versus 64.7%, respectively (Craske et al. 1988). Yet, individuals with obsessions are known to consistently struggle against the intrusive ideation, and this appears to be one of the defining characteristics of the condition.

Discussion. Whereas the terms *worry* and *rumination* refer to repetitive thoughts that are typically related to normal experiences of everyday living, obsessions frequently appear in the form of thoughts, images, and impulses. In addition, obsessions tend to be related to themes of dirt/contamination, religion, sex, and aggression as opposed to the issues related to family, money, and work that are frequently identified as topics of worry in GAD patients. Both OCD and GAD patients may report concerns related to health or illness. Although worry and obsessions are reported to be experienced as uncontrollable, and both may be related to disturbance in mood, worry does not appear to be as intrusive as obsessions, and worry does not appear to be experienced as ego-dystonic. Thus, the major differences between worry and obsessionality appear to be in the form and content of the cognitive processes rather than in the individual's response to the process itself.

There is some confusing use of terminology related to rumination, worry, and obsessions, making it somewhat difficult to ascertain exactly what is being described in some studies. With respect to the relationship of worry to obsessions, one must conclude that, despite some similarities, worry, particularly as it is associated with GAD, refers to a substantially different cognitive process than that in characteristic obsessions. Further research with normal and patient populations is needed, however, before the distinction between these apparently different cognitive processes can be sharpened.

Hypochondriasis and OCD[2]

A systematic review of the psychiatric and psychological literature was completed on the following topics: 1) all empirical studies of hypochondriasis dating back to 1960, 2) all empirical studies of OCD and its relationship to hypochondriacal symptoms dating back to 1960, 3) all empirical studies of panic disorder and its relationship to hypochondriacal symptoms dating back to 1960, and 4) all empirical studies of depression and its relationship to hypochondriacal symptoms dating back to 1960. These reviews included a Medline search on each topic that covered the time span of 1970–1989. The searches were extended to 1960 through the use of cross-referencing of relevant articles. Citations were limited to articles and books published in the English language about human subjects. No studies were excluded on the basis of their definition of hypochondriasis, but the criteria provided in each study were recorded.

In addition, results were drawn from an as yet unpublished study of 575 patients meeting DSM-III-R criteria for OCD who had primary somatic obsessions accompanied by checking compulsions and the need to ask or confess (Goodman et al. 1989a). These patients were drawn from 20 geographically distinct sites (for details, see DeVeaugh-Geiss et al. 1989). Patients were required to have had OCD for at least 1 year prior to entrance into the study to meet inclusion criteria. Patients with concurrent Axis I pathology including a diagnosis of primary major depression, panic disorder, or Tourette's syndrome were excluded as were patients with significant medical problems.

Studies of the clinical features of hypochondriasis. Most of these studies have been directed toward the question of whether there is a distinct clinical entity of primary hypochondriasis. In a retrospective study, Kenyon (1964) found that of 512 patients who were given a diagnosis of hypochondriasis, 301 were primary (58%). Another large sample of inpatients with prominent hypochondriacal symptoms contained only a small percentage who had primary hypochondriasis without another concomitant diagnosis (Ladee 1966). Pilowsky (1970) interviewed 147 psychiatric inpatients and outpatients whose dominant presenting clinical problem was an overriding concern or fear about health or disease: 45% were classified as having primary hypochondriasis, and 55% were felt to be secondary to other Axis I diagnoses. Obsessional symptoms were present in 29% of the primary and 17% of the secondary hypochondriacal patients. In the only clinical study of hypochondriasis that attempted to use DSM-III (American Psychiatric Association 1980)

---

[2]Rasmussen and Goodman.

diagnoses, Kellner (1986) found that 13 of 36 patients had hypochondriasis alone, whereas 23 of 36 had concomitant Axis I disorders.

Two recent studies have examined the validity of the DSM-III criteria for hypochondriasis. Barsky et al. (1986) assessed 92 consecutive outpatients with the Whitely Index, the MMPI, SCL-90, and the Beck Depression Inventory. The major DSM-III-R criteria for hypochondriasis, disease conviction, disease fear, and bodily preoccupation were confirmed and showed a significant degree of intercorrelation. In a more recent study, Kellner et al. (1989) compared 21 patients meeting DSM-III criteria for hypochondriasis with matched groups of psychiatric control subjects: patients drawn from a general medical practice and hospital employees. The hypochondriacal patients were found to have significantly greater somatic and anxiety-related symptoms than the control groups.

Studies of hypochondriacal symptoms in other anxiety and affective disorders. Several studies have noted that there is a high frequency of hypochondriacal symptoms in patients with primary diagnoses of OCD, panic disorder, phobic disorders, and major depression. The significant comorbidity and the difficulty in determining which symptoms are primary or dominant complicate the differential diagnosis. This is particularly true with major depression, where many of the depressions are likely to be secondary to the emotional and cognitive consequences of the hypochondriacal fears and beliefs. In a study of 105 patients who had primary depression, 18% were also found to have an illness phobia (Stenback and Jalava 1962). A subsequent analysis of data from 143 paranoid psychotic patients with mixed diagnoses found that 15% had hypochondriacal fears (Stenback and Rimon 1964). Sheehan et al. (1980) found that in a consecutive series of 100 patients meeting criteria for panic disorder, 63% had fears of physical illness and 83% had fears of losing their minds and going crazy. Finally, Rasmussen and Tsuang (1986) reported that 35% of patients meeting DSM-III criteria for OCD had somatic obsessions. The frequency of hypochondriacal symptoms in two much larger unpublished studies of OCD patients is reported below.

Relationship of hypochondriasis to OCD. The fear or belief that one is developing a serious illness can be seen as a type of obsession. Recent studies in OCD psychotic patients have pointed to the fact that resistance and insight are on a continuum and that they can vary in degree not only between individuals but also in a given individual's course of illness. Thus, the conviction that one has a serious illness (Insel and Akiskal 1986) found in hypochondriasis can also be seen in OCD. To date, there has been no study of primary hypochondriasis that has determined the incidence of other obsessions and compulsions in that population. Evidence has recently become available from two large databases that the incidence of somatic obsessions in OCD is high. A smaller percentage of these patients had somatic obsessions as their principal presenting symptoms. Analysis of data from more than 900 patients with a DSM-III-R diagnosis of OCD (575 patients from Goodman et al. [1989a] and 325 patients from Rasmussen's clinic at Brown University) have shown that 20%–30% have somatic obsessions. Of that subgroup, 3%–4% have somatic obsessions as their presenting symptom. These patients meet criteria for both OCD and hypochondriasis. These data could lead one to hypothesize that the entity known as primary hypochondriasis should be subcategorized under the anxiety disorders or even under OCD. However, due to the lack of empirical studies on hypochondriasis since the introduction of DSM-III, any such changes for DSM-IV would be at best premature.

Discussion.   If the clinical entity of primary hypochondriasis exists, what is its relationship to OCD? Most of the articles and books that were reviewed give little or no attention to this topic. As media attention has brought many heretofore untreated OCD patients to obsessive disorders clinics, more patients with somatic obsessions have come to clinical attention. It is possible that patients who have been diagnosed as having hypochondriasis in the past are truly obsessive-compulsive or obsessive-compulsive with psychotic features. The ambiguity about whether this might be true is heightened by the similarity in definitions for obsessions and hypochondriasis. For hypochondriasis, the essential feature is preoccupation with the fear of having or the belief that one has a serious disease. If the hypochondriacal fear/thought is resisted, then it would meet the criteria for an obsession. If the belief is irrational and the patient is convinced that it is true, it would meet criteria for delusional disorder or OCD with psychotic features. Although we know that obsessive-compulsive patients can present as having primary somatic obsessions with checking compulsions, we do not know whether patients who were previously defined as having primary hypochondriasis also manifested other signs and symptoms consistent with either OCD or delusional disorder. No study of hypochondriacal patients has examined whether they have other symptoms of panic, OCD, or generalized anxiety. In summary, although there appears to be a marked similarity in the description of hypochondriasis and OCD in DSM-III-R, more empirical data are needed to define the relationship between the two disorders.

Body Dysmorphic Disorder and Its Relationship to OCD[3]

A search was conducted of the psychiatric and psychological literature for all studies concerned with body dysmorphic disorder. The review included a computer search

---

[3]Hollander.

with Medline, Psychlit, and Medlars II with terms such as *body dysmorphic disorder*, *monosymptomatic hypochondriasis*, and *dysmorphophobia* covering the period from 1974 to 1989. The computer search was confined to research concerning human subjects. The reference lists of recent review articles were also reviewed.

The review included studies that provided data on diagnostic issues, clinical course, treatment, etiology, and relationship to OCD and other disorders. The review revealed that research on body dysmorphic disorder is still in a primitive state with no existing large controlled studies of body dysmorphic disorder or of comparisons with OCD. The bulk of the literature consists of anecdotal case reports and a few analogue studies in nonclinical populations.

Relationship to OCD.   Patients with body dysmorphic disorder have repetitive, persistent thoughts about their perceived body defects. Because obsessions are defined as persistent ideas or thoughts that are experienced, at least initially, as intrusive or senseless, this definition could conceivably include patients with body dysmorphic disorder. However, some body dysmorphic patients experience their overvalued beliefs as ego-syntonic rather than ego-dystonic. This is somewhat problematic because OCD typically, but not always, is characterized by ego-dystonic obsessions.

However, this issue of ego-dystonic versus ego-syntonic may also be related to issues of uncertainty versus certainty. A review and phenomenological analysis of OCD suggested that delusions (ego-syntonic certainty) can arise in the course of this illness (Insel and Akiskal 1986). These delusions do not signify a schizophrenic diagnosis but represent generally transiently reactive affective or paranoid psychoses. The authors argued that OCD represented a psychopathological spectrum varying along a continuum of insight, with patients at the extreme end having an "obsessive-compulsive psychosis." Hollander et al. (1989) argued the same for body dysmorphic disorder, that is, that patients lie along a continuum of insight or uncertainty. Patients at the extreme end who are currently classified as delusional disorder, somatic subtype, or as hypochondriacal psychosis may be considered as body dysmorphic disorder psychosis. These patients would experience ego-syntonic symptoms.

Some have suggested that "obsessive-compulsiveness" is a main factor in dysmorphophobia (Hunecke and Bosse 1985). As noted above, obsessional or compulsive traits are a hallmark of this disorder. However, obsessive-compulsive personality and obsessive-compulsive traits differ from OCD. Most patients with OCD do not have coexistent obsessive-compulsive personality disorder. In addition, most patients with obsessive-compulsive personality do not go on to develop OCD (Rasmussen and Tsuang 1986). Finally, obsessive-compulsive symptoms or traits may be identical to features of OCD but differ in terms of severity, because they do not cause distress or interfere with functioning. Nevertheless, there seems to be a high rate of OCD, obsessive-compulsive symptoms, and obsessive-compulsive personality traits described in cases of body dysmorphic disorder patients with chronic monosymptomatic psychogenic eye pain who failed to respond to a wide variety of treatments and killed themselves (Bebbington 1976).

In a 15-year follow-up study of 187 patients who had a rhinoplasty, those patients who had the operation for aesthetic reasons had a significantly higher rate of severe neurosis or schizophrenia than those who had the operation following disease or injury (Connolly and Gipson 1978). Of 86 patients who had the operation for aesthetic reasons, 32 were severely neurotic and 6 were schizophrenic at follow-up, suggesting that dysmorphophobia was an ominous symptom.

Follow-up studies of OCD are also limited, but one study reported that the course of OCD could be divided into three categories: 1) unremitting and chronic, 2) phasic with periods of complete remission, and 3) episodic with incomplete remissions (Goodwin et al. 1969). DSM-III-R states that the course is usually chronic with waxing and waning symptoms. Thus, both disorders appear to have a chronic course.

It has been noted that life events that cause distress are associated with the development of hypochondriacal concerns (Kellner et al. 1983). OCD also seems to arise during certain developmental stages associated with distress.

Patients with OCD are felt to manifest abnormality of central serotonergic functions based on pharmacological response (Thoren et al. 1980a) and cerebrospinal fluid (Thoren et al. 1980b), and peripheral platelet (Flament et al. 1985) findings. Furthermore, administration of oral m-chlorophenyl-piperazine (m-CPP), a selective 5-HT agonist, has been shown to transiently exacerbate OCD symptoms (Zohar et al. 1987). If body dysmorphic disorder patients respond preferentially to serotonin reuptake inhibitors, this is consistent with possible serotonergic dysregulation. There have been reports of exacerbation of body dysmorphic symptoms of delusional intensity with smoking of marijuana (Hollander et al. 1989), which has central 5-HT effects. However, this is not a selective 5-HT provocative test, because marijuana affects several other neurotransmitter systems, including acetylcholine. A fascinating case report of a woman who developed body dysmorphic disorder following chronic abuse of cyproheptadine, a serotonin antagonist, does make a serotonergic etiology intriguing (Craven and Rodin 1987).

An alternative hypothesis is that OCD involves organic disturbance. In particular, there are reports of the onset of OCD following encephalitis and meningitis (Grimshaw 1964; Schilder 1938). There are also reports of body dysmorphic disorder occurring following infection in children (Carek and Santos 1984) and following subacute sclerosing panencephalitis in early adulthood (Salib 1988).

Discussion.   A hallmark of body dysmorphic disorder is an obsessive preoccupation with an imagined body defect, sometimes coupled with compulsive checking behavior. Thus, it makes some clinical sense that there might be a relationship between body dysmorphic disorder and OCD. The data described above document the potential clinical importance of determining obsessive-compulsive symptoms in patients with body dysmorphic disorder, as well as in looking for body dysmorphic symptoms in patients with OCD.

At first glance, the notion of including body dysmorphic disorder as a subgroup of OCD or noting the relationship between the disorders might appear to meet some of the criteria for change for DSM-IV outlined previously:

1. Clarifying the relationship between body dysmorphic disorder and OCD might enhance communication regarding the notion of OCD-related disorders.

2. In terms of clinical utility, a number of clinicians have noted that obsessive-compulsive symptoms or traits are present in, and in fact are a hallmark of, body dysmorphic disorder. Furthermore, the classification of body dysmorphic disorder as a somatoform disorder and as a delusional disorder, somatic subtype, makes it awkward to classify individual patients. Their diagnosis may change from a somatoform to a delusional disorder as they progress through different stages of the same illness.

3. The lack of systematic studies of body dysmorphic disorder makes it difficult to assess the validity of body dysmorphic disorder as a subgroup of OCD. However, in terms of predicting the clinical course of illness, body dysmorphic disorder appears to have a chronic course if untreated, whereas the course of OCD varies from chronic to fluctuating. Thus, the occurrence of body dysmorphic disorder might be predictive of a chronic course of illness. However, both body dysmorphic disorder and OCD are frequently confounded by coexisting affective, anxiety, and personality disorders, which might alter the clinical course.

4. External validators, such as age at onset, clinical course, comorbidity, impairment, prevalence, treatment implications, and possible etiologies do suggest a close relationship between the disorders.

Obsessions, Overvalued Ideas, and Delusions in OCD[4]

A literature search for the years 1983–1988 was conducted with the following key words: *overvalued ideation, delusions and OCD, OCD and schizophrenia,* and *OCD*

---

[4]Kozak and Foa.

and psychosis. Of the 22 articles identified, 11 were judged to be relevant to this issue. Additional articles were identified from the references cited in these articles. Two unpublished manuscripts were also included. Special weight was given to papers that included data that had been collected systematically and to seminal writings on the topic. Little weight was afforded to papers drawing conclusions from anecdotal evidence or to brief letters to the editor.

Clarification of concepts. According to DSM-III-R, obsessions are persistent ideas, thoughts, impulses, or images that are experienced initially as intrusive and senseless. They are recognized by patients as products of their own minds and are often resisted. Overvalued ideation (OVI) is described as an "almost unshakable" belief that can be acknowledged as potentially unfounded only after considerable discussion. Delusions are not defined, but at least one distinguishing characteristic is implied—that they are usually fixed convictions that cannot be shaken.

These concepts are quite ambiguous. For example, the distinction between OVI and delusions seems to rest on a subtle difference in the "shakability" of the belief and cannot be easily established. DSM-III-R also provides no formal way to distinguish obsessions from OVI. The absence of such a distinction is important because OCD patients present a continuum of strength of belief in the senselessness of their obsessions and compulsions. Therefore, the point at which obsessions become overvalued ideas can be empirically difficult to ascertain.

The ambiguities in the DSM-III-R approach to obsessions, OVI, and delusions reflect the difficulties with these concepts that exist in the psychiatric literature. The concept of the overvalued idea was developed by Wernike (1900), who construed it as a solitary belief that was felt to be justified and that strongly determined actions. Subsequently, Jaspers (1959) defined OVI as understandable (*verständlich*) convictions that are wrongly taken to be true. He distinguished OVI from delusions, the content of which is not reasonably understandable (*undverständlich*). Fish (in Hamilton 1974) similarly distinguished between OVI and delusions but also emphasized a discrepancy between belief and action in delusions versus a concordance between belief and action in OVI.

As examples of OVI, McKenna (1984) listed the querulous paranoid state, morbid jealousy, hypochondriasis, and anorexia nervosa. Whereas these phenomena are examples that illustrate that OVI is nonintrusive, unresisted, and not seen as senseless, they leave unclear McKenna's distinction between OVI and delusion. This is especially troublesome because he seems to embrace Jaspers's notion that delusions are characterized by an "undefinable but easily recognizable alien quality" (McKenna 1984, p. 583). This traditional view that delusions have an important "undefinable" quality that distinguishes them from OVI constitutes an unsatisfactory resolution of this issue.

Psychotic manifestations and OCD.   Janet (1908) and Schneider (1925) offered clear criteria for OCD: 1) subjective feeling of being forced or compelled to think, feel, or act; 2) content of the obsession is perceived as absurd or nonsensical and ego-alien; 3) the obsession is resisted.

Clinicians recognize that many obsessive-compulsive patients do not "fit" this definition. Following Lewis (1935), Solyom et al. (1985) noted that not all obsessive patients report the subjective feeling of forced thoughts or action, nor do all OCD patients recognize the senselessness of their obsessions or rituals. They further noted Schneider's (1925) observation that insight was present only "upon quiet reflection." According to Solyom et al. 1985, "when the resistance becomes zero, the content of the thought is accepted and the obsession becomes a delusion" (p. 177).

In the DSM-III-R, a major diagnostic criterion for psychosis is impaired reality testing, and the presence of delusions constitute a strong indicator of such impairment. Thus, OCD patients who perceive their obsessions as sensible and do not resist them would be considered delusional and therefore psychotic. The observation that some OCD patients have psychotic features has also been made by Insel and Akiskal (1986). On the basis of case reports, they argued that psychotic experiences belong to the severe end of the obsessive-compulsive spectrum.

Solyom et al. (1985) studied 45 OCD patients, 8 of whom differed from typical OCD patients in that they had severely debilitating main obsessions "bordering on the delusional" but showed no schizophrenic symptoms. Differences in etiology and prognosis between the typical and atypical groups were examined via structured interviews and standardized questionnaires. Because debilitation was a criterion for the atypical group, symptom severity could not be separated from the presence of delusion-like symptoms, and this makes their conclusions about the contribution of delusions questionable. Furthermore, patients were assigned to a variety of treatments, according to symptom severity, and many of the treatments have no established record of effectiveness with OCD (e.g., thought stopping, aversion relief, imipramine, phenothiazines). Despite these shortcomings, the study yielded the following suggestive findings for the atypical group: earlier onset and poorer prognosis. Whereas poor prognosis may have been consequent to symptom severity, delusion-like thinking may have been a contributor.

In a more recent investigation, Eisen and Rasmussen (1993) identified 67 of 475 OCD patients with psychotic symptoms, including delusions, hallucinations, and/or thought disorder. OCD patients with psychotic symptoms (atypical) were compared to more typical OCD patients on demographics and clinical features. Heterogeneity of psychotic symptoms was apparent: 18 patients met criteria for OCD and schizophrenia, 8 for OCD and delusional disorder, 14 for OCD and schizotypal personality, and 27 for OCD without insight into the irrationality of their obsessions and compulsions. Patients with both OCD and psychotic features were more likely to be male and single, to have a deteriorative course, and to have been younger at the time of first professional contact.

Rather than dividing patients into typical versus atypical OCD patients, Lelliott et al. (1988) and Basoglu et al. (1988) used a structured interview about the patients' beliefs to examine delusional qualities. Beliefs were rated by an independent assessor on four dimensions: 1) fixity—how strongly is the obsessive belief held, 2) bizarreness—how valid is the belief, 3) resistance—frequency of attempts to resist urges, and 4) controllability—ease with which patient can control compulsive urges. The fixity dimension has three subscales: 1) strength of belief in feared consequence, 2) patient's perceived absurdity of belief in feared consequences, and 3) response to evidence contradicting the obsessional belief. Of 45 patients, 33% believed that, without their rituals, feared consequences would occur, 12% never tried to resist their compulsions, and 43% had no control over intrusive thoughts and urges to ritualize. Furthermore, patients were distributed over the whole range of the scales. These results strongly contradict Schneider's and Janet's traditional notions that the obsessional beliefs are recognized by patients as senseless, are resisted, and are "ego-alien."

The above method of assessing insight and resistance to obsessions was adopted by Insel and Akiskal (1986). They rated four aspects of OCD ideas in 23 patients: 1) perceived validity, 2) resistance, 3) strength of belief in harmful consequences, and 4) perceived absurdity compared to culturally accepted norms. Most patients perceived their obsessions as absurd, but many were nevertheless quite confident that harmful consequences would occur if they did not perform rituals. Additionally, more than half the patients reported that only sometimes did they try to resist obsessive ideas. Interestingly, resistance often varied within patients, depending on environmental situation and fatigue.

OVI, delusions, and outcome of therapy.   Distinctions among the types of thinking that characterize OCD are useful to the extent that they are related to etiology and/or treatment. The prognosis of OCD with OVI has been a focus of attention since Foa (1979) reported the failure of behavior therapy for four OCD patients with strong convictions in the validity of their obsessive beliefs. In contrast, Lelliott and Marks (1987) and Salkovskis and Wernike (1985) reported successful outcomes with single cases of OCD with strongly held beliefs. Also contradicting Foa's observation is a subsequent study of 49 OCD patients with a range of obsessive conviction: 12% defended their obsessions so strongly that they made no attempt to resist urges to ritualize. Patients with strong convictions responded as well to treatment as those whose obsessions were recognized as senseless (Lelliott et al. 1988). Using a different statistical analysis of the same data, Basoglu et al. (1988)

reported no correlation between pretreatment degree of conviction and outcome immediately posttreatment and a weak ($r = -.3$) relationship at 1-year follow-up. However, it is premature to conclude that the strength of the obsessional conviction is unrelated to outcome simply because no linear relationship was found in the above studies. It is conceivable that only patients with extreme conviction would be resistant to treatment. Such nonlinear relationships may not be detected by linear regression procedures.

Another approach to evaluating the relationship of obsessional thinking to treatment outcome is studying schizotypal personality and OCD. Several DSM-III criteria of schizotypy refer to disordered thinking: 1) magical thinking, 2) ideas of reference, and 3) suspiciousness. In a retrospective study, Jenike et al. (1986) examined 43 "treatment-resistant" OCD patients and found that those with concomitant schizotypal personality disorder had a high rate of failure: of 29 treated nonschizotypal OCD patients, 26 (90%) improved at least moderately; only 1 of 14 (7%) schizotypal patients improved. Inspection of the data suggests that the presence of ideas of reference and paranoia/suspiciousness is more predictive of poor outcome than are magical ideas, which occurred in both treatment successes and failures for both schizotypal and nonschizotypal patients. Perhaps ideas of reference and paranoia are peculiar to schizophrenic-spectrum disorders, whereas magical thinking and delusions are not, and it is the schizophrenic spectrum that predicts poor outcome. Jenike et al.'s results converge with the findings of Eisen and Rasmussen (1989), who reported that "atypical" OCD patients with concomitant schizophrenia or schizotypy responded more poorly to pharmacological treatment for OCD than did patients with obsessional delusions.

Discussion.   In the psychiatric literature on OCD, distinctions among obsessions, delusions, and overvalued ideas are not sufficiently clear to be of diagnostic utility. In principle, the contrast of obsessions versus delusions and overvalued ideas is comprehensible. Obsessions are viewed by the patients as senseless and to be resisted. Overvalued ideas and delusions, on the other hand, are perceived by the individual as sensible and valid. However, the distinction between delusions and overvalued ideas is, at best, vague; the two concepts have often been used interchangeably. It seems that the impetus to maintain such a distinction stems from the seeming contradiction between the classification of OCD as a neurosis and the observation that OCD patients can manifest psychotic delusional thinking. To reduce this dissonance, the concept of overvalued ideas was embraced.

Although the distinction between obsessions and delusions/overvalued ideas is comprehensible, clinical observations and research findings cast doubt on its usefulness. OCD patients vary greatly in their degree of insight and resistance. It is evident that the beliefs of OCD patients cannot be dichotomized into senseless and sensible. As suggested by Insel and Akiskal (1986), the notion of a continuum better represents OCD phenomenology. Interestingly, Hollander et al. (1989) arrived at the same conclusion with regard to body dysmorphia.

DSM-III-R implies that OVI evolves from obsessions. No controlled studies directly addressed this issue. The available relevant clinical observations do not support this view. Patients alternate between periods of insight and periods of delusional beliefs. Moreover, clinical observation suggests that the degree of conviction may be situation dependent. Patients are more likely to display insight in the therapist's office than when confronted with a feared situation.

In addition to the limited validity of the dichotomy between "senseless" and "sensible" belief, its usefulness is also questionable in light of treatment outcome findings. Whereas some clinical observations suggested that OCD patients with overvalued ideas are less responsive to behavioral treatment, several reports found such patients quite responsive to treatment by drugs and/or behavior therapy. Thus, the relationship between strength of conviction and outcome remains unresolved.

Are there mental compulsions?   According to DSM-III-R, to be diagnosed with OCD, an individual must have either obsessions or compulsions.

> *Obsessions* are persistent ideas, thoughts, impulses, or images that are experienced, at least initially, as intrusive and senseless . . . The person attempts to ignore or suppress such thoughts or impulses or to neutralize them with some other thought or action. The person recognizes that the obsessions are a product of his or her own mind, and are not imposed from without. (p. 245)

> *Compulsions* are repetitive, purposeful, and intentional behaviors that are performed in response to an obsession, according to certain rules, or in a stereotyped fashion. The behavior is designed to neutralize or to prevent discomfort or some dreaded event or situation. However, either the activity is not connected in a realistic way with what it is designed to neutralize or prevent, or it is clearly excessive . . . The person recognizes that his or her behavior is excessive or unreasonable (this may not be true for young children and may no longer be true for people whose obsessions have evolved into overvalued ideas). (p. 245)

Three traditional views have influenced the language of DSM-III-R. Traditionally, obsessions are construed as mental events such as thoughts, images, or impulses. Compulsions, on the other hand, are observable, overt behaviors such as washing, checking, repeating actions, or ordering. However, the distinction between obsessions and compulsions on the basis of the modality in which they are expressed conflicts with a current view about OCD that emphasizes a dynamic functional relationship between obsessions and compulsions. According to this view, obsessions are mental events that elicit distress, such as thoughts of being contaminated, thoughts of being responsible for a catastrophe, impulse to kill one's child, or blasphemous images. Compulsions are viewed as overt behaviors or mental events that are performed to reduce the distress associated with the obsessions. These include overt behaviors such as washing to offset contamination distress and also covert rituals such as silent checking or counting to offset obsessional distress or bad luck. Both the behaviors and the thoughts in these examples aim at reducing obsessional distress, and, therefore, both can be viewed as compulsions. The distress-reducing thoughts can be termed *cognitive compulsions*. The traditional view that obsessions are mental and compulsions are behavioral conflicts with a current view that certain thoughts are designed to neutralize other thoughts or impulses and therefore constitute compulsions. This leads to confusion in DSM-III-R because, although the compulsions criteria do not encompass neutralizing thoughts, the obsessions criteria specify that attempts to neutralize obsessions are made with "some other thought or action."

Recommendations

1. Definition of Obsessions as Distressing

There are results from several sources (i.e., both physiological and self-report) that obsessions are accompanied by distress. Furthermore, the effective behavioral treatment procedures aim to reduce distress. Notably, the reduction of distress following behavior therapy is related to overall improvement in OCD symptoms. Therefore, it is important to distinguish obsessions from appetitive preoccupations (e.g., sexual). Thus, it is recommended that the criteria for obsessions should explicitly define obsessions as distressing.

2. Distinctions Between Obsessions and Worries, Hypochondriacal Preoccupations, and Body Dysmorphic Concerns

The review of the literature on similarities and differences between obsessions and worries considered both process and content. More research is required to understand differences in cognitive processes in worries and obsessions. Regarding content, however, the existing literature suggests that the contents of worries are predominantly exaggerations of ordinary concerns, such as career, finance, or family, whereas the content of obsessions tends to be more unusual, such as acting on unacceptable impulses or spreading dangerous contamination. When compulsions are clearly present, the distinction between the associated ideas and "worries" is not troublesome, however, the differential diagnosis between GAD and OCD can be more difficult for those with "pure" obsessions. Therefore, it is recommended that the criteria for obsessions be amended to include language that specifies that obsessions are not simply worries about realistic events.

The DSM-III-R definition of hypochondriasis has succeeded in clearly delineating the diagnostic differences between hypochondriasis, delusional disorder, and the remaining somatoform disorders. However, it is now somewhat more difficult to distinguish primary hypochondriasis from the anxiety disorders, particularly OCD and GAD. A major difference between hypochondriacal patients and those with OCD that has been emphasized in the past is the fact that OCD patients experience their obsessions as senseless and that they therefore have the insight to resist them. However, accumulating evidence has shown that resistance, as well as conviction and belief, lie on a continuum in OCD. In OCD, there may be primary somatic obsessions with checking rituals or the compulsive need to ask for reassurance. However, there are almost invariably other types of obsessions and compulsions present in addition to the somatic obsessions. Patients who exhibit hypochondriacal fears with checking rituals should be classified as having OCD and not hypochondriasis. Checking rituals should not just include numerous visits to the doctor.

Body dysmorphic disorder shares many similarities with OCD in terms of phenomenology, demographic and associated features, etiology, and treatment response. However, the existing evidence stems from a collection of anecdotal case reports, and there remains a paucity of large, systematic studies. There is real difficulty with the current diagnostic system with respect to body dysmorphic disorder. There appears to be even less evidence linking body dysmorphic disorder to other somatoform disorders than to OCD. Furthermore, as individual patients progress through the course of their illness, their diagnosis may shift from a somatoform to a delusional disorder. Whereas one could argue that body dysmorphic disorder should be classified a subgroup of OCD, the evidence is not definitive. Nevertheless, the close relationship between the two disorders is worthy of mention in the text of DSM-IV. If larger and more systematic studies become available, this issue may be reconsidered for DSM-V.

3. Specifying That Obsessions Must Be Recognized by the Patient as Senseless, Unreasonable, or Excessive

The DSM-III-R assertion that most people with OCD perceive their symptoms as senseless is not supported by the two available studies about this issue. Rather, the data indicate a broad range of recognition of senselessness. However, the number of patients in these studies was too small to afford a strong conclusion. The field study will examine the range of recognition of senselessness in OCD patients and its relationship to behavioral and pharmacological treatments. If most patients state that at sometime during the course of the disorder they recognized their symptoms as senseless, then the emphasis on senselessness should remain in the DSM-IV. On the other hand, if patients are broadly distributed on the recognition of sense-lessness continuum, then the idea that obsessions are viewed as senseless should be de-emphasized in DSM-IV. If the data indicate natural groupings in the distribution of recognition of senselessness and that these groups are related to outcome of treatment, subtypes corresponding to such groupings will be indicated. For example, if patients on the extreme end of the continuum respond poorly to treatment, a subtype of OCD with delusions will be indicated.

4. Specifying That Compulsions Can Be Either Behavioral or Mental Acts

The distinction between obsessions and compulsions has not been delineated clearly. Therefore, studies of cognitive compulsions are unavailable. The Yale-Brown Obsessive-Compulsive Scale (Y-BOCS) (Goodman et al. 1989b), a widely accepted measure of OCD, lists many items for overt compulsions and only one for mental compulsions. Clinical observations suggest that certain mental events can have the same functional relationship to obsessions as behavioral rituals (i.e., both aim at reducing obsessional distress). Thus, it is desirable to specify this in the criteria for compulsions. The unavailability of systematic studies of the issue of mental rituals, however, leads to the recommendation that relevant data be collected in a field trial. If the results indicate that mental rituals occur with some frequency, it will be recommended that the criteria for compulsions be changed to reflect this.

A field study conducted at six sites will examine the incidence of cognitive compulsions and whether they are intended to neutralize harm or reduce distress in the same way that behavioral compulsions are. It will also investigate how many patients with so-called "pure obsessions" evidence cognitive compulsions and thus can be viewed as having both obsessions and compulsions.

5. Should ICD-10 Subcategories of a) Obsessions, b) Compulsions, and c) Obsessions and Compulsions Be Adopted for DSM-IV?

Clinical observations suggest that patients who exhibit mostly obsessions respond differently to behavioral treatment than do those with compulsions. However, systematic studies of this observation are unavailable, making it difficult to evaluate the validity of the ICD-10 subcategories. Therefore, it is recommended that relevant data be gathered in the field trial.

The proposed field trial will investigate the usefulness of such subcategories by examining the following issues: 1) What is the frequency of obsessions alone, compulsions alone, and the combination? 2) If the three groups exist, do they differ systematically on other variables such as types of obsessions and compulsions and response to psychosocial and pharmacological treatment?

Recommendations about whether DSM-IV should incorporate the ICD-10 subcategories will depend on the results of the trial.

References

Akhtar S, Wig NH, Verna VK, et al: A phenomenological analysis of symptoms in obsessive-compulsive neuroses. Br J Psychiatry 127:342–348, 1975

American Psychiatric Association: Diagnostic and Statistical Manual of Mental Disorders, 3rd Edition. Washington, DC, American Psychiatric Association, 1980

American Psychiatric Association: Diagnostic and Statistical Manual of Mental Disorders, 3rd Edition, Revised. Washington, DC, American Psychiatric Association, 1987

Barlow, DH: Anxiety and Its Disorders. New York, Guilford, 1988

Barsky AJ, Wyshak G, Klerman GL: Hypochondriasis: an evaluation of the DSM-III criteria in medical outpatients. Arch Gen Psychiatry 43:493–500, 1986

Basoglu M, Lax T, Kasvikis Y, et al: Predictors of improvement in obsessive-compulsive disorder. J Anx Disord 2:299–317, 1988

Bebbington PE: Monosymptomatic hypochondriasis, abnormal illness behavior and suicide. Br J Psychiatry 128:475–478, 1976

Beech HR: Obsessional States. London, Methuen, 1974

Borkovec TD, Robinson E, Pruzinsky T, et al: Preliminary exploration of worry: some characteristics and processes. Behav Res Ther 21:9–16, 1983

Borkovec TD, Shadick RN, Hopkins M: The nature of normal versus pathological worry, in Chronic Anxiety: Generalized Anxiety Disorders and Mixed Anxiety Depression. New York, Guilford, 1991

Boulougouris JC, Rabavilas AD, Stefanis C: Psychophysiological responses in obsessive-compulsive patients. Behav Res Ther 15:221–230, 1977

Carek DJ, Santos AB: Atypical somatoform disorder following infection in children: a depressive equivalent? J Clin Psychiatry 45:108–111, 1984

Connolly FH, Gipson M: Dysmorphophobia: a long term study. Br J Psychiatry 132:568–570, 1978

Craske MG, Rapee RM, Jackel L, et al: Qualitative dimensions of worry in DSM-III generalized anxiety disorder subjects and nonanxious controls. Behav Res Ther 27:397–402, 1988

Craven JL, Rodin GM: Cyproheptadine dependence associated with an atypical somatoform disorder. Can J Psychiatry 32:143–145, 1987

DeVeaugh-Geiss J, Landau P, Katz R: Treatment of OCD with clomipramine. Psychiatric Annals 19:97–101, 1989

Edwards S, Dickerson M: Intrusive unwanted thoughts: a two-stage model of control. Br J Med Psychol 60:317–328, 1987

Eisen JL, Rasmussen SA: Obsessive-compulsive disorder with psychotic features. J Clin Psychiatry 54:373–379, 1993

England SL, Dickerson M: Intrusive thoughts: unpleasantness not the major cause of uncontrollability. Behav Res Ther 26:279–282, 1988

Flament MF, Rapoport JL, Berg CL, et al: Clomipramine treatment of childhood obsessive-compulsive disorder, a double blind controlled study. Arch Gen Psychiatry 42:977–986,1985

Foa EB: Treatment of obsessive-compulsives with prolonged exposure and strict response prevention. Archives of Greek Association for Behavioral Modification and Research 1:5–17, 1979

Foa EB, Tillmanns A: The treatment of obsessive-compulsive neurosis, in Handbook of Behavioral Interventions: A Clinical Guide. Edited by Goldstein A, Foa EB. New York, Wiley, 1980, pp 416–500

Goodman WK, Rasmussen SA, McDougale CS, et al: Drug response in obsessive compulsive subtypes. Paper presented at the ACNP, Maui, HI, December 1989a

Goodman WK, Price L, Rasmussen S: The Yale Brown obsessive-scale (Y BOCS): past development, use, and reliability. Arch Gen Psychiatry 46:1006–1016, 1989b

Goodwin DW, Guze SB, Robins E: Follow-up studies in obsessional neurosis. Arch Gen Psychiatry 20:182–187, 1969

Grimshaw L: Obsessional disorder and neurological illness. J Neurol Neurosurg Psychiatry 27:229–231, 1964

Hamilton M: Fish's Clinical Psychopathology. Bristol, John Wright, 1974

Hodgson RJ, Rachman S: The effects of contamination and washing in obsessional patients. Behav Res Ther 10:111–117, 1972

Hollander E, Liebowitz MR, Winchel R, et al: Treatment of body dysmorphic disorder with serotonin reuptake blockers. Am J Psychiatry 146:768–770, 1989

Hoogduin K: On the diagnosis of obsessive-compulsive disorder. Am J Psychother 40:36–51,1986

Hornsveld RHJ, Kraaimaat FW, van dam Baggen RMJ: Anxiety/discomfort and handwashing in obsessive-compulsive and psychiatric control patients. Behav Res Ther 17:223–228, 1979

Hunecke P, Bosse K: Dysmorphophobia as casus pro diagnosi. Z Hautkr 60:1986–1989, 1985

Insel TR, Akiskal H: Obsessive-compulsive disorder with psychotic features: a phenomenologic analysis. Am J Psychiatry 12:1527–1533, 1986

Janet P: Les Obsessions et la Psychosthenie (Second Edition). Paris, Bailliere, 1908

Jaspers K: General Psychopathology (1959). Translated by Hoenig J, Hamilton MW. Manchester, Manchester University Press, 1963

Jenike MA, Baer L, Minichiello WE, et al: Concomitant obsessive-compulsive disorder and schizotypal personality disorder. Am J Psychiatry 143:530–532, 1986

Kellner R: Somatization and Hypochondriasis. New York, Praeger, 1986

Kellner R, Abbot D, Pathak W, et al: Hypochondriacal beliefs and attitudes in family practice and psychiatric patients. Int J Psychiatry Med 13:127–139, 1983

Kellner R, Abbott P, Winslow W, et al: Anxiety, depression , and somatization in DSM-III hypochondriasis. Psychosomatics 30:57–64, 1989

Kenyon FE: Hypochondriasis: a clinical study. Br J Psychiatry 110:478–488, 1964

Khanna S, Channabasavanna SM: Phenomenology of obsessions in obsessive-compulsive neurosis. Psychopathology 21:12–18, 1988

Kozak MJ, Foa EB, Steketee G: Process and outcome of exposure treatment with obsessive-compulsives: psychophysiological indicators of emotional processing. Behavior Therapy 19:157–169, 1988

Ladee GA: Hypochondriacal Syndromes. New York, Elsevier, 1966

Lelliott P, Marks I: Management of obsessive compulsive rituals associated with delusions, hallucinations, and depression: a case report. Behav Psychother 15:77–87, 1987

Lelliott PT, Noshirvani HF, Basoglu M, et al: Obsessive-compulsive beliefs and treatment outcome. Psychol Med 18:697–702, 1988

Lewis A: Problems of obsessional illness. Proc R Soc Med 29:325–336, 1935

Liebert RM, Morris LW: Cognitive and emotional components of test anxiety: a distinction and some initial data. Psychological Reports 20:975–978, 1967

Likierman H, Rachman SJ: Spontaneous decay of compulsive urges: cumulative effects. Behav Res Ther 18:387–394, 1980

Mavissakalian MR: Functional classification of obsessive-compulsive phenomena. J Behav Assess 1:271–279, 1979

McKenna PJ: Disorders with overvalued ideas. Br J Psychiatry 145:579–585, 1984

Pilowsky I: Primary and secondary hypochondriasis. Acta Psychiatr Scand 46:273–285, 1970

Rabavilas AD, Boulougouris JC: Physiological accompaniments of ruminations, flooding, and thought-stopping in obsessive patients. Behav Res Ther 12:239–243, 1974

Rachman SJ, Hodgson R: Obsessions and Compulsions. Englewood Cliffs, NJ, Prentice Hall, 1980

Rachman S, de Silva P: Abnormal and normal obsessions. Behav Res Ther 16:233–248, 1978

Rasmussen SA, Tsuang MT: The epidemiology of obsessive-compulsive disorder. J Clin Psychiatry 45:450–457, 1984

Rasmussen SA, Tsuang MT: Clinical characteristics and family history in DSM-III obsessive-compulsive disorder. Am J Psychiatry 143:317–322, 1986

Salib EA: Subacute sclerosing panencephalitis (SSPE) presenting at the age of 21 as a schizophrenia-like state with bizarre dysmorphophobic features. Br J Psychiatry 152:709–710, 1988

Salkovskis PM: Obsessional compulsive problems: a cognitive behavioral analysis. Behav Res Ther 23:571–583, 1985

Salkovskis PM, Harrison J: Abnormal and normal obsessions—a replication. Behav Res Ther 22:549–552, 1984

Salkovskis PM, Wernike HMC: Cognitive therapy of obsessive-compulsive disorder: treating treatment failures. Behav Psychother 13:243–255, 1985

Sanderson WC, Barlow DH: Domains of worry within the proposed DSM-III Revised generalized anxiety disorder category: reliability and description. Paper presented at the Association for Advancement of Behavior Therapy Annual Meeting, Chicago, November 1986

Schilder P: The organic background of obsessions and compulsions. Am J Psychiatry 94:1397–1416, 1938

Schneider K: Schwangs zus tande un Schizophrenie. Archiv fur Psychiatrie und Nervenkrankheiten 74:93–107, 1925

Sheehan DV, Ballenger J, Jacobson G: Treatment of endogenous anxiety with phobia, hysterical, and hypochondriacal symptoms. Arch Gen Psychiatry 37:51–59, 1980

Solyom L, Sookman D, Solyom C, et al: Behavior therapy versus drug therapy in the treatment of obsessional illness. Unpublished manuscript, 1985

Stenback A, Jalava V: Hypochondria and depression. Acta Psychiatr Scand Suppl 37:240–246, 1962

Stenback A, Rimon R: Hypochondria and paranoia. Acta Psychiatr Scand Suppl 40:379–385, 1964

Thoren P, Asberg M, Bertilsson L, et al: Clomipramine treatment of obsessive compulsive disorder, II: biochemical aspects. Arch Gen Psychiatry 37:1289–1294, 1980a

Thoren P, Asberg M, Chronholm B, et al: Clomipramine treatment of obsessive compulsive disorder: a controlled clinical trial. Arch Gen Psychiatry 40:605–612, 1980b

Wernike C: Gundriss der Psychiatrie. Leipzig, Verlag von Georg Thieme, 1900

Westphal C: Zwengsvor stellungen. Arch Psychiat Nervenkr 8:734–750, 1878

Woodruff RA, Goodwin DW, Guze SB: Psychiatric diagnosis. New York, Oxford University Press, 1974

World Health Organization: ICD-10 Chapter V: Mental and Behavioral Disorders: Diagnostic Criteria for Research. Geneva, Switzerland, World Health Organization, 1990

Zohar J, Mueller EA, Insel TR, et al: Serotonergic responsivity in obsessive compulsive disorder. Arch Gen Psychiatry 44:946–951, 1987

Chapter 19

Posttraumatic Stress Disorder

Jonathan Davidson, M.D., Edna B. Foa, Ph.D.,
Arthur S. Blank, M.D., Elizabeth A. Brett, Ph.D.,
John Fairbank, Ph.D., Bonnie L. Green, Ph.D.,
Judith L. Herman, M.D., Terence M. Keane, Ph.D.,
Dean L. Kilpatrick, Ph.D., John S. March, M.D., M.P.H.,
Richard J. McNally, Ph.D., Roger K. Pitman, M.D.,
Heidi S. Resnick, Ph.D., and Barbara O. Rothbaum, Ph.D.

Introduction

The Posttraumatic Stress Disorder (PTSD) sub-Work Group identified eight principal areas for review with respect to developing criteria for DSM-IV. These topics, which are listed sequentially throughout this chapter, are 1) the stressor criterion, 2) the cohesiveness of the syndrome across groups, 3) the classification of PTSD, 4) the relevance of biological research, 5) longitudinal course and subtypes of PTSD, 6) duration and subtypes of PTSD and overlap with adjustment disorder, 7) epidemiology of PTSD, and 8) evidence for an additional, more complex, syndrome following chronic and repeated trauma.

Statement of the Issues

The Stressor Criterion in DSM-IV

The stressor criterion (criterion A) serves as a gatekeeper to the diagnosis of PTSD. Is the definition satisfactory as it stands? Should it be broadened to include events of lesser magnitude or those that are more commonplace? Should subjective appraisal form part of the definition? Should event characteristics be included in the definition?

Symptomatology of PTSD: Studies in Crime Victims, Combat Veterans, Disaster Victims, and Children

In DSM-III (American Psychiatric Association 1980), the symptom groupings for PTSD were chosen on the basis of clinical tradition and earlier pre-DSM-II (American Psychiatric Association 1968) studies. In DSM-III-R (American Psychiatric Association 1987), three symptom clusters were identified: intrusive, avoidant/denial, and hyperarousal symptoms. The validity of this grouping was unknown at the time and is examined to some extent in these reviews. There have also been concerns as to the desired number of PTSD symptoms that should be required for the diagnosis (previously defined arbitrarily), along with the overall coherence of symptoms into a clinical syndrome. Other important questions include frequency of symptom occurrence, how frequently they occur, and their diagnostic sensitivity and specificity.

Classification of PTSD in DSM-IV: Anxiety Disorder, Dissociative Disorder, or Stress Disorder?

Controversy exists as to the current position of PTSD in DSM-III-R. Although the evidence strongly supports classifying PTSD as an anxiety disorder, other points of view need to be entertained. These alternatives include 1) viewing PTSD as a dissociative disorder or 2) creating a new category of stress- or trauma-related psychiatric illnesses, in which PTSD would be included.

Biological Aspects of PTSD

How can biological findings from PTSD research inform 1) the proper location of the disorder in DSM-IV and 2) the diagnostic criteria?

Longitudinal Course of PTSD

This review concerns the natural history of PTSD and includes the information available from 1980 to 1991 about the longitudinal course of PTSD. Such information was not sufficiently addressed in the DSM-III or DSM-III-R formulations of the diagnosis of PTSD.

PTSD Subtypes and Duration of Symptoms

This review examines the evidence for subtyping PTSD, the issue of symptom duration, and the overlap with adjustment disorder.

Epidemiology of PTSD

Large population samples derived from those who did not seek treatment should be taken into account in the comprehensive description of a disease. Reliance on clinically derived samples will likely provide unrepresentative findings.

This review describes several recent epidemiological studies of PTSD, that are grouped into populations "at risk" and those who are "not at risk." Issues addressed are 1) prevalence rates, 2) duration of symptoms, 3) co-morbidity patterns, 4) pretrauma risk factors, 5) relationship between trauma characteristics and PTSD, 6) interactions between premorbid risk factors and trauma, 7) characteristic symptoms, 8) differences between acute and chronic PTSD, and 9) construct validity of PTSD.

Effects of Prolonged and Repeated Trauma: Evidence for a Complex Posttraumatic Syndrome (DESNOS)

The current diagnostic formulation of PTSD derives largely from observations of survivors of relatively circumscribed traumatic events such as combat, disaster, or rape. It has been suggested that this formulation does not capture the protean manifestations of prolonged, repeated trauma, or the extensive alterations of personality that follow prolonged captivity. This review addressed the evidence for a more complex form of posttraumatic disorder following prolonged, repeated trauma. A preliminary formulation of this syndrome is currently under consideration for inclusion in DSM-IV.

Significance of the Issues

Stressor Criterion in DSM-IV

A DSM-III-R diagnosis of PTSD does not rest on symptoms alone but also on an event having occurred that meets specified criteria. The event must be judged 1) to be outside usual human experience and 2) to be markedly distressing to almost anybody. The following concerns have been expressed about criterion A in its present form: 1) victims of events of lesser magnitude or that are more commonplace should be allowed to receive the diagnosis of PTSD if they otherwise meet the required number of symptoms in clusters B, C, and D; 2) subjective appraisal of the event is important, as is already recognized in the text; and 3) certain objective properties of the event may determine whether it is traumatogenic.

Symptomatology of PTSD: Studies in Crime Victims, Combat Veterans, Disaster Victims, and Children

At least one intrusive symptom, three avoidant symptoms, and two hyperarousal symptoms are needed to meet criteria for a diagnosis of PTSD. Some evidence suggests that the number of required avoidant symptoms is excessive and that requiring three avoidance symptoms may preclude traumatized victims with clinically significant disturbance (e.g., those who meet the required number of B and D criteria but only have one or two avoidance symptoms) from receiving the diagnosis.

Finally, if evidence exists that the PTSD symptom clusters differ significantly across victim groups, this should be acknowledged in DSM-IV, as it would to some extent undermine the assumed cohesiveness of the disorder across different traumata.

Classification of PTSD in DSM-IV: Anxiety Disorder, Dissociative Disorder, or Stress Disorder?

Although psychiatric classification in DSM-III-R is largely atheoretical and based on descriptive phenomenology, the classification of disease ultimately aspires to an etiological basis. In PTSD, we know at least something about etiology, namely that it is derived from a traumatic event. At the same time, if the clinical and research evidence supports the view that PTSD is an anxiety disorder or a form of dissociation, then this cannot be ignored in the deliberation over where PTSD should be classified.

Biological Aspects of PTSD

Biological data might help to clarify the relationships between PTSD and anxiety, dissociative, or other disorders with which it overlaps. The data may also illuminate the question about whether PTSD should be classified separately. Psychophysiological procedures have some potential as a diagnostic test for PTSD and might have a place within the diagnostic criteria, thereby introducing the laboratory as part of psychiatric diagnosis in DSM-IV.

Longitudinal Course of PTSD

What is the longitudinal course of PTSD and what are its patterns with respect to subtypes? Is there a "normal" posttraumatic stress reaction distinguishable from PTSD? How do symptoms vary over time, especially with reference to intrusion, avoidance, and hyperarousal symptoms? How do types of trauma affect course? What factors may be associated with intensification or amelioration during the disorder? What are the effects of secondary gain on the course of PTSD, and what are the effects of PTSD over time on functioning? What are some of the limitations of recently published studies and what are the key problems in investigating longitudinal course?

PTSD Subtypes and Duration of Symptoms

PTSD is the only anxiety disorder for which the occurrence of an external event is specified in the diagnostic criteria. As such, its delineation includes etiological aspects. Because it is expected that a traumatic event would always elicit emotional distress, it is important to distinguish between normal and pathological reactions. One important aspect related to this is duration of symptoms. Because the diagnosis of adjustment disorder rests in part on the duration of symptoms following a stressor, this review also attempts to clarify the overlap between PTSD and adjustment disorder.

Patterns of posttraumatic response vary across individuals. Although some individuals become acutely distressed following the incident, others may not develop symptoms until later. Accordingly, DSM-III distinguished the acute and chronic or delayed subtypes. The utility of these is addressed.

Epidemiology of PTSD

The epidemiological literature is significant because of limitations inherent in drawing conclusions from studies based only on treatment seekers. Large community-based samples also provide a better opportunity to uncover associated characteristics that might not be detectable in smaller clinically based samples.

Effects of Prolonged and Repeated Trauma: Evidence for a Complex Posttraumatic Syndrome (DESNOS)

Strong evidence in favor of a complex posttraumatic syndrome, following traumata of the kinds described, would lend support to the creation of a new category of psychological disorders related to trauma.

Methods

Various issues were assigned to individual committee members as follows: 1) definition of the stressor criterion (criterion A): John S. March, M.D.; 2) cohesiveness of symptomatology across victim groups: T. Keane, Ph.D. (combat veterans), B. Green, Ph.D. (disaster victims), D. Kilpatrick, Ph.D., and H. Resnick, Ph.D. (crime victims), and R. McNally, Ph.D. (children); 3) the classification of PTSD: E. A. Brett, Ph.D.; 4) the relevance of biological research on PTSD to DSM-IV: R. Pitman, M.D.; 5) the longitudinal course of PTSD: A. S. Blank, M.D.; 6) duration and subtypes of PTSD: B. Rothbaum, Ph.D., and E. B. Foa, Ph.D.; 7) the epidemiology of PTSD: J. Davidson, M.D., and J. Fairbank, Ph.D.; 8) the effects of chronic traumatization: J. Herman, M.D.

Results

Stressor Criterion (Criterion A)

This review examines the definition of criterion A, as well as the possible relevance of subjective appraisal and event characteristics to PTSD.

A Medline search was conducted of English language articles published between 1966 and 1989, using appropriate key words. Personal communications and opinions and unpublished articles were also solicited. Almost all articles reviewed employed DSM-III or DSM-III-R criteria. Written input was obtained from other committee members in response to this review, and final recommendations were made after these were taken into account.

In most studies examined, stressor magnitude was directly proportional to the risk of developing PTSD regardless of stressor type and methodological variations (Green et al. 1985; Laufer et al. 1985; Shore et al. 1986; Solomon et al. 1988; Speed et al. 1989). A direct relationship was not found in all studies, however (Madakasira and O'Brien 1987; Zeiss and Dickman 1989). There was no evidence for a "threshold effect," but no guidelines exist to help distinguish between an event that is inside or outside the range of usual experience. Only limited support exists to suggest that low-magnitude events give rise to PTSD (Burstein 1985), but this issue has not been adequately studied.

Many reports examined qualitative characteristics of the event. Injury was correlated with PTSD in some studies (Kilpatrick et al. 1989; Pitman et al. 1989; Speed et al. 1989) but not in all (Green et al. 1989; Madakasira and O'Brien 1987). Bereavement was positively related in most studies (Breslau and Davis 1987; Green et al. 1985; Helzer et al. 1987) but was unrelated in one (Green et al. 1989). Being involved in atrocities and exposure to grotesque death were positively related to PTSD (Breslau et al. 1987; Green et al. 1989). Witnessing death and hearing about death were also positively related to PTSD in some studies (Saigh 1989; Speed et al. 1989). Rape, torture, life threat, and property damage were also related in some studies (Green et al. 1985; Kilpatrick et al. 1987; Shore et al. 1986; Speed et al. 1989). Dimensions of threat to life, severe physical harm, exposure to grotesque death or atrocity, and loss or injury to a loved one are modestly correlated with the development of PTSD.

With respect to subjective appraisal, or impact of the event, there was weak evidence to suggest a possible relationship between PTSD and perception of low controllability (helplessness), fear, perceived threat to life, or perceived threat of violence. Several methodological problems were identified with regard to the validity of these findings.

Cohesiveness of PTSD Symptomatology (Criteria B, C, D)

Four reviews examined symptom frequency, cohesiveness, and factor structure in different victim groups: traumatized children, victims of crime and assault, and veterans of combat. Reviews were conducted in four different victim groups: children (McNally), disaster victims (Green), combat veterans (Keane), crime victims (Kilpatrick and Resnick). Searches employed Medline and PsycInfo, reference lists from articles so identified, reprints of unpublished data, ongoing research, and specific journal searches. DSM-III criteria were used in most instances, but when studies using DSM-III-R criteria were available, they were also included.

Results

Disaster victims. In studies of disaster victims, the data revealed that all symptoms occur to some extent in most samples, with the exception of survivor guilt, which was in any event deleted in DSM-III-R (Maida et al. 1989; Shore 1986; Smith and North 1988; Solomon and Canino 1990; Steinglass and Gerrity 1990). In one of the few studies that evaluated the DSM-III-R criteria, recurrent dreams, numbing, irritability, and flashbacks were relatively uncommon at the 14-year follow-up point, whereas avoidance of thoughts about the trauma was the most common symptom in this community sample (Green et al. 1990).

Numbing symptoms were not observed as frequently (except for the study referenced above), and some surveys noted the difficulties in operationalizing some of the avoidance items, as well as problems arising from interviews in which the symptoms had to be linked to the event by the subject (Solomon and Canino 1990). Avoidance of thoughts or activities are common in some studies.

Symptoms showed good internal consistency, with coefficient alpha being 0.57 for intrusion, 0.81 for denial, 0.78 for hyperarousal, and 0.86 for overall DSM-III-R symptoms in a single study (Green et al. 1990).

Related symptoms and symptom profiles were similar among flood, disaster, and Vietnam combat survivors with PTSD, although social isolation was higher in the latter group. With respect to sex, most (Green et al. 1990; Steinglass and Gerrity 1990; Wilkinson 1983) but not all (Smith and North 1988) studies found that PTSD or PTSD symptoms occur more frequently in women. Men and women showed similar symptom profiles in the Buffalo Creek survivors group.

Combat veterans. Among Vietnam veterans, a review by Keane showed that the DSM-III-R criteria for PTSD, as measured by the Structured Clinical Interview for Diagnosis (SCID) (Spitzer and Williams 1985), produced four factors closely in line with the present conceptualization of the disorder. Factor 1 comprised symptoms of intrusive reexperiencing, reliving, hypervigilance, and constricted affect. Factor 2 extracted items of hypervigilance, startle, and avoidance. Factor 3 included irritability and impaired concentration. Factor 4 contained reduced interest. Four factors emerged in the self-rated Mississippi PTSD (M-PTSD) scale (Keane et al. 1988): reexperiencing items (Factor 1); numbing, restricted affect, anger, and irritability (Factor 2); impulse control problems (Factor 3); poor concentration and reduced interest (Factor 4). Therefore, although the factor structure does not correspond exactly with the DSM-III-R groupings, the factors are generally supportive of them. Cronbach's alpha was 0.93, indicating high internal consistency and unity of dimension for this disorder. The item-subtotal score correlations averaged 0.70, ranging from 0.54 to 0.85. With the M-PTSD, Cronbach's alpha was 0.89, with a mean item-subtotal score correlation of 0.47.

Crime victims. Kilpatrick and Resnick (1993) reported on three samples of criminally victimized individuals in the community who were assessed for PTSD by DSM-III-R criteria. These samples included a group of female rape victims ($n = 33$), a criminal justice sample ($n = 128$), and the national probability adult female sample ($n = 1,101$). All three studies showed highest frequency for intrusive and hyperarousal symptoms but lower frequency of avoidant symptoms. Constricted affect and psychogenic amnesia were uncommon. Among the criminal justice sample, all symptoms performed well with respect to predictive value/correctness of classification (range 0.75 to 0.89), although amnesia, foreshortened future, and being made worse on reminder of the trauma were not examined.

The effect of varying the minimum required number of avoidance items was studied. In two samples (Kilpatrick and Resnick 1993; Kilpatrick et al. 1989), lifetime prevalence rates of PTSD were 60.6% and 40.6% when three avoidance symptoms were required, with the rates increasing to 75.8% and 57.0%, respectively, when the threshold was reduced to two required symptoms.

Children. With respect to the symptomatology in childhood, McNally reviewed the literature on child victims of sexual abuse, natural disaster, war, violent crime, and burns (e.g., Beck and van der Kolk 1987; Browne and Finkelhor 1986; Burke et al. 1982; Kinzie et al. 1989; Lyons 1987; Malmquist 1986; Stoddard et al. 1989). There was no indication that the criteria as currently used should be modified on the basis of these reviews, but data do not exist, or are inconsistent, concerning the extent to which children experience flashbacks, amnesia, irritability, and foreshortened future.

Classification of PTSD

This review assesses the pros and cons of classifying PTSD as an anxiety disorder, a dissociative disorder, or separately in a new category of trauma-related psychological disorders.

Four hundred fifty articles were abstracted from Medline, covering 1985–1989. Additional journal sources were examined, including five major psychiatric and psychological journals. All papers reviewed made use of structured diagnostic interviewing.

PTSD as an anxiety disorder. Comorbidity data from epidemiological studies showed high levels of comorbidity between PTSD and other forms of anxiety, although comorbidity with other illnesses was equally frequent (Davidson et al. 1985a, 1991; Escobar et al. 1983; Green et al. 1989; Helzer et al. 1987; Sierles et al. 1983).

A specific association was found between PTSD and comorbid panic disorder in conjunction with war zone stress. Special assignment duties, in which elements of fear and terror were common, led to an associated picture of panic disorder and PTSD, whereas such stresses were less predictive of comorbid depression (Green et al. 1989).

With respect to psychophysiological studies, the two chief findings are 1) stimuli resembling the trauma cause sympathetic hyperactivity, and 2) high resting sympathetic hyperactivity is probably a response to the original stress (Pitman 1993).

Further evidence for a link between PTSD and anxiety is described by Barlow, Brown, Jones, and Prins's Commentary on Brett's Proposition of PTSD as a Stress Response Disorder (report prepared for DSM-IV Committee). They point out that 1) dissociative and intrusive symptoms can occur in other forms of anxiety disorder; 2) psychic numbing could be an avoidance response to unpleasant affects in PTSD; 3) behavioral and cognitive avoidance occur in both PTSD and panic disorder (Craske and Barlow 1989; Jones and Barlow 1990); 4) in a survey of PTSD patients who were interviewed with a structured questionnaire, the Anxiety Disorder Interview Schedule (ADIS) (DiNardo and Barlow 1988), 50% had panic disorder, 32% had social phobia, and 18% had panic disorder with agoraphobia; and 5) many effective approaches to PTSD treatment have been derived from theoretical models of anxiety.

Classifying PTSD as a dissociative disorder. In favor of classifying PTSD within the dissociative disorders group are 1) the fact that PTSD and the dissociative disorders share a proclivity for dissociative mechanisms and symptoms, such as amnesia and flashbacks (Loewenstein and Putnam 1988; Spiegel et al. 1988; Stutman and Bliss 1985); 2) the principal intrusive and numbing symptoms of PTSD have been regarded by some as dissociative; and 3) the dissociative disorders are believed to be reactions to severe stress, although this has not been absolutely established.

Against classifying PTSD as a dissociative disorder are 1) the justification for viewing intrusion and numbing as primarily dissociative in nature is not entirely convincing, and an equally strong case has been made for seeing these as manifestations of severe anxiety with avoidance; 2) the relationship of dissociative disorders to extreme stress has not been established as clearly as has been the association between PTSD and severe stress; and 3) although PTSD and the dissociative disorders may be shown to be responses to severe stress, this could also argue in favor of creating a new stress reaction category.

Classifying PTSD in a new category: stress response disorder.　　Two solutions have been considered by the committee. The first is to create a category for stress response disorders, comprising acute distress disorder, PTSD, pathological grief, uncomplicated bereavement, and adjustment disorders.

Horowitz (1989), in a brief outline, emphasized the importance of counseling for some individuals undergoing normal grief reactions. He also felt it important to differentiate normal grief from abnormal (pathological) grief reactions. This was proposed for inclusion as a clinical entity, because symptoms somewhat resembling PTSD would occur but would not amount to the full syndrome.

This proposal has the advantage that reactions to stress are classified on an etiological basis and that having one category for stress reactions facilitates the differential diagnostic process following severe stress. The disadvantages of such a proposal are: 1) the work distinguishing and relating bereavement, pathological grief, PTSD, and other potential disorders involving not only different syndromes but stressors of varying severity is not sufficiently advanced to justify reclassification at this time; and 2) a comprehensive stress response category would have to include groups of disorders such as dissociative disorders and dream anxiety disorders that are currently classified elsewhere with a fair degree of nosological comfort.

Classifying PTSD in a new category: disorders of extreme stress not elsewhere classified.　　A second alternative to the more comprehensive stress response category is creating a more narrowly defined category containing the following three disorders: acute stress disorder, PTSD, and disorders of extreme stress not otherwise specified (DESNOS). This would include the acute stress response disorder (brief reactive dissociative disorder) currently proposed by Spiegel and Spitzer and under examination as part of the field trial process for DSM-IV. The second disorder in this category, PTSD, is self-evident. The third proposed category would be DESNOS, a residual category to be tested in the field trials. Among the questions examined are its reliability, validity, internal consistency, and overlap with PTSD. This category could be used as a residual classification for responses following trauma that do not meet the criteria for acute stress reactions or PTSD. Much of the thinking that gave rise to this proposal derived from observations made in victims of chronic psychological and/or physical trauma who were not thought to meet the criteria for PTSD.

The advantages of the second option are 1) etiology is used as a basis for classification; 2) stressors of different levels of intensity are not placed in the same category which remains selective for unusual events (although this notion itself is to be tested in the field trials); 3) for each of the three disorders in this category, the other two will most often be the ones that the clinician is concerned about differentiating; 4) although this category recognizes that other disorders may be precipitated by extreme stress, it allows them to remain classified according to descriptive symptomatology at the present time; 5) the inclusion of acute stress disorder as well as PTSD makes DSM-IV more comparable to ICD-10, as indeed does the inclusion of a separate category of disorders of psychological trauma; and 6) the development of a stress disorder category recognizes and facilitates work in the field of stress studies.

Disadvantages of this proposal are 1) classification by etiology is not in keeping with the descriptive nature of DSM-IV; 2) it is recognized that, in most instances, more is required than the trauma itself to induce PTSD (i.e., the trauma is necessary but not sufficient); and 3) inclusion of DESNOS will lead to the diagnosis of disorders that are simply cases of mild PTSD.

Biological Findings and PTSD

The questions addressed are: How can biological research on PTSD provide information relevant to 1) the proper classification of PTSD and 2) the criteria for PTSD? Sources of information include a MEDLARS search from 1980 to 1988 and published articles in the major journals in 1989, a book source, presentations at meetings, and oral communications.

Results

Tonic (i.e., enduring) and phasic (i.e., intermittent) aspects of PTSD were addressed.

Tonic aspects. Tonic autonomic arousal occurs in some populations of traumatized individuals (Davidson and Baum 1986; Malloy et al. 1983; Pitman et al. 1987), with the evidence indirectly suggesting that it results from the experience itself rather than being an antecedent (Pitman 1993). However, data are far from conclusive in this regard, and an unresolved methodological issue concerns whether baseline measures really represent a tonic state or whether they reflect the effect of anticipatory anxiety.

Lowered indices of sympathetic activity were found with respect to platelet and lymphocyte cyclic AMP signal transductions and platelet monoamine oxidase and α_2-adrenergic receptor activities (Davidson et al. 1985b; Lerer et al. 1987; Perry et al. 1987). Hypothalamic-pituitary-adrenal (HPA) axis activity is altered, albeit inconsistently (Mason et al. 1990; Pitman et al. 1990). However, DST and CRF studies suggest that whereas PTSD has only a loose relationship with depression, it has a closer tie with panic disorder (Kudler et al. 1987; Smith et al. 1989). The same may be said with respect to studies of sleep disturbance and PTSD (Van Kammen et al. 1990).

Phasic aspects.   Greater autonomic arousal occurred in response to combat cues among combat veterans with PTSD than in those with other forms of anxiety disorder, or in control groups (Blanchard et al. 1982; Malloy et al. 1983; Pitman et al. 1987). Also, in such PTSD patients, the aroused affect was as likely to be anger or depression as anxiety. Psychophysiological indices reveal a two-thirds frequency of hypersensitivity in patients with PTSD and near-zero rate in those without PTSD (i.e., less-than-perfect diagnostic sensitivity but excellent specificity).

Longitudinal Course of PTSD

This review addresses the longitudinal course of PTSD and possible variations therein. It concludes with suggestions as to subtypes of PTSD.

A computer search of the PTSD literature from 1970 to 1989 was used, including key terms such as *course, longitudinal course, follow-up,* and *outcome.* In addition, personal communications between the author and other researchers in the PTSD field were used, as well as information available from the staff of the Department of Veterans Affairs Veterans Centers. Studies were catalogued with respect to time from trauma to study, diagnostic criteria and method used, whether repeated measures were used, type of sample, number of subjects, type of trauma, mean age of subjects, male-to-female ratio, and typical response rate.

Results

1. Posttraumatic stress symptoms not amounting to full PTSD are quite common in response to traumatic stress, may represent a normal response to extreme or catastrophic situations, may fade in a short time, may persist as such, or may develop into PTSD. They should be reflected in some form in DSM-IV (Blank 1993a).

2. There is ample evidence for acute, delayed, chronic, intermittent, recurrent, and reactivated forms of PTSD with respect to course.

3. The correlation between length, severity, and complexity of trauma is partial and not absolute.

4. Relative proportions of intrusion, avoidance, and hyperarousal symptoms probably vary over time in some cases. Recent studies indicate that, on a group basis, intrusion symptoms may be more prominent initially, whereas avoidance symptoms may become more prominent later. However, these data are preliminary.

5. In some cases, PTSD symptoms diminish over time, probably in association with many differing factors. In other cases they do not diminish and may worsen in the absence of treatment.

6. Whereas acute symptoms often precede a chronic condition, delayed PTSD may appear a significant time after the traumatic stress, there having been few or no symptoms soon after the stress.

7. Comorbidity of PTSD with other psychiatric disorders may change over time.

8. A wide variety of factors may affect the course of PTSD, including coping mechanisms, social support, type and duration of stress, later stress, family functioning, and personality and other disorders.

Duration and Subtypes of PTSD

Validity of the acute and chronic subtypes of PTSD are assessed, along with the relationship between PTSD and adjustment disorder.

A literature search was conducted of psychological, psychiatric, nursing, and social work journals for articles concerning the aftermath of trauma. Key words included *posttraumatic stress disorder, trauma, stress, war, rape, fire, disaster,* and *accident.* Unpublished data were also included, and PTSD researchers were contacted for recent data that had not yet been presented. Clinical impressions of experienced clinicians were also included. Particular attention was given to studies assessing PTSD symptoms at several points starting soon after the trauma.

Results

1) **Duration.** Eight studies evaluated the course of symptoms following the trauma (Kilpatrick and Resnick 1993; Kilpatrick et al. 1987, 1988; McFarlane 1988a, 1988b; Nader et al. 1990; Pynoos et al. 1987; Rothbaum and Foa 1993; Saigh 1988). Following rape and criminal assault, it is evident that the frequency of PTSD is very high in the first few months, reaching as high as 94%. By 3–4 months, the prevalence rates had dropped to approximately 45%–50%. At 1 year, prevalence rates ranged

from 11% to 47%, according to population. Following rape, as many as 17% still fulfilled diagnostic criteria at an average of 15 years postassault. Following aggravated assault, 10% met diagnostic criteria at an average of 10 years postassault. However, following wartime shelling, civilians who develop acute reactions generally improve, and the rate of continued distress is extremely low.

The course of PTSD in children appears to be similar to that in adults. In one prospective follow-up study (Nader et al. 1990) following a sniper attack on a school playground, 74% of children who were close to the scene of the trauma still manifested PTSD 14 months later, as opposed to 19% of those who were not in the immediate vicinity.

2) Subtypes.   The subtypes of PTSD have not received extensive study, but the available evidence suggests that there are no significant differences between acute-onset and delayed-onset PTSD subtypes (Watson et al. 1988). No cases of delayed PTSD exist in the literature on schoolchildren. Some experts (e.g., McFarlane 1988a) regard the definitions of acute-onset, delayed-onset, and chronic PTSD as "an arbitrary generalization based on clinical experience" (p. 34).

3) Overlap between PTSD and adjustment disorder.   In DSM-III-R, PTSD symptoms must persist at least 1 month for the diagnosis to be made. One would therefore assume that many acutely stressed individuals who have dysfunctional symptoms would receive an alternative diagnosis of adjustment disorder in the interim. In the one study that undertook follow-up evaluations of patients diagnosed with adjustment disorder, none of the patients received a subsequent diagnosis of PTSD (Andreasen and Hoenk 1982). This would suggest that adjustment disorder is not an acute form of PTSD and that little overlap exists. From the study of combat stress reaction (CSR) in Israeli veterans, it appears that combat stress reaction or some similar form of acute stress response would be a more appropriate interim diagnosis for patients who subsequently develop PTSD (Solomon et al. 1988).

Epidemiology of PTSD

The study of large populations that did not seek treatment can provide more comprehensive characteristics of a disorder than it is possible to obtain from the treatment-seeking population described above.

The review was based on studies identified by Medline and PSYCH searches of the English language literature, along with inclusion of numerous other published and unpublished reports known to us. To be included, studies were required to have used structured interviews for DSM-III or DSM-III-R criteria for PTSD.

Results

1) **Prevalence.** In community samples that were not at risk for PTSD, the lifetime prevalence of PTSD ranged from 1% to 2.6%, with a further 6.6%–15% exhibiting subthreshold symptoms of PTSD (Davidson et al. 1991; Helzer et al. 1987; Shore et al. 1986). All major community studies have used the Diagnostic Interview Schedule (DIS) (Robins et al. 1981), which almost certainly underestimates the true prevalence. Prevalence rates in samples at risk through exposure to trauma, including firefighters, combat veterans, victims of sexual assault, those who have experienced a volcanic eruption, and traumatized schoolchildren, all show increased prevalence rates compared with samples that are not at risk, with values ranging from 3.1% to 14% in studies using the DIS (Centers for Disease Control 1988; Helzer et al. 1987; Shore et al. 1989), and from 19% to 58% in studies using other more diagnostically sensitive interviews (Card 1987; Kulka et al. 1988; Pynoos et al. 1987).

2) **Duration of illness.** All except one survey found that PTSD remained present for at least 1 year in approximately 50% of cases, indicating that it becomes a chronic illness in a large number of victims.

3) **Comorbidity.** Rates of comorbid psychiatric illness range from 62% to 98% in chronic PTSD. There is no consistency with regard to type of illness, nor is it always possible to detect the sequence in which illnesses unfolded. In general, depression, obsessive-compulsive disorder, generalized anxiety disorder, and alcohol/substance abuse were the most frequently associated disorders, but this may also reflect the fact that these were the disorders most frequently inquired about (Davidson et al. 1991; Helzer et al. 1987; Kulka et al. 1988; Shore et al. 1986). As an isolated condition, chronic PTSD is extremely rare.

4) **Pretrauma risk factors.** The following factors were most frequently found to be related to a subsequent risk of developing PTSD: family psychiatric illness, parental poverty, traumatization in childhood, early parental separation, childhood behavior disorder, neuroticism, introversion, previous psychiatric disorder, other adverse life events, and being female.

5) **Relationship between trauma and diagnosis.** A number of studies indicate a positive relationship between the risk of developing PTSD and the intensity of, or the individual's propinquity to, the trauma. Physical injury increased the risk of developing PTSD following combat and sexual assault. Similar relationships were noted in traumatized children and in victims of a fire or a natural disaster. The

epidemiological literature supports the view that PTSD risk increases in proportion to the intensity of the trauma.

6) **Interaction of vulnerability factors with trauma.**   Data from the National Vietnam Veterans Readjustment Study (NVVRS) lead to the conclusion that premorbid risk factors and intensity of trauma both contribute independently and interactively to the risk of developing PTSD (Kulka et al. 1988). Studies show that after the eruption of Mount St. Helens, premorbid risk factors became less important once the degree of trauma had exceeded a certain threshold (Shore et al. 1986).

7) **Differences between acute and chronic PTSD.**   Chronic PTSD is associated with more frequent social phobia and somatization disorder, as well as more prominent avoidance symptoms and behaviors (Davidson et al. 1991). Predictors of chronicity include neuroticism, adverse events before the trauma, previous treatment for psychiatric disorder, and avoidance of thinking about the trauma (McFarlane 1989).

8) **Construct validity.**   PTSD was one of only a few psychiatric disorders to increase in the community after a natural disaster or in association with earlier sexual assault (Shore et al. 1986; Winfield et al. 1990). Epidemiological studies support the view that severe trauma, as understood by DSM-III-R, is more than a nonspecific stress that can give rise to a broad range of psychiatric illness.

Effects of Prolonged and Repeated Trauma

This review examines the evidence for a complex posttraumatic stress syndrome that, it is believed, is not adequately accounted for by the PTSD criteria.

The usual methods for systematic literature search could not be employed, because the proposed diagnosis has not been previously named. The literature reviewed included first-person accounts of survivors themselves, descriptive clinical literature, and rigorously designed clinical studies. Particular attention was focused on those observations of the sequelae of prolonged victimization that did not fit readily into the existing PTSD criteria.

Results

Clinical recognition of a DESNOS-like entity.   Several leading writers have proposed an expanded diagnostic concept to encompass the extensive characterological changes seen in survivors of prolonged and repeated trauma. These writers include clinicians working with adult survivors of childhood abuse, political refugees, prisoners of war, and survivors of the Nazi Holocaust (Gelinas 1983;

Goodwin 1988; Horowitz 1986; Kolb 1989; Kroll et al. 1989; Niederland 1968).

Clinical observations identify three broad areas of disturbance that transcend simple PTSD: 1) pleomorphic symptom picture, 2) characterological changes, and 3) vulnerability to repeated harm.

Symptomatic sequelae of prolonged traumatization. Many studies have documented a polysymptomatic syndrome, with high distress in multiple domains including somatization, depression, anxiety, interpersonal sensitivity, paranoia, and transient cognitive changes. The triad of multiple somatic complaints, persistent affective dysregulation, and marked dissociative symptomatology is frequently noted (e.g., Browne and Finkelhor 1986; Bryer et al. 1987; Hoppe 1968; Kroll et al. 1989; Spiegel 1990; Tennant et al. 1986).

Characterological sequelae of prolonged traumatization. *Pathological changes in relationship:* Chronic, repetitive trauma can occur only when the victim is in a state of captivity, unable to escape, or under the control of the perpetrator. As a result, the psychology of the victim is shaped by the actions and beliefs of the perpetrator. The methods of the perpetrator involve the systematic use of terror, enforced helplessness, and isolation of the victim (Amnesty International 1973). Under these conditions, erosion of the victim's previous personality structure may occur, and a pathological attachment, sometimes described as "traumatic bonding," may be formed with the perpetrator (Dutton and Painter 1981; Graham et al. 1988; Symonds 1982). The victim may show constriction of initiative and planning, with apparent passivity and dependence on the perpetrator (Flannery 1987; Walker 1979). Even following release or escape, the survivor may remain preoccupied with the perpetrator. Disturbances in other relationships are also seen following release from captivity. The survivor may oscillate between suspicious withdrawal from others and desperate search for a "special," dependent relationship with an idealized rescuer (Melges and Swartz 1989; Zanarini et al. 1990).

Pathological changes in identity: Subjection to a coercive relationship produces marked alterations in the victim's identity. All structures of the self, including body image, ego ideals, and moral values are invaded and systematically broken down. The resulting deformed identity may include a sense of the self as contaminated, guilty, or evil (Niederland 1968). Fragmentation in the sense of self is common (Rieker et al. 1986), reaching its most extreme expression in survivors of prolonged childhood abuse. The combination of identity fragmentation and elaborate dissociative psychopathology can be seen in multiple personality disorder, with the formation of named alters. Lesser but still marked identify diffusion is found in borderline personality disorder. Both disorders are strongly associated with early, severe, and prolonged childhood abuse (Herman et al. 1989; Putnam 1989).

Repetition of harm following repeated traumatization. Deliberate self-injury, rarely seen after a single acute trauma, is often seen in individuals with a history of prolonged traumatization (van der Kolk 1989). Such behavior is found most commonly in victims whose abuse began early in childhood. Survivors of prolonged early trauma may also be at high risk for repeated victimization in later life (Russell 1986). After prolonged abuse, some survivors may re-enact early traumatic experiences by harming others. Male survivors in particular appear to be at risk of abusing others, whereas female survivors are more likely to harm themselves or to become passive accomplices of abusive men (Burgess et al. 1984; Carmen et al. 1984; Goodwin et al. 1982). It should be noted that the great majority of survivors do not become perpetrators or accomplices in crimes against others (Herman 1988; Kaufman and Zigler 1987).

Discussion

Stressor Criterion

Preferred and alternative proposals for the stressor criterion are described in this section. There are several possibilities, although not all are considered feasible.

1. Eliminate criterion A altogether, basing judgment on subjective appraisal that the event was traumatic. This places the burden of diagnostic sensitivity on criterion B, which, by demonstrating 100% sensitivity, would serve as the entry criterion. This would present a problem because criteria C and D, which are not uniformly applied, would be unlikely to hold anywhere near 100% specificity, thus leading to numerous false-positive diagnoses.

2. To adopt a narrower view, events could be limited to those that have traditionally been described in the literature. This would minimize diagnostic heterogeneity and would preserve the assumed construct validity, that is, that certain events do present a challenge with which the majority of individuals are unprepared to cope and would be regarded by most as unusual experiences. On the other hand, too narrow a definition could lead to false-negative diagnoses.

3. Adopt a definition that eliminates reference to the unusualness of the event or the universality of distress but emphasizes characteristics of the event and continues to retain some degree of restrictiveness.

4. Include a definition that refers to subjective appraisal.

5. Adopt the ICD-10 definition.

6. Leave the criteria unchanged.

Symptoms Across Groups

The results of the four reviews of PTSD in different victim groups presented in this chapter agree in not supporting any major change in the composition or content of the B, C, and D symptom criteria.

One reasonable proposal for change would be to recommend a reduction in the minimum number of avoidance (C) items from three to two for reasons discussed above. Additional support for this proposal comes from a recent publication by Solomon and Canino (1990). The effect this change will have (e.g., on prevalence or possible difference in characterization between groups with two and three avoidance symptoms) will be examined in a field trial.

A second proposal arises from the finding that criterion C items do not emerge as one common factor. Specifically, loss of interest/alienation does not group with avoidance of thoughts about the trauma. Because one of these groups is PTSD-specific (avoidance of thoughts or actions concerning the trauma), whereas the other is not (foreshortened future, reduced interest, detachment from others, constricted affect), a second proposal is to employ a polythetic approach that would require that at least one of the two (or three) criterion C items be either avoidance of thoughts or situations reminiscent of the trauma or psychogenic amnesia (i.e., C1, C2, and C3 in the current criteria).

A third proposal arising from Keane's review of the literature, and supported by Pitman's review of the psychophysiology of PTSD, is to recommend that symptom D6 (physiological hyperresponsivity on exposure to reminders of the event) be moved from the generalized hyperarousal cluster (the D symptoms) into the PTSD-specific intrusive symptoms (B cluster).

Last, Green's literature review of disaster victims and Herman's review of chronic and prolonged traumatization suggest that more emphasis be placed on the occurrence of somatic symptoms (e.g., headache, upset stomach), although evidence is perhaps insufficient to justify including this as a new criterion.

Biological Findings

Biological data are compatible with a causal role for trauma in the development of PTSD. Although the findings are not extensive, they are coherent. Psychophysiological studies indicate a specific link between a traumatic event and the subsequent development of PTSD symptomatology in combat veterans. The other major finding of tonic sympathetic hyperarousal is probably an effect of the traumatic event.

Classical conditioning models are supported by the literature, and it is suggested that these could apply to many affects and not merely to anxiety. Sleep and neuroendocrine studies suggest a closer link with anxiety than with depression.

Data do support a weak link with dissociative disorder, basically derived from a study in combat veterans of stress-induced opiate-mediated analgesia, which can be reversed by naloxone (van der Kolk et al. 1989).

Course of PTSD

It would be very useful to provide guidance regarding the different PTSD subtypes. Awareness that the disorder may diminish with time promotes therapeutic optimism, but recognition that it may recur will also help to maintain a proper perspective concerning the reality of the condition.

It is important to note that the onset of PTSD can be delayed and to amplify this point in the text. This will lessen the tendency to miss the disorder when a longer time has passed since the trauma.

Although the designation of subtypes of a disorder is usually reserved for forms of a disorder that are distinctly different in one way or another, or in which different treatments would be indicated, it is unclear to what extent these considerations apply in the case of PTSD. It is recommended that both subtype designations and text describing the subtypes be included in DSM-IV.

Subtypes and Duration

There might be a higher rate of diagnosis of (acute) PTSD if the 1-month duration requirement were eliminated. On the other hand, requiring a minimum duration before a diagnosis of PTSD could be made might reduce help-seeking behavior as well as reimbursement for treatment. Several studies suggest that the presence of PTSD at 3 months posttrauma is a good predictor of the chronic state.

The DSM-III subtypes of acute versus delayed PTSD relied on uncontrolled clinical observations. Although some individuals do have delayed PTSD, it is an extremely rare diagnosis; however, there may still be some advantage to preserving it, because it does exist.

If a duration criterion is required for PTSD, the dilemma that arises concerns the fact that an individual's initial PTSD reaction (i.e., prior to meeting minimum duration) may be so severe that a psychiatric diagnosis is warranted. We have found that adjustment disorder is an inappropriate interim diagnosis. This may support the value of reintroducing the concept of acute PTSD, which had been dropped in DSM-III-R. Other alternative diagnoses could also be used (i.e., posttraumatic stress reaction, DESNOS, or uncomplicated posttraumatic stress reaction with a V-code).

Epidemiology

The epidemiological literature provides construct validity for the link between traumatic stress and the PTSD symptom cluster, although at this time no data are available to indicate whether the same symptom cluster might also follow less severe stressors. PTSD is a common illness; it often becomes chronic and by that time is almost always associated with other comorbid psychiatric illness. Premorbid risk factors do exist that contribute independently to the development of PTSD. However, trauma intensity and quality of trauma also contribute directly to the risk of the disorder.

Recommendations

Stressor Criterion

The Work Group recommends the third proposal and proposes that the fourth and fifth proposals be experimentally tested in field trials. This would be performed by uncoupling criterion A from criteria B, C, and D. Previous research in PTSD has always included criterion A with the symptomatology (i.e., it assumed the DSM-III-R criteria set but never evaluated the relationship between criterion A and the symptoms). We will also test the relationship between symptoms and stressors of different magnitudes (i.e., low- and high-magnitude events). Three options for the stressor criterion are proposed:

1. "The person has experienced, witnessed or been confronted with an event or events that involve actual or threatened death or injury, or a threat to the physical integrity of oneself or others" (option A1 in *DSM-IV Options Book,* American Psychiatric Association, 1991).
2. Adopt a two-part definition of criterion A as follows: "(i) The person has experienced, witnessed, or been confronted with an event, or events, that involve actual or threatened death or injury, or a threat to the physical integrity of oneself or others. (ii) The person's response involved intense fear, distress, helplessness or horror." In this definition, both parts would be required (option A2 in *DSM-IV Options Book*).
3. "Exposure to an exceptional mental or physical stressor, either brief or prolonged." This is the proposed ICD-10 definition (option A3 in *DSM-IV Options Book*).

Symptomatology of PTSD

Several options concerning the PTSD symptomatology criteria have been proposed: 1) not changing the symptom criteria, 2) reducing the number of required avoidance symptoms from three to two, 3) an alternative proposal to option 2 would be to require two symptoms but insist that one of these should be specific to PTSD (i.e., avoidance of thoughts related to the trauma, avoidance of situations that remind the victim of the trauma, or psychogenic amnesia), 4) removing the physiological reactivity symptom from the D cluster and inserting it in the B cluster, 5) emphasizing the frequency of somatization in PTSD in the text section dealing with "Associated Features."

Classification of PTSD

The committee recommends that PTSD be assigned to a separate category of "disorders related to psychological trauma" and that this category include the proposed acute stress response (also known as brief reactive dissociative disorder) and, if the field trials are supportive, DESNOS. This would not only bring DSM-IV in line with ICD-10, but it would also promote the well-founded notion that classification should reflect etiology when this is known and would assign the concept of trauma-related disorders to a level of nosological importance that many people feel is deserved.

The second recommendation would be that, if no separate category of stress response disorders is established, PTSD remain within the anxiety disorders section, because the evidence to support this, while not overwhelming, remains strong.

Biological Findings

The available data support an independent, separate, etiologically based classification of PTSD. Such a classification would have the merit of emphasizing prevention of traumatic (etiological) events in public health considerations. Should there be strong reasons not to so classify PTSD, then its retention as an anxiety disorder receives strong support.

With regard to the diagnostic criteria, based on the review, the committee concluded that a prominent place is warranted for physiological hyperactivity in response to reminders of the trauma. Because it is diagnostically specific, it is recommended that this item be moved from the general hyperarousal criterion (criterion D) into the PTSD-specific intrusive features (criterion B). It may be regarded as a diagnostically sufficient feature, although not a necessary one. Tonic sympathetic hyperarousal, on the other hand, is necessary but not sufficient. In the current state of understanding, it would be inappropriate to recommend inclusion of positive psychophysiological laboratory findings as a diagnostic criterion.

Course and Subtypes

1. A specific recommendation is given for describing the course of PTSD in the DSM-IV text. For this, the reader is referred to the DSM-IV text itself.

2. A recommended text for "uncomplicated posttraumatic stress reaction to traumatic stress" is given for inclusion as a V-code. Such a category would facilitate access to treatment for individuals with subthreshold PTSD yet avoid the possible stigmatizing effects of a psychiatric disorder in situations where the reaction to extreme stress is itself normal (Blank 1993b).

3. It has been proposed that the 1-month minimum duration of symptoms be dropped as a requirement because a severe disorder is no less important because of brevity, and documentation of a prior brief episode may provide important information in the event of recurring symptoms in the future (Blank 1993b).

4. It has been proposed that 1 month should elapse following the initial trauma before the diagnosis can be made.

Duration

It is proposed that no minimum duration of symptoms be required for the diagnosis of PTSD but that the acute form of PTSD would be assigned to an individual for the first 3 months of symptoms, and the chronic form of PTSD would be assigned for individuals with symptoms beyond the 3-month point. If PTSD symptoms do not arise until at least 3 months after the trauma, the term *delayed PTSD* would be used.

The use of adjustment disorder is not an appropriate interim diagnosis. Whether adjustment disorder would be included in a new category of traumatic psychological disorder is open to debate.

Epidemiology

The epidemiological data will be used chiefly to inform the text in the sections describing associated features, comorbidity, risk factors, and prevalence. The review also concludes that epidemiological support exists for the separate classification of PTSD in DSM-IV but does not provide any evidence that the criteria themselves should change.

Effects of Prolonged and Repeated Trauma

The review of the literature offers extensive but unsystematized support for the concept of a complex posttraumatic syndrome (DESNOS) in survivors of prolonged, repeated victimization. This syndrome appears to be distinct from simple PTSD and warrants systematic empirical testing.

The current draft of DESNOS was developed primarily by clinicians working with survivors of domestic and sexual abuse. A more representative depiction of this syndrome would require inclusion of data from survivors of political torture and imprisonment as well.

If field trials validate the concept of DESNOS, this would provide further support for the recommendation set forth in other position papers for the establishment of a group of posttraumatic disorders as a separate category in DSM-IV.

References

American Psychiatric Association: Diagnostic and Statistical Manual of Mental Disorders, 2nd Edition. Washington, DC, American Psychiatric Association, 1968

American Psychiatric Association: Diagnostic and Statistical Manual of Mental Disorders, 3rd Edition. Washington, DC, American Psychiatric Association, 1980

American Psychiatric Association: Diagnostic and Statistical Manual of Mental Disorders, 3rd Edition, Revised. Washington, DC, American Psychiatric Association, 1987

Amnesty International: Report on Torture. New York, Farrar, Strauss & Giroux, 1973

Andreasen NC, Hoenk PR: The predictive value of adjustment disorders: a follow-up study. Am J Psychiatry 139:584–590, 1982

Beck JC, van der Kolk BA: Reports of childhood incest and current behavior of chronically hospitalized psychotic women. Am J Psychiatry 144:1474–1476, 1987

Blanchard EB, Mold LC, Pallmeyer TP, et al: A psychophysiological study of posttraumatic stress disorder in Vietnam veterans. Psychiatr Q 54:220–229, 1982

Blank AS: The longitudinal course of posttraumatic stress disorder, in Posttraumatic Stress Disorder: DSM-IV and Beyond. Edited by Davidson JRT, Foa EB. Washington, DC, American Psychiatric Press, 1993a, pp 3–20

Blank AS: Suggested recommendations for DSM-IV on course and subtypes, in Posttraumatic Stress Disorder: DSM-IV and Beyond. Edited by Davidson JRT, Foa EB. Washington, DC, American Psychiatric Press, 1993b, pp 237–240

Breslau N, Davis G: Post traumatic stress disorder: the etiologic specificity of wartime stressors. Am J Psychiatry 144:578–583, 1987

Browne A, Finkelhor D: Impact of child sexual abuse: a review of the literature. Psychol Bull 99:66–67, 1986

Bryer JB, Nelson BA, Miller JB, et al: Childhood sexual and physical abuse as factors in adult psychiatric illness. Am J Psychiatry 144:1426–1430, 1987

Burgess AW, Hartman CR, McCausland MP, et al: Response patterns in children and adolescents exploited through sex rings and pornography. Am J Psychiatry 141:656–662, 1984

Burke JD Jr, Burns JF, Burns BJ, et al: Changes in children's behavior after a natural disaster. Am J Psychiatry 139:1010–1014, 1982

Burstein A: Post traumatic stress disorder (letter). J Clin Psychiatry 46:554, 1985

Card JJ: Epidemiology of PTSD in a national cohort of Vietnam veterans. J Am Psychol 43:6–17, 1987

Carmen EH, Rieker PP, Mills T: Victims of violence and psychiatric illness. Am J Psychiatry 141:378–383, 1984

Centers for Disease Control: Health status of Vietnam veterans: psychosocial characteristics. JAMA 259:2701–2707, 1988

Craske MG, Barlow DH: Nocturnal panic. J Nerv Ment Dis 177:160–167, 1989

Davidson JRT, Swartz M, Storck M, et al: A diagnostic and family study of post-traumatic stress disorder. Am J Psychiatry 142:90–93, 1985a

Davidson JRT, Lipper SL, Kilts CD, et al: Platelet MAO activity in post traumatic stress disorder. Am J Psychiatry 142:1341–1343, 1985b

Davidson JRT, Hughes DL, Blazer DG, et al: Post traumatic stress disorder in the community: an epidemiological study. Psychol Med 21:713–721, 1991

Davidson LM, Baum A: Chronic stress and post traumatic stress disorders. J Consult Clin Psychol 54:303–308, 1986

DiNardo PA, Barlow DH: Anxiety Disorders Interview Schedule, Revised. Albany, NY, Center for Stress and Anxiety Disorders, The University at Albany, State University of New York, 1988

Dutton D, Painter SL: Traumatic bonding: the development of emotional attachments in battered women and other relationships of intermittent abuse. Victimology 6:139–155, 1981

Escobar JI, Randolph ET, Puente G, et al: Post traumatic stress disorder in Hispanic Vietnam veterans: clinical phenomenology and sociocultural characteristics. J Nerv Ment Dis 171:585–596, 1983

Flannery R: From victim to survivor: a stress management approach in the treatment of learned helplessness, in Psychological Trauma. Edited by van der Kolk BA. Washington, DC, American Psychiatric Press, 1987, pp 216–232

Gelinas D: The persistent negative effects of incest. Psychiatry 46:312–332, 1983

Goodwin J: Evaluation and treatment of incest victims and their families: a problem oriented approach, in Modern Perspectives in Psycho-Social Pathology. Edited by Howells JG. New York, Brunner/Mazel, 1988

Goodwin J, McMarty T, DiVasto P: Physical and sexual abuse of the children of adult incest victims, in Sexual Abuse: Incest Victims and Their Families. Edited by Goodwin J. Boston, MA, John Wright, 1982, pp 139–154

Graham DL, Rawlings E, Rimini N: Survivors of terror: battered women, hostages, and the Stockholm syndrome, in Feminist Perspectives on Wife Abuse. Edited by Yllo K, Bograd M. Beverly Hills, CA, Sage, 1988, pp 217–233

Green B, Grace M, Gleser G: Identifying survivors at risk, long term impairment following the Beverley Hills Supper Club fire. J Consult Clin Psychol 53:672–678, 1985

Green BL, Lindy JD, Grace MC, et al: Multiple diagnosis in post traumatic stress disorder: the role of war stressors. J Nerv Ment Dis 177:329–335, 1989

Green BL, Lindy JD, Grace MC, et al: Buffalo Creek Survivors in the second decade: stability of stress symptoms. Am J Orthopsychiatry 60:43–54, 1990

Helzer JE, Robins LN, McEvoy L: Post-traumatic stress disorder in the general population: findings of the Epidemiologic Catchment Area Study. N Engl J Med 317:630–634, 1987

Herman J: Considering sex offenders: a model of addiction. Signs: Journal of Women in Culture and Society 13:695–724, 1988

Herman JL, Perry JC, van der Kolk BA: Childhood trauma in borderline personality disorder. Am J Psychiatry 146:490–495, 1989

Hoppe KD: Resomatization of affects in survivors of persecution. Int J Psychoeval 49:324–326, 1968

Horowitz M: Stress Response Syndromes. Northridge, NJ, Jason Aronson, 1986

Horowitz M: Contributions to DSM-IV, separate category on stress response syndromes: the description of normal and pathological grief reactions. Unpublished report to DSM-IV sub-Work Group, 1989

Jones JC, Barlow DH: The etiology of post-traumatic stress disorder. Clin Psychol Rev 10:299–328, 1990

Kaufman J, Zigler E: Do abused children become abusive parents? Am J Orthopsychiatry 57:186–192, 1987

Keane TM, Caddell JM, Taylor KL: Mississippi scale for combat-related posttraumatic stress disorder: three studies in reliability and validity. J Consult Clin Psychol 56:85–90, 1988

Kilpatrick DG, Resnick HS: Posttraumatic stress disorder associated with exposure to criminal victimization in clinical and community populations, in Posttraumatic Stress Disorder: DSM-IV and Beyond. Edited by Davidson JRT, Foa EB. Washington, DC, American Psychiatric Press, 1993, pp 113–143

Kilpatrick DG, Saunders BE, Veronen LJ, et al: Criminal victimization: lifetime prevalence, reporting to police and psychological impact. Crime and Delinquency 33:479–489, 1987

Kilpatrick DG, Amick A, Resnick HS. Preliminary research data on post traumatic stress disorder following murders and drunk driving crashes. Paper presented at National Organization for Victims Assistance 14th Annual Meeting, Tucson, AZ, September 1988

Kilpatrick D, Saunders B, Amick-McMillan A, et al: Victim and crime factors associated with the development of posttraumatic stress disorder. Behavior Therapy 20:199–214, 1989

Kinzie JD, Sack W, Angell R, et al: A three-year follow-up of Cambodian young people traumatized as children. J Am Acad Child Adolesc Psychiatry 28:501–504, 1989

Kinzie JD, Boehnlein JK, Leung PK, et al: The prevalence of post traumatic stress disorder and its clinical significance among Southeast Asian refugees. Am J Psychiatry 147:913–917, 1990

Kolb LC: Letter to editor. Am J Psychiatry 146:811–812, 1989

Kroll J, Habericht M, McKenzie T, et al: Depression and post traumatic stress disorders in Southeast Asian refugees. Am J Psychiatry 146:1592–1597, 1989

Kudler HS, Davidson JRT, Meador K, et al: The DST and posttraumatic stress disorder. Am J Psychiatry 144:1068–1071, 1987

Kulka RA, Schlenger WE, Fairbank JA, et al: Contractual Report of Findings from the National Vietnam Veterans Readjustment Study. Research Triangle Park, NC, Research Triangle Institute, November 7, 1988

Laufer R, Brett EB, Gallops M: Dimensions of post traumatic stress disorder among Vietnam veterans. J Nerv Ment Dis 173:538–545, 1985

Lerer B, Ebstein RP, Shestatsky M, et al: Cyclic AMP signal transduction in post-traumatic stress disorder. Am J Psychiatry 144:1324–1327, 1987

Loewenstein RJ, Putnam FW: A comparison study of dissociative symptoms in patients with complex partial seizures, multiple personality disorder and post traumatic stress disorder. Dissociation 1:17–23, 1988

Lyons JA: Posttraumatic stress disorder in children and adolescents: a review of the literature. Develop Behav Pediatrics 8:349–356, 1987

Madakasira S, O'Brien K: Acute post traumatic stress disorder in victims of a natural disaster. J Nerv Ment Dis 175:256–290, 1987

Maida CA, Gordon NS, Steinberg A, et al: Psychosocial impact of disasters: victims of the Baldwin Hills Fire. J Traumatic Stress 2:37–48, 1989

Malloy PF, Fairbank JA, Keane TM: Validation of a multimethod assessment of post-traumatic stress disorders in Vietnam veterans. J Consult Clin Psychol 51:488–494, 1983

Malmquist CP: Children who witness parental murder: posttraumatic aspects. J Am Acad Child Adolesc Psychiatry 25:320–325, 1986

Mason JW, Giller EL, Kosten TR, et al: Psychoendocrine approaches to the diagnosis and pathogenesis of post traumatic stress disorder, in Biological Assessment and Treatment of Post Traumatic Stress Disorder. Edited by Giller EL Jr. Washington, DC, American Psychiatric Press, 1990, pp 165–186

McFarlane AC: The longitudinal course of posttraumatic morbidity: the range of outcomes and their predictors. J Nerv Ment Dis 176:30–39, 1988a

McFarlane AC: The phenomenology of posttraumatic stress disorders following a natural disaster. J Nerv Ment Dis 176:22–29, 1988b

McFarlane AC: The aetiology of post traumatic morbidity: predisposing, precipitating and perpetrating factors. Br J Psychiatry 154:221–228, 1989

Melges FT, Swartz MS: Oscillations of attachment in borderline personality disorder. Am J Psychiatry 146:1115–1120, 1989

Nader K, Pynoos R, Fairbanks L, et al: Children's PTSD reactions one year after a sniper attack on their school. Am J Psychiatry 147:1526–1530, 1990

Niederland WG: Clinical observations on the "survivor syndrome." Int J Psychoanal 49:313–315, 1968

Perry BD, Giller EL, Southwick SM: Altered platelet alpha-2 adrenergic receptor affinity states in post-traumatic stress disorder. Am J Psychiatry 144:1511–1512, 1987

Pitman R: Biological findings in PTSD: implication for the DSM-IV classification, in Posttraumatic Stress Disorder: DSM-IV and Beyond. Edited by Davidson JRT, Foa EB. Washington, DC, American Psychiatric Press, 1993, pp 173–190

Pitman RK, Orr SP, Forgue DF, et al: Psychophysiologic assessment of post traumatic stress disorder imagery in Vietnam combat veterans. Arch Gen Psychiatry 44:970–975, 1987

Pitman R, Altman B, Macklin M: Prevalence of post-traumatic stress disorder in wounded Vietnam veterans. Am J Psychiatry 175:286–290, 1989

Putnam FW: Diagnosis and Treatment of Multiple Personality Disorder. New York, Guilford, 1989

Pynoos RS, Frederick C, Nader K, et al: Life threat and post traumatic stress in school-age children. Arch Gen Psychiatry 44:1057–1063, 1987

Rieker PP, Carmen E, Hilberman E: The victim-to-patient process: the disconfirmation and transformation of abuse. Am J Orthopsychiatry 56:360–370, 1986

Robins LN, Helzer JE, Croughan JL, et al: National Institute of Mental Health Diagnostic Interview Schedule: its history, characteristics, and validity. Arch Gen Psychiatry 38:381–389, 1981

Rothbaum BO, Foa EB: Subtypes of posttraumatic stress disorder and duration of symptoms, in Post Traumatic Stress Disorder: DSM-IV and Beyond. Edited by Davidson JRT, Foa EB. Washington DC, American Psychiatric Press, 1993, pp 23–36

Russell DEH: The Secret Trauma. New York, Basic Books, 1986

Saigh PA: Anxiety, depression and assertion across alternating intervals of stress. J Abnorm Psychol 97:338–341, 1988

Saigh P: The development of post traumatic stress disorder pursuant to different modes of traumatization. Paper presented at 97th Annual Convention of the American Psychological Association, New Orleans, 1989

Shore JH: Psychiatric reactions to disaster: the Mount St. Helen's experience. Am J Psychiatry 143:590–595, 1986

Shore JH, Tatum E, Vollmer WM: Evaluation of mental health effects of disaster: Mt. St. Helen's eruption. Am J Publ Health 76 (suppl):76–83, 1986

Shore JH, Vollmer WM, Tatum EL: Community patterns of post traumatic stress disorders. J Nerv Ment Dis 177:681–685, 1989

Sierles FS, Chen JJ, McFarland RE, et al: Post-traumatic stress disorder and concurrent psychiatric illness: a preliminary report. Am J Psychiatry 140:1177–1179, 1983

Smith MA, Davidson JRT, Ritchie JC, et al: The corticotropin-releasing hormone test in patients with post traumatic stress disorder. Biol Psychiatry 26:349–355, 1989

Smith EM, North CS: Aftermath of a disaster: psychological response to the Indianapolis Ramada jet crash. Quick Response Research Report #23. Boulder, CO, Natural Hazards Research and Applications Information Center, 1988

Solomon S, Canino GJ: Appropriateness of the DSM-III-R criteria for post traumatic stress disorder. Compr Psychiatry 31:227–237, 1990

Solomon Z, Benbenisty R, Mikulincer M: A follow-up of Israeli casualties of combat stress reaction ('battle shock') in the 1982 Lebanon war. Br J Clin Psychol 27:125–135, 1988

Speed N, Engdahl B, Schwartz J, et al: Post traumatic stress disorder as a consequence of the POW experience. J Nerv Ment Dis 177:1447–1530, 1989

Spiegel D: Trauma dissociation and hypnosis, in Incest-Related Syndromes of Adult Psychopathology. Edited by Kluft RP. Washington, DC, American Psychiatric Press, 1990

Spiegel D, Hunt T, Dondeshine HE: Dissociation and hypnotizability in post traumatic stress disorder. Am J Psychiatry 145:301–305, 1988

Spitzer RL, Williams JBW: Structured Clinical Interview for DSM-III (SCID). New York, Biometrics Research Department, New York State Psychiatric Institute, 1985

Steinglass P, Gerrity E: Natural disasters and post traumatic stress disorder: short-term vs long-term recovery in two disaster affected communities. J Appl Soc Psychol 20:1746–1765, 1990

Stoddard FJ, Norman DK, Murphy JM, et al: Psychiatric outcome of burned children and adolescents. J Am Acad Child Adolesc Psychiatry 28:589–595, 1989

Stutman RK, Bliss EL: Post traumatic stress disorder, hypnotizability and imagery. Am J Psychiatry 142:741–743, 1985

Symonds M: Victim responses to terror: understanding and treatment, in Victims of Terrorism. Edited by Ochberg FM, Soskis DA. Boulder, CO, Westview, 1982, pp 95–103

Task Force on DSM-IV: DSM-IV Options Book: Work in Progress. Washington, DC, American Psychiatric Association, 1991

Tennant CC, Goulston KJ, Dent OF: The psychological effects of being a prisoner of war. Am J Psychiatry 145:618–622, 1986

van der Kolk BA: Compulsion to repeat the trauma: re-enactment, revictimization, and masochism. Psychiatr Clin North Am 12:389–411, 1989

van der Kolk BA, Greenberg MS, Orr SP: Endogenous opioids, stress induced analgesia, and post-traumatic stress disorder. Psychopharmacol Bull 25:416–421, 1989

van Kammen WB, Christiansen C, Van Kammen DP, et al: Sleep and the prisoner of war experience—40 years later, in Biological Assessment and Treatment of Posttraumatic Stress Disorder. Edited by Giller EL Jr. Washington, DC, American Psychiatric Press, 1990, pp 159–172

Walker L: The Battered Woman. New York, Harper & Row, 1979

Watson CG, Kucala T, Manifold V, et al: Differences between post traumatic stress disorder patients with delayed and undelayed onsets. J Nerv Ment Dis 176:568–572, 1988

Wilkinson CB: Aftermath of a disaster: the collapse of the Hyatt Regency Hotel Skywalks. Am J Psychiatry 140:1134–1139, 1983

Winfield I, George LK, Swartz M, et al: Sexual assault and psychiatric disorders among a community sample of women. Am J Psychiatry 147:335–341, 1990

Zanarini M, Gunderson J, Frankenburg F, et al: Discriminating borderline personality disorder from other Axis II disorders. Am J Psychiatry 146:161–167, 1990

Zeiss R, Dickman H: PTSD 40 years later: incidence and person-situation correlates in former POWs. J Clin Psychol 45:80–87, 1989

Chapter 20

Generalized Anxiety Disorder

Karla Moras, Ph.D., T. D. Borkovec, Ph.D.,
Peter A. DiNardo, Ph.D., Ronald Rapee, Ph.D.,
John Riskind, Ph.D., and David H. Barlow, Ph.D.

Statement of the Issues

Four literature reviews were done on generalized anxiety disorder (GAD) (Borkovec et al. 1989; DiNardo 1990; Rapee 1989; Riskind et al. 1989). Three of the reviews were focused on two issues: 1) the reliability of the GAD diagnosis and 2) evidence that GAD can be discriminated from other diagnoses (i.e., dysthymia, the somatoform disorders, and psychophysiological disorders such as irritable bowel syndrome). Thus, two main issues were the reliability and discriminant validity of GAD. A third issue examined by Borkovec et al. (1989) in the fourth literature review was features that distinguish pathological and normal worry.

Subsequent to the preparation of the four reviews cited above for the DSM-IV Task Force, three of them became the bases of chapters published in Rapee and Barlow (1991), Borkovec et al. (1991), Barlow and DiNardo (1991), and Riskind et al. (1991). The reader is referred to these chapters for more extensive presentations of the original reviews.

Significance of the Issues

Issue 1: Reliability of GAD

The reliability with which any psychiatric diagnosis can be made is central to evaluating its validity and potential utility (Blashfield and Livesley 1991). The reliability of the GAD diagnosis was the focus of a review because the DSM-III (American Psychiatric Association 1980) criteria for GAD were found to have low reliability relative to the other anxiety disorders (DiNardo et al. 1983). In addition, a study based on partial DSM-III-R (American Psychiatric Association 1987) GAD criteria found that the reliability of the current GAD criteria was in the poor range (kappa = .27) (Mannuzza et al. 1989).

Issue 2: Validity of GAD—Its Discriminability From Other DSM-III-R Disorders

GAD was first defined in DSM-III. Several considerations converged, leading to the creation of GAD (Moras 1991). For example, GAD was regarded mainly as a residual category when it was originally conceived (Barlow et al. 1986). It was a diagnosis for people who had somatic symptoms that were regarded as manifestations of anxiety but who did not meet the diagnostic criteria for any of the specific phobic or anxiety disorders included in DSM-III, such as simple phobia, social phobia, and panic disorder (Barlow et al. 1986).

GAD's history as a residual category contributed to concern that it might not identify a distinct and discrete syndrome. Specifically, the discriminability of GAD from the DSM-III-R mood disorder of dysthymia has been questioned, in part because both are associated with chronic dysphoric affect. Thus, one of the main issues regarding GAD was its validity, particularly in terms of its ability to be distinguished from certain DSM-III-R mood disorders (e.g., Breslau and Davis 1985b). Another specific discriminant validity question was whether GAD could be distinguished from DSM-III-R hypochondriasis and other somatoform disorders. The question emerged in part because a person can worry excessively about his or her health. When this happens, can a diagnostician distinguish between the health concern that constitutes a GAD sphere of worry versus health worries that are a key diagnostic feature of hypochondriasis?

Issue 3: What Features Distinguish Pathological From Normal Worry?

Evidence concerning this issue was reviewed because the key diagnostic feature of DSM-III-R GAD is unrealistic and excessive worry about at least two different topics such as the safety of one's children and being able to pay one's bills. Because worry is a common human experience, it is necessary to identify features that distinguish normal worry from worry that is beyond normal limits and that merits identification as a symptom of a disorder within the DSM system.

Method

Issue 1

Peter DiNardo, Ph.D., reviewed empirical findings on the reliability with which DSM-III-R GAD can be diagnosed. DiNardo's review also attempted to identify sources of disagreement that might contribute to the lower-than-desirable reliability of GAD.

Issue 2

John Riskind, Ph.D., and colleagues reviewed the empirical evidence on the relationship of GAD to mood disorders. Ronald Rapee, Ph.D., reviewed the empirical evidence on the discriminability of GAD from DSM-III-R somatoform disorders and from psychophysiological disorders such as irritable bowel syndrome.

Issue 3

T. D. Borkovec, Ph.D., and colleagues reviewed the empirical evidence on differences between normal and pathological worry.

Results

Issue 1: Reliability of GAD

Methods and results. DiNardo (1990) conducted a literature search using the PsycLit CD-ROM system. The system is based on information in *Psychological Abstracts* and the PsycInfo database, which covers January 1983 to June 1989. Key words used in the search were obtained from the *Thesaurus of Psychological Index Terms.* They were *psychodiagnosis, anxiety neurosis, psychodiagnostic interview,* and *reliability.* The terms *generalized anxiety* and *generalized anxiety disorder* were used in combination with the Thesaurus terms. Through contacts with members of the DSM-IV Task Force, DiNardo obtained articles and manuscripts in press or in preparation. Finally, the reference sections of the articles obtained through these methods were examined for additional relevant citations.

This review examined the reliability of the DSM-III-R GAD diagnosis and the reliability of the GAD diagnostic criterion D, i.e., the requirement of 6 of 18 symptoms from three areas: motor tension, autonomic hyperactivity, and vigilance and scanning. The focus of the review was reliability findings from two companion studies (Fyer et al. 1989; Mannuzza et al. 1989) and from the Center for Stress and Anxiety Disorders (CSAD), University at Albany, State University of New York. Mannuzza et al. (1989) and Fyer et al. (1989) reported findings from two independent test-retest diagnostic interviews done 60 days or less apart on 104 patients using the Schedule for Affective Disorders and Schizophrenia, Lifetime Version (modified for the study of anxiety disorders) (SADS-LA) (Fyer et al. 1985) at the New York State Psychiatric Institute (NYSPI). The CSAD findings were based on 164 patients who received independent test-retest diagnostic interviews separated by ≤ 42 days using the Anxiety Disorders Interview Schedule—Revised (ADIS-R) (DiNardo and Barlow 1988).

The findings reviewed indicated that the reliability of GAD varied from poor to good, following conventions commonly used to interpret kappa coefficients (Cicchetti and Sparrow 1981; Landis and Koch 1977). For DSM-III-R GAD, Mannuzza et al. (1989) obtained poor reliability (.27). However, a kappa of .54 was obtained in the CSAD data for DSM-III-R GAD as a principal diagnosis. A higher kappa (.64) was obtained for presence versus absence of GAD as either a principal or additional diagnosis in the CSAD data.

Regarding sources of disagreement that could contribute to the less-than-desirable reliability figures for GAD, DiNardo (1990) suggested that diagnosticians might be unable to reliably distinguish GAD worry from worry that is an associated feature of other Axis I disorders. For example, it might be difficult to classify illness concerns as being in the GAD worry sphere as opposed to being a preoccupation with serious illness, which is a diagnostic criterion of hypochondriasis. Regarding the GAD criterion requiring 6 of 18 symptoms, DiNardo (1990) concluded that the reliability of ratings of the 18 symptoms generally is poor. The kappas reported by Fyer et al. (1989) ranged from .08 to .48 for the 18 symptoms; Pearson correlations for the CSAD data ranged from .05 to .63. No symptom showed consistent reliability across the NYSPI and the CSAD samples.

Discussion.   Two of DiNardo's (1990) recommendations are summarized here. First, he stated that additional studies were needed to determine the reliability of the GAD diagnosis and of the symptom criterion (criterion D) because the results of only two data sets were available for his review. Second, DiNardo (1990) recommended modification of the DSM-III-R GAD criterion D. He noted that the Fyer et al. (1989) data and the CSAD data did not suggest how the criterion could be modified, because none of the 18 symptoms showed consistently poor or good reliability across the two studies.

Given the lack of empirically based evidence on useful ways to modify criterion D, DiNardo suggested that general symptom areas of the type used in the DSM-III definition of GAD (e.g., motor tension, autonomic hyperactivity, and vigilance and scanning) could be reintroduced. DiNardo did not discuss the possibility of completely dropping the symptom criterion for GAD.

Issue 2: Validity of GAD—Its Discriminability From Dysthymia and Dysthymic Disorder

Methods and results.   Riskind et al. (1989) searched the psychiatric and psychological literature for empirical studies that compared GAD and dysthymia or dysthymic disorder. Searches were done of the Medline and PsycLit databases using terms such as *generalized anxiety, dysthymic disorder, anxiety and depression, anxiety neurosis,* and *GAD.* The years covered were 1980 to the time of the search in the fall of 1989. The search was focused on English language articles involving human subjects.

The shelf copies of the following selected journals of 8 years prior to the year of the review were reviewed manually: *Journal of Affective Disorders, Archives of General Psychiatry, Journal of Abnormal Psychology, American Journal of Psychiatry, British Journal of Psychiatry, Journal of Nervous and Mental Disease, Comprehensive Psychiatry, Journal of Clinical Psychiatry, Psychiatric Clinics of North America,* and *Journal of Anxiety Disorders.* Additional sources were explored by reviewing the bibliographic references in recent empirical articles and review papers. Finally, eight known investigators or groups were contacted about analyses, manuscripts, or data sets that were pertinent to the review.

Riskind et al. (1989) observed that previous research has provided considerable evidence that GAD is related to depression. In fact, the argument was advanced that DSM-III GAD and major depressive disorder were so closely related that they could not be meaningfully distinguished (Breier et al. 1984). However, a few studies done at Beck's Center for Cognitive Therapy (CCT) that compared DSM-III-R GAD and major depression suggested that significant differences do exist (Beck et al. 1987; Riskind et al. 1987).

The main focus of the Riskind et al. (1989) review was GAD and dysthymia. The two diagnostic categories are of particular interest because they may be harder to distinguish than GAD and major depression, because both are low-grade affective disturbances that display chronicity and are cross-situational rather than "uni-situational" in nature. Furthermore, some data suggest that anxiety symptoms are an important part of the symptom profile in a subgroup of patients with dysthymia, as they are for patients with major depression.

Although previous studies have raised important issues, they have not provided the data required to resolve questions regarding the discriminability of GAD and dysthymia. Because of the lack of existing data, Riskind et al. (1989) analyzed relevant data from Beck's CCT. The analyses compared GAD and dysthymia (GAD alone = "pure GAD," $n = 26$; dysthymia alone = "pure dysthymia," $n = 31$; GAD as principal, second, or third diagnosis and no dysthymia = "mixed GAD," $n = 156$; dysthymia as principal, second, or third diagnosis and no GAD = "mixed dysthymia," $n = 104$). Riskind et al. (1989) also reviewed an unpublished study that included GAD patients ($n = 15$) from Barlow's CSAD and dysthymia patients ($n = 15$) from other settings (Benshoof et al. 1989). The patients in the Benshoof et al. (1989) groups were categorized by principal diagnosis. However, 4 of the 15 dysthymia patients had GAD as an additional diagnosis. DSM-III diagnoses were used by Benshoof et al. (1989), whereas the data from Beck's CCT included patients diagnosed with DSM-III and DSM-III-R.

Discussion. A major limitation of existing data is that very few cases of pure GAD and pure dysthymia (as defined above) have been studied. The lack of pure case data makes it impossible to draw definitive conclusions at this time regarding the extent to which GAD and dysthymia can be distinguished. Results of Riskind et al.'s (1989) analyses of the CCT data offered provisional evidence for the validity of the distinction between DSM-III-R GAD and dysthymia. However, the results of the DSM-III–based study from CSAD (Benshoof et al. 1989) were less supportive of the distinctiveness of the two categories.

1. Discriminability of GAD and dysthymia: empirical findings from clinical samples. Although Riskind et al.'s (1989) analyses of the CCT data indicated that GAD and dysthymia differed significantly on many symptoms, the results of Benshoof et al. (1989) only partially replicated the Riskind et al. (1989) findings. Thus, findings from additional data sets are required before firm conclusions can be drawn about the distinctiveness of GAD and dysthymia in terms of symptomatology (e.g., item ratings from the Hamilton Anxiety Rating Scale [HARS, Hamilton 1959] and the Hamilton Rating Scale for Depression [HRSD, Hamilton 1960]). However, Riskind et al. (1989) concluded that the existing evidence converges on one conclusion: GAD and dysthymia are distinguished on severity of certain symptoms of depression (depressed mood, suicidality, impairment in work/activities, hopelessness, helplessness).

2. Methodological issues. Data are needed from patient samples that have been reliably diagnosed with structured interviews such as the Anxiety Disorders Interview Schedule—Revised (ADIS-R) (DiNardo and Barlow 1988) or the Structured Clinical Interview for DSM-III-R (SCID) (Spitzer et al. 1987). In addition, the studies should include symptom measures of anxiety and depression that do not contain overlapping item content like the original HARS and HRSD do, because the presence of depression items (e.g., depressed mood) on the HARS and vice versa might partially account for the failure to distinguish GAD and mood disorders at the symptom level. For example, some evidence exists that the revised scoring system developed by Riskind et al. (1987) for the HARS and HRSD discriminates GAD and dysthymia better than the original Hamilton scales do.

Longitudinal studies could also help elucidate the distinctiveness of GAD and dysthymia. For example, Roth et al. (1972) reported that episodic anxiety is found in depression, but persistent anxiety characterizes anxiety disorders. Similarly, they concluded that episodic depression appears in anxiety disorders such as GAD, but persistent depression characterizes disorders in which the primary distress involves depression.

3. Diagnostic issues: heterogeneity of GAD and dysthymia populations and co-morbidity. Both GAD and dysthymia show substantial heterogeneity in symptoms and associated characteristics. Consequently, it is of interest to determine whether differences between the two disorders are obtained over potential subtypes of each category. For example, Hoehn-Saric and McLeod (1985) proposed a difference between one subtype of GAD patients, those who show extensive autonomic arousal (e.g., elevation of heart rate, skin conductance) and muscle tension after stress, and another subtype who show only muscle tension. It is of interest to know whether only the former subtype of GAD patients exhibit higher levels of autonomic and cardiovascular symptoms than dysthymia patients because the two symptom domains were the major sources of differences between GAD and dysthymia in the analyses done for the Riskind et al. (1989) review. In other words, the Riskind et al. (1989) analyses suggested that the GAD subtype without autonomic symptoms in response to stress would be harder to distinguish from dysthymia patients than the GAD subtype that showed autonomic reactivity. Of course, it is also of interest to replicate Hoehn-Saric and McLeod's (1985) evidence for a "nonautonomic" subtype of GAD and, if replicated, to determine how these patients differ from dysthymia patients on anxiety symptoms.

Another potentially important question is the discriminability of GAD from early-onset (before age 25) versus late-onset (age 25 or older) dysthymia. Klein et al. (1988) reported differences in the rate of comorbid anxiety disorders among persons who have early- versus late-onset dysthymia. Patients with early-onset dysthymia were more likely to have comorbid anxiety disorders than patients with late-onset dysthymia. Such findings imply that early-onset dysthymia might be relatively difficult for diagnosticians to distinguish from GAD, whereas late-onset dysthymia is not.

The actual comorbidity rates of GAD and dysthymia provide relevant evidence on the discriminability of the two disorders. Tables from the Moras (1989) review of comorbidity findings for DSM-III and DSM–III-R anxiety and mood disorders are presented in the integrative review chapter on mixed anxiety depression (see Moras et al., Chapter 21, this volume). The median comorbidity percentage for an additional diagnosis of dysthymia or major depression with principal GAD was 33% (range 0%–42%); the median comorbidity percentage for additional GAD with principal dysthymia or major depression was 23% (range 17%–60%). Moras (1989) noted the "symmetry" of the comorbidity percentages (i.e., similar percentages regardless of whether GAD or a mood disorder was the principal diagnosis). The symmetrical comorbidity could indicate that GAD is less distinguishable from the mood disorders than most of the other DSM-III-R anxiety disorders, but there are alternative interpretations for the symmetrical comorbidity percentages. For example, they could simply indicate that GAD symptoms and depressive symptoms often co-occur.

4. Affect and cognitive variables that distinguish GAD and dysthymia. It would be useful to explore affect and cognitive variables that might discriminate GAD and dysthymia. For example, one could examine whether the constructs of negative and positive affect (as developed by Tellegen [1985] and Clark and Watson [1991]) discriminate GAD and dysthymia. Existing research suggests that cognitive processing variables can help sharpen the discrimination between GAD and mood disorders in general. For example, MacLeod et al. (1986) suggest that vigilance and scanning discriminate GAD and dysthymia. One question that merits further study is whether cognitive characteristics such as apprehensive expectation (worry) that are key features of DSM-III-R GAD are sometimes nonspecific and apply to dysthymia and to mood disorders in general.

Issue 2. Validity of GAD: Its Discriminability From Somatoform Disorders and From Psychophysiological Disorders

Methods and results. Rapee's (1989) literature review was preceded by a two-phase search. First, *Psychological Abstracts* between 1970 and 1989 inclusive and Index Medicus between 1970 and 1989 inclusive were searched. Key words included *generalized anxiety disorder, chronic anxiety, anxiety neurosis, anxiety disorder, hypochondriasis, somatization, colonic diseases, functional, headache, irritable bowel syndrome, psychophysiological disorders, stress,* and *psychosomatic disorders.* Any abstracts that referred to both a GAD-like disorder and another disorder of interest to the review were examined for possible relevance. Second, a total of 12 clinics and laboratories around the world known to be involved in research on one of three kinds of disorders (GAD, somatoform, psychophysiological) were contacted and asked to supply unpublished or recently submitted findings. Researchers specifically were asked if they had data on any of seven issues: 1) medical record data, medical presentations of GAD; 2) comorbidity of GAD, somatoform, and psychophysiological disorders; 3) mean number, type, and intensity of somatic symptoms associated with GAD; 4) clinical features of GAD, somatoform, and psychophysiological disorder populations; 5) associated Axis II disorders; 6) self-report questionnaire scores and physiological measures; and 7) treatment response.

The Rapee (1989) review focused on the discriminability of DSM-III and DSM–III-R GAD, hypochondriasis, and irritable bowel syndrome because, of the DSM-III-R somatoform and psychophysiological disorders, the last two disorders have been the most extensively researched and appear to show the greatest clinical similarity to GAD. Research on the discriminability of GAD and somatization disorder was not reviewed because the DSM-III-R criteria for somatization disorder and for GAD seem sufficiently distinct that diagnostic confusion is unlikely.

Rapee's (1989) main conclusion was that insufficient empirical data exist to make specific recommendations on whether changes in diagnostic criteria are needed to enhance the discriminability of GAD and hypochondriasis, or GAD and psychophysiological disorders such as irritable bowel syndrome. No well-controlled studies were found that compared either GAD and hypochondriasis or GAD and irritable bowel syndrome. However, Rapee (1989) observed that modifying diagnostic criteria could facilitate differential diagnosis. For example, distinguishing between GAD and hypochondriasis can be difficult due to symptom overlap across the two disorders: GAD patients can report many somatic symptoms, as do hypochondriasis patients; a key feature of GAD is worry, which also is a typical presenting feature of hypochondriasis. By definition, hypochondriasis patients worry about health, and health is one of the spheres of worry typically identified by patients who meet diagnostic criteria for GAD (Craske et al. 1989; Sanderson and Barlow 1990).

Discussion.   Based on the foregoing observations, Rapee (1989) concluded that clarification of the GAD and/or hypochondriasis diagnostic criteria is needed to help diagnosticians determine when health worry is a GAD sphere of worry and when it should be classified as a symptom of hypochondriasis. As one solution, Rapee (1989) cited Pilowsky's (1967) identification of three dimensions in hypochondriasis: disease fear, bodily preoccupation, and disease conviction. Rapee noted that GAD patients clinically appear to have the first two dimensions but perhaps not the third. DSM-III-R states that hypochondriasis should be given if either fear *or* conviction of disease is present. Rapee (1989) suggested that modifying the hypochondriasis criteria to emphasize or require *disease conviction* might help distinguish it from health concerns that could be classified as a GAD sphere of worry. Rapee (1989) also suggested that lack of response to reassurance also might help distinguish GAD from hypochondriasis, with lack of response being more characteristic of hypochondriasis.

   The distinction between GAD and psychophysiological disorders (e.g., DSM-III-R psychological factors affecting physical condition [PFAPC]) can also be difficult. Rapee (1989) stated that the studies he reviewed consistently showed that GAD patients often have physical conditions such as gastrointestinal symptoms and recurrent headaches (e.g., Anderson et al. 1984; Breslau and Davis 1985a; Rapee 1985). Such symptoms are likely to be exacerbated by external stressors, contributing to differential diagnostic problems. For example, a patient could meet criteria for GAD and also have recurrent headaches (recorded on Axis III). Two weeks after losing a job, the headaches might worsen. Technically, the person would meet criteria for comorbid diagnoses of GAD and PFAPC. However, it can be argued that the comorbid diagnoses are an unnecessary complication, because the original diagnoses (Axis I and III) adequately capture the clinical picture. The foregoing argument suggests that the PFAPC diagnosis might often be unnecessary. Drawing implications from the foregoing rationale, Rapee suggested that hierarchical rules be created for PFAPC so that it would be given only when no other Axis I diagnosis applies.

Issue 3. What Features Distinguish Pathological From Normal Worry?

Methods and results. Borkovec et al. (1989) conducted a computer search based on the PsycInfo system to identify articles in the psychological and psychiatric literature from January 1966 to April 1989 relevant to normal and/or pathological worry. Key words used in the search included *worry, apprehensive expectation, chronic anxiety, generalized anxiety, generalized anxiety disorder,* and *intrusive thoughts.* Research on intrusive thought was included because of the probable overlap of the phenomenon with worry, but research on obsessive thoughts, images, and impulses was specifically excluded because another review paper was being prepared on that topic. The search include all theoretical and empirical articles on human subjects in the English, German, and Spanish languages.

A second search was done with the above key words with the PsycLit CD-ROM system based on *Psychological Abstracts.* The time interval covered was January 1983 to August 1989. References from identified articles were also inspected for relevant publications. The last 2 years of the following selected journals were manually examined to update the computer searches: *Behaviour Research and Therapy, Behavior Therapy, Cognition and Emotion, Clinical Psychology Review, Journal of Abnormal Psychology, Journal of Anxiety Disorders, Journal of Behavior Therapy and Experimental Psychiatry,* and *Journal of Consulting and Clinical Psychology.* Letters were written to researchers interested in GAD and in worry to solicit unpublished material.

The main purpose of Borkovec et al.'s (1989) review was to identify features that distinguish normal worry from pathological worry. With regard to distinguishing normal and pathological worry, the basic issues are 1) the threshold at which normal worry becomes a diagnosable GAD worry, 2) definition of the terms *excessive* and "unrealistic, 3) specification of the content of "spheres of worry," and 4) similarities and differences in the worry process manifested by normal versus psychiatric groups.

Borkovec et al. (1989) found that little research on worry in psychiatric samples exists. Thus, it was not possible to draw firm conclusions about the four foregoing issues at the time of the review. Borkovec et al.'s (1989) conclusions were based on their review of what was currently known about the nature of worry in normal samples and the limited amount of research on psychiatric samples. Due to the lack of empirical data, Borkovec et al. (1989) made the goal of their review the identification of fruitful areas of research on worry.

Borkovec et al. (1989) found three basic themes in the literature on normal and clinical worry: 1) spheres, or content domains, of worry; 2) salient dimensions of worry such as frequency, intensity, uncontrollability, and disruptiveness; and 3) the relationship of worry to somatic aspects of anxiety. The reviewers' general conclusion was that worry in GAD involves an excess of the same process found in normal subjects, although they underlined the fact that their conclusion was based on limited data.

Discussion.   All of Borkovec et al.'s (1989) recommendations were for further research designed to identify the features that characterize pathological worry.

1. Spheres of worry.   The number of current worries might be one useful dimension of worry to explore because GAD patients tend to report more specific worries than nonanxious control subjects (unpublished data, Penn State GAD therapy trial). A second useful issue to examine is change in content of worry over time. Existing evidence suggests that the content of GAD worry tends to be highly variable, with no particular content being specific to the disorder (Craske et al. 1989; Sanderson and Barlow 1990; unpublished data, Penn State GAD therapy trial). Data are needed to adjust or further support the foregoing evidence. Research on number of worries and change over time should be preceded by the development of improved methods of measurement, because the findings will depend on the reliability of the content categories. Furthermore, greater standardization of the operational definitions of each category and more thorough and systematic interviewing methods that specify the source of worry are required before meaningful data can be obtained from classifications of content of worry.

2. Excessive and/or unrealistic worry.   Additional research is needed on the criteria that interviewers and patients use to judge spheres of worry as unrealistic and/or excessive. Research of this type could lead to a more valid definition of pathological worry.

3. Frequency, intensity, uncontrollability, and disruptiveness.   Existing evidence suggested that uncontrollability might be a central dimension that distinguishes pathological from normal worry (Borkovec et al. 1983; Craske et al. 1989). Further research on the uncontrollability of worry in GAD compared to other diagnostic groups seems particularly promising (Borkovec et al. 1983; Metzger et al. 1990). Disruptiveness of the worry process also appears to distinguish pathological and normal worry. However, because of the general absence of resources in clinical situations to measure disruptiveness, it would be useful to develop interview and self-report assessment methods that focus on the ways in which and the degree to

which worry interferes with a patient's daily functioning. Promising preliminary results suggest that assessor ratings of interference with daily functioning may discriminate GAD from other anxiety disorders, although separation of the effects of interference due specifically to "worry," as distinguished from "anxiety and tension," needs to be done.

Discussion and Recommendations

Issue 1. Reliability of GAD

Because existing evidence strongly indicates that the GAD diagnostic criterion D (i.e., the presence of 6 of 18 specified symptoms) has low reliability, additional research was recommended by the DSM-IV Anxiety Disorders Work Group to explore ways to modify criterion D. DiNardo received MacArthur Foundation funding to do relevant studies. Pilot studies were conducted at CSAD by DiNardo, Moras, and Barlow to determine 1) which, if any, of the 18 symptoms could be reliably assessed by diagnosticians and 2) which, if any, reliably rated symptoms distinguished patients with a principal diagnosis of GAD from patients with other anxiety disorders. The results of the pilot studies led to option 3, criterion E, in the *DSM-IV Options Book* draft. The results of this data reanalysis will be given in more detail in a report to be published in Volume 4 of the *DSM-IV Sourcebook.*

Issue 2. Validity of GAD: Its Discriminability From Other DSM-III-R Disorders

The DSM-IV Anxiety Disorders Work Group acknowledged that the discriminability of GAD from dysthymia is a contested issue but did not recommend revision of any of the GAD criteria based on existing evidence. The main conclusion, based on Riskind et al.'s (1989) review, was that essentially no published studies of clinical samples exist on the discriminability of DSM-III-R GAD from dysthymia and major depression, except the comorbidity data from clinical samples summarized by Moras (1989). However, the comorbidity data in themselves do not provide evidence that can be definitively interpreted in terms of the distinctiveness of GAD compared with dysthymia and major depression.

Rapee's (1989) observations about the difficulty of determining when worry about one's health is a diagnostic criterion for hypochondriasis versus a GAD sphere of worry were incorporated in the *DSM-IV Options Book* (Task Force on DSM-IV 1991) draft of GAD criterion D. The criterion states that a focus of worry that is related to another Axis I disorder that is present (e.g., concern about having a serious illness as in hypochondriasis) should not be regarded as a symptom of GAD worry.

Issue 3. What Features Distinguish Pathological From Normal Worry?

Borkovec et al.'s (1989) conclusion that uncontrollability and disruptiveness might be dimensions that distinguish pathological from normal worry led to the recommended inclusion of a diagnostic criterion which states that the worry is "difficult to control" and interferes with focusing attention on tasks at hand (criterion C, *DSM-IV Options Book*).

References

American Psychiatric Association: Diagnostic and Statistical Manual of Mental Disorders, 3rd Edition. Washington, DC, American Psychiatric Association, 1980

American Psychiatric Association: Diagnostic and Statistical Manual of Mental Disorders, 3rd Edition, Revised. Washington, DC, American Psychiatric Association, 1987

Anderson DJ, Noyes R Jr, Crowe RR: A comparison of panic disorder and generalized anxiety disorder. Am J Psychiatry 141:572–575, 1984

Barlow DH, DiNardo PA: The diagnosis of generalized anxiety disorder: development, current status, and future directions, in Chronic Anxiety, Generalized Anxiety Disorder, and Mixed Anxiety-Depression. Edited by Rapee RM, Barlow DH. New York, Guilford, 1991, pp 95–118

Barlow DH, Blanchard EB, Vermilyea JA, et al: Generalized anxiety and generalized anxiety disorder: description and reconceptualization. Am J Psychiatry 143:40–44, 1986

Beck AT, Brown G, Steer RA, et al: Differentiating anxiety and depression: a test of the content-specificity hypothesis. J Abnorm Psychol 96:179–183, 1987

Benshoof BB, Moras K, DiNardo P, et al: A comparison of symptomatology in anxiety and depressive disorders. Unpublished manuscript, Albany, State University of New York, Center for Stress and Anxiety Disorders, 1989

Blashfield RK, Livesley WJ: Metaphorical analysis of psychiatric classification as a psychological test. J Abnorm Psychol 100:262–270, 1991

Borkovec TD, Robinson E, Pruzinsky T, et al: Preliminary exploration of worry: some characteristics and processes. Behav Res Ther 21:9–16, 1983

Borkovec TD, Shadick RN, Hopkins M: The nature of normal versus pathological worry. Review paper for the DSM-IV Generalized Anxiety Disorder and Mixed Anxiety Depression Work Group. Pennsylvania State University, 1989

Borkovec TD, Shadick RN, Hopkins M: The nature of normal versus pathological worry, in Chronic Anxiety, Generalized Anxiety Disorder, and Mixed Anxiety-Depression. Edited by Rapee RM, Barlow DH. New York, Guilford, 1991, pp 29–51

Breier A, Charney DS, Heninger GR: Major depression in patients with agoraphobia and panic disorder. Arch Gen Psychiatry 41:1129–1135, 1984

Breslau N, Davis GC: DSM-III generalized anxiety disorder: an empirical investigation of more stringent criteria. Psychiatry Res 14:231–238, 1985a

Breslau N, Davis GC: Further evidence on the doubtful validity of generalized anxiety disorder. Psychiatry Res 16:177–179, 1985b

Cicchetti DV, Sparrow SS: Developing criteria for establishing the interrater reliability of specific items in a given inventory: applications to assessment of adaptive behavior. American Journal of Mental Deficiency 86:127–137, 1981

Clark LA, Watson D: Tripartite model of anxiety and depression: psychometric evidence and taxonomic implications. J Abnorm Psychol 100:316–336, 1991

Craske MG, Rapee RM, Jackel L, et al: Qualitative dimensions of worry in DSM-III-R generalized anxiety disorder subjects and nonanxious controls. Behav Res Ther 27:397–402, 1989

DiNardo PA: Diagnostic reliability of DSM-III-R generalized anxiety disorder. Review paper for the DSM-IV Generalized Anxiety Disorder and Mixed Anxiety Depression Work Group. Albany, State University of New York, 1990

DiNardo PA, Barlow DH: Anxiety Disorders Interview Schedule-Revised (ADIS-R). Albany, NY, Phobia and Anxiety Disorders Clinic, Center for Stress and Anxiety Disorders, 1988

DiNardo PA, O'Brien GT, Barlow DH, et al: Reliability of DSM-III anxiety disorder categories using a new structured interview. Arch Gen Psychiatry 40:1070–1075, 1983

Fyer AJ, Endicott J, Mannuzza S, et al: Schedule for Affective Disorders and Schizophrenia: Lifetime Version (modified for the study of anxiety disorders). New York, Anxiety Disorders Clinic, New York State Psychiatric Institute, 1985

Fyer AJ, Mannuzza S, Martin LY, et al: Reliability of anxiety assessment, II: symptom agreement. Arch Gen Psychiatry 46:1102–1110, 1989

Hamilton M: The assessment of anxiety states by rating. Br J Med Psychol 32:50–59, 1959

Hamilton M: A rating scale for depression. J Neurol Neurosurg Psychiatry 23:56–62, 1960

Hoehn-Saric R, McLeod DR: Generalized anxiety disorder. Psychiatr Clin North Am 8:73–87, 1985

Klein DN, Taylor EB, Dickstein S, et al: The early-late onset distinction in DSM-III-R dysthymia. J Affect Disord 14:25–33, 1988

Landis JR, Koch GG: The measurement of observer agreement for categorical data. Biometrics 33:159–174, 1977

MacLeod C, Mathews A, Tata P: Attentional bias in emotional disorders. J Abnorm Psychol 95:15–20, 1986

Mannuzza S, Fyer A, Martin LY, et al: Reliability of anxiety assessment: diagnostic agreement. Arch Gen Psychiatry 46:1093–1101, 1989

Metzger RL, Miller M, Cohen M, et al: Worry changes decision making: the effect of negative thoughts on cognitive processing. J Clin Psychol 46:78–88, 1990

Moras K: Diagnostic comorbidity in the DSM-III and DSM-III-R anxiety and mood disorder: implications for the DSM-IV. Review paper for the DSM-IV Generalized Anxiety Disorder and Mixed Anxiety Depression Work Group. Center for Stress and Anxiety Disorders, University at Albany, State University of New York, 1989

Moras K: The assessment of generalized anxiety disorder. Unpublished manuscript, University at Albany, State University of New York, Center for Stress and Anxiety Disorders, 1991

Pilowsky I: Dimensions of hypochondriasis. Br J Psychiatry 113:89–93, 1967

Rapee RM: Distinctions between panic disorder and generalised anxiety disorder: clinical presentation. Aust N Z J Psychiatry 19:227–232, 1985

Rapee RM: Generalized anxiety disorder boundary issues: GAD and somatoform disorders; GAD and psychophysiological disorders. Review paper for the DSM-IV Generalized Anxiety Disorder and Mixed Anxiety Depression Work Group. St. Lucia, Queensland, Australia, University of Queensland, Department of Psychology, 1989

Rapee RM, Barlow DH (eds): Chronic Anxiety, Generalized Anxiety Disorder, and Mixed Anxiety-Depression. New York, Guilford, 1991

Riskind JH, Beck AT, Brown G, et al: Taking the measure of anxiety and depression: validity of the reconstructed Hamilton Scales. J Nerv Ment Dis 22:474–478, 1987

Riskind JH, Hohmann AA, Harman B, et al: The relation between generalized anxiety disorder and depression and dysthymic disorder in particular. Paper for the DSM-IV Generalized Anxiety Disorder and Mixed Anxiety Depression Work Group. Fairfax, VA, George Mason University, and Philadelphia, PA, Center for Cognitive Therapy, 1989

Riskind JH, Hohmann AA, Beck AT, et al: The relation of generalized anxiety disorder to depression in general and dysthymic disorder in particular, in Chronic Anxiety, Generalized Anxiety Disorder, and Mixed Anxiety-Depression. Edited by Rapee RM, Barlow DH. New York, Guilford, 1991, pp 153–171

Roth M, Gurney C, Garside RF, et al: Studies in the classification of affective disorders: relationship between anxiety states and depressive illness. Br J Psychiatry 121:147–161, 1972

Sanderson WC, Barlow DH: A description of patients diagnosed with DSM-III-Revised generalized anxiety disorder. J Nerv Ment Dis 178:558–591, 1990

Spitzer RL, Williams JBW, Gibbon M: Structured Clinical Interview for DSM-III-R—Patient Version (4/1/87). New York: New York State Psychiatric Institute, 1987

Task Force on DSM-IV: DSM-IV Options Book: Work in Progress. Washington, DC, American Psychiatric Association, 1991

Tellegen A: Structures of mood and personality and their relevance to assessing anxiety, with an emphasis on self-report, in Anxiety and the Anxiety Disorders. Edited by Tuma AH, Maser JD. Hillsdale, NJ, Erlbaum, 1985, pp 681–706

Chapter 21

Mixed Anxiety-Depression

Karla Moras, Ph.D., Lee Anna Clark, Ph.D., Wayne Katon, M.D.,
Peter Roy-Byrne, M.D., David Watson, Ph.D., and
David H. Barlow, Ph.D.

Statement of the Issues

Issue 1. A principal reason for undertaking literature reviews on mixed anxiety-depression was the DSM-IV Task Force's aim to make the DSM system more compatible with ICD-10 (World Health Organization 1988). A diagnosis of mixed anxiety and depression in the ICD-10 prompted consideration of adding a similar diagnosis to the DSM-IV. The ICD-10 diagnosis identifies cases with symptoms of anxiety and depression that are "mild or moderate" but not "severe" and that do not meet any of the ICD-10 anxiety or depressive disorder diagnoses.

Issue 2. A second principal issue was whether the DSM nomenclature should be revised 1) to more adequately describe the substantial overlap between symptoms of anxiety and depression and/or 2) to include a new category of mixed anxiety-depression that would, in effect, combine DSM-III-R anxiety and mood disorder diagnoses that typically co-occur. The issue was raised largely because the co-occurrence of symptoms of anxiety and depression and of DSM-III (American Psychiatric Association 1980) and DSM-III-R (American Psychiatric Association 1987) mood and anxiety disorders has often been observed clinically and empirically over the years (see, e.g., Kendall and Watson's 1989 book on this issue; Downing and Rickels 1974; Maser and Cloninger 1990; Roth et al. 1972).

Issue 3. A third issue was the utility of reintroducing the diagnostic construct of neurasthenia into the DSM system. The issue arose in part because the proposed ICD-10 included a syndrome called neurasthenia among the neurotic disorders. An excellent historical review of neurasthenia was provided by Morey and Kurtz (1989). The review indicated that neurasthenia, as defined in ICD-10, is focused on symptom clusters that are not central to prevailing conceptualizations of mixed anxiety and depression (i.e., feelings of physical weakness and exhaustion). Therefore, the neurasthenia-related issues were not considered further within the context of mixed anxiety-depression and are not discussed further in this summary of the literature reviews that were done for the generalized anxiety disorder (GAD) and mixed anxiety-depression subgroup of the DSM-IV Anxiety Disorders Work Group.

For the sake of clarity, note that Issue 1 concerns creating a diagnosis that would classify people whose symptoms of anxiety and depression do not meet definitional thresholds for anxiety or mood disorders in the DSM-III-R nomenclature. Issue 2 goes beyond issue 1 and concerns the feasibility of creating one or more new diagnostic categories that would, in effect, redefine certain DSM-III-R anxiety and mood disorder diagnoses that typically occur together.

Significance of the Issues

Issue 1. Compatibility of ICD-10 and DSM-IV: Should a diagnosis of mixed anxiety-depression be created that would identify patients whose symptoms are below the definitional threshold for a disorder in the DSM-III-R system?

Compatibility of ICD-10 and DSM-IV would foster cross-cultural communication within psychiatry and related disciplines. Compatible diagnostic systems would facilitate clinical communication and research of all types including treatment efficacy studies, psychopathology research, and classification research. Furthermore, the addition to DSM-IV of a diagnosis of mixed anxiety-depression that was compatible with the ICD-10 diagnosis could identify patients who have symptoms of anxiety and depression that currently are "subclinical" according to the DSM-III-R system but are commonly seen in primary care settings and might benefit from systematic intervention.

Issue 2. Should one or more diagnoses of mixed anxiety-depression be created for DSM-III-R mood and anxiety disorders that frequently co-occur?

The co-occurrence of symptoms of anxiety and depression is among the earliest clinical observations. For example, Akiskal (1990) cites Hippocrates's description of a case in which symptoms of anxiety and depression co-occurred. As Akiskal (1990) points out, Hippocrates also noted that symptoms of anxiety can be followed by symptoms of depression.

The relationship between anxiety and depression was the focus of much study before the introduction of DSM-III. Moreover, repeated findings of comorbidity between the DSM-III and DSM-III-R anxiety and mood disorders suggest that

DSM-III-R might artificially separate all anxiety and mood disorders when, in fact, at least one type of mixed anxiety-depression disorder exists (i.e., a syndrome in which symptoms of anxiety and depression always co-occur).

Overview

Subsequent to the preparation of the three DSM-IV Task Force reports on mixed anxiety-depression, two of them were published as articles in a special series in the *Journal of Abnormal Psychology* (Clark and Watson 1991b; Katon and Roy-Byrne 1991). This chapter contains abbreviated summaries of the original Task Force reviews. For more extensive presentations of the Clark and Watson (1989) and Katon and Roy-Byrne (1989) reviews, the reader is referred to the published articles.

Method

Issue 1

Wayne Katon, M.D., and Peter Roy-Byrne, M.D., reviewed the empirical evidence that patients exist who have clinically significant (i.e., associated with subjective distress and/or impairment of functioning) symptoms of anxiety and depression that do not meet criteria for specific DSM-III-R diagnoses. The review was to examine both the 1) prevalence of anxiety and depression in nonpsychiatric samples and 2) evidence that such patients meet the basic DSM criterion for a disorder (i.e., subjective distress and/or functional impairment).

Issue 2

Lee Anna Clark, Ph.D., and David Watson, Ph.D., reviewed the evidence on the relationship between symptoms of anxiety and depression and drew implications from their review for the creation of a new diagnostic category of mixed anxiety-depression.

Karla Moras, Ph.D., reviewed evidence on the comorbidity of anxiety and mood disorders. The purpose of the review was to identify any DSM-III-R anxiety and mood disorders that tend to co-occur and that would therefore be obvious candidates for a revised diagnostic category of mixed anxiety-depression.

Results

Issue 1: Compatibility of the ICD-10 and DSM-IV: Should a diagnosis of mixed anxiety-depression be created that would identify patients whose symptoms are below the definitional threshold for a disorder in the DSM-III-R system?

Method and results. Katon and Roy-Byrne's (1989) literature review was based on empirical studies of patients with symptoms of anxiety and depression. Studies were identified with a Medline search with selection terms such as *anxiety, depression,* and *affective illness.* Studies from 1988 to the time of the review in fall 1989 were requested. Additional references were drawn from the bibliographies of papers selected from the Medline search. The Medline search focused on English language journal articles involving human subjects. In addition, the shelf copies of the following selected journals for the past 10 years were reviewed manually: *American Journal of Psychiatry, Archives of General Psychiatry, British Journal of Psychiatry, Journal of Nervous and Mental Disease, Journal of Clinical Psychiatry, Comprehensive Psychiatry,* and *Journal of Affective Disorders.* Finally, 10 investigators and groups were contacted about data sets or manuscripts that might be pertinent to the review.

Findings were reviewed from community, primary care, and psychiatric samples. Some genetic evidence on anxiety and depression also was reviewed briefly but is not summarized here. An overview of Katon and Roy-Byrne's (1989) findings and conclusions from studies of community, primary care, and psychiatric samples follows.

Community samples. The studies reviewed suggest that a disparity exists between the prevalence of mood disorders such as major depression and dysthymia in epidemiological samples (about 3%–8% in the Epidemiologic Catchment Area study [Myers et al. 1984]), and the prevalence of depressive symptoms that are not accompanied by all the diagnostic criteria required for a mood disorder (13%–20% [Boyd and Weissman 1981; Weissman and Boyd 1983]). Findings on the clustering of depressive symptoms in a community sample also were reviewed. Blazer et al. (1988) found a mixed anxiety-depressive symptom cluster that appeared to be characteristic of community subjects with moderate to severe depressive symptoms. Of 406 persons with depressive symptoms, 9.9% had a high probability (greater than 0.50 loading) of having mixed anxiety-depressive symptoms, in contrast to 1.7% who had a high probability of having multiple major depression symptoms (Blazer et al. 1988). Many of the subjects would not meet DSM-III criteria for an affective or anxiety disorder because they did not have enough symptoms.

Based on their review of findings from community samples (e.g., Blazer et al. 1988; Brown et al. 1986; Eaton et al. 1989), Katon and Roy-Byrne (1989) speculated that the gap between the prevalence of depressive symptoms and the lower prevalence of mood disorder diagnoses might be narrowed by either including a subgroup of mixed anxiety-depression in DSM-IV or, alternatively, by lowering the number of symptoms required for major depressive disorder.

Primary care samples. Katon and Roy-Byrne (1989) indicated that several studies of primary care samples reported higher rates of distress (i.e., symptoms of anxiety and depression) using screening scales such as the General Health Questionnaire (GHQ) (Goldberg 1978), the Beck Depression Inventory (Beck et al. 1988), the Zung Self-Rating Depression Scale (Zung 1965), and the SCL-90 (Derogatis et al. 1974) than of disorders classified by structured diagnostic interviews. For example, Von Korff et al. (1987) found that 39.3% of primary care patients had a score of 5 or greater on the GHQ, the suggested cutoff that is sensitive and specific to psychiatric diagnoses. Of the same patients, 25% met DSM-III criteria for a psychiatric disorder, based on the National Institute of Mental Health (NIMH) Diagnostic Interview Schedule (DIS) (Robins et al. 1981). Thus, approximately 14% of the patients were found to be distressed but did not meet diagnostic criteria for a disorder.

A study by Barrett et al. (1988) used the SCL-90 (Derogatis et al. 1974) to screen general practice patients for distress. The Schedule for Affective Disorders and Schizophrenia (SADS) (Endicott and Spitzer 1978) was used to diagnose patients according to the Research Diagnostic Criteria (Spitzer et al. 1978). Several distressed patients did not readily fit into a diagnostic category. Of the total sample, 4.1% had mixed anxiety and depressive symptoms; 6.4% had suspected depression. Barrett et al. (1988) noted that both groups had definite symptomatology and some impairment in occupational or social functioning.

Additional evidence of symptomatic distress in patients who did not meet criteria for a psychiatric disorder was reported by Katon et al. (1987). They studied the prevalence of panic attacks and panic disorder in a primary care sample. A "large" (specific figures are not given) subgroup of primary care patients had infrequent panic attacks that never met severity criteria for panic disorder (i.e., they never had three panic attacks in a 3-week period, as required by DSM-III). The patients with infrequent panic had higher anxiety and depression scores on psychological tests, more simple phobias, and a higher lifetime risk for affective disorder than patients who said they never had a panic attack.

Psychiatric samples. Two papers that outline possible typologies for patients presenting with symptoms of depression or depression and anxiety (Davidson et al. 1988; Tyrer 1985) were the focus of this section of the Katon and Roy-Byrne (1989) review. Tyrer (1985) suggested that a large subgroup of distressed persons with chronic symptoms of anxiety and depression meet criteria for a "general neurotic syndrome." Such patients have a core of anxiety and depressive symptoms that might meet criteria for DSM GAD or dysthymia and that are longitudinally stable. Panic disorder, major depression, or both occur in the context of acute stressful life events. The disorders resolve, but the chronic anxiety and/or depressive symptoms remain. Tyrer presented operational criteria for the general neurotic syndrome that he described based on a longitudinal study of patients.

Davidson et al. (1988) used multivariate statistical techniques to examine depression and the relationship between anxiety and depression in 190 psychiatric patients who met Research Diagnostic Criteria (Spitzer et al. 1978) for major or minor depression. A "pure type III" category was found that had many characteristics of the mixed anxiety-depressive cluster described in community studies. The category also resembled "atypical depression," i.e., the presence of panic attacks, agoraphobia, hyperphagia, weight gain, childhood anxiety, and predominant outpatient presentation. The type III depression was characterized by mild degrees of symptomatology on most items of the Hamilton Rating Scale for Depression (Hamilton 1960), with the exception that 85% of the patients in the group experienced severe psychic anxiety.

Discussion.   Katon and Roy-Byrne (1989) concluded that existing data strongly suggest that there is a subgroup of people who have mixed anxiety and depressive symptoms but do not have enough symptoms of either disorder to meet DSM-III-R diagnostic thresholds (e.g., Brown et al. 1986; Sireling et al. 1985). Moreover, studies suggest that such patients have impairments in social and vocational functioning (e.g., Barrett et al. 1988), and some evidence exists that people with mixed anxiety and depressive symptoms might represent a population at risk for more severe mood and anxiety disorders when exposed to life stresses (e.g., Brown et al. 1986). Katon and Roy-Byrne (1989) made several recommendations for research that is needed prior to the creation of a new diagnosis for symptoms of anxiety and depression that currently are subclinical and for the development of diagnostic criteria. The recommendations they made that focused most directly on issues that need to be considered to create a new diagnostic category follow:

1. To develop diagnostic criteria for a new category of subclinical mixed anxiety-depression, empirical evidence is needed on the types of symptoms that would define the category, required duration of symptoms, and required signs of functional impairment. Regarding the latter point, an index of functional impairment must be included in the diagnostic criteria to aid in the determination of caseness for the diagnosis. Measures of disability such as those used in the Medical Outcomes Study (e.g., Wells et al. 1989) could be helpful.

2. The relative advantages of defining a new category of mixed anxiety-depression versus lowering the criteria for caseness of existing related disorders such as major depression should be explored.

3. Longitudinal studies are needed to determine a) the presence of increased risk for more severe syndromes in patients who have features of subthreshold mixed anxiety and depression and b) whether a nonchronic subgroup exists that improves without treatment.

Issue 2. Should one or more diagnoses of mixed anxiety-depression be created for DSM-III-R mood and anxiety disorders that frequently co-occur?

Two reviews addressed this issue. One, by Clark and Watson (1989), drew conclusions based on the extensive psychometric literature on the measurement of anxiety and depression. The second review, by Moras (1989), tallied existing comorbidity findings for anxiety and mood disorders in samples diagnosed by DSM-III and DSM-III-R. The two reviews are summarized separately in the sections that follow.

Conclusions Based on a Review of Psychometric Issues Associated With Measurement of Anxiety and Depression

Method and results.   Clark and Watson's (1989) literature search was initiated by "treeing" through reference lists, prior reviews, and bibliographies. The strategy yielded 166 relevant articles, books, or book chapters. In addition, a letter soliciting reprints was sent to 53 active researchers, yielding 46 papers (29 published; 17 unpublished, under review, or in press) from 18 researchers. Finally, a PsycLit computer search of articles published since 1983 was made using the joint descriptors *anxiety* and *depression*, which yielded more than 1,200 entries. A subset of the entries was selected that included the root terms *measure-* or *assess-*. Non-English-language reports were excluded, as were primarily pharmacological, pediatric, and treatment studies. A final database of 181 potentially relevant articles was produced. The articles were systematically reviewed. Searches on specific topics (e.g., the reliability of clinical rating scales) were carried out as needed.

The Clark and Watson (1989) review was organized around two major topics: 1) properties of measures of anxiety and depression, including the reliability and convergent/discriminant validity of self-report and clinical ratings of depression and anxiety in both clinical and nonclinical samples; and 2) evidence for general and specific factors in anxiety and depression, including analyses of how context and scale content influence ratings, factor analytic studies, and an examination of the role of low positive affect in depression. Clark and Watson's (1989) review of psychometric findings on measures of anxiety and depression was very comprehensive (e.g., 23 pages of the review were devoted to convergent and discriminant validity findings for anxiety and depression measures). Due to space limitations here, only a few of the more representative psychometric findings are described (the interested reader is referred to Clark and Watson 1991b for a more complete presentation). The remainder of the summary presents Clark and Watson's (1989) rationale and proposal for a major revision of the DSM-III-R anxiety and mood disorder categories, based on a model of the structure of affect that is consistent with the psychometric findings on anxiety and depression.

Self-report measures. Test-retest reliabilities of self-report symptom measures of anxiety and depression are adequate to good, especially in nonclinical samples. For example, the median test-retest reliability of the Beck Depression Inventory (Beck et al. 1988) was .78 in eight nonclinical samples with a median test-retest interval of 2 weeks. Substantial levels of convergent validity also have been found. Convergent correlations for self-report measures of anxiety and depression average .71 or higher in both clinical and nonclinical samples (see reviews by Beck et al. 1988; Dobson 1985; Gotlib 1984). However, discriminant validity findings for self-report measures are weak. In fact, the discriminant correlations between self-report depression and anxiety often approach the levels found for convergent validity indices (e.g., .62 and above for discriminant indices). (Clark and Watson stated that 21 studies were reviewed that provided discriminant validity evidence, but specific studies were not cited.)

Clark and Watson (1989) concluded that the overlap in self-report measures of anxiety and depression is consistent with the possibility that a strong nonspecific distress factor, which they call "negative affect," dominates self-ratings of anxiety and depression. Clark and Watson (1989) recommended that the existence of a substantial nonspecific component of these syndromes should be explicitly acknowledged in DSM IV.

Clinical rating measures. Clinical ratings of anxiety and depression scales are both reliable and convergent within affect (i.e., .70 or higher) when 1) the raters are similarly and adequately trained, 2) the rating criteria are clearly specified and the ratings are based on the same information, and 3) there is adequate within-sample variation (see reviews by Clark 1989; Deluty et al. 1986; Maier et al. 1988). Use of global rating scales, unstructured and/or separate interviews, untrained raters, and homogeneous samples all lower reliability and validity (Clark 1989).

Based on several studies that provide findings on the relationship between clinical ratings of anxiety and depression (e.g., Deluty et al. 1986; Eaton and Ritter 1988), Clark and Watson (1989) concluded that a discriminant coefficient in the low .40s represents a reasonable estimate of the correlation between clinical ratings of anxiety and depression. They described the overlap as "substantial" but noted that a greater level of discrimination is found in clinical ratings compared with self-ratings. Clark and Watson (1989) suggested that the greater discrimination in clinical ratings may be because clinicians give more weight than patients do to factors distinguishing anxiety from depression.

Discussion. Clark and Watson's (1989) basic conclusion was that convergent and discriminant validity findings on measures of anxiety and depression (both self-report and clinical ratings) and factor analytic studies of symptoms (see reviews by Clark and Watson 1991a; Beck 1972) are consistent with a tripartite model of the relationship between anxiety and depression. The model described by Clark and Watson (1989, 1991b; Watson et al. 1988) is an elaboration of Tellegen's (1985) earlier work on negative and positive affect. The three elements of the tripartite model are nonspecific general distress, features specific to anxiety, and features specific to depression. The general distress factor posited by Clark and Watson (1989) accounts for the fact that moderate to high correlations are consistently found between symptom measures of anxiety and depression. The second factor, features specific to anxiety, consists of physiological symptoms of hyperarousal that consistently tend to distinguish anxious and depressed diagnostic groups. The third factor, which is posited to be specific to depression, is lack of positive affect. Symptoms that indicate lack of positive affect are those associated with pervasive anhedonia such as loss of interest/pleasure, apathy, hopelessness, and fatigue. In essence, the tripartite model implies that a complete description of the affective domain observed in anxious and depressed syndromes requires measurement of both the common and unique elements of the syndromes (i.e., general distress, features specific to anxiety, and features specific to depression).

Based on their review of psychometric data, Clark and Watson offered several recommendations for revisions of the DSM-III-R nomenclature that would affect the anxiety and mood disorder categories. The revisions that they recommended are based on the following rationale: Elevated levels of the nonspecific general distress component of affective syndromes will nearly always be evident in anxious or depressed patients. Nonspecific general distress essentially signals the presence of the disorders. Therefore, the presence of a high negative-affect level suggests the relevance of anxiety and depressive diagnoses (and perhaps other diagnoses as well) but in and of itself offers no basis for finer discrimination. The two specific factors (i.e., physiological hyperarousal and pervasive anhedonia) provide an appropriate basis for the needed discrimination. Based on a simple dichotomous high/low scheme that would characterize a patient's scores on each of the three factors, Clark and Watson (1989) identified four relatively distinct syndromes for which they recommended that diagnostic criteria be developed.

1. Generalized affective (or mood) disorder. Many patients will show low levels of both specific factors; that is, neither marked physiological symptoms nor anhedonia will be particularly salient aspects of their symptom presentation. Such patients' predominant symptoms will therefore be nonspecific (e.g., distress, demoralization, irritability, mild disturbances of sleep and appetite, distractibility, vague somatic complaints) according to the tripartite model. For such patients, the development of a new diagnostic category was recommended: "generalized affective disorder" or "generalized mood disorder." The disorder would be expected to embrace most patients currently diagnosed with GAD, dysthymia, and atypical depression. Patients with the diagnosis would probably be most prevalent in general medical populations but would not be uncommon in psychiatric settings.

2. *Major depressive disorder.* Patients who report subjective distress and other nonspecific symptoms, and who also experience the pervasive anhedonia and low positive-affect characteristic of major depression (e.g., loss of interest/pleasure, retardation, extreme fatigue or loss of energy, social withdrawal) but do not report the psychophysiological arousal that is more characteristic of anxiety disorders would receive a diagnosis of major depression. During severe episodes (i.e., melancholia), low positive affect may dominate the symptom picture.

3. *Major anxiety syndrome(s).* Patients who report substantial levels of clear somatic symptomatology (e.g., tachycardia, shakiness, other autonomic signs, chest pain, dizziness) and high negative affect but who do not report significant decrements in positive affect would be diagnosed as having an anxiety syndrome (without depression). Because the anxiety disorders are more heterogeneous than the depressive disorders, this broad category would need to be further differentiated by specifying other defining characteristics, such as distress level, the temporal pattern of symptoms, or the relation (if any) of symptoms to situational cues.

A separate diagnosis, perhaps like DSM-III-R GAD, might be needed for patients who present with chronically high levels of both distress/anxious mood and physiological tension/hyperarousal, but without depressive symptomatology or panic attacks. About one-third of those currently diagnosed with GAD have been found to fit this symptom picture (Breslau and Davis 1985). Finally, persons with specific phobias can also be placed within this framework (i.e., relatively low in general distress, with marked anxiety, physiological and otherwise, in target situations).

4. *Mixed anxiety-depression.* Finally, the development of a new diagnosis, "mixed anxiety-depression," was recommended for patients who report significant levels of both anhedonia and psychophysiological distress. Akiskal (1990) labeled a comparable syndrome "panic-depressive disorder." Another label for the diagnosis could be "mixed mood disorder." Each component diagnosis could be assigned independently, but creating a "mixed" category would recognize the apparent synergistic quality of the dual diagnosis. Such a diagnosis would represent a lifetime diagnosis, as bipolar disorder does currently, because episodes of marked

anxiety and anhedonic depressive episodes do not necessarily occur simultaneously in these patients (Breier et al. 1984). Following the bipolar analogy, alternate forms such as "mixed anxiety-depression, depressed" could be used to designate the current episode.

Clark and Watson's (1989) recommended classification system would require some reorganization of the DSM. Specifically, the current mood and anxiety disorders would need to be combined into a higher-order affective (or mood) disorders category, with three subgroupings: depressive disorders, anxiety disorders, and mixed affective disorders. Related disorders (e.g., obsessive-compulsive disorder [OCD], posttraumatic stress disorder [PTSD], phobias) that have their own distinctive features could continue to be listed separately, within the most appropriate subgroup. Comorbidity among the various newly redefined affective disorders would not disappear under the system (e.g., the comorbidity of panic disorder and phobias would be unchanged, OCD would sometimes coexist with major depression). However, certain of the more common comorbidity problems would be resolved.

In summary, the psychometric data on anxiety and depression provide a framework for understanding affective syndromes in terms of their specific and nonspecific components. In particular, Clark and Watson (1989) concluded that the data strongly support the development of a new diagnostic category that formally recognizes the importance of the pervasive and highly general trait of neuroticism/negative affectivity. The factor emerged repeatedly in psychometric data from clinical and nonclinical samples. Clark and Watson (1989) suggested that the often-unrecognized presence of such a nonspecific general distress factor in affective disorders is impeding efforts to forge a satisfactory diagnostic taxonomy in this area.

Conclusions Based on Review of Comorbidity of DSM-III and DSM-III-R Anxiety and Mood Disorders

Method and results.   Moras (1989) identified relevant studies using two basic methods. First, a PsycLit computer search of articles published between 1983 and 1989 was done with the PsycLit classification code *mental disorders* and the joint descriptors *anxiety and depression*. The search yielded 616 articles that were inspected for relevance to the relationship between anxiety and depression in patients meeting DSM-III or DSM-III-R criteria for an anxiety or mood disorder. Second, reference lists of review papers on anxiety and depression (e.g., Dobson 1985; Foa and Foa 1982; Lesse 1982; Stavrakaki and Vargo 1986) and reference lists of chapters in edited books on anxiety and depression (Kendall and Watson 1989; Maser and Cloninger 1990; Racagni and Smeraldi 1987) were searched for relevant studies. No systematic attempt was made to locate unpublished studies, although a few were found while conducting the search.

The review only included studies in which DSM-III or DSM-III-R criteria were used to diagnose the patient samples, because implications for modifying the DSM nomenclature can be drawn most directly and accurately from such studies. Thus, for example, relevant studies based on Research Diagnostic Criteria (Spitzer et al. 1978) were not reviewed (e.g., Weissman et al. 1984). Furthermore, any study was excluded that appeared not to use all the DSM-III or DSM-III-R criteria to diagnose disorders (e.g., Breslau and Davis 1985 used an early draft of the DSM-III-R criteria for GAD that did not include the final criterion of two spheres of worry).

Studies in which lifetime diagnoses were used to assess comorbidity (e.g., Breier et al. 1984; Hiller et al. 1989; Raskin et al. 1982) were excluded because a central aim of the review was to examine the discriminant validity of the DSM-III-R anxiety and mood disorder diagnostic criteria, as a basis for making recommendations to the DSM-IV Task Force for modifying the criteria to create one or more mixed anxiety-depression diagnoses. Data on current (cross-sectional) comorbidity are directly relevant to the discriminant validity of diagnostic criteria, whereas lifetime comorbidity data are not, unless one is seeking evidence for a mixed anxiety-depression disorder that involves course criteria like bipolar disorder does, a possibility suggested by Clark and Watson (1989). Lastly, studies of comorbid anxiety and depression in children and adolescents were excluded.

The review was focused only on anxiety and mood disorder diagnostic data. However, Moras's (1989) conclusions were informed by findings from syndromal ratings (e.g., ratings on the Hamilton Anxiety Rating Scale [Hamilton 1959] and on the Hamilton Rating Scale for Depression [Hamilton 1960]) and from self-report data (i.e., patients' responses to questionnaires) as reviewed by Clark (1989) and by Gotlib and Cane (1989), for example.

Although comorbidity patterns of anxiety and mood disorders have been examined in many studies (for review, see Clark 1989), DSM-III or DSM-III-R diagnostic criteria were used in only a small subgroup of studies. Only 10 were found for the Moras (1989) review: Barlow et al. (1986); Benshoof et al. (1989); Dealy et al. (1981); de Ruiter et al. (1989); DiNardo and Barlow (1990); Harris et al. (1983); Lesser et al. (1988); Riskind et al. (1987); Sanderson et al. (1990a, 1990b).

Two mood disorders, major depression and dysthymia, generally have been examined in comorbidity studies of DSM-III and DSM-III-R anxiety and mood disorders. The Moras (1989) review focused on major depression and dysthymia from the DSM mood disorders. Thus, for example, comorbidity findings for bipolar disorder with anxiety disorders were not included.

Comorbidity findings were located for all of the DSM anxiety disorders with mood disorders, although the sample sizes for some anxiety disorders were small. For example, only 1 case of principal PTSD and only 36 cases of principal OCD were reported in the 10 studies reviewed. The small sample sizes probably reflected the low prevalence of the two disorders in the settings where DSM-III and DSM-III-R comorbidity data have been obtained.

Tables 21–1 and 21–2 summarize the comorbidity findings reported in the 10 studies reviewed. Comorbidity percentages were tabulated for additional mood disorders with principal anxiety disorders (Table 21–1), as well as for additional anxiety disorders with principal mood disorders (Table 21–2). (The term *principal diagnosis* refers to the DSM-III or DSM-III-R condition that is the main focus of treatment and/or the major source of impairment or distress at the time of evaluation. An "additional" diagnosis is any other disorder for which a patient also meets criteria). Comorbidity studies of samples diagnosed with principal major depression or dysthymia by DSM-III-R were extremely rare; only one study of this type was found (Sanderson et al. 1990b).

Tables 21–1 and 21–2 show comorbidity percentages when major depression and dysthymia are considered separately and when major depression and dysthymia are combined. For example, Barlow et al. (1986) reported that in a sample of patients with a principal diagnosis of agoraphobia, 15% had an additional diagnosis of major depression and 24% had an additional diagnosis of dysthymia. In Table 21–1, the median percentages for major depression and dysthymia counted separately are shown in addition to the percentages when major depression and dysthymia were combined. Thus, the value Barlow et al. (1986) used to calculate median percentage with major depression and/or dysthymia for Table 21–1 was that 39% of patients with a principal diagnosis of agoraphobia had an additional mood disorder.

Are the comorbidity percentages for major depression and dysthymia separately or combined more relevant for determining whether creating a mixed anxiety-depression disorder is indicated? For an index of the discriminant validity of the DSM-III and DSM-III-R anxiety and mood disorders, the separate percentages are more relevant. For an index of the extent to which the various anxiety disorders are associated with a mood disorder, the percentages for major depression and dysthymia combined are more relevant.

Inspection of the comorbidity percentages led to three main observations:

1. The comorbidity percentages for most of the disorders were quite variable across studies, as indicated by the ranges shown in Tables 21–1 and 21–2. For example, the range of comorbid mood disorder with principal OCD is 7%–67%; the range of comorbid GAD with principal major depression or dysthymia is 17%–60% (Table 21–2). The variable percentages across samples

Table 21–1. Comorbidity rates of mood disorders with principal anxiety disorders

	Principal anxiety disorders with comorbid mood disorders						
	AG with Dep	PD with Dep	GAD with Dep	OCD with Dep	SOC with Dep	SIM with Dep	PTSD with Dep
% of cases with ≥1 comorbid depressive disorder(s) range	7–50	7–36	0–42	7–67	0–25	0–12	(0)[a]
Median % major depression	11	9.5	10	33	4.5	6	
Median % dysthymia	18	17	17	20	17.5	8	
Median % major depression or dysthymia	24	18	33	66	24	16	
n[b]	742	92	98	36	94	51	1
n studies	6	3	5	4	4	3	1

Note. DSM-III or DSM-III-R diagnoses. Results of 10 studies were aggregated to provide percentages: Barlow et al. 1986; Benshoof et al. 1989; Dealy et al. 1981; deRuiter et al. 1989; DiNardo and Barlow 1990; Harris et al. 1983; Lesser et al. 1988; Riskind et al. 1987; Sanderson et al. 1990a, 1990b. AG = generalized anxiety disorder. PD = panic disorder without agoraphobia. GAD = generalized anxiety disorder. OCD = obsessive-compulsive disorder. SOC = social phobia. SIM = simple phobia. PTSD = posttraumatic stress disorder. Dep = depression or dysthymic disorder/dysthymia.

[a]Percentage based on small n.
[b]Sum of sample sizes of aggregated studies.

Table 21–2. Comorbidity rates of anxiety disorders with principal mood disorders

	Principal mood disorders with comorbid anxiety disorders						
	MD or D with AG	MD or D with PD	MD or D with GAD	MD or D with OCD	MD or D with SOC	MD or D with SIM	MD or D with PTSD
% Comorbidity range	0–33	0–18	17–60	0–7	0–44	2–50	0
Median % for MD[a]	9	15	17	2	12	24	
Median % for D[a]	3	3	27	0	33	27	
Median % for MD or D[a]	6.5	10.5	23	1.5	21.5	25	
n[b]	316	316	341	316	316	316	260
n studies	4	4	5	4	4	4	1

Note. DSM-III or DSM-III-R diagnoses. Results of 10 studies were aggregated to provide percentages: Barlow et al. 1986; Benshoof et al. 1989; Dealy et al. 1981; deRuiter et al. 1989; DiNardo and Barlow 1990; Harris et al. 1983; Lesser et al. 1988; Riskind et al. 1987; Sanderson et al. 1990a, 1990b. AG = panic disorder or panic attacks with agoraphobia or agoraphobia without history of panic attacks. PD = panic disorder without agoraphobia. GAD = generalized anxiety disorder. OCD = obsessive-compulsive disorder. SOC = social phobia. SIM = simple phobia. PTSD = posttraumatic stress disorder. Dep = major depression or dysthymic disorder/dysthymia. MD = major depression. D = dysthymia.
[a]Principal diagnosis.
[b]Sum of sample sizes of aggregated studies.

were obtained both when the principal diagnosis was a mood disorder and when it was an anxiety disorder.

2. The median comorbidity percentages for major depression or dysthymia with a principal anxiety disorder and vice versa (a comorbid anxiety disorder with principal major depression or dysthymia) provided evidence for the discriminant validity of the DSM-III and DSM-III-R anxiety disorders and mood disorders major depression and dysthymia. The median comorbidity percentages shown in the tables are not excessively high, using an arbitrary 50% as the criterion for "excessive." For example, when major depression and dysthymia were considered separately, the two highest median percentages were 33% for comorbid depression with principal OCD and 33% for comorbid social phobia with principal dysthymia. The percentages suggest that there are more cases in which the disorders do not co-occur than vice versa, which provides some evidence for the discriminant validity of the specific DSM-III and DSM-III-R anxiety and mood disorders that were examined in the studies reviewed.

3. The median comorbidity percentages summed across major depression and dysthymia suggest that of all the anxiety disorders, a mood disorder is most likely to be associated with principal OCD (66%) (Table 21–1). A mood disorder is about equally likely to co-occur with a principal diagnosis of agoraphobic disorder (24%), social phobia (24%), and GAD (33%). Simple phobia may be least likely to be associated with a mood disorder (the median percentage was 16%).

The median comorbidity percentages for the anxiety disorders with a principal mood disorder were generally lower than those for an additional mood disorder with a principal anxiety disorder. For example, the median percentage of comorbid depression with principal OCD was 66%, but the median percentage of comorbid OCD with a principal mood disorder was 1.5%. GAD and social phobia were two anxiety disorders that tended to show the most symmetry (similarity) in terms of frequency of comorbid mood disorder, regardless of which type of disorder was the principal diagnosis (e.g., the median percentage of comorbid major depression and/or dysthymia with principal social phobia was 24%; median percentage of social phobia with principal major depression or dysthymia was 21.5%).

Discussion.   Moras's (1989) main conclusion was that existing comorbidity data do not clearly indicate that the diagnostic criteria of any of the DSM-III-R diagnoses considered in the review should be revised to create one or more new categories of mixed anxiety-depression. The disorders included in the review were panic disorder with agoraphobia, panic disorder without agoraphobia, GAD, OCD, PTSD, simple phobia, social phobia, major depression, and dysthymia.

Two caveats to the preceding conclusion were made. First, the studies reviewed included only one case of principal PTSD. Thus, not enough data existed to evaluate the extent to which PTSD might co-occur with a mood disorder (i.e., major depression or dysthymia). The second caveat was that certain disorders (GAD and social phobia) manifest symmetrical comorbidity with major depression and dysthymia. That is, the frequency with which major depression or dysthymia is present when either GAD or social phobia is the principal diagnosis is comparable to the frequency with which GAD and social phobia appear as coexisting disorders with principal major depression and dysthymia. This symmetrical comorbidity can be interpreted as evidence that GAD and social phobia tend to be associated with a mood disorder. However, GAD and social phobia only co-occurred with major depression or dysthymia in about one-quarter to one-third of the cases.

Four main reasons supported Moras's (1989) basic conclusion that the existing comorbidity data did not provide an empirical basis for revising DSM-III-R diagnostic criteria for any of the anxiety disorders to create one or more new diagnoses of mixed anxiety-depression. First, the median comorbidity percentages for a mood disorder with each DSM-III or DSM-III-R principal anxiety disorder and vice versa were not excessively high (i.e., all were $\leq 33\%$; median % = 14) and thus were generally consistent with the conclusion that the anxiety disorders and major depression and dysthymia can be discriminated. Second, the comorbidity percentages were quite variable across the 10 relevant studies reviewed. Variable findings fail to provide cumulative evidence that any specific anxiety disorder is consistently associated with major depression or dysthymia. Third, interjudge reliabilities were not reported for the diagnoses made in most of the studies. Hence, the reproducibility of the existing findings could not be assumed. Fourth, much of the comorbidity data on samples with principal diagnoses of an anxiety disorder by DSM-III or DSM-III-R are from one setting, the Center for Stress and Anxiety Disorders in Albany.

Recommendations

Issue 1. Compatibility of ICD-10 and DSM-IV: Should a diagnosis of mixed anxiety-depression be created that would identify patients whose symptoms are below the definitional thresholds for a disorder in the DSM-III-R system?

The conclusion of the DSM-IV Anxiety Disorders Work Group was that existing empirical data supported the examination and exploration of the possibility of creating a new diagnostic category of mixed anxiety-depression that would identify symptoms of anxiety and depression that 1) are associated with distress and/or impairment and 2) are below definitional thresholds for anxiety and/or mood disorders in the DSM-III-R system. Based on the foregoing conclusion, a field trial was recommended to investigate possible sets of diagnostic criteria for a category of mixed anxiety-depression that would identify patients who 1) would not meet DSM-III-R criteria for a mood or anxiety disorder, although they have symptoms of anxiety and depression; and 2) demonstrate impairment severe enough to qualify for the designation of a disorder. It was also recommended that the field trial examine the possibility that patients have been identified in existing community and primary care samples as having anxiety and depression *but not* meeting anxiety and/or mood disorder criteria, because diagnostic assessors in nonpsychiatric settings are relatively unfamiliar with the DSM system.

Issue 2. Should one or more diagnoses of mixed anxiety-depression be created for DSM-III-R mood and anxiety disorders that frequently co-occur?

The DSM-IV Anxiety Disorders Work Group concurred with the conclusion of the Moras (1989) review that the existing comorbidity data on DSM-III and DSM-III-R anxiety and mood disorders do not support the creation of one or more new diagnostic categories of mixed anxiety-depression. However, Clark and Watson's (1989) review of psychometric data on symptoms of anxiety and depression and their recommended integration and reorganization of the DSM-III-R mood and anxiety disorder categories based on a tripartite model of affect (nonspecific general distress, physiological arousal, lack of positive affect) was closely considered by the Work Group. The recommendation of the Work Group was that Clark and Watson's (1989) model for the DSM mood and anxiety disorders be part of a research agenda in preparation for DSM-V. The model was not accepted for DSM-IV primarily because empirical evidence on their proposed diagnostic categories was not yet available.

References

Akiskal HS: Toward a clinical understanding of the relationship of anxiety and depressive disorders, in Comorbidity of Mood and Anxiety Disorders. Edited by Maser JD, Cloninger CR. Washington, DC, American Psychiatric Press, 1990

American Psychiatric Association: Diagnostic and Statistical Manual of Mental Disorders, 3rd Edition. Washington, DC, American Psychiatric Association, 1980

American Psychiatric Association: Diagnostic and Statistical Manual of Mental Disorders, 3rd Edition, Revised. Washington, DC, American Psychiatric Association, 1987

Barlow DH, DiNardo PA, Vermilyea BB, et al: Comorbidity and depression among anxiety disorders: issues in diagnosis and classification. J Nerv Ment Dis 174:63–72, 1986

Barrett JE, Barrett JA, Oxman TE, et al: The prevalence of psychiatric disorders in general practice. Arch Gen Psychiatry 45:1100–1106, 1988

Beck AT: The phenomena of depression: a synthesis, in Modern Psychiatry and Clinical Research. Edited by Offer D, Freedman DX. New York, Basic Books, 1972

Beck AT, Steer RA, Garbin MG: Psychometric properties of the Beck Depression Inventories: twenty-five years of evaluation. Clin Psychol Rev 8:77–100, 1988

Benshoof BB, Moras K, DiNardo P, et al: A comparison of symptomatology in anxiety and depressive disorders. Unpublished manuscript, Albany, State University of New York, Center for Stress and Anxiety Disorders, 1989

Blazer D, Schwartz M, Woodbury M, et al: Depressive symptoms and depressive diagnoses in a community population. Arch Gen Psychiatry 45:1078–1084, 1988

Boyd JH, Weissman MM: Epidemiology of affective disorders: a reexamination and future directions. Arch Gen Psychiatry 38:1039–1046, 1981

Breier A, Charney DS, Heninger GR: Major depression in patients with agoraphobia and panic disorder. Arch Gen Psychiatry 41:1129–1135, 1984

Breslau N, Davis G: DSM-III Generalized Anxiety Disorder: an empirical investigation of more stringent criteria. Psychiatry Res 14:231–238, 1985

Brown GW, Bifulco A, Harris T, et al: Life stress, chronic subclinical symptoms and vulnerability to clinical depression. J Affect Disord 11:1–19, 1986

Clark LA: The anxiety and depressive disorders: descriptive psychopathology and differential diagnosis, in Anxiety and Depression: Distinctive and Overlapping Features. Edited by Kendall PC, Watson D. San Diego, CA, Academic Press, 1989

Clark LA, Watson D: Psychometric issues relevant to a potential DSM-IV category of mixed anxiety-depression. Review paper for the DSM-IV Generalized Anxiety Disorder and Mixed Anxiety Depression Work Group, Southern Methodist University, Dallas, TX, 1989

Clark LA, Watson D: Theoretical and empirical issues in differentiating depression from anxiety, in Psychosocial Aspects of Mood Disorders. Edited by Becker J, Kleinman A. Hillsdale, NJ, Erlbaum, 1991a

Clark LA, Watson D: Tripartite model of anxiety and depression: psychometric evidence and taxonomic implications. J Abnorm Psychol 100:337–345, 1991b

Davidson J, Woodbury MA, Pelton S, et al: A study of depressive typologies using grade of membership analysis. Psychol Med 18:179–189, 1988

Dealy RS, Ishiki DM, Avery DH, et al: Secondary depression in anxiety disorders. Compr Psychiatry 22:612–618, 1981

Deluty BM, Deluty RH, Carver CS: Concordance between clinicians' and patients' ratings of anxiety and depression as mediated by private self-consciousness. J Pers Assess 50:93–106, 1986

Derogatis LR, Lipman RS, Rickels K, et al: The Hopkins Symptom Checklist (HSCL): a self-report symptom inventory. Behav Sci 19:1–15, 1974

de Ruiter C, Ruken H, Garssen B, et al: Comorbidity among the anxiety disorders. J Anx Disord 3:57–68, 1989

DiNardo PA, Barlow DH: Syndrome and symptom comorbidity in the anxiety disorders, in Comorbidity of Anxiety and Mood Disorders. Edited by Maser JD, Cloninger CR. Washington, DC, American Psychiatric Press, 1990

Dobson KS: The relationship between anxiety and depression. Clin Psychol Rev 5:307–324, 1985

Downing RW, Rickels K: Mixed anxiety-depression: fact or myth? Arch Gen Psychiatry 30:312–317, 1974

Eaton WW, Ritter C: Distinguishing anxiety and depression with field survey data. Psychol Med 18:155–166, 1988

Eaton WW, McCutcheon A, Dryman A, et al: Latent class analysis of anxiety and depression. Sociological Methods and Research 18:104–125, 1989

Endicott J, Spitzer RL: A diagnostic interview: the Schedule for Affective Disorders and Schizophrenia. Arch Gen Psychiatry 35:837–844, 1978

Foa EB, Foa UG: Differentiating depression and anxiety: Is it possible? Is it useful? Psychopharmacol Bull 18:62–68, 1982

Goldberg D: Manual of the General Health Questionnaire. Slough, UK, National Foundation for Educational Research, 1978

Gotlib IH: Depression and general psychopathology in university students. J Abnorm Psychol 93:19–30, 1984

Gotlib IH, Cane DB: Self-report assessment of depression and anxiety, in Anxiety and Depression: Distinctive and Overlapping Features. Edited by Kendall PC, Watson D. San Diego, CA, Academic Press, 1989

Hamilton M: The assessment of anxiety states by rating. Br J Med Psychol 32:50–55, 1959

Hamilton M: A rating scale for depression. J Neurol Neurosurg Psychiatry 23:56–62, 1960

Harris EL, Noyes R, Crowe RR, et al: Family study of agoraphobia: report of a pilot study. Arch Gen Psychiatry 40:1061–1064, 1983

Hiller W, Zaudig M, Bose M: The overlap between depression and anxiety on different levels of psychopathology. J Affect Disord 16:223–231, 1989

Katon W, Roy-Byrne PP: Mixed anxiety and depression in primary care studies. Review paper for the DSM-IV Generalized Anxiety Disorder and Mixed Anxiety Depression Work Group. Seattle, University of Washington School of Medicine, 1989

Katon W, Roy-Byrne PP: Mixed anxiety depression. J Abnorm Psychol 100:337–345, 1991

Katon W, Vitaliano P, Russo J, et al: Panic disorder: spectrum of severity and somatization. J Nerv Ment Dis 175:12–19, 1987

Kendall PC, Watson D (eds): Anxiety and Depression: Distinctive and Overlapping Features. San Diego, CA, Academic Press, 1989

Lesse S: The relationship of anxiety to depression. Am J Psychother 36(3):332–349, 1982

Lesser IM, Rubin RT, Pecknold JC, et al: Secondary depression in panic disorder and agoraphobia, 1: frequency, severity, and response to treatment. Arch Gen Psychiatry 45:437–443, 1988

Maier W, Buller R, Philipp M, et al: The Hamilton Anxiety Scale: reliability, validity and sensitivity to change in anxiety and depressive disorders. J Affect Disord 14:61–68, 1988

Maser JD, Cloninger CR (eds): Comorbidity of Anxiety and Mood Disorders. Washington, DC, American Psychiatric Press, 1990

Moras K: Diagnostic comorbidity in the DSM-III and DSM-III-R anxiety and mood disorders: implications for the DSM-IV. Review paper for the DSM-IV Generalized Anxiety Disorder and Mixed Anxiety Depression Work Group. Center for Stress and Anxiety Disorders, University of Albany, State University of New York, 1989

Morey LC, Kurtz JE: The place of neurasthenia in the DSM-IV. Review paper for the DSM-IV Generalized Anxiety Disorder and Mixed Anxiety Depression Work Group. Nashville, TN, Vanderbilt University, 1989

Myers JK, Weissman MM, Tischler GL, et al: Six-month prevalence of psychiatric disorder in three communities, 1980 to 1982. Arch Gen Psychiatry 41:959–967, 1984

Racagni G, Smeraldi E (eds): Anxious Depression: Assessment and Treatment. New York, Raven, 1987

Raskin M, Peeke HVS, Dickman W, et al: Panic and generalized anxiety disorders: developmental antecedents and precipitants. Arch Gen Psychiatry 39:687–689, 1982

Riskind JH, Beck AT, Berchick RJ, et al: Reliability of DSM-III diagnoses for major depression and generalized anxiety disorder using the structured clinical interview for DSM-III. Arch Gen Psychiatry 44:817–820, 1987

Robins LN, Helzer JE, Croughan J, et al: National Institute of Mental Health Diagnostic Interview Schedule: its history, characteristics, and validity. Arch Gen Psychiatry 38:381–389, 1981

Roth M, Gurney C, Garside RF, et al: Studies in the classification of affective disorders: relationship between anxiety states and depressive illness. Br J Psychiatry 121:147–161, 1972

Sanderson WC, DiNardo PA, Rapee RM, et al: Syndrome co-morbidity in patients diagnosed with a DSM-III-Revised anxiety disorder. J Abnorm Psychol 99:308–312, 1990a

Sanderson WC, Beck AT, Beck J: Syndrome co-morbidity in patients with major depression or dysthymia: prevalence and temporal relationships. Am J Psychiatry 147:1025–1028, 1990b

Sireling LI, Paykel ES, Freeling P, et al: Depression in general practice: case thresholds and diagnosis. Br J Psychiatry 147:113–119, 1985

Spitzer RL, Endicott J, Robins E: Research Diagnostic Criteria: rationale and reliability. Arch Gen Psychiatry 35:773–782, 1978

Stavrakaki C, Vargo B: The relationship of anxiety and depression: a review of the literature. Br J Psychiatry 149:7–16, 1986

Tellegen A: Structures of mood and personality and their relevance to assessing anxiety, with an emphasis on self-report, in Anxiety and the Anxiety Disorders. Edited by Tuma AH, Maser JD. Hillsdale, NJ, Erlbaum, 1985

Tyrer P: Neurosis divisible? Lancet 1:685–688, 1985

Von Korff M, Shapiro S, Burke JD, et al: Anxiety and depression in a primary care clinic: comparison of Diagnostic Interview Schedule, General Health Questionnaire and practitioner assessments. Arch Gen Psychiatry 44:152–156, 1987

Watson D, Clark LA, Carey G: Positive and negative affect and their relation to anxiety and depressive disorders. J Abnorm Psychol 97:346–353, 1988

Weissman MM, Boyd JH: The epidemiology of affective disorders: rates and risk factors, in Psychiatry Update: American Psychiatric Association Annual Review, Vol 2. Edited by Grinspoon L. Washington DC, American Psychiatric Press, 1983

Weissman MM, Leckman JF, Merikangas KR, et al: Depression and anxiety disorders in parents and children. Arch Gen Psychiatry 41:845–852, 1984

Wells KB, Stewart A, Hays RD: The functioning and well-being of depressed patients: results from the Medical Outcomes Study. J Am Med Assoc 262:914–919, 1989

World Health Organization: ICD-10 Chapter V. Mental and Behavioral Disorders. Diagnostic Criteria for Research. Geneva, Switzerland, World Health Organization, 1988

Zung W: A self-rating depression scale. Arch Gen Psychiatry 12:63–70, 1965

Section IV

Personality Disorders

Introduction to Section IV

Personality Disorders

John Gunderson, M.D.

This introduction provides a summary of the major issues that the DSM-IV Work Group on personality disorders addressed and the process by which it developed options and then ultimately made its proposals. Findings from the ongoing DSM-IV field trials that relate to the diagnoses of antisocial personality disorder and depressive personality disorder and MacArthur reanalyses related to the diagnosis of schizotypal personality disorder are not included in this overview but will be presented in later volumes of the *DSM-IV Sourcebook*.

Magnitude and Basis for Change

From the start, the DSM-IV Work Group on Personality Disorders was confronted with a major question concerning the extent of the changes that it should propose. More radical change was considered because the existing criteria for most of the personality disorders (DSM-III [American Psychiatric Association 1980]; DSM-III-R [American Psychiatric Association 1987]) were derived by a committee that, for the most part, lacked clinical expertise with the disorders and that had virtually no empirical database as a guide. This history led to numerous criticisms about both the content and the lack of empirical justification for the Axis II categories (Caplan 1987; Gunderson 1983; Kaplan 1983; Kernberg 1984; Michaels 1984; Millon 1981; Perry 1990). Problems evident for most of the personality disorders concern coverage and descriptive validity (Widiger et al. 1988). The prevalence rates reported for some of the personality disorder diagnoses have been inconsistent with clinical and theoretical expectations. Some occur at excessive rates, whereas

The chapters provided within this section were published previously in the *Journal of Personality Disorders* (1991, pp. 122–209 and pp. 337–398, and 1993, pp. 28–85). They are reprinted with permission by Guilford Press. Updated versions with critical commentaries are also provided in Livesley (1995).

others have been inordinately rare. Table 1 provides the rates of occurrence reported in 12 studies published through 1988. In addition, there are substantial co-occurrence and overlap among the personality disorder diagnoses (Blashfield and Breen 1989). The average number of personality disorder diagnoses per patient in inpatient samples has ranged from 2.8 (Zanarini et al. 1987) to 4.6 (Skodol et al. 1988). The weak evidentiary base for the existing definitions and the documentation of problems with overlap and coverage were reasons for the committee to consider making radical changes.

Some changes introduced in DSM-III-R in 1985 resulted from better-informed clinical input (e.g., histrionic and schizoid personality types). Other changes involved modifications in format, most notably making all criteria sets polythetic. The effect of these changes was to make criteria more congruent with informed clinical opinions, but the changes also led to increased rates of prevalence and comorbidity (Morey 1988) and were disruptive to emerging and ongoing research. So, when work began on DSM-IV in 1988, the anticipation of any further revisions to the personality disorders section was already cause for concern (Blashfield et al. 1990; Caplan 1991; Zimmerman 1988).

In another sense, the question of how much DSM-IV should change Axis II involved questions about whether the evidentiary basis for diagnostic changes could still be derived from informed expert clinical judgments or whether more scientifically acquired justifications should be required. For the Personality Disorders Work Group, this question was influenced on the one hand by the fact that the categories originally failed to reflect informed expert clinical judgment and, on the other, by the sudden explosion of empirical research that had developed based on DSM-III's flawed descriptions. The Work Group attempted to balance these two sides.

Historically, psychiatry has never had an empirically based system for classifying personality disorders. Outside of psychiatry's clinical descriptive tradition, there have been multiple attempts to develop classification systems based on theoretical models from the framework of biogenetics, traits, or psychological organizations (i.e., psychodynamics) (Gunderson 1992). Specifically, DSM-III and DSM-III-R had several categories that were considered biogenetic variants of Axis I disorders (i.e., cyclothymia and schizotypal personality disorder) that were inconsistently managed (i.e., one was placed on Axis I, the other on Axis II). DSM-III and DSM-III-R also included some disorders that could primarily be conceptualized as extreme variants of normally occurring traits (i.e., dependent and avoidant types). Indeed, as the DSM-IV Work Group pursued its tasks, it wrestled with the question of whether the admixture of types derived from these models in DSM-III-R categories should be simplified or made more consistent. Related to this were discussions about whether to retain the cluster system found in DSM-III and DSM-III-R. That cluster system (odd/eccentric, dramatic, and anxious) was based

Table 1. Rates of personality disorder diagnoses in 12 studies

Study	N	PPD	SZPD	STPD	ASPD	BPD	HPD	NPD	AVPD	DPD	OCPD	PAP
Alneas and Torgersen 1988	298	.05	.02	.06	.00	.15	.14	.05	.55	.47	.20	.10
Dahl 1986	103	.01	.03	.22	.18	.20	.19	.02	.09	.02	.01	.02
Frances et al. 1984	76	.08	.01	.13	.03	.34	.22	.16	.21	.25	.09	.09
Hyler and Lyons 1988	358	.02	.02	.02	.02	.21	.06	.06	.06	.09	.11	.06
Kass et al. 1985	609	.05	.01	.04	.02	.11	.06	.03	.05	.08	.02	.02
Loranger et al. 1987	60	.03	.01	.33	.12	.30	.15	.05	.07	.05	.08	.00
Morey 1988	291	.07	.01	.17	.06	.32	.22	.06	.11	.14	.09	.08
Pfohl et al. 1986	131	.01	.01	.09	.04	.22	.19	.04	.11	.13	.05	.14
Skodol et al. 1988	97	.35	.05	.18	.08	.52	.26	.16	.49	.35	.18	.12
Standage and Ladha 1988	20	.30	.00	.20	.20	.70	.15	.35	.50	.55	.20	.05
Widiger et al. 1987	84	.20	.08	.64	.37	.63	.45	.11	.33	.48	.02	.52
Zanarini et al. 1987	43	.12	.00	.35	.23	.60	.42	.16	.35	.30	.12	.19

Note. PPD = paranoid personality disorder. SZPD = schizoid personality disorder. STPD = schizotypal personality disorder. ASPD = antisocial personality disorder. BPD = borderline personality disorder. HPD = histrionic personality disorder. NPD = narcissistic personality disorder. AVPD = avoidant personality disorder. DPD = dependent personality disorder. OCPD = obsessive-compulsive personality disorder. PAPD = passive-aggressive personality disorder.
Source. Reprinted from Widiger T: "DSM-IV and Personality Disorders: Introduction to Special Series." *Journal of Personality Disorders* 5:122–134, 1991. Used with permission.

on descriptive similarities. It received some empirical support (Hyler and Lyons 1988; Kass et al. 1985; Morey et al. 1985; Zimmerman and Coryell 1990) but also was subject to conceptual and empirically based criticisms (Gunderson 1992; Millon 1981; Widiger et al. 1987). In particular, consideration was given to developing new clusters for the personality disorders; possibilities included clusters based on spectrum conditions (biogenetic model), extreme self-distortions (intrapsychic model), or dimensions with normality (trait model).

Three factors led the Work Group to adopt a conservative strategy. First, they foresaw the possibility that the long tradition of factor analytic approaches in academic psychology, although largely performed with normal populations and tied to a dimensional approach, might eventually yield a more scientific means of classifying personality disorders. Second, the very diversity of models by which the Axis II system might be reorganized reflected the lack of any prevailing consensus. Third, the Work Group believed that the many studies of Axis II disorders done with systematic structured interview assessments might already provide sufficient empirical support to guide changes and might even shape new and more compelling models for the organization of the personality disorders.

Adoption of Dimensional Model

Although medical practice has always used a categorical model (i.e., a disorder is considered either present or absent), this model may not be as appropriate for personality disorders, because the boundaries with normal personality, and to some extent with each other, are inherently blurred. Proposals considered by the Axis II Work Group included adding an alternative dimensional schema derived from factor analytic studies of normal populations. This model identified seven dimensions: extraversion, neuroticism, constraint, agreeableness, openness, reward dependence, and cognitive disorganization. Another alternative was to classify existing personality disorders along dimensions of severity (either according to how many criteria were met or by descriptors such as *absent, threshold,* or *prototypic*). However, because clinicians already fail to use more than one category (despite instructions in DSM-III and DSM-III-R to do so), the Work Group concluded that they would be unlikely to accept added diagnostic complexity. The more clinically familiar categorical format (and types) are therefore proposed because they remain the standards on which the clinical literature and clinical judgments are based.

How to Improve Descriptive Validity

To ensure that the definitions of the categories reflect informed clinician judgment, the Work Group identified clinicians with recognized expertise for each disorder and invited them to help develop and revise proposals. Seventy-eight advisers were involved in this process.

Data were also obtained with respect to the prototypicality and face validity of each of the DSM-III and DSM-III-R personality disorder criteria. Blashfield (1988) provided unpublished results concerning the frequency with which each of the DSM-III-R personality disorder criteria are confused with and misassigned to other diagnoses. Prototypicality ratings and data on face validity were obtained from publications by Blashfield and Haymaker (1988), Burns (1986), Hilbrand and Hirt (1987), and Livesley et al. (1987). In addition to the prototypicality ratings offered by the data, and by Blashfield in particular, the Work Group solicited detailed reviews from Lorna Benjamin to take advantage of her empirically derived perspectives on the interpersonal basis for each disorder. A third resource was an ad hoc Work Group of the American Psychoanalytic Association chaired by Arnold Cooper. That committee offered perspectives derived from observations of intrapsychic organizing characteristics.

In recognition that clinicians do not approach diagnosis with a polythetic model but search for and give added weight to specific features, we discussed departing from the polythetic format. Because of the uncertain effects of such a reversal and the research advantages of retaining the polythetic format (i.e., the capacity to build on earlier findings and use earlier databases), the Work Group found other ways to make the criteria more compatible for clinicians. One way was to focus extra attention on the definition of an essential feature for each category and to underscore its presentation at the start of each criteria set. A second way was to present the criteria in the rank order of their diagnostic importance as measured by their diagnostic efficiency credentials (i.e., most notably their phi coefficients but with special reference to their specificity). Third, an effort was made to provide a more clinically rich and compelling narrative explication for each of the diagnoses enhanced by the contributions from the advisers cited above.

How to Reduce Overlap

As noted earlier, neither the DSM-III nor the DSM-III-R system successfully identifies distinguishable categories of personality disorder. In DSM-III and DSM-III-R, this was handled by encouraging clinicians to document all the disorders for which criteria are met, which is inconsistent with clinical practice, however (Pfohl et al. 1986; Widiger and Frances 1985).

One strategy the Work Group considered to diminish excessive overlap was to implement a hierarchical strategy whereby some Axis II disorders would be given diagnostic priority. For example, if a patient met criteria for paranoid personality disorder, it would be considered redundant and irrelevant if that patient also met criteria for avoidant personality disorder. Similarly, if a patient met criteria for borderline personality disorder, it would be of no value or interest to clinicians to note that the patient has met criteria for dependent personality disorder. The principle underlying such a hierarchical strategy is that some of the personality disorders have sufficiently overriding prognostic and therapeutic implications so that the presence of other clearly less severe diagnoses is not meaningful. Although everyone agreed that such a hierarchy would make Axis II more compatible (user friendly) with clinical practices, there were concerns that operationalizing such a system would be premature (i.e., that before adopting any such system, its conformity with clinical practice needs to be empirically demonstrated). The Work Group thus concluded that a hierarchy would not be proposed but that clinicians would be encouraged to identify the personality disorder they considered primary, with documentation of others being given secondary significance.

The main approach that the Work Group used to reduce overlap was revision of criteria to increase the differentiation among the personality disorders. A search was therefore conducted to obtain results from studies that reported 1) co-occurrence among all of the personality disorders or 2) the sensitivity, specificity, positive predictive power, and/or negative predictive power rates for the criteria sets. Table 2 provides a list of the studies that were published through 1988 and their methodological features. Because few of these studies had published data on DSM-III-R or reported co-occurrence rates for all the personality disorders, researchers were solicited to provide additional results from their unpublished data sets. Dubro (1988), Malow and Donnelly (1988), McGlashan and Fenton (1988), and Reich (1988) provided data regarding individual personality disorders. Freiman and Widiger (1989), Millon and Tringone (1989), Morey and Heumann (1988), Pfohl and Blum (1990), Skodol (1989), and Zanarini et al. (1989) provided data on all of the personality disorders, including 1) co-occurrence rates for all the DSM-III-R personality disorders and 2) the sensitivity, specificity, positive and negative predictive power, and phi coefficients for every DSM-III-R personality disorder criterion. These data were helpful in verifying empirically the degree and direction of overlap among the personality disorders at different research sites and in identifying empirically which criteria were the most and least useful to the respective diagnoses.

It became apparent, however, that additional information was necessary to determine which items contributed to the overlap among the personality disorders. For example, the co-occurrence tables indicated substantial overlap between histrionic and borderline personality disorders, but it was not known which items were making the principal contributions to this overlap. One might assume that the histrionic item involving exaggerated emotion was one of the criteria that was primarily responsible, but it was unknown whether there was any consistent

Table 2. Diagnostic efficiency studies

Study	N	Nomenclature	Methodology	Location	Institution	Comparison group	Percentage male	Published?
Clarkin et al. 1983	76	DSM-III	ST	O	MC	PD	21	P
Cowdry et al. 1985	59	DSM-III	CI	I	MC	DEP	–	P
Dahl 1986	1.3	DSM-III	SI	I	MC	PD	58	P
Dubro 1988	56	DSM-III	SI	I	VA	PD/Nm	93	U
First and Spitzer 1989	284	DSM-III-R	SI	Mxd	Mxd	Mxd	–	U
Freiman and Widiger 1989	50	DSM-III-R	SI	I	PUB	PD	70	U
Jacobsberg et al. 1986	64	DSM-III	SI	O/I	MC	PD	39	P
Kass 1987	367	DSM-III-R	CS	O	PP/CL	–	39	P
Kass et al. 1986	59	DSM-III-R	CS	O	PP/CL	Mxd	36	P
Malow and Donnelly 1988	163	DSM-III	SI	I	VA	DRG	100	U
McGlashan and Fenton 1988	109	DSM-III	CT	I	PRH	BPD/STPD	36	U
Millon and Tringone 1989	614	DSM-III-R	CI	Mxd	Mxd	–	46	U
Modestin 1987	129	DSM-III	CI	I	MC	PD	50	P
Morey and Goodman 1989[a]	291	DSM-III-R	CI	Mxd	Mxd	PD	44	U
Nurnberg et al. 1986	37	DSM-III	SI	I	MC	NOR	46	P
Perry et al. 1984	19	DSM-III	SI	O	Mxd	BPD/BAD	–	P
Pfohl and Blum 1990	112	DSM-III-R	SI	Mxd	Mxd	Mxd	29	U
Pfohl et al. 1986	137	DSM-III	SI	Mxd	MC	PF	24	P
Plakun 1987	63	DSM-III	CT	I	PRH	NPD	38	P
Reich 1988	159	DSM-III	INV	O	Mxd	Mxd/Anx	37	U

(continued)

Table 2. Diagnostic efficiency studies (*continued*)

Study	N	Nomenclature	Methodology	Location	Institution	Comparison group	Percentage male	Published?
Ronningstam and Gunderson 1988	51	Mixed	SI	Mxd	PRH	–	51	P
Skodol 1989	97	DSM-III-R	SI	I	MC	PD	–	U
Spitzer et al. 1979	1,616	DSM-III	CI	Mxd	Mxd	Mxd	64	P
Spitzer et al. 1989	444	DSM-III-R	CI	Mxd	Mxd	PD	41	P
Spitzer et al. 1989	1,391	DSM-III-R	CI	Mxd	Mxd	BPD/DPD	37	P
Widiger et al. 1986	84	DSM-III	SI	I	PUB	PD	–	P
Zanarini et al. 1989	253	DSM-II	SI	Mxd	Mxd	Mxd	42	U

Note. Methodologies: SI = semistructured interview. CI = clinical interview. CT = chart review. INV = self-report inventory.

Locations: I = inpatient. O = outpatient. Mxd = mixed).

Institutions: MC = medical center. VA = Veterans Administration hospital. PUB = public hospital. PP = private practice. CL = community clinic. PRH = private hospital. Mxd = mixed.

Comparison groups: PD = personality disorders. DEP = depressed. NOR = normal. DRG = drug abuse. BPD = borderline personality disorder. STPD = schizotypal personality disorder. BAD = bipolar affective disorder. NPD = narcissistic personality disorder. ANX = anxiety disorder. Mxd = mixed. P = published. U = unpublished.

Source. Reprinted from Widiger T: "DSM-IV and Personality Disorders: Introduction to Special Series." *Journal of Personality Disorders* 5:122–134, 1991.
[a]Morey and Heumann 1988 involves the same data set as Morey and Goodman 1989.

empirical support across research programs for this assumption. Relevant information would include the sensitivity, specificity, positive and negative predictive power, phi coefficient, and point biserial correlations of each DSM-III-R criterion to every other personality disorder diagnosis. With the support of the MacArthur Foundation, these results were provided for all of the personality disorder criteria by First and Spitzer (1989), Freiman and Widiger (1989), Millon and Tringone (1989), Morey and Goodman (1989), Pfohl and Blum (1990), Skodol (1989), and Zanarini (1989). Findings from these analyses were particularly informative with respect to developing proposals to diminish problematic overlap between Axis II categories.

Schizotypal Personality Disorder

Schizotypal personality disorder (STPD) entered our nosology in DSM-III. It is the first personality disorder defined in part by its genetic relationship to an Axis I disorder, i.e., chronic schizophrenia. The major issues addressed by the Work Group were: 1) Should STPD be included with other schizophrenia-related disorders on Axis I? 2) Can modifications in the STPD criteria improve the strength of the genetic relationship with schizophrenia? 3) Can changes be made in the STPD criteria to diminish overlap with other Axis II disorders, particularly with borderline personality disorder?

Although the strength and specificity of the relationship between STPD and chronic schizophrenia in clinical settings has not been well studied (there has been a problem identifying schizotypal patients within clinical settings), multiple studies do confirm this relationship with family history, biological characteristics, outcome, and treatment response. These studies confirm a relationship that argues for the inclusion of STPD on Axis I among the schizophrenia-related disorders. Nonetheless, the Work Group felt that moving STPD to Axis I would set a problematic precedent because there are other stable psychopathological characteristics of Axis II disorders that represent biogenetically related variants of other Axis I conditions. In a sense, such a move would foreclose the possible development of an Axis II classification system based on biogenetic factors or temperaments, a direction in which the Axis II classification might and possibly should move. The ICD-10 (World Health Organization 1990) code number F21 reflects the association of STPD with Axis I.

In view of growing evidence that it is the social and interpersonal deficits that provide the strongest link to a schizophrenic genotype, these characteristics are given due emphasis in the proposed description of the essential feature of the disorder: "A pervasive pattern of social and interpersonal deficits marked by acute discomfort with, and reduced capacity for, close relationships as well as by cognitive or perceptual distortions and eccentricities of behavior." To improve the discrimination from borderline personality disorder, a preamble statement is proposed to indicate that the criteria should not be limited to discrete periods of mood symptomatology. Moreover, we propose that the disturbed perceptual experiences of schizotypal patients (to be described in criterion 3 of DSM-IV) be exemplified as somatosensory (bodily) illusions rather than illusions related to sensing a person's presence, because the latter are more characteristic of borderline personality disorder.

Although we recognized that there are high levels of overlap between STPD and paranoid and schizoid personality disorders, the Work Group did not go to great lengths to try to distinguish them because of the perception that they represent a valid cluster, due to both their relatedness to psychotic conditions and their unity around the central characteristic of social detachment.

Paranoid Personality Disorder

A few changes are proposed to make criteria more distinctly characteristic of this disorder, namely, by indicating that both the "tendency to counterattack" (DSM-IV criterion 6) and the "suspicions of infidelity" (DSM-IV criterion 7) occur in response to misperceptions of others.

Schizoid Personality Disorder

To reduce redundancy in the criteria and give added weight to the characteristic of anhedonia, it is proposed that DSM-IV criterion 4 be changed from a description of more general emotional flatness (an absence of strong emotions) to a lack of pleasure from activities.

Antisocial Personality Disorder

A significant reworking of the criteria for this disorder was prompted by the lengthy, complicated, and potentially culturally biased criteria used in DSM-III and DSM-III-R.

A field trial was conducted to identify crosswalks to the personality traits used in ICD-10 and in research on psychopathology. This has resulted in a proposed shortened criteria set that more closely resembles the format of criteria for other personality diagnoses but preserves, to a considerable extent, the construct that was present in previous research using DSM-III or DSM-III-R criteria for antisocial personality disorder.

Borderline Personality Disorder

Over 300 empirical articles have been published about borderline personality disorder (BPD) since 1980, reflecting the widespread interest in this disorder. Approximately 25 people outside of the Work Group with established expertise in this disorder actively advised about the changes being proposed.

The two major issues that concerned the Work Group were: 1) Do the high prevalence and overlap rates for this disorder reflect an artifact of an overly inclusive definition? and 2) Will the construct be better reflected by including a criterion related to the cognitive-perceptual problems of these patients?

Studies on the overlap of BPD with other Axis II disorders confirmed significant overlaps with antisocial, narcissistic, histrionic, and, surprisingly, avoidant personality disorders. Other literature indicated significant overlap of BPD with mood disorders and posttraumatic stress disorder. Such work indicated the boundaries where BPD's definition could helpfully become more distinct.

Growing evidence suggested that the overlap with affective disorders was partly a definitional artifact and was unlikely to reflect a more basic relationship in the etiologies of these disorders (Gunderson and Phillips 1991). Rather, evidence points toward the importance of the impulse regulatory problem as a major component of borderline psychopathology (Silverman et al. 1991) and the importance of childhood trauma as a component of this pathogenesis. These shifts in the borderline construct led to a proposed alteration in the description of the essential feature for the disorder, so that the word *mood* would be replaced by *affects* and *control over impulses* would be added as a pattern of instability. Moreover, it is proposed that the criterion that reflects affective instability be altered from a description of *marked shifts* of mood to *marked reactivity* of mood to highlight the degree to which the affective instability is related to identifiable events as opposed to the autonomous internal lability seen in primary mood disorders. A change is also proposed for the criterion on identity disturbance, which had poor reliability and specificity. To improve it and to narrow the construct and make this criterion more consistent with both the essential feature and the trauma history, the revised version would emphasize gross distortions in self-image.

After a systematic review of the considerable data and much advice, the Work Group adopted a proposal to add a ninth criterion, "transient, stress-related severe dissociative symptoms or paranoid ideation." Although the addition of this criterion runs the risk of confusing state-related symptoms with enduring state-independent traits, it captures a characteristic that has been found to be a pattern in the majority of borderline patients and that has a very useful clinical implication. Hence, this change won the endorsement of virtually all the advisers. As with the affective instability criterion, a study stimulated by the Work Group showed that it is the reactive, stress-related nature of the dissociative or paranoid symptoms that can help distinguish BPD, most notably from STPD (Sternbach et al. 1992).

Histrionic Personality Disorder

The relatively few changes proposed for this disorder were intended to reduce overlap with borderline, antisocial, and narcissistic personality disorders. Special attention was given to the danger of a sex-bias in the criteria (i.e., of pathologizing normal or adaptive feminine behaviors). It was proposed that one criterion ("seeks reassurance or praise") be omitted because of its low specificity.

Narcissistic Personality Disorder

A few changes are proposed to help reduce the overlap with other personality disorders (especially antisocial and histrionic personality disorders). In addition, one DSM-III-R criterion ("reacts to criticism with feelings of rage, shame, or humiliation") is proposed for deletion because of its low specificity and a new criterion ("arrogant, haughty behaviors or attitudes") is proposed for addition because of its usefulness in distinguishing this disorder from other personality disorders. The major issue for which no solution was found is that the current criteria set probably overlooks less aggressive and observable forms of narcissistic personality psychopathology (Cooper 1987).

Avoidant Personality Disorder

A major issue that concerned the Work Group about avoidant personality disorder was the nature of the construct that the criteria are intended to reflect. This concern can be traced to the emergence of this category in DSM-III without a significant clinical tradition or literature. Its use has thus been confused with schizoid personality disorder and with the phobic character (Fenichel 1945). The changes made in the criteria for this disorder in DSM-III-R greatly enlarged its coverage and its usage. The Work Group used the available empirical evidence to try to modify the criteria to diminish overlap with other personality disorders. It was also proposed that two DSM-III-R criteria with particularly low specificity be deleted. The Work Group also considered the clinical and conceptual overlap with generalized social phobia and worked with the Anxiety Disorders Work Group to distinguish traits belonging on Axis II from symptoms belonging on Axis I.

Dependent Personality Disorder

A major issue concerning this category was the definition of its underlying central construct. The Work Group was concerned that, although the six new criteria added in DSM-III-R reduced unnecessary overlap, they also confounded the disorder's construct. The Work Group therefore gave special attention to defining the essential feature of this disorder and proposed changing that from "a pervasive pattern of dependent and submissive behavior" to "a pervasive and excessive need to be taken care of, which leads to submissive and clinging behavior and fears of separation." The Work Group also proposed modifications in the criteria to reflect both the attachment component of a dependency disorder that relates to the emotional reliance on another person and the more general component related to lack of social self-confidence (Hirschfeld et al. 1976; Livesley et al. 1990). Special attention was given to make criteria free of sex bias.

Obsessive-Compulsive Personality Disorder

The few changes in the criteria for this disorder are proposed to improve the discrimination from other personality disorders and to increase compatibility with ICD-10. It is proposed that the criterion "indecisiveness" be omitted because of its low specificity and lack of clustering with the other items.

Passive-Aggressive Personality Disorder

Several issues have been raised about this disorder: 1) it is too narrowly defined, with redundant items; 2) it is too situation specific; and 3) it is a single symptom or dynamic rather than a personality disorder. Because of the relatively low prevalence of this disorder and the absence of any strong empirical verification of its clinical utility or validity, the Work Group proposed that it be omitted and that a related construct, negativistic personality disorder, be developed for the appendix. This negativistic personality disorder construct would have broader coverage and would reflect both the same pattern of passive resistance and a more general negativistic attitude. If included in the appendix, this category would then be available so that its possible clinical applications could be tested and its merits evaluated. In the meantime, the proposed negativistic personality disorder, despite its lineage from passive-aggressive personality disorder, lacks the necessary clinical and empirical support to justify inclusion.

Appendix Categories

As noted in the preceding section, although the Work Group proposed deleting passive-aggressive personality disorder from DSM-IV, they also proposed that a somewhat broader version of this entity called negativistic personality disorder be included in the appendix to DSM-IV for disorders requiring further study. The Work Group also proposed two other categories, self-defeating personality disorder and depressive personality disorder, for inclusion in the appendix. It is notable that all three of these disorders identify persons who have problems with the direct expression of their aggression or with their assertiveness. Beyond this overriding similarity, the disorders have quite different theoretical and clinical traditions. Negativistic personality disorder was developed by the Work Group as a way of preserving what was best out of the passive-aggressive category. As such, its origins had to do with resistance within social situations to external structures and authority. Self-defeating personality disorder is a disorder arising out of psychoanalytic theory (i.e., moral masochism) that is intended to describe a pattern of relationships in which a person persistently accepts unpleasant or demeaning treatment from others without leaving or taking other recourse, despite its apparent availability. Depressive personality disorder comes out of the descriptive psychiatric tradition in which it was first identified as a temperament and, more recently, has been conceptualized as a spectrum disorder (i.e., the personalogic variant of and predisposing vulnerability for major depressive disorders). As such, its endorsement by the Work Group follows on the decision to endorse the continued inclusion of schizotypal personality disorder on Axis II despite its well-documented biogenetic and therapeutic relationship with chronic schizophrenia. Quite polarized views surround both self-defeating personality disorder and depressive personality disorder, testifying to the importance of the issues and the need for more empirical data before conclusions are reached about their inclusion in the official diagnostic system. The major objection to self-defeating personality disorder has been that it is used to pathologize normative and even adaptive aspects of female psychology such as the attribution of "excessive self-sacrifice" and that it may be misused to pathologize victims within abusive relationships. The opposition to the inclusion of a depressive personality disorder is more complicated. Part of it reflects a concern that its inclusion on Axis II would lead clinicians away from the appropriate use of medications. In part, opposition comes from those who accept the concept of an early-onset, personalogic variant of depressive disorders but feel it should be included on Axis I.

The final issue related to appendix categories involved sadistic personality disorder, a category introduced in DSM-III-R. Because there is little evidence of its clinical utility and because of the fact that most of the few persons who meet the criteria for sadistic personality disorder also meet criteria for either antisocial personality disorder or narcissistic personality disorder, it was decided to omit this category.

Personality Change Categories

As part of the effort to align DSM-IV categories with those used in ICD-10, the Work Group considered the addition of two new categories related to personality change. The review of evidence supported the adoption of a category for personality change resulting from catastrophic experience. Because the construct includes an etiological component and because it has adult and relatively rapid onset, the Work Group did not, however, recommend its inclusion in DSM-IV as part of Axis II. A review of the evidence for the category personality change resulting from another mental disorder was deemed insufficient to support inclusion of it.

References

Alnaes R, Torgerson S: The relationship between DSM-III symptom disorders (Axis I) and personality disorders (Axis II) in an outpatient population. Acta Psychiatr Scand 78:485–492, 1988

American Psychiatric Association: Diagnostic and Statistical Manual of Mental Disorders, 3rd Edition. Washington, DC, American Psychiatric Association, 1980

American Psychiatric Association: Diagnostic and Statistical Manual of Mental Disorders, 3rd Edition, Revised. Washington, DC, American Psychiatric Association, 1987

Blashfield R: Similarity matrix for personality disorders. Unpublished raw data, Gainesville, University of Florida, 1988

Blashfield R, Breen M: Face validity of the DSM-III-R personality disorders. Am J Psychiatry 146:1575–1579, 1989

Blashfield R, Haymaker D: A prototype analysis of the diagnostic criteria for DSM-III-R personality disorders. Journal of Personality Disorders 2:272–280, 1988

Blashfield R, Sprock J, Fuller A: Suggested guidelines for including/excluding categories in the DSM-IV. Journal of Personality Disorders 31:15–19, 1990

Burns T: Use of the term "borderline patient" by Swedish psychiatrists. Int J Soc Psychiatry 32:32–39, 1986

Caplan P: The psychiatric association's failure to meet its own standards: the dangers of "self-defeating personality disorder." Journal of Personality Disorders 1:178–182, 1987

Caplan P: How do they decide who is normal? The bizarre, but true, tale of the DSM process. Can Psychol 32:162–170, 1991

Clarkin J, Widiger T, Frances A, et al: Prototypic typology and the borderline personality disorder. J Abnorm Psychol 92:263–275, 1983

Cooper A: Histrionic, narcissistic and compulsive personality disorders, in Diagnosis and Classification in Psychiatry. Edited by Tischler G. New York, Cambridge University Press, 1987, pp 290–299

Cowdry R, Pickar D, Davies R: Symptoms and EEG findings in the borderline syndrome. Int J Psychiatry Med 15:201–211, 1985

Dahl A: Some aspects of the DSM-III personality disorders illustrated by a consecutive sample of hospitalized patients. Acta Psychiatr Scand 73:61–66, 1986

Dubro A: Diagnostic efficiency statistics for borderline personality disorder. Unpublished raw data, White Plains, NY, Cornell University Medical Center, 1988

Fenichel O: The Psychoanalytic Theory of Neuroses. New York, Norton, 1945

First M, Spitzer R: Diagnostic efficiency statistics. Unpublished raw data, New York State Psychiatric Institute, 1989

Frances A, Clarkin J, Gilmore M, et al: Reliability of criteria for borderline personality disorder: a comparison of DSM-III and the Diagnostic Interview for Borderline Patients. Am J Psychiatry 141:1080–1084, 1984

Freiman K, Widiger T: Co-occurrence and diagnostic efficiency statistics. Unpublished raw data, Lexington, University of Kentucky, 1989

Gunderson J: DSM-III diagnosis of personality disorders, in Current Perspectives on Personality Disorders. Edited by Frosch J. Washington, DC, American Psychiatric Press, 1983, pp 20–39

Gunderson JG: Diagnostic controversies, in American Psychiatric Press Review of Psychiatry, Vol 11. Edited by Tasman A, Riba MB. Washington, DC, American Psychiatric Press, 1992, pp 9–24

Gunderson JG, Phillips KA: Borderline personality disorder and depression: a current overview of the interface. Am J Psychiatry 148:967–975, 1991

Hilbrand M, Hirt M: The borderline patient: an empirically developed prototype. Journal of Personality Disorders 1:299–306, 1987

Hirschfeld RM, Klerman GL, Chodoff P, et al: Dependency—self-esteem—clinical depression. J Am Acad Psychoanal 41:610–618, 1976

Hyler S, Lyons M: Factor analysis of the DSM-III personality disorder clusters: a replication. Compr Psychiatry 29:304–308, 1988

Jacobsberg L, Hymowitz P, Barasch A, et al: Symptoms of schizotypal personality disorder. Am J Psychiatry 143:1222–1227, 1986

Kaplan M: A woman's view of DSM-III. Am Psychol 38:786–792, 1983

Kass F: Self-defeating personality disorder: an empirical study. Journal of Personality Disorders 1:168–173, 1987

Kass F, Skodol A, Charles E, et al: Scaled ratings of DSM-III personality disorders. Am J Psychiatry 142:627–630, 1985

Kass F, MacKinnon R, Spitzer R: Masochistic personality: an empirical study. Am J Psychiatry 143:216–218, 1986

Kernberg O: Severe Personality Disorders. New Haven, CT, Yale University Press, 1984

Livesley WJ (ed): The DSM-IV Personality Disorders. New York, Guilford, 1995

Livesley W, Reiffer L, Sheldon A, et al: Prototypicality ratings of DSM-III criteria for personality disorders. J Nerv Ment Dis 175:395–401, 1987

Livesley WJ, Schroeder ML, Jackson DN: Dependent personality disorder and attachment problems. Journal of Personality Disorders 4:232–240, 1990

Loranger AW, Susman VL, Oldham JM, et al: The personality disorders examination: a preliminary report. Journal of Personality Disorders 1:1–13, 1987

Malow R, Donnelly J: Diagnostic efficiency statistics for borderline personality disorder. Unpublished raw data, New Orleans, LA, Veterans Administration Medical Center, 1988

McGlashan T, Fenton W: Diagnostic efficiency of DSM-III borderline personality disorder and schizotypal disorder, in Axis II: New Perspectives on Validity. Symposium conducted by the 141st annual meeting of the American Psychiatric Association, Montreal, Canada, May 1988

Michaels R: First rebuttal. Am J Psychiatry 141:548–551, 1984

Millon T: Disorders of Personality. DSM-III: Axis II. New York, Wiley, 1981

Millon T, Tringone R: Co-occurrence and diagnostic efficiency statistics. Unpublished raw data, Miami, FL, University of Miami, 1989

Modestin J: Quality of interpersonal relationships: the most characteristic DSM-III BPD criterion. Compr Psychiatry 28:397–402, 1987

Morey L: Personality disorders in DSM-III and DSM-III-R: convergence, coverage, and internal consistency. Am J Psychiatry 145:573–577, 1988

Morey L, Goodman R: Diagnostic efficiency statistics. Unpublished raw data, Nashville, TN, Vanderbilt University, 1989

Morey L, Heumann K: Co-occurrence and diagnostic efficiency statistics. Unpublished raw data, Nashville, TN, Vanderbilt University, 1988

Morey LC, Waugh MH, Blashfield RK: MMPI scales for DSM-III personality disorders: their derivation and correlates. J Pers Assess 49:245–251, 1985

Nurnberg H, Feldman A, Hurt S, et al: Core criteria for diagnosing borderline patients. Hillside Journal of Clinical Psychiatry 8:111–131, 1986

Perry C: Challenges in validating personality disorders: beyond description. Journal of Personality Disorders 4:273–289, 1990

Perry J, O'Connell M, Drake R: An assessment of the schedule for schizotypal personalities and the DSM-III criteria for diagnosing schizotypal personality disorder. J Nerv Ment Dis 172:674–680, 1984

Pfohl B, Blum N: Internal consistency statistics for the DSM-III-R personality disorder criteria. Unpublished raw data, Iowa City, University of Iowa, 1990

Pfohl B, Coryell W, Zimmerman M, et al: DSM-III personality disorders: diagnostic overlap and internal consistency of individual DSM-III criteria. Compr Psychiatry 27:21–34, 1986

Plakun E: Distinguishing narcissistic and borderline personality disorders using DSM-III criteria. Compr Psychiatry 28:437–443, 1987

Reich J: Diagnostic efficiency statistics for personality disorders. Unpublished raw data, Brockton, MA, Brockton VA Medical Center, 1988

Ronningstam E, Gunderson J: Narcissistic traits in psychiatric patients. Compr Psychiatry 29:545–549, 1988

Silverman JM, Pinkham L, Horvath TB, et al: Affective and impulsive personality disorder traits in the relatives of patients with borderline personality disorder. Am J Psychiatry 148:1378–1385, 1991

Skodol A: Co-occurrence and diagnostic efficiency statistics. Unpublished raw data, New York, New York State Psychiatric Institute, 1989

Skodol A, Rosnick L, Kellman D, et al: Validating structured DSM-III-R personality disorder assessments with longitudinal data. Am J Psychiatry 145:1297–1299, 1988

Spitzer R, Endicott J, Gibbon M: Crossing the border into borderline personality and borderline schizophrenia. Arch Gen Psychiatry 36:17–24, 1979

Spitzer R, Williams J, Kass F, et al: National field trial of the DSM-III-R diagnostic criteria for self-defeating personality disorder. Am J Psychiatry 146:1561–1567, 1989

Standage K, Ladha N: An examination of the reliability of the PDE and a comparison with other methods of identifying personality disorders in a clinical sample. Journal of Personality Disorders 2:267–271, 1988

Sternbach S, Judd A, Sabo A, et al: Cognitive and perceptual distortions in borderline personality disorder and schizotypal personality disorder in a vignette sample. Compr Psychiatry 33:186–189, 1992

Widiger T: DSM-IV and personality disorders: introduction to special series. Journal of Personality Disorders 5:122–134, 1991

Widiger T, Frances A: The DSM-III personality disorders: perspectives from psychology. Arch Gen Psychiatry 42:615–623, 1985

Widiger T, Frances A, Warner L, et al: Diagnostic criteria for the borderline and schizotypal personality disorders. J Abnorm Psychol 95:43–51, 1986

Widiger TA, Trull TJ, Hurt SW, et al: A multidimensional scaling of the DSM-III personality disorders. Arch Gen Psychiatry 44:557–563, 1987

Widiger T, Frances A, Spitzer R, et al: The DSM-III personality disorders: an overview. Am J Psychiatry 145:786–795, 1988

World Health Organization: ICD-10 Chapter V: Mental and Behavioral Disorders: Diagnostic Criteria for Research. Geneva, Switzerland, World Health Organization, 1990

Zanarini MC, Frankenburg FR, Chauncey DL, et al: The diagnostic interview for personality disorders: interrater and test-retest reliability. Compr Psychiatry 28:467–480, 1987

Zanarini MC, Frankenburg F, Chauncey D, et al: Co-occurrence and diagnostic efficiency statistics. Unpublished raw data, Boston, MA, McLean Hospital, 1989

Zimmerman M: Why are we rushing to publish DSM-IV? Arch Gen Psychiatry 45:1135–1138, 1988

Zimmerman M, Coryell WH: DSM-III personality disorder dimensions. J Nerv Ment Dis 178:686–692, 1990

Chapter 22

Paranoid Personality Disorder

David P. Bernstein, Ph.D., David Useda, B.A., and
Larry J. Siever, M.D.

Introduction

Since the time of Kraepelin (1921), the defining feature of paranoid personality disorder (PPD) has been considered to be a pervasive and unwarranted mistrust of others. Other clinical characteristics that have figured prominently in the descriptive literature on this disorder are the paranoid individual's hypersensitivity to criticism (Cameron 1943, 1963; Kretschmer 1925), antagonism and aggressiveness (Schneider 1923; Sheldon 1940; Sheldon and Stevens 1942), rigidity (Shapiro 1965), hypervigilance (Cameron 1963; Shapiro 1965), and excessive need for autonomy (Millon 1969, 1981). This body of clinical literature formed the basis of the diagnostic criteria for PPD that were incorporated in DSM-III (American Psychiatric Association 1980). DSM-III required that patients meet three criteria for suspiciousness, two for hypersensitivity, and two for restricted affectivity to receive a diagnosis of PPD. In DSM-III-R (American Psychiatric Association 1987), the grouping of diagnostic criteria into sets was replaced by a truly polythetic system in which no single feature (or group of features) was required, and any combination of four of seven criteria was sufficient for a PPD diagnosis.

In this chapter, some of the major nosological issues concerning PPD are discussed in the light of current research findings. Particular emphasis is placed on research pertaining to the development of diagnostic criteria for PPD in DSM-IV.

Statement and Significance of the Issues

A central issue regarding PPD is its status as a possible "schizophrenia spectrum" disorder. Kraepelin (1921) observed that premorbid "paranoid personalities" were often present in individuals who later developed paranoid psychoses, including dementia praecox. Subsequent writers also considered premorbid traits such as suspiciousness and hostility to be predisposing factors in the emergence of later delusional illness, particularly in the "late paraphrenias" of old age (Herbert and Jacobson 1967). Historically, then, PPD has been thought of by some authors as a possible precursor of other more severe paranoid conditions. More recent speculations based on the current diagnostic nomenclature have concerned the position of PPD on a hypothetical "schizophrenia spectrum" (Siever and Davis 1991) that includes DSM-III-R Axis I schizophrenia and Axis II schizoid personality disorder and schizotypal personality disorder (STPD).

The conceptualization of PPD as a possible schizophrenia spectrum disorder raises issues concerning syndromal boundaries: 1) What is the relationship between PPD and STPD, an Axis II disorder with which PPD shares certain diagnostic features such as suspiciousness? The high rate of diagnostic overlap between these disorders raises questions about their discriminant validity and suggests the possibility of subsuming PPD within a broadly redefined schizotypal category. 2) What is the relationship between PPD and Axis I delusional disorder? The differential diagnosis between PPD and delusional disorder rests on the absence of systematized delusions in the former, yet "true" delusions are sometimes difficult to distinguish from the cognitive distortions of patients with PPD, and delusional beliefs may appear in individuals with long-standing paranoid personality traits. These findings raise the possibility of a spectrum that encompasses both PPD and delusional disorder, and that is distinct from or only partially overlapping with the schizophrenia-related disorders.

An additional set of issues concerns the development of the DSM-IV diagnostic criteria for PPD. 3) Which of the DSM-III-R PPD criteria are candidates for modification or elimination in DSM-IV, as indicated by their diagnostic efficiency (e.g., sensitivity and specificity)? 4) To what extent can North American approaches to the definition of the disorder (i.e., DSM-III-R) be made compatible with other diagnostic systems, particularly the World Health Organization's upcoming ICD-10 (World Health Organization 1990)? Increasing compatibility between the two systems would have the desirable effect of facilitating international communication and collaboration regarding both research and clinical practice.

The resolution of these nosological issues will require studies employing diagnostic validators, such as phenomenology, family history, laboratory findings, and treatment response; however, research on the validation of PPD has been limited. This report therefore attempts to reach some preliminary conclusions based on the empirical studies that have been conducted to date.

Methods

These issues were addressed with a computer-assisted search of the published literature on PPD, supplemented by a review of unpublished data sets made available to the DSM-IV Work Group on Personality Disorders. This review process was not intended to be exhaustive but rather to focus on issues germane to the refinement of the PPD diagnostic criteria.

Results

Epidemiology

Paranoid ideation has long been reported to be especially prevalent among groups such as prisoners (Faergeman 1963; Slater and Roth 1969), refugees and immigrants (Eitinger 1959; Mezey 1960), the elderly (Christenson and Blazer 1984; Fish 1960; Post 1966; Roth 1955), and the hearing impaired (Kay and Roth 1961). However, the extent to which these groups are truly at risk for PPD is uncertain, because the variable methodologies and diagnostic criteria employed in these studies, most of which were conducted before DSM-III, make their findings difficult to evaluate. Furthermore, many of these studies failed to distinguish paranoid personality traits, which may accompany a variety of psychiatric or physical conditions, from PPD or to determine whether PPD was primary or secondary to organic causes (e.g., as in hearing impairment).

Most clinically based studies have reported a preponderance of PPD in males (Alnaes and Torgersen 1988a; Reich 1987), although the sex distribution of PPD in the general population has not been established. Whereas overall prevalences of PPD in clinically based studies have varied widely (Table 22–1), it appears that the extensive revision of the PPD diagnostic criteria in DSM-III-R has resulted in an increased diagnostic prevalence of this disorder compared with DSM-III. Prevalences of PPD in 11 studies employing DSM-III criteria ranged from less than 1% to 20%, with a median prevalence of 5.5% (Alnaes and Torgerson 1988a, 1988b; Clarkin et al. 1983; Dahl 1986; Kass et al. 1985; Khantzian and Treece 1985; Koenigsberg et al. 1985; Mellsop et al. 1982; Pfohl et al. 1986; Reich 1987; Widiger et al. 1986; Zanarini 1989), whereas in the four studies using DSM-III-R criteria, prevalences of PPD ranged from 1% to 30%, with a median prevalence of 18% (Freiman and Widiger 1989; Millon and Tringone 1989; Morey and Heumann 1988; Skodol et al. 1988). The prevalence of PPD in the general population is unknown, although one epidemiological study has estimated it to be 3.3% in young adults ages 18–21 (Bernstein et al. 1993), an estimate that is slightly higher than that obtained in four published studies of adult nonpsychiatric control subjects (range, 0.5%–2.3%; median prevalence, 1.4%) (Baron et al. 1985; Coryell and Zimmerman 1989; Drake and Valliant 1985; Kendler and Gruenberg 1982).

Table 22–1. Comorbidity among Axis II disorders in six clinical studies

	SZPD	STPD	HPD	NPD	BPD	ASPD	AVPD	DPD	OCPD	PAPD	SDPD	SAD
Percentage with PPD receiving indicated diagnosis												
Widiger et al. 1986	18	71	23	2	41	29	18	12	0	53	—	—
Morey 1988	23	25	28	36	48	8	48	30	8	17	—	—
Skodol et al. 1988[a]	0	43	14	57	93	14	86	57	50	29	43	—
Zanarini 1989	0	50	56	38	100	13	56	31	19	50	—	—
Millon and Tringone 1989[b]	8	17	8	75	0	25	8	0	33	17	0	0
Freiman and Widiger 1989	33	33	27	47	53	33	60	27	0	40	13	27
Percentage with indicated diagnosis receiving PPD												
Widiger et al. 1986	43	25	10	22	13	16	11	5	0	20	—	—
Morey 1988	47	59	29	36	32	28	39	29	22	3	—	—
Skodol et al. 1988[a]	0	38	12	38	21	25	31	24	33	67	30	—
Zanarini 1989	0	10	8	13	9	2	17	7	17	14	—	—
Millon and Tringone 1989[b]	0	12	1	4	3	0	0	0	0	1	0	6
Freiman and Widiger 1989	62	46	44	64	47	36	47	33	0	75	50	44

Note. SZPD = schizoid personality disorder. STPD = schizotypal personality disorder. HPD = histrionic personality disorder. NPD = narcissistic personality disorder. BPD = borderline personality disorder. ASPD = antisocial personality disorder. AVPD = avoidant personality disorder. DPD = dependent personality disorder. OCPD = obsessive-compulsive personality disorder. PAPD = passive-aggressive personality disorder. SDPD = self-defeating personality disorder. SAD = sadistic personality disorder.

[a]Prevalence of STPD in this table based on the Personality Disorder Examination (PDE). Skodol et al. (1988) also reported prevalences based on other diagnostic instruments.

[b]Prevalence of STPD in this table based on the Millon Clinical Multiaxial Inventory (MCMI). Millon and Tringone (1989) also reported prevalences based on other diagnostic instruments.

Criteria Performance

Only a handful of studies have systematically examined the diagnostic efficiency of the clinical features of PPD, by DSM-III or DSM-III-R diagnostic criteria. Two studies (Livesley 1986; Zanarini 1989) have called into question the diagnostic efficiency of the DSM-III PPD features grouped under the heading "restricted affectivity" (appears cold and unemotional, presents himself or herself as objective and rational, lacks a sense of humor, and absence of tender feelings towards others). These criteria have been eliminated in the revised edition of DSM-III.

Most of the DSM-III-R PPD diagnostic criteria have exhibited satisfactory sensitivity and specificity in the few clinical studies that have examined their diagnostic efficiency (Freiman and Widiger 1989; Millon and Tringone 1989; Morey and Heumann 1988). However, PPD criterion 6, "is easily slighted," was found to be the least specific of any in the paranoid criteria set (range, .62–.64; median, .63), whereas another PPD feature, "questions the fidelity of spouse or sexual partner" (criterion 7), exhibited poor sensitivity in two of the three studies surveyed (range, .17–.60; median, .38). Although the diagnostic efficiency of PPD criteria 6 and 7 is sufficient to warrant their continued inclusion in the PPD criteria set, these criteria may be candidates for modification in DSM-IV.

Comparison of DSM-III-R and ICD-10 Diagnostic Criteria

The DSM-III-R criteria set for PPD was found to only partially overlap with the proposed PPD items in the ICD-10, based on a meeting between American Psychiatric Association and World Health Organization representatives (Michael First, M.D., personal communication). Corresponding ICD-10 items were found for DSM-III-R criteria 4 (ICD-10 item 3), 5 (ICD-10 item 2), 6 (ICD-10 item 3), and 7 (ICD-10 item 5), but not for DSM-III-R criteria 1, 2, or 3. Four additional items were included in the ICD-10 criteria set that were unrepresented in DSM-III-R: ICD-10 items 1 (excessive sensitiveness to setbacks and rebuffs), 4 (a combative and tenacious sense of personal rights out of keeping with the actual situation), 6 (a tendency to experience excessive self-importance, manifest in a persistent self-referential attitude), and 7 (preoccupation with unsubstantiated conspiratorial explanations of events around the subject or in the world at large). At this time, there are no empirical data that might help resolve these discrepancies.

Comorbidity

Fewer than 25% of PPD patients in clinically based samples are free of other personality disorder diagnoses (Millon and Tringone 1989; Zanarini 1989). Table 22–1 presents rates of overlap between PPD and other Axis II disorders reported in six clinically based studies. Rates of overlap with specific Axis II disorders varied considerably across the studies. For example, the percentage of patients with PPD receiving comorbid diagnoses of STPD ranged from 17% (Millon and Tringone 1989) to 71% (Widiger et al. 1986) in the six studies surveyed. In most of the studies, however, PPD overlapped extensively with STPD, with which it shares diagnostic criteria for paranoid ideation. PPD also exhibited high rates of overlap with several other Axis II disorders, particularly narcissistic, borderline, avoidant, and passive-aggressive personality disorders.

Few studies with DSM-III or DSM-III-R criteria have reported rates of diagnostic overlap between PPD and Axis I disorders. In a study of 298 psychiatric outpatients, Alnaes and Torgersen (1988b) found that patients with PPD were 3.5 times more likely to receive a DSM-III Axis I diagnosis of agoraphobia without panic than would be expected on the basis of the prevalence of this disorder in the total sample. No other Axis I diagnosis was significantly associated with PPD. Coryell and Zimmerman (1989) examined the relationship between DSM-III Axis I and Axis II disorders in a combined sample of 797 relatives of psychiatric and nonpsychiatric control probands. Compared with relatives without personality disorder diagnoses, those with PPD were at significantly increased lifetime risk for Axis I diagnoses of alcohol and drug abuse/dependence, schizophrenia, obsessive-compulsive disorder, phobic disorder, and bulimia, and for history of attempted suicide. However, compared with relatives with other personality disorders, those with PPD were at greater risk only for Axis I diagnoses of bulimia.

Family/Genetic Studies

Studies reporting on the familial aggregation of PPD in the relatives of schizophrenic probands have produced mixed results. Although PPD appears to be slightly more prevalent in the relatives of schizophrenics than in the family members of control subjects, statistically significant findings have been reported in only two (Baron et al. 1985; Kendler and Gruenberg 1982) of five published studies (Baron et al. 1985; Coryell and Zimmerman 1989; Kendler and Gruenberg 1982; Kendler et al. 1985; Stephens et al. 1975).

There is some evidence that PPD may share a stronger familial relationship with Axis I delusional disorder than with schizophrenia. Kendler et al. (1985) reported a morbid risk of PPD that was significantly greater in the first-degree relatives of probands with delusional disorder (4.8%) compared with both the relatives of schizophrenics (0.8%) and medical control subjects (0%). Furthermore, there is some evidence that schizophrenia and delusional disorder do not share a substantial genetic basis. For example, Kendler and Hays (1981) found that cases of schizophrenia were significantly less common in the first- and second-degree relatives of probands with delusional disorder (0.6%) than in the relatives of schizophrenic probands (3.8%). Thus, PPD and delusional disorder may share a genetic basis with each other that is stronger than or distinct from the one they share with schizophrenia. In contrast, schizophrenia may share a genetic basis with Axis II schizotypal personality disorder, because an excess of relatives with STPD has been found in many (Baron et al. 1985; Siever et al. 1990) but not all (Coryell and Zimmerman 1989) studies in which schizophrenic patients have served as probands.

Discussion

Evidence from phenomenological studies offers some tentative support for the diagnostic validity of PPD and does not appear to warrant subsuming PPD within a broadly redefined schizotypal diagnostic category. Whereas PPD and STPD exhibit a high rate of overlap in clinically based studies, a substantial proportion of paranoid patients do not qualify for a schizotypal diagnosis. Furthermore, patients with PPD frequently share the clinical characteristics of several other Axis II disorders, particularly narcissistic, borderline, avoidant, and passive-aggressive personality disorders. Phenomenologically, PPD appears to be a heterogeneous diagnostic category whose members may share none, some, or many schizotypal diagnostic features.

Family/genetic studies have also supported the discriminant validity of PPD. Whereas research has largely supported the hypothesis of STPD as a schizophrenia spectrum disorder, findings regarding the relationship between PPD and schizophrenia have been less consistent. There is also evidence that PPD and Axis I delusional disorder may share a genetic basis with each other that is more substantial than the one they share with schizophrenia. However, at this early stage of family/genetic research, it would be premature to characterize PPD as either a schizophrenia spectrum or a delusional spectrum disorder.

Although few studies have assessed the diagnostic efficiency of the DSM-III or DSM-III-R criteria for PPD, it appears that criterion 6 ("is easily slighted and is quick to react with anger or to counterattack") may warrant modification to increase its diagnostic specificity, and criterion 7 ("questions, without justification, fidelity of spouse or sexual partner") may need alteration to increase its sensitivity.

It appears that there are substantial differences between the PPD criteria included in the DSM-III-R and those proposed for ICD-10. However, empirical studies comparing these criteria sets are needed before these discrepancies can be resolved.

Recommendations

Slight changes are recommended in PPD criteria 6 and 7. It is suggested that criterion 6 be modified to read, "*Perceives attacks on his or her character or reputation that are not apparent to others* and is quick to react with anger or to counterattack (altered text is italic). This modification indicates that the defensive outbursts of paranoid individuals are a response to perceived attacks, providing greater differentiation from similar reactions based on wounded self-esteem (e.g., as in dependent and avoidant personality disorders) or impulsivity and/or affective lability (e.g., as in borderline and histrionic personality disorder). Criterion 7 has been modified as follows: "*Recurrent suspicions, without justification, regarding* fidelity of spouse or sexual partner." This proposed modification emphasizes the intensity and pervasiveness of the paranoid individual's pathological jealousy with the aim of increasing the item's sensitivity.

It is also recommended that the "stem" for the seven PPD inclusion criteria be changed as follows: "A. A pervasive *distrust and suspiciousness of others such that their motives are interpreted as malevolent,* beginning by early adulthood and present in a variety of contexts, as indicated by at least four of the following." This proposed modification emphasizes the fact that suspiciousness and mistrust of others are the central defining features of the PPD syndrome.

While it is premature to propose substantial changes in the DSM-III-R or ICD-10 criteria sets in order to increase their compatibility, the following slight modification of DSM-III-R criterion 5 is recommended to increase compatibility with ICD-10 item 2: "*tendency to* bear grudges *persistently, i.e., to be* unforgiving of insults, *injuries,* or slights."

References

Alnaes R, Torgersen S: DSM-III symptom disorder (Axis I) and personality disorders (Axis II) in an outpatient population. Acta Psychiatr Scand 78:348–355, 1988a

Alnaes R, Torgersen S: The relationship between DSM-III symptom disorders (Axis I) and personality disorders (Axis II) in an outpatient population. Acta Psychiatr Scand 78:485–492, 1988b

American Psychiatric Association: Diagnostic and Statistical Manual of Mental Disorders, 3rd Edition. Washington, DC, American Psychiatric Association, 1980

American Psychiatric Association: Diagnostic and Statistical Manual of Mental Disorders, 3rd Edition, Revised. Washington, DC, American Psychiatric Association, 1987

Baron M, Gruen R, Rainer JD, et al: A family study of schizophrenic and normal control probands: implications for the spectrum concept of schizophrenia. Am J Psychiatry 142:447–454, 1985

Bernstein DP, Cohen P, Velez CN, et al: The prevalence and stability of the DSM-III-R personality disorders in a community-based survey of adolescents. Am J Psychiatry 150:1237–1243, 1993

Cameron N: The paranoid pseudo-community. American Journal of Sociology 49:32–38, 1943

Cameron N: Personality Development and Psychopathology. Boston, MA, Houghton Mifflin, 1963

Christenson R, Blazer D: Epidemiology of persecutory ideation in an elderly population in the community. Am J Psychiatry 141:1088–1091, 1984

Clarkin JF, Widiger TA, Frances A, et al: Prototypic typology and the borderline personality disorder. J Abnorm Psychol 92:263–273, 1983

Coryell WH, Zimmerman M: Personality disorder in the families of depressed, schizophrenic, and never-ill probands. Am J Psychiatry 146:496–502, 1989

Dahl A: Some aspects of the DSM-III personality disorders illustrated by a consecutive sample of hospitalized patients. Acta Psychiatr Scand Suppl. 328:61–67, 1986

Drake R, Valliant G: A validity study of Axis II of DSM-III. Am J Psychiatry 142:553–558, 1985

Eitinger L: The incidence of mental disease among refugees in Norway. J Ment Sci 105:326–338, 1959

Faergeman P: Psychogenic Psychoses. London, Butterworths, 1963

Fish F: Senile schizophrenia. J Ment Sci 106:938–946, 1960

Freiman K, Widiger T: Co-occurrence and diagnostic efficiency statistics. Unpublished raw data, Lexington, University of Kentucky, 1989

Herbert ME, Jacobson S: Late paraphrenia. Br J Psychiatry 113:461–469, 1967

Kass F, Skodol AE, Charles E, et al: Scaled ratings of DSM-III personality disorders. Am J Psychiatry 142:627–630, 1985

Kay DWK, Roth M: Environmental and hereditary factors in the schizophrenias of old age ("late paraphrenia") and their bearing on the general problem of causation in schizophrenia. J Ment Sci 107:649–686, 1961

Kendler KS, Gruenberg AM: Genetic relationship between paranoid personality disorder and the "schizophrenic spectrum" disorders. Am J Psychiatry 139:1185–1186, 1982

Kendler KS, Hays P: Paranoid psychosis (delusional disorder) and schizophrenia: a family history study. Arch Gen Psychiatry 38:547–551, 1981

Kendler KS, Masterson CC, Davis KL: Psychiatric illness in first-degree relatives of patients with paranoid psychosis, schizophrenia and medical illness. Br J Psychiatry 147:524–531, 1985

Khantzian EJ, Treece C: DSM-III psychiatric diagnosis of narcotic addicts: recent findings. Arch Gen Psychiatry 42:1067–1071, 1985

Koenigsberg HW, Kaplan RD, Gilmore MM, et al: The relationship between syndrome and personality disorder in DSM-III: experience with 2,462 patients. Am J Psychiatry 142:207–212, 1985

Kraepelin E: Manic-Depressive Insanity and Paranoia. Edinburgh, UK, Livingstone, 1921

Kretschmer E: Korperbau und Charakter. Berlin, Springer-Verlag, 1925. Physique and character (English translation). London, Kegan Paul, 1926

Livesley WJ: Trait and behavioral prototypes of personality disorder. Am J Psychiatry 143:728–732, 1986

Mellsop G, Varghese F, Joshua S, et al: The reliability of Axis II of DSM-III. Am J Psychiatry 139:1360–1361, 1982

Mezey A: Personal background, emigration and mental disorder in Hungarian refugees. J Ment Sci 106:618–627, 1960

Millon T: Modern Psychopathology: A Biosocial Approach to Maladaptive Learning and Functioning. Philadelphia, PA, WB Saunders, 1969

Millon T: Disorders of Personality: DSM-III Axis II. New York, Wiley, 1981

Millon T, Tringone R: Co-occurrence and diagnostic efficiency statistics. Unpublished raw data, Miami, FL, University of Miami, 1989

Morey L: Personality disorders in DSM-III and DSM-III-R: convergence, coverage, and internal consistency. Am J Psychiatry 145:573–577, 1988

Morey L, Heumann K: Co-occurrence and diagnostic efficiency statistics. Unpublished raw data, Nashville, TN, Vanderbilt University, 1988

Pfohl B, Coryell W, Zimmerman M, et al: DSM-III personality disorders: diagnostic overlap and internal consistency of individual DSM-III criteria. Compr Psychiatry 27:21–34, 1986

Post F: Persistent Persecutory States of the Elderly. Oxford, UK, Pergamon, 1966

Reich J: Sex distribution of DSM-III personality disorders in psychiatric outpatients. Am J Psychiatry 144:485–488, 1987

Roth M: The natural history of mental disorder in old age. J Ment Sci 101:281–301, 1955

Schneider K: Die psychopathischen Personlichkeiten. Vienna, Deuticke, 1923

Shapiro D: Neurotic Styles. New York, Basic Books, 1965

Sheldon WH: The Varieties of Human Physique: An Introduction to Constitutional Psychology. New York, Harper, 1940

Sheldon WH, Stevens SS: The Varieties of Temperament: A Psychology of Constitutional Differences. New York, Harper, 1942

Siever LJ, Davis K: A psychobiologic perspective on the personality disorders. Am J Psychiatry, 148:1647–1658, 1991

Siever LJ, Silverman JM, Horvath TB, et al: Increased morbid risk for schizophrenic-related disorders in relatives of schizotypal personality disordered patients. Arch Gen Psychiatry 47:634–640, 1990

Skodol AE, Rosnick L, Kellman D, et al: Validating structured DSM-III-R personality disorder assessments with longitudinal data. Am J Psychiatry 145:1297–1299, 1988

Slater E, Roth M: Clinical Psychiatry. Baltimore, MD, Williams & Wilkins, 1969

Stephens DA, Atkinson MW, Kay DWK, et al: Psychiatric morbidity in parents and sibs of schizophrenics and non-schizophrenics. Br J Psychiatry 127:97–108, 1975

Widiger TA, Frances A, Warner L, et al: Diagnostic criteria for the borderline and schizotypal personality disorders. J Abnorm Psychol 95:43–51, 1986

World Health Organization: ICD-10 Chapter V: Mental and Behavioral Disorders: Diagnostic Criteria for Research. Geneva, Switzerland, World Health Organization, 1990

Zanarini M: Co-occurrence and diagnostic efficiency statistics. Unpublished raw data, Boston, MA, McLean Hospital, 1989

Chapter 23

Schizoid Personality Disorder

Oren Kalus, M.D., David P. Bernstein, Ph.D., and
Larry J. Siever, M.D.

Introduction

Schizoid personality disorder (SZPD) is distinguished from the other DSM-III-R (American Psychiatric Association 1987) "odd cluster" personality disorders, schizotypal personality disorder (STPD) and paranoid personality disorder (PPD), chiefly by the prominence of social, interpersonal, and affective deficits (i.e., negative symptoms) and the absence of psychotic-like positive symptoms.

DSM-III (American Psychiatric Association 1980) attempted to sharpen the boundaries of this historically heterogeneous disorder by the addition of STPD and PPD within the odd cluster and the addition of avoidant personality disorder (AVPD) within the "anxious cluster." Evidence of extensive criteria overlap, as well as comorbidity, with these personality disorders raises serious concerns about the boundaries and separateness of the SZPD diagnosis, however. Whereas modifications of the SZPD diagnostic criteria in DSM-III-R appear to have increased the prevalence of the diagnosis, the scarcity of empirical data on either DSM-III or DSM-III-R SZPD remains a significantly limiting factor.

Statement and Significance of the Issues

There are several key issues in resolving the nosological status of SZPD.

First, the extent of SZPD's overlap with and separation from other personality disorders, particularly STPD and AVPD. This concern arises from evidence that a number of the key features of SZPD, such as social isolation, pursuit of solitary activities, absence of intimate relationships, and restricted affectivity, may be shared with STPD and PPD. Extensive comorbidity between SZPD, STPD, PPD, and AVPD raises the possibility that SZPD may have been annexed by these other disorders.

The distinction between SZPD and AVPD is also problematic, given the extensive overlap between these presumably mutually exclusive diagnoses. While both share the features of prominent social isolation, they are also theoretically distinguishable by the avoidant individual's intimacy needs and rejection sensitivity. That distinction may not be as clear-cut in the clinical setting as prominent concerns about intimacy such as ambivalence and fear of engulfment, which may also characterize SZPD (Akhtar 1987). In addition, social anxiety (Overholser 1989) may also be involved in SZPD's social isolation. Finally, SZPD has rarely been diagnosed using DSM-III criteria. Although the prevalence of SZPD appears to have increased using DSM-III-R criteria, its low prevalence casts additional doubt on whether it remains a valid diagnosis. Taken together, these concerns raise the question of whether SZPD should be retained or deleted as a separate diagnosis in DSM-IV.

Second, the similarities between SZPD and the residual and prodromal phases of schizophrenia suggest that some schizophrenic patients may have been misdiagnosed as SZPD. A related issue is the extent to which SZPD is genetically and familially related along a continuum to schizophrenia. Although STPD has specifically been singled out as having a genetic/familial relation to schizophrenia, this has not been adequately addressed with respect to SZPD. The evidence supporting genetic transmission of negative rather than positive symptoms in schizophrenia, and the prominence of negative symptoms in SZPD suggests a possible link between schizophrenia and SZPD (Gunderson et al. 1983).

Several features reported by Akiskal (1987) to describe chronically dysthymic individuals (i.e., introversion, anhedonia, and psychomotor inertia) bear a resemblance to SZPD, raising the issue of an additional overlap and/or comorbidity with the affective disorders.

Third, a number of the proposed revisions to the schizoid criteria were motivated in part by a desire to increase compatibility with the World Health Organization's ICD-10 (World Health Organization 1990) because increased compatibility would facilitate international clinical and research efforts.

Methods

A literature search was conducted that focused on 1) review articles describing historical (pre-DSM-III) and clinical information on SZPD that might cast light on some of the diagnostic questions for DSM-IV and 2) more recent (post-DSM-III and -DSM-III-R) empirical, clinical, and prevalence studies of SZPD with a Medline search that addressed the issue of clinical overlap and possible annexation of SZPD by AVPD and STPD. Finally, recent unpublished data sets on personality disorder criterion performance and prevalence assembled by the DSM-IV Personality Disorders Work Group were studied for information on the diagnostic efficiency of DSM-III and DSM-III-R SZPD criteria and implications for criteria modifications in DSM-IV.

Results

Historical/Clinical Literature

The term *schizoid* was originated by Bleuler (1924) to describe a tendency to turn inward, the absence of emotional expressiveness, and simultaneous contradictory dullness and sensitivity. Although most historical descriptions of SZPD appear consistent with DSM-III-R criteria, there are some discrepancies. Kretschmer (1926) posited the simultaneous presence of "hyperesthetic and anaesthetic" qualities, that contrasted overt insensitivity with inner hypersensitivity. That DSM-III separated these contrasting behaviors into the SZPD and AVPD categories may not be entirely justified. Thus the apparent interpersonal indifference and emotional detachment in schizoid personality disorder may mask a marked inner sensitivity (Heston 1970; Wolff and Chick 1980), highlighting the problem of inferring subjective experience from a purely "objective" descriptive manifestation.

Observations by Terry and Rennie (1938) and others of deviant sexuality in the individual with SZPD (e.g., compulsive masturbation and perverse sexuality), although consistent with the DSM-III criteria of absent heterosexual relationships, are not consistent with the absence of sexual desire. Other clinical features either not reported or de-emphasized in DSM-III include autistic thinking, fragmented self-identity, disembodiment, and symptoms of derealization/depersonalization (Guntrip 1969).

Several revisions of the DSM-III criteria in DSM-III-R appear to have improved on these limitations, including expanding the number of criteria from three to seven and providing a richer and potentially more sensitive description (Akhtar 1987). The use of a polythetic system that does not require any one single feature added further flexibility and may increase the sensitivity of the diagnosis.

Prevalence

Estimates of the prevalence of SZPD in the general population based on community survey (Reich et al. 1989), nonpsychiatric control subjects (Drake and Valliant 1985), and relatives of psychiatric patients (Zimmerman and Coryell 1990) have ranged from 0.5% to 7%. In a longitudinal epidemiological study of adolescents and children, using DSM-III-R criteria, Bernstein (1990), reported prevalence rates

Table 23–1.   Prevalence of DSM-III and DSM-III-R schizoid personality disorder in
                  14 clinical studies

Study	N	Diagnostic nomenclature	Type of sample	Prevalence n	%
Mellsop et al. 1982	77	DSM-III	Inpatient	8	10
Clarkin et al. 1983	76	DSM-III	Outpatient	6	8
Kass et al. 1985	609	DSM-III	Outpatient	30	5
Khantzian and Treece 1985	87	DSM-III	Outpatient	2	2
Koenigsberg et al. 1985	2,462	DSM-III	Mixed	11	1
Dahl 1986	103	DSM-III	Inpatient	1	1
Pfohl et al. 1986	131	DSM-III	Outpatient	1	1
Widiger et al. 1986	84	DSM-III	Inpatient	17	20
Reich 1987	170	DSM-III	Outpatient	11	6
Morey 1988	291	DSM-III-R	Mixed	64	22
Skodol et al. 1988	97	DSM-III-R	Inpatient	14	14
Alnaes and Torgerson 1988b	298	DSM-III	Outpatient	15	5
Zanarini et al. 1989	253	DSM-III	Mixed	16	6
Millon and Tringone 1989	809	DSM-III-R	Mixed	12	1
Freiman and Widiger 1989	50	DSM-III-R	Inpatient	15	30

of 1.7% for SZPD, 1.2% for STPD, and 4.1% for PPD.

Considerable variation in the prevalence rates in clinical settings is apparent,
although studies using DSM-III-R criteria generally report higher prevalence rates
than those using DSM-III criteria (Table 23–1). Morey (1988), for example, compared DSM-III with DSM-III-R SZPD diagnoses in the same group of 291 personality disorder patients and reported a substantially higher prevalence of the
diagnosis using DSM-III-R criteria (1.4% versus 11.0%). For studies using DSM-III
criteria, prevalence rates ranged from 0% to 5%, with a median of 1%, whereas in
those using DSM-III-R criteria, the rates ranged from 1% to 16%, with a median
of 8.5%.

Criteria Performance

In three studies examining the performance of the DSM-III-R criteria for SZPD
(Freiman and Widiger 1989 [N = 8]; Millon and Tringone 1989 [N = 26]; Morey

and Heumann 1988 [*N* = 32]), results were divergent, but some trends were apparent. Of the three SZPD criteria reflecting impaired capacity for interpersonal relationships, only criterion 1 (neither desires nor enjoys close relationships) demonstrated high sensitivity and specificity and was considered prototypical by clinicians. Criterion 2 (prefers solitary activities) had high sensitivity and was judged to be prototypical but had moderate sensitivity. Although criterion 6 (no close friends) also demonstrated high sensitivity, it had the lowest specificity (median, .67) of all the SZPD criteria. The low specificity of criterion 6 and possibly criterion 2 indicates that other personality disorders share these characteristics as well.

In contrast to the high sensitivity and low to moderate specificity of the preceding criteria, criterion 3 (rarely experiences strong emotion), 4 (little desire for sex), and 5 (indifferent to praise or criticism) demonstrated low sensitivity and low prototypicality but high specificity. These criteria may define a subgroup of SZPD patients dominated by deficits in affective responsivity and capacity for pleasure. Retaining them in DSM-IV despite their low sensitivity may be justified by their possible ability to identify atypical cases. Criterion 5 (indifferent to praise or criticism) had the lowest sensitivity of all the SZPD criteria (range, .00–.34; median, .13); thus modifying this item may be justified on the basis of its low frequency. Criterion 7 (constricted affect) demonstrated intermediate sensitivity, specificity, and prototypicality.

DSM-III-R Compatibility With ICD-10

Revisions in DSM-III-R SZPD criteria appear to have significantly increased compatibility with the ICD-10, and proposed revisions in DSM-IV may further enhance their correspondence. DSM-III-R criteria 1, 2, 3, 5, 6, and 7 are closely matched with the corresponding ICD-10 criteria (6, 5, 4, 6, 3, and 2, respectively). DSM-III-R criterion 4 ("rarely, if ever, claims or appears to experience strong emotions, such as anger or joy") diverges from the corresponding ICD-10 criterion 1, which emphasizes lack of pleasure ("incapacity to experience pleasure"). ICD-10 criterion 7 ("marked difficulty in recognizing and adhering to social convention, resulting in eccentricity of behavior") does not have a corresponding DSM-III-R item.

Comorbidity

Rates of comorbidity of SZPD with other personality disorders are listed in Table 23–2. Among the highest was the comorbidity with STPD, perhaps reflecting the high degree of criteria overlap between the two (e.g., social isolation, restricted affect). AVPD also demonstrated high comorbidity with SZPD. Lesser degrees of comorbidity were demonstrated with PPD, antisocial PD, borderline PD, dependent PD, and passive-aggressive PD.

Table 23–2. Comorbidity of schizoid personality disorder with other Axis II disorders: percentage of criterion group receiving schizoid diagnosis

	PPD	STPD	ASPD	BPD	HPD	NPD	AVPD	DPD	OCPD	PAPD
Dahl 1986	0	80	40	20	20	0	60	0	0	0
Morey 1988	47	38	3	19	9	28	53	19	16	19
Freiman and Widiger 1989	62	62	25	38	0	38	88	0	0	50
Skodol et al. 1988	40	60	0	60	0	20	80	20	20	0
Millon and Tringone 1989										
Clinical interview	4	27	0	0	0	8	23	15	8	0
Diagnostic checklist	0	32	0	0	0	4	46	7	7	4
MCMI	0	2	0	0	0	7	39	20	17	11

Note. PPD = paranoid personality disorder. STPD = schizotypal personality disorder. ASPD = antisocial personality disorder. BPD = borderline personality disorder. HPD = histrionic personality disorder. NPD = narcissistic personality disorder. AVPD = avoidant personality disorder. DPD = dependent personality disorder. OCPD = obsessive-compulsive personality disorder. PAPD = passive-aggressive personality disorder. MCMI = Millon Clinical Multiaxial Inventory.

In a study examining Axis I/Axis II comorbidity, Alnaes and Torgerson (1988a) reported that the eccentric personality disorders as a group showed high comorbidity with dysthymic disorder, social phobia, and agoraphobia. Of seven relatives of psychiatric patients diagnosed with SZPD, Zimmerman and Coryell (1989) reported a 14.3% rate of mania, and rates of 28.6% of alcohol abuse/dependence, and 14.3% of drug abuse/dependence.

Genetic/Family Studies

Some family/genetic studies suggest that the boundaries of schizophrenia-related disorders may extend beyond STPD to include SZPD and PPD (Baron et al. 1985; Gunderson et al. 1983), whereas others suggest that the relationship is specific to STPD and not SZPD (Baron et al. 1985). Some of the studies examining the genetic characteristics of the schizophrenic spectrum may also have been confounded by a failure to clearly distinguish between SZPD and STPD. That negative rather than positive symptoms are associated with increased heritability in schizophrenia (Dworkin and Lenzenweger 1984) would theoretically support a familial/genetic link with the predominantly negative-symptom SZPD.

Discussion

Delineating the boundaries of SZPD from the other phenomenologically similar personality disorders in the odd cluster and AVPD remains a key concern. Whether the issue is one of a more refined differential diagnosis or of diagnostic validity will require additional research; however, the high comorbidity of SZPD, particularly with STPD, suggests that more discriminating diagnostic features are needed. Nearly all the current SZPD criteria with high specificity demonstrated unsatisfactory sensitivity, whereas those with high sensitivity had generally low specificity. Although SZPD shares a number of the social deficit symptoms with STPD, SZPD should be separable on the basis of the absence of positive-like psychotic symptoms. STPD also appears to have clearer familial and genetic links to schizophrenia than SZPD.

Although some studies suggest that SZPD can be empirically distinguished from AVPD (Trull et al. 1987) on the basis of intimacy needs and rejection sensitivity, contrasting historical descriptions of coexisting sensitivity/insensitivity in SZPD and more recent empirical studies suggesting indistinguishable anxiety and other clinical symptomatology (Overholser 1989) call for additional investigation. The poor performance of "insensitivity to criticism" as an SZPD criterion is consistent with this concern. The discrepancy between appearance and experience of sensitivity also highlights the need for more reliable and sensitive behavioral measures beyond mere clinical observation.

These concerns, along with the low prevalence of SZPD using DSM-III criteria, raise the question of whether SZPD should be retained as an independent diagnosis in DSM-IV. However, the increased prevalence of SZPD using DSM-III-R criteria, as well as historical and more recent clinical evidence in favor of a separate SZPD distinct from AVPD and STPD, argues for its present inclusion.

Although the DSM-III-R SZPD criteria demonstrate increased compatibility with the ICD-10, some discrepancies remain. Revising DSM-III-R criterion 4 relating to experience and expression of emotion toward an emphasis on lack of pleasure (anhedonia) as is done in ICD-10 criterion 1 might be considered to further increase compatibility. In contrast, it is unlikely that ICD-10 criterion 7 ("eccentricity of behavior") would be adopted because of its close correspondence to the DSM-III-R STPD criteria.

Determining whether SZPD may be related to schizophrenia on a continuum of schizophrenic spectrum disorders will also require additional investigation. Future research should incorporate biological markers such as deviant eye tracking and attentional deficits that have been identified in STPD and schizophrenia.

Recommendations

A few modifications in the SZPD diagnostic criteria are recommended for clarification and increased compatibility with ICD-10. In the stem of criterion A, it is proposed to replace *indifference to* social relationships with *detachment from,* and restricted range of *emotional experience and expression* with *expression of emotions in interpersonal settings.* The first modification emphasizes a more objective behavioral description (rather than an inferred subjective state) and the second modification provides increased specificity for the context in which emotional expression is absent. Criterion A4 would be modified to emphasize the individual's difficulty in taking pleasure in everyday activities (emphasizing anhedonia, rather than difficulty in experience and expression of a broader range of emotions). Criterion A6 would be modified to include individuals who appear indifferent to praise or criticism but who may indeed have an underlying sensitivity. It is recommended that items A3, A4, A5, and A7 be modified to increase compatibility with ICD-10.

References

Akhtar S: Schizoid personality disorder: a synthesis of developments, dynamic, and descriptive features. Am J Psychother 41:499–518, 1987

Akiskal H: The clinical management of affective disorders, in Psychiatry. Edited by Michels R. New York, Basic Books, 1987, pp 1–15

Alnaes R, Torgerson S: DSM-III symptom disorders (Axis I) and personality disorders (Axis II) in an outpatient population. Acta Psychiatr Scand 78:348–355, 1988a

Alnaes R, Torgerson S: The relationship between DSM-III symptom disorders (Axis I) and personality disorders (Axis II) in an outpatient population. Acta Psychiatr Scand 78:485–492, 1988b

American Psychiatric Association: Diagnostic and Statistical Manual of Mental Disorders, 3rd Edition. Washington, DC, American Psychiatric Association, 1980

American Psychiatric Association: Diagnostic and Statistical Manual of Mental Disorders, 3rd Edition, Revised. Washington, DC, American Psychiatric Association, 1987

Baron M, Gruen R, Rainer JD, et al: A family study of schizophrenic and normal control probands: implications for the spectrum concept of schizophrenia. Am J Psychiatry 142:447–454, 1985

Bernstein DP: The prevalence and stability of the DSM-III-R personality disorders in adolescence. Unpublished doctoral dissertation, New York, New York University, 1990

Bleuler E: Textbook of Psychiatry. Translated by Brill AA. New York, Macmillan, 1924

Clarkin JF, Widiger TA, Frances A, et al: Prototypic typology and the borderline personality disorder. J Abnorm Psychol 92:263–273, 1983

Dahl A: Some aspects of the DSM-III personality disorders illustrated by a consecutive sample of hospitalized patients. Acta Psychiatr Scand 73 (Suppl 228):61–66, 1986

Drake R, Valliant G: A validity study of Axis II of DSM-III. Am J Psychiatry 142:553–558, 1985

Dworkin R, Lenzenweger M: Symptoms and the genetics of schizophrenia: implications for diagnosis. Am J Psychiatry 141:1541–1546, 1984

Freiman K, Widiger T: Co-occurrence and diagnostic efficiency statistics. Unpublished raw data, Lexington, University of Kentucky, 1989

Gunderson JG, Siever LJ, Spaulding E: The search for a schizotype: crossing the border again. Arch Gen Psychiatry 40:15–22, 1983

Guntrip H: Schizoid Phenomena, Object Relations and the Self. New York, International Universities Press, 1969

Heston LL: The genetics of schizophrenia and schizoid disease. Science 167:249–256, 1970

Kass F, Skodol AE, Charles E, et al: Scaled ratings of DSM-III personality disorders. Am J Psychiatry 142:627–630, 1985

Khantzian EJ, Treece C: DSM-III psychiatric diagnosis of narcotic addicts: recent findings. Arch Gen Psychiatry 42:1067–1071, 1985

Koenigsberg HW, Kaplan RD, Gilmore MW, et al: The relationship between syndrome and personality disorder in DSM-III: experience with 2,462 patients. Am J Psychiatry 142:207–212, 1985

Kretschmer E: Korperbau und Charakter. Berlin, Springer-Verlag, 1925. Physique and Character (English translation), London, Kegan Paul, 1926

Mellsop G, Varghese F, Joshua S, et al: The reliability of Axis II of DSM-III. Am J Psychiatry 139:1360–1361, 1982

Millon T, Tringone R: Co-occurrence and diagnostic efficiency statistics. Unpublished raw data, Miami, FL, University of Miami, 1989

Morey L: Personality disorders in DSM-III and DSM-III-R: convergence, coverage, and internal consistency. Am J Psychiatry 145:573–577, 1988

Morey L, Heumann K: Co-occurrence and diagnostic efficiency statistics. Unpublished raw data, Nashville, TN, Vanderbilt University, 1988

Overholser JC: Differentiation between schizoid and avoidant personalities: an empirical test. Can J Psychiatry 34:785–790, 1989

Pfohl B, Coryell W, Zimmerman M, et al: DSM-III personality disorders: diagnostic overlap and internal consistency of individual DSM-III criteria. Compr Psychiatry 27:21–34, 1986

Reich J: Sex distribution of DSM-III personality disorders in psychiatric outpatients. Am J Psychiatry 144:485–488, 1987

Reich J, Yates W, Nduaguba M: Prevalence of DSM-III personality disorders in the community. Soc Psychiatry Epidemiol 24:12–16, 1989

Skodol AE, Rosnick L, Kellman D, et al: Validating structured DSM-III-R personality disorder assessments with longitudinal data. Am J Psychiatry 145:1297–1299, 1988

Terry GC, Rennie T: Analysis of Paraergasia. Am J Orthopsychiatry 9:817–818, 1938

Trull TJ, Widiger TA, Frances A: Covariation of criteria sets for avoidant, schizoid, and dependent personality disorders. Am J Psychiatry 144:767–771, 1987

Wolff S, Chick J: Schizoid personality in childhood. Psychol Med 10:85–101, 1980

Widiger T, Frances A, Warner L, et al: Diagnostic criteria for the borderline and schizotypal personality disorders. J Abnorm Psychol 95:43–51, 1986

World Health Organization: ICD-10 Chapter V. Mental and Behavioral Disorders. Diagnostic Criteria for Research. Geneva, Switzerland, World Health Organization, 1990

Zanarini M, Frankenburg F, Chauncey D, et al: Co-occurrence and diagnostic efficiency statistics. Unpublished raw data, Boston, MA, McLean Hospital, 1989

Zimmerman M, Coryell WH: DSM-III personality disorder diagnoses in a nonpatient sample. Arch Gen Psychiatry 46:682–689, 1989

Zimmerman M, Coryell WH: Diagnosing personality disorders in the community: a comparison of self-report and interview measures. Arch Gen Psychiatry 47:527–531, 1990

Chapter 24

Schizotypal Personality Disorder

Larry J. Siever, M.D., David P. Bernstein, Ph.D., and
Jeremy M. Silverman, Ph.D.

The schizotypal, paranoid, and schizoid personality disorders constitute the "odd cluster" of the DSM-III-R personality disorders. All are characterized by a degree of social detachment and odd or idiosyncratic behavior that can be observed in much more extreme form in the schizophrenic disorders. Schizotypal personality disorder (STPD) is characterized by eccentricity and cognitive/perceptual distortions, paranoid personality disorder by suspiciousness and mistrust of others, and schizoid personality disorder by a preference for solitary activities without necessarily involving distortions in perceptions of reality.

STPD is the most recently adopted disorder in this cluster. It also represents the first personality disorder defined in part by its genetic relationship to chronic schizophrenia. For these reasons, the inclusion of STPD in DSM-III (American Psychiatric Association 1980) has provided the stimulus for investigation of this disorder and its relationship both to other personality disorders and to the schizophrenic disorders. Increasingly compelling evidence suggests that STPD is related to schizophrenia in terms of common phenomenological (Kendler 1985; Siever and Gunderson 1983), genetic (Kendler 1985; Kendler et al. 1981; Torgerson 1985), biological (Siever 1985), outcome (McGlashan 1986), and treatment-response (Goldberg et al. 1986; Serban and Siegel 1984) characteristics.

Statement and Significance of the Issues

The major issues regarding the odd cluster personality disorders center around the extent to which they overlap with each other, with the other personality disorders, and with the Axis I psychotic disorders, specifically the schizophrenic and paranoid disorders. There are four main issues.

1) Should STPD and possibly the other odd cluster diagnoses be included with other schizophrenia-related disorders on Axis I? The schizophrenia-related disorders appear to represent a continuum from severe, chronic "Kraepelinian" schizophrenia to the milder schizophrenia-related personality disorders, of which STPD is the prototype. Investigations suggesting that STPD is closely related to schizophrenia have sharpened questions regarding the relation of the Axis I to the Axis II disorders and prompted questions as to whether STPD would more properly be placed with the Axis I disorders. On the other hand, the Axis II disorders are defined in terms of "enduring patterns of perceiving, relating to, and thinking about the environment and oneself" (American Psychiatric Association 1987). The criteria for STPD reflect persistent disturbances in perception/cognition and in relatedness between self and others, so that STPD would appear to fully meet the definition for an Axis II disorder.

2) Could the substantial overlap between borderline personality disorder and STPD be reduced by refining the criteria for STPD, particularly the psychotic-like criteria? The well-documented overlap between STPD and borderline personality disorder could be a function of random overlap, an artifact of the inclusion of psychotic-like symptoms solely in STPD criteria, or genuine synergism in pathophysiological antecedents to these disorders. To the extent overlap might be reduced by sharpening criteria, how should criteria for STPD be revised to be more specific?

3) Could the specificity of the relation of STPD to schizophrenia as opposed to the affective disorders be enhanced by modifying the STPD criteria? The offspring and relatives of affective disorder and schizophrenic disorder patients show comparably increased prevalences of STPD (Ingraham 1989; Squires-Wheeler et al. 1988), prompting questions about whether some of the criteria for STPD encompass affective-related characteristics and whether criteria changes would increase the specificity of the relationship between STPD and schizophrenia.

4) An additional issue concerns the compatibility of the DSM-III-R STPD criteria with the World Health Organization's proposed diagnostic criteria for the ICD-10 (World Health Organization 1990). Increasing compatibility between the two systems would help facilitate international clinical and research efforts.

To clarify these issues and potential paradoxes, the relationship between STPD and schizophrenia and other personality disorders is reviewed from phenomenological, genetic, biological, outcome, and treatment-response viewpoints.

Methods

The issues were approached by reviewing published studies and, where available, unpublished data sets pertaining to STPD and highlighting results of studies germane to these issues. These included clinical studies of the reliability and diagnostic efficiency of the criteria, overlap with other personality disorders, and comorbidity with the Axis I disorders. Studies using external validators such as family history or family study, biological indices, outcome, and response to treatment were emphasized.

Results

Phenomenological Studies

The impetus for the designation of STPD as a new diagnostic category in DSM-III emerged from concerns on the part of Spitzer and other architects of DSM-III that the definition of borderline conditions had become too diffuse, including both affectively unstable and schizophrenia-related personality disorders, whereas the criteria for schizoid personality disorder were too broadly defined to specifically characterize individuals with enduring psychotic-like traits (Spitzer et al. 1979). To define a prototypic personality disorder with the chronic psychotic-like characteristics observed in the relatives of chronic schizophrenic patients, the case histories of individuals diagnosed as "borderline" or "latent" and uncertain schizophrenia by Kety et al. (1975) in the Danish adoptive studies were reviewed and provided the basis for the DSM-III criteria for STPD. Because the diagnoses in the Kety et al. studies had a demonstrable genetic relation to chronic schizophrenia, STPD represents the only Axis II disorder to be defined empirically on the basis of a genetic relationship with an Axis I disorder.

However, while the individual latent or uncertain schizophrenic case histories selected from the Danish adoptive studies included biological relatives of chronic schizophrenic patients, they also included relatives and probands with no demonstrated genetic relationship to chronic schizophrenia (Gunderson et al. 1983). The criteria selected for DSM-III may therefore not have defined personality characteristics reflective of a genetic relationship with schizophrenia as precisely as possible. Furthermore, it was not the intention of Spitzer and colleagues to restrict the definition to a personality disorder that was necessarily specifically related to schizophrenia but rather to use the adoptive studies as a starting point to define a personality disorder with chronic psychotic-like characteristics associated with social withdrawal rather than with affective instability, as in contemporary definitions of borderline personality (Spitzer et al. 1979). To further this aim, they refined the defining characteristics on the basis of a questionnaire sent to members of the American Psychiatric Association to differentiate STPD from "unstable personality disorder," which included impulsive and affectively unstable but not psychotic-like characteristics, (since changed to borderline personality disorder). Thus, although STPD was defined in part on the basis of a genetic relationship with chronic schizophrenia, it was conceived by its architects as a clinical personality disorder characterized by chronic psychotic-like characteristics rather than specifically as a milder schizophrenia-related disorder.

In fact, relatives of schizophrenics from the Danish adoptive studies (Gunderson et al. 1983) and from the Iowa non-500 study (Kendler et al. 1985) appear more likely to manifest the negative symptoms of STPD such as social isolation, poor rapport, and eccentricity rather than the positive psychotic-like symptoms of magical thinking, referential ideation, and perceptual distortion. In contrast, clinically defined STPD patients may be specifically defined by their positive psychotic-like characteristics (Jacobsberg et al. 1986; Widiger et al. 1986). Frances (1985) has argued, on the basis of such studies, that STPD should be defined as a clinical personality disorder that may not necessarily be the same as the schizophrenia-related personality disorders observed in the relatives of chronic schizophrenic patients.

Sensitivity and Specificity of Criteria

Attempts to identify symptoms that are sensitive to and specific for STPD have used comparisons between STPD and other personality disorder patients, particularly patients with borderline personality disorder. In a review of the studies of schizotypal criteria, McGlashan (1987) suggested that odd communication, suspiciousness/paranoid ideation, and social isolation represent the most characteristic or core criteria for STPD, whereas illusions/depersonalization/derealization is not characteristic in his sample. Although undue social anxiety is nearly universal among schizotypal patients (Pfohl et al. 1986), it is not particularly specific for this disorder. The discriminating power of positive symptoms such as odd communication, ideas of reference, magical thinking, and illusions are emphasized by Jacobsberg et al. (1986) in a study comparing schizotypal and borderline patients. In a similarly designed study, Widiger et al. (1986) found ideas of reference, odd speech, and paranoid ideation to be most closely correlated with the total number of schizotypal symptoms. Although these studies have not been entirely consistent and have employed different clinical populations and analytic tools, most tend to support social withdrawal, odd/eccentric speech and behavior, and suspicious/paranoid ideation as central disturbances in the schizotypal patient.

Although studies comparing borderline and schizotypal patients have tended to specifically identify positive symptoms as discriminators of the schizotypal diagnosis, these results may reflect the fact that the schizotypal-borderline overlap patients may be characterized by prominent psychotic symptoms, whereas borderline patients without a schizotypal diagnosis are unlikely to have positive symptoms, or they would have met the schizotypal criteria. Recent phenomenological, family history, and biological data suggest that the overlap group may represent variants of borderline personality disorder with psychotic-like symptoms but not necessarily related to schizophrenia per se (Siever et al. 1987b). Alternatively, they may represent the synergistic effects of biogenetic and psychosocial precursors to each disorder.

Comorbidity

The overlap between STPD and Axis I disorders has not been extensively studied, but a substantial overlap with major depressive disorder has been found in several studies. McGlashan (1983) retrospectively assigned DSM-III Axis II diagnoses to former patients at the Chestnut Lodge and found that, at the time of hospital admission, 9% of the 75 patients diagnosed with STPD were also given a diagnosis of mania, and 29% received a diagnosis of depression. Pfohl et al. (1984) reported that of 78 patients with major depressive disorder, 9% also met DSM-III criteria for STPD. L. J. Siever (unpublished data set) found that 49% of patients with STPD also met criteria for major depressive disorder at the time of the study, and 63% had a history of at least one major depressive episode. Conversely, 51% of the patients presenting with major depressive disorder also received a schizotypal diagnosis.

Because personality disorders are rarely diagnosed in the presence of more florid schizophrenic symptomatology, few studies have examined the comorbidity of schizophrenia and the Axis II disorders. McGlashan (1983) found that 44% of the 75 Chestnut Lodge patients retrospectively diagnosed with STPD also qualified for a diagnosis of schizophrenia. No other personality disorder showed a comparably high rate of overlap with schizophrenia.

STPD often coexists with other personality disorders, as do all of the Axis II personality disorders. These associations do not appear to be random but may occur in two patterns. On the one hand, STPD co-occurs with the other odd cluster diagnoses and personality disorders from other clusters that reflect social isolation and detachment such as obsessive-compulsive and avoidant personality disorders (Kass et al. 1985; Siever 1985). On the other hand, many patients meeting DSM-III criteria for STPD also carry a concurrent borderline personality disorder diagnosis (Jacobsberg et al. 1986; McGlashan 1987). In seven clinical studies reporting rates of diagnostic overlap among all DSM-III or DSM-III-R Axis II disorders (Table 24–1), the percentage of patients with STPD receiving comorbid borderline diagnoses ranged from 33% (Skodol 1989) to 91% (Zanarini et al. 1989; median comorbidity = 50%), whereas that of borderline patients given comorbid schizotypal diagnoses ranged from 0% (Millon and Tringone 1989) to 53% (Freiman and Widiger 1989; median comorbidity = 23%).

Table 24–1. Comorbidity among Axis II disorders in seven clinical studies

	SZPD	PPD	HPD	NPD	BPD	ASPD	AVPD	DPD	OCPD	PAPD	SDPD	SAD
Percentage with STPD receiving indicated diagnosis												
Dahl 1986	10	2	15	2	41	32	15	0	0	0	—	—
Pfohl et al. 1986	0	0	33	8	50	8	58	0	17	50	—	—
Morey 1988	44	59	18	33	33	4	59	30	11	15	—	—
Skodol 1989[a]	0	38	12	44	88	19	88	62	31	12	50	0
Zanarini et al. 1989	0	10	71	29	91	38	29	39	8	32	—	—
Millon and Tringone 1989[b]	12	12	0	3	47	3	68	15	0	9	26	3
Freiman and Widiger 1989	46	46	0	45	54	46	54	46	0	50	18	27
Percentage with indicated diagnosis receiving STPD												
Dahl 1986	80	100	17	33	45	38	35	0	0	0	—	—
Pfohl et al. 1986	0	0	13	20	21	20	47	0	29	33	—	—
Morey 1988	38	25	8	14	9	6	20	12	13	11	—	—
Skodol 1989[a]	0	43	12	33	23	38	36	30	24	33	40	0
Zanarini et al. 1989	0	50	48	51	40	29	43	45	33	45	—	—
Millon and Tringone 1989[b]	8	17	8	75	0	25	8	0	33	17	0	0
Freiman and Widiger 1989	33	33	27	47	53	33	60	27	0	40	13	27

Note. SZPD = schizoid personality disorder. PPD = paranoid personality disorder. HPD = histrionic personality disorder. NPD = narcissistic personality disorder. BPD = borderline personality disorder. ASPD = antisocial personality disorder. AVPD = avoidant personality disorder. DPD = dependent personality disorder. OCPD = obsessive-compulsive personality disorder. PAPD = passive-aggressive personality disorder. SDPD = self-defeating personality disorder. SAD = sadistic personality disorder. STPD = schizotypal personality disorder.

[a]Prevalence of STPD in this table based on the Personality Disorder Examination (PDE). Skodol (1989) also reported prevalences based on other diagnostic instruments.

[b]Prevalence of STPD in this table based on the Millon Clinical Multiaxial Inventory (MCMI). Millon and Tringone (1989) also reported prevalences based on other diagnostic instruments.

Compatibility Between DSM-III-R and ICD-10

DSM-III-R criteria for STPD appear to overlap substantially with the proposed ICD-10 criteria, based on discussion between American Psychiatric Association and World Health Organization representatives (M. First, M.D., personal communication, 1991). Corresponding ICD-10 items were found for all DSM-III-R STPD features, although the match between criteria was not always one-to-one, and slight differences were found in the wording of corresponding items. DSM-III-R criteria 1 and 2 were matched by ICD-10 item 4, DSM-III-R criterion 3 by ICD-10 item 6, DSM-III-R criterion 4 by ICD-10 item 7, DSM-III-R criterion 5 by ICD-10 item 4, DSM-III-R criterion 6 by ICD-10 item 1, DSM-III-R criterion 7 by ICD-10 item 2, and DSM-III-R criteria 8 and 9 by ICD-10 item 3. In addition, no corresponding DSM-III-R criteria were found for two of the ICD-10 items: ICD-10 item 5 ("obsessive ruminations without inner resistance, often with dysmorphophobic, sexual, or aggressive contents") and item 8 ("occasional transient quasi-psychotic episodes with intense illusions, auditory or other hallucinations and delusion-like ideas, usually occurring without external provocation"). A final difference between the two criteria sets is the placement of the ICD-10 criteria in the section with schizophrenia and other psychotic disorders, whereas the DSM-III-R groups STPD with the personality disorders on Axis II (the placement of STPD may be modified in DSM-IV, increasing its compatibility with ICD-10 [see Recommendations]).

Genetic/Family Studies

Adoptive studies (Gunderson et al. 1983; Kendler 1985; Kendler et al. 1981; Torgerson 1985) and familial studies (Baron et al. 1985; Schulz et al. 1986; Soloff and Millward 1983; Stone 1977) are consistent in suggesting a common genetic diathesis for schizophrenia and STPD. Although phenomenologically oriented psychiatrists since the time of Bleuler have observed that the family members of schizophrenic patients are often eccentric and socially isolated, the first definitive evidence for a genetic relationship between chronic schizophrenia and STPD derives from the adoptive studies of Kety et al. (1975) and subsequent reanalyses of the case histories in these studies using DSM-III criteria. STPD was found to be more common among the biological relatives of schizophrenic patients than among their adoptive relatives or than among the biological or adoptive relatives of control subjects (Gunderson et al. 1983; Kendler 1985). In fact, STPD has been diagnosed more frequently than chronic schizophrenia itself in the relatives of the schizophrenic probands, raising the possibility that schizotypal symptoms may represent a more common phenotypic expression than chronic schizophrenia of an underlying diathesis to the schizophrenia-related disorders.

Further support for a relationship between STPD and chronic schizophrenia is provided by studies of the first-degree relatives, siblings, and cotwins of chronic schizophrenic probands (Torgerson 1985). Preliminary results of a more recent direct-interview family study suggests that STPD is more prevalent in the relatives of schizophrenic probands than in those of control subjects and that schizotypal signs were more discriminating than schizotypal symptoms (Kendler et al. 1989). Studies identifying schizotypal patients as probands and psychiatrically evaluating their relatives (Baron et al. 1985; Schulz et al. 1986; Soloff and Millward 1983; Stone 1977) or cotwins (Torgerson 1985) suggest familial transmission of STPD as part of a continuum of schizophrenia-related disorders. The cumulative risk for schizophrenia-related disorders is greater in the relatives of STPD probands than in the relatives of probands with other non-schizophrenia-related personality disorders, whereas the cumulative risk for other psychiatric disorders, including major affective disorders, antisocial disorders, and other personality disorders, does not differ between groups (Silverman et al. 1986). Indications of a reciprocal familial/genetic relationship between STPD and chronic schizophrenia have been reported (Schulz et al. 1986; Soloff and Millward 1983), although sample sizes to date have been too small to establish or disconfirm this hypothesis. Thus, these studies support the relationship between STPD and schizophrenia and even more strongly support familial/genetic transmission of STPD itself.

The genetic specificity of current definitions of STPD is less clearly established. Biological relatives of adopted major affective disorder patients may also demonstrate schizotypal characteristics (S. Kety, personal communication, 1987), although it is not clear whether these represent the core or positive symptoms. Schizotypal patients in the clinical setting frequently present with depressive symptoms, and such patients have an increased familial cumulative risk for major affective disorders (Silverman et al. 1988). Relatives of schizotypal/borderline patients have an increased morbid risk for schizophrenia-related disorders, primarily schizophrenia-related personality disorders, but also for personality disorders with marked affective and impulsive features (Silverman et al. 1987). Could the psychotic-like symptoms and broad social dysfunction as represented in current criteria for STPD be related to affective and impulsive disorders in some cases? Would the symptoms of such individuals differ in character from the truly schizophrenia-related schizotypal personality?

Biological Studies

Biological correlates of chronic schizophrenia may also be abnormal in at least some forms of STPD. Impaired smooth-pursuit eye movements (SPEM) have been reported in 60%–80% of schizophrenic patients and approximately half of their relatives, in contrast to a much smaller proportion of the relatives of manic-depressive patients (Holzman et al. 1984; Lipton et al. 1983). SPEM impairment has been specifically associated with STPD but not with other types of psychopathology in volunteer subjects (Siever et al. 1984, 1989), personality disorder patients (Siever et al. 1990), and the offspring of schizophrenic parents (P. S. Holzman, personal communication, 1988), supporting a biological association between STPD and schizophrenia. Performance on a backward masking task, an information processing test, shows abnormalities in STPD patients that are similar to, although milder than, those observed in schizophrenic patients (Braff 1986). Some of these measures have been found to be abnormal in affective disorder patients as well, raising issues of specificity, but the abnormalities appear more likely to be state dependent in affective disorders and may differ in character from those found in schizophrenic patients (Siever 1985). Decreased activity of platelet monoamine and/or plasma amine oxidase has been reported in schizotypal volunteers and schizotypal relatives of schizophrenic patients (Baron and Levitt 1980; Baron et al. 1980, 1983), but seems more closely related to sensation seeking and affective symptomatology in other studies (Buchsbaum et al. 1976). Abnormalities in galvanic skin-orienting response and evoked potential responses similar to those observed in schizophrenic patients have been reported in college volunteers who were selected by a psychological test profile similar to that observed in schizophrenic patients (Siever 1985; Simons 1981, 1982) and in preliminary studies of STPD patients. Computerized tomographic (CT) scan studies have shown increases in the ventricular-brain ratio (VBR) in schizophrenic patients (Shelton and Weinberger 1986) and schizotypal patients (Siever et al. 1987a). These studies cumulatively suggest that schizotypal individuals and at least a subgroup of clinically defined patients with STPD demonstrate biological/psychophysiological abnormalities characteristic of chronic schizophrenia. Thus, biological studies complement genetic studies in supporting a relationship between STPD and schizophrenia that extends to include clinically defined schizotypal patients.

These biological correlates (e.g., SPEM impairment, increased VBR, backward masking) are often associated with chronic attentional/cognitive dysfunction apparently reflecting structural alteration of the central nervous system. These biological factors tend to be correlated with the negative or deficit symptoms of schizophrenia, whereas neurochemical variables that may be more state-related such as the catecholamine metabolites tend to be associated with the positive psychotic-like symptoms of schizophrenia. Plasma homovanillic acid (HVA), the major metabolite of dopamine, has been found to be correlated with psychotic symptoms in drug-free schizophrenic patients (Davis et al. 1985) and diminishes in parallel with psychotic symptoms with neuroleptic treatment (Pickar et al. 1986). Preliminary studies of schizotypal patients suggest that cerebrospinal fluid (CSF) and plasma HVA are increased in schizotypal patients compared with control subjects with other personality disorders and that these increases may be partially associated with increased psychotic-like symptoms (Siever et al. 1991). Some preliminary evidence suggests that patients with a more prototypic schizotypal profile emphasizing the core deficit features without concomitant borderline features may be more likely to evidence biological correlates related to schizophrenia than do the schizotypal-borderline group (Siever 1985; Siever et al. 1987a), although larger samples with measures that are relatively more specific for schizophrenic versus affective disorders are required to clarify this issue.

Outcome

Schizotypal patients have also been shown to have a long-term outcome that is more similar to that of chronic schizophrenia than to that of another severe personality disorder—borderline personality disorder (McGlashan 1986). The premorbid and illness characteristics of the schizotypal patients, however, were more similar to the other personality disorder groups than to the schizophrenics with the exception of their premorbid social adjustment and their frequency of social contacts. Most specific outcome measures fell between those of the schizophrenic patients and the personality disorder groups. The overlap schizotypal-borderline patients were more socially related than the pure schizotypal patients and functioned more like borderline patients, although their capacity for more intimate relationships seemed poorer than did that of the pure borderline personality disorder patients.

The proportion of patients with STPD who actually go on to develop chronic schizophrenia is not clear, although as many as 25% of one sample of schizotypal patients were reported to have satisfied criteria for schizophrenia on follow-up 2 years later (Schulz and Soloff 1987), and 17% of the Chestnut Lodge sample received a later schizophrenic diagnosis (Fenton and McGlashan 1989). This proportion was substantially lower in a sample of male veterans, and in patients diagnosed as having schizophrenia on follow-up in the study of male veterans, at least two may have had schizophrenic symptoms that they were concealing on initial evaluation (L. J. Siever, unpublished data). In the Chestnut Lodge outcome study, symptoms of paranoid ideation, social isolation, and magical thinking were good predictors of the later onset of schizophrenia in character disorder patients (Fenton and McGlashan 1989). In summary, the course of STPD is similar to, although not quite as severely impaired as, that of chronic schizophrenia, particularly with respect to social relatedness; paranoid symptomatology and social impairment may be associated with worse outcome.

Treatment Response

Like schizophrenic patients, STPD patients respond positively to neuroleptics such as thiothixene and haloperidol (Goldberg et al. 1986; Serban and Siegel 1984). Psychotic-like and anxiety symptoms (i.e., illusions, ideas of reference, psychoticism, obsessive-compulsive symptoms, and phobic anxiety) responded specifically to the neuroleptic treatment (Goldberg et al. 1986). Although antidepressants such as monoamine oxidase inhibitors, tricyclics, and lithium carbonate have been reported to cause symptomatic improvement in diagnoses that were forerunners to the schizotypal diagnosis such as pseudoneurotic schizophrenia (Klein 1967; Rifkin et al. 1972), they have not been proven to have benefit in rigorously diagnosed schizotypal patients. Thus, schizotypal patients resemble chronic schizophrenic patients in their response to neuroleptics, particularly with respect to reduction of psychotic-like symptoms. However, patients with borderline personality disorder have also been reported to respond to neuroleptic medications (Soloff et al. 1986).

Controlled studies of the treatment response of STPD to psychotherapy are not available. However, Frosch (1983), Hoch and Polatin (1949), Knight (1954), and Searles (1965) discuss problems encountered in treating patients with characteristics similar to current criteria for STPD. Such patients tend to decompensate in the setting of unmodified analytic treatment but may respond to a psychotherapeutic approach with reality testing, attention to interpersonal boundaries, and educative interventions (Stone 1985), if the goals are not too ambitious. The psychotherapeutic approach to schizotypal patients thus incorporates techniques used in the treatment of both schizophrenic patients and patients with severe personality disorders.

Discussion

1) STPD: Axis I or Axis II?

The common features of chronic schizophrenia and STPD described in the previous section suggest that the boundaries of the schizophrenia spectrum extend beyond chronic schizophrenia to include at least a substantial subset of schizotypal individuals. Although the strength and specificity of this relationship for schizotypal patients identified in a clinical setting require further investigation, initial results of studies evaluating family history, biological characteristics, outcome, and treatment response of schizotypal patients support the existence of such a relationship. These considerations argue for the inclusion of STPD as one of the schizophrenia-related disorders, which are currently placed among the Axis I disorders.

However, genetic and epidemiological studies suggest that schizophrenia-related personality disorders may be more common manifestations of genotypes predisposing to the schizophrenia-related disorders than chronic schizophrenia itself (i.e., that the schizophrenia spectrum may include more individuals with Axis

II than with Axis I disorders). The multiaxial system of DSM-III does not easily accommodate or acknowledge the existence of spectrum disorders that may include both the episodic, symptomatic disorders included on Axis I and the stable psychopathological characteristics of the Axis II disorders. However, as our knowledge of the genetics, biology, outcome, and treatment response of both the Axis I and Axis II disorders increases, it seems likely that there will be increasing evidence not only for a schizophrenia spectrum but also for an affective spectrum, anxiety spectrum, and impulse disorder spectrum, with manifestations varying from symptoms that have periods of exacerbation and remission to more persistent character traits. To simply remove STPD from Axis II and include it on Axis I might set a problematic precedent. It would raise questions as to whether schizoid or paranoid personality disorder as defined in DSM-III-R should also be included with the Axis I schizophrenic disorders, whether avoidant personality disorder should be included with the Axis I phobic anxiety disorders, whether borderline personality disorder should be included with the Axis I impulse disorders, or depressive/self-defeating personality disorder with the Axis I affective disorders. Whereas these relationships are less clearly established than that between STPD and schizophrenia, these personality disorders have been less intensively investigated using the approaches applied to STPD. Available evidence, however, suggests that at least some of these personality disorders will be found to be related to the corresponding Axis I disorders.

One potential solution to this dilemma in DSM-IV that would not involve restructuring the multiaxial format would be to explicitly acknowledge STPD on both Axes I and II. The concept of spectrums could be introduced in the introduction to and explanation of the multiaxial system to clarify why STPD is noted with both the Axis I and the Axis II disorders. This solution would alert the clinician that STPD should be potentially considered a schizophrenia-related disorder, but that it does satisfy all the criteria for an Axis II disorder (i.e., an enduring constellation of traits that describes an individual's interpersonal, cognitive, and affective style and may not invariably, at least according to current criteria, define a disorder related to chronic schizophrenia). Investigators should be encouraged to examine a larger range of characteristics than those included in DSM-III-R or even DSM-IV, to better refine which schizotypal characteristics are most specific for the personality disorders related to schizophrenia as opposed to those schizotypal criteria (e.g., possibly some variants of psychotic-like symptoms) with etiologies unrelated to schizophrenia. Such an endeavor would not only be important in furthering our understanding of the schizophrenia-related disorders but could have important implications for the diagnosis, prognosis, and treatment of the severe personality disorders. Premature closure of the status of STPD in a dichotomous Axis I/Axis II framework might impair further research in the areas of both schizophrenic and personality disorders, which has been quite productive with the present framework, whereas the acknowledgment of a spectrum of schizophrenia-related disorders that includes both Axis I and Axis II disorders might enhance both clinicians' and investigators' appreciation of the relationship between these two axes.

2) Overlap Between STPD and Borderline Personality Disorder

Available data raise the possibility that some of the overlap between STPD and borderline personality disorder may be an artifact of criteria describing less specific psychotic-like symptoms that may occur with both of these disorders. The resolution of this question requires larger empirical studies that attempt to define more discriminating criteria that might reduce the overlap between these two disorders. Ultimately, external validating studies will be required to determine whether STPD patients with a concomitant borderline personality disorder differ from pure schizotypal patients in genetic, biological, outcome, and treatment-response parameters. Preliminary studies suggest that patients with STPD and borderline personality disorder have characteristics that fall between those of pure STPD patients and pure borderline patients, suggesting that there is some genuine overlap in addition to the artifactual overlap.

3) Specificity of Relationship Between STPD and Schizophrenia

Affective characteristics, which may be observed both in borderline patients and relatives of affective disorder patients, may lead to cognitive/perceptual distortions, difficulty in maintaining relationships, suspiciousness and projection under stress, and social anxiety. However, these characteristics would be expected to be most prominent in altered affective states. Again, studies attempting to refine the criteria for STPD, as well as studies of external validators, are needed to finally resolve this question.

4) Compatibility Between DSM-III-R STPD and ICD-10

There appears to be substantial correspondence between DSM-III-R and ICD-10 schizotypal diagnostic criteria, although slight alterations in wording might further increase their compatibility. A more substantive difference concerns the placement of ICD-10 schizotypal criteria with other putative schizophrenia-related disorders—an option that is also being considered for DSM-IV.

Recommendations

Proposed modifications in the diagnostic criteria for STPD in DSM-IV are directed toward reducing the frequently high degree of diagnostic overlap between STPD and other personality disorders that are considered to fall outside of the schizo-phrenia spectrum, particularly borderline personality disorder. Phenomenological studies have suggested that the occurrence of psychotic-like symptomatology in non-schizophrenia related personality disorders may be an important source of this diagnostic overlap. The recommended changes in the schizotypal criteria set are directed toward improving the specificity of the schizotypal criteria by taking into account the persistence of psychotic-like symptomatology outside of the context of discrete periods of affective symptoms. It is hypothesized that the appearance of psychotic-like symptomatology among predominantly borderline patients will be associated with these periods (e.g., depression, anxiety, and anger), whereas psy-chotic-like features will be persistent and relatively independent of affective symp-toms in schizotypal patients. It is therefore proposed that the DSM-IV schizotypal criteria set include the requirement that schizotypal *"signs and symptoms should not be limited to discrete periods of mood symptomatology (e.g., depression, anxiety, anger)."*

Additional options to be considered for DSM-IV concern items 8 (social isolation) and 9 (social anxiety). The following addition is proposed for item 8: "no close friends or confidants (or only one) other than first-degree relatives *due primarily to lack of desire, pervasive discomfort with others, or eccentricities."* Thus a patient who avoids or otherwise lacks close friendships because of past troubles associated with their intensity, instability, or emotional turmoil would not receive the proposed item. Alternatively, a patient who has never held any interest in establishing a close connection with others would be given this item. The following addition is proposed for item 9: "excessive social anxiety (e.g., extreme discomfort in social situations *that does not diminish with familiarity and tends to be associated with paranoid fears rather than negative judgments about self."* This proposed revision would thus exclude those socially anxious individuals who are able to "warm up" to novel social situations over time or who are primarily concerned that they will be judged negatively (e.g., being seen as "unattractive" or "a jerk").

It is also recommended that the following modifications be made to DSM-III-R items 3, 4, 6, and 7, to increase compatibility with corresponding ICD-10 criteria (altered text is shown in italics): item 3, "unusual perceptual experiences, *including somatosensory (bodily) illusions*; item 4, "odd *thinking and* speech (without loosen-ing of associations or incoherence) (e.g., vague, *circumstantial, metaphorical, over-elaborate, or stereotyped)*"; item 6, "inappropriate or constricted affect (e.g., *appears cold* and aloof)"; and item 7, "behavior or appearance that is odd, eccentric, or peculiar" (deletion of previous text only).

It is also suggested that the stem for the nine STPD inclusion criteria be modified as follows: "A pervasive pattern of *social and interpersonal* deficits *marked by acute discomfort with, and reduced capacity for, close relationships as well as by cognitive or perceptual distortions and eccentricities of behavior,* beginning by early adulthood, and present in a variety of contexts, as indicated by at least five of the following:" This proposed modification emphasizes the presence of both negative (i.e., interpersonal deficit) and positive (i.e., cognitive/perceptual distortion) symptoms in STPD.

A final option concerns the placement of STPD on Axis I or Axis II in the DSM-IV, with the former alternative acknowledging its relationship with other schizophrenia spectrum disorders and the latter its emphasis on enduring and pathological personality characteristics. To accommodate both of these perspectives, it is proposed that DSM-IV STPD be listed on both axes, with its diagnostic code given on Axis I and its explication and diagnostic criteria presented on Axis II. This arrangement will also facilitate compatibility with ICD-10, which groups STPD with other schizophrenia-related disorders.

References

American Psychiatric Association: Diagnostic and Statistical Manual of Mental Disorders, 3rd Edition. Washington, DC, American Psychiatric Association, 1980

American Psychiatric Association: Diagnostic and Statistical Manual of Mental Disorders, 3rd Edition, Revised. Washington, DC, American Psychiatric Association, 1987

Baron M, Levitt M: Platelet monoamine oxidase activity: relation to genetic load of schizophrenia. Psychiatry Res 3:69–74, 1980

Baron M, Levitt M, Perlman R: Low platelet monoamine oxidase activity: a possible biochemical correlate of borderline schizophrenia. Psychiatry Res 3:329–335, 1980

Baron JM, Gruen R, Asnis L, et al: Familial relatedness of schizophrenia and schizophrenia and schizotypal states. Am J Psychiatry 140:1437–1442, 1983

Baron M, Gruen R, Rainer JD, et al: A family study of schizophrenic and normal control probands: implications for the spectrum concept of schizophrenia. Am J Psychiatry 142:447–454, 1985

Braff DL: Impaired speed of information processing in nonmedicated schizotypal patients. Schizophr Bull 7:499–508, 1986

Buchsbaum MS, Coursey RD, Murphy DL: The biochemical and high-risk paradigm: behavioral and familial correlates of low platelet monoamine oxidase activity. Science 193:339–341, 1976

Dahl A: Some aspects of the DSM-III personality disorders illustrated by a consecutive sample of hospitalized patients. Acta Psychiatr Scand Suppl 328:61–67, 1986

Davis KL, Davidson M, Mohs RC, et al: Plasma HVA concentrations correlate with the severity of schizophrenic illness. Science 227:1601–1602, 1985

Fenton TS, McGlashan TH: Risk of schizophrenia in character disordered patients. Am J Psychiatry 146:1280–1284, 1989

Frances A: Validating schizotypal personality disorders: problems with the schizophrenia connection. Schizophr Bull 11:595–597, 1985

Freiman K, Widiger T: Co-occurrence and diagnostic efficiency statistics. Unpublished raw data, Lexington, University of Kentucky, 1989

Frosch J: The Psychotic Process. New York, International Universities Press, 1983

Goldberg SC, Schulz SC, Schulz PM, et al: Borderline and schizotypal personality disorders treated with low-dose thiothixene vs. placebo. Arch Gen Psychiatry 43:680–686, 1986

Gunderson JG, Siever LJ, Spaulding E: The search for a schizotype: crossing the border again. Arch Gen Psychiatry 40:15–22, 1983

Hoch PH, Polatin P: Pseudoneurotic forms of schizophrenia. Psychiatr Q 23:248–276, 1949

Holzman PS, Solomon CM, Levin S, et al: Pursuit eye movement dysfunctions in schizophrenia. Arch Gen Psychiatry 41:136–140, 1984

Ingraham LJ: Genetic factors in schizophrenia and schizophrenia-like illness from a national sample of adopted individuals and their families. Abstracts of the 28th annual meeting of the American College of Neuropsychopharmacology, Las Vegas, NV, 1989

Jacobsberg L, Hymowitz P, Barasch A, et al: Symptoms of schizotypal personality. Am J Psychiatry 143:1222–1227, 1986

Kass F, Skodol AE, Charles E, et al: Scaled ratings of DSM-III personality disorders. Am J Psychiatry 142:627–630, 1985

Kendler K: Diagnostic approaches to schizotypal personality disorder: a historical perspective. Schizophr Bull 11:538–553, 1985

Kendler KS, Gruenberg AM, Strauss JS: An independent analysis of the Copenhagen sample of the Danish adoption study of schizophrenia. Arch Gen Psychiatry 38:982–987, 1981

Kendler KS, Gruenberg AM, Tsuang MT: Psychiatric illness in first degree relatives of schizophrenic and surgical control patients: a family study using DSM-III criteria. Arch Gen Psychiatry 42:770–779, 1985

Kendler KS, Walsh D, Su Y, et al: The Roscommon family and linkage study of schizophrenia: preliminary report. Abstracts of the 28th annual meeting of the American College of Neuropsychopharmacology, Las Vegas, NV, 1989

Kety SS, Rosenthal D, Wender PH, et al: Mental illness in the biological and adoptive families of adopted individuals who have become schizophrenic, in Genetic Research in Psychiatry. Edited by Fieve RR, Rosenthal D, Brill H. Baltimore, MD, Johns Hopkins University Press, 1975, pp 147–165

Klein DF: Importance of psychiatric diagnosis in prediction of clinical drug effects. Arch Gen Psychiatry 16:118–126, 1967

Knight RP: Management and psychotherapy of the borderline schizophrenic patient, in Psychoanalytic Psychiatry and Psychology. Edited by Knight RP, Friedman CR. New York, International Universities Press, 1954, pp 110–122

Lipton RB, Levin S, Holzman PS, et al: Eye movement dysfunctions in psychiatric patients: a review. Schizophr Bull 9:13–32, 1983

McGlashan TH: The borderline syndrome, II: is it a variant of schizophrenia or affective disorder? Arch Gen Psychiatry 40:1319–1323, 1983

McGlashan TH: Schizotypal personality disorder, Chestnut Lodge follow-up study, VI: long-term follow-up perspective. Arch Gen Psychiatry 43:329–334, 1986

McGlashan TH: Testing DSM-III symptom criteria for schizotypal and borderline personality disorders. Arch Gen Psychiatry 44:15–22, 1987

Millon T, Tringone R: Co-occurrence and diagnostic efficiency statistics. Unpublished raw data, Miami, FL, University of Miami, 1989

Morey L: Personality disorders in DSM-III and DSM-III-R: convergence, coverage, and internal consistency. Am J Psychiatry 145:573–577, 1988

Pfohl B, Stangl D, Zimmerman H: The implications of DSM III personality disorders for patients with major depression. J Affect Disord 7:299–315, 1984

Pfohl B, Coryell W, Zimmerman M, et al: DSM-III personality disorders: diagnostic overlap and internal consistency of individual DSM-III criteria. Compr Psychiatry 27:21–34, 1986

Pickar D, Labarca R, Doran A, et al: Longitudinal measurement of plasma homovanillic acid levels in schizophrenic patients. Arch Gen Psychiatry 43:669–676, 1986

Rifkin A, Quitkin F, Carrillo C: Lithium carbonate in emotionally unstable character disorder. Arch Gen Psychiatry 27:519–523, 1972

Schulz PM, Schulz SC, Goldberg SC, et al: Diagnoses of the relatives of schizotypal outpatients. J Nerv Ment Dis 174:457–463, 1986

Schulz PM, Soloff PH: Still borderline after all these years. Paper presented at the 140th annual meeting of the American Psychiatric Association, Chicago, IL, May 1987

Searles HF: Collected Papers on Schizophrenia and Related Subjects. New York, International Universities Press, 1965

Serban G, Siegel S: Response of borderline and schizotypal patients to small doses of thiothixene and haloperidol. Am J Psychiatry 141:1455–1458, 1984

Shelton RC, Weinberger DR: X-ray computerized tomography studies of schizophrenia: a review and synthesis, in The Neurology of Schizophrenia. Edited by Nasrallah HA, Weinberger DR. Amsterdam, Elsevier Science Publishers, 1986, pp 325–348

Siever LJ: Biological markers in schizotypal personality disorder. Schizophr Bull 11:564–575, 1985

Siever LJ, Gunderson JG: The search for a schizotypal personality: historical origins and current status. Compr Psychiatry 24:199–212, 1983

Siever LJ, Coursey RD, Alterman IS, et al: Impaired smooth pursuit eye movement: vulnerability markers for schizotypal personality disorder in a volunteer population. Am J Psychiatry 141:1560–1565, 1984

Siever LJ, Coccaro EF, Zemishlany Z, et al: Psychobiology of personality disorder: pharmacologic implications. Psychopharmacol Bull 23:333–336, 1987a

Siever LJ, Klar H, Coccaro EF, et al: Schizotypal and borderline personality overlap. Abstracts of the American Psychiatric Association, Chicago, IL, May 1987b

Siever LJ, Coursey RD, Alterman IS, et al: Clinical, psychophysiological, and neurological characteristics of volunteers with impaired smooth pursuit eye movements. Biol Psychiatry 26:35–51, 1989

Siever LJ, Keefe R, Bernstein DP, et al: Eye tracking impairment in clinically identified schizotypal personality disorder patients. Am J Psychiatry 147:740–745, 1990

Siever L, Amin F, Coccaro E, et al: Plasma homovanillic acid in schizotypal personality disorder. Am J Psychiatry 148:1246–1248, 1991

Silverman JM, Mohs RC, Siever LJ, et al: Heritability for schizophrenia-spectrum disorder in schizophrenia and schizophrenia-related personality disorder. Clin Neuropharmacol 9 (suppl 4):271–273, 1986

Silverman JM, Siever LJ, Mohs RC, et al: Risk for affective and personality disorders in relatives of personality disordered patients. Abstracts of the Society of Biological Psychiatry, 1987

Silverman JM, Siever LJ, Pinkham L, et al: Risk for affective, schizophrenia-related and personality disorders in relatives of depressed personality disordered patients. Abstracts of the annual convention of the Society of Biological Psychiatry, 1988

Simons RF: Electrodermal and cardiac orienting in psychometrically high risk subjects. Psychiatry Res 4:347–356, 1981

Simons RF: Physical anhedonia and future psychopathology: a possible electrocortical continuity. Psychophysiology 19:433–441, 1982

Skodol A: Co-occurrence and diagnostic efficiency statistics. Unpublished raw data, New York, New York State Psychiatric Institute, 1989

Soloff PH, Millward JW: Psychiatric disorders in the families of borderline patients. Arch Gen Psychiatry 40:37–44, 1983

Soloff PH, George A, Nathan RS: Progress in pharmacotherapy of borderline disorders. Arch Gen Psychiatry 43:698–700, 1986

Spitzer RL, Endicott J, Gibbon M: Crossing the border into borderline personality and borderline schizophrenia: the development of criteria. Arch Gen Psychiatry 36:17–24, 1979

Squires-Wheeler E, Skodol AE, Friedman D, et al: The specificity of DSM-III schizotypal personality traits. Psychol Med 18:757–765, 1988

Stone M: The borderline syndrome: evolution of the term, genetic aspects and prognosis. Am J Psychother 31:345–365, 1977

Stone M: Schizotypal personality psychotherapeutic aspects. Schizophr Bull 11:576–589, 1985

Torgerson S: Relationship of schizotypal personality disorder to schizophrenia: genetics. Schizophr Bull 11:554–563, 1985

Widiger TA, Frances A, Warner L, et al: Diagnostic criteria for the borderline and schizotypal personality disorders. J Abnorm Psychol 95:43–51, 1986

World Health Organization: ICD-10 Chapter V. Mental and Behavioral Disorders. Diagnostic Criteria for Research. Geneva, Switzerland, World Health Organization, 1990

Zanarini M, Frankenburg F, Chauncey D, et al: Co-occurrence and diagnostic efficiency statistics. Unpublished raw data, Boston, MA, McLean Hospital, 1989

Chapter 25

Antisocial Personality Disorder

Thomas A. Widiger, Ph.D., and Elizabeth M. Corbitt, Ph.D.

Statement and Significance of the Issues

The issues considered in this review are whether the DSM-III-R (American Psychiatric Association 1987) criteria for antisocial personality disorder (ASPD) should be revised 1) to place more emphasis on personality traits of psychopathy (or less emphasis on behaviorally specific acts) and 2) to be simpler to use.

The DSM-III (American Psychiatric Association 1980) and DSM-III-R criteria for ASPD have received more criticism than any other personality disorder diagnosis (e.g., Frances 1980; Gunderson 1983; Hare et al. 1991; Kernberg 1989; Millon 1981, 1983; Perry 1990; Reid 1987; Rogers and Dion 1991; Skodol 1989; Vaillant 1984; Wulach 1983). Much of this criticism has suggested that the ASPD criteria placed an overemphasis on overt criminal acts and related behaviors while neglecting more general personality traits of psychopathy and that this contributes to 1) a failure to adequately represent traditional concepts of psychopathy, 2) an overdiagnosis of ASPD in criminal and forensic settings, 3) an underdiagnosis of ASPD in various noncriminal settings, 4) difficulties in the differentiation of ASPD from substance use disorders, and 5) an overly complex and cumbersome criteria set.

Methods

We considered all papers and studies on ASPD identified through 1) prior reviews of the personality disorders, 2) a systematic review of the table of contents of 12 journals from 1988 to 1991, and 3) a Medline computer search confined to the

A more detailed version of this chapter is provided by Widiger and Corbitt (1993). We express our appreciation to Drs. Blum, Freiman, Heumann, Millon, Morey, Pfohl, Tringone, and Zanarini for providing unpublished data.

English language from 1980 to 1991 using the index term *antisocial personality disorder* (which identified 1,105 citations).

Results

Representation of Clinical Tradition

Hare et al. (1991), Kernberg (1989), Millon (1981, 1983), and others have suggested that the DSM-III and DSM-III-R criteria for ASPD are discrepant with historical and clinical tradition. The description of ASPD presented in DSM-II (American Psychiatric Association 1968) was closer to the original formulations of psychopathy developed by Cleckley (1941) and others than the DSM-III-R diagnostic criteria, and the DSM-III and DSM-III-R criteria were based primarily on the criteria sets developed by Feighner et al. (1972), Robins (1966), and Spitzer et al. (1978). Livesley et al. (1987) reported higher prototypicality ratings by the clinicians they surveyed for such traits as unstable interpersonal relationships, failure to learn from experience, disregard for consequences, egocentricity, manipulativeness, and disregard for the feelings of others than were obtained for many of the DSM-III ASPD criteria. Blashfield and Breen (1989) also suggested, on the basis of their survey, that clinicians do not consider such behaviorally specific items as unemployment for 6 months, traveling from place to place without a prearranged job, and a child's illness resulting from minimal hygiene to adequately reflect antisocial personality traits. Tennent et al. (1990) obtained ratings from British psychiatrists, psychologists, and probation officers. The items that were consistently rated as the most important and/or essential were an age at onset no later than the early 20s, impulsivity, pathological egocentricity, little response to special consideration or kindness, callous unconcern for others, behavior unaffected by punishment, lacking sense of responsibility, chronically or currently antisocial, inability to experience guilt, and unable to form meaningful relationships. Tennent et al. noted in particular that many of the DSM-III-R items "were not rated as being of any great help" (p. 44). Comparable results were obtained by Davies and Feldman (1981) in a survey of British forensic specialists.

Hare and associates reported weak convergent validity for the DSM-III and DSM-III-R ASPD criteria with global ratings of psychopathy across a series of studies (Hare 1991; Hare et al. 1991). DSM-III and DSM-III-R ASPD, however, has obtained at least adequate agreement between clinicians' diagnoses and semistructured and/or self-report inventory assessments (e.g., Hyler et al. 1989; Skodol et al. 1991), suggesting perhaps that the DSM-III and DSM-III-R criteria are consistent with clinicians' diagnoses. However, clinical diagnoses of ASPD could simply reflect an adherence to the official nomenclature rather than clinicians' preferred formulations.

Overdiagnosis Within Prison and Forensic Settings

Most of the critiques of DSM-III and DSM-III-R ASPD have suggested that the criteria set results in an overdiagnosis of ASPD within criminal and forensic settings. Frances (1980) and Wulach (1983) cited Guze et al. (1969) as indicating that 80% of criminals would be diagnosed with ASPD. Guze et al. followed 223 convicted male felons from 1959 through 1968; of these, 79% met their research criteria for "sociopathy" at intake (but on follow-up only 52% of the remaining 176 subjects continued to meet the same criteria). The criteria for sociopathy used by Guze et al. do have a historical relation to DSM-III and DSM-III-R ASPD, but they are also more inclusive than DSM-III and DSM-III-R. The Guze et al. criteria consist of a history of police trouble (other than traffic arrests) plus any two of five items (history of excessive fighting, school delinquency, poor job record, period of wanderlust, or running away from home; prostitution could substitute for any of these five for female subjects).

Hare (1980) reported that 76% of 146 prison inmates satisfied (initial draft) DSM-III criteria for ASPD, compared to only 33% who met research criteria for psychopathy. In three subsequent studies (Hare 1983, 1985; Hart and Hare 1989), Hare and colleagues reported prevalence rates of 50%, 49%, and 50% for ASPD within prison settings using the DSM-III and DSM-III-R criteria, compared to 35%, 33%, and 12.5%, respectively, using the Psychopathy Checklist (PCL) and Psychopathology Checklist-Revised (PCL-R) (Hare 1991). Hare (1991) summarized the association of the PCL and the PCL-R with DSM-III and DSM-III-R across 10 data sets (all prison or forensic settings). The point-biserial correlation of the ASPD diagnoses with total PCL or PCL-R scores varied between .54 and .63 for 7 of the data sets (each with a sample size greater than 100). The lowest correlations occurred with the smaller samples. The two lowest findings were point-biserial correlations of only .13 and .08, and in both cases, the base rate for ASPD was around 80%. Cote and Hodgins (1990) administered the Diagnostic Interview Schedule (DIS) (Robins et al. 1981) to a random sample of 495 male inmates of Quebec penitentiaries. ASPD was diagnosed in 61.5% of these subjects. Similar findings were reported by Bland et al. (1990).

Robins et al. (1991) suggested that, if the criticism that ASPD "medicalizes" criminality were warranted, then most persons with an ASPD diagnosis would have a criminal history. On the basis of the National Institute of Mental Health (NIMH) Epidemiologic Catchment Area (ECA) data, they reported that only 47% of those who met the DSM-III ASPD criteria had a significant arrest record ($N = 628$). "Rather than criminality, the adult symptoms that typify the antisocial personality are job troubles (found in 94%), violence (found in 85%), multiple moving traffic offenses (found in 72%), and severe marital difficulties (desertion, multiple separations or divorces, multiple infidelities, found in 67%)" (p. 260). In addition, the occurrence of a significant arrest record was not predictive of an ASPD diagnosis. Only 37% of those with multiple non-traffic arrests (40% for males) met the DSM-III ASPD criteria. The ECA sample also included prisoners, and based on these data, Robins et al. suggested that "only about half of all prison residents meet criteria for the DSM-III ASPD disorder" (p. 289). This prevalence estimate within a prison setting is comparable to the results reported by Hare (1983, 1985), but Robins et al. suggested that a 50% base rate for ASPD within a prison is within theoretical and clinical expectations.

Underdiagnosis Within Other Nonclinical Settings

Critical reviews of the DSM-III and DSM-III-R ASPD criteria have also suggested that the behaviorally specific criteria may contribute to an underdiagnosis of ASPD/psychopathy within nonclinical settings other than prison and forensic institutions. To the extent that the DSM-III and DSM-III-R criteria emphasize criminal and delinquent activity, psychopathic persons who operate within the letter of the law would not be diagnosed as having an antisocial personality disorder.

However, there are few empirical data that pertain directly to this hypothesis. Robins et al. (1984) reported an ASPD lifetime prevalence of 2.1%, 2.6%, and 3.3% in three of the ECA sites (New Haven, CT; Baltimore, MD; and St. Louis, MO; respectively). Bland et al. (1988) reported a lifetime rate of 3.7% based on a sample of 3,258 Edmonton, Alberta, Canada, urban community residents. Regier et al. (1988) reported 1-month prevalence rates from five ECA sites of .3% (New Haven), .5% (Baltimore), .8% (St. Louis), .4% (Durham, NC), and .4% (Los Angeles, CA). Zimmerman and Coryell (1989) reported that 3.3% of 797 relatives of patients and normal subjects met the DSM-III criteria for ASPD, the highest rate for any personality disorder. Interpretation of these findings, however, is complicated by the absence of any theoretical or clinical consensus for what the rate of psychopathy/ASPD should be within a community.

Widom (1977) lamented sometime ago that "we have no knowledge of the extent to which psychopathy remains undetected in the general population or even whether the concept is a meaningful one outside the prison or psychiatric hospital" (p. 675). She therefore placed advertisements in a Boston counterculture newspaper seeking, for example, "adventurous carefree people who've led exciting impulsive lives" (p. 675). Seventy-three persons responded, and 28–30 subjects participated in a series of tests and interviews. The psychopaths she identified, however, may not have been appreciably different from those who would be sampled in clinical or prison settings. Of these, 61% reported some form of psychiatric experience, 46% had been in outpatient treatment, 21% had been inpatients, and 29% had a history of suicide attempts. They were somewhat distinct from a prison/forensic sample. Although 74% had been arrested, only 18% of those arrested had ever been convicted (50% had been incarcerated but only 25% for longer than 2 weeks). Of most interest to this review, however, was the finding that 79% met the Robins (1966) criteria for the diagnosis of sociopathy (e.g., 79% had a poor work history, 68% used excessive drugs, and 43% had school problems or truancy). Similar results were provided in a subsequent report by Widom and Newman (1985). One qualification to these findings, however, is that the Robins criteria may have influenced the selection of subjects.

Sutker and Allain (1983) used the Minnesota Multiphasic Personality Inventory (MMPI) (Hathaway and McKinley 1970) to identify "adaptive sociopaths" within a medical student population. Only 2.4% of the 450 students met the MMPI criteria for sociopathy; 8 of the male sociopaths were studied in more detail. None of them met the DSM-III criteria for ASPD, although 5 of them did meet the ASPD conduct disorder criterion. Before the age of 15 years, 50% had repeated sexual intercourse in a casual relationship (versus none of 8 comparison males), 63% acknowledged vandalism (versus 25%), 63% acknowledged chronic violations of rules at home and/or at school (versus 13%), and 50% acknowledged the initiation of fights (versus 0%). By adulthood, at least half admitted to difficulties in maintaining an enduring sexual relationship, honoring financial obligations, and refraining from recklessness, and 88% admitted to being arrested (versus 25% of the comparison males), but none of the subjects met a sufficient number of criteria to receive a DSM-III ASPD diagnosis. Sutker and Allain suggested that these were indeed psychopathic persons who exhibited (in laboratory testing) impulsive errors, disregard for details of instruction, and exaggerated needs for excitement seeking, but that "strong desires for the rewards often associated with respectable professional status motivated and sustained adaptiveness" (p. 77).

Coolidge et al. (1990) assessed the prevalence of the DSM-III-R criteria for ASPD among purportedly normal college students. In one study, 39% of 89 males met the DSM-III-R conduct disorder criteria, and in the other, 5% of 170 males met the full ASPD criteria and 37% met the conduct disorder criteria. These findings are opposite to the concern that the behaviorally specific DSM-III-R ASPD criteria would underdiagnose ASPD in nonclinical, noncriminal settings, but they may also reflect limitations of the self-report methodology. For example, 34% of the male subjects answered true to the item of deliberately destroying property before age 15. It is possible that further inquiry would have indicated that the destruction was inconsequential and normative.

Additional research is necessary to determine whether the DSM-III-R ASPD criteria would or should identify the successful and/or adaptive psychopath.

Widom (1977) suggested that her approach was useful in identifying "the more 'successful' psychopath who may be arrested frequently but convicted infrequently" (p. 682). However, one might question whether these persons were really successful given their history of inpatient and/or outpatient treatment, history of arrests, difficulties in school, suicide attempts, and poor work history. A psychopathic lawyer, politician, or businessperson without a significant history of unemployment, childhood conduct disorder, arrests, and defaults on debts would probably fail to meet the DSM-III-R ASPD criteria, but it is then questionable whether these persons should receive a mental disorder diagnosis. The threshold for the diagnosis of a personality disorder is largely arbitrary and difficult to define, and it will be of particular interest in future research to explore whether the successful, adaptive psychopath does indeed have a clinically significant personality disorder.

Differentiation of ASPD From Substance Use Disorders

A variety of studies have indicated a substantial association of ASPD with various substance use disorders (Grande et al. 1984). Interpretation of this research, however, has been complicated by the questionable independence of the diagnoses (Gerstley et al. 1990).

For example, the DSM-III-R ASPD diagnosis includes an inability to sustain consistent work behavior, failure to conform to social norms with respect to lawful behavior, failure to honor financial obligations, failure to plan ahead, recklessness in regard to safety, and inability to function as a responsible parent. The DSM-III-R diagnosis of substance dependence includes hazardous behavior, theft, and the failure to fulfill major role obligations at home, school, or work. Some of the diagnostic criteria are almost equivalent; as a result, it is difficult to determine which (if any) direction of causality has occurred when one assesses the covariation of the presence of at least 4 of any of the 10 adult antisocial criteria (the threshold for an ASPD diagnosis), with at least 3 of any of the 9 substance dependence criteria (the threshold for the substance dependence diagnosis), even with the requirement of the childhood antisocial criterion.

In using the Research Diagnostic Criteria (RDC) for ASPD (Spitzer et al. 1978), raters count only those manifestations of ASPD that cannot clearly be attributed to a drug use disorder. In DSM-III, it was stated that the ASPD criteria would count "regardless of the extent to which some of the antisocial behavior may be a consequence of the Substance Use Disorder, e.g., illegal selling of drugs, or the assaultive behavior associated with Alcohol Intoxication" (p. 319). No revision to this statement occurred in DSM-III-R. Williams and Spitzer (1982) suggested that the RDC and DSM-III ASPD criteria sets would identify virtually the same group of persons. Hesselbrock et al. (1982) did report a kappa of .79 for the agreement between RDC and DSM-III (assessed by the DIS) in a sample of 42 alcoholic inpatients, but Hasin and Grant (1987) reported a kappa of only .05 in a sample of 120 substance abuse patients. Rounsaville et al. (1983), however, reported that 54% of 533 opiate dependents met the DSM-III criteria for ASPD, whereas only 27% did so with the RDC. Rounsaville et al. concluded "that the key difference in the two systems . . . is in the RDC requirement that antisocial activity be independent of the need to obtain drugs" (p. 38). Woody et al. (1985) likewise reported that 45% of their 110 opiate-dependent subjects met the DSM-III criteria for ASPD, but only 19% met the RDC criteria.

Alterman and Cacciola (1991) and Gerstley et al. (1990) suggested that the DSM-III and DSM-III-R ASPD criteria overdiagnose ASPD in substance use patients due to a "focus on behavioral patterns rather than underlying personality dynamics" (Gerstley et al. 1990, p. 173) (as well as the absence of an exclusion criterion to rule out substance abuse). They recommended, as an alternative, using the Psychopathy Checklist, which places relatively more emphasis on psychopathic personality traits. Additional emphasis on more general traits (e.g., lack of remorse or guilt, superficial charm, and callous lack of empathy) would presumably be more successful in assessing antisocial/psychopathic personality traits independent of a substance use disorder than an emphasis on more specific behaviors (e.g., the DSM-III-R item for being reckless regarding safety as indicated by driving while intoxicated). On the other hand, it is also possible that, in the assessment of such personality traits as manipulativeness, poor behavior control, and proneness to boredom (Hare 1991), one might still use specific acts and behaviors (e.g., driving while intoxicated) that are secondary to a substance use disorder (Widiger and Shea 1991). Cooney et al. (1990) compared the DIS ASPD and the PCL psychopathy assessments in a sample of 118 alcoholic inpatients. The point-biserial correlation between total PCL scores and DIS ASPD diagnoses was insignificant ($r = .14$). These results, however, may not have been due to an overdiagnosis of ASPD by the DIS, because only 25% of the subjects met the DSM-III criteria.

Complexity of the DSM-III and DSM-III-R ASPD Criteria Set

Hare et al. (1991), Rogers and Dion (1991), and Vaillant (1984) have suggested that the increased behavioral specificity of the ASPD criteria has been problematic to clinical utility. It is no coincidence that the criteria set that is the most specific is also the longest and most complex. The DSM-III-R ASPD criteria set consists of 10 adult items and 1 childhood item, with the childhood item including 12 subitems. Three of the 10 adult items also involve subitems (parental irresponsibility includes 6 subitems). A diagnosis of ASPD therefore involves the consideration of 30 items.

The DSM-III and DSM-III-R criteria for ASPD may have been constructed primarily for the benefit and concerns of the researcher rather than for the practicing clinician (Frances et al. 1990). Researchers will have little difficulty with lengthy and complex criteria sets, but it is unlikely that clinicians could adhere closely to the DSM-III-R ASPD criteria during routine clinical practice. A systematic and comprehensive assessment of the personality disorders can require 2 hours of interviewing; as a result, clinicians may often fail to closely follow the criteria when making their diagnoses (Morey and Ochoa 1989). Ford and Widiger (1989) suggested that sex biases in the diagnosis of ASPD were due in part to a failure of clinicians to adhere closely to the diagnostic criteria.

One might be able to simplify the ASPD criteria by deleting or collapsing items to construct a more practical and user-friendly set that would not result in any change in who is diagnosed. For example, in studies of the DSM-III-R ASPD criteria by Freiman and Widiger (1989), Millon and Tringone (1989), Morey and Heumann (1988), and Pfohl and Blum (1990), the item with the lowest correlation with the diagnosis of ASPD was typically irresponsibility as a parent (phi coefficients equal to .03, −.03, .22, and −.02, respectively), due in large part to its low sensitivity (e.g., it cannot be scored if the person is not a parent and it is difficult to document as present when the person is a parent). The next worst item was usually failure to sustain a monogamous relationship (phi coefficients equal to .04, .13, .25, and −.03, respectively). The worst-performing item in a study by Zanarini et al. (1989) using DSM-III criteria was also irresponsibility as a parent (phi coefficient = .27). It is conceivable that this item (and others) could be deleted without significantly affecting who receives the diagnosis.

Simplification without any effect on diagnosis would appear to be an unassailable proposal. On the other hand, if specific criteria do provide an overly narrow representation of the construct (Hare et al. 1991), resulting in the need to include a substantial number of items to fully represent the construct, it may not be possible to reduce the number of items without affecting the diagnosis. A brief list of very specific items would provide an even more narrow representation of psychopathy than is provided by the 30 DSM-III-R items.

Empirical support for the perception that the DSM-III and DSM-III-R criteria set is cumbersome and unwieldy may also be somewhat limited. The finding that ASPD is the only personality disorder diagnosis to consistently obtain adequate to good levels of interrater reliability in routine clinical practice and adequate to good convergent validity with semistructured interview and self-report assessments (Hyler et al. 1989; Skodol et al. 1991) suggests that practicing clinicians may be able to use the criteria set in a consistent and valid manner. Robins et al. (1981) compared lay diagnoses of ASPD using the DIS with psychiatrists' ASPD diagnoses using DSM-III criteria and reported that the psychiatrists did not feel constrained or dissatisfied with the specific and explicit criteria (in only 7% of 204 cases did they indicate doubts about their diagnoses).

Morey and Ochoa (1989) reported that clinicians' diagnoses were often in disagreement with the diagnoses that would be given if the diagnoses had been based on the same clinicians' own assessments of each of the DSM-III personality disorder criteria. This disagreement was lowest for the borderline and antisocial diagnoses (the clinicians diagnosed 6.8% of 291 cases with ASPD, whereas 5.8% would be diagnosed with ASPD based on their ratings of the ASPD criteria; kappa = 53, $P < .001$), but Morey and Ochoa (1989) did conclude that "a history of criminal acts may lead a diagnostician to assign the antisocial diagnosis even though other criteria are not met" (p. 190). In other words, clinicians may not find the criteria set to be particularly cumbersome because they focus on only a subset of the criteria (e.g., overt criminal acts), resulting in the high reliability, consistent usage, and convergent validity with other measures that have a similar emphasis.

Discussion

A review of the empirical literature does provide support for some of the criticisms regarding DSM-III-R ASPD. The two most viable alternatives to the DSM-III-R ASPD criteria set are provided by the PCL-R (Hare 1991) and the ICD-10 research criteria for dyssocial personality disorder (World Health Organization 1990), both of which place more emphasis on such personality traits as lack of remorse or guilt, callous lack of empathy, and failure to accept responsibility for one's actions.

Compatibility with the forthcoming ICD-10 is both desirable and to some extent necessary (Frances et al. 1990). Deviations from the international nomenclature should at least be supported by empirical documentation. This concern is particularly important in the case of ASPD, given the relatively greater emphasis that the ICD-10 will place on personality traits of psychopathy. Hare and his colleagues have consistently obtained good to excellent interrater reliability in the assessment of these traits (Hare 1991; Hare et al. 1991), a finding replicated by independent researchers (e.g., Raine 1985; Smith and Newman 1990). There is also substantial empirical support for the PCL and PLC-R formulation of psychopathy (Hare 1991; Hart et al., in press). For example, Hart et al. (1988) reported that the PCL was more predictive of recidivism subsequent to prison release than the DSM-III ASPD diagnosis. The PCL predicted postrelease behavior in their sample of 231 federal offenders even when prior criminal history, previous conditional-release violations, and demographic variables were controlled. Similar findings were reported by Serin et al. (1990). Laboratory tests of hypothesized correlates of psychopathy, including abnormal processing of the affective components of language, selective attention, and disinhibition and passive-avoidance learning have also consistently supported the construct validity of the PCL(-R) (Hart et al., in press).

However, the research reviewed above concerning the overdiagnosis, under-diagnosis, and differential diagnosis of DSM-III and DSM-III-R ASPD has not been consistently negative. In addition, DSM-III and DSM-III-R ASPD has substantial empirical support, including epidemiological, psychophysiological, longitudinal, childhood antecedent, family history, and treatment studies (Robins et al. 1991; Sutker et al. 1993). Research cited in support of the DSM-III and DSM-III-R diagnosis has at times concerned studies that used previous and/or alternative diagnostic criteria, but the empirical support includes many studies that used the DSM-III, DSM-III-R, or comparable criteria (e.g., Cadoret et al. 1985; Grove et al. 1990; Lewis et al. 1985; Regier et al. 1988; Robins et al. 1984). Finally, DSM-III and DSM-III-R ASPD is the only personality disorder to consistently obtain at least adequate to good levels of interrater reliability in clinical practice (Mellsop et al. 1982). Any revision of the ASPD criteria set that required more subjective judgment and inferences could undermine the most clinically reliable personality disorder diagnosis (Skodol et al. 1991).

Recommendations

The proposals to simplify the ASPD criteria and to place more emphasis on psychopathic personality traits are reasonable options to consider for DSM-IV. They are responsive to criticisms of DSM-III and DSM-III-R ASPD and to the empirical literature. However, the threshold for revisions to the nomenclature are necessarily higher for DSM-IV than was the case for DSM-III or DSM-III-R (Frances et al. 1990). The DSM-III-R criteria set for ASPD is lengthy and complex and fails to provide substantial representation of the personality traits of psycho pathy included within the ICD-10 and the PCL-R, but it has performed well in clinical practice, it is supported by empirical data, and any revision would likely be disruptive to both research and clinical practice. It is therefore particularly important to field test any proposed revisions to document that the proposed revisions do in fact represent an improvement. The field trial being conducted for DSM-IV is comparing four criteria sets: 1) the current DSM-III-R ASPD criteria; 2) a simplified version (generated through item analyses of the current criteria set); 3) the seven-item research criteria for the ICD-10 dyssocial personality disorder; and 4) a 10-item criteria set developed through data reanalyses of the PCL-R by Hare et al. (1991) (i.e., glib and superficial, inflated and arrogant self-appraisal, lacks remorse, lacks empathy, deceitful and manipulative, early behavior problems, adult antisocial behavior, impulsive, poor behavioral controls, and irresponsible). Details regarding the field trial are provided in Widiger et al. (1991).

References

Alterman AI, Cacciola JS: The antisocial personality disorder diagnosis in substance abusers: problems and issues. J Nerv Ment Dis 179:401–409, 1991

American Psychiatric Association: Diagnostic and Statistical Manual of Mental Disorders, 2nd Edition. Washington, DC, American Psychiatric Association, 1968

American Psychiatric Association: Diagnostic and Statistical Manual of Mental Disorders, 3rd Edition. Washington, DC, American Psychiatric Association, 1980

American Psychiatric Association: Diagnostic and Statistical Manual of Mental Disorders, 3rd Edition, Revised. Washington, DC, American Psychiatric Association, 1987

Bland RC, Orn H, Newman SC: Lifetime prevalence of psychiatric disorders in Edmonton. Acta Psychiatr Scand 77:24–32, 1988

Bland RC, Newman SC, Dyck RJ, et al: Prevalence of psychiatric disorders and suicide attempts in a prison population. Can J Psychiatry 35:407–413, 1990

Blashfield RK, Breen MJ: Face validity of the DSM-III-R personality disorders. Am J Psychiatry 146:1575–1579, 1989

Cadoret RJ, O'Gorman TW, Troughton E, et al: Alcoholism and antisocial personality: interrelationships, genetic and environmental factors. Arch Gen Psychiatry 42:161–167, 1985

Cleckley H: The Mask of Sanity. St. Louis, MO, Mosby, 1941

Coolidge FL, Merwin MM, Wooley MJ, et al: Some problems with the diagnostic criteria of the antisocial personality disorder in DSM-III-R: a preliminary study. Journal of Personality Disorders 4:407–413, 1990

Cooney NL, Kadden RM, Litt MD: A comparison of methods for assessing sociopathy in male and female alcoholics. J Stud Alcohol 51:42–48, 1990

Cote G, Hodgins S: Co-occurring mental disorders among criminal offenders. Bull Am Acad Psychiatry Law 18:271–281, 1990

Davies W, Feldman P: The diagnosis of psychopathy by forensic specialists. Br J Psychiatry 138:329–331, 1981

Feighner JP, Robins E, Guze SB, et al: Diagnostic criteria for use in psychiatric research. Arch Gen Psychiatry 26:57–63, 1972

Ford MR, Widiger TA: Sex bias in the diagnosis of histrionic and antisocial personality disorders. J Consult Clin Psychol 57:301–305, 1989

Frances AJ: The DSM-III personality disorders section: a commentary. Am J Psychiatry 137:1050–1054, 1980

Frances AJ, Pincus HA, Widiger TA, et al: DSM-IV: work in progress. Am J Psychiatry 147:1439–1448, 1990

Freiman K, Widiger TA: Co-occurrence and diagnostic efficiency statistics. Unpublished raw data, Lexington, University of Kentucky, 1989

Gerstley LJ, Alterman AI, McLellan AT, et al: Antisocial personality disorder in patients with substance abuse disorders: a problematic diagnosis? Am J Psychiatry 147:173–178, 1990

Grande TP, Wolf AW, Schubert DS, et al: Associations among alcoholism, drug abuse, and antisocial personality: a review of the literature. Psychol Rep 55:455–474, 1984

Grove WM, Eckert ED, Heston L, et al: Heritability of substance abuse and antisocial behavior: a study of monozygotic twins reared apart. Biol Psychiatry 27:1293–1304, 1990

Gunderson JG: DSM-III diagnoses of personality disorders, in Current Perspectives on Personality Disorders. Edited by Frosch J. Washington, DC, American Psychiatric Press, 1983, pp 20–39

Guze SB, Goodwin DW, Crane JB: Criminality and psychiatric disorders. Arch Gen Psychiatry 20:583–591, 1969

Hare RD: A research scale for the assessment of psychopathy in criminal populations. Personality and Individual Differences 1:111–117, 1980

Hare RD: Diagnosis of antisocial personality disorder in two prison populations. Am J Psychiatry 140:887–890, 1983

Hare RD: A comparison of procedures for the assessment of psychopathy. J Consult Clin Psychol 53:7–16, 1985

Hare RD: The Hare Psychopathy Checklist-Revised. Toronto, Multi-Health Systems, 1991

Hare RD, Hart SD, Harpur TJ: Psychopathy and the DSM-IV criteria for antisocial personality disorder. J Abnorm Psychol 100:391–398, 1991

Hart SD, Hare RD: Discriminant validity of the Psychopathy Checklist in a forensic psychiatric population. Psychol Assess: J Consult Clin Psychol 1:211–218, 1989

Hart SD, Kropp PR, Hare RD: Performance of male psychopaths following conditional release from prison. J Consult Clin Psychol 56:227–232, 1988

Hart SD, Hare RD, Harpur TJ: The Psychopathy Checklist: an overview for researchers and clinicians, in Advances in Psychological Assessment, Vol 8. Edited by Rosen J, McReynolds P. New York, Plenum (in press)

Hasin DS, Grant BF: Psychiatric diagnosis of patients with substance abuse problems: a comparison of two procedures, the DIS and the SADS-L. J Psychiatr Res 21:7–22, 1987

Hathaway SR, McKinley JC: Minnesota Multiphasic Personality Inventory, Revised. Minneapolis, University of Minnesota, 1970

Hesselbrock V, Stabenau J, Hesselbrock MN, et al: A comparison of two interview schedules. Arch Gen Psychiatry 39:674–677, 1982

Hyler SE, Rieder RO, Williams JBW, et al: A comparison of clinical and self-report diagnoses of DSM-III personality disorders in 552 patients. Compr Psychiatry 30:170–178, 1989

Kernberg OF: The narcissistic personality disorder and the differential diagnosis of antisocial behavior. Psychiatr Clin North Am 12:553–570, 1989

Lewis CE, Rice J, Andreasen N, et al: Alcoholism in antisocial and nonantisocial men with unipolar major depression. J Affect Disord 9:253–263, 1985

Livesley WJ, Reiffer LI, Sheldon AER, et al: Prototypicality ratings of DSM-III criteria for personality disorders. J Nerv Ment Dis 175:395–401, 1987

Mellsop G, Varghese FTN, Joshua S, et al: Reliability of Axis II of DSM-III. Am J Psychiatry 139:1360–1361, 1982

Millon T: Disorders of Personality, DSM-III: Axis II. New York, Wiley, 1981

Millon T: The DSM-III: an insider's perspective. Am Psychol 38:804–818, 1983

Millon T, Tringone R: Co-occurrence and diagnostic efficiency statistics. Unpublished raw data, Miami, FL, University of Miami, 1989

Morey L, Heumann K: Co-occurrence and diagnostic efficiency statistics. Unpublished raw data, Nashville, TN, Vanderbilt University, 1988

Morey LC, Ochoa ES: An investigation of adherence to diagnostic criteria: clinical diagnosis of the DSM-III personality disorders. Journal of Personality Disorders 3:180–192, 1989

Perry JC: Challenges in validating personality disorders: beyond description. Journal of Personality Disorders 4:273–289, 1990

Pfohl B, Blum N: Internal consistency statistics for the DSM-III-R personality disorder criteria. Unpublished raw data, Iowa City, University of Iowa, 1990

Raine A: A psychometric assessment of Hare's checklist for psychopathy on an English prison population. Br J Clin Psychol 24:247–258, 1985

Regier DA, Boyd JH, Burke JD, et al: One-month prevalence of mental disorders in the United States. Arch Gen Psychiatry 45:977–986, 1988

Reid WH: Antisocial personality, in Psychiatry. Edited by Michels R, Cavenar JO. Philadelphia, PA, JB Lippincott, 1987, pp 1–13

Robins LN: Deviant Children Grown Up. Baltimore, MD, Williams & Wilkins, 1966

Robins LN, Helzer JE, Croughan J, et al: The NIMH Diagnostic Interview Schedule: its history, characteristics, and validity. Arch Gen Psychiatry 38:381–389, 1981

Robins LN, Helzer JE, Weissman MM, et al: Lifetime prevalence of specific psychiatric disorders in three sites. Arch Gen Psychiatry 41:949–958, 1984

Robins LN, Tipp J, Przybeck T: Antisocial personality, in Psychiatric Disorders in America. Edited by Robins LN, Regier D. New York, Free Press, 1991, pp 258–290

Rogers R, Dion K: Rethinking the DSM-III-R diagnosis of antisocial personality disorder. Bull Am Acad Psychiatry Law 19:21–31, 1991

Rounsaville BJ, Eyre SL, Weissman MM, et al: The antisocial opiate addict, in Psychosocial Constructs: Alcoholism and Substance Abuse. Edited by Stimmeo B. New York, Haworth Press, 1983, pp 29–42

Serin R, Peters RD, Barbaree HE: Predictors of psychopathy and release outcome in a criminal population. Psychol Assess: J Consult Clin Psychol 2:419–422, 1990

Skodol AE: Problems in Differential Diagnosis: From DSM-III to DSM-III-R in Clinical Practice. Washington, DC, American Psychiatric Press, 1989

Skodol AE, Oldham JM, Rosnick L, et al: Diagnosis of DSM-III-R personality disorders: a comparison of two structured interviews. Methods in Psychiatric Research 1:13–26, 1991

Smith SS, Newman JP: Alcohol and drug abuse-dependence disorders in psychopathic and nonpsychopathic criminal offenders. J Abnorm Psychol 99:430–439, 1990

Spitzer RL, Endicott J, Robins E: Research diagnostic criteria: rationale and reliability. Arch Gen Psychiatry 35:773–778, 1978

Sutker PB, Allain AN: Behavior and personality assessment in men labeled adaptive sociopaths. J Behav Assess 5:65–79, 1983

Sutker PB, Bugg F, West JA: Antisocial personality disorder, in Comprehensive Handbook of Psychopathology, 2nd Edition. Edited by Sutker PB, Adams H. New York, Plenum, 1993, pp 337–369

Tennent G, Tennent D, Prins H, et al: Psychopathic disorder: a useful clinical concept? Med Sci Law 30:39–44, 1990

Vaillant GE: The disadvantages of DSM-III outweigh its advantages. Am J Psychiatry 141:542–545, 1984

Widiger TA, Corbitt EM: Antisocial personality disorder: proposals for DSM-IV. Journal of Personality Disorders 7:63–77, 1993

Widiger TA, Shea T: Differentiation of Axis I and Axis II disorders. J Abnorm Psychol 100:399–406, 1991

Widiger TA, Frances AJ, Pincus HA, et al: Toward an empirical classification for the DSM-IV. J Abnorm Psychol 100:280–288, 1991

Widom CS: A methodology for studying noninstitutionalized psychopaths. J Consult Clin Psychol 45;674–683, 1977

Widom CS, Newman JP: Characteristics of noninstitutionalized psychopaths, in Current Research in Forensic Psychiatry and Psychology, Vol 2. Edited by Gunn J, Farrington D. New York, Wiley, 1985, pp 57–80

Williams JBW, Spitzer RL: Research Diagnostic Criteria and DSM-III: an annotated comparison. Arch Gen Psychiatry 39:1283–1289, 1982

Woody GE, McLellan AT, Luborsky L, et al: Sociopathy and psychotherapy outcome. Arch Gen Psychiatry 42:1081–1086, 1985

World Health Organization: ICD-10 Chapter V. Mental and Behavioral Disorders. Diagnostic Criteria for Research. Geneva, Switzerland, World Health Organization, 1990

Wulach JS: Diagnosing the DSM-III antisocial personality disorder. Prof Psychol Res Pract 14:330–340, 1983

Zanarini M, Frankenburg F, Chauncey D, et al: Co-occurrence and diagnostic efficiency statistics. Unpublished raw data, Boston, MA, McLean Hospital, 1989

Zimmerman M, Coryell W: DSM-III personality disorder diagnoses in a nonpatient sample. Arch Gen Psychiatry 46:682–689, 1989

Chapter 26

Borderline Personality Disorder

John Gunderson, M.D., Mary C. Zanarini, Ed.D., and
Cassandra L. Kisiel, B.A.

In this chapter, we review the available literature and data that bear on the question of whether the DSM-III-R (American Psychiatric Association 1987) criteria for borderline personality disorder (BPD) should undergo change for DSM-IV. A more extended version of this review is provided by Gunderson et al. (1991). The emphasis is on empirical evidence assembled since the introduction of this category in DSM-III (American Psychiatric Association 1980), but the review necessarily moves into the earlier literature that led to the recognition of the disorder and into the nonempirical resources offered by the accumulated expertise of advisers. Questions of revision need to reconcile the value of sustaining an existing definition of BPD that has now received partial validation with the value of modifications that might better reflect the BPD construct.

Statement and Significance of the Issues

The following issues are addressed in this chapter:

1. Is the diagnosis distinct from other disorders? (Gunderson 1984; Nurnberg et al. 1987; Zanarini et al. 1990b)
2. Are the criteria effective in identifying this disorder? (Nurnberg et al. 1987; Pfohl et al. 1986; Widiger and Frances 1989; Zanarini et al. 1990b)
3. Do the criteria accurately identify the intended constructs? (Morey and Ochoa 1989; Pfohl et al. 1986; Zanarini et al. 1990b, 1991)

Appreciation is due to Drs. Freiman, Goodman, Millon, Morey, Skodol, Tringone, Trull, Widiger, and Zanarini for providing access to their unpublished data.

4. Are the criteria congruent with the descriptive literature? (Gunderson 1984; Widiger and Frances 1989)
5. Are the polythetic format and current threshold appropriate? (Widiger and Frances 1989; Widiger et al. 1986b)
6. Should the essential feature be altered? (Gunderson and Zanarini 1987)

Methods

Potential sources were identified through a computer search of all English language journal articles published between 1975 and 1990 using the index terms *borderline personality, borderline conditions,* and *borderline states,* a review of the table of contents over the past 8 years of 15 major psychiatry and psychology journals, and a review of major review articles and books (e.g., Gunderson 1984; Gunderson and Zanarini 1987; Skodol and Spitzer 1987). From the resulting list of approximately 1,300 articles, chapters, or books, the sources were reduced by deleting those that concerned primarily children and/or adolescents, that were not empirical, that sampled fewer than five cases, or that failed to address descriptive issues. In reports that involved identical or overlapping data sets (approximately 7% of the total), preference was given to the results based on the largest sample size and to results based on DSM-III-R criteria. In addition, researchers who had developed structured interviews for the diagnosis of the DSM-III or DSM-III-R personality disorders and/or those who had previously published research on the performance characteristics of the criteria were solicited to offer us access to any relevant descriptive validity data that had not yet been published. Table 1 in the introduction to this section gives background information on the major data sources that are used in this review to address the issues of overlap and diagnostic efficiency.

In addition to these efforts to canvas the relevant data and literature, input from a range of advisers was invited (see Table 26–1). Efforts were made to include individuals with varied professional, conceptual, and clinical orientations.

Results and Discussion

Is the Diagnosis Distinct From Other Disorders?

The comorbidity with other Axis II disorders observed in 10 samples of borderline patients indicates that BPD was rarely the only personality disorder diagnosis. The percentage of cases with a single diagnosis ranged from a low of 3% (Dahl 1986) to a high of only 10% (Millon and Tringone 1989; Pfohl et al. 1986).

Table 26–1. Advisers for borderline personality disorder

Gerald Adler	Paul Links
Salman Akhtar	Michael Lyons
Lorna Smith Benjamin	James Masterson
Mark Berelowitz	Thomas McGlashan
Roger Blashfield	Leslie Morey
John Clarkin	Joel Paris
Alv Dahl	Christopher Perry
John Frosch	James Reich
Judith Herman	Kenneth Silk
Jeffrey Jonas	Paul Soloff
Otto Kernberg	Robert Spitzer
Donald Klein	Michael Stone
Harold Koenigsberg	Marvin Swartz
Jerome Kroll	Alex Tarnopolsky
Marsha Linehan	Mary Zanarini

In the studies using DSM-III criteria, the most serious overlap was with histrionic personality disorder (HPD) (Table 26–2). Three investigators found that more than 50% of the patients who met criteria for BPD also met criteria for HPD (Dahl 1986; Pfohl et al. 1986; Zanarini 1989). As intended, the changes in the DSM-III-R definitions of the disorders significantly lowered the levels of overlap with HPD. In seven studies using DSM-III-R criteria, the mean overlap fell to 23%.

Table 26–2 also shows that the overlap with antisocial personality disorder (ASPD) was reduced in DSM-III-R—based studies. On the other hand, DSM-III-R introduced new overlap issues vis-à-vis self-defeating personality and avoidant personality disorder (AVPD). The increased levels of overlap with AVPD may be partly due to a change in one BPD criterion (i.e., DSM-III's intolerance of aloneness criterion for BPD may have been more able to distinguish borderline from avoidant patients than its DSM-III-R replacement, abandonment fears). However, the more likely cause for the increased overlap in DSM-III-R is the radical shifts that took place in the AVPD conceptualization and criteria (Millon 1991), which greatly increased the number of patients who met its diagnostic requirements (Morey 1988).

The assembled data were next examined from the reverse overlap perspective (i.e., which other types of Axis II disorder most frequently also fulfill criteria for BPD). From this perspective, self-defeating personality disorder often emerged as being comorbid with BPD and, to a lesser extent, so did schizotypal personality disorder (STPD). These studies on overlap with other Axis II disorders show that DSM-IV might usefully sharpen the boundaries (i.e., improve the discriminability) of BPD and that this is most important vis-à-vis the other dramatic cluster types and with the avoidant, schizotypal, and self-defeating types.

The data sources shown in Table 1 of the introduction to this section do not address the overlap of BPD with Axis I diagnoses; however extensive literature has arisen regarding the overlap of BPD with mood disorders (Gunderson and Elliot 1985). This literature indicates that it would be useful if DSM-IV could more clearly distinguish the affective problems seen in borderline patients from those that belong on Axis I. Another conceptually complex overlap involves posttraumatic stress disorder (Herman et al. 1989). Here, too, the DSM-IV criteria should aspire to help clinicians make this distinction.

Table 26–2. Percentage of borderline personality disorder patients with a diagnosis of other selected personality disorders

Study	Criteria	N	ASPD	HPD	NPD	AVPD	STPD	SDPD
Dahl 1986[a]	DSM-III	38	68	61	5	3	45	—
Pfohl et al. 1986[b]	DSM-III	29	14	69	14	21	21	—
Zanarini et al. 1989[c]	DSM-III	179	46	62	24	24	40	—
Morey 1988[d]	DSM-III-R	96	8	36	31	9	36	—
Skodol et al. 1988a[e]	DSM-III-R	61	10	25	34	59	23	30
Skodol et al. 1988b[f]	DSM-III-R	60	13	35	23	55	20	50
Freiman and Widiger 1989[g]	DSM-III-R	17	59	24	29	59	35	24
Millon and Tringone 1989[h]	DSM-III-R	118	7	14	7	9	3	19
Millon and Tringone 1989[d]	DSM-III-R	95	2	12	2	12	9	22
Millon and Tringone 1989[i]	DSM-III-R	40	20	15	5	25	3	38

Note. Different subsets of patients are provided from same data sets because diagnoses were provided by different methods. Diagnoses made by [a]Schedule for Affective Disorders and Schizophrenia (SADS) (Dahl 1986), [b]Structured Interview for the Diagnosis of Personality Disorders (SIDP) (Stangl et al. 1985), [c]Diagnostic Interview for Personality Disorders (DIPD) (Zanarini et al. 1987), [d]clinicians, [e]Personality Disorder Examination (PDE) (Loranger 1988), [f]Structured Interview for DSM-III-R (SCID-II) (Spitzer et al. 1990), [g]Personality Interview Questions—II (PIQ-II) (Widiger et al. 1989), [h]Checklist, and Millon Clinical Multiaxial Inventory (MCMI) (Millon 1987).

Are the Criteria Effective in Identifying This Disorder?

The large number of studies providing evidence for the generally high diagnostic efficiency of all the criteria (Table 26–3) argue for a conservative approach to the consideration of change. Nonetheless, two other considerations (i.e., the overlap problems noted above and the potential advantages of new criteria) justify examining each criterion's psychometric efficiency in more detail.

Item (criterion)-by-diagnosis analyses indicate that the first four criteria (unstable/intense relationships, impulsivity, affective instability, inappropriate/intense anger) contribute heavily to the overlap with other "dramatic cluster" disorders and that criterion 6 (affective instability) is especially problematic. Affective instability is very prevalent in borderline samples but lacks specificity. It contributes heavily to overlap problems with respect to schizotypal, histrionic, and self-defeating types. It also seems likely that criterion 6 has contributed to the overlap with depression and bipolar disorders. To retain the focus on affective instability but diminish these overlap problems, a revision is proposed (Table 26–4) that continues to cite the presence of anxiety and irritability but replaces depression with "dysphoria" and emphasizes that the affects are reactive. These changes should help differentiate the unstable affects in BPD from the mood lability seen in cyclothymic disorder, while also improving the discrimination between borderline patients and unipolar depressive patients.

Do the Criteria Accurately Identify the Intended Constructs?

Criterion 3 (identity problems) has been found to be the least reliable criterion for assessment (Widiger and Frances 1989). It was considered too unclear and/or hard to assess by the ICD representatives. It now reads like Erikson's identity crisis of adolescence and has the generalizability that Kernberg (1967) suggested typifies all forms of serious personality disorder. In particular, vacillations in sexual orientation, goals, careers, values, and types of friends are all aspects of more general identity problems that lack specificity for BPD. This criterion was originally included because of the centrality it was given in Kernberg's seminal description of borderline personality organization (Kernberg 1967; Spitzer et al. 1979); however, this construct was meant to characterize all serious personality disorders, not BPD specifically. Accordingly, item-by-diagnosis analyses show that it is common in most other Axis II disorders and, most notably, in the antisocial, narcissistic, and self-defeating categories, where the need for better differentiation is documented. Although identity problems are prevalent in borderline samples, the criterion lacks specificity. One factor in favor of omitting this criterion is that a strong candidate for a new criterion exists that could replace criterion 3 and offer better specificity (see below). The most telling argument for retaining criterion 3 is the hope that a

Table 26–3.   Phi coefficients of borderline personality disorder criteria

	N	UIR	IMP	AFF	ANG	PSD	IDD	EMP	INT
DSM-III studies									
Clarkin et al. 1983	20	.59	.63	.55	.43	.57	.46	.59	.34
Cowdry et al. 1985	59	.14	.66	.35	.40	.42	—	.57	.32
Dahl 1986	38	.64	.43	.59	.27	.41	.52	.33	.29
Dubro 1988	10	.37	.59	.57	.57	.47	.51	.54	.21
Jacobsberg									
et al. 1986	22	.18	.14	.30	.33	.46	.20	.16	.28
McGlashan and									
Fenton 1988	99	.29	.43	.44	.39	.34	.36	.31	.21
Malow and									
Donnelly 1988	38	.56	.29	.57	.56	.41	.50	.43	—
Modestin 1987	33	.45	.44	.42	.38	.34	.39	.35	.48
Morey 1985	21	.28	.67	.32	.32	.61	.45	.14	.13
Morey and									
Heumann 1988	97	.50	.52	.50	.35	.54	.47	.55	.42
Nurnberg et al. 1986	17	.84	.84	.46	—	.56	.68	.56	—
Pfohl et al. 1986	29	.63	.66	.53	.54	.77	.63	.51	.28
Plakun 1987	44	.30	.52	.36	.35	.36	.35	.30	.34
Spitzer et al. 1979	808	.12	.11	.08	.11	.11	.11	.09	.05
Widiger et al. 1986a	53	.39	.53	.06	.44	.58	.36	.41	.30
Zanarini et al. 1989	179	.66	.47	.42	.50	.36	.33	.40	.33
Prototype studies									
Burns 1986	467	—	.20	—	.06	.20	.71	.58	—
Hilbrand and									
Hirt 1987	30	.73	.50	.70	.60	.53	<.50	.57	<.50
Livesley et al. 1987	45	6.3	5.3	5.5	5.9	5.6	6.0	5.6	4.9
								4.8	
DSM-III-R studies[a]									
Millon and									
Tringone 1989	118	.28	.43	.44	.21	.46	.29	.19	.14
Freiman and									
Widiger 1989	17	.32	.38	.41	.30	.36	.32	.43	.47
Morey and									
Goodman 1989	97	.51	.52	.51	.36	.50	.48	.53	.41
Prototype studies									
Blashfield and									
Haymaker 1988	61	.79	.75	.73	.50	.84	.80	.84	45

Note.   UIR = unstable/intense relationships. IMP = impulsivity. AFF = affective instability.
ANG = inappropriate/intense anger. PSD = physically self-damaging acts. IDD = identity disturbance.
EMP = emptiness or boredom. INT = intolerance of being alone.
[a]Criteria as in DSM-III except PSD changed to SCD = recurrent, suicidal threats, etc.; and INT
changed to ABN = avoid abandonment.

significant revision might greatly help its reliability and specificity. The proposed revision (Table 26–4) is derived from the clinical experience of the DSM-IV Work Group and its expert advisers. The revision highlights that aspect of identity that is introduced as part of the essential features for BPD (i.e., instability of self-image) and gives more specific examples.

Another proposal for change involves dropping the reference to chronic boredom from DSM-III-R criterion 7 (chronic feelings of emptiness and boredom). Boredom was linked to emptiness because they were combined into one characteristic in the original version of the Diagnostic Interview for Borderline Patients (DIB), which was shown to be discriminating (Gunderson and Kolb 1978; Gunderson et al. 1981). It subsequently became clear to users of the DIB that boredom was not particularly useful. As a result, a specific analysis (comparing 43

Table 26–4.   DSM-III-R criteria for borderline personality disorder

---

A pervasive pattern of instability of interpersonal relationships, self-image, and [MOOD] **poor control of impulses and affects** beginning by early adulthood and present in a variety of contexts, as indicated by at least six of the following:

1) frantic efforts to avoid real or imagined abandonment (Do not include suicidal or self-mutilating behavior covered in criterion 5.)

2) a pattern of unstable and intense interpersonal relationships characterized by alternating between extremes of [OVER]idealization and devaluation

3) [omit or] **identity disturbance: persistent and markedly disturbed, distorted, or unstable self-image and/or sense of self, e.g., he/she may feel like he/she does not exist or embodies evil** [MARKED AND PERSISTENT IDENTITY DISTURBANCE MANIFESTED BY UNCERTAINTY ABOUT AT LEAST TWO OF THE FOLLOWING: SELF-IMAGE, SEXUAL ORIENTATION, LONG-TERM GOALS OR CAREER CHOICE, TYPE OF FRIENDS DESIRED, PREFERRED VALUES]

4) impulsiveness in at least two areas that are potentially self-damaging (e.g., spending, sex, substance use, shoplifting, reckless driving, binge eating) (Do not include suicidal or self-mutilating behavior covered in criterion 5.)

5) recurrent suicidal threats, gestures, or behavior or self-mutilating behavior

6) affective instability: **marked reactivity of mood (e.g., intense episodic dysphoria, irritability, or anxiety),** [MARKED SHIFTS FROM BASELINE MOOD TO DEPRESSION, IRRITABILITY, OR ANXIETY] usually lasting a few hours and only rarely more than a few days

7) chronic feelings of emptiness [OR BOREDOM]

8) inappropriate, intense anger or lack of control of anger (e.g., frequent displays of temper, constant anger, recurrent physical fights)

9) **transient, stress-related, severe dissociative experiences or paranoid ideation**

Note.   Contents of DSM-III-R whose omission is proposed are [CAPITALIZED AND BRACKETED]. Contents that are proposed for addition in DSM-IV are printed in **bold type.**

BPD patients to 58 patients with other personality disorders) was conducted. It revealed that emptiness is highly discriminating for the BPD diagnosis ($P < .001$) whereas boredom is not (cf., M. C. Zanarini, personal communication, 1990). Because boredom is more prevalent in narcissistic or antisocial patients than in borderline patients, its removal from the borderline criteria set should aid differentiation.

Are the Criteria Congruent With the Descriptive Literature?

A criterion describing brief psychotic regressive experiences was advocated for the DSM-III definition of BPD because of its centrality in seminal descriptions of borderline patients (Friedman 1975; Kernberg 1967; Knight 1953; Masterson 1972; Zetzel 1971) and its initial empirical support (Grinker 1968; Gunderson and Kolb 1978; Sheehy et al. 1980; Singer and Larsen 1981). The decision to include stress-related psychotic symptoms only as an associated feature stirred controversy (Rosenthal 1979; Siever and Gunderson 1979; Spitzer and Endicott 1979). Since then, nine studies (Table 26–5) have shown that cognitive-perceptual dysfunctions are common among borderline patients (most studies indicating about 75%) and statistically discriminated borderline patients from others in six of the eight controlled studies. Whereas dissociative experiences and nondelusional paranoia are the most common symptomatology of this sort, about 20%–40% of borderline patients experience transient, circumscribed, and/or atypical delusions and hallucinations (Silk et al. 1989; Widiger et al. 1987; Zanarini et al. 1990a). The latter type of cognitive-perceptual dysfunction is nearly pathognomonic (i.e., rarely found in any other diagnostic group) (Zanarini et al. 1990a, 1990b).

This literature shows that borderline patients have cognitive-perceptual problems that can be distinguished from the psychotic experiences found in other diagnostic groups. This empirical evidence for the diagnostic efficiency of such a feature joins with the clinical importance of the loss of reality testing in unstructured contexts to support the addition of a cognitive-perceptual criterion to the BPD definition. Indeed, when asked about such an addition, 15 of 21 advisers endorsed this plan. Most of the advocates, in line with the arguments by Gunderson (1979, 1984) and Frosch (1988), felt strongly that this feature is central to the borderline construct and that its addition would likely capture one of the most discriminating features of the disorder and thereby diminish the current overuse of this diagnosis.

The controversy surrounding the addition of such a criterion is reflected in reactions from the remaining six advisers. Only two objected because this feature did not conform to their concept or usage of BPD; the other four objected because they felt that better empirical substantiation was needed. The most telling empirical objection is that the cognitive-perceptual disturbances seen in borderline patients may be caused by comorbid STPD. This argument is supported by the fact that, in all four studies that compared "pure" borderline patients to those who were "mixed" (borderline plus schizotypal) and/or to pure schizotypal patients, it was found that the pure borderline patients had fewer cognitive difficulties than either the mixed or pure schizotypal samples (George and Soloff 1986; McGlashan 1987; Perry 1988; Widiger et al. 1987).

Currently, three initiatives are under way to address the issue of whether the cognitive-perceptual problems observed in borderline patients can be differentiated from those that typify STPD. First, a series of vignettes describing the cognitive-perceptual problems of either pure borderline or pure schizotypal patients were solicited and subjected to careful ratings by clinicians (Sternbach et al. 1992). The second initiative is a multisite effort to prospectively assess whether the cognitive-perceptual problems of schizotypal patients are more stable and chronic and those in BPD are more affective and interpersonally reactive (Silverman et al., in press). The third initiative is a reanalysis of existing data sets (Silk et al. 1990; Zanarini et al. 1990b) to determine the effect of the more circumscribed concept of STPD found in DSM-III-R on the prevalence rates of cognitive difficulties in pure borderline patients versus both mixed samples and pure schizotypal patients.

Table 26–5. Prevalence of cognitive perceptual symptoms in borderline personality disorder samples

Cognitive/perceptual problem	Study[a]	Range (%)
Depersonalization	1,3,5,7,8,9	30–85
Derealization	1,3,4,7,8,9	30–92
Paranoid experiences	3,5,6,7,8,9	32–100
Hope/worthlessness	3,7,8	77–88
Visual illusions	4,5,6,7,9	24–42
Muddled thinking	4	52
Magical thinking	5,6,9	34–68
Ideas of reference	5,6,9	49–74
Odd speech	5,6	30–59
Disturbed thoughts	2,9	39–68

[a]1 = Frances et al. 1984. 2 = Pope et al. 1985. 3 = Chopra and Beatson 1986. 4 = George and Soloff 1986. 5 = Jacobsberg et al. 1986. 6 = Widiger et al. 1987. 7 = Links et al. 1988. 8 = Silk et al. 1989. 9 = Zanarini et al. 1990a.

Are the Polythetic Format and Current Threshold Appropriate?

The generally high diagnostic efficiency of all eight of the criteria in both the DSM-III and the DSM-III-R data sets is impressive. The high performance characteristics of the criteria are also reflected in the series of studies that have reported that a smaller set of criteria, three to five, can attain the same efficiency as the entire set of eight (McGlashan and Fenton 1991; Nurnberg et al. 1987; Reich 1990). Regrettably, because the preferred subgroup of criteria found in each of these studies is different, they fail to distinguish certain core criteria that should receive heavier weighting. These results argue for the retention of a polythetic format for the borderline criteria set, which corresponds to the current era of diverse theories about the nature of that core feature. The results also indicate that dropping any criterion would have little effect on "caseness."

The overlap with other disorders presumably could be reduced by increasing the diagnostic threshold from five to six criteria. However, the possible effect of such a change on the construct has only been assessed in one study (Zanarini et al. 1991). Because the initial threshold for this category was one of the few derived from empirical results, it seems improvident to change it unless criterion 9 is adopted. In that case, the increase in the threshold to six will be a desirable way to keep the category from losing specificity.

Should the Essential Feature Be Altered?

The essential feature identified in DSM-III-R is "a pervasive pattern of instability of self-image, interpersonal relationships, and mood." Nineteen experts responded to the request for a critique of it. A minority of the advisers favored the following alternative essential feature: "fear of and angry intolerance for being alone—typically leading to repetitive self-destructiveness, substance abuse, promiscuity, and other desperate impulsive actions." Those who favored this alternative did so because it offers more explanation for the interrelationship of the descriptive characteristics (Adler 1985; Gunderson 1984; Masterson 1971), conveys more meaning in terms of both etiology and treatment, and because it could usefully help differentiate BPD from posttraumatic stress disorder, narcissistic personality disorder, and depression. Nonetheless, the majority of the advisers felt that the existing definition's emphasis on instability links it with an atheoretical descriptive tradition, that it is satisfactorily apt, and that any change should await empirical validation of what is the core concept.

Nevertheless, the essential feature should correspond to what the empirical evidence indicates is central to the diagnosis. As noted, the existing essential feature highlights three aspects, two of which (i.e., unstable self-image and mood) were problematic criteria where revisions are now proposed (i.e., criterion 6, affective instability, and criterion 3, identity problems) because they lacked specificity and/or reliability. Criterion 3 is even considered for omission. Moreover, because of growing evidence that dyscontrol over impulses (as reflected in criteria 4, 5, and 8) may be essential to this diagnosis (Gunderson and Zanarini 1989; Zanarini 1993), it is proposed that impulsivity should be added to the description of the essential feature of the disorder. Given the growing evidence of a nonspecific relationship with affective disorders (Gunderson and Phillips 1991), the instability of mood emerges as a questionable component.

Recommendations

The existing studies highlight the need to sharpen the boundaries between BPD and other disorders. Multiple diagnoses are accepted in DSM-III-R, but the extent of overlap is problematic to establishing their validity, and it clearly does not reflect clinical practice (Dahl 1986; Morey and Ochoa 1989; Pfohl et al. 1986; Zanarini et al. 1987). More specifically, the results point to the value of increasing the differentiation between BPD and other dramatic cluster disorders and between BPD and the schizotypal and self-defeating types. Less obvious from this review but apparent to most readers of the literature is the need to clarify the boundary between BPD and recurrent and labile mood disorders (Akiskal et al. 1985; Gunderson and Elliott 1985). The proposed options for revision of criteria 3, 6, and 7 are designed to help sharpen these boundaries.

The addition of criterion 9 is expected to have direct usefulness for clinicians, and it is likely to reduce overlap with other disorders. Yet, despite the overwhelming consensus of the advisers and its imposing empirical support, this proposal is the most controversial. Because it touches on the nature of the borderline construct itself, there is an ongoing effort to investigate the issues empirically.

This entire review should be understood within its historical perspective. Borderline personality is a new disorder within psychiatric classification. It has engendered far more study than any other new category, perhaps more than all the others combined. It represents a melding of psychiatry's dynamic traditions with its newer empiricism. In this process, the clinical base for the diagnosis may be ignored and/or lost. Many clinicians believe the diagnosis of BPD is indiscriminately overused and that the nonspecificity of the DSM-III-R definition contributes to this. The question as to whether the proposed changes will help refine the usage to a more discrete and specific diagnostic entity remains to be seen.

References

Adler G: Borderline Psychopathology and Its Treatment. New York, Jason Aronson, 1985

Akiskal HS, Chen SE, Davis GC, et al: Borderline: an adjective in search of a noun. J Clin Psychiatry 46:41–48, 1985

American Psychiatric Association: Diagnostic and Statistical Manual of Mental Disorders, 3rd Edition. Washington, DC, American Psychiatric Association, 1980

American Psychiatric Association: Diagnostic and Statistical Manual of Mental Disorders, 3rd Edition, Revised. Washington, DC, American Psychiatric Association, 1987

Blashfield R, Haymaker D: A prototype analysis of the diagnostic criteria for DSM-III-R personality disorders. Journal of Personality Disorders 2:272–280, 1988

Burns T: Use of the term "borderline patient" by Swedish psychiatrists. Int J Soc Psychiatry 32:32–39, 1986

Chopra HD, Beatson JA: Psychotic symptoms in borderline personality disorder. Am J Psychiatry 143:1605–1607, 1986

Clarkin J, Widiger T, Frances A, et al: Prototypic typology and the borderline personality disorder. J Abnorm Psychol 92:263–275, 1983

Cowdry R, Pickar D, Davies R: Symptoms and EEG findings in the borderline syndrome. Int J Psychiatry Med 15:201–211, 1985

Dahl A: Some aspects of the DSM-III personality disorders illustrated by a consecutive sample of hospitalized patients. Acta Psychiatr Scand 73:61–66, 1986

Dubro A: Diagnostic efficiency statistics for borderline personality disorder. Unpublished raw data, White Plains, NY, Cornell University Medical Center, 1988

Frances A, Clarkin J, Gilmore M, et al: Reliability of criteria for borderline personality disorder: a comparison of DSM-III and the Diagnostic Interview for Borderline Personality Disorder. Am J Psychiatry 141:1080–1084, 1984

Freiman K, Widiger TA: Co-occurrence and diagnostic efficiency statistics. Unpublished raw data, Lexington, University of Kentucky, 1989

Friedman H: Psychotherapy of borderline patients: influences of theory and technique. Am J Psychiatry 132:1048–1052, 1975

Frosch J: Psychotic character versus borderline (Part 1). Int J Psychoanal 69: 347–357, 1988

George A, Soloff P: Schizotypal symptoms in patients with borderline personality disorders. Am J Psychiatry 143:212–215, 1986

Grinker R: The Borderline Syndrome. New York, Basic Books, 1968

Gunderson JG: The relatedness of borderline and schizophrenic disorders. Schizophr Bull 5:17–22, 1979

Gunderson JG: Borderline Personality Disorder. Washington, DC, American Psychiatric Press, 1984

Gunderson JG, Elliot G: The interface between borderline personality and affective disorder. Am J Psychiatry 142:277–288, 1985

Gunderson JG, Kolb JE: Discriminating features of borderline patients. Am J Psychiatry 135:792–796, 1978

Gunderson JG, Phillips KA: Borderline personality disorder and depression: a current overview of the interface. Am J Psychiatry 148:967–975, 1991

Gunderson JG, Zanarini MC: Current overview of the borderline diagnosis. J Clin Psychiatry 48:5–11, 1987

Gunderson JG, Zanarini MC: Pathogenesis of borderline personality, in The American Psychiatric Press Review of Psychiatry, Vol 8. Edited by Frances AJ, Hales RE, Tasman A. Washington, DC, American Psychiatric Press, 1989, pp 25–48

Gunderson JG, Kolb JE, Austin V: The diagnostic interview for borderline patients. Am J Psychiatry 138:896–903, 1981

Gunderson JG, Zanarini MC, Kisiel CK: Borderline personality disorder: a review of data on DSM-III-R descriptions. Journal of Personality Disorders 5:340–352, 1991

Herman J, Perry C, van der Kolk B: Childhood trauma in borderline personality disorder. Am J Psychiatry 4:490–495, 1989

Hilbrand M, Hirt M: The borderline patient: an empirically developed prototype. Journal of Personality Disorders 1:299–306, 1987

Jacobsberg L, Hymowitz P, Barasch A, et al: Symptoms of schizotypal personality disorder. Am J Psychiatry 143:1222–1227, 1986

Kernberg O: Borderline personality organization. Am J Psychiatry 15:641–685, 1967

Knight R: Borderline states. Bull Menninger Clin 17:1–12, 1953

Links PS, Steiner M, Offord D, et al: Characteristics of borderline personality disorder: a Canadian study. Can J Psychiatry 33:336–340, 1988

Livesley W, Reiffer L, Sheldon A, et al: Prototypicality ratings of DSM-III criteria for personality disorders. J Nerv Ment Dis 175:395–401, 1987

Loranger AW: Personality Disorder Examination (PDE) Manual. Yonkers, NY, DV Communications, 1988

Malow R, Donnelly J: Diagnostic efficiency statistics for borderline personality disorder. Unpublished raw data, New Orleans, LA, VA Medical Center, 1988

Masterson J: Treatment of the adolescent with borderline syndrome (a problem in separation-individuation). Bull Menninger Clin 35:5–18, 1971

Masterson J: Treatment of the Borderline Adolescent: a Developmental Approach. New York, Wiley, 1972

McGlashan TH: Testing DSM-III symptom criteria for schizotypal and borderline personality disorders. Arch Gen Psychiatry 44:143–148, 1987

McGlashan TH, Fenton W: Diagnostic efficiency statistics for borderline and schizotypal personality disorders. Unpublished raw data, New Haven, CT, Yale University Medical Center, 1988

McGlashan TH, Fenton W: Diagnostic efficiency of DSM-III borderline personality disorder and schizotypal disorder, in Personality Disorders: New Perspectives on Validity. Edited by Oldham J. Washington, DC, American Psychiatric Press, 1991, pp 121–143

Millon T: Manual for the MCMI-II, 2nd Edition. Minneapolis, MN, National Computer Systems, 1987

Millon T: Avoidant personality disorder: a review of the data on DSM-III-R descriptions. Am J Psychiatry 5:353–362, 1991

Millon T, Tringone R: Co-occurrence and diagnostic efficiency statistics. Unpublished raw data, Miami, FL, University of Miami, 1989

Modestin J: Quality of interpersonal relationships: the most characteristic DSM-III BPD criterion. Compr Psychiatry 28:397–402, 1987

Morey LC: A psychometric analysis of five DSM-III categories. Personality and Individual Differences 6:323–329, 1985

Morey LC: Personality disorder under DSM-III and DSM-III-R: an examination of convergence, coverage, and internal consistency. Am J Psychiatry 145:573–577, 1988

Morey L, Goodman R: Diagnostic efficiency statistics. Unpublished raw data, Nashville, TN, Vanderbilt University, 1989

Morey L, Heumann K: Co-occurrence and diagnostic efficiency statistics. Unpublished raw data, Nashville, TN, Vanderbilt University, 1988

Morey LC, Ochoa E: An investigation of adherence to diagnostic criteria: clinical diagnosis of the DSM-III personality disorders. Journal of Personality Disorders 3:180–192, 1989

Nurnberg H, Feldman A, Hurt S, et al: Core criteria for diagnosing borderline patients. Hillside Journal of Clinical Psychiatry 8:111–131, 1986

Nurnberg H, Hurt S, Feldman A, et al: Efficient diagnosis of borderline personality disorder. Journal of Personality Disorders 1:307–315, 1987

Perry JC: A prospective study of life stress, defenses, psychotic symptoms, and depression in borderline and antisocial personality disorders and bipolar type II affective disorder. Journal of Personality Disorders 2:49–59, 1988

Pfohl B, Coryell W, Zimmerman M, et al: DSM-III personality disorders: diagnostic overlap and internal consistency of individual DSM-III criteria. Compr Psychiatry 27:21–34, 1986

Plakun E: Distinguishing narcissistic and borderline personality disorders using DSM-III criteria. Compr Psychiatry 28:437–443, 1987

Pope H, Jonas J, Hudson J, et al: An empirical study of psychosis in borderline personality disorder. Am J Psychiatry 142:1285–1290, 1985

Reich J: Diagnostic efficiency statistics for personality disorders. Unpublished raw data, Brockton, MA, Brockton VA Medical Center, 1988

Reich J: Criteria for diagnosing DSM-III borderline personality disorders. Annals of Clinical Psychiatry 2:189–197, 1990

Rosenthal D: Was Thomas Wolfe a borderline? Schizophr Bull 5:87–94, 1979

Sheehy M, Goldsmith L, Charles E: A comparative study of borderline patients in a psychiatric outpatient clinic. Am J Psychiatry 137:1374–1379, 1980

Siever L, Gunderson JG: Genetic determinants of borderline conditions. Schizophr Bull 1:59–86, 1979

Silk K, Lohr N, Westen D, et al: Psychosis in borderline patients with depression. Journal of Personality Disorders 3:92–100, 1989

Silk K, Westen D, Lohr N, et al: DSM-III and DSM-III-R schizotypal symptoms in borderline personality disorder. Compr Psychiatry 31:103–110, 1990

Silverman JM, Siever L, Zanarini MC: DSM-IV field trials for schizotypal personality disorder, in DSM-IV Sourcebook, Vol 4. Edited by Widiger TA, Frances AJ, Pincus HA, et al. Washington, DC, American Psychiatric Press (in press)

Singer M, Larson D: Borderline personality and the Rorschach test. Arch Gen Psychiatry 38:693–702, 1981

Skodol A, Spitzer R (eds): An Annotated Bibliography of DSM-III. Washington, DC, American Psychiatric Press, 1987

Skodol A, Rosnick L, Kellman D, et al: Validating structured DSM-III-R personality disorder assessments with longitudinal data. Am J Psychiatry 145:1297–1299, 1988a

Skodol A, Rosnick L, Kellman D, et al: The validity of structured assessments of Axis II. Paper presented at the 141st annual meeting of the American Psychiatric Association, Montreal, Quebec, May 11, 1988b

Spitzer R, Endicott J: Justification for separating schizotypal and borderline personality disorders. Schizophr Bull 5:95–104, 1979

Spitzer R, Endicott J, Gibbon M: Crossing the border into borderline personality and borderline schizophrenia: the development of criteria. Arch Gen Psychiatry 36:17–24, 1979

Spitzer RL, Williams JBW, Gibbon M, et al: User's Guide for the Structured Clinical Interview for DSM-III-R (SCID). Washington, DC, American Psychiatric Press, 1990

Stangl D, Pfohl B, Zimmerman M, et al: A structured interview for DSM-III personality disorder. Arch Gen Psychiatry 42:591–596, 1985

Sternbach S, Judd A, Sabo A, et al: Cognitive and perceptual distortions in borderline personality disorder and schizotypal personality disorder in a vignette sample. Compr Psychiatry 33:186–189, 1992

Widiger TA, Frances AJ: Epidemiology, diagnosis and comorbidity of borderline personality disorder, in The American Psychiatric Press Review of Psychiatry, Vol 8. Edited by Frances A, Hales R, Tasman A. Washington DC, American Psychiatric Press, 1989

Widiger T, Frances A, Warner L, et al: Diagnostic criteria for the borderline and schizotypal personality disorders. J Abnorm Psychol 95:43–51, 1986a

Widiger T, Sanderson C, Warner L: The MMPI, prototypal typology, and borderline personality disorder. J Pers Assess 50:540–553, 1986b

Widiger TA, Trull T, Hurt S, et al: A multidimensional scaling of the DSM-III personality disorders. Arch Gen Psychiatry 44:557–563, 1987

Widiger TA, Frances AJ, Trull TJ: Personality disorders, in Clinical and Diagnostic Interviewing. Edited by Craig R. Northvale, NJ, Jason Aronson, 1989, pp 231–236

Zanarini MC: Co-occurrence and diagnostic efficiency statistics. Unpublished raw data, Belmont, MA, McLean Hospital, 1989

Zanarini MC: BPD as an impulse spectrum disorder, in Borderline Personality Disorder: Etiology and Treatment. Edited by Paris J. Washington, DC, American Psychiatric Press, 1993, pp 67–85

Zanarini MC, Frankenburg FR, Chauncey DL, et al: The Diagnostic Interview for Personality Disorders: interrater and test-retest reliability. Compr Psychiatry 28: 467–480, 1987

Zanarini MC, Frankenburg F, Chauncey D, et al: Co-occurrence and diagnostic efficiency statistics. Unpublished raw data, Boston, MA, McLean Hospital, 1989

Zanarini MC, Gunderson JG, Frankenburg FR: Cognitive features of borderline personality disorder. Am J Psychiatry 147:57–63, 1990a

Zanarini MC, Gunderson JG, Frankenburg FR, et al: Discriminating borderline personality disorder from other Axis II disorders. Am J Psychiatry 147:161–167, 1990b

Zanarini MC, Gunderson JG, Frankenburg FR, et al: The face validity of the DSM-III and DSM-III-R criteria sets for borderline personality disorder. Am J Psychiatry 148:870–874, 1991

Zetzel E: A developmental approach to the borderline patient. Am J Psychiatry 128:867–871, 1971

Chapter 27

Histrionic Personality Disorder

Bruce Pfohl, M.D.

Statement of the Issues

The concerns noted most often in the literature and by the Personality Disorder Work Group members and consultants relate to the extent to which the histrionic personality disorder (HPD) diagnosis is sex biased (Blashfield et al. 1990; Chodoff 1982; Kaplan 1983), to how adequately it represents the clinical concept of hysterical personality (Cooper 1987; Gunderson 1983; Kernberg 1988), and to the fact that it may lack adequate descriptive validity (Pfohl et al. 1986; Siever and Klar 1986) and is somewhat different from ICD-10 (World Health Organization 1992) histrionic personality disorder (PD). These issues can be operationalized as follows: Are criteria congruent with the descriptive literature? Are criteria internally consistent? Are criteria supported by external validators? Is the diagnosis applied prejudicially to patients, especially women? Is the diagnosis distinct from other disorders? Can the DSM-III-R (American Psychiatric Association 1987) and ICD-10 criteria for HPD be reconciled?

Significance of the Issues

The DSM-III-R criteria for HPD represent the current state of a concept that has evolved over many decades. The concept was first officially recognized by DSM-II (American Psychiatric Association 1968), which defined "hysterical personality." DSM-III (American Psychiatric Association 1980) drew on the DSM-II concept to produce operational criteria, which were modified in DSM-III-R to reduce overlap with borderline PD. Thus, DSM-III-R omitted criteria referring to craving for excitement, angry outbursts, and suicide attempts. DSM-III-R added two new criteria: "inappropriately sexually seductive" and "speech that is excessively impressionistic." Before considering any further changes, it is important to examine the empirical support for the current criteria set.

In this review, priority was given to issues raised in the literature that have a direct bearing on the validity of the diagnosis of HPD and its overlap and relationship to other disorders because the value of separating patients into different diagnostic categories ultimately lies in showing that different diagnoses carry different implications. Although agreement with ICD-10 is not a validity issue per se, future empirical research can be greatly facilitated by a common language for communication between psychiatrists in different countries.

Methods

A Medline search was conducted on literature published between the introduction of DSM-III in 1980 and the beginning of 1991 on the search term *histrionic personality disorder*. This yielded 229 papers. Closer scrutiny was given to those that contained empirical data. In addition, review papers associated with terms such as *hysteria* or *hysterical* were also scanned, going back 25 years. Investigators with relevant data sets were asked to provide information on internal consistency of the criteria and overlap with other psychiatric disorders. Advisers were invited to express any general concerns about the criteria or underlying constructs.

Results

Are Criteria Congruent With the Descriptive Literature?

Although clinical tradition and theoretical constructs do not establish validity, they do provide a useful starting point. The roots of histrionic personality can be traced to cases of hysterical neurosis described by Freud (Kernberg 1988). Easser and Lesser (1965) comment, "The terms, hysteria, hysterical character, etc., are so loosely defined and applied so promiscuously that their application to diagnostic categories has become meaningless" (p. 392). In a similar vein, Lazare (1971) wrote, "Hysterical is commonly used in a pejorative sense to describe a patient who is self-engrossed, incapable of loving deeply, lacking depth, emotionally shallow, fraudulent in affect, immature, emotionally incontinent, and a great liar. . . . The presence, of just one of these traits together with a tired resident, may result in the diagnosis of 'just hysterical'" (p. 131).

Table 27–1 indicates a variety of different but overlapping descriptive traits and features that have been used to describe histrionic (or hysterical) personality. Kernberg (1967) attempted to outline features that distinguished HPD from related disorders. Several of these are not represented by the current DSM-III-R criteria

Table 27–1. Prototypic traits for histrionic personality disorder (HPD)

- **DSM-III-R HPD criteria**
  Seeks reassurance/approval
  Seductive
  Concerned with physical attractiveness
  Exaggerated expression of emotion
  Uncomfortable if not center of attention
  Shifting/shallow expression of emotion
  Self-centered/immediate gratification
  Vague speech

- **Kernberg 1967**
  Emotional lability
  Overinvolvement (superficial resonance with others)
  Dependent and exhibitionistic needs
  Pseudohypersexuality
  Sexual inhibition[a]
  Competitiveness (oedipal rivalry)[a]
  Masochism (strict punitive superego)[a]

- **Lazare et al. 1966 (literature review)**
  Dependence[a]
  Egocentricity
  Emotionality
  Exhibitionism
  Fear of sexuality[a]
  Sexual provocativeness
  Suggestibility[a]

- **Lazare 1971**
  Healthier (genital) histrionic
  Seductive
  Ambitious, competitive[a]
  Buoyant and energetic[a]
  Experiences guilt (punitive superego) and obsessional traits[a]
  Stable object relations although sexually frigid[a]

  Sicker (oral) histrionic
  Self-absorption[a]
  Crude socially disapproved sexual behavior[a]
  Generalized impulsivity[a]

  Generalized lability
  Weaker superego, little guilt[a]
  Unstable object relations[a]

- **Lazare et al. 1966, 1970 (factor analysis)**
  Aggression[a]
  Emotionality
  Oral aggression[a]
  Exhibitionism
  Egocentricity
  Sexual provocativeness
  Dependence
  Obstinacy[a]

- **Suggested additions by Work Group advisers[a]**
  Naive
  Denial of dysphoric affects
  Disingenuous interpersonal interaction
  Desire to be taken care of by strong but controllable person
  Manipulative suicide gestures
  Disinterest in developing personal competence in tasks or logic
  Helplessness and dependency
  Profound lack of self-esteem

- **ICD-10 HPD**
  Self-dramatization, theatricality, exaggerated expression of emotions
  Suggestibility, easily influenced by others or by circumstances[a]
  Shallow and labile affectivity
  Continual seeking for excitement, appreciation by others, and activities in which the patient is the center of attention
  Inappropriate seductiveness in appearance or behavior
  Overconcern with physical attractiveness

[a]Traits not currently represented by DSM-III-R HPD criteria.

for HPD. The next entry summarizes traits from a comprehensive review of the literature on hysterical personality before 1966 by Lazare et al. (1966). In a later publication, Lazare (1971) notes that psychoanalytic theorists often distinguished between a healthier (genital) and sicker (oral) hysteric personality. Several traits of the sicker variant appear to overlap with DSM-III-R borderline PD.

Lazare et al. (1966, 1970) were the first to systematically examine the clustering of traits in hysterical personality using factor analysis. They began with a series of traits representing the oral, obsessive, and hysterical personality constructs and used a 200-item self-report rating scale to operationalize measurement of the underlying traits. The scale (later called the Lazare-Klerman Trait Scale [LKTS]) was given to a series of female psychiatric patients. A hysterical factor emerged that included aggression, emotionality, oral aggression, exhibitionism, egocentricity, and sexual provocativeness (Table 27–1). Dependence and obstinacy had a moderate loading on this factor. The hypothesized association with fear of sexuality, suggestibility, superego, and lack of perseverance did not load on this self-report–based hysterical factor. Similar results were obtained by Torgersen (1980) using the same instrument, this time with a mixed-sex, nonpatient sample.

Are Criteria Internally Consistent?

Internal consistency is used here to describe how well the components of a criteria set cluster together in individual patients and discriminate from other syndromes. Rather than referring to external validators, this analysis represents a bootstrap procedure in which the criteria as a whole are assumed to approximate a real diagnostic entity, and patients are categorized as cases or noncases according to the criteria set taken as a whole. Individual criteria can be examined according to their frequency among cases (sensitivity) and rarity among noncases (specificity).

Only limited data are available for DSM-III-R. Data from four unpublished data sets are discussed. The Freiman and Widiger (1989) data set is based on a study of 50 hospitalized psychiatric patients who received a structured interview for personality assessment. The Millon and Tringone (1989) data set is based on 584 patients described by clinicians as part of a mail survey. DSM-III-R criteria were paraphrased in this study. The Morey and Heumann (1988) data set is based on a mixed group of 291 patients who received an unstructured clinical interview. The Pfohl data set (Pfohl and Blum 1990) is based on the Structured Interview for DSM-III-R Personality (SIDP-R) (Pfohl et al. 1989) of a mixed group of 112 nonpsychotic inpatients, outpatients, and normal control subjects.

Statistics for these four studies are presented in Table 27–2. Sensitivity for all eight criteria averaged approximately 0.5 or better across the four studies, with the possible exception of criterion 8 (impressionistic speech). Given that only four criteria are required for diagnosis, this should be more than adequate.

The first criterion for HPD in DSM-III-R reads, "Constantly seeks or demands reassurance, approval, or praise." Compared with the other seven criteria, this criterion had the lowest specificity in the Morey and Heumann study (0.71) and the second lowest in the Freiman and Widiger study (0.63), the Millon and

Table 27–2. Internal-consistency–based diagnostic statistics for DSM-III-R histrionic personality disorder criteria

	Frequency[a]	A1	A2	A3	A4	A5	A6	A7	A8
Sensitivity									
Freiman and Widiger 1989	9	0.56	0.78	0.67	0.56	0.78	(0.33)	0.89	(0.44)
Millon and Tringone 1989	44	0.77	0.55	(0.32)	0.55	—	0.55	0.68	(0.34)
Morey and Heumann 1988	63	0.75	0.65	(0.60)	0.68	(0.54)	0.73	0.81	0.71
Pfohl and Blum 1990	26	0.92	(0.54)	0.62	0.73	(0.54)	0.81	0.81	(0.23)
Specificity									
Freiman and Widiger 1989	9	(0.63)	0.95	0.98	0.76	0.81	0.98	(0.51)	0.85
Millon and Tringone 1989	44	(0.78)	0.88	0.87	0.85	—	0.85	0.74)	0.91
Morey and Heumann 1988	63	(0.71)	0.91	0.85	0.86	0.94	0.93	(0.74)	0.78
Pfohl and Blum 1990	26	(0.66)	0.87	0.79	0.83	0.98	0.84	(0.59)	0.98
Positive predictive value									
Freiman and Widiger 1989	9	(0.25)	0.78	0.86	0.33	0.47	0.75	(0.29)	0.40
Millon and Tringone 1989	44	0.22	0.26	(0.18)	0.23	—	0.23	(0.18)	0.24
Morey and Heumann 1988	63	(0.42)	0.67	0.53	0.58	0.72	0.73	(0.46)	0.47
Pfohl and Blum 1990	26	(0.45)	0.56	0.47	0.56	0.88	0.60	(0.38)	0.75

Note. Numbers in parentheses indicate the two worst-performing items in each study.
A1 = demands reassurance. A2 = sexually seductive. A3 = physical attractiveness. A4 = exaggerated emotion. A5 = center of attention. A6 = shifting and shallow emotions. A7 = self-centered. A8 = impressionistic speech.
[a]Frequency of histrionic personality disorder diagnosis in each study. Total sample size was 50 in Freiman and Widiger, 584 in Millon and Tringone, 291 in Morey and Heumann, and 112 in Pfohl and Blum.

Tringone study (0.78), and the Pfohl and Blum study (0.66). Positive predictive value ranged from 0.22 to 0.45 across the four studies. The Pfohl and Blum study reported this criterion in 92% of histrionic patients, 88% of dependent PD patients, 80% of borderline PD patients, and 79% of passive-aggressive PD patients.

Criterion 7 in DSM-III-R reads, "is self-centered, actions being directed toward obtaining immediate satisfaction; has no tolerance for the frustration of delayed gratification." Compared with the other seven criteria, this criterion had the lowest specificity in the Freiman and Widiger (0.51), the Pfohl and Blum (0.59), and the Millon and Tringone (0.74) studies and the second-lowest specificity in the Morey and Heumann study (0.74). In the Pfohl and Blum study, this criterion was present among 81% of HPD patients, 85% of borderline PD patients, 83% of passive-aggressive PD patients, and 80% of dependent PD patients.

The evaluation of criterion 7 is complicated because it contains two separate items—self-centered and no tolerance for delayed gratification. The latter is captured to some extent by a phrase in the Millon and Tringone study, "has penchant for momentary excitements," which received a moderately high specificity of 0.87. The phrase was scored positive in 48% of histrionic, 36% of antisocial, and 31% of narcissistic cases. In contrast, the factor-analytic studies by Lazare et al. (1966, 1970) found no evidence of a negative loading for "perseverance" on the hysterical factor. The old DSM-III criterion "egocentric, self-indulgent, and inconsiderate of others" captures the essence of self-centered. This criterion had a specificity of 0.60 in a study by Pfohl et al. (1986) and 0.75 in a study by Zanarini et al. (1989). These results place the self-centered concept in the average range for both studies. However, these two studies used DSM-III rather than DSM-III-R criteria to define HPD.

With the exception of criteria 1 and 7, the remaining HPD criteria appeared to have reasonable internal consistency. To the extent that overlap between the personality disorder diagnoses is viewed as undesirable, the performance of criteria 1 and 7 must be considered a weakness in the diagnostic criteria.

Are the Criteria Supported by External Validators?

Only a limited number of studies examined predictive validity and other external validators for the DSM-III or DSM-III-R criteria for HPD. Therefore, studies using other assessment schemes are considered briefly.

Pollak (1981) reviewed empirical research supporting the construct of hysterical personality. Most of the studies used some type of self-report measure to assess hysterical personality, such as the LKTS (Lazare et al. 1966) or the Hysterioid-Obsessoid Questionnaire (HOQ) (Caine and Hawkins 1963). Compared with control subjects, individuals who score high on hysterical personality are more likely to have depression and somatization symptoms and emotional lability rated prospectively over a 2-week period, are less likely to perform well in a learning task involving sexual words when tested by a flirtatious examiner, and are more sensitive to unfavorable judgments made about their sex-role adequacy. Pollak concludes that the research literature is "rather modest in size and scope" (p. 96) but that it would be premature to dismiss the concept.

Since 1981, there has been a modest increase in empirical studies of the histrionic dimension (Magaro et al. 1983; Slavney and Chase 1985; Standage et al. 1984; Von der Lippe and Torgersen 1984), including a positive twin study (Torgersen 1980).

Is the Diagnosis Used in a Manner Prejudicial to Patients?

Historically, the typical patient with hysterical personality has been described as female, and there is concern that the diagnosis may be prejudicial to women (Chodoff 1982; Chodoff and Lyons 1958). This raises several questions. Are women truly at higher risk for receiving this diagnosis than men? Are any sex-related differences in rates of diagnosis accounted for by sex-related differences in underlying psychopathology? Does the diagnosis result in inappropriate treatment of the patient?

Depending on the approach to diagnosis, it is not clear that women are at higher risk than men for a DSM-III or DSM-III-R diagnosis of HPD. Reich et al. (1987) assessed DSM-III personality diagnosis using a variety of instruments in nonpsychotic nonorganic psychiatric outpatients. In this sample, 64% of the patients were women. Of 31 cases diagnosed as HPD by the SIDP-R (Pfohl et al. 1989), 20 (65%) were women, indicating no sex bias. Using the same interview, Zimmerman and Coryell (1989) reported similar results with a series of 797 relatives of inpatients of whom 56% were women. Twenty-five received a diagnosis of HPD, and 58% of these were women. Nestadt et al. (1990) reported one of the few interview-based epidemiological studies of HPD and found the disorder about equally prevalent among men and women.

The method of diagnosis (clinical assessment versus structured interview) may account for many of the conflicting findings regarding sex bias (Ford and Widiger 1989; Slavney and Chase 1985; Thompson and Goldberg 1987; Warner 1978).

Is the Diagnosis Distinct From Other Disorders?

This raises the question as to whether the criteria are too broadly or too narrowly defined. Does HPD overlap so often with other diagnoses that it is not a clearly distinguishable entity? Is HPD better conceptualized as being on a continuum with other disorders? Freud initially described hysterical personality features in women with conversion symptoms. There is current evidence that somatization disorder and histrionic personality are more frequently comorbid than would be expected

Table 27–3.   Percentage of histrionic patients with comorbid Axis II cluster B diagnoses

Study	Criteria	N	Antisocial	Borderline	Narcissistic
Pfohl et al. 1986	DSM-III	131	10	67	13
Zanarini et al. 1989	DSM-III	253	49	95	34
Dahl 1986	DSM-III	103	36	64	8
Freiman and Widiger 1989	DSM-III-R	50	44	44	33
Skodol 1989	DSM-III-R	97	31	94	44

by chance (Kaminsky and Slavney 1983; Lilienfeld et al. 1986; Pollak 1981).

In several studies that used a structured approach to ensure that all diagnostic criteria were evaluated on their own merits, a great deal of overlap was found between HPD and other Axis II personality disorders using DSM-III and DSM-III-R criteria. This is not necessarily true of studies where clinicians apply the criteria in a global manner. In Table 27–3, the overlap of histrionic and borderline personality ranges from 44% to 95%, although the design of several of these studies could be expected to select for more severe cases with higher overlap. This finding is compatible with at least two different hypotheses. Either borderline PD and HPD are distinct entities with operational criteria that provide inadequate discrimination, or the two disorders represent slightly different manifestations of the same underlying psychopathology. Some have suggested that disorders such as borderline PD and HPD might represent part of a continuum of personality pathology (Kernberg 1988; Stone 1981). No empirical studies have compared borderline PD to HPD on such variables as childhood history of sexual abuse and other significant events, family history of psychiatric disorder, rates of comorbid Axis I disorders, social and occupational functioning, and other variables that might validate the independence of these two diagnoses.

Can DSM-III-R and ICD-10 Be Reconciled?

Most of the DSM-III-R criteria for HPD are represented in the ICD-10 criteria for HPD. ICD-10 criterion 4 (Table 27–1) includes the concept of excitement seeking, which is not present in DSM-III-R. The remaining components of this criterion combine the concepts of approval seeking and need to be the center of attention, which are two separate criteria in DSM-III-R. The suggestibility criteria in ICD-10 is not present in DSM-III-R criteria. A meeting between representatives of the DSM-IV and ICD-10 committees may be necessary to determine whether some compromise is possible in the interest of easing the way for future international collaboration. In cases where the same concept is worded differently, it may be possible to reach a consensus based on clarity and cross-cultural appropriateness. For example, the ICD-10 criterion "self-dramatization, theatricality, exaggerated expression of emotions" may provide sufficient precision without the same risk of cross-cultural bias inherent in the examples given in the equivalent DSM-III-R criteria. Other adjustments such as including the criteria of suggestibility in DSM-IV may be more problematic, because there are data suggesting that this trait may not cluster with other histrionic traits (Lazare et al. 1966, 1970).

Discussion and Recommendations

Enough empirical research exists to suggest that the diagnosis of HPD has fair internal consistency and at least some external validity. The biggest problem with the current criteria is the overlap with other personality disorders. Another is the limited test-retest reliability, especially when general clinical interview rather than structured clinical interview is used. There appear to be important sex-related differences in the application of this diagnosis, but the clinical implications of this are not clear.

Although there is reason to conclude that improvements are needed, there is disagreement about how much data should be accumulated before a change is accepted as justified. A relatively high threshold for justifying changes is adopted here because frequent disruptions to the diagnostic system complicate both teaching and research. The following proposals should be considered options for further consideration:

1. Because criterion 1 (constantly seeks or demands reassurance, approval, or praise) was found to be very frequent among patients without a diagnosis of HPD, the proposal has been made that the criterion be dropped from the criteria but mentioned in the text as a common feature.

2. Because criterion 7 is also frequent among other disorders, and it incorporates two different concepts (self-centered and no tolerance for frustration), the suggestion has been made to change this criterion to "is excessively intolerant of, or frustrated by, situations involving delayed gratification."

3. To maintain a total of eight criteria, many of the consultants judged the following new criterion as reasonably characteristic: "views relationships as possessing greater intimacy than is actually the case" (e.g., refers to someone he/she recently met as a "dear, dear friend"; uses first name and talks about "special" relationship when referring to a doctor known on a casual professional level).

4. Representatives from the ICD-10 and DSM-IV committees should meet and

attempt to reconcile any differences in criteria to promote a common language for psychiatric disorder.

5. Field trials and other studies would be highly desirable to determine whether the proposed changes improve internal consistency and external validity for this disorder.

More extensive discussion of these proposed changes and a more detailed review is provided elsewhere (Pfohl 1991).

References

American Psychiatric Association: Diagnostic and Statistical Manual of Mental Disorders, 2nd Edition. Washington, DC, American Psychiatric Association, 1968

American Psychiatric Association: Diagnostic and Statistical Manual of Mental Disorders, 3rd Edition. Washington, DC, American Psychiatric Association, 1980

American Psychiatric Association: Diagnostic and Statistical Manual of Mental Disorders, 3rd Edition, Revised. Washington, DC, American Psychiatric Association, 1987

Blashfield R, Sprock J, Fuller A: Suggested guidelines for including/excluding categories in the DSM-IV. Compr Psychiatry 31:15–19, 1990

Caine T, Hawkins L: Questionnaire measure of the hysteroid/obsessoid component of personality. J Consult Clin Psychol 27:206–209, 1963

Chodoff P: Hysteria and women. Am J Psychiatry 139:545–551, 1982

Chodoff P, Lyons H: Hysteria: personality in hysterical conversion. Am J Psychiatry 114:734–740, 1958

Cooper A: Histrionic, narcissistic, and compulsive personality disorders, in Diagnosis and Classification in Psychiatry. Edited by Tischler G. Washington, DC, American Psychiatric Press, 1987, pp 20–39

Dahl A: Some aspects of the DSM-III personality disorders illustrated by a consecutive sample of hospitalized patients. Acta Psychiatr Scand 73:61–66, 1986

Easser B, Lesser S: Hysterical character and psychoanalysis. Psychoanal Q 34:390–405, 1965

Ford M, Widiger T: Sex bias in the diagnosis of histrionic and antisocial personality disorders. J Consult Clin Psychol 57:301–305, 1989

Freiman K, Widiger T: Co-occurrence and diagnostic efficiency statistics. Unpublished raw data, Lexington, University of Kentucky, 1989

Gunderson J: DSM-III diagnosis of personality disorders, in Current Perspectives on Personality Disorders. Edited by Frosch J. Washington, DC, American Psychiatric Press, 1983, pp 20–39

Kaminsky M, Slavney P: Hysterical and obsessional features in patients with Briquet's syndrome (somatization disorder). Psychol Med 13:111–120, 1983

Kaplan M: A woman's view of DSM-III. Am Psychol 38:786–792, 1983

Kernberg O: Borderline personality organization. J Am Psychoanal Assoc 15:641–685, 1967

Kernberg O: Hysterical and histrionic personality disorders, in The Personality Disorders and Neuroses. Edited by Cooper A, Frances A, Sacks M. Philadelphia, PA, JB Lippincott, 1988, pp 231–241

Lazare A: The hysterical character in psychoanalytic theory. Arch Gen Psychiatry 25:131–137, 1971

Lazare A, Klerman G, Armor D: Oral, obsessive and hysterical personality patterns. Arch Gen Psychiatry 14:624–630, 1966

Lazare A, Klerman G, Armor D: Oral, obsessive and hysterical personality patterns: replication of factor analysis in an independent sample. J Psychiatr Res 7:275–279, 1970

Lilienfeld S, Van Valkenburg C, Larntz K, et al: The relationship of histrionic personality disorder to antisocial personality and somatization disorder. Am J Psychiatry 143:718–722, 1986

Magaro P, Smith P, Ashbrook R: Personality style differences in visual search performance. Psychiatry Res 10:131–138, 1983

Millon T, Tringone R: Co-occurrence and diagnostic efficiency statistics. Unpublished raw data, Lexington, University of Kentucky, 1989

Morey L, Heumann K: Co-occurrence and diagnostic efficiency statistics. Unpublished raw data, Nashville, TN, Vanderbilt University, 1988

Nestadt G, Romanoski AJ, Merchant CA, et al: An epidemiological study of histrionic personality disorder. Psychol Med 20:413–422, 1990

Pfohl B: Histrionic personality disorder: a review of available data and recommendations for DSM-IV. Journal of Personality Disorders 5:150–166, 1991

Pfohl B, Blum N: Internal consistency statistics for the DSM-III-R personality disorder criteria. Unpublished raw data, Iowa City, University of Iowa, 1990

Pfohl B, Coryell W, Zimmerman M, et al: DSM-III personality disorders: diagnostic overlap and internal consistency of individual DSM-III criteria. Compr Psychiatry 27:21–34, 1986

Pfohl B, Blum N, Zimmerman M, et al: Structured Interview for DSM-III-R Personality (SIDP-R). Iowa City, University of Iowa College of Medicine, 1989

Pollak J: Hysterical personality: an appraisal in light of empirical research. Genet Psychol Monogr 104:71–105, 1981

Reich J: Sex distribution of DSM-III personality disorders in psychiatric outpatients. Am J Psychiatry 144:485–488, 1987

Siever L, Klar H: A review of DSM-III criteria for the personality disorders, in Psychiatry Update. Edited by Frances A, Hales R. Washington, DC, American Psychiatric Press, 1986, pp 279–314

Skodol AE: Co-occurrence and diagnostic efficiency statistics. Unpublished raw data. New York, New York State Psychiatric Institute, 1989

Slavney P, Chase G: Clinical judgments of self-dramatization: a test of the sexist hypothesis. Br J Psychiatry 146:614–617, 1985

Standage K, Bilsbury C, Subhash J, et al: An investigation of role-taking in histrionic personalities. Can J Psychiatry 29:407–411, 1984

Stone M: Borderline syndromes: a consideration of subtypes and an overview, directions for research. Psychiatr Clin North Am 4:3–24, 1981

Thompson D, Goldberg D: Hysterical personality disorder: the process of diagnosis in clinical and experimental settings. Br J Psychiatry 150:241–245, 1987

Torgersen S: The oral, obsessive and hysterical personality syndromes: a study of hereditary and environmental factors by means of the twin method. Arch Gen Psychiatry 37:1272–1277, 1980

Von der Lippe A, Torgersen S: Character and defense: relationships between oral, obsessive and hysterical character traits and defense mechanisms. Scand J Psychol 25:258–264, 1984

Warner R: The diagnosis of antisocial and hysterical personality disorders: an example of sex bias. J Nerv Ment Dis 166:839–845, 1978

World Health Organization: The ICD-10 Classification of Mental Disorders and Behavioral Disorders: Clinical Descriptions and Diagnostic Guidelines. Geneva, Switzerland, World Health Organization, 1992

Zanarini M, Frankenburg F, Chauncey D, et al: Co-occurrence and diagnostic efficiency statistics. Unpublished raw data, Boston, MA, McLean Hospital, 1989

Zimmerman M, Coryell W: DSM-III personality disorder diagnoses in a nonpatient sample. Arch Gen Psychiatry 46:682–689, 1989

Chapter 28

Narcissistic Personality Disorder

John Gunderson, M.D., Elsa Ronningstam, Ph.D., and
Lauren E. Smith, B.A.

Introduction

Narcissistic personality disorder (NPD) was introduced into our diagnostic system in DSM-III (American Psychiatric Association 1980). There was no precedent in earlier DSMs or in the ICD for a narcissistic category. The stimulus for its inclusion derived from the widespread use of the term by psychodynamically informed clinicians. The DSM-III definition of NPD arose out of that committee's summary of the pre-1978 literature and was modified for DSM-III-R (American Psychiatric Association 1987) after additional expert input (Table 28–1).

Notable in the changes that occurred from DSM-III to DSM-III-R were the following:

1. The format for the criteria were changed from a mixed polythetic-monothetic criteria set to a polythetic set.
2. DSM-III included interpersonal relationship features as one criterion with the requirement that patients have two of the four listed options. In DSM-III-R, these four options were made into three separate criteria; namely, criterion 2 (exploitative), criterion 6 (entitlement), and criterion 8 (lack of empathy). The fourth option in DSM-III, "relationships characterized by idealization and devaluation," was dropped in DSM-III-R because it overlapped with a similar criterion for borderline personality disorder (BPD).
3. Criterion 3 in DSM-III related to both grandiosity and uniqueness. It was

Appreciation is due to Drs. Freiman, Goodman, Millon, Morey, Skodol, Tringone, Widiger, and Zanarini for providing access to their unpublished data.

subdivided into two criteria in DSM-III-R: criterion 3 retained the focus on grandiosity per se, and a second criterion (criterion 4 in DSM-III-R) took up the focus on uniqueness.

4. A new criterion (criterion 9) concerning preoccupation with feelings of envy was added in DSM-III-R.

Table 28–1.   DSM-III-R criteria for narcissistic personality disorder and proposed changes for DSM-IV

A pervasive pattern of grandiosity (in fantasy or behavior), **need for admiration** [HYPERSENSITIVITY TO THE EVALUATION OF OTHERS], and lack of empathy beginning by early adulthood and present in a variety of contexts, as indicated by at least five of the following:

1) has grandiose sense of self-importance (e.g., exaggerates achievements and talents, expects to be **recognized as superior without commensurate achievements** [NOTICED AS "SPECIAL" WITHOUT APPROPRIATE ACHIEVEMENT] (DSM-III-R criterion 3)

2) is preoccupied with fantasies of unlimited success, power, brilliance, beauty, or ideal love (DSM-III-R criterion 5)

3) believes that [HIS OR HER PROBLEMS ARE UNIQUE] **he or she is** "special" **and unique** and can be understood only by, **or should be associated with,** other special **or high-status** people **(or institutions)** (DSM-III-R criterion 4)

4) requires [CONSTANT] **excessive** admiration [AND ATTENTION, E.G., KEEPS FISHING FOR COMPLIMENTS] (DSM-III-R criterion 7)

5) has a sense of entitlement: unreasonable expectation of especially favorable treatment **or automatic compliance with his or her expectations** [E.G., ASSUMES THAT HE OR SHE DOES NOT HAVE TO WAIT IN LINE WHEN OTHERS MUST DO SO] (DSM-III-R criterion 6)

6) is interpersonally exploitative: takes advantage of others to achieve his or her own ends (DSM-III-R criterion 2)

7) lack of empathy: inability to recognize [AND EXPERIENCE HOW OTHERS FEEL] **or identify with** the feelings **and needs** of others [E.G., ANNOYANCE AND SURPRISE WHEN A FRIEND WHO IS SERIOUSLY ILL CANCELS A DATE] (DSM-III-R criterion 8)

8) is [PREOCCUPIED WITH FEELINGS OF ENVY] **often envious of others or believes that others are envious of him or her (e.g., often resents others who have privileges, achievements, or loyalties that they feel are better deserved by themselves)**

9) **arrogant, haughty behaviors or attitudes** (new criterion proposed for DSM-IV) [REACTS TO CRITICISM WITH FEELINGS OF RAGE, SHAME, OR HUMILIATION (EVEN IF NOT EXPRESSED)] (DSM-III-R criterion 1)

Note. Contents of DSM-III-R whose omission is proposed are [CAPITALIZED AND BRACKETED]. Contents that are proposed for addition in DSM-IV are printed in **bold type.** Criteria appear in the order proposed for DSM-IV.

Statement and Significance of the Issues

This review examines available empirical data about both the DSM-III and DSM-III-R descriptions of NPD with respect to the following issues: 1) Prevalence: does this disorder apply to a significant subsample in clinical populations? 2) Overlap (comorbidity): can the disorder, as currently defined, be distinguished from other disorders? 3) Criterion performance (diagnostic efficiency): what is the relative contribution of the existing criteria to capturing prototypic features and/or to the problems in overlap? 4) Phenomenological studies: are there alternative criteria that perform as well or better than the existing ones? 5) Essential feature: is it clearly stated and congruent with the literature and does it capture the most prototypic features of the disorder?

Based on this review, the problems that DSM-IV should address are identified, and revisions are proposed.

Methods

The review of the literature began with the already published reviews and commentaries on the DSM-III-R description of NPD (Akhtar 1989; Akhtar and Thomson 1982; Bursten 1982, 1989; Cooper 1982, 1987; Emmons 1987; Frances 1980; Goldstein 1985; Gunderson 1983; Kernberg 1984, 1987; Lerner 1985; Ronningstam 1988; Vaillant and Perry 1985; Widiger et al. 1988). The literature search was then extended by a computer search of Medline using the key term *narcissism* with modifiers that included *pathological, personality,* and *character,* covering the period from 1978 to 1989. This search for the relevant post-DSM-III literature located 789 documents on narcissism, 397 on narcissistic personality, 77 on narcissistic personality disorder, 64 on narcissistic character, and 45 on pathological narcissism. It indicated that, despite the continued widespread interest in this category, much of the literature continues to be theoretical and therapeutic, with relatively few descriptive examinations.

Nonpublished sources for this review included 46 major contributors to the personality disorder literature who were invited to provide advice about the essential features of this disorder. A smaller group of advisers with special interest in this disorder offered comments and/or references relevant to its possible revision in DSM-IV (Table 28–2). In addition, 20 researchers who had collected relevant data were solicited to provide unpublished data that could be used in conjunction with the published reports to examine overlap, diagnostic efficiency, and item-by-diagnosis analyses.

Table 28–2. Initial advisers for narcissistic personality disorder

Gerald Adler	Donald Klein
Salman Akhtar	James Masterson
Roger Blashfield	Les Morey
Benjamin Bursten	Elsa Ronningstam
Arnold Cooper	Eric Plakun
Otto Kernberg	Lorna Smith-Benjamin

Results

Prevalence

The use of NPD as the primary clinical diagnosis is probably relatively unusual in both outpatient and inpatient settings. The shifts from DSM-III to DSM-III-R greatly increased the number of patients diagnosable by the NPD criteria (Morey 1988a). In studies assessing clinical populations, the prevalence of patients meeting criteria varies from 2.0% (Dahl 1986) to 16% (Frances et al. 1984; Skodol 1989; Zanarini et al. 1987). Given the extensive literature within psychoanalytic or psychotherapeutic journals, its usage would likely be substantial in outpatient private practice settings. Its prevalence in the general population is estimated to be less than 1% (Reich et al. 1989; Zimmerman and Coryell 1990).

Comorbidity

Data from 11 studies (Blashfield and Breen 1989; Dahl 1986; Frances et al. 1984; Freiman and Widiger 1989; Loranger et al. 1987; Millon and Tringone 1989; Morey 1988a; Pfohl et al. 1986; Skodol 1989; Widiger et al. 1987; Zanarini et al. 1987) using structured DSM-III or DSM-III-R assessments indicate that only rarely do patients meet criteria for this disorder and not also criteria for other Axis II disorders. The highest rate of a single diagnosis of NPD was found in the data from Millon and Tringone (1989), in which the single diagnosis of NPD appeared in 21% of patients receiving personality disorder diagnoses. These studies also indicate that patients meeting requirements for NPD have especially high overlap with other dramatic cluster disorders; the overlap actually exceeded 50% in most studies. When DSM-III-R criteria were used, the overlap with "dramatic cluster" disorders fell about 25% and was never above 50%, but other personality types that emerged with significant overlap included passive-aggressive, schizotypal, and paranoid. The fact that these high rates of overlap with other personality disorders derived from all three clusters reflects the diversity of overlap in personality disorders. The degree to which the overlap varied from study to study reflects the power of idiosyncrasies in the samples or in the assessment instruments.

Although many studies on clinical populations have documented the prevalence of patients who meet criteria for NPD, these studies do not provide evidence about whether this prevalence agrees with the rate at which the NPD diagnosis is given in clinical settings, which was the incentive for including the NPD diagnosis in DSM-III. Work by Morey and Ochoa (1989) showed that clinicians used the NPD diagnosis twice as often as the patients met DSM-III criteria. Both Millon and Tringone (1989) and Ronningstam and Gunderson (1990) reported that even the more inclusive DSM-III-R criteria frequently fail to identify patients who are given a primary NPD diagnosis clinically. In the latter study, only 10 of 24 prototypic NPD patients met the threshold for the DSM-III-R diagnosis of NPD.

In general, these results indicate that the correspondence between DSM-III-R criteria for NPD and clinical diagnosis of the disorder is not very high and that the distinction between NPD and other Axis II disorders, especially the dramatic cluster disorders, needs to be sharpened.

Criteria Performance Characteristics (Diagnostic Efficiency)

The phi coefficients ("hit rates") for the individual NPD criteria were similar in the two DSM-III–based studies (Plakun 1987; Zanarini et al., unpublished data 1989) insofar as both found that the three worst criteria were poor response to criticism, alternating attitudes, and lack of empathy (Table 28–3). The overriding criterion about disturbed interpersonal relationships (i.e., requiring two of the four interpersonal features) was the best in one study (Zanarini et al. 1987) but untested in the other. Three other studies using DSM-III-R criteria (Freiman and Widiger 1989; Millon and Tringone 1989; Morey and Heumann 1988) found that criteria 3 (grandiose self-importance), 5 (fantasies of unlimited success), and 7 (attention and admiration) had the best phi coefficients (see Table 28–3). As with the DSM-III–based studies, the criteria related to "reactions to criticism" (criterion 1) and "lack of empathy" (criterion 8) were among the worst performers; the new DSM-III-R criterion 9 (feelings of envy) that had replaced the previous poor performer ("alternating attitudes") also performed poorly. In general, these studies showed considerable variability in the quality of NPD criteria, but they highlighted the fact that criteria related to grandiosity were usually the best performers, whereas criteria 1, 8, and 9 performed poorly.

DSM-III-R criterion 1 (reaction to criticism) was a sufficiently poor performer that omission or radical revision is indicated. Item-by-diagnosis analyses indicate that the criterion has similar (or higher) sensitivity, specificity, positive predictive power, and phi for paranoid personality disorder (First and Spitzer 1989; Morey and Goodman 1989; Skodol 1989) and BPD (Freiman and Widiger 1989; Morey and Goodman 1989; Skodol 1989). Morey (1988b) also found a high point biserial correlation for this criterion with paranoid personality disorder and BPD. Adviser input and the work by Ronningstam and Gunderson (1990) suggest that adding defeat and rejection to criticism as precipitants for the narcissistic reactions could help the performance of this criterion. Moreover, "rage" as a type of reactive feeling does not differentiate narcissistic patients from other dramatic cluster personality disorders, whereas "disdain," along with the shame and humiliation already noted in this criterion, is likely to be more pathognomonic (Morey and Goodman 1989). These observations suggested that the criteria could possibly be improved as follows: "Reacts to criticism, defeat, or rejection with sustained feelings of disdain, shame, or humiliation (even if not expressed)." This effort to salvage "narcissistic injury," a prototypic feature in the analytic literature (Kernberg 1984; Kohut 1972), ultimately gave way to the advantages of adding a new criterion (see below).

Criterion 8 (lack of empathy) reflects a frequently cited feature of narcissistic persons in the clinical literature (Kohut 1971). Whatever its clinical utility, Ron-

Table 28–3. Phi coefficients of narcissistic personality disorder criteria

	N	GUI	GRF	EXH	CRT	DRL	ENT	EXP	ALT	EMP
DSM-III study[a]										
Plakun 1987	19	.74	.54	.70	.46	—	.52	.58	.16	.41
Zanarini et al. 1989	45	.53	.44	.58	.24	.64	.44	.37	.32	.30

	N	CRT	EXP	IMP	UNQ	GRF	ENT	ATT	EMP	ENV
DSM-III-R study[b]										
Millon and Tringone 1989	49	.03	.38	.41	—	.26	.31	.19	.20	.05
Freiman and Widiger 1989	11	.26	.10	.46	.31	.61	.45	.57	.16	.25
Morey and Heumann 1988	64	.28	.36	.57	.30	.64	.45	.46	.41	.32

[a]GUI = grandiose uniqueness/self-importance. GRF = grandiose fantasies. EXH = exhibitionism. CRT = poor response to criticism. DRL = two of the disturbed relationships. ENT = entitlement. EXP = exploitativeness. ALT = alternating attitudes. EMP = lack of empathy.
[b]CRT = reaction to criticism. EXP = exploitative. IMP = grandiose self-importance. UNQ = unique problems. GRF = grandiose fantasies. ENT = entitlement. ATT = attention and admiration. EMP = lack of empathy. ENV = feelings of envy.

ningstam and Gunderson (1989) argue that it is sufficiently difficult to achieve valid judgments about the presence or absence of this criterion from single interviews that it should be ignored or omitted when rated from single assessments or research-based diagnoses. A closer examination of its poor efficiency using item-by-diagnosis analyses shows that it is equally associated with antisocial and passive-aggressive personalities (First and Spitzer 1989; Morey 1988b; Skodol 1989). Point biserial correlations show significant convergence with antisocial, histrionic, passive-aggressive, and schizoid personality disorders (Morey 1988b). This indicates that revision might diminish problematic overlap by distinguishing between the problems of individuals with antisocial personality disorder that are due to uncaring callousness and those of individuals with passive-aggressive personality disorder that are due to obstructionism. In contrast, it is proposed that the revised criterion for NPD should specify that the empathic failures of those with NPD are due to an unwillingness, not an inability, to identify with the feelings and needs of others (see Table 28–1).

Existing research indicates that the third problematic criterion, number 9 (envy), is not found that often and is not necessarily found in NPD subjects. In one study, more than half of a sample of clinicians assigned this criterion to other categories (Blashfield and Breen 1989). The item-by-diagnosis analyses show that this criterion has high performance characteristics for histrionic personality disorder (First and Spitzer 1989) and avoidant personality disorder (Morey and Goodman 1989). Point biserial correlations show significant association with seven of the other personality disorders (Morey 1988b). These problems seem related to the particular wording of the criterion and difficulty in its assessment. Ronningstam and Gunderson (1990) found that, whereas "preoccupation with envy" was not useful in distinguishing a prototypic NPD sample, such people frequently inferred envy about themselves in others. NPD advisers agreed that such patients might more readily acknowledge resentment than envy per se toward others who have privileges, achievements, or loyalties that they feel are better deserved by themselves. Hence, revisions in the envy criterion are proposed to increase the likelihood of positive responses and perhaps the specificity (see Table 28–1).

Phenomenological Studies

Several investigators have evaluated features related to pathological narcissism beyond those found in DSM-III-R. Those features that functioned better than some (or all) of the existing NPD criteria are noted as possible additions or replacements.

Using a structured Diagnostic Interview for Narcissism (DIN) (Gunderson et al. 1990) to assess 33 characteristics imputed to narcissistic personality from the literature, three features emerged as helpful non-DSM criteria: 1) "boastful and/or pretentious behavior," 2) "arrogant and haughty attitude or behavior," and 3) "self-centered, self-referential" (Ronningstam et al. 1990). Morey's (1988a) survey of how DSM-III and DSM-III-R personality disorder criteria corresponded with clinician diagnoses of NPD in a sample of 291 personality disordered patients pointed toward the advantages of the following alternative characteristics: 1)"egocentricity," 2) "dominance," 3) "interpersonal disdain," 4) "preoccupation with status," 5) "petulant anger," and 6) "fragile self-concept" (L. C. Morey, personal communication, 1989). Millon and Tringone (1989) used the Millon Personality Disorder Checklist (MPDC) (Millon 1987) to evaluate four existing DSM-III-R criteria (1, 2, 5, and 6) in a sample of 49 patients diagnosed with NPD. This work supported the possible use of four new features: 1) "acts arrogantly self-assured and confident," 2) "has sense of high self-worth," 3) "viewed as vain and self-indulgent," and 4) "views self as gregarious and charming."

These studies suggest that an alternative criterion to be considered for DSM-IV is "arrogant, haughty behaviors and/or attitudes" (Table 28–1). This criterion has both cognitive and interpersonal dimensions. It captures the personal disdain or even contempt toward others that is indirectly reflected in the "entitlement" and "insensitivity toward others" criteria (DSM-III-R criteria 6 and 8, respectively). Ronningstam and Gunderson (1990) found that this observable behavior was useful in distinguishing narcissistic patients and could be more readily identified in single interviews than several existing criteria (i.e., DSM-III-R criteria 8 or 9). A related item, "acts arrogantly self-assured and confident," was clearly the best item in the Millon and Tringone (1989) survey to assess pathological narcissism, surpassing even the very good DSM criteria (DSM-III-R criterion 2, interpersonally exploitative, and the part of criterion 3 related to grandiose self-image) (Millon and Tringone 1989). It helps to differentiate NPD from histrionic, antisocial, and borderline personality disorders in which individuals are respectively self-centered but coquettish, distant but callous, and entitled but needy.

A number of small revisions are identifiable that may incorporate some of these alternatives while clarifying the clinical phenomena belonging to NPD in ways that will help diminish overlap, especially with histrionic personality disorder. For example, although criterion 3 (grandiose) is generally an excellent performer, item-by-diagnosis analyses indicate that this criterion has similar performance characteristics for histrionic personality disorder (First and Spitzer 1989; Morey and Goodman 1989; Zanarini et al. 1989). Furthermore, point biserial correlates show a high convergence with histrionic, passive-aggressive, and antisocial personality disorders (Morey 1988b). Replacing "expects to be noticed as 'special' " with "as superior," seems likely to diminish the overlap with HPD while capturing a descriptor more tightly aligned with the grandiosity construct (see Table 28–1). "Superiority" was the best-performing item on studies using the DIN (Ronningstam and Gunderson 1990) and also using the MPDC (Millon and Tringone 1989).

Moreover, removing "special" from this criterion and combining it with the feature noted in DSM-III-R criterion 4 (uniqueness of problems) seems like a close conceptual union that would help move the criterion away from the clinical situation into a more general narcissistic trait. Likewise, although DSM-III-R criterion 7 (requires attention and admiration) is not a notably weak performer, the attention component encourages the overlap noted earlier with both histrionic and borderline personality disorders and the example ("fishing for compliments") implies more manifest insecurity than is typical for those with NPD. In fact, according to item-by-diagnosis analyses (First and Spitzer 1989; Freiman and Widiger 1989; Morey and Goodman 1989; Skodol 1989) and the point biserial correlations (Morey 1988b), this criterion regularly correlates and predicts histrionic personality disorder better than it does NPD. Thus, omitting attention promises to help the performance of this criterion (Table 28–1).

Essential Feature

The existing description of the essential feature for NPD is "a pervasive pattern of grandiosity (in fantasy or behavior), lack of empathy, and hypersensitivity to the evaluation of others." The responses from 20 advisers about the essential feature(s) of this disorder generally supported the current statement. Concern was expressed that grandiosity may not be overt and thereby may easily be overlooked by descriptors that do not attend to subjective experience, internal fantasies, and more covert behaviors. An alternative that was considered was "A persistent and unrealistic overevaluation of one's own importance and achievements." This simpler and more restrictive version gave centrality to grandiosity, a feature that is central to many descriptions of NPD (e.g., Kernberg 1984; Kohut 1971; Masterson 1981) and that emerged as the source of the most discriminating features for patients with this diagnosis (see above); however, it was not considered preferable by most advisers. Concern was expressed that groups with other diagnoses such as hypomania and obsessive-compulsive disorder can also be grandiose. There was no clear consensus about any other direction an alternative should take. When it became clear that the "hypersensitivity" component reflected a very poorly performing criterion that is proposed for omission (see above), the committee suggested the phrase be replaced by "needs the admiration of others."

Discussion and Recommendations

The available empirical data related to the DSM-III and DSM-III-R definitions of NPD represent significant progress in efforts to describe this disorder. Nonetheless, these data are marked by two fundamental limitations. Although the criteria that appeared in DSM-III and DSM-III-R were meant to capture and reflect what informed clinical judgments would identify as narcissistic psychopathology, the vast majority of the research that has been done has utilized the criteria without reference to this intention. With few exceptions, research on NPD has not tested or demonstrated that the existing DSM criteria and cutoff capture the patients about whom the clinical literature on narcissistic personality has been written. To do this requires employing clinicians with expertise on narcissistic psychopathology as the standards of reference or, at least, using the "longitudinal, expert, all data (LEAD)" standard as proposed by Spitzer (1983). The other major failure of the existing research is the absence of validating studies. Research has not yet broached the important questions as to whether identification of patients as having NPD can provide information on etiological and/or pathogenetic origins or predict course and/or treatment responsivity. In the absence of such studies, the value of including this category in DSM rests solely on the attributions of clinical utility from a widely recognized, psychodynamically informed clinical literature and tradition.

The existing data largely bear on the descriptive validity of the NPD category. Moreover, much of these data derive from systematic assessments of patient populations using the structured clinical interviews that assess all of the Axis II disorders. These data, gathered from several thousand patients, indicate that NPD as defined in DSM rarely occurs in patients who do not fulfill criteria for other Axis II disorders. Although DSM-III-R made significant progress in diminishing the very high levels of overlap with the other dramatic cluster disorders, these disorders, and particularly histrionic and antisocial types, remain major differential diagnostic problems. The diagnostic efficiency assessments have especially highlighted the problems found in DSM-III-R criteria 1, 8, and 9. Item-by-diagnosis analyses have indicated that these criteria are important sources for the overlap problems with other Axis II disorders. The phenomenological studies, as well as adviser input, have suggested ways in which the revision of these problematic criteria may increase their specificity. Phenomenological studies have also identified more subtle ways in which changes can be introduced to other criteria to heighten their specificity. This review therefore highlights a series of specific revisions, shown in Table 28–2, that might profitably be made in DSM-IV.

References

Akhtar S: Narcissistic personality disorder: descriptive features and differential diagnosis. Psychiatr Clin North Am 12:505–529, 1989

Akhtar S, Thomson J: Overview: narcissistic personality disorder. Am J Psychiatry 139:12–20, 1982

American Psychiatric Association: Diagnostic and Statistical Manual of Mental Disorders, 3rd Edition. Washington, DC, American Psychiatric Association, 1980

American Psychiatric Association: Diagnostic and Statistical Manual of Mental Disorders, 3rd Edition, Revised. Washington, DC, American Psychiatric Association, 1987

Blashfield RK, Breen MJ: Face validity of the DSM-III-R personality disorders. Am J Psychiatry 146:1575–1579, 1989

Bursten B: Narcissistic personalities in DSM-III. Compr Psychiatry 23:409–420, 1982

Bursten B: The relationship between narcissistic and antisocial personalities. Psychiatr Clin North Am 12:571–584, 1989

Cooper A: Narcissistic disorders within psychoanalytic theory, in Psychiatry 1982, Vol 1. Edited by Grinspoon L. Washington, DC, American Psychiatric Press, 1982, pp 487–498

Cooper A: Histrionic, narcissistic, and compulsive personality disorders, in Diagnosis and Classification in Psychiatry: A Critical Appraisal of DSM-III. Edited by Tischler G. New York, Cambridge University Press, 1987, pp 290–299

Dahl F: Some aspects of the DSM-III personality disorders illustrated by a consecutive sample of hospitalized patients. Acta Psychiatr Scand 73 (Suppl 328):61–66, 1986

Emmons R: Narcissism: theory and measurement. J Pers Soc Psychol 52:11–17, 1987

First M, Spitzer R:. Diagnostic efficiency statistics. Unpublished raw data. New York, New York State Psychiatric Institute, 1989

Frances A: The DSM-III personality disorders section: a commentary. Am J Psychiatry 137:1050–1054, 1980

Frances A, Clarkin J, Gilmore M, et al:. Reliability of criteria for borderline personality disorder: a comparison of DSM-III and the Diagnostic Interview for Borderline Personality Disorder. Am J Psychiatry 141:1080–1084, 1984

Freiman K, Widiger TA: Co-occurrence and diagnostic efficiency statistics. Unpublished raw data, Lexington, University of Kentucky, 1989

Goldstein W: DSM-III and the narcissistic personality. Am J Psychother 39:4–16, 1985

Gunderson J: DSM-III diagnosis of personality disorders, in Current Perspectives on Personality Disorders. Edited by Frosch J. Washington, DC, American Psychiatric Press, 1983, pp 20–39

Gunderson J, Ronningstam E, Bodkin A: The Diagnostic Interview for Narcissistic Patients. Arch Gen Psychiatry 47:676–680, 1990

Kernberg O: Problems in the classification of personality disorders, in Severe Personality Disorders. New Haven, CT, Yale University Press, 1984, pp 77–94

Kernberg O: Narcissistic personality disorder, in Psychiatry, Vol 1. Edited by Michels R, Cavenar J. Philadelphia, PA, JB Lippincott, 1987, pp 1–17

Kohut H: The Analysis of the Self. New York, International Universities Press, 1971

Kohut H: Thoughts on narcissism and narcissistic rage. Psychoanal Study Child 27:360–400, 1972

Lerner P: Current psychoanalytic perspectives on the borderline and narcissistic concepts. Clin Psychol Rev 5:199–214, 1985

Loranger AW, Susman VL, Oldham JM, et al: The Personality Disorder Examination: a preliminary report. Journal of Personality Disorders 1:1–13, 1987

Masterson JF: The Narcissistic and Borderline Disorders. New York, Brunner/Mazel, 1981

Millon T: Millon Clinical Multiaxial Inventory-II: Manual. Minneapolis, MN, National Computer Systems, 1987

Millon T, Tringone R: Co-occurrence and diagnostic efficiency statistics. Unpublished raw data, Miami, FL, University of Miami, 1989

Morey LC: Personality disorders in DSM-III and DSM-III-R: convergence, coverage, and internal consistency. Am J Psychiatry 145:573–577, 1988a

Morey L: A psychometric analysis of the DSM-III-R personality disorder criteria. Journal of Personality Disorders 2:109–124, 1988b

Morey L, Goodman R: Diagnostic efficiency statistics. Unpublished raw data, Nashville, TN, Vanderbilt University, 1989

Morey L, Heumann K: Co-occurrence and diagnostic efficiency statistics. Unpublished raw data, Nashville, TN, Vanderbilt University, 1988

Morey LC, Ochoa ES: An investigation of adherence to diagnostic criteria: clinical diagnosis of the DSM-III personality disorders. Journal of Personality Disorders 3:180–192, 1989

Pfohl B, Coryell W, Zimmerman M, et al: DSM-III personality disorders: diagnostic overlap and internal consistency of individual DSM-III criteria. Compr Psychiatry 27:21–34, 1986

Plakun E: Distinguishing narcissistic and borderline personality disorders using DSM-III criteria. Compr Psychiatry 28:437–443, 1987

Reich J, Yates W, Nduaguba M: Prevalence of DSM-III personality disorders in the community. Soc Psychiatry Psychiatr Epidemiol 24:12–16, 1989

Ronningstam E: Comparing three systems for diagnosing narcissistic personality disorder. Psychiatry 51:300–311, 1988

Ronningstam E, Gunderson J: Descriptive studies on narcissistic personality disorder. Psychiatr Clin North Am 12:585–601, 1989

Ronningstam E, Gunderson J: Identifying criteria for NPD. Am J Psychiatry 147:918–922, 1990

Skodol A: Co-occurrence and diagnostic efficiency statistics. Unpublished raw data, New York, New York State Psychiatric Institute, 1989

Spitzer RL: Psychiatric diagnosis: are clinicians still necessary? Compr Psychiatry 24:399–411, 1983

Vaillant G, Perry C: Personality disorders, in Comprehensive Textbook of Psychiatry, Vol 1, 4th Edition. Edited by Kaplan H, Sadock B. Baltimore, MD, Williams & Wilkins, 1985, pp 958–986

Widiger T, Trull T, Hurt S, et al: A multidimensional scaling of the DSM-III personality disorders. Arch Gen Psychiatry 44:557–563, 1987

Widiger T, Frances A, Spitzer R, et al: The DSM-III-R personality disorders: an overview. Am J Psychiatry 145:786–795, 1988

Zanarini M, Frankenburg F, Chauncey D, et al: The diagnostic interview for personality disorders: interrater and test-retest reliability. Compr Psychiatry 28:467–480, 1987

Zanarini M, Frankenburg F, Chauncey D, et al: Co-occurrence and diagnostic efficiency statistics. Unpublished raw data. Boston, MA, McLean Hospital, 1989

Zimmerman M, Coryell W: Diagnosing personality disorders in the community: a comparison of self-report and interview measures. Arch Gen Psychiatry 47:527–531, 1990

Chapter 29

Avoidant Personality Disorder

Theodore Millon, Ph.D.

Introduction

Avoidant personality disorder (AVPD) represents a category named and included for the first time in DSM-III (American Psychiatric Association 1980), although parallels may be found in the writings of numerous early and more recent clinical theorists (Bleuler 1911; Burnham et al. 1969; Fenichel 1945; Horney 1945; Kretschmer 1925; Millon 1969).

Statement of the Issues

The major issues surrounding AVPD may be separated into five questions:

1. What prototypal traits should be selected to represent the category's essential features?
2. As a new category, does AVPD display evidence of adequate prevalence level or diagnostic usage?
3. Can AVPD be differentiated from other disorders with which it shares certain features?
4. Do the DSM-III-R (American Psychiatric Association 1987) AVPD criteria achieve satisfactory levels of diagnostic efficiency and validity?
5. Are there DSM-III-R criteria that should be omitted, modifications that may perform better, and alternate criteria that may add important features beyond those on the current list?

Significance of the Issues

Because AVPD was recently introduced into the nomenclature, several clinicians and investigators have asked whether it represents a distinct personality disorder (PD) (e.g., Kernberg 1984; Livesley et al. 1985; Trull et al. 1987) and whether it exists as an entity separate from certain Axis I disorders, most notably social phobia (Liebowitz et al. 1985; Turner et al. 1986). These issues continue to be discussed in the literature, suggesting the need for the Personality Disorders Work Group to fully clarify distinctions between the AVPD and both other Axis II disorders and Axis I disorders (e.g., Herbert et al. 1992; Holt et al. 1992; Turner et al. 1992; Widiger 1992).

Methods

Dialog Information Services provided Medline and other less medically oriented computer-based literature searches to locate articles, chapters, and books from 1978 to 1990 in which the term *avoidant personality* was included; other references, employing the terms *shy* and *phobic,* for example, were likewise provided. Related clinical references (mostly under the designation *schizoid*) before this period were also obtained. Owing to its recent introduction, the literature using the label *avoidant personality* is quite sparse; only a few studies were empirical. A total of 284 articles were identified, the majority reflecting earlier literature on the schizoid designation.

Forthcoming articles on a wide range of relevant issues were recommended by advisers and consultants. Unpublished data relevant to prevalence and descriptive validity were also supplied by numerous investigators (Blashfield 1988; Dahl 1986; First and Spitzer 1989; Freiman and Widiger 1989; Millon and Tringone 1989; Morey and Heumann 1988; Pfohl and Blum 1990; Reich 1988; Skodol 1989; Zanarini et al. 1989).

Results and Discussion

This section is organized into five parts in accordance with the five issues noted previously.

1. What prototypic criteria should be used for the category's essential features? The following characteristics were proposed by the Work Group's advisers: 1) "There is intense fear of social derogation, humiliation, and rejection. The baseline position is to avoid social contact, to wall off socially, and to tightly restrain self-expression"; 2) "There is fearful avoidance of situations in which one is observed by others and in which there is a risk of failure, rejection, or revelation of strong feelings"; 3) "Accompanying the fearful avoidance is a strong desire for interpersonal affiliation"; 4) "Important . . . is the wish for relationships to help distinguish it from the schizoid"; 5) "The essential feature is low self-esteem and a chronic state of social anxiety, especially in situations where there is a risk of rejection or failure. . . . These fearful and self-demeaning attitudes coexist with strong desires for affection and acceptance"; 6) "[There] is the simultaneous existence . . . of strong wishes for relationships and challenges and of fearful avoidance of people and situations where there is a risk of failure, rejection, or strong feelings, resulting in a pervasive pattern of social discomfort, fear of negative evaluation and timidity."

As a final guide, the Work Group examined the following criteria formulated for the anxious (avoidant) PD for the fourth revision of ICD-10 (World Health Organization 1990):

(1) persistent and pervasive feelings of tension and apprehension; (2) habitual self-consciousness and feelings of insecurity and inferiority; (3) continuous yearning to be liked and accepted; (4) hypersensitivity to rejection and criticism; (5) refusal to enter into relationships unless receiving strong guarantees of uncritical acceptance; very restricted personal attachments; (6) habitual proneness to exaggerate the potential dangers or risks in everyday situations, to the extent of avoiding certain activities, not amounting to phobic avoidance; (7) restricted lifestyle because of need to have certainty and security. (p. 105)

In contrast to decisions regarding the specific items in the diagnostic criteria, where efficiency and validity statistics could be drawn on, judgments concerning the essential features of the disorder were of a qualitative nature. The proposed description of essential features for this disorder was phrased as follows: "A pervasive pattern of social discomfort and reticence, low self-esteem, and hypersensitivity to negative evaluation."

2. Does AVPD achieve a satisfactory prevalence level and frequency of diagnostic usage? One issue raised in some quarters after the publication of DSM-III pertained to whether cases described as AVPD were, in fact, found in clinical settings (e.g., Kernberg 1984). As of this date, the Personality Disorders Work Group does not have a fully representative PD epidemiological study among the general population or among patients (Weissman 1990). However, a review of several studies on DSM-III and DSM-III-R PD prevalence reported in Table 1 of the introduction to this section indicates that the range for AVPD is extensive, from .05 to .55. Excluding the upper extremes, where multiple diagnoses were encouraged, AVPD prevalence clusters around 10%. The advent of AVPD (and also schizotypal PD) has resulted, however, in a decline in the prevalence of schizoid PD, sufficient to raise questions as to the latter's viability as a diagnosable entity.

3. Can AVPD be differentiated from other disorders with which it shares certain features? Empirically based data on comorbidity from several studies have been analyzed. Although these data are based on diverse methodologies and patient samples, a measure of consistency does appear. Excluding borderline PD, where overlap can be attributed to that disorder's high prevalence in many studies, AVPD shows up most frequently with schizoid, schizotypal, dependent, paranoid, and self-defeating PDs—a wide variety—but each understandable in terms of particular shared features.

To expect each PD to be a wholly distinct entity with defining features (or diagnostic criteria) that do not overlap with those of other PDs is to expect a level of symptomatological uniqueness rarely found in medicine at large. Numerous "diseases" share symptoms yet may be differentiated by the unique configuration of their symptoms. Individuals with prototypal AVPD share the characteristic of "social withdrawal" with individuals with both prototypal schizoid and schizotypal PDs; they share the characteristic of "low self-esteem" (as per DSM-III) with individuals with dependent PD, "social anxiety" with individuals with social phobia, and so on. It may be useful to briefly elaborate on this theme as it applies to this latter, somewhat problematic, Axis I syndrome.

Social phobia is an anxiety disorder in which the defining feature is a persistent fear of and immediate anxiety reaction to social situations (circumscribed or generalized). Social phobia may covary with AVPD, but the two may be distinguished on several grounds. First, AVPD consists of several traits and behaviors, of which the essential feature of social phobia is but one. AVPD exhibits a wider range of anxiety precipitants than social phobia. Persons with social phobia may have a multitude of satisfying social/personal relationships with others; the individual with AVPD is socially withdrawn, has few close relationships, and desires close relationships but does not trust others sufficiently to relate closely without assurances of acceptance. AVPD is essentially a problem of relating to persons; social phobia has been formulated largely as a problem of performing in situations. The individual with prototypic AVPD has low self-esteem; the social phobia concept implies no such self-critical judgment. Nevertheless, recent studies indicate that the DSM-III-R criteria for these two disorders result in considerable overlap and differential diagnostic difficulties (Herbert et al. 1992; Holt et al. 1992; Turner et al. 1992).

The overlap problem between AVPD and social phobia was created in part by the actions of the DSM-III-R PD committee; their decisions, it should be noted, were not guided by empirical data but rather by an epistemological reversal in DSM principles, namely that of favoring a particular theoretical viewpoint. Trait criteria considered central to the DSM-III avoidant formulation (e.g., "desire for acceptance" and "low self-esteem") were deleted; at the same time, several new criteria were added, such as "fear of saying something inappropriate" and "fear of being embarrassed by blushing." The latter changes not only represented a theoretically based shift, but they also created an overlap with the expanded construct of social phobia. By dropping DSM-III criteria for AVPD that differentiated it and introducing common "phobia" criteria, the DSM-III-R committees inadvertently made AVPD and social phobia highly comparable, a similarity further compounded by the decision to introduce a "generalized type" of social phobia. However, several studies (e.g., Greenberg and Stravynski 1983; Turner et al. 1986) had suggested that AVPD and social phobia could be distinguished on clinical grounds based on DSM-III criteria; individuals with AVPD were seen as being more severely impaired and showing greater deficits in social skills, interpersonal sensitivity, and avoidant behaviors, as well as experiencing greater distress, anxiety, and depression. The planned changes for DSM-IV avoidant criteria were guided by the need to strengthen distinctions that were blurred in DSM-III-R.

Turning to other Axis II disorders, both AVPD and dependent PD are characterized by low self-esteem (Reich 1991). However, in dependent PD, this stems from a feeling of inadequate competence that leads to a fear of performing on one's own. Individuals with dependent PD do not share the broad-ranging fear of relating to others found in AVPD; on the contrary, they feel most secure when they do affiliate. The general level of anxiety in dependent PD is not a notable feature, as it is in AVPD. Most central to the anxieties in dependent PD is interpersonal loss, in contrast to the avoidant individual's anxieties, which derive from fears of becoming interpersonally too close (Trull et al. 1987).

Although schizoid and avoidant PDs share the trait of social disengagement or distancing, this feature stems from opposite sources (Millon 1981). In the individual with schizoid PD, it reflects interpersonal indifference; in the individual with AVPD it reflects interpersonal anxiety. Whereas the individual with AVPD desires (but does not trust) affection and closeness, the individual with schizoid PD has little interest in affection and closeness. The person with AVPD devalues himself and has low self-esteem; the person with schizoid PD does not. The person with AVPD is self-conscious and hyperalert to the meaning of others' communications; the person with schizoid PD is unselfconscious and insensitive to the feelings and intents conveyed in the communications of others.

Diagnostic problems could be avoided by having the Work Group rewrite the criteria for AVPD to more clearly differentiate them from similar criteria for schizoid PD, dependent PD, social phobia, and other disorders.

4. Do the criteria selected to represent AVPD in DSM-III-R achieve satisfactory levels of diagnostic efficiency and validity? The studies provided to the Work Group (First and Spitzer 1989; Freiman and Widiger 1989; Millon and Tringone 1989; Morey and Heumann 1988; Pfohl and Blum 1990; Reich 1988; Skodol 1989) show certain common results, although differences are notable as well. Diagnostic efficiency statistics, both internal and external, suggest that the criterion "easily hurt by criticism/disapproval" is not only highly consistent with other avoidant criteria but does not overlap appreciably with the criteria for other disorders. It fares poorly, however, when examined against clinician AVPD diagnoses (low specificity is the problem). "No close friends/confidants" shows high consistency with AVPD but also with schizoid and schizotypal PDs; in fact, using this gauge, it is a superior item for the latter two. As far as external validity is concerned, it proves reasonably efficient. "Unwilling to get involved" is an excellent item in that it is both highly consistent internally and shows good external validity. "Avoids social/occupational interpersonal contact" overlaps somewhat with schizoid and schizotypal but shows better internal consistency with AVPD than with the former two. Its strength is its excellent correspondence with external diagnoses of AVPD. "Reticent/fears looking foolish in public" proved a poor item both internally and externally, as did "fears of being embarrassed." Although "exaggerates difficulties outside routine" obtained reasonable results, it proved the weakest criterion on the important sensitivity statistic.

Although the overall efficiency statistics for AVPD are adequate, revisions in the form of criterion condensations, sharpening distinctions from overlapping disorders, greater concordance with the ICD-10 avoidant/anxious PD, and the addition of trait criteria that broaden the descriptive range of AVPD would be a reasonable undertaking.

5. Are there DSM-III-R criteria that should be omitted, modifications that may perform better, and alternate criteria that may add important diagnostic features beyond those on the current list? Turning first to the third consideration just noted, a major DSM-III criterion, "low self-esteem," was inadvisedly deleted from DSM-III-R according to several Work Group consultants. Evidence favoring the reintroduction of this general criterion was also obtained in a study of new diagnostic criteria (Millon and Tringone 1989). Moreover, this characteristic is related to a new ICD-10 criterion, "habitual self-consciousness and feelings of insecurity and inferiority." In their discussions, the Personality Disorders Work Group considered data, advisor input, descriptive literature, and consonance with ICD-10 in fashioning a proposed new AVPD criterion for DSM-IV phrased "belief that one is socially inept, personally unappealing, or inferior to others."

As far as the option of pruning the current DSM-III-R list because of the high overlap and weak diagnostic efficiency statistics of some items, it was proposed that two criteria be combined, criterion 6, "fears being embarrassed by blushing," and criterion 7 "exaggerates the potential difficulties . . . in doing something ordinary, but outside . . . usual routine." The following synthesis should also reduce overlap with the social phobic clinical syndrome attributable to highly similar criteria. The new criterion is phrased "is unusually reluctant about taking personal risks or engaging in any new activities because they may prove embarrassing."

Recommendations

The following paragraphs outline the suggestions (and the rationale for those suggestions) made by the Work Group to further increase the diagnostic clarity of the DSM-III-R criteria and to improve their effectiveness in distinguishing AVPD from similar disorders and syndromes. The listing follows the sequence of DSM-III-R; the sequence for DSM-IV will differ because it will be arranged according to the Work Group's judgment of the most prominent to the least prominent criterion item.

Criterion A(1): *Is easily hurt by criticism and disapproval.*

Proposal for change: To reduce overlap and to draw attention to the anticipatory and ruminative character of the sensitivity in AVPD, the following modification was suggested in Work Group discussions: *Preoccupation with being criticized or rejected in social situations.*

Criterion A(2): *Has no close friends or confidants (or only one) other than first degree relatives.*

Proposal for change: To differentiate the discontent over lack of friends in AVPD from, for example, the indifference seen in schizoid PD, the Work Group evolved the following alternative, which has similarities to the planned AVPD ICD-10 criterion that speaks of a "continuous yearning to be liked and accepted": *Has few friends despite the desire to relate to others.*

Criterion A(3): *Is unwilling to get involved with people unless certain of being liked.* No change proposed.

Criterion A(4): *Avoids social or occupational activities that involve significant interpersonal contact, e.g., refuses a promotion that will increase social demands.*

Proposal for change: Work Group discussions suggested that the example given in the criterion ("refuses a promotion") was too infrequent and unauthentic an event to be useful. The following alternative was proposed: *Avoids social or occupational activities that involve significant interpersonal contact, because of fears of criticism, disapproval, or rejection.*

Criterion A(5): *Is reticent in social situations because of a fear of saying something inappropriate or foolish or of being unable to answer a question.*

Proposal for change: To further distinguish AVPD from social phobia, the Work Group concluded that the quality that AVPD possesses beyond mere reticence in social situations is a fear of establishing intimate personal relationships. The following phrasing attempts to capture this distinction: *development of intimate relationships is inhibited (despite desire for them) owing to the fear of being foolish and ridiculed or being exposed and shamed.*

The Work Group also recommended that criteria 6 and 7 be combined because of the high overlap and weak diagnostic efficiency of these items. The following phrasing is proposed to reduce overlap with social phobia: *is unusually reluctant about taking personal risks or engaging in any new activities because they may prove embarrassing.*

These recommendations were made to sharpen distinctions, to be consistent with current clinical research, and to enhance correspondence with the forthcoming ICD-10.

References

American Psychiatric Association: Diagnostic and Statistical Manual of Mental Disorders, 3rd Edition. Washington, DC, American Psychiatric Association, 1980

American Psychiatric Association: Diagnostic and Statistical Manual of Mental Disorders, 3rd Edition, Revised. Washington, DC, American Psychiatric Association, 1987

Blashfield R: Similarity matrix for personality disorders. Unpublished raw data, 1988

Bleuler E: Dementia Praecox. New York, International Universities Press, 1911

Burnham DL, Gladstone AO, Gibson RW: Schizophrenia and the Need-Fear Dilemma. New York, International Universities Press, 1969

Dahl A: Some aspects of the DSM-III personality disorders illustrated by a consecutive sample of hospitalized patients. Acta Psychiatr Scand 73:1–66, 1986

Fenichel O: The Psychoanalytic Theory of the Neurosis. New York, Norton, 1945

First M, Spitzer R: Diagnostic efficiency statistics. Unpublished raw data, New York, New York State Psychiatric Institute, 1989

Freiman K, Widiger TA: Co-occurrence and diagnostic efficiency statistics. Unpublished raw data, Lexington, University of Kentucky, 1989

Greenberg D, Stravynski A: Social phobia. Br J Psychiatry 143:526, 1983

Herbert JD, Hope DA, Bellack AS: Validity of the distinction between generalized social phobia and avoidant personality disorder. J Abnorm Psychol 101:332–339, 1992

Holt CS, Heinberg RG, Hope DA: Avoidant personality disorder and the generalized subtype in social phobia. J Abnorm Psychol 101:318–325, 1992

Horney K: Our Inner Conflicts. New York, Norton, 1945

Kernberg O: Problems in the classification of personality disorders, in Severe Personality Disorders. New Haven, CT, Yale University Press, 1984, pp 77–94

Kretschmer E: Physique and Character. London, Kegan Paul, 1925

Leibowitz MR, Gorman JM, Fryer AJ, et al: Social phobia. Arch Gen Psychiatry 43:729–736, 1985

Livesley WJ, West M, Tanney A: Historical comment on the DSM-III schizoid and avoidant personality disorders. Am J Psychiatry 143:1344–1347, 1985

Millon T: Modern Psychopathology. Philadelphia, PA, WB Saunders, 1969

Millon T: Disorders of personality, DSM-III: Axis II. New York, Wiley, 1981

Millon T, Tringone R: Co-occurrence and diagnostic efficiency statistics. Unpublished raw data, Miami, FL, University of Miami, 1989

Morey L, Heumann K: Co-occurrence and diagnostic efficiency statistics. Unpublished raw data, Nashville, TN, Vanderbilt University, 1988

Pfohl B, Blum N: Internal consistency statistics for the DSM-III-R personality disorder criteria. Unpublished raw data, Iowa City, University of Iowa, 1990

Reich J: Diagnostic efficiency statistics for personality disorders. Unpublished raw data, Brockton, MA, Brockton VA Medical Center, 1988

Reich J: The relationship between DSM-III avoidant and dependent personality disorders. Psychiatry Res 29:131–139, 1991

Skodol A: Co-occurrence and diagnostic efficiency statistics. Unpublished raw data, New York, New York State Psychiatric Institute, 1989

Trull TJ, Widiger TA, Frances A: Covariation of criteria sets for avoidant, schizoid and dependent personality disorder. Am J Psychiatry 144:767–772, 1987

Turner SM, Beidel DC, Dancu CV, et al: Psychopathology of social phobia and comparison to avoidant personality disorder. J Abnorm Psychol 95:389–394, 1986

Turner SM, Beidel DC, Townsley RM: Social phobia: a comparison of specific and generalized subtypes and avoidant personality disorder. J Abnorm Psychol 101:326–331, 1992

Weissman MM: The epidemiology of personality disorder: a 1990 update. Paper presented at the Conference on the Personality Disorders, Williamsburg, VA, 1990

Widiger T: Generalized social phobia versus avoidant personality disorder: a commentary on three studies. J Abnorm Psychol 101:340–343, 1992

Widiger TA, Trull TJ, Hurt SW, et al: A multidimensional scaling of the DSM-III personality disorders. Arch Gen Psychiatry 44:557–563, 1987

World Health Organization: ICD-10 Chapter V. Mental and Behavioral Disorders. Diagnostic Criteria for Research. Geneva, Switzerland, World Health Organization, 1990

Zanarini M, Frankenburg F, Chauncey D, et al: Co-occurrence and diagnostic efficiency statistics. Unpublished raw data, Boston, MA, McLean Hospital, 1989

Chapter 30

Dependent Personality Disorder

Robert M. A. Hirschfeld, M.D., M. Tracie Shea, Ph.D., and
K. M. Talbot, B.S.

Introduction

The concept of dependency has its roots in psychoanalytic theory, social psychological theory, and ethological theory (Hirschfeld et al. 1976). Psychoanalytic theory emphasizes the attainment of instinctual aims through interaction with social objects, such as the mother, as the source of dependency. Social learning theories consider dependency to be a learned behavior, that is, one acquired in experience rather than being instinctual in the organism. More specifically, dependency refers to a class of behaviors, stemming from the infant's initial reliance on the mother; subsequently, these learned behaviors generalize to interpersonal relationships in general. In ethological theory, the concept of attachment has been proposed to refer to the affectional bond that one person forms with another specific individual. This bond is manifested by behaviors fostering proximity to and contact with the love object and by behavioral disruptions if separation occurs.

These theoretical sources have contributed to the concept of dependent personality disorder (DPD), as defined in DSM-III and DSM-III-R (American Psychiatric Association 1980, 1987). The core feature of this mental disorder has been abnormal dependency that causes subjective distress and/or impairment in functioning for the individual.

Statement of the Issues

The major issues to be addressed in considering revisions to the criteria for DPD were

1. To what extent does DPD overlap conceptually with other personality disorders (PDs)?
2. To what extent does DPD overlap empirically with other disorders?
3. How do the individual criteria for DPD perform (e.g., sensitivity and specificity)?
4. Is DPD characterized by single or multiple components?
5. Is there sex bias in the application of DPD?
6. Are the criteria compatible with those of ICD-10?

Methods

In a National Library of Medicine Medline computer search performed on journal articles published from January 1980 through May 1990, 47 articles appeared under the direct subject heading *dependent personality disorder.* An additional 38 articles from this source, found by combining terms, were determined to be relevant to the review. Other information and data were collected from book chapters on the topic, journal articles not abstracted on Medline, and reports of unpublished data.

Results and Discussion

Conceptual Overlap

Conceptual overlap of features of DPD can be found with features of borderline, avoidant, and histrionic PDs.

Borderline PD. Both dependent and borderline PDs are characterized by fear of abandonment. However, the behavioral patterns of these two disorders are quite different. Fear of abandonment elicits rage and manipulation in borderline PD, whereas it elicits submissive and clinging behavior in DPD. Whereas borderline PD patients have difficulty being alone under any circumstances, for those with DPD the issue is more the need to be attached or have access to a strong other person on whom they can rely for care and support.

Avoidant PD. Both dependent and avoidant PDs are characterized by feelings of inadequacy, sensitivity to criticism, and need for reassurance. However, DPD patients can be distinguished by their quite distinct behavior patterns. Avoidant PD is based on a fear of humiliation and rejection that results in social timidity and withdrawal. At the heart of DPD is an excessive need for attachment that leads to fears of separation and submissive and clinging behavior.

Histrionic PD.   Both dependent and histrionic PDs are characterized by a need for reassurance and approval. For histrionic PD, however, the need is for approval and praise in and of itself, whereas for DPD, the need is more for reassurance due to doubt about one's judgment and ability (i.e., to be assured by others that one's actions are correct).

Empirical Overlap

Studies have shown considerable diagnostic overlap between both DSM-III and DSM-III-R DPD and other PDs, particularly borderline PD (Table 30–1). More than 50% of patients with DPD also had borderline PD in two of four studies using DSM-III criteria (Morey 1988; Zanarini et al. 1987) and all three studies using DSM-III-R criteria (Morey 1988; Skodol et al. 1988). The second most frequent overlap was with avoidant PD, although there was also frequent overlap with histrionic and schizotypal PDs. Relatively few patients met criteria for DPD and for no other Axis II conditions. The percentage of PD patients with a single diagnosis of DPD ranged from 7% to 47%, with a median of 20%, in five studies (Table 30–1).

Performance of Criteria

Widiger (1991) provided data from five studies (First and Spitzer 1989; Freiman and Widiger 1989; Morey and Goodman 1989; Pfohl and Blum 1990; Skodol 1989) on the relationship between specific DSM-III-R criteria and the diagnosis of DPD. Criterion 9 (easily hurt by criticism or disapproval) performs particularly poorly in all the studies because it is not specific to DPD.

A. W. Loranger (personal communication, 1990) provided data on criteria performance in a sample of 136 nonpsychotic, nonbipolar patients who were assessed using the Personality Disorder Examination (Loranger 1988). Criterion 7 (feels devastated or helpless when a close relationship ends) and criterion 9 (easily hurt by criticism or disapproval) did particularly poorly in two ways. First, the endorsement rate of each was very high in patients who had no PD. Second, the endorsement rate on each was extremely high (usually over 80%) in almost all PDs, including dependent. These two criteria, therefore, were not at all specific to DPD. The item with the lowest endorsement rate for DPD was criterion 5 (volunteers to do things that are unpleasant or demeaning to get other people to like him or her).

Unitary Concept

Whether dependency is characterized by a single dimension or multiple dimensions has received considerable attention (Birchnell 1988; Hirschfeld et al. 1976; Livesley et al. 1990). Several investigations (Hirschfeld et al. 1976, 1977; Livesely et al. 1990) have assessed composite traits in normal and clinical samples and have examined them psychometrically. The findings have been consistent and have identified two

Table 30–1. Percentage of dependent personality disorder subjects who met the diagnostic criteria for other Axis II disorders

	PPD	SZPD	STPD	HPD	NPD	BPD	ASPD	AVPD	OCPD	PAPD	SING
DSM-III											
Pfohl et al. 1986	—	—	—	29	—	41	—	18	6	28	47
Zanarini et al. 1987	7	—	45	54	22	86	30	25	9	25	7
Dahl 1986	—	—	—	25	—	25	—	75	—	—	—
Morey 1988	29	9	23	29	26	51	3	49	9	17	—
Trull et al. 1987	—	0	—	—	—	—	—	50	—	—	—
DSM-III-R											
Morey 1988	29	9	12	29	26	51	3	49	9	17	—
Skodol et al. 1988	24	—	30	30	58	85	15	73	30	12	—
Skodol et al. 1988	36	3	24	33	21	79	3	70	27	18	—

Note. PPD = paranoid personality disorder. SZPD = schizoid personality disorder. STPD = schizotypal personality disorder. HPD = histrionic personality disorder. NPD = narcissistic personality disorder. BPD = borderline personality disorder. ASPD = antisocial personality disorder. AVPD = avoidant personality disorder. OCPD = obsessive-compulsive personality disorder. PAPD = passive-aggressive personality disorder. SING = percentage with dependent personality disorder only.

distinguishable components of DPD, attachment (or reliance on a single other person) and general dependency (or lack of social self-confidence). The implication of these findings is that the diagnostic criteria for DPD should access both concepts.

Sex Bias

The issue of potential sex bias in diagnosis has been hotly debated in psychiatry, particularly for DPD (Brown 1986; Frances and Widiger 1987; Gunderson 1983; Kaplan 1983; Williams and Spitzer 1983). Unfortunately, there has been far more rhetoric than research on this issue, with a few exceptions. Widiger and Spitzer (1991) have recently completed a scholarly investigation of the issue, in which they distinguished between sex differences and sex bias in terms of etiology, sampling, diagnosis, assessment procedures, and criteria.

Three studies have reported data relevant to the question of whether the criteria for DPD are biased toward diagnosing more women than men (Kass et al. 1983; Reich 1987; Reich et al. 1988). Although the findings from these studies are far from conclusive, the results suggest that when standardized assessment measures are used for diagnosis, disparities in diagnostic frequency by sex are substantially reduced. In fact, in one study (Reich 1987) using three standardized diagnostic interviews (Structured Interview for DSM-III Personality Disorders [Stangl et al. 1985], Personality Diagnostic Questionnaire [Hyler and Rieder 1987], and Millon Inventory [Millon 1983]), Reich found that the percentage of DPD among female outpatients in his study was not significantly different from the percentage of men within the male outpatients.

Compatibility/Congruency With ICD-10

The items for DPD in the two nomenclatures, DSM and ICD-10, are very similar. In fact, three of the criteria are almost identical. This similarity followed a meeting between representatives of those working to develop the two nomenclatures, the purpose of which was to address differences between the systems and to resolve them where possible.

Recommendations

The goal for DSM-IV is to consider the following issues as carefully and completely as possible to improve the definition of DPD:

1. With regard to the conceptual overlap, especially with borderline, avoidant, and histrionic PDs, the Personality Disorders Work Group proposes to include the conceptual core of DPD as a necessary criterion for this disorder. There-

fore, an individual with DPD must demonstrate a pervasive and excessive need to be taken care of, which leads to submissive and clinging behavior and fears of separation.

2. The Work Group views DPD as composed of both excessive attachment needs and excessive instrumental dependency needs. Criteria assessing these qualities are included.

3. Criteria that have been found to perform poorly or are ambiguous have been modified or deleted.

4. The Work Group has examined all the criteria from the vantage of sex bias and has endeavored to make all criteria free of sex bias. This, of course, may not lead to equal distribution between the sexes but rather will not cause artifactual differences.

It is the intention of the Work Group that these changes will sharpen the concept and the diagnosis of DPD, will reduce overlap with other disorders, and will address sex bias issues.

Options for Revision of DSM-III-R

The Work Group's proposal for change in criteria follows. Each criterion section lists the current proposal for DSM-IV and the rationale for the proposed modification.

Essential feature: The essential feature of DPD is a pervasive and excessive need to be taken care of, which leads to submissive and clinging behavior and fears of separation.

Proposed criterion 1: *Is unable to make everyday decisions without an excessive amount of advice and reassurance from others.* Rationale: The underscore of "everyday" is to distinguish it from criterion 2, which deals with important decisions.

Proposed criterion 2: *Allows others to make most of his/her important decisions, e.g., where to live, what job to take, having children, getting married, and getting divorced.* Rationale: The underscore of "important" is to distinguish it from criterion 1, which deals with everyday decisions.

Proposed criterion 3: *Has difficulty expressing disagreement with others because of fear of their anger or loss of support.* Rationale: It is not the rejection per se that motivates the compliance but rather the consequences of rejection (i.e., the loss of care and support). The change emphasizes the fear of anger or loss of support.

Proposed criterion 4: *Has difficulty independently initiating projects or doing things on his or her own. This is due to a lack of self-confidence in judgment and not to a lack of motivation or energy.* Rationale: The change emphasizes that it is lack of confidence in judgment and/or abilities that results in difficulty in independent initiation rather than a lack of energy or motivation.

Proposed criterion 5: *Goes to excessive lengths to obtain nurturance and support from others, to the point of volunteering to do things that are unpleasant.* Rationale: This change emphasizes the reason for the behavior to distinguish it from self-defeating behavior. In self-defeating PD, the motivation for volunteering for unpleasant tasks is to induce guilt or to martyr and/or devalue oneself.

Proposed criterion 6: *Feels uncomfortable or helpless when alone, because of exaggerated fears of inability to care for himself or herself.* Rationale: The change emphasizes the reason for the feelings of discomfort and helplessness when alone and helps to distinguish this criterion from Criterion 8 of borderline PD, "frantic attempts to avoid real or imagined abandonment."

Proposed criterion 7: *When close relationships end, undiscriminatingly seeks another relationship to provide nurturance and support.* Rationale: Because of the high endorsement rate for the criterion "feels devastated and helpless when a close relationship ends," both in other PDs and in other psychiatric disorders, an attempt has been made to make the criterion more specific to DPD. In particular, this change addresses the overlap with avoidant PD. In addition, because immediate seeking of another relationship may be a common expression of dependency in males, this broadening of the criterion may improve the sensitivity of the criteria set for males with abnormal dependency.

Proposed criterion 8: *Is frequently preoccupied with fears of being left to take care of himself or herself.* Rationale: The change emphasizes the fear of being without support, and distinguishes this criterion from the "fear of abandonment" in borderline PD.

Proposed Criterion 9: It is proposed to drop the item "is easily hurt by criticism or disapproval." Rationale: This symptom is found in other PDs and other psychiatric disorders and is not specific to DPD.

References

American Psychiatric Association: Diagnostic and Statistical Manual of Mental Disorders, 3rd Edition. Washington, DC, American Psychiatric Association, 1980

American Psychiatric Association: Diagnostic and Statistical Manual of Mental Disorders, 3rd Edition, Revised. Washington, DC, American Psychiatric Association, 1987

Birchnell J: Defining dependence. Br J Med Psychol 61:222–223, 1988

Brown L.S: Gender role analysis: a neglected component of psychological assessment. Psychotherapy 23:243–248, 1986

Dahl AA: Some aspects of the DSM-III personality disorders illustrated by a consecutive sample of hospitalized patients. Acta Psychiatr Scand Suppl 328:61–67, 1986

First M, Spitzer RL: Co-occurrence and diagnostic efficiency statistics. Unpublished raw data, New York, New York State Psychiatric Institute, 1989

Frances A, Widiger T: A critical review of four DSM-III personality disorders: borderline, avoidant, dependent, and passive-aggressive, in Diagnosis and Classification in Psychiatry. Edited by Tischler G. New York, Cambridge University Press, 1987, pp 269–289

Freiman K, Widiger TA: Co-occurrence of diagnostic efficiency statistics. Unpublished raw data, Lexington, University of Kentucky, 1989

Gunderson, J: DSM-III diagnosis of personality disorders, in Current Perspectives on Personality Disorders. Edited by Frosch J. Washington, DC, American Psychiatric Press, 1983, pp 20–39

Hirschfeld RMA, Klerman GL, Chodoff P, et al: Dependency-self-esteem-clinical depression. J Am Acad Psychoanal 4:373–388, 1976

Hirschfeld RMA, Klerman GL, Gough HG, et al: A measure of interpersonal dependency. J Pers Assess 41:610–618, 1977

Hyler SE, Rieder RO: Personality Diagnostic Questionnaire, Revised (PDQ-R). New York, New York State Psychiatric Institute, 1987

Kaplan M: A woman's view of DSM-III. Am Psychol 38:786–792, 1983

Kass F, Spitzer FL, Williams JBW: An empirical study of the issue of sex bias in the diagnostic criteria of DSM-III Axis II personality disorders. Am Psychol 38:799–801, 1983

Livesley WJ, Schroeder ML, Jackson DN: Dependent personality disorder and attachment problems. Journal of Personality Disorders 4:232–240, 1990

Loranger AW: Personality Disorder Examination (PDE) Manual. Yonkers, NY, DV Communications, 1988

Millon T: Millon Clinical Multiaxial Inventory Manual, 3rd Edition. Minneapolis, MN, National Computer Systems, 1983

Morey LC: Personality disorders in DSM-III and DSM-III-R: convergence, coverage, and internal consistency. Am J Psychiatry 145:573–577, 1988

Morey LC, Goodman R: Diagnostic efficiency statistics. Unpublished raw data, Nashville, TN, Vanderbilt University, 1989

Pfohl B, Blum N: Internal consistency statistics for the DSM-III-R personality disorder criteria. Unpublished data, Iowa City, University of Iowa, 1990

Pfohl B, Coryell W, Zimmerman M, et al: DSM-III personality disorders: diagnostic overlap and internal consistency of individual DSM-III criteria. Compr Psychiatry 27:21–34, 1986

Reich J: Sex distribution of DSM-III personality disorders in psychiatric outpatients. Am J Psychiatry 144:485–488, 1987

Reich J, Nduaguba M, Yates W: Age and sex distribution of DSM-III personality traits in a community population. Compr Psychiatry 29:298–303, 1988

Skodol AE: Co-occurrence and diagnostic efficiency statistics. Unpublished raw data, New York, New York State Psychiatric Institute, 1989

Skodol AE, Rosnick L, Kellman D, et al: Validating structured DSM-III-R personality disorder assessments with longitudinal data. Am J Psychiatry 145:1297–1299, 1988

Stangl D, Pfohl B, Zimmerman M, et al: A structured interview for the DSM-III personality disorders: a preliminary report. Arch Gen Psychiatry 42:591–596, 1985

Trull TJ, Widiger TA, Frances A: Covariation of criteria sets for avoidant, schizoid, and dependent personality disorders. Am J Psychiatry 144:767–771, 1987

Widiger T: DSM-IV and personality disorders: introduction to special series. Journal of Personality Disorders 5:122–134, 1991

Widiger TA, Spitzer RL: Sex bias in the diagnosis of personality disorders: conceptual and methodological issues. Clin Psychol Rev 11:1–22, 1991

Williams JBW, Spitzer RL: The issue of sex bias in DSM-III: a critique of "A Woman's View of DSM-III" by Marie Kaplan. Am Psychol 38:793–798, 1983

Zanarini MC, Frankenburg FR, Chauncey DL: The diagnostic interview for personality disorders: interrater and test-retest reliability. Compr Psychiatry 28:467–480, 1987

Chapter 31

Obsessive-Compulsive Personality Disorder

Bruce Pfohl, M.D.

Statement of the Issues

The following issues were considered in the course of the review of obsessive-compulsive personality disorder (OCPD): Are criteria congruent with the descriptive literature? Are criteria internally consistent? Are criteria supported by external validators? How is OCPD related to obsessive-compulsive disorder (OCD) and other Axis I disorders? Is OCPD distinct from other personality disorders (PDs)? Are the structure of the diagnostic criteria and the threshold for diagnosis appropriate? Can differences between the DSM-III-R (American Psychiatric Association 1987) criteria for OCPD and ICD-10 (World Health Organization 1990) criteria for anankastic PD be reconciled?

Significance of the Issues

The DSM-III-R criteria for OCPD represent an attempt to capture a historical concept whose implications and validity are largely untested. In his classic 1908 paper, Freud (1908/1959) outlines the anal character as arising from a defense against anal eroticism and said such individuals are "orderly, parsimonious and obstinate. . . . Orderly covers the notion of bodily cleanliness, as well as conscientiousness in carrying out small duties and trustworthiness. . . . Parsimony may [include] . . . avarice; and obstinacy can go over into defiance, to which rage and revengefulness are easily joined" (p. 169).

The criteria in the first DSM (American Psychiatric Association 1952) for compulsive personality and the nearly identical DSM-II (American Psychiatric Association 1968) criteria for obsessive-compulsive personality (abstracted in Table 31–1) emphasized the "orderly" component of this personality type. DSM-III

Table 31–1.   Prototypic traits for obsessive-compulsive personality disorder (PD)

- **DSM-III-R obsessive-compulsive PD criteria**

  Perfectionism

  Preoccupation with details, rules, order, organization

  Insistence that others submit to exactly his or her way of doing things

  Excessive devotion to work

  Indecisiveness

  Overconscientiousness, scrupulousness, and inflexibility (not in DSM-III)

  Restricted expression of affection

  Lack of generosity (not in DSM-III)

  Inability to discard worn-out or worthless objects (not in DSM-III)

- **DSM-II obsessive-compulsive personality**

  Excessive concern with conformity and adherence to standards of conscience

  Rigid, overinhibited, overconscientious

  Unable to relax easily

- **ICD-9 anankastic PD**

  Rigidity

  Personal insecurity and doubt[a]

  Conscientiousness, checking, stubbornness, and caution

  Perfectionism and meticulous accuracy

  Unwelcome thoughts and impulses (not as severe as in obsessional neurosis)[a]

- **Freud's (1908/1959) anal character**

  Orderliness: bodily cleanliness, conscientiousness in carrying out small duties, trustworthy

  Parsimony: may include greed

  Obstinacy: argumentative, perhaps to the point of rage and revengefulness[a]

- **Abraham's (1921/1966) anal character**

  Pleasure in indexing, compiling lists, and arranging things symmetrically

  Superficial fastidiousness masking disarray underneath

  Pleasure in possession, inability to throw away worn-out or worthless objects

  Tendency to postpone every action and unproductive perseverance

  Preoccupation with preserving correct social appearances

  In close personal relationships, refuses to accommodate others, expects compliance

  Exaggerated criticism of others, insists on controlling interactions with others[a]

  Generally morose or surly attitude[a]

- **Lazare (from Lazare-Klerman Scale) (Lazare et al. 1966, 1970)**

  Orderliness

  Strong superego

  Perseverance

  Obstinacy

  Rigidity

  Parsimony

  Emotional constriction

  Rejection of others[a,b]

  Self-doubt[a,b]

- **ICD-10 anankastic PD**

  Feelings of excessive doubt and caution

  Preoccupation with details, rules, lists, order, organization, or schedule

  Perfectionism that interferes with task completion

  Conscientiousness and preoccupation with productivity to the exclusion of relationships

  Excessive pedantry and adherence to social convention

  Rigidity and stubbornness

  Insistence that others submit to his or her way

  Intrusion of insistent and unwelcome thoughts or impulsesa

[a]Traits not currently represented by DSM-III-R obsessive-compulsive PD criteria.
[b]Not included consistently across the factor analyses.

expanded the description with five operational criteria, of which four were required for diagnosis. DSM-III-R made relatively minor changes to the five criteria and added four more, requiring five of nine criteria to make the diagnosis. It is important to consider how past changes affected the scope of the diagnosis and the overlap with other PDs (Morey 1988).

In this review, priority was given to issues raised in the literature that have a direct bearing on the validity of the diagnosis of OCPD (Pollak 1979) and its overlap with and relation to other disorders (Rasmussen and Tsuang 1986), because the value of separating patients into different diagnostic categories ultimately rests in showing that different diagnoses carry different implications. Although agreement with ICD-10 is not a validity issue per se, future empirical research can be greatly facilitated by a common language for communication between psychiatrists in different countries.

Methods

A Medline search was conducted on literature published between the introduction of DSM-III in 1980 and the beginning of 1991 on the search term *compulsive personality disorder*. This yielded 88 papers. Closer scrutiny was given to those that contained empirical data. In addition, review papers associated with terms such as *compulsivity* and *anal personality* were scanned going back 25 years. Investigators with relevant data sets were asked to provide information on internal consistency of the criteria and overlap with other psychiatric disorders.

Results

Are Criteria Congruent With the Descriptive Literature?

Because there is only limited empirical research supporting the DSM-III-R criteria for OCPD, it is worth investigating whether the criteria at least capture those traits that have historically been associated with this personality type. Traits elucidated by Freud (1908/1959) and Abraham (1921/1966) are summarized in Table 31–1 and have been reviewed by Oldham and Frosch (1988).

Lazare et al. (1966) were the first to systematically examine psychoanalytic concepts of personality, using factor analysis to determine whether the theoretically derived components truly clustered together (Lazare et al. 1966, 1970). They began with a series of traits representing the oral, obsessive, and hysterical personality constructs and used a 200-item self-report rating scale to operationalize the measurement of the underlying traits. An "obsessional" dimension emerged, characterized by orderliness, strong superego, perseverance, obstinacy, rigidity, rejection of others, parsimony, and emotional constriction (see Table 31–1).

There have been at least two replication studies, one by Lazare et al. (1970) and one by Torgersen (1980). "Self-doubt" (including difficulty in making decisions) was not consistently associated with the obsessional dimension in the three studies. "Rejection of others" was associated with the obsessional dimension in the study by Lazare et al. and among men but not among women in the study by Torgersen (1980). The DSM-III-R criteria include virtually all the traits that have been consistently supported by the factor-analytic studies.

Are Criteria Internally Consistent?

Internal consistency refers to how well the components of a criteria set appear to cluster together in individual patients and how well they discriminate from other syndromes. The analysis becomes a type of bootstrap procedure in which the criteria as a whole are assumed to approximate a real diagnostic entity, and patients are categorized as cases or noncases according to the criteria set taken as a whole. Individual criteria can then be examined according to their frequency among cases (sensitivity), rarity among noncases (specificity), and the frequency of the diagnosis when the criterion is present (positive predictive value).

Only limited data are available for DSM-III-R. Data from four unpublished data sets are discussed. The Freiman and Widiger (1989) data set is based on a study of 50 hospitalized psychiatric patients who received a structured interview for personality assessment. The Millon and Tringone (1989) data set is based on 584 patients described by clinicians as part of a mail survey. DSM-III-R criteria were paraphrased in this study. The Morey and Heumann (1988) data set is based on a mixed group of 291 patients who received an unstructured clinical interview. The Pfohl and Blum (1990) data set is based on the Structured Interview for the DSM-III-R Personality Disorders (SIDP-R) of a mixed group of 112 nonpsychotic inpatients, outpatients, and normal control subjects.

The statistics for these four studies are presented in Table 31–2. Parentheses indicate the two worst-performing criteria in each category. Results varied across studies, suggesting the need for cautious interpretation. The sensitivity for the nine criteria averaged approximately 0.5 or better across the three informative studies, with the exception of criteria 8 and 9. Given that these two criteria had very high specificity scores and that only five criteria are required for diagnosis, this may not be a problem.

Criterion 3, "unreasonable insistence that others submit to exactly his or her way of doing things, or unreasonable reluctance to allow others to do things because of the conviction that they will not do them correctly," showed low specificity in

Table 31–2. Internal-consistency–based diagnostic statistics for DSM-III-R obsessive-compulsive personality disorder criteria

	Frequency[a]	A1	A2	A3	A4	A5	A6	A7	A8	A9
Sensitivity										
Freiman and Widiger 1989	0	—	—	—	—	—	—	—	—	—
Millon and Tringone 1989	60	0.47	0.47	(0.27)	0.75	(0.17)	0.50	0.47	—	—
Morey and Heumann 1988	23	0.65	0.78	0.74	0.61	0.74	0.54	0.96	(0.30)	(0.22)
Pfohl and Blum 1990	31	0.87	0.87	0.74	(0.42)	0.87	0.58	0.55	(0.29)	0.48
Specificity										
Freiman and Widiger 1989	0	0.88	0.92	0.78	0.92	(0.56)	0.96	(0.64)	0.90	0.86
Millon and Tringone 1989	60	0.87	0.90	0.82	0.81	(0.64)	0.85	(0.74)	—	—
Morey and Heumann 1988	23	0.86	0.88	(0.53)	0.90	(0.56)	0.84	0.71	0.90	0.97
Pfohl and Blum 1990	31	0.74	(0.62)	0.72	0.91	(0.69)	0.78	0.74	0.86	0.78
Positive predictive value										
Freiman and Widiger 1989	0	—	—	—	—	—	—	—	—	—
Millon and Tringone 1989	60	0.29	0.36	(0.15)	0.31	(0.06)	0.28	0.17	—	—
Morey and Heumann 1988	23	0.29	0.35	(0.12)	0.35	(0.13)	0.22	0.22	0.21	0.36
Pfohl and Blum 1990	31	0.56	0.47	0.50	0.65	0.52	0.50	(0.45)	(0.45)	(0.45)

Note. Numbers in parentheses indicate the two worst-performing items in each study. A1 = perfectionism. A2 = preoccupation with details. A3 = insistence that others submit. A4 = devotion to work. A5 = indecisiveness. A6 = overconscientiousness. A7 = restricted affection. A8 = lack of generosity. A9 = inability to discard.
[a]Frequency of obsessive-compulsive personality disorder diagnosis in each study. Total sample size was 50 in Freiman and Widiger, 584 in Millon and Tringone, 291 in Morey and Heumann, and 112 in Pfohl and Blum.

one study and very low positive predictive value in two of three studies (Table 31–2). In the Morey and Heumann study, this criterion was present in 74% of the OCPD cases, 81% of the histrionic PD cases, 77% of the narcissistic PD cases, and 83% of the passive-aggressive PD cases. In the Pfohl and Blum study, this criterion was present in 74% of the OCPD cases, 75% of the narcissistic PD cases, and 60% of the borderline PD cases. Given the lack of consistency across studies, more data would be desirable.

Criterion 5, "indecisiveness: decision making is either avoided, postponed, or protracted" showed low sensitivity in one of three studies and low specificity in all of four studies. The positive predictive value was very low in two of three studies. In the Morey and Heumann study, this criterion was present in 74% of the OCPD cases, 78% of the dependent PD cases, 71% of the avoidant PD cases, and 63% of the schizotypal PD cases. In the Pfohl and Blum study, this criterion was present in 87% of the OCPD cases, 71% of the paranoid PD cases, 64% of the dependent PD cases, 62% of the avoidant PD cases, and 67% of the schizotypal PD cases. Thus, there is fair agreement across studies that this criterion does not discriminate well.

The remaining criteria appeared to have acceptable internal consistency statistics or at least a lack of any consistent evidence of weakness across studies.

Are the Criteria Supported by External Validators?

Although almost no data are available using DSM-III-R criteria for OCPD, note that external validators are the most desirable basis for revising criteria. Potential validators might include family history of OCPD and other disorders, biological markers, attitudes of parents regarding discipline during childhood, occupational preference, and specific types of problems in occupational and social functioning.

How Is OCPD Related to OCD and Other Axis I Disorders?

The overlap between OCPD and OCD deserves special attention, since the similarity in names implies similar or related disorders and may lead to confusion. According to DSM-III-R, individuals with OCD view the associated thoughts and behaviors as "intrusive and senseless" whereas patients with OCPD view the associated personality traits as desirable. It is not clear whether this distinction is supported by any external validators. Before the introduction of DSM-III criteria, Pollak (1979) reviewed studies that examined the co-occurrence of obsessive-compulsive neurosis and OCPD (Ingram 1961; Rosenberg 1967; Sandler and Hazari 1960). He summarizes, "Clearly there is no necessary one-to-one relationship between obsessional personality and obsessional neurosis, despite the occasional findings that more obsessive-compulsive neurotics than would be expected by chance show evidence of a premorbid obsessional personality" (p. 232).

Rasmussen and Tsuang (1986) assessed a series of 44 outpatients with DSM-III

OCD using a clinical interview and checklist to rate DSM-III criteria for personality disorder; of these, 24 (55%) met criteria for DSM-III compulsive personality disorder. There was no control group. The next most common personality diagnosis was histrionic PD (9%). Baer et al. (1990) used a structured personality interview to assess DSM-III personality criteria in a series of 96 patients with OCD: 6 (6%) of the patients met criteria for compulsive personality disorder; 44 (45%) met criteria for other personality diagnoses, with mixed, dependent, and histrionic PDs being the most common.

In a preliminary report of a collaborative project, Pfohl et al. (1988) compared the rates of OCPD across several diagnostic groups using the SIDP (Pfohl et al. 1982). DSM-III compulsive personality disorder was diagnosed in 22 (19%) of 114 OCD patients, 5 (6%) of 78 patients with major depression, and 7 (8%) of 83 patients with panic disorder. Two other personality diagnoses were more common than compulsive personality in the patients with OCD: avoidant PD (22%) and dependent PD (21%). In a smaller series of patients interviewed using the SIDP-R (Pfohl et al. 1989), we found that criteria for DSM-III-R OCPD were met in 7 (31%) of 22 patients with OCD, 7 (35%) of 20 patients with generalized anxiety disorder, 6 (30%) of a mixed group of 20 nonpsychotic inpatients with other diagnoses (most often major depression), and none of the 10 normal control subjects.

There are even fewer data regarding the association between OCPD and other Axis I disorders. The data presented above indicate that OCPD is not uncommon among patients with affective and anxiety disorders. Although there are references in the literature to various measures of obsessional character traits predisposing to depression (Kendell and Discipio 1970; Matussek et al. 1983; Perris et al. 1984), there are other studies that fail to find such an association (Hirschfeld et al. 1983, 1989).

In summary, available studies suggest that the majority of patients with OCD do not meet criteria for OCPD. Among patients with OCD who do have a PD, several other PDs may be just as common or more common than OCPD. The relationship between OCPD and other Axis I disorders is even less clear.

Is OCPD Distinct From Other PDs?

We have found some inconsistent and surprising overlaps with other PDs across studies. Table 31–3 presents the rates of other comorbid personality diagnoses that are unexpectedly high across several studies. Whereas it might be reasonable to expect that diagnoses such as paranoid PD would be associated with many OCPD traits, others such as borderline PD are theoretically at the opposite end of the spectrum.

The findings may relate to the fact that individuals with other PDs may have similar behaviors, although for different reasons. For example, unreasonable insis-

Table 31–3. Percentage of obsessive-compulsive personality disorder (OCPD) patients with selected comorbid personality disorder diagnoses

Study	Criteria	OCPD cases (n)	N	Paranoid	Histrionic	Borderline	Narcissistic	Avoidant
Pfohl et al. 1986	DSM-III	7	131	0	43	29	14	29
Zanarini et al. 1989	DSM-III	17	253	17	39	72	28	50
Morey and Heumann 1988	DSM-III-R	23	291	22	13	9	30	56
Skodol 1989	DSM-III-R	21	97	33	24	86	48	62
Pfohl and Blum 1990	DSM-III-R	31	112	52	36	26	16	52
Pfohl and Blum 1990	Modified[a]	19	112	68	37	16	26	47

[a]The modified criteria are identical to DSM-III-R criteria except that criterion 5 was deleted from the compulsive personality disorder criteria, and five of the remaining eight criteria were required for diagnosis.

tence that others submit to their wishes, indecisiveness, and lack of generosity may all exist in other PDs, although the motivation for these behaviors may differ in ways not easily captured by the criteria. One possibility may be to modify the criteria to draw a distinction between similar traits. For example, lack of generosity could by rephrased to indicate that the individual is miserly toward both self and others.

Are the Structure of the Diagnostic Criteria and the Threshold for Diagnosis Appropriate?

As noted previously, the DSM-III criteria for compulsive PD required four of five criteria to make the diagnosis. The DSM-III-R Personality Advisory Group chose to expand the description to nine criteria, of which only five were required (see Table 31–1). The nine criteria were thought to better represent the full domain of traits represented in the clinical descriptions of OCPD, and the requirement of only five of nine criteria allowed for greater variation between patients in how the PD was expressed. It is to be expected that such a major change in the structure of the criteria would have some effect on the rate of diagnosis. A review of the data in Table 31–3 suggests that studies using DSM-III-R are diagnosing OCPD at roughly twice the rate of studies using DSM-III criteria.

The best way to clearly delineate the impact of the changes from DSM-III to DSM-III-R is to apply both criteria sets to the same set of patients. Pfohl and Blum (1990) assessed a mixed group of 72 nonpsychotic inpatients and outpatients with normal intellectual functioning using the SIDP for DSM-III personality diagnoses and the SIDP-R for DSM-III-R diagnoses. Eleven (15%) patients met DSM-III criteria and 20 (27%) met DSM-III-R criteria for OCPD. Of the 11 patients who met DSM-III criteria, 9 met DSM-III-R criteria. Morey (1988) assessed DSM-III and DSM-III-R in the same set of patients using a mail survey instrument filled out by volunteer clinicians. He found no difference in the rates of OCPD diagnoses under the two systems. Although it would be desirable to collect more data to determine the effects of changes in criteria on rates of diagnosis, it is difficult to develop objective criteria for deciding what rate of diagnosis is appropriate.

As noted above, one problem with the current criteria is the unexpectedly high overlap with other PDs. The elimination of criteria with low specificity (i.e., those frequently present in other PDs) represents one approach to decreasing overlap that can be immediately tested with existing data sets. An example of this approach is represented in the bottom row of Table 31–3. If criterion 5 is eliminated and five of the remaining eight criteria are required for diagnosis, the rate of diagnosis in the Pfohl and Blum data set drops from 31 (28%) to 19 (17%). The overlap with borderline PD drops from 26% to 16%, but the overlap with several other PDs actually increases. This is probably due to the fact that requiring five of fewer criteria (eight) selects for more severe cases and more severe cases may be more likely to score positive on a variety of dimensions.

Can DSM-III-R and ICD-10 Criteria Be Reconciled?

The term *anankastic* is used in ICD-10 for the equivalent PD. Although the use of this term might help reduce confusion with the Axis I diagnosis of OCD, the term is not one that is meaningful to many clinicians in the United States. The label *perfectionistic PD* has been suggested as a compromise by some advisers.

The ICD-10 criteria for anankastic PD include most of the concepts in DSM-III-R except for the criteria involving lack of generosity and inability to discard worn-out objects. The ICD-10 criteria "rigidity and stubbornness" and "intrusion of insistent and unwelcome thoughts or impulses" are not represented in the equivalent DSM-III-R PD criteria. There is concern that the inclusion of the latter would weaken the distinction between OCPD and OCD.

Whereas it may be possible for the DSM-IV and ICD-10 committees to reconcile some of the arbitrary differences in wording, more major differences in content may be more difficult to resolve, because the implications are not trivial.

Discussion and Recommendations

OCPD represents an attempt to operationalize a concept that has long been part of the psychiatric literature. The criteria generally possess good content validity with respect to the descriptive literature including the factor-analytic work of Lazare et al. (1966, 1970). Problems with this disorder include the high degree of overlap with other PDs and the lack of empirical studies that provide external validity for the current criteria. The relationship between OCD and OCPD is apparently weak, and it is unfortunate that the similarity in names may lead to confusion.

Based on the review of the literature described in this chapter, the following recommendations are made for DSM-IV:

1. Because criterion 3 as currently worded fails to discriminate well from other disorders, the following change in wording is proposed to further highlight the unique features of this trait in OCPD: "reluctant to delegate tasks or to work with others unless they submit to exactly his or her way of doing things."
2. Because criterion 5 (indecisiveness) shows poor discrimination in recent studies and weak association with the disorder in factor-analytic studies, the recommendation has been made that this criterion be dropped.
3. Because the rate of diagnosis of this disorder may have increased using DSM-III-R compared with DSM-III criteria, consideration should be given to ad-

justing the number of criteria required for diagnosis of this disorder.

4. Representatives from the ICD-10 and DSM-IV committees should meet and attempt to reconcile any differences in criteria to promote a common language for psychiatric disorders.

5. Field trials and other studies would be highly desirable to determine whether the proposed changes improve internal consistency and external validity for this disorder.

References

Abraham K: Contributions to the theory of the anal character (1921), in On Character and Libido Development. New York, Basic Books, 1966, pp 370–341

American Psychiatric Association: Diagnostic and Statistical Manual: Mental Disorders. Washington, DC, American Psychiatric Association, 1952

American Psychiatric Association: Diagnostic and Statistical Manual of Mental Disorders, 2nd Edition. Washington, DC, American Psychiatric Association, 1968

American Psychiatric Association: Diagnostic and Statistical Manual of Mental Disorders, 3rd Edition. Washington, DC, American Psychiatric Association, 1980

American Psychiatric Association: Diagnostic and Statistical Manual of Mental Disorders, 3rd Edition, Revised. Washington, DC, American Psychiatric Association, 1987

Baer L, Jenike MA, Ricciardi J: Standardized assessment of personality disorders in obsessive-compulsive disorder. Arch Gen Psychiatry 47:826–830, 1990

Freiman K, Widiger TA: Co-occurrence and diagnostic efficiency statistics. Unpublished raw data, Lexington, University of Kentucky, 1989

Freud S: Character and anal-eroticism (1908), in The Standard Edition of the Complete Psychological Works of Sigmund Freud, Vol 9. Translated and edited by Strachey J. London, Hogarth Press, 1959, pp 167–175

Hirschfeld RMA, Klerman GL, Clayton PJ, et al: Personality and depression. Arch Gen Psychiatry 40:993–998, 1983

Hirschfeld RMA, Klerman GL, Lavori P, et al: Premorbid personality assessments of first onset of major depression. Arch Gen Psychiatry 46:345–350, 1989

Ingram IM: The obsessional personality and obsessional illness. Am J Psychiatry 117:1016–1019, 1961

Kendell RE, Discipio WJ: Obsessional symptoms and obsessional personality traits in patients with depressive illness. Psychol Med 1:65–72, 1970

Lazare A, Klerman G, Armor DJ: Oral, obsessive and hysterical personality patterns. Arch Gen Psychiatry 14:624–630, 1966

Lazare A, Klerman G, Armor DJ: Oral, obsessive and hysterical personality patterns: replication of factor analysis in an independent sample. J Psychiatr Res 7:275–279, 1970

Matussek P, Feil BF: Personality attributes of depressive patients. Arch Gen Psychiatry 40:783–790, 1983

Millon T, Tringone R: Co-occurrence and diagnostic efficiency statistics. Unpublished raw data, Miami, FL, University of Miami, 1990

Morey LC: Personality disorders in DSM-III and DSM-III-R: convergence, coverage, and internal consistency. Am J Psychiatry 145:573–577, 1988

Morey LC, Heumann K: Co-occurrence and diagnostic efficiency statistics. Unpublished raw data, Nashville, TN, Vanderbilt University, 1988

Oldham JM, Frosch WA: Compulsive personality disorder, in Psychiatry. Edited by Michels R, Cavenar JO, Brodie HKH, et al. Philadelphia, PA, JB Lippincott, 1988

Perris C, Eisemann M, von Knorring L: Personality traits in former depressed patients and healthy subjects without past history of depression. Psychopathology 17:178–186, 1984

Pfohl B, Blum N: Co-occurrence and diagnostic efficiency statistics. Unpublished raw data, Iowa City, University of Iowa, 1990

Pfohl B, Stangl D, Zimmerman M: The Structured Interview for DSM-III Personality Disorders (SIDP). Iowa City, University of Iowa College of Medicine, 1982

Pfohl B, Coryell W, Zimmerman M, et al: DSM-III personality disorders: diagnostic overlap and internal consistency of individual DSM-III criteria. Compr Psychiatry 27:21–34, 1986

Pfohl B, Black D, Noyes R: Axis I/Axis II comorbidity findings. Paper presented at the 141st annual meeting of the American Psychiatric Association, Montreal, Canada, May 1988

Pfohl B, Blum N, Zimmerman M, et al: Structured Interview for DSM-III-R Personality (SIDP-R). Iowa City, University of Iowa College of Medicine, 1989

Pollak JM: Obsessive-compulsive personality: a review. Psychol Bull 86:225–241, 1979

Rasmussen SA, Tsuang MT: Clinical characteristics and family history in DSM-III obsessive compulsive disorder. Am J Psychiatry 143:317–322, 1986

Rosenberg CM: Personality and obsessional neurosis. Br J Psychiatry 113:471–477, 1967

Sandler J, Hazari A: The "obsessional": on the psychological classification of obsessional character traits and symptoms. Br J Med Psychol 33:113–122, 1960

Skodol A: Co-occurrence and diagnostic efficiency statistics. Unpublished raw data. New York, New York State Psychiatric Institute, 1989

Torgersen S: The oral, obsessive and hysterical personality syndromes: a study of hereditary and environmental factors by means of the twin method. Arch Gen Psychiatry 37:1272–1277, 1980

World Health Organization: ICD-10 Chapter V: Mental and Behavioral Disorders: Diagnostic Criteria for Research. Geneva, Switzerland, World Health Organization, 1990

Zanarini MC, Frankenburg F, Chauncey D, et al: Co-occurrence and diagnostic efficiency statistics. Unpublished raw data, Boston, MA, McLean Hospital, 1989

Chapter 32

Personality Disorder Dimensional Models

Thomas A. Widiger, Ph.D.

Statement of the Issues

The issues for this review are whether DSM-IV should provide a formal recognition of the dimensional model for the classification of the personality disorders and, if so, what form this should take.

Significance of the Issues

The question of whether mental disorders are optimally classified categorically or dimensionally is a long-standing issue that is particularly pertinent to the personality disorders (Frances 1982). The categorical approach to the diagnosis of personality disorders has received substantial criticism, with a variety of authors recommending a change to a dimensional approach (e.g., Adamson 1989; Cloninger 1989; Eysenck 1987; Grove and Tellegen 1991; Tyrer 1988; Widiger 1992). Others, however, have argued in favor of the categorical approach (e.g., Frances 1990; Gunderson et al. 1991; Millon 1981).

Method

A Medline computer search for journal articles in the English language from the years 1975 through June 1989, using the index term *personality disorders,* yielded 1,160 citations. Additional references were obtained through prior reviews, clinical and empirical papers and by soliciting information from persons who have authored related papers (Drs. Benjamin, Blashfield, Clark, Cloninger, Costa, Eysenck, Frances, Gunderson, Kiesler, Livesley, McCrae, Millon, Morey, Siever,

Spitzer, Tellegen, and Wiggins). A more detailed presentation of this review has been published elsewhere (Widiger 1991).

Results

Advantages of the Categorical Approach

Ease in conceptualization and communication.   A categorical approach can be easier to use than a dimensional one. It is easier to consider and discuss the presence of one, two, or three disorders than a profile of the degree to which all of the various disorders are present. One category (e.g., borderline) can communicate a great deal of vivid information. Categorical diagnoses require only one decision: whether the patient does or does not have the disorder. Diagnoses within a dimensional model would require more specific and detailed assessments. To the extent that a dimensional model retains more information, it requires that more information initially be obtained and communicated. A systematic and comprehensive assessment of only five to seven dimensions, however, could require less time and effort than a comprehensive assessment of the 11 DSM-III-R (American Psychiatric Association 1987) diagnostic categories (Widiger 1991).

Familiarity.   The categorical system is more familiar to clinicians. All prior and current diagnoses within the DSM have been categorical. It would provide a major shift in clinical practice to convert to a dimensional system (Frances 1990). The categorical approach is also consistent with the neo-Kraepelinian emphasis on identifying homogeneous, distinct syndromes (Robins and Helzer 1986). For many clinicians, the concept of disorder implies the presence of distinct syndromes that are qualitatively distinct from normality (Gunderson et al. 1991).

Consistency with clinical decisions.   Clinical decisions tend to be categorical. If treatment, insurance, forensic, and other clinically relevant decisions involved shades of gray, then a more quantitative nomenclature might have developed. Many clinicians would convert a dimensional profile to categories to facilitate their decisions. There may be little advantage to increasing the complexity of diagnosis by requiring ratings along a continuum that might be used rarely in clinical practice.

Advantages of the Dimensional Approach

Classificatory dilemmas.   One difficulty with the categorical approach is identifying nonarbitrary boundaries. Only the cutoff points for the schizotypal and borderline personality disorders were based on empirical data (Spitzer et al. 1979), and there is little basis to assume that these thresholds provide the optimal cutoff points for treatment decisions, family history, and other external validators (Kendler 1990). Persons who fall near the boundaries may not be adequately described by the designation of having or not having the disorder. Patients may also meet the criteria for as many as five, six, seven, or even more diagnoses, with the average approximately four (e.g., Skodol et al. 1991). The frequency of multiple diagnoses compromises the utility and validity of the categorical model (Cloninger 1989). To the extent that the categorical distinctions are arbitrary, clinicians are being required to make distinctions for which there is no correct answer. It is therefore not surprising that there is substantial disagreement and poor reliability (Heumann and Morey 1990).

Retention of information. The members of a specific diagnostic category are not homogeneous with respect to the criteria that were used to assign that diagnosis, nor are nonmembers of a diagnostic category homogeneous with respect to the criteria for that diagnosis that were not met. There are 93 different ways to meet the DSM-III-R criteria for borderline personality disorder and more than 848 ways to meet the criteria for antisocial personality disorder, yet only one diagnostic label is given to characterize all these cases (Widiger 1991, 1992). There are also 162 different possible combinations of borderline symptomatology in persons who would not meet the DSM-III-R criteria for this disorder, and all of these cases are labeled as being without the disorder. The presence of personality disorder pathology in persons who do not meet the arbitrary threshold for a diagnosis is problematic for treatment and research (McGlashan 1987).

Categories do provide vivid, clear descriptions, but, to the extent that the patient is not a prototypic case, the description can be misleading and stereotyping (Cantor and Genero 1986). The categorical format can be easier to use, but this simplicity may be obtained at the cost of not recognizing the complexity that actually exists. A dimensional model would diminish stereotyping and provide more precise information.

Flexibility. The advantages of a categorical approach can be retained in a dimensional model by providing cutoff points. The reverse translation is not possible because, once the categorical diagnosis is provided, the ability to return to a more precise classification cannot be recovered. The dimensional model would also allow the option of different cutoff points for different decisions and situations (Kendler 1990).

Empirical Support for the Categorical
and Dimensional Models

Most authors within the published literature prefer the dimensional model (Widiger 1992). It is not clear which format is preferred by clinicians. The categorical format is more familiar for the diagnosis of personality disorders, but the dimensional format is more familiar for the description of personality (Millon 1981). A variety of surveys regarding DSM-III (American Psychiatric Association 1980) and DSM-III-R have been conducted, but none has considered the preference for a dimensional versus categorical format for the personality disorders. Kass et al. (1985) indicated that feedback from staff and trainees during their study suggested that a four-point severity scale would be feasible and acceptable in routine clinical practice.

A dimensional variable will obtain reduced relations with external validators when it is dichotomized, whereas a dichotomous variable will show decreased relations or at least no change when it is dimensionalized (Miller and Thayer 1989). The former occurs as a result of the loss of information (e.g., measuring height simply by a short versus tall distinction); the latter as a result of the inclusion of irrelevant, invalid information (e.g., making differentiations or distinctions that are unnecessary and irrelevant). Widiger (1992) indicated that in 15 of 16 studies in which the data were analyzed both categorically and dimensionally, the reliability and/or validity data were better for the dimensional model (e.g., Heumann and Morey 1990). This suggests that reliable and valid information is being lost by converting a continuum to a simplistic, black-white distinction.

Factor and cluster analyses are useful for identifying and confirming the substance of particular dimensions and categories (e.g., Morey 1988), but both techniques can create dimensions or categories even when the alternative model is more valid or closer to the truth (Grove and Andreasen 1989). An application of factor analysis that is relevant to the validity of the dimensional model is the comparison of factor solutions across groups purportedly distinct with respect to a latent class taxon. Measures that are highly discriminating between such groups should not correlate substantially within the groups and the factor solution of the intercorrelation among such measures would not replicate across groups (Eysenck 1987). Both Livesley (1991) and Tyrer and Alexander (1979) used this approach to assess the validity of personality disorder categorical distinctions and concluded that their results favored the dimensional model.

Neither multimodality nor a distinct break in the distribution of personality disorder scores has ever been obtained. Frances et al. (1984), Kass et al. (1985), Nestadt et al. (1990), and Zimmerman and Coryell (1990) concluded that the distributions they obtained were most consistent with the dimensional model.

Admixture analysis examines the distribution of canonical coefficient scores derived from a discriminant function analysis for evidence of bimodality. Cloninger (1989) applied admixture analysis to personality disorder data and concluded that the results supported the dimensional model. Maximum covariation analysis capitalizes on the fact that the covariation between any two signs of a categorical variable will be minimized in groups of subjects who share the class membership and will be maximized in mixed groups, whereas no such variation in covariation will be found across levels of a dimensional variable. Maximum covariation analysis has suggested the presence of a latent class taxon for a "schizoid" group that would subsume the schizotypal, schizoid, and other personality disorders but not for individual personality disorders such as borderline (Trull et al. 1990).

Alternative Dimensional Models

Research contrasting the dimensional and categorical approaches appears to favor the dimensional. Research with respect to which dimensional model is preferable is more controversial. A variety of models have been proposed. Space limitations prohibit a detailed summary of each viable alternative; a more detailed summary is presented elsewhere (Widiger and Frances 1994). The major alternatives are the five-factor model (neuroticism, extraversion, openness, agreeableness, and conscientiousness; Costa and McCrae 1992); the three dimensions identified by Eysenck (1987) (neuroticism, extraversion, and psychoticism); the three clusters provided in DSM-III-R (odd-eccentric, dramatic-emotional, and anxious-fearful); the four spectra identified by Siever and Davis (1991) (cognitive disorganization, affective instability, impulsivity, and anxiety); the three dimensions identified by Cloninger (1987) (harm avoidance, novelty seeking, and reward dependence); the interpersonal circumplex dimensions of affiliation and power (Kiesler 1986); and the three dimensions of negative emotionality, positive emotionality, and constraint emphasized by Clark (1990) and Tellegen and Waller (in press). More complex dimensional models are offered by Livesley (1991) and Clark (1990).

Discussion

Deleting the existing diagnostic categories would provide a severe and very disruptive shift in clinical practice and research. However, there are a variety of options for providing some recognition of the dimensional approach in DSM-IV. The three major options are 1) to include in the text of DSM-IV a uniform terminology and criteria for converting the existing categories to a more dimensional format, 2) to provide more explicit criteria for the rating of severity, and 3) to include a dimensional model in an appendix to DSM-IV or within the introductory section to the personality disorders.

Provide a Conversion Table

Table 32–1 presents a proposal for converting existing categories to a more dimensional format. Six levels are provided: absent, traits, subthreshold, threshold, moderate, and prototypic. The rating in each case is compatible with the current format. "Absent" means an absence of any symptoms. "Traits" means that there are simply one to three symptoms (DSM-III-R currently recommends that the clinician code personality disorder "traits" on Axis II when a patient meets some but not enough of the criteria to be given the diagnosis). "Subthreshold" means that the person is only one symptom short of having the disorder. "Threshold" means that the person just barely meets the criteria for the disorder. "Moderate" means that the person has more than enough of the criteria. "Prototypic" means that all of the diagnostic features are present.

This coding is compatible with the current categorical format while providing uniform terminology and criteria for describing the extent to which the person has each disorder. The terminology and criteria would facilitate uniform discussion among clinicians and researchers who want to indicate the extent to which the disorder is present, without disrupting the current diagnostic system.

Revise Criteria for Severity Rating

DSM-III-R includes a specification of mild, moderate, or severe "to indicate the severity of the current disorder . . . at the time of the evaluation when all of the diagnostic criteria are met" (American Psychiatric Association 1987, p. 24). The

Table 32–1. Converting diagnostic categories to dimensional ratings

Personality disorder	Number of criteria					
	Absent	Traits	Subthreshold	Threshold	Moderate	Prototypic
Paranoid	0	1–2	3	4	5–6	7
Schizoid	0	1–2	3	4	5–6	7
Schizotypal	0	1–3	4	5–6	7–8	9
Antisocial[a]	0	1–2	3	4–5	6–9	10
Borderline	0	1–3	4	5	6–7	8
Histrionic	0	1–2	3	4–5	6–7	8
Narcissistic	0	1–3	4	5–6	7–8	9
Compulsive	0	1–3	4	5–6	7–8	9
Passive-aggressive	0	1–3	4	5–6	7–8	9

[a]Confined to items occurring since age 15 years.

rating considers level of impairment in social and occupational functioning secondary to the respective disorder. One could facilitate the use of this rating by including explicit criteria within the Personality Disorders section.

A severity rating, however, concerns a level of functioning for persons who have a (categorically diagnosed) disorder. A person with only a few borderline symptoms could be much more severely dysfunctional than a person with all of the compulsive symptoms. The severity rating does not indicate the degree to which a person represents a prototypic case. It is also questionable whether a specific severity rating could be made reliably. A person will typically meet the criteria for more than one personality disorder or for both an Axis I and Axis II disorder, and it will be difficult to differentiate their respective contributions to social and occupational dysfunction (e.g., whether a marital difficulty was due to the borderline, dependent, avoidant, or histrionic traits).

Include a Dimensional Model in an Appendix or Introduction

A third proposal is to provide a dimensional model in an appendix to DSM-IV or within the introduction to the Personality Disorders section. Providing only one model would be theoretically biased, whereas including all of them would provide considerable redundancy and confusion. A compromise is to represent each of the major models by one or two dimensions, indicating in each case how the dimensions from the other models relate to the dimension that is included. The advantage of this approach is that it would represent all of the major formulations in a succinct and balanced fashion yet preserve their distinctive features.

The proposal consists of seven dimensions: extraversion, neuroticism, constraint, antagonism (versus agreeableness), openness, reward dependence, and cognitive disorganization (developed in consultation with Drs. Cloninger, Costa, Eysenck, McCrae, Siever, Tellegen, and Wiggins). The definition of extraversion would be based on Eysenck's (1987) model, but it would also represent the extraversion dimension of the five-factor model and the interpersonal circumplex dimension of affiliation, the self-other dimension from Millon (1981), and the positive affectivity dimension (Clark 1990; Tellegen and Waller, in press). The neuroticism dimension would be defined by Eysenck's model, but it would also represent the neuroticism dimension of the five-factor model (Costa and McCrae 1992), negative emotionality (Clark 1990; Tellegen and Waller, in press), harm avoidance (Cloninger 1987), and anxious-fearfulness from the DSM-III-R clusters and the spectra emphasized by Siever and Davis (1991). Constraint would be defined by Tellegen and Waller's model, but it would also represent the psychoticism dimension of Eysenck, conscientiousness from the five-factor model, novelty seeking from Cloninger, and impulsivity from Siever and Davis. Antagonism (versus agreeableness) would be defined by the five-factor model but it would also represent the interpersonal circumplex dimension of dominance (versus submission; Kiesler 1986). Openness to experience would represent the five-factor model, reward dependence would represent Cloninger's model, and cognitive disorganization would represent the model of Siever and Davis.

There are, however, limitations to this proposal. One difficulty is that the clinical utility of the dimensions will not be readily apparent to many clinicians. The relevance of reward dependence and openness to experience to clinical practice is not as obvious as the relevance of the histrionic and borderline diagnoses. It is also unclear how one would apply the dimensions in clinical practice. Most of the dimensional models are assessed by self-report inventories. There are no explicit guidelines for the assessment of neuroticism, constraint, or extraversion via a clinical interview.

An additional issue is the inclusion of normal traits within the diagnostic nomenclature. The DSM is a manual for the diagnosis of mental disorders, not normal functioning; however, the extent that personality disorders involve extreme, exaggerated, or maladaptive variants of normal personality traits, it is perhaps appropriate for a classification of abnormal personality to involve normal personality traits. Their inclusion would also provide a more comprehensive description of a patient's entire personality, consistent with the spirit of a comprehensive multiaxial assessment.

Recommendations

The consensus of the Personality Disorders Work Group is that the three options represent reasonable proposals for DSM-IV. Each was therefore acknowledged in the *DSM-IV Options Book* (Task Force on DSM-IV 1991). Support within the Work Group for each of the proposals is at best mixed, however. The final recommendation of the Personality Disorders Work Group will be based on further review of the issues and data presented in this review and in reviews forwarded to the Work Group in response to the publication of the *DSM-IV Options Book*.

References

Adamson J: An appraisal of the DSM-III system. Can J Psychiatry 34:303–310, 1989

American Psychiatric Association: Diagnostic and Statistical Manual of Mental Disorders, 3rd Edition. Washington, DC, American Psychiatric Association, 1980

American Psychiatric Association: Diagnostic and Statistical Manual of Mental Disorders, 3rd Edition, Revised. Washington, DC, American Psychiatric Association, 1987

Cantor N, Genero N: Psychiatric diagnosis and natural categorization: close analogy, in Contemporary Directions in Psychopathology. Edited by Millon T, Klerman G. New York, Guilford, 1986, pp 233–256

Clark L: Toward a dimensional model of assessment in personality disorder, in Advances in Personality Assessment, Vol 8. Edited by Butcher J, Spielberger C. Hillsdale, NJ, Erlbaum, 1990, pp 243–266

Cloninger CR: A systematic method for clinical description and classification of personality variants. Arch Gen Psychiatry 44:573–588, 1987

Cloninger CR: Establishment of diagnostic validity in psychiatric illness: Robins and Guze's method revisited, in The Validity of Psychiatric Diagnosis. Edited by Robins L, Barrett J. New York, Raven, 1989, pp 9–18

Costa PT, McCrae RR: The five-factor model of personality and its relevance to personality disorders. Journal of Personality Disorders 6:343–359, 1992

Eysenck H: The definition of personality disorders and the criteria appropriate for their description. Journal of Personality Disorders 1:211–219, 1987

Frances A: Categorical and dimensional systems of personality diagnosis: a comparison. Compr Psychiatry 23:516–527, 1982

Frances A: Conceptual Problems of Psychiatric Classification. Paper presented at the 143rd annual meeting of the American Psychiatric Association, New York, May 1990

Frances A, Clarkin J, Gimore M, et al: Reliability of criteria for borderline personality disorder: a comparison of DSM-III and the Diagnostic Interview for Borderline Patients. Am J Psychiatry 42:591–596, 1984

Grove W, Andreasen N: Quantitative and qualitative distinctions between psychiatric disorders, in The Validity of Psychiatric Diagnosis. Edited by Robins L, Barrett J. New York, Raven, 1989, pp 127–141

Grove WM, Tellegen A: Problems in the classification of personality disorders. Journal of Personality Disorders 5:31–41, 1991

Gunderson JG, Links PS, Reich JH: Competing models of personality disorders. Journal of Personality Disorders 5:60–68, 1991

Heumann K, Morey L: Reliability of categorical and dimensional judgments of personality disorder. Am J Psychiatry 147:498–500, 1990

Kass F, Skodol A, Charles E, et al: Scaled ratings of DSM-III personality disorders. Am J Psychiatry 142:627–630, 1985

Kendler KS: Toward a scientific psychiatric nosology: strengths and limitations. Arch Gen Psychiatry 47:969–973, 1990

Kiesler D: The 1982 Interpersonal Circle: an analysis of DSM-III personality disorders, in Contemporary Directions in Psychopathology. Edited by Millon T, Klerman G. New York, Guilford, 1986, pp 571–597

Livesley WJ: Classifying personality disorders: ideal types, prototypes, or dimensions? Journal of Personality Disorders 5:52–59, 1991

McGlashan T: Borderline personality disorder and unipolar affective disorder: long-term effects of comorbidity. J Nerv Ment Dis 175:467–473, 1987

Miller M, Thayer J: On the existence of discrete classes in personality: is self-monitoring the correct joint to carve? J Pers Soc Psychol 57:143–155, 1989

Millon T: Disorders of Personality. DSM-III: Axis II. New York, Wiley, 1981

Morey LC: The categorical representation of personality disorder: a cluster analysis of DSM-III-R personality features. J Abnorm Psychol 97:314–321, 1988

Nestadt G, Romanoski A, Chahal R, et al: An epidemiological study of histrionic personality disorder. Psychol Med 20:413–422, 1990

Robins L, Helzer J: Diagnosis and clinical assessment: the current state of psychiatric diagnosis. Annu Rev Psychol 37:409–432, 1986

Siever LJ, Davis KL: A psychobiological perspective on the personality disorders. Am J Psychiatry 148:1647–1658, 1991

Skodol A, Rosnick L, Kellman D, et al: Development of a procedure for validating structured assessments of Axis II, in Personality Disorders: New Perspectives on Diagnostic Validity. Edited by Oldham J. Washington, DC, American Psychiatric Press, 1991, pp 41–70

Spitzer R, Endicott J, Gibbon M: Crossing the border into borderline personality and borderline schizophrenia. Arch Gen Psychiatry 36:17–24, 1979

Task Force on DSM-IV: DSM-IV Options Book: Work in Progress. Washington, DC, American Psychiatric Association, 1991

Tellegen A, Waller N: Exploring personality through test construction: development of the Multidimensional Personality Questionnaire, in Personality Measures: Development and Evaluation, Vol 1. Edited by Briggs S, Cheeks J. Greenwich, CT, JAI Press (in press)

Trull T, Widiger T, Guthrie P: The categorical versus dimensional status of borderline personality disorder. J Abnorm Psychol 99:40–48, 1990

Tyrer P: What's wrong with DSM-III personality disorders? Journal of Personality Disorders 2:281–291, 1988

Tyrer P, Alexander J: Classification of personality disorder. Br J Psychiatry 135:163–167, 1979

Widiger TA: Personality disorder dimensional models proposed for DSM-IV. Journal of Personality Disorders 5:386–398, 1991

Widiger TA: Categorical versus dimensional classification: implications from and for research. Journal of Personality Disorders 6:287–300, 1992

Widiger TA, Frances AJ: Toward a dimensional model for the personality disorders, in Personality Disorders and the Five-Factor Model of Personality. Edited by Costa P, Widiger T. Washington, DC, American Psychological Association, 1994, pp 19–39

Zimmerman M, Coryell W: DSM-III personality disorder dimensions. J Nerv Ment Dis 178:686–692, 1990

Chapter 33

Depressive Personality Disorder

Katharine A. Phillips, M.D., Robert M. A. Hirschfeld, M.D.,
M. Tracie Shea, Ph.D., and John Gunderson, M.D.

Introduction

The concept of the depressive personality has a long and rich history (Phillips et al. 1990). It has been described by diverse clinical theorists under a variety of names, beginning with Hippocrates' and Aristotle's description of a "black gall" or melancholic, temperament thousands of years ago. It has also been referred to as depressive character, typus melancholicus, dysthymic temperament, characterologic depression, subaffective dysthymia, dysthymic psychopathy, and anankastic personality disorder (PD) with depressive features.

Emil Kraepelin (1921) is among several German phenomenologists (also Kretschmer 1925; Tellenbach 1961) who described a depressive temperament consisting of a predominantly despondent and despairing mood. These individuals were also serious, burdened, guilt ridden, self-reproaching, self-denying, and lacking in self-confidence. Kraepelin considered this personality type to be inherited and perceptible in youth and to predispose to, and be a temperamental underpinning of, major depression and mania.

Kurt Schneider (1959), who first described modern PDs, included the depressive personality among them. Like Kraepelin, he considered these individuals to be gloomy, pessimistic, serious, and incapable of enjoyment or relaxation; quiet; skeptical; worrying; duty bound; and self-doubting. However, unlike Kraepelin, he did not posit a relationship between this disorder and major mood disorder.

Several psychoanalysts (Berliner 1966; Kahn 1975; Simons 1986) also described a depressive personality. Among them was Kernberg (1987), who has

We thank Kathleen Talbot for extensive contributions to this manuscript.

proposed that these individuals have the following characteristics: 1) overly serious, somber, burdened, responsible, conscientious, and highly critical of themselves and others (traits reflecting an excessively severe superego); 2) overdependent on the support and acceptance of others (although they may appear counterdependent); and 3) difficulty expressing aggression, so they often do not overtly express their critical and harsh judgments of others.

Although cognitive and behavioral theorists have not described a depressive personality per se, some of their work on enduring, depressogenic beliefs may have relevance to this disorder. For example, Beck (1967) and Alloy et al. (1988) believe that individuals prone to major depression have chronically distorted negative cognitions that predispose to the development of more severe depressive episodes. However, these theories focus primarily on the premorbid features of major depression rather than on a depressive personality type that may or may not predispose to major depressive episodes.

Statement of the Issues

The purpose of this review was to make a recommendation about whether depressive PD should be included in DSM-IV and, if so, whether it should be included in the main body of the manual or in an appendix for disorders requiring further investigation. To do this, the following specific questions were considered:

1. To what extent does depressive PD overlap conceptually with other PDs and Axis I mood disorders?
2. To what extent does depressive PD overlap empirically with other PDs and Axis I mood disorders?
3. How do the individual criteria for depressive PD perform?

Significance of the Issues

Despite depressive personality's long and rich historical tradition, it has received little empirical attention. Thus, there are many unanswered questions about this disorder, many of which focus on nosological issues. In particular, it has been suggested that the depressive personality may be a redundant concept, overlapping excessively with other PDs, such as self-defeating, dependent, obsessive-compulsive, and avoidant. Others question whether depressive personality might overlap significantly with Axis I mood disorders such as dysthymia; a related concern is that patients with chronic mood disorder might be misdiagnosed with a PD and consequently receive inadequate somatic treatment (although a PD diagnosis should not rule out the use of medication). For all of these reasons, the depressive personality remains a controversial entity in need of further empirical study.

Methods

The psychiatric literature was searched for all references related to depressive personality, which included a Medline computer search that used index terms such as *dysthymia* and *depression and personality;* this search generated approximately 50 relevant references. Historical references on depressive personality that were known to the authors were also reviewed, and additional sources were obtained from the bibliographies of these books and articles. Finally, 10 researchers and advisers with an interest in depressive PD (both advocates and individuals with a neutral stance) identified relevant historical or empirical sources, provided feedback on its descriptive features, and commented on its possible inclusion in DSM-IV. This review is based on those references that most directly inform the issues listed above.

Results

Conceptual Overlap

It has been suggested that depressive PD may overlap conceptually with several PDs, primarily self-defeating (Kernberg 1984), dependent (Kernberg 1984), obsessive-compulsive (Schneider 1959), and avoidant (Standage 1986) PDs. Some of the conceptual similarities and differences between depressive PD, other PDs, and dysthymia are discussed below.

Self-defeating PD.   Unlike in depressive PD, in self-defeating PD, individuals take an active role in producing and maintaining their symptoms, choosing people and situations that lead to disappointment and failure. As Simons (1986) suggested, patients with self-defeating PD unconsciously torture and blackmail others, provoking retaliation; in contrast, individuals with depressive PD internalize their conflict, which leads to self-torture and self-defeat in the absence of provoked retaliation from others. Whereas individuals with self-defeating PD actively reject opportunities for pleasure and have a negative reaction when positive events occur, those with depressive PD simply find it difficult to get any enjoyment or pleasure out of such opportunities and events. In contrast to individuals with self-defeating

PD, who often fail to accomplish tasks crucial to their success, those with depressive PD may be overly conscientious, responsible, and self-disciplining (Laughlin 1967).

Dependent PD.   Unlike the German phenomenologists, several psychoanalysts feature dependency in their description of depressive PD (Kahn 1975; Kernberg 1987). Kernberg (1990), however, believes that, although these individuals are overly dependent on the approval of others, they are not overtly clinging and often appear counterdependent. As such, they tend to reject others before they can be rejected to avoid feeling disappointed and frustrated when their dependency needs are not met.

Obsessive-compulsive PD.   Conscientious, duty bound, and self-disciplining are traits of obsessive-compulsive PD that have been proposed to characterize depressive PD (Akiskal 1989; Kernberg 1987; Laughlin 1967; Schneider 1959; Simons 1986; Tellenbach 1961). However, these disorders differ in that individuals with obsessive-compulsive PD are more constricted in their expression of affection and are not necessarily persistently gloomy (Kernberg 1990). Also, in contrast to the controlling interpersonal style of individuals with obsessive-compulsive PD, those with depressive PD are often passive and unassertive (Kernberg 1990).

Avoidant PD.   Although it has been proposed that depressive PD, like avoidant PD, is characterized by shyness and introversion (Akiskal 1989; Schneider 1959; Simons 1986), individuals with depressive PD are less reluctant to enter into relationships and hence have more and better relationships with others (Kernberg 1984). According to Kernberg, individuals with depressive PD in fact have an enormous sense of personal responsibility and therefore attempt to relate well to others, which may result in good surface relations at the cost of tension and doubts that they deserve others' love and friendship (Kernberg 1984). In addition, individuals with avoidant PD are not necessarily chronically gloomy and unhappy.

Borderline PD.   In borderline PD, mood is unstable and disturbed by outbursts of anger, which tend to be unexpressed in depressive PD. Relationships in borderline PD are also often unstable, with alternation between extremes of idealized expectations and the perception of bitter betrayals, whereas in depressive PD, relationships are more stable and more consistently involve unexpressed negative thoughts about others (Kernberg 1984). The severe identity disturbance marked by vacillation and a sense of extreme badness seen in borderline PD is not characteristic of the stable low self-esteem seen in depressive PD. And individuals with depressive PD tend toward behavioral constriction and constraint, unlike the impulsiveness of those with borderline PD (Kernberg 1990).

Passive-aggressive PD. The negativism of passive-aggressive PD is often directed toward authority figures, expressed in response to demands, and obstructive. In contrast, individuals with depressive PD are often compliant and particularly anxious to please authority figures (Laughlin 1967). In addition, individuals with passive-aggressive PD are not necessarily persistently gloomy and dysphoric.

Negativistic PD. Depressive PD and the newly proposed negativistic PD share the features of pessimism and criticism of others. However, the criticism of negativistic PD (like that of passive-aggressive PD) is preferentially directed at authority figures, whereas that of depressive PD is not; in addition, individuals with depressive PD may be more likely to inhibit expression of critical, hostile, or aggressive thoughts or feelings. They are also more likely to feel guilty and to blame themselves rather than others, and their mood is generally gloomy and unhappy rather than sullen, irritable, and angry.

Dysthymia. It has also been suggested that depressive PD may overlap excessively with Axis I mood disorder, in particular dysthymia (Kocsis 1991). However, by definition, dysthymia is a mild, chronic form of mood disorder, not a PD. Thus, its central pathology primarily involves mood dysregulation, not interpersonal relationships, cognitions, or self-concept. Other, more specific theoretical differences between depressive PD and dysthymia include the following:

1. Depressive PD is of early onset, beginning by early adulthood, whereas dysthymia can begin at any age.
2. Depressive PD is chronic and persistent, whereas dysthymia can remit.
3. Depressive PD is characterized primarily by personality traits rather than symptoms.
4. Many depressive PD traits are cognitive and interpersonal, in contrast to those of dysthymia, which are largely somatic depressive symptoms.

Dysthymia is a broader and more heterogeneous category than depressive PD; for example, dysthymia can occur at any age and can be primary or secondary (e.g., it can occur in response to medical illness) (Akiskal 1989). Further research is needed to determine whether depressive PD and dysthymia are distinct disorders or whether depressive PD corresponds to a subtype of dysthymia as it is currently defined, specifically, the early-onset, primary type of dysthymia.

Empirical Overlap

Several researchers have investigated the overlap between depressive personality and other psychiatric disorders, in particular, personality and mood disorders.

Standage (1986), using Schneider's concept of the depressive personality, assessed this disorder's overlap with DSM-III (American Psychiatric Association 1980) PDs in four patients. He found that one patient had a diagnosis of avoidant PD, one had avoidant traits, and two had a mixed PD, in addition to the diagnosis of depressive PD.

Klein (1990) empirically assessed the overlap between depressive PD and DSM-III schizotypal and borderline PDs and mood disorders. He studied 177 outpatients with high scores on the General Behavior Inventory (GBI, a measure of chronic hypomanic and depressive symptoms; Depue et al. 1989), assessing them at baseline and 6-month follow-up with an expanded version of the Schedule for Affective Disorders and Schizophrenia (Endicott and Spitzer 1978), the Family History Research Diagnostic Criteria interview (Andreasen et al. 1977), and Akiskal's (1983) criteria for depressive PD (Table 33–1). A significantly greater proportion of patients meeting (23%) than not meeting (7%) criteria for depressive PD received a diagnosis of schizotypal PD ($P < .01$), but the two groups did not differ significantly on rates of borderline PD.

Regarding the overlap between depressive PD and Axis I dysthymia, significantly more patients with than without depressive PD also met criteria for DSM-III dysthymia, but the two disorders appeared to be distinct; only 30% of patients met criteria for both depressive PD and dysthymia (kappa = .22). Compared with patients with dysthymia, patients with depressive PD had less severe depression (as measured by the GBI [Depue et al. 1989] and Beck Depression Inventory [Beck et

Table 33–1.   Akiskal's 1989 criteria for depressive personality (subaffective dysthymia)[a]

Indeterminate early onset (<21 years old)

Habitually long sleeper (>9 hours of sleep)

Psychomotor inertia that is typically worse in the morning

At least five of the following traits:

1. Gloomy, pessimistic, humorless, or incapable of fun
2. Quiet, passive, and indecisive
3. Skeptical, hypercritical, or complaining
4. Brooding and given to worry
5. Conscientious or self-disciplining
6. Self-critical, self-reproaching, and self-derogatory
7. Preoccupied with inadequacy, failure, and negative events to the point of morbid enjoyment of one's failures

[a]This is an updated version of Akiskal's 1983 criteria and, like the 1983 criteria, is based on a modification of Schneider's description of the depressive personality.

al. 1979]) and fewer relatives with unipolar depression. However, patients with depressive PD had more severe depression and significantly more family members with bipolar disorder or hospitalization for mood disorder than outpatients without depressive PD. In another study, Klein et al. (1988) found a similar familial relationship between depressive PD and major mood disorder; depressive PD was more common in offspring of patients hospitalized for major depression than in offspring of normal control subjects or patients hospitalized for medical disorders. Similarly, Wetzel et al. (1980) found that depressive personality traits are more likely than other traits to occur in relatives of patients with major depression. Klein concluded that, although depressive PD appears to be distinct from dysthymia, it may nonetheless be related to major mood disorder and dysthymia, perhaps being a less symptomatic, more trait-like variant of mood disorder than dysthymia. This "spectrum relationship" posited for depressive PD and major mood disorder is similar to that documented for schizotypal PD and schizophrenia (Baron et al. 1983; Gunderson and Siever 1985).

Akiskal's work similarly suggests that depressive PD can be differentiated from the heterogeneous concept of dysthymia. Yerevanian and Akiskal (1979) prospectively studied 150 outpatients with "characterologic depression," a mild, chronic, depressive illness of early insidious onset that is similar to DSM's early-onset dysthymia. They found that early-onset dysthymia consists of two subtypes, depressive personality (Table 33–1) and character-spectrum disorder (Akiskal 1983; Akiskal et al. 1980). Patients with depressive personality (subaffective dysthymia) shared features with a unipolar depressed control group: shortened rapid eye movement (REM) latency, family history of unipolar or bipolar mood disorder, relatively normal developmental history and good social outcome, more frequent superimposed and melancholic major depressive episodes, and good response to antidepressant medications, lithium, and social skills training.

In contrast, character-spectrum disorder (a heterogeneous mix of PDs, primarily histrionic and antisocial, with secondary dysphorias) was characterized by normal REM latency; family history of alcoholism and sociopathy but not mood disorder; childhood parental loss, separation, or divorce; poor social outcome; nonmelancholic major depressive episodes; poor response to antidepressant medication; and polysubstance and alcohol abuse.

Hauri and Sateia (1984) replicated Akiskal's REM latency findings, and Rhimer (1990) subsequently found that patients with depressive PD but not character-spectrum disorder had abnormal dexamethasone suppression test results and responded to sleep deprivation. Akiskal, like Klein, concluded that depressive personality is a variant of classic mood disorder that is chronic, subsyndromal, and trait-like (rather than episodic, symptomatic, and state-like) and thus warrants classification as a PD. He also concluded that, like major mood disorder, depressive

PD can improve with antidepressant medication, underscoring the fact that a PD diagnosis should not rule out the use of medication. Finally, Akiskal believes depressive PD is a subset of early-onset dysthymia and that it differs from other forms of dysthymia, such as the late-onset type and the character-spectrum subtype of early-onset dysthymia (Akiskal 1989).

The work cited above, although preliminary, suggests that depressive PD may be distinct from existing mood disorders and PDs. Although, like all disorders, it has some overlap with other diagnostic categories, the overlap appears to be incomplete. However, further research is needed to assess depressive PD's relationship with a broader range of Axis I and Axis II disorders.

Performance of Criteria

In several studies (Klein 1990; Klein et al. 1988), Akiskal's 1983 criteria had good interrater reliability for both the number of depressive personality traits ($r = .86$) and the presence or absence of the diagnosis (kappa = .82). Another study, using Schneider's description of depressive PD (Standage 1979), also found a high interrater reliability (kappa = .75) for the disorder's presence or absence.

The depressive PD criteria have also been shown to have an acceptable internal consistency (alpha = .61) that is comparable to that of other DSM-III-R (American Psychiatric Association 1987) PDs (Morey 1988). In this study, the one item that did not correlate highly with the others was conscientiousness. Regarding test-retest stability over a 6-month interval, Klein (1990) found that the number of depressive PD traits rated as present in the initial and follow-up evaluations correlated .43 ($P < .001$) and that there was a 71% concordance on the presence or absence of the diagnosis (kappa = .41).

Discussion and Recommendations

Should the depressive personality be included in DSM-IV? In support of its inclusion are its long historical tradition, its advocacy by expert clinicians from diverse theoretical perspectives, and some empirical evidence. However, more data are needed, especially data establishing its discriminability from other disorders, such as dysthymia and near-neighbor PDs. Field trials are under way to evaluate the proposed criteria set for depressive PD and the comorbidity of depressive PD with Axis I disorders, and other ongoing studies are assessing its overlap with Axis II disorders.

In the meantime, the Work Group on Personality Disorders for DSM-IV has considered several options: this disorder might be included on Axis II, included in the appendix of proposed diagnoses requiring further study, or omitted from DSM altogether. In light of the depressive PD's strong historical tradition and preliminary empirical support, the Personality Disorder Work Group supports its inclusion in DSM-IV. This recommendation reflects the Work Group's belief that certain Axis II disorders may be on a spectrum with certain Axis I disorders (i.e., that certain PDs may be early-onset, enduring, trait-like variants of the more episodic and severely symptomatic Axis I disorders and may share similar family history, treatment response, and perhaps etiology). Such a link has been demonstrated for schizophrenia and schizotypal PD and may also exist for Axis I mood disorders and depressive PD, as has been suggested by the work of Akiskal and Klein.

Nonetheless, the Work Group has some concerns about including depressive PD on Axis II at this time. In particular, as is noted above, this disorder's delineation from other Axis II disorders and from dysthymia is not yet clear. Some groups have expressed the concern that, if depressive PD is actually a type of dysthymia but is placed on Axis II, patients may not receive adequate somatic treatment. Although this concern may have some validity, it reflects the false assumption that PDs are devoid of biological underpinnings and should not be treated with medication; in fact, as is suggested by the spectrum concept, certain PDs, including depressive PD, are likely to be at least partly biological in origin and may warrant such treatment. Another concern of the Work Group is that, if such a personality type exists, it may be a temperamental or constitutional variant of normal personality rather than a PD with associated distress and impairment. Because of these concerns, depressive PD is thought to be a good candidate for inclusion in the DSM-IV appendix, as a proposed diagnosis warranting further study, rather than on Axis II. However, if strong evidence in support of this disorder emerges from the DSM-IV Mood Disorder Field Trial in progress, depressive PD might instead warrant inclusion on Axis II.

Another option was to recommend that depressive PD and Axis I dysthymia be combined, as has been proposed for ICD-10 (World Health Organization 1990). Although depressive PD was a separate disorder (a type of affective PD) in ICD-9, it is subsumed under dysthymia in the proposed ICD-10, a category that includes both affective symptoms (e.g., insomnia and poor concentration) and some of the personality traits characteristic of depressive PD (pessimism, brooding, and feelings of inadequacy). Similarly, the proposed DSM-IV criteria for dysthymia have been somewhat broadened to include not only the primarily affective and somatic symptoms of DSM-III-R dysthymia but also several depressive PD characteristics (pessimism, brooding, and feelings of inadequacy). However, at this time, there appears to be insufficient empirical support for combining these disorders; indeed, what preliminary evidence is available suggests they may be distinct but related disorders. If they do overlap, such overlap would be expected only with the primary, early-onset subtype of dysthymia.

Proposed Criteria for DSM-IV

The following proposed criteria represent characteristics of depressive personality commonly described in the clinical and empirical literature. Because the symptoms of a major depressive episode might produce some of the features listed below, it is important to ascertain that these features do not occur exclusively during major depressive episodes; that is, they should not be symptoms (state-like) but should be characteristic of the individual's personality (trait-like). Thus, they should be pervasive, of late-adolescent or early-adult onset, and persistent and stable rather than short lived and episodic and should cause either significant distress or impairment in functioning.

Proposed Criteria

Essential Feature: Excessive negative, pessimistic beliefs about oneself and other people.

A1: *Usual mood is characterized by dejection, gloominess, cheerlessness, joylessness, unhappiness.* Rationale: The predominant mood of individuals with depressive PD is dysphoric, in particular, gloomy and unhappy. Although the mood may fluctuate, it is fairly persistently negative and somber (Akiskal 1989; Kraepelin 1921; Laughlin 1967; Schneider 1959; Simons 1986). These individuals are often overly serious, lack a sense of humor, and feel they do not deserve to have fun or be happy (Kernberg 1990; Laughlin 1967).

A2: *Prominent self-concepts center around beliefs of inadequacy, worthlessness, and low self-esteem.* Rationale: Individuals with depressive PD feel inferior and tend to doubt and undervalue their self-worth and abilities (Akiskal 1989; Arieti and Bemporad 1980; Berliner 1966; Kahn 1975; Kraepelin 1921; Schneider 1959; Simons 1986).

A3: *Is critical, blaming, derogatory, and punitive toward oneself.* Rationale: Individuals with depressive PD are harsh in their self-judgments, tending to be self-critical and disparaging of their accomplishments, performance, and conduct (Akiskal 1989; Arieti and Bemporad 1980; Berliner 1966; Kahn 1975; Kraepelin 1921; Laughlin 1967; Simons 1986; Tellenbach 1961).

A4: *Is brooding and given to worry.* Rationale: Individuals with depressive PD tend to ruminate about and persistently dwell on negative and unhappy thoughts (Akiskal 1989; Laughlin 1967; Schneider 1959; Simons 1986).

A5: *Is negativistic, critical, and judgmental toward others.* Rationale: Individuals with depressive PD tend to judge others as harshly as they judge themselves. They tend to see and expect the worst in others and focus on others' failings rather than their positive attributes (Akiskal 1989; Berliner 1966; Kernberg 1987; Simons 1986).

A6: *Is pessimistic.* Rationale: Individuals with depressive PD tend to have negative expectations for the future, see life as futile, and anticipate the worst

(Akiskal 1989; Laughlin 1967; Schneider 1959; Simons 1986).

A7: *Is prone to feeling guilt.* Rationale: Individuals with depressive PD have a tendency to feel remorseful about their behavior and excessively blame themselves for their failings (Berliner 1966; Kahn 1975; Kernberg 1987; Kraepelin 1921; Laughlin 1967; Schneider 1959; Tellenbach 1961).

B: *Does not occur exclusively during major depressive episodes.*

Additional criteria, proposed by some clinicians and researchers, may be added to those listed above if supported by data from ongoing studies of depressive personality and the DSM-IV field trial. These proposed criteria include

1. Quiet, introverted, passive, and unassertive (Akiskal 1989; Berliner 1966; Laughlin 1967; Schneider 1959; Simons 1986)
2. Conscientious, duty bound, self-disciplining (Akiskal 1989; Kernberg 1987; Laughlin 1967; Schneider 1959; Simons 1986; Tellenbach 1961)
3. The following addition to criterion 5: "although such thoughts are often difficult to express and often kept to themselves" (Berliner 1966; Kahn 1975; Kernberg 1987; Laughlin 1967)

References

Akiskal HS: Dysthymic disorder: psychopathology of proposed chronic depressive subtypes. Am J Psychiatry 140:11–20, 1983

Akiskal HS: Validating affective personality types, in The Validity of Psychiatric Diagnosis. Edited by Robins L, Barrett J. New York, Raven, 1989

Akiskal HS, Rosenthal TL, Haykal RF, et al: Characterological depressions: clinical and sleep EEG findings separating "subaffective dysthymia" from "character spectrum disorders." Arch Gen Psychiatry 37:777–783, 1980

Alloy LB, Abramson LY, Metalsky GI, et al: The hopelessness theory of depression: attributional aspects. Br J Clin Psychology 27:5–21, 1988

American Psychiatric Association: Diagnostic and Statistical Manual of Mental Disorders, 3rd Edition. Washington, DC, American Psychiatric Association, 1980

American Psychiatric Association: Diagnostic and Statistical Manual of Mental Disorders, 3rd Edition, Revised. Washington, DC, American Psychiatric Association, 1987

Andreasen NC, Endicott J, Spitzer RL, et al: The family history method using diagnostic criteria. Arch Gen Psychiatry 34:1229–1235, 1977

Arieti S, Bemporad JR: The psychological organization of depression. Am J Psychiatry 137:1360–1365, 1980

Baron M, Gruen R, Asnis L, et al: Familial relatedness of schizophrenia and schizotypal states. Am J Psychiatry 140:1437–1442, 1983

Beck AT: Depression: Causes and Treatment. Philadelphia, University of Pennsylvania Press, 1967

Beck AT, Rush AJ, Shaw BF, et al: Cognitive Therapy of Depression. New York, Guilford, 1979

Berliner B: Psychodynamics of the depressive character. Psychoanal Forum 1:244–251, 1966

Depue RA, Krauss S, Spoont MR, et al: General Behavior Inventory identification of unipolar and bipolar affective conditions in a nonclinical university population. J Abnorm Psychol 98:117–126, 1989

Endicott J, Spitzer RL: A diagnostic interview: the Schedule for the Affective Disorders and Schizophrenia. Arch Gen Psychiatry 35:837–844, 1978

Gunderson JG, Siever L: Relatedness of schizotypal to schizophrenic disorders. Schizophr Bull 11:532–537, 1985

Hauri P, Sateia MJ: REM sleep in dysthymic disorders. Sleep Res 13:119, 1984

Kahn E: The depressive character. Folia Psychiatr Neurol Jpn 29:291–303, 1975

Kernberg O: Severe Personality Disorders: Psychotherapeutic Strategies. New Haven, CT, Yale University Press, 1984

Kernberg O: Clinical dimensions of masochism, in Masochism: Current and Psychotherapeutic Contributions. Edited by Glick RA, Meyers DI. Hillsdale, NJ, Analytic Press, 1987, pp 61–79

Kernberg O: Differential diagnosis of the depressive-masochistic personality disorder. Presented at the American Psychiatric Association, 143rd annual meeting, New York, May 16, 1990

Klein DN: Depressive personality: reliability, validity, and relation to dysthymia. J Abnorm Psychol 99:412–421, 1990

Klein DN, Clark DC, Dansky L, et al: Dysthymia in the offspring of parents with primary unipolar affective disorder. J Abnorm Psychol 97:265–274, 1988

Kocsis JH: Resolved: depressive personality is a useful construct that should be included in DSM-IV. CME Syllabus and Proceedings Summary. American Psychiatric Association, 144th annual meeting, New Orleans, LA, May 1991

Kraepelin E: Manic-Depressive Insanity and Paranoia. Translated by Barclay RM, edited by Robertson GM. Edinburgh, UK, E & S Livingstone, 1921

Kretschmer E: Physique and Character. New York, Harcourt Brace, 1925

Laughlin HP: The Neuroses. Stoneham, MA, Butterworths, 1967

Morey LC: The categorical representation of personality disorder: a cluster analysis of DSM-III-R personality features. J Abnorm Psychol 97:314–321, 1988

Phillips KA, Gunderson JG, Hirschfeld RMA, et al: A review of the depressive personality. Am J Psychiatry 147:830–837, 1990

Rhimer Z: Dysthymia: a clinician's perspective, in Dysthymic Disorder. Edited by Burton SW, Akiskal HS. London, Gaskell (Royal College of Psychiatrists), 1990, pp 112–125

Schneider K: Clinical Psychopathology. Translated by Hamilton MW. London, Grune & Stratton, 1959

Simons RC: Psychoanalytic contributions to psychiatric nosology: forms of masochistic behavior. J Am Psychoanal Assoc 35:583–608, 1986

Standage KF: The use of Schneider's typology for the diagnosis of personality disorders: an examination of reliability. Br J Psychiatry 135:238–242, 1979

Standage K: A clinical and psychometric investigation comparing Schneider's and the DSM-III typologies of personality disorders. Compr Psychiatry 27:35–45, 1986

Tellenbach H: Melancholy: History of the Problem, Endogeneity, Typology, Pathogenesis, Clinical Considerations. Pittsburgh, PA, Duquesne University Press, 1961

Wetzel RD, Cloninger CR, Hong B, et al: Personality as a subclinical expression of the affective disorders. Compr Psychiatry 21:197–205, 1980

World Health Organization: ICD-10 Chapter V: Mental and Behavioral Disorders: Diagnostic Criteria for Research. Geneva, Switzerland, World Health Organization, 1990

Yerevanian BI, Akiskal HS: "Neurotic," characterological, and dysthymic depressions. Psychiatr Clin North Am 2:595–617, 1979

Chapter 34

Negativistic (Passive-Aggressive) Personality Disorder

Theodore Millon, Ph.D.

Introduction

With the exception of the two new personality disorders (PDs) included in the appendix to DSM-III-R (American Psychiatric Association 1987), passive-aggressive PD was one of the two or three PDs from the original group in DSM-III (American Psychiatric Association 1980) that elicited considerable discussion at Work Group meetings and within the post–DSM-III critical literature. Questions have been raised about the very legitimacy of passive-aggressive PD as a PD and about whether an expansion of its rather narrow range of diagnostic criteria to that of a more broadly based negativistic PD would enhance its viability in this regard (Frances and Widiger 1987; Millon 1981).

The descriptive features that characterize the disorder have been portrayed in considerable detail by numerous distinguished clinicians for close to a century under a variety of different designations. Its most recent revival, termed as the passive-aggressive personality *trait disturbance* in DSM-I (American Psychiatric Association 1952), represented the manner in which the disorder was expressed in the Armed Forces during World War II. However, numerous early clinical theorists portrayed diversely labeled "dispositions" and "characters" whose features included those of passive-aggressive PD but paralleled even more closely the broadly formulated outline for the proposed negativistic PD. For example, Kraepelin (1913) wrote about individuals with constitutions that incline them to "take all things hard and feel the unpleasantness in every occurrence" (p. 219), as well as to show an "extraordinarily fluctuating emotional equilibrium . . . often in an unpleasant way" (p. 222). Bleuler (1924) spoke of these personalities as being irritable of mood, and Aschaffenburg (1922) described them as dissatisfied personalities who go through life as if they were perpetually wounded. Hellpach (1920) depicted them as fussy people of sour disposition, and Schneider (1923) referred to them as "ill-tempered depressives" and characterized them as nagging, spiteful, malicious, and likely to be "doggedly pessimistic and rejoice when things go wrong" (p. 81). Basing his observations on Abraham's (1924) concept of the "oral-biting" character, where "envy, hostility, and jealousy" are prominent, Menninger (1940) portrayed such a personality as "inclined to blame the world for everything unpleasant that happens to him . . . (to be) cantankerous, contemptuous, petulant . . . inclined to find everything wrong . . . (to be) emotionally soured (and) perpetually discontented" (pp. 393–394).

Statement of the Issues

Based on the literature, past and recent, as well as Work Group discussions and input from consultants, there appear to be five main questions that need to be answered:

1. Should the prototypal traits that were selected to represent the passive-aggressive category's essential features in DSM-III-R be modified to include the features of a more broadly conceived negativistic PD?
2. Despite their problematic character, do prevalence data for passive-aggressive PD give evidence that a broadened negativistic PD would achieve an adequate prevalence level or diagnostic usage?
3. Can the precursor to negativistic PD, an expanded version of passive-aggressive PD, be differentiated from PDs with which it shares certain important traits?
4. On the basis of its current DSM-III-R formulation, do the more limited clinical features of passive-aggressive PD demonstrate acceptable levels of diagnostic reliability, internal consistency, and external validity?
5. Can DSM-III-R passive-aggressive PD be expanded to comprise a more full-range negativistic PD based on the historic clinical literature that suggests additional and diverse trait criteria?

Significance of the Issues

Passive-aggressive PD was first introduced into the nomenclature in a War Department technical bulletin in 1945 to describe military personnel who expressed their opposition to authority figures in an indirect, "subverting" manner rather than openly and directly. The term was carried over into both the U.S. Joint Armed Services and Standard VA Classification systems shortly thereafter and included as part of the first DSM in 1952 (American Psychiatric Association 1952). Although recognized in that manual as one of several subtypes of aggressive expression, it has not been accepted internationally; it has never been included in the International Classification of Diseases (ICD). It was reluctantly included in DSM-II (American Psychiatric Association 1968), owing to its narrow scope as a PD, and in DSM-III, with the stipulation that its diagnosis not be made in conjunction with any other PD—the only PD restricted in this manner. It has achieved minimal clinical usage (a meager case history or theoretical literature) and has prompted a very small body of empirical studies. In recent critical reviews of DSM (Kernberg 1984; Zimmerman 1988), passive-aggressive PD has been noted as among those DSM-III-R categories that are least supportable for inclusion in DSM-IV (see, in particular, Blashfield et al. 1990).

Although the form of expression, indirect or passive hostility, is undoubtedly a feature of this personality style, it is usually one of several covariant features, a number of which were well described in the pre-World War II literature, where oppositional and negativistic expression included cognitive, interpersonal, self-image, affective, and behavioral characteristics.

The main issue, therefore, is whether a more comprehensive formulation, negativistic PD, inclusive of multiple criterion domains (a defining feature of a PD) would achieve greater acceptance by the profession, prove to be more clinically useful, and stimulate greater empirical research than its more narrowly focused passive-aggressive forerunner.

Methods

Dialog Information Services provided Medline and other less medically oriented computer searches of the 1978–1990 literature and were guided by terms such as *passive-aggressive personality, oppositional behavior, negativism, aggression,* and the like. References before that period were also examined, because the disorder has forerunners in the clinical literature going back to the 1920s. The literature specific to the label *passive-aggressive PD,* however, is sparse. Empirical studies associated with DSM-III and DSM-III-R formulations do include passive-aggressive PD but rarely as a primary focus; where found, it is primarily included simply as one of the Axis II group. A total of 17 articles and chapters were located that contained more than just passing reference to the designation.

Comments from advisers and consultants also were not extensive. A coordinated body of diagnostic criteria and comorbidity data for all the PDs, including passive-aggressive PD, were, however, generously supplied by numerous investigators (Blashfield 1988; Dahl 1986; First and Spitzer 1989; Freiman and Widiger 1989; Millon and Tringone 1989; Morey and Heumann 1988; Pfohl and Blum 1990; Reich 1988; Skodol 1989; Zanarini et al. 1989).

Results and Discussion

The five issues noted previously frame the commentary and data.

1. *Should the prototypal traits that were selected to represent the passive-aggressive category's essential features in DSM-III-R be modified to include features of a more broadly conceived negativistic PD?*

As briefly noted in prior pages, clinical theorists of an earlier period (Kraepelin, Abraham, Bleuler, Schneider) described "character types" similar to passive-aggressive PD that predated the official World War II passive-aggressive PD designation; their conceptions, however, encompassed a wider range of clinical features than the singular element of resistance to external demands. More contemporary researchers seeking to identify a core or essential set of features have also found a similar but again wider range of elements that typify the construct. Small et al. (1970) found that those categorized as having passive-aggressive PD were notable by the "stormy nature of their personal relationships." Whitman et al. (1954) observed earlier that among the distinctive features of this PD was the "conflict between their dependency needs and guilt feelings," resulting in "pseudo-aggression" and "fears of external retaliation." Although Livesley et al. (1987) reported that "resistance to demands of adequate performance" was central to the disorder, he also found features such as stubbornness and procrastination. To Kiesler (1986), the core element of the passive-aggressive construct is the combination of both quarrelsomeness and submissiveness. Work Group members and advisers suggested additional characterizing features, such as "sullen affect and deliberate rudeness," "resentfully argumentative," "irritable," and "feelings of victimization." Because of the Work Group's desire to broaden the characterization of this disorder, the following phrase was proposed for the essential feature description of the negativistic PD: a pervasive pattern of argumentativeness, oppositional behavior, and negative and defeatist attitudes.

2. *Do prevalence data for passive-aggressive PD give evidence that a broadened negativistic PD would achieve an adequate prevalence level and/or diagnostic usage?* A truly representative DSM epidemiological study of the PDs has yet to be carried out (Weissman 1990). Nevertheless, as summarized in a series of studies reported to the Work Group, passive-aggressive PD prevalences range from .00 to .52 (Widiger 1991). This lack of consensus may reflect a lack of uniform standards and

methodologies (e.g., whether second and third diagnoses were included). In studies with larger Ns the clinical usage rate ranged from .02 to .08. In those cases in which a secondary, co-occurrent PD diagnosis was assigned, the frequency at which passive-aggressive PD was used as a secondary diagnosis was roughly 10% (Millon and Tringone 1989). Despite questions concerning its adequacy as currently conceived, clinicians appear to use the diagnosis. It appears reasonable to assume, therefore, that a more comprehensive formulation, as is proposed for negativistic PD, would prove at least equally useful and discriminating.

3. *Can the passive-aggressive precursor to negativistic PD be differentiated from other PDs with which it shares certain traits?* Diagnostic overlap statistics do not indicate an unusual pattern of comorbidities for passive-aggressive PD, a fact that may reflect the early DSM-III proscription against codiagnosing this PD. At best, there is a weak indication of a correspondence between passive-aggressive PD and borderline PD (perhaps reflecting their shared ambivalence about many matters), as well as a more unexpected covariance with narcissistic PD (Morey 1988). Among the studies with larger Ns (Millon and Tringone 1989), there are minor correspondences between passive-aggressive PD and self-defeating and sadistic PDs, suggesting that the passive-aggressive PD dynamic is composed of both timorous and hostile qualities. As the passive-aggressive PD construct is broadened into negativistic PD, with a more diverse set of traits, both its prevalence and pattern of comorbidity may shift. This is one of the reasons why the Work Group believes that the negativistic construct should be placed in the DSM-IV appendix rather than in the manual's main text.

4. *On the basis of its current DSM-III-R formulation, do the more limited clinical features of passive-aggressive PD demonstrate acceptable levels of diagnostic reliability, internal consistency, and external validity?* Poor reliability statistics have been found for this disorder. Kappas with the DSM-III set were especially unimpressive. This in part reflected the fact that the disorder had been characterized by essentially one trait; reliability figures are usually poor for constructs composed of a "small item pool." The Work Group has not yet been able to develop reliability statistics on either the broadened DSM-III-R passive-aggressive or the proposed negativistic PD construct; the self-report Millon Clinical Multiaxial Inventory—II (MCMI-II) passive-aggressive PD scale, associated with the DSM-III-R formulation and aspects of the negativistic pattern, does show an improvement over its pre–DSM-III version (Millon 1987). Perhaps this signifies that a more comprehensive set of criteria for this disorder will lead to improved reliability.

Large unpublished studies carried out by Work Group members and consultants (e.g., Freiman and Widiger 1989; Millon and Tringone 1989; Morey and Heumann 1988) have furnished data (sensitivity, specificity, positive predictive power, negative predictive power, Phi) on each of the DSM-III-R passive-aggressive

PD criteria. Additional studies concerning the expanded scope of the negativistic PD criteria are under way but still incomplete.

A brief review of these data is in order, despite the Work Group's proposal that passive-aggressive PD and the majority of its criteria be replaced by the negativistic PD formulation. In general, the various studies show similar results, although the magnitude of validity numbers is appreciably higher in some projects than in others. These data show relatively weak discriminability among passive-aggressive PD criteria; they overlap appreciably with antisocial PD and somewhat less with narcissistic PD criterion scores. Strong criteria overlap may be seen in some studies with paranoid PD and, where it was included, with DSM-III-R sadistic PD.

Internal consistency statistics for passive-aggressive PD may be spuriously high. This may reflect the fact that many DSM-III-R passive-aggressive PD criteria say the same thing, or something close to the same thing; for example, "A1: procrastination" and "A3: work(s) deliberately slowly" may be indistinguishable. So too may "A2: sulky . . . when asked to do something he or she does not want to do," "A4: protests . . . that others make unreasonable demands," and "A7: resents useful suggestions from others."

5. *Can DSM-III-R passive-aggressive PD be expanded to comprise a more full-range negativistic PD, based on the historic clinical literature that suggests additional and diverse trait criteria?* A major issue raised by several Work Group consultants was related to whether passive-aggressive PD is a "true" PD, or whether it is merely a single trait, essentially a defense mechanism whose presence is based on a psychodynamic inference (Perry and Flannery 1982). Phrased differently, one may ask whether passive-aggressive PD should exist at all as a PD in DSM-IV. It has never achieved acceptance in Europe, was not included in ICD-9 (World Health Organization 1978), and it is not scheduled for inclusion in ICD-10 (World Health Organization 1990). Moreover, the scarcity of literature on the disorder may indicate a lack of both clinical and research interest; if so, should it be deleted from the list of Axis II disorders (Blashfield et al. 1990)?

On the other hand, is it possible that these problems arise from the manner in which the disorder has been formulated, both before and after DSM-III? Might there be a more valid and clinically useful diagnostic entity (more in line with the descriptions of Kraepelin, Abraham, Bleuler, Schneider, and Menninger) than that which World War II military psychiatrists fashioned in highly restrictive terms? If the Work Group were to enlarge the scope of this diagnostic entity's "criteria" to include a multiple domain set of character traits, would both the clinical usage and research literature grow?

Although the DSM-III-R list was improved over that of DSM-III, would it be further enhanced if a wider range of trait domains were tapped, such as several of the following, derived from a number of diverse sources (e.g., Cameron 1951;

Horney 1945; Kraepelin 1913; Millon 1981; Reich 1933; Schneider 1923; Shapiro 1965): frequently irritable and erratically moody; a tendency to report being easily frustrated and angry; discontented self-image, as expressed in feeling misunderstood and unappreciated by others; characteristically pessimistic, disgruntled, and disillusioned with life; interpersonal ambivalence, as seen in a struggle between acting dependently acquiescent and being assertively independent; the use of unpredictable and sulking behaviors to provoke discomfort in others; sullen malcontents and perennial complainers; anguished and discontented with themselves; but never satisfied with others either.

Dissatisfaction with the passive-aggressive designation itself has been raised in both the literature and in Work Group deliberations. In exploring a more broadened, "civilian," and neutral nomenclature for this disorder, a number of authors have suggested alternative designations. To quote from one review of these alternatives (Frances and Widiger 1987):

> 1. "Passive-aggressive personality disorder" emphasizes the ambivalent coexistence of dependence and oppositionalism; but it has the problems of etiological connotation and previous misuse in military settings.
> 2. "Oppositional personality disorder" provides continuity with the section on childhood disorders and is interpersonally descriptive, but has an excessively narrow connotation that captures only the interpersonal aspect of the syndrome.
> 3. "Negativistic personality disorder" is appealingly broad and clearly descriptive, and it captures both interpersonal and intrapsychic aspects of behavior, but is a new term without tradition. This term does suggest less about underlying dynamics than the term "passive-aggressive," and opens a broader scope for the introduction of new and appropriate criteria. (p. 284)

Recommendations

It was the Work Group's view that there were grounds for maintaining the key criteria from DSM-III-R. However, many of the criteria are highly specific and essentially redundant and should be collapsed into a few general trait descriptors. On the other hand, the current scope of the DSM-III-R criteria appears to be narrowly restricted to the label's origins in military settings. A decision was made to enlarge the scope of the criteria to encompass nondynamic behavioral, cognitive, and affective features that the historic clinical literature indicates often coexist in syndromal form with the "passive-aggressive" element. Two options were discussed. The first and more conservative stance would be to retain but refine the current list of criteria for the passive-aggressive PD personality construct. The second option, favored by the Work Group, is to introduce a new category to replace or supplement passive-aggressive PD (which would be dropped from DSM). This new PD would encompass a broader range of "oppositional" trait features in line with the clinical literature, would be termed *negativistic PD,* and would be placed in the appendix to permit clinicians and researchers to evaluate its utility and efficiency.

Passive-aggression would continue as one significant component of the disorder. However, the new designation would permit the introduction of new criteria of a more cognitive and affective nature, a set of clinical features that may coexist in syndromal form with the core passive-aggressive behaviors but agree better with the established pre–World War II literature.

The following criteria for negativistic PD were developed by the Work Group and its advisers and consultants:

1. Passively resists fulfilling routine social and occupational tasks (e.g., behaviorally procrastinates, is inefficient)
2. Complains of being victimized, misunderstood, and unappreciated by those with whom he or she lives and works
3. Sullen, irritable, and argumentative, especially in reaction to the wishes or expectations of others
4. Unreasonably criticizes and scorns authority
5. Communicates a pervasive mix of angry and pessimistic attitudes toward numerous and diverse events (e.g., cynically notes the potentially troublesome aspects of situations that are going well)
6. Expresses envy and resentment toward those apparently more fortunate
7. Claims to be luckless, ill-starred, and jinxed in life; personal discontent is more a matter of whining and grumbling than of feeling forlorn or despairing
8. Alternates between hostile assertions of personal autonomy and independence, and acting contrite and dependent

Such a reformulation might fit better with a designation such as negativistic PD, thereby providing a behaviorally less overt and indirectly expressed adult variant of the childhood/adolescent oppositional defiant disorder.

References

Abraham K: The influence of oral eroticism on character formation, in Selected Papers on Psychoanalysis. London, Hogarth, 1924, pp 127–161

American Psychiatric Association: Diagnostic and Statistical Manual: Mental Disorders. Washington, DC, American Psychiatric Association, 1952

American Psychiatric Association: Diagnostic and Statistical Manual of Mental Disorders, 2nd Edition. Washington, DC, American Psychiatric Association, 1968

American Psychiatric Association: Diagnostic and Statistical Manual of Mental Disorders, 3rd Edition. Washington, DC, American Psychiatric Association, 1980

American Psychiatric Association: Diagnostic and Statistical Manual of Mental Disorders, 3rd Edition, Revised. Washington, DC, American Psychiatric Association, 1987

Aschaffenburg G: Constitutional psychopathies, in Handbook of Medical Practice, Vol 4. Leipzig, Germany, Barth, 1922, pp 12–28

Blashfield R: Similarity matrix for personality disorders. Unpublished raw data, 1988

Blashfield R, Sprock J, Fuller A: Suggested guidelines for including/excluding categories in the DSM-IV. Compr Psychiatry 31:15–19, 1990

Bleuler E: Textbook of Psychiatry (English translation). New York, Macmillan, 1924

Cameron N: Personality Development and Psychopathology. Boston, MA, Houghton Mifflin, 1951

Dahl A: Some aspects of the DSM-III personality disorders illustrated by a consecutive sample of hospitalized patients. Acta Psychiatr Scand 73:61–66, 1986

First M, Spitzer R: Diagnostic efficiency statistics. Unpublished raw data, New York, New York State Psychiatric Institute, 1989

Frances A, Widiger T: A critical review of four DSM-III personality disorders, in Diagnosis and Classification in Psychiatry. Edited by Tischer G. New York, Cambridge University Press, 1987, pp 269–289

Freiman K, Widiger TA: Co-occurrence and diagnostic efficiency statistics. Unpublished raw data, Lexington, University of Kentucky, 1989

Hellpach W: Amphithymia. Zietschrift fuer die gesamte. Neurol Psychiatr 52:136–152, 1920

Horney K: Our Inner Conflicts. New York, Norton, 1945

Kernberg OF: Problems in the classification of personality disorders, in Severe Personality Disorders. New Haven, CT, Yale University Press, 1984, pp 77–94

Kiesler DJ: The 1982 Interpersonal Circle, in Contemporary Directions in Psychopathology. Edited by Millon T, Klerman G. New York, Guilford, 1986, pp 571–597

Kraepelin E: Psychiatre: Ein Lehrbach, 8th Edition. Leipzig, Germany, Barth, 1913

Livesley WJ, Reiffer LI, Sheldon AE, et al: Prototypicality ratings of DSM-III criteria for personality disorders. J Nerv Ment Dis 175:395–401, 1987

Menninger K: Character disorders, in The Psychodynamics of Abnormal Behavior. Edited by Brown JE. New York, McGraw-Hill, 1940, pp 384–403

Millon T: Disorders of Personality: DSM-III: Axis II. New York, Wiley, 1981

Millon T: Manual, MCMI-II. Minneapolis, MN, National Computer Systems, 1987

Millon T, Tringone R: Co-occurrence and diagnostic efficiency statistics. Unpublished raw data, Miami, FL, University of Miami, 1989

Morey L, Heumann K: Co-occurrence and diagnostic efficiency statistics. Unpublished raw data, Nashville, TN, Vanderbilt University, 1988

Perry JC, Flannery RB: Passive-aggressive personality disorder: treatment implications of a clinical typology. J Nerv Ment Dis 170:164–173, 1982

Pfohl B, Blum N: Internal consistency statistics for the DSM-III-R personality disorder criteria. Unpublished raw data, Iowa City, University of Iowa, 1990

Reich J: Diagnostic efficiency statistics for personality disorders. Unpublished raw data, Brockton, MA, Brockton VA Medical Center, 1988

Reich W: Charakteranalyse. Leipzig, Germany, Sexpol Verlag, 1933

Schneider K: Psychopathic Personalities. London, Cassell, 1923

Shapiro D: Neurotic Styles. New York, Basic Books, 1965

Skodol AE: Co-occurrence and diagnostic efficiency statistics. Unpublished raw data, New York, New York State Psychiatric Institute, 1989

Small IF, Small JG, Alig VB, et al: Passive-aggressive personality disorder: a search for a syndrome. Am J Psychiatry 126:973–981, 1970

Weissman MM: The epidemiology of personality disorder: a 1990 update. Paper presented at the Conference on the Personality Disorders, Williamsburg, VA, 1990

Whitman R, Trosman H, Koenig R: Clinical assessment of passive-aggressive personality. Arch Neurol Psychiatry 72:540–549, 1954

Widiger TA: DSM-IV reviews of the personality disorders: introduction to special series. Journal of Personality Disorders 5:136–148, 1991

World Health Organization: Mental Disorders: Glossary and Guide to Their Classification in Accordance With the Ninth Revision of the International Classification of Diseases. Geneva, World Health Organization, 1978

World Health Organization: ICD-10 Chapter V: Mental and Behavioral Disorders: Diagnostic Criteria for Research. Geneva, Switzerland, World Health Organization, 1990

Zanarini M, Frankenburg F, Chauncey D, et al: Co-occurrence and diagnostic efficiency statistics. Unpublished raw data, Boston, MA, McLean Hospital, 1989

Zimmerman M: Why are we rushing to publish DSM-IV? Arch Gen Psychiatry 45:1135–1138, 1988

Chapter 35

Sadistic Personality Disorder

Susan J. Fiester, M.D., and Martha Gay, M.D.

Statement and Significance of the Issues

During the process of developing DSM-III-R, sadistic personality disorder (SPD) was suggested for inclusion by several psychiatrists who felt there was a clinical need for a category to describe persons, usually seen in forensic settings, who demonstrated a long-standing maladaptive pattern of cruel, demeaning, and aggressive behavior toward others but whose personality disturbance did not fit any other DSM-III-R diagnosis. They saw this disorder as distinct from the other personality disorders, including antisocial personality disorder. As a result of discussions with the Advisory Committee on Personality Disorders, eight criteria were subsequently developed along with an exclusion criterion. These criteria were subsequently approved for inclusion in an appendix of the DSM-III-R titled "Proposed Diagnostic Categories Needing Further Study."

There was substantial controversy about including this diagnostic category in DSM-III-R (Spitzer et al. 1991). These controversies are outlined and discussed after a summary and critical review of data on prevalence, sex bias, comorbidity, differential diagnosis, clinical phenomenology, treatment, and course and prognosis relevant to resolving these controversies. The following critical questions are addressed in the review, as indicated previously in Fiester and Gay (1991):

1. Is SPD a discrete entity distinguishable from other existing personality disorder diagnoses, or is there significant overlap of SPD with other personality disorder categories?
2. Do the SPD diagnosis and criteria have good reliability?
3. Does the SPD diagnostic category have descriptive validity, and is it supported by external validators?
4. Is there sex bias in the SPD diagnostic criteria or in the application of the criteria?
5. Are there problems in applying the SPD criteria (i.e., is a high degree of inference required to determine presence or absence of criteria)?

6. Does the SPD diagnostic category have clinical utility?
7. Will the inclusion of SPD result in harmful consequences for any particular populations?

Methods

The literature review for SPD included published articles, chapters, or books on sadism or SPD. Other than for conceptual, theoretical, or historical purposes, all sources that did not involve empirical data were excluded (e.g., case studies). The studies were identified through a computer search of English language journal articles published from 1960 through 1990. The index terms used were *sadism, sadomasochism, sadistic personality,* and *sadistic personality disorder.* Information was solicited from researchers who had data sets with relevant data on SPD, including unpublished articles and reports. Input was also solicited from a wide range of advisers with varied theoretical, clinical, and research backgrounds.

Results

Prevalence/Clinical Utility

Several empirical studies have examined the prevalence of SPD. Gay (1989) reported on a sample of 235 adults accused of child abuse referred by the juvenile court system for psychiatric evaluation of fitness to parent, 12 of whom (5%) met criteria for a diagnosis of SPD. Freiman and Widiger (1989), in a study using the Personality Interview Questions—II (PIQ-II) (Widiger et al. 1989), found that 18% of a sample of 50 inpatients, primarily male, in a public psychiatric hospital were diagnosed as having SPD.

Millon and Tringone (1989), in a study using an outpatient sample from a wide variety of settings, found that 3% met criteria for SPD. Spitzer et al. (1991) found that approximately 2.5% of all cases evaluated by forensic psychiatrists over the past year met criteria for SPD. One recent study using the Personality Disorder Examination (Loranger 1988) found a high prevalence rate (33%) in a group of 21 sex offenders (pedophiles and rapists), most of whom were in prison (Berger 1991).

Thus, three of five studies found a relatively low prevalence of the disorder (2.5%–5%), whereas two other studies found much higher prevalence rates (18%–33%). Note that the highest prevalence was found in a very specialized forensic population where the disorder might be expected to be much more prevalent than in the general population.

Several factors may partially account for the low prevalence rates. In discussion with consultants and advisers, particularly in the forensic field, it was generally felt that it may at times be difficult to determine the presence of SPD criteria, because the person must admit to a wide variety of socially unacceptable behaviors such as cruel and aggressive behavior, lying, and frightening and intimidating others. In addition, the disorder may be relatively rare in general practice settings, because individuals with SPD do not often voluntarily seek treatment.

Regarding the utility of this diagnostic category, in the Spitzer et al. (1991) survey, only 19% of psychiatrists indicated that the diagnosis was not useful for any particular purpose. Respondents felt the diagnosis was useful for the following purposes: 75% for describing the individual's pattern of behavior, 65% for predicting the individual's likely future pattern of behavior, 61% for use in providing the court with information that will be relevant in sentencing, 55% for making treatment or management decisions, and 51% for evaluating a parent's fitness for custody. Only 11% noted that it would be useful as a psychiatric defense in mitigating responsibility for a crime. Thus, a majority of the respondents who had at some time evaluated individuals with the diagnosis of SPD believe that it has value in both clinical and forensic settings.

Phenomenological Studies

There are few descriptive data except for those from a study by Gay (1989) and from a survey by Spitzer et al. (1991). In the Gay study, 75% of the subjects with SPD had a history of physical abuse during childhood, 42% reported a history of significant emotional abuse, 16% had experienced early childhood sexual abuse, and 8% reported a history of significant neglect. There was also a very high frequency (25%) of loss of parental figure by death during childhood or adolescence or significant childhood losses (75%). Spitzer et al. also found high prevalence of childhood abuse and loss (90% emotional abuse, 76% physical abuse, 52% multiple losses, and 41% sexual abuse).

Gay (1989) found that subjects with SPD were surprisingly high functioning, with 66% having steady employment and few having legal problems. In addition, they tended to have intense, long-lasting attachments to their chosen partners, which were extremely difficult to break. Subjects with SPD also demonstrated considerable remorse and sadness about the separations and losses precipitated by their violence.

Abuse behaviors exhibited by the subjects in the Gay (1989) study ranged from verbally demeaning the other to threats of killing the victim to actual beating and killing. Abuse of the spouse in addition to the children was frequent (75%), as was abuse toward others outside the immediate family.

Gay (1989) also found that there was a very poor prognosis in most cases of

SPD, with no recurrence of the child abuse in only two cases (17%) when the child was returned to the home. In both these cases, the person was provided with in-house modeling of improved parenting skills. Unfortunately, these subjects were reluctant to acknowledge their problems and therefore reluctant to seek or receive any type of treatment unless it was remanded by the justice system. She felt that persons with SPD often saw their behaviors as egosyntonic and consistent with culturally accepted sexist patriarchal values.

Comorbidity

Several studies have examined the degree of overlap of SPD with other personality disorders. Freiman and Widiger (1989) found the highest overlap of SPD with narcissistic (56%), paranoid (44%), and antisocial (44%) personality disorders and a moderate amount of overlap with schizotypal, borderline, histrionic, and passive-aggressive personality disorders (33% in each case). Millon and Tringone (1989) used three different means of diagnosing personality disorders (clinical diagnosis, diagnostic checklist, and the Millon Clinical Multiaxial Inventory [MCMI]) and found the greatest overlap of SPD with antisocial (17%–30%), passive-aggressive (15%–60%), and narcissistic (8%–42%) personality disorders. A small degree of overlap was found with borderline and paranoid personality disorders. Interestingly, some overlap was also found with self-defeating personality disorder (2%–15%).

Spitzer et al. (1991) found that 37%–47% of cases of SPD were also diagnosed as having narcissistic personality disorder, and 67%–75% were diagnosed with antisocial personality disorder. Gay (1989) found only a small amount of overlap in her study, with 8% of subjects with SPD receiving an additional diagnosis of narcissistic personality disorder. Finally, Berger (1991) found SPD to be comorbid with avoidant (43%), borderline (29%), antisocial (24%), and paranoid (24%) personality disorders. He found no overlap with self-defeating personality disorder. In a survey study (Spitzer et al. 1991), 76% of the respondents thought it would be useful to note both SPD and antisocial personality disorder diagnoses primarily because SPD indicated specific features that were usually not present in antisocial personality disorder alone.

Blashfield and Breen (1989) supplied clinicians with case histories on computer and asked the clinicians to give DSM-III-R diagnoses for the cases. In this study, 73% of the clinicians attributed the SPD diagnosis to the SPD cases. The most frequent other personality disorder diagnoses given to these SPD cases were antisocial (11%) and paranoid (6%) personality disorders.

Regarding the overlap of SPD with Axis I disorders, Gay (1989) found that 16% met criteria for alcohol dependence. One-third had a prior history of mixed substance abuse, and 8% met criteria for current substance abuse. There were no other comorbid Axis I disorders present. Spitzer et al. (1991) found that 27% of cases with SPD also had comorbid major depressive disorder or dysthymia, and 61% had comorbid psychoactive substance abuse or dependence.

The high comorbidity of SPD with narcissistic and antisocial personality disorders, as well as several other personality disorders across a number of studies, raises the concern that SPD may not be a distinct entity. However, the simple presence of overlap or comorbidity does not necessarily imply that the disorder is not distinct from other personality disorders or that it is not a valid category.

Performance Characteristics

Three studies have examined the performance characteristics of the individual SPD criteria (Blashfield and Breen 1989; Freiman and Widiger 1989; Millon and Tringone 1989). Overall, the characteristic with the best phi (the correlation of the presence/absence of the criterion with the presence/absence of the disorder) is criterion 6. Criteria 3 and 7 had extremely low phi. There was a moderately high positive predictive power (PPP) for nearly all criteria and a high negative predictive power (NPP) for nearly all the criteria. Very high sensitivity was found for criteria 1, 4, 5, and 6. Fairly high sensitivity was found for nearly all criteria in both studies, except for criterion 3, which had very poor sensitivity.

Spitzer et al. (1991) examined the sensitivity (frequency/100) and specificity (100 − frequency in noncases/100) of each of the SPD criteria for the entire group. Sensitivities ranged from .65 to .94, with the highest sensitivity for criteria 1, 2, 4, and 6 and the lowest for 5. Specificities ranged from .93 to .99.

In summary, criteria 3 ("harsh discipline") and 7 ("restricts autonomy") appear to have the poorest face validity. Criterion 1 ("physical cruelty or violence") appears to perform quite well, as does criterion 4 ("amusement or pleasure in suffering"). Overall, the studies found consistently good performance for nearly all the criteria with remarkably high specificity and generally high sensitivity.

Reliability

There is only one study that examined test-retest or interrater reliability for SPD. Freiman and Widiger (1989) found a high (85%) interrater reliability for SPD using Master's level clinical psychologists for ratings.

External Validity

No studies to date have examined external validators such as biochemical variables, response to treatment, course of illness, or family history.

Problems in Applying the Criteria

No studies were located that examined difficulties in determining the presence or absence of particular SPD criteria. The criteria are clear and behaviorally based.

Several criteria require some degree of inference to determine their presence. For example, criterion 5 requires determining the motivation for lying, criterion 3 requires a judgment about what constitutes "unusually harsh" discipline, and criterion 4 requires a determination of the subjects' affective state in relation to the suffering of others (amusement or pleasure).

Sex Bias

Several studies examined differences in the prevalence of SPD in men and women. Gay (1989) found a 2:1 male-female ratio (67% male versus 33% females). Widiger and Freiman (1989) found that 100% of the cases of SPD in their study population (which was 70% male) were male. In Spitzer et al.'s (1991) survey, 98% of the cases of SPD were male. Thus, empirical data are consistent with the theoretical literature and clinical case reports that have suggested that sadistic behavior is much more common among men than among women.

Only one study (Sprock et al. 1990) examined issues related to differential assignment of the SPD diagnosis to males versus females. In this study, 49 undergraduate students, primarily female, who were not familiar with the DSM-III-R were presented with stimuli consisting of 142 DSM-III-R criteria for the 11 personality disorders plus self-defeating personality disorder and SPD. It is not clear whether the raters were asked to evaluate whether the personality characteristics described as primarily male represented a normal male or not. Exclusion criteria were not presented, nor was the central trait for each disorder listed.

The stimuli were presented in random order, and subjects were asked to sort the cards along a dimension of sex from features most characteristic of males to those most characteristic of females. SPD was seen as most typical of males, followed by antisocial and schizoid personality disorders. All criteria associated with SPD were rated in a direction consistent with their overall mean. Male and female raters did not differ in their mean ratings for the diagnosis or for individual symptoms.

The symptoms seen as most strongly associated with male or female stereotypes were examined, and an attempt was made to construct a prototypic male and prototypic female personality disorder. The result was a sadistic male who was cruel, angry, and aggressive, suggesting that SPD is strongly linked to stereotypical male behaviors. All of the symptoms from the male stereotype came from SPD except for one that came from borderline personality disorder. Because the masculine personality disorder prototype is close to the stereotypical role for males in society, this raises concern about the potential for labeling normal men as having personality disorder.

Other Controversies

Critics of the SPD category feel that it was created as a "companion" personality disorder category to justify the inclusion of self-defeating personality disorder by having a comparable sex-role stereotyped category that applied primarily to men rather than to women. It was suspected that this might neutralize criticism regarding self-defeating personality disorder. However, the stimulus for the development of the disorder arose primarily from the clinical observations by forensic psychiatrists who felt there was a gap in the diagnostic system that lacked a category to describe sadistic persons.

Another concern involves the potential use of SPD to mitigate responsibility for violent crime. There was a feeling that diminished responsibility or not-guilty by reasons of insanity defenses might be used in the defense of a spouse abuser or a person engaging in other violent behavior. In the Spitzer et al. (1991) survey, although 11% of the survey respondents felt that the diagnosis of SPD might be used as a psychiatric defense in mitigating responsibility for a crime, only 1% were familiar with instances in which it had been misused. Other forensic experts who responded to inquiries about the use of the SPD diagnosis as a defense strategy reported that this rarely occurs in their experience. However, this low frequency of use may simply reflect the fact that the diagnosis, not being an official personality disorder, has been infrequently used.

Of the respondents in the Spitzer et al. (1991) survey, 76% believed that, if SPD were to become an official personality diagnosis, it would have significant potential for being misused, either in forensic or clinical settings, for mitigating criminal responsibility in spouse or child abuse cases. As one eloquent respondent of the survey noted, "The medicalization of evil deeds becomes an avenue of excuses" (p. 877). However, concern about misuse of a diagnostic category within the judicial system should not necessarily lead to exclusion of that category from the diagnostic nomenclature if it is indeed a useful and valid category. Many diagnoses carry the potential for misuse in forensic settings; it is thus in part the responsibility of the judicial system to develop guidelines and procedures for appropriate use of psychiatric evaluation and testimony within its domain. As an example, Oregon has passed a statute that disallows a personality disorder as the basis for an insanity defense, thus limiting the potential abuse of personality disorder diagnoses in the legal arena.

Another concern involves the possible stigmatization of a patient labeled with SPD. One respondent of the survey (Spitzer et al. 1991) felt that patients labeled with an SPD diagnosis might be abused by correctional or police officers. Finally, labeling a person with an SPD in a treatment setting might beget a "blame the perpetrator" attitude, which could interfere with effective treatment.

Discussion

There are relatively few studies of SPD, with little systematic data collection. Unfortunately, the few studies that have been carried out have significant limitations, involving the use of small samples from highly selected populations and other methodological flaws. In a few cases, SPD has been included in the data sets from larger studies examining all the personality disorders. However, in most studies of this type, it is generally not included, in part because of its status as an "unofficial" personality disorder.

From the existing data, SPD appears to be relatively uncommon (2%–5%), although it may have a higher prevalence in special forensic populations. There is significant comorbidity with antisocial, narcissistic, and a number of other personality disorders, thus raising questions about the distinctiveness of the disorder. There is a high male-female ratio (approximately 5:1) for the diagnosis, and the disorder is highly associated with sex-role stereotyped masculine behavior.

Phenomenologically, there appears to be a very high prevalence of childhood physical, sexual, and emotional abuse and of parental death and other significant losses in the history of individuals with SPD. Whether this may be etiologically related to the disorder is not known at this time. There are no studies that lend external validation to the diagnostic category.

There is generally very high specificity for the criteria and excellent sensitivity. The criteria are behaviorally based, do not appear to be particularly ambiguous, and require little inference in determining their presence or absence.

Although many psychiatrists feel the category has utility, a large number are also concerned about potential misuse of this personality disorder category in forensic or clinical settings. However, there are few actual data on abuse or misuse of this diagnosis in clinical or legal settings.

Future Research

It is surprising that the inclusion of this category in the DSM-III-R appendix has led to little new research. Clearly, more research is needed to determine whether this is a useful and valid category of personality disorder. Some additional data on SPD will be collected as part of a multisite field trial of several antisocial personality disorder criteria sets proposed for DSM-IV. Data from this trial will be preliminary but might provide some additional information on the prevalence of SPD in a variety of settings (e.g., inpatient and outpatient psychiatric settings, correctional settings). Studies to determine the prevalence of SPD in other populations such as spouse abusers would also be informative.

A better understanding of the phenomenology of the disorder (e.g., childhood antecedents and subsequent intrapsychic dynamics) might allow for the development of effective interventions for persons with SPD who are willing and/or able to be engaged in treatment. To make an analogy, individuals with antisocial personality disorder constitute a group that was previously felt to be difficult to engage in treatment and to have a poor prognosis. However, recent research has resulted in the identification of a subgroup of patients who are able to form a therapeutic alliance and who actually benefit from psychotherapy (Woody et al. 1985). Treatment of subgroups of persons with SPD, such as the child abusers with SPD who were provided in-home modeling to help change their abusive behavior, could result in alleviation of distress and suffering in victims and might provide an approach toward addressing the widespread societal problem of domestic violence and abuse (Hamberger and Hastings 1988).

Recommendations

Regarding the fate of SPD, one of two alternatives may be appropriate. The current data do not support elevating this disorder to the status of an official DSM-IV personality disorder. The disorder could thus remain in the current appendix in the hope that its continued presence will stimulate future research that will help in deciding its ultimate fate. Alternatively, because the "scientific" basis for including SPD is weak given the poverty of research that has been carried out, the disorder could be dropped from the nomenclature and included in the *DSM-IV Sourcebook*.

References

Berger P: Unpublished raw data, 1991

Blashfield RK, Breen MJ: Face validity of the DSM-III-R personality disorders. Am J Psychiatry 146:1575–1579, 1989

Fiester SJ, Gay M: Sadistic personality disorder: a review of data and recommendations for DSM-IV. Journal of Personality Disorders 5:376–385, 1991

Freiman K, Widiger TA: Co-occurrence and diagnostic efficiency statistics. Unpublished raw data, Lexington, University of Kentucky, 1989

Gay M: Personality disorders among child abusers. Symposium on Psychiatric Diagnosis, Victimization and Women. Scientific Proceedings, American Psychiatric Association annual meeting, Washington, DC, 1989

Hamberger LK, Hastings J: Characteristics of male spouse abusers consistent with personality disorders. Hosp Community Psychiatry 39:763–770, 1988

Loranger AW: Personality Disorder Examination (PDE) Manual. Yonkers, NY, DV Communications, 1988

Millon T, Tringone R: Co-occurrence and diagnostic efficacy statistics. Unpublished raw data, Miami, FL, University of Miami, 1989

Spitzer RL, Fiester S, Gay M, et al: Results of a survey of forensic psychiatrists on the validity of the sadistic personality disorder diagnosis. Am J Psychiatry 148:875–879, 1991

Sprock J, Blashfield RK, Smith B: Gender weighting of DSM-III-R personality disorder criteria. Am J Psychiatry 147:586–590, 1990

Widiger TA, Frances AJ, Trull TJ: Personality disorders, in Clinical and Diagnostic Interviewing. Edited by Craig R. Northvale, NJ, Jason Aronson, 1989, pp 231–236

Woody GE, McLellan AT, Luborsky L, et al: Sociopathy and psychotherapy outcome. Arch Gen Psychiatry 42:1081–1086, 1985

Chapter 36

Self-Defeating Personality Disorder

Susan J. Fiester, M.D.

Statement and Significance of the Issues

Since it was first proposed as a diagnostic category, there has been ongoing controversy and heated debate about the inclusion of self-defeating personality disorder (SDPD) in DSM-III-R (American Psychiatric Association 1987), with much opposition to its inclusion (Caplan 1985, 1987; Kaplan 1983; Rosewater 1987; Walker 1987; Widiger and Frances 1989). Masochistic personality disorder (MPD) was first proposed as a category for DSM-III-R in 1983 based on a presumed clinical utility (Kass et al. 1989). After discussion at a 1984 meeting of the Advisory Committee on Personality Disorders of the Work Group to Revise DSM-III, a draft version consisting of nine criteria was developed and published in October 1985 (Work Group to Revise DSM-III 1986).

Concerns were subsequently raised by the American Psychiatric Association Committee on Women about potential problems with the MPD diagnosis (e.g., sex-bias, association with the psychoanalytic concept of masochism, issues regarding the potential misuse of the disorder in the context of victimization and abuse, and others that are discussed in depth in later sections of this chapter). As a result, the criteria were further revised, exclusion criteria were added (Work Group to Revise DSM-III 1986), and the name of the category was changed to "self-defeating personality disorder." A discussion by the Board of Trustees of the American Psychiatric Association at first approved SDPD for inclusion in the main body of DSM-III-R but later decided to place it in an appendix titled "Proposed Diagnostic Categories Needing Further Study."

The major issues and controversies surrounding this disorder are noted in the form of eight questions listed below. These questions are addressed in a summary and critical review of research data relevant to resolving the controversies.

1. How prevalent is SDPD?
2. Is SDPD a discrete entity distinguishable from existing personality disorder (PD) diagnoses, or is there significant overlap?
3. Do the SDPD diagnosis and criteria have good reliability and internal consistency?
4. Is SDPD a valid diagnostic category?
5. Are there problems in applying the criteria (e.g., a high degree of inference required to determine presence or absence of criteria)?
6. Is there sex bias in the diagnostic criteria or in the application of the criteria?
7. Has the inclusion of SDPD resulted in harmful consequences for women, and/or might it result in harmful consequences in the future?
8. Does SDPD overlap with mood disorders?

Methods

The literature review for SDPD covered published articles, chapters, and books on masochism and on masochistic or self-defeating PD. Other than for conceptual, theoretical, or historical purposes, all sources that did not involve empirical data (e.g., case studies) were excluded. Empirical studies were included if they used the criteria for the originally proposed MPD or the final revised criteria for SDPD. Studies using the earlier criteria were included because of the paucity of research on the disorder and the importance of reviewing all empirical data that were in any way relevant to determining the fate of SDPD.

The sources of data were identified through a computer search of English language journal articles published between 1960 and 1989. The index terms used were *masochism, self-defeating behavior,* and *masochistic or self-defeating personality disorder.* Information was solicited from researchers who had data sets with relevant data on SDPD, including unpublished articles and reports. Input was also solicited from a wide range of advisers with varied theoretical, clinical, and research backgrounds, including critics of the proposed diagnosis.

Results

Prevalence

Several studies have shown empirical support for SDPD by demonstrating high prevalence rates in samples of psychiatric patients. Because of space limitations, descriptions of the studies and their specific findings on prevalence are presented in detail in a review by Fiester (1991).

To summarize the findings, several studies found a surprisingly high prevalence (14%–22%) of SDPD (Kass 1987; Kass et al. 1986; Nurnberg et al. 1991; Reich 1987; Skodol et al. 1988; Spitzer et al. 1989), with two outlying studies showing very high rates of 37% and 42% (Skodol et al. 1988; Spitzer et al. 1989). A number of other studies found much lower prevalence rates (5%–8%) (Freiman and Widiger 1989; Millon and Tringone 1989; Pfohl 1990; Spitzer et al. 1989). One study (Reich 1987) found a prevalence rate of 5% in a sample of "normal" volunteers, which was not significantly different from the rate in the patient sample. Note that many of these studies suffer from serious methodological problems such as limited, nonrandom, and relatively homogeneous samples; use of only one scale (usually self-report) to diagnose PD; and other significant flaws described in further detail by Caplan (1985) and Fiester (1991). It remains to be seen whether the higher or lower prevalence rates will hold up in more methodologically sound studies of larger and more heterogeneous samples. Finally, simply identifying a prevalence rate does not necessarily lend credence to the existence or validity of the disorder.

Distinctiveness From Other Disorders/Comorbidity

Regarding whether a need for the SDPD category is perceived among clinicians, Spitzer et al. (1989) conducted a survey of 2,000 psychiatrists with a special interest in PDs. Half (620) of the respondents felt there was a need for SDPD in DSM-III-R. However, if there was a differential return rate, according to whether the psychiatrists felt the category was useful or not, this could have led to a significant bias in the data. There was no relationship between endorsement of the diagnosis and the psychiatrist's sex, type of clinical practice, or years of experience.

A number of studies have addressed the issue of whether MPD/SDPD is an entity distinct from the other PDs. Fuller (1986) used 10 case descriptions of patients with MPD, including prototypic and nonprototypic cases. Ten clinicians using the DSM-III (American Psychiatry Association 1980) PD criteria could not consistently assign any PD diagnosis to even the nonprototypic "masochism" case descriptions. However, another group of 10 clinicians who applied DSM-III-R criteria to the same case histories could reliably identify the prototypic masochism cases as MPD.

In a second study (Fuller and Blashfield 1989), 150 mental health professionals were asked to diagnose 15 case descriptions generated from the scientific literature which included prototypic and nonprototypic borderline, passive-aggressive, antisocial, dependent, and masochistic PDs using DSM-III categories. They did not assign other personality diagnoses with high rates of agreement to the prototypic masochistic cases when they were asked to use DSM-III Axis II diagnoses (MPD was not a possible diagnosis). For the three prototypic masochistic cases, the diagnoses most commonly given were "mixed" or "other" PD. Dependent was given most commonly (58%) for one nonprototypic case, and avoidant was given most commonly (36%) for the other nonprototypic case.

When clinicians were asked to assign DSM-III-R diagnoses to the cases, they most commonly assigned MPD to each of the prototypic cases (regardless of the sex of the case), whereas the nonprototypic cases most commonly received diagnoses of dependent, avoidant, or not-otherwise-specified PDs. The results did not support the idea that the masochistic cases described could be subsumed under the already existing DSM-III PD diagnoses. Finally, Blashfield and Breen (1989) supplied clinicians with case histories and asked them to make DSM-III-R diagnoses. In this study, 71% of the clinicians gave a diagnosis of SDPD when presented with a case containing the SDPD criteria. Rarely were SDPD cases assigned other PD diagnoses.

Examining comorbidity of the diagnosis, Spitzer et al. (1989) found that SDPD had considerable overlap with other PD categories, being the sole diagnosis in only 3.8% of cases. In 6% of the cases, it was comorbid with dependent, in 5% with borderline, and in 22% with both PDs. A principal-components factor analysis resulted in three factors that did not match the domains of the three PDs studied. Three self-defeating PD criteria were contained in the "borderline" factor, and four dependent PD criteria were contained in the "self-defeating" factor, further suggesting problems with the concept of SDPD as a separate construct.

Several other studies investigated the degree of overlap or comorbidity of MPD/SDPD with other PDs (Table 36–1). A study by Freiman and Widiger (1989) of 50 subjects, only 4 of whom were diagnosed as having SDPD, showed significant overlap of SDPD with other PDs, with the greatest overlap occurring with borderline, avoidant, antisocial, and dependent PDs. A study by Skodol et al. (1988), using the Personality Disorder Examination (PDE) (Loranger 1988) and the Structured Clinical Interview for DSM-III-R (SCID-II) (Spitzer et al. 1990), also found a significant overlap between SDPD and other PDs, with the greatest overlap occurring with borderline, avoidant, and dependent PDs. For the PDE alone, there was also high overlap with narcissistic and obsessive-compulsive PDs.

Millon and Tringone (1989) used three different methods of diagnosing PDs (clinical diagnosis, a diagnostic checklist, and the Millon Clinical Multiaxial Inventory [MCMI; Millon 1987]) and examined comorbidity among all the PDs. For all three methods of diagnosis, they found the highest overlap between SDPD and dependent, avoidant, and borderline PDs. There was also a high degree of overlap using the MCMI with passive-aggressive PD.

Reich (1987) used the Personality Diagnostic Questionnaire (PDQ), MCMI, and the Structured Interview for DSM-III Personality Disorder (SIDP) (Stangl et al. 1985) as diagnostic instruments and found greatest overlap (greater than 50%

Table 36–1. Comorbidity percentages

Study	N	PPD	SZPD	STPD	ASPD	BPD	HPD	NPD	AVPD	DPD	OCPD	PAPD	SAD
Frieman and Widiger 1989	4	50	50	50	75	100	25	25	100	75	0	25	0
Skodol et al. 1988													
PDE	20	30	0	40	20	90	30	50	55	65	55	10	0
SCID-II	36	43	9	23	11	86	29	26	57	51	23	17	—
Millon and Tringone 1989													
Clinical diagnosis[a]	27	0	0	0	0	19	7	0	19	41	4	7	4
Diagnostic checklist[b]	31	0	3	0	0	32	3	0	19	74	3	3	0
MCMI[c]	40	0	8	0	0	20	15	0	55	43	0	35	3
Reich 1987													
PDQ	17	12	12	65	12	71	35	0	53	76	59	6	—
MCMI	17	0	53	12	6	35	6	0	59	82	6	53	—
SIDP	15	0	0	20	7	53	53	7	33	73	27	0	—
Blashfield and Breen 1989	—	1	3	0	1	3	0	2	2	3	3	5	2
Spitzer et al. 1989[d]	—	—	—	—	—	5	—	—	6	6	—	—	—

Note. PPD = paranoid personality disorder. SZPD = schizoid personality disorder. STPD = schizotypal personality disorder. ASPD = antisocial personality disorder. BPD = borderline personality disorder. HPD = histrionic personality disorder. NPD = narcissistic personality disorder. AVPD = avoidant personality disorder. DPD = dependent personality disorder. OCPD = obsessive-compulsive personality disorder. PAPD = passive-aggressive personality disorder. SAD = sadistic personality disorder. PDE = Personality Disorder Examination. SCID-II = Structured Clinical Interview for DSM-III-R. PDQ = Personality Diagnostic Questionnaire. MCMI = Millon Clinical Multiaxial Inventory. SIDP = Structured Interview for DSM-III Personality Disorder.

[a]No cases received only diagnosis of self-defeating personality disorder (SDPD).

[b]13% of cases received only diagnosis of SDPD.

[c]5% of cases received only diagnosis of SDPD.

[d]3.8% of cases received only diagnosis of SDPD; 22% comorbid with both DPD and BPD.

on two of the three instruments) with dependent, avoidant, and borderline PDs. Nurnberg et al. (1991) found high (75%) overlap with avoidant and obsessive-compulsive PDs and somewhat lower overlap with dependent PD.

Reich's (1987) study is the only study that examined overlap of MPD or SDPD with Axis I disorders. He found that 15 of 17 MPD patients had Axis I disorders: 53% major depressive disorder, 7% minor depression, 7% schizoaffective-depressed, 7% panic disorder, 20% phobia, 13% obsessive-compulsive disorder, 13% generalized anxiety disorder, 13% alcohol abuse, and 7% drug abuse.

In summary, these studies present mixed data, some supporting the concept of SDPD as a distinct entity (Blashfield and Breen 1989; Fuller 1986; Fuller and Blashfield 1989) and others suggesting significant overlap with a number of other PDs (Freiman and Widiger 1989; Millon and Tringone 1989; Nurnberg 1991; Reich 1987; Skodol et al. 1988; Spitzer et al. 1989). Interestingly, the studies using case histories that were diagnosed by clinicians tended to suggest the distinctiveness of SDPD, whereas the studies using various instruments to diagnose actual subjects tended to show significant overlap, arguing against the distinctiveness of SDPD.

Over all studies and all instruments, the greatest comorbidity for MPD/SDPD was found with borderline, avoidant, and dependent PDs. Almost no overlap was found with sadistic PD and very little with antisocial, paranoid, schizoid, schizotypal, and narcissistic PDs. However, it should be noted that overlap or comorbidity does not necessarily imply that the disorder is not distinct from other PD categories or that it is not a valid category. Finally, the studies cited have numerous methodological problems that account for the somewhat contradictory results and may limit the conclusions that can be drawn from the data.

Reliability/Internal Consistency/Validity

Two studies examined the test-retest or interrater reliability for SDPD. Spitzer et al. (1989) in the SCID-II (Spitzer et al. 1990) reliability study found test-retest reliability for SDPD of only .33, one of the lowest for any of the PDs. Freiman and Widiger (1989) found an interrater reliability for SDPD of .49, again one of the lowest for any of the PDs.

There are few studies that address the question of the validity of SDPD, and most of these address only the descriptive validity. Three studies examined the internal consistency of the criteria for MPD/SDPD. Kass (1987) found only moderate correlations between each MPD criterion and the mean of the other eight masochistic criteria (mean, .35; range, .27–.40). His 1986 study (Kass et al. 1986) found slightly higher correlations (mean, .44; range, .24–.64). Correlation of each MPD criterion with the 13 nonmasochistic PD criteria ranged from .07 to .29. For six of the nine criteria, correlations with other masochistic criteria were significantly higher than correlations with the mean score for the presence or absence of the 13 nonmasochistic traits. Thus, Kass showed fairly good internal consistency for MPD criteria.

Spitzer et al. (1989) found moderate to high internal consistencies for each of the criteria sets (borderline, dependent, and self-defeating) with a Cronbach's alpha of .70 for SDPD. However, intercorrelations among the criteria sets, when corrected for attenuation due to measurement error, were also quite high indicating a relative lack of independence, particularly between dependent PD and self-defeating PD.

In a further survey (Spitzer et al. 1989), 222 psychiatrists provided information about two patients they knew well, one with SDPD and a "control" with any other DSM-III PD. Although each of the SDPD criteria was significantly more common in the SDPD patients, all eight SDPD criteria were relatively common in the control patients as well (present in 29%–51% of cases).

Very few data are available on the external validation of SDPD by clinical description, delineation from other disorders, biochemical parameters, response to treatment, course of illness, and family history (genetic factors). Reich (1989a) found that patients with SDPD did not differ from outpatients without SDPD on demographic factors such as sex, age, marital status, or education. Reich (1989b), however, did find a higher prevalence of SDPD in first-degree relatives of patients with SDPD, thus providing the only validity data to date that use family history. Pfohl (1990) reported a significantly greater frequency of childhood sexual abuse in persons with SDPD compared with those with other PDs (with the exception of borderline). There has been no research on course, response to treatment, outcome, or biological factors. Thus, there is no information to support the utility of this category in informing decisions regarding clinical management or choice of treatment or in predicting treatment outcome. However, adequate external validation studies have been carried out for only a few of the PDs.

Problems in Applying Criteria

One criticism frequently leveled at the PDs is that determining the presence or absence of some criteria involves a high degree of inference. A number of the SDPD criteria appear to require a high degree of inference to determine their presence or absence, for example, criterion 8, "engages in excessive self-sacrifice that is unsolicited by the intended recipients of the sacrifice." Different clinicians/researchers might have very different perceptions of thresholds for "excessive" self-sacrifice. In addition, in a society that tends to encourage self-sacrificing behavior on the part of women as one aspect of the stereotyped feminine role, it is not clear how one would determine what constitutes excessive self-sacrifice. Would the threshold for excessive self-sacrifice differ for men and women given that the normative behaviors for the male versus female sex roles differ? Likewise it might be difficult to determine whether the self-sacrifice was solicited or unsolicited by the intended recipient. Although self-sacrifice might not be explicitly encouraged, more subtle communication of such an expectation could be present.

A high degree of inference is also required to determine whether the person "rejects people who consistently treat him/her well." What constitutes "treated well" may differ by sex, social class, ethnic or cultural group, and/or race. Finally, for "chooses people and situations that lead to disappointment, failure, or mistreatment even when better options are clearly available," it is unclear how one would adequately judge whether "better options are clearly available." For example, a patient of low socioeconomic level who lives in an environment and culture of poverty, substance abuse, violence, and general deprivation might be involved with people or situations leading to disappointment, failure, or mistreatment. Given certain external conditions or limitations, it might be unclear whether other "better options" are in fact available and are realistic options for the person. Unfortunately, no studies have been carried out to determine whether the degree of inference required poses an actual problem in making the diagnosis of SDPD.

Sex Bias

The issue of sex bias is a complex one and is discussed in depth in several papers (Kaplan 1983; Kass et al. 1983; Williams and Spitzer 1983). Sprock et al. (1990) point out that apparent sex differences in the frequency of assigning a particular diagnosis can result from 1) inherent sex bias in the diagnostic criteria (i.e., bias within the criteria themselves that reflects sex-role stereotypes [societal prescriptions about which types of behavior are healthy versus pathological for males versus females]); 2) sex bias in the way clinicians apply the criteria; 3) real differences in the prevalence of the disorders in males and females as a reflection of different susceptibilities to the disorder based on psychological, biological, genetic, social, and/or environmental factors; or 4) any combination of these three factors. So whereas there are differing female-male ratios in the prevalence of a number of PDs other than SDPD (higher prevalence of histrionic, dependent, and borderline PDs in women; higher prevalence of antisocial, schizoid, passive-aggressive, and paranoid PDs in men), it is not clear why this is the case. Furthermore, the occurrence of a disorder in women may have different implications than the occurrence of the disorder in men.

Several studies have addressed the issue of differences in the frequencies of diagnosis of SDPD in men and women. In Kass et al. (1986), six of the eight patients diagnosed as having MPD were female (75%). The correlation of the mean of the 10 masochistic traits (absent versus present) with the sex of the patients (male versus female) was not statistically significant; however, the small samples in both studies (Kass 1987; Kass et al. 1986) limit the conclusions that can be drawn from the data. In Kass's 1987 study, there was a higher-than-expected female-male ratio for five of the nine MPD criteria. Interestingly, no association was found between social class and the presence of masochistic criteria, except for one criterion. Spitzer et al. (1989) found a 1.5:1 female-male ratio (42% versus 28%) for SDPD.

In another study reported in Spitzer et al. (1989), 62% of patients with SDPD versus 55% of patients with other PDs were female. In the study by Reich (1987), 58% of the subjects with MPD were women, which was not significantly different from the percentage of women in the overall patient population. Reich also examined sex differences in the prevalence of individual criteria and found a significantly higher prevalence in women of two criteria ("sacrifices own needs for the needs of others," and "taken advantage of and not complaining," which is no longer a criterion). However, over all criteria, there was no significant difference. Spitzer et al. (1989) regressed the diagnosis of SDPD on the eight diagnostic criteria using sex as a covariate. No item showed a significant interaction by sex. Finally, Nurnberg et al. (1991) found a prevalence of SDPD of 55% in women and 45% in men, not significantly different from the sex ratio of the overall sample.

Additional studies have examined potential bias in the assignment of the SDPD diagnosis using ratings of case histories rather than diagnosis of actual subjects. Fuller and Blashfield (1989) selected 15 case histories to present to clinicians for diagnosis of DSM-III-R PD. Five cases represented MPD, with three of these being prototypal cases. Three groups participated (150 psychiatrists, 150 psychologist clinicians, and 150 clinicians of various training). Reversing the sex of the cases did not affect the diagnoses for either the prototype or the nonprototype cases. When the investigators examined the impact of the sex of the clinician performing the ratings, no significant differences were found, except for one case in which the female clinicians were more likely to diagnose the case as MPD when the case was presented as a female, whereas male clinicians were more likely to use the MPD diagnosis when the case was written as a male. Thus, the authors concluded that the data did not support a hypothesis of sex bias.

In another study (Sprock et al. 1990), 49 undergraduate students who were unfamiliar with DSM-III-R were presented with 142 cards, each containing one of the criteria for the DSM-III-R PDs, including self-defeating and sadistic PDs, in random order. They were instructed to sort the cards along a dimension of sex from features most characteristic of males to those most characteristic of females. Dependent PD was seen as the most characteristically female, followed by histrionic and avoidant PDs. Sadistic PD was seen as most typical of males, followed by antisocial and schizoid PDs. SDPD fell near the mean. Males and females did not differ in their mean ratings for diagnoses or for individual symptoms. Although subjects did associate criteria used to define DSM-III-R PD with stereotyped sex roles, SDPD was viewed as equally applicable to males and females.

In summary, the available empirical data suggest that, overall, SDPD is diagnosed more frequently in women than in men and that a few individual SDPD criteria may occur more frequently in women than in men. Experimental studies have not found a sex bias in the application of the diagnosis to identical male versus female cases when diagnosed by either male or female clinicians. Furthermore, one prototype study (Sprock et al. 1990) found that the prototype PD for females was closest to the dependent PD and not the SPD. The answer to the question of whether there are real differences in the prevalence of SDPD in females versus males awaits further research.

Another concern regarding sex bias involves the potential diagnosis of SDPD in women who are merely exhibiting behaviors that conform to the societal expectations for the female sex role. Walker (1987) points out that some behaviors consistent with SDPD criteria might actually be adaptive (e.g., in terms of enhancing a woman's desirability for marriage and motherhood or enhancing the probability of survival in a violent encounter), thus leading to the possible characterization of normal women in traditional roles as having PDs. Although Sprock et al.'s (1990) research found the feminine PD prototype to be close to the stereotypical role of a normal female in society, this seems to be more of a concern for dependent PD than SDPD, because the feminine PD prototype was of a dependent female, not a self-defeating one. In addition, Reich (1987) found that only 5% of his "normal" sample received the diagnosis of SDPD. If there were a real potential for the diagnosis to be applied to women who are merely exhibiting behaviors that conform to the expected female sex role, then one would expect a far greater rate of SDPD in the general population. Finally, a body of psychological research suggests that various types of self-defeating behaviors are relatively common in the general population in both men and women (Bauermeister and Scher 1988; Berglas 1985; Curtis 1989).

Misapplications of SDPD Diagnosis: "Blame the Victim" and "Misuse in Abuse" Situations

Critics of SDPD have suggested that the inclusion of the SDPD diagnosis will have widespread negative effects in many arenas for women (Caplan 1985, 1987; Kaplan 1983; Rosewater 1987; Walker 1987; Widiger and Frances 1989). One concern is with the potential misapplication of the SDPD diagnosis in the forensic setting. For example, in cases in which women are prosecuted for harming their physically abusive spouses, SDPD might be used by the prosecution to "blame" the woman for remaining in the abusive relationship and turn attention away from the use of a legitimate psychiatric diagnosis in the defense (e.g., posttraumatic stress syndrome [battered woman syndrome]). Furthermore, there is concern that SDPD might lead to women being deprived of custody of their children in cases where "fitness" to parent is an issue. There is also concern regarding potential harmful effects in treatment settings where therapists might conclude that women are responsible for their predicaments ("blame the victim") and assume a negative therapeutic stance that could result in a negative outcome. Alternatively, SDPD may have utility in helping conceptualize specific treatment approaches for different subtypes of patients with SDPD (those who fear success, those who pursue victory through defeat, and those who desire secondary gain through sadomasochistic relationships).

No research or clinical reports were located that addressed the issue of actual harm that has occurred to women in clinical, forensic, or other settings as a result of the use of SDPD. In addition, no anecdotal information was obtained from the various consultants and forensic experts regarding specific instances of misuse or abuse of the disorder in forensic settings. There are reports in the literature that suggest the potential for misuse (Snell et al. 1964). A broader survey or another form of data collection might be helpful in determining if this is a realistic concern.

Another major concern involves the potential inappropriate application of the SDPD diagnosis to women in abusive situations. There is concern that the behaviors included as criteria in SDPD may be characteristic of women who are physically, sexually, and/or psychologically abused and that this could lead to misdiagnosis of a PD in persons who have a "chronic" posttraumatic disorder as a result of prior victimization. Critics of the SDPD feel that many self-defeating behaviors represent accommodation or response to various types of physical and/or psychological victimization and decrease in frequency or disappear if the abuse is eliminated (Walker 1987). In line with this, Frances (1980) notes that it is often difficult on cross-sectional evaluation to determine whether current behaviors represent enduring, lifelong patterns or whether they are primarily a function of the patient's current clinical state and/or role expectations.

To address this criticism, the DSM-III-R Personality Disorder Committee added an exclusion criterion that the diagnosis could not be made when the behaviors occurred exclusively in response to, or in anticipation of, being physically, sexually, or psychologically abused. However, as Walker (1987) notes, interviewers or clinicians frequently do not attempt to assess the history of or presence of current abuse. Even when they do inquire, abuse may be denied by the victim.

The problem is further complicated by the fact that some women may have suppressed knowledge of earlier abuse, and recall of the abuse experiences may occur only during treatment (Herman and Schatzow 1987). Herman and Schatzow (1987) found a relationship between the severity and duration of the abuse and the degree to which memory of the abuse had been suppressed, suggesting that those women most severely affected by the impact of previous abuse are those least likely to recall and/or report the abuse during a diagnostic assessment. Thus, it may be difficult to determine whether self-defeating behaviors have occurred only in the context of an abusive situation.

Relation to Affective Disorder Spectrum

Another controversy centers around the proposition that SDPD is really a disorder on the spectrum of affective disorders, not a PD. There is a clinical and theoretical tradition supporting the concept of a depressive-masochistic personality. This is perhaps best described by Kernberg (1984), who also briefly reviews the origin of the concept in the writings of early psychoanalysts such as Kraepelin, Schneider, Fenichel, and others. Akiskal (1983) also proposes a "character spectrum" disorder as a chronic depressive subtype based on his research on dysthymic disorder. Furthermore, empirically, many of the criteria for SDPD are present in patients who have depression (e.g., guilty responses to positive events, rejecting opportunities for pleasure, failing to accomplish tasks, rejecting others who treat the person well). Thus, in some cases, it may be difficult to tease apart whether the self-defeating behaviors reflect maladaptive personality traits or are a manifestation of current or more long-standing depressive illness of either a characterological or syndromal nature.

Examining the SDPD criteria, there is some overlap with traits described in the clinical literature as being characteristic of the "depressive personality." However, there is little overlap with the criteria currently being proposed for a depressive PD (see Phillips et al., Chapter 33, this volume). Of interest in relation to this issue are data from the Reich (1987) study, which showed a high level of comorbidity between Axis I diagnoses and MPD (53% of patients with MPD had major depression and 7% minor depression) before the exclusion criterion for depression was added.

In summary, it appears that there is confusion regarding the nature of the relationship between SDPD and the affective disorders. However, it is not clear that SDPD could be satisfactorily subsumed under a depressive personality category, at least as this category is currently being conceived.

Discussion and Recommendations

Since the inclusion of SDPD in the appendix of DSM-III-R, a number of studies have been carried out to investigate its prevalence, internal consistency, clinical utility, validity, overlap with other PDs, and potential sex bias in the criteria and their clinical application. Although there has been progress in the attempt to elucidate the nature of SDPD, the small body of research that has been carried out over the past several years has significant limitations, as previously noted. Data from existing studies show a relatively high prevalence, a slightly higher female-male ratio, good internal consistency, significant overlap with several other PDs (particularly borderline, dependent, and avoidant PDs), some possible inherent sex bias in the criteria, and an apparent lack of sex bias in the application of the criteria by clinicians. Few data are available to address the issue of external validity (e.g., associated features, impairment, complications, predisposing factors, family history, and biological markers), except for one study showing increased prevalence of SDPD in relatives of SDPD probands and another showing a high frequency of childhood sexual abuse in persons with SDPD. There are no formal data on the potential harmful effects of use of the disorder in clinical, forensic, or other settings. There is little or no information about whether the diagnosis implies something about the course of illness or prognosis or helps inform decisions regarding treatment. In addition, significant concerns exist about the potential negative consequences of including the disorder in DSM-IV.

In summary, although there is a historical tradition and some support for the clinical utility of SDPD, data are lacking to support its inclusion in the DSM-IV PD section. It was the consensus of the Work Group that it should not receive formal recognition in DSM-IV. In the absence of methodologically sound data, the Work Group recommended that SDPD either continue to be included in an appendix of disorders requiring further study, with the intention that future research will help resolve the question of its ultimate fate, or be deleted entirely from the manual. The Work Group proposed that, if it is decided to continue to include SDPD in the appendix to DSM-IV, the following changes in the criteria be made:

1. Increase emphasis on the pervasiveness of the disorder by specifying that the behavior be present in more than one area of functioning

2. Omit DSM-III-R criterion 8 ("engages in excessive self-sacrifice that is unsolicited by the intended recipients of the sacrifice") because of the potential for gender, cultural, and religious bias inherent in the judgment of what constitutes "excessive" self-sacrifice

3. Add an additional criterion describing cognitive aspects of the disorder: "perceives himself or herself as undeserving of being treated well"

References

Akiskal H: Dysthymic disorder: psychopathology of proposed chronic depressive subtypes. Am J Psychiatry 140:11–20, 1983

American Psychiatric Association: Diagnostic and Statistical Manual of Mental Disorders, 3rd Edition. Washington, DC, American Psychiatric Association, 1980

American Psychiatric Association: Diagnostic and Statistical Manual of Mental Disorders, 3rd Edition, Revised. Washington, DC, American Psychiatric Association, 1987

Bauermeister RF, Scher SJ: Self-defeating behavior patterns among normal individuals: review and analysis of common self-destructive tendencies. Psychol Bull 104:3–22, 1988

Berglas S: Self-handicapping and self-handicappers: a cognitive/attributional model of interpersonal self-protective behavior. Perspectives in Personality 1:235– 270, 1985

Blashfield RK, Breen MJ: Face validity of the DSM-III-R personality disorders. Am J Psychiatry 146:1575–1579, 1989

Caplan PJ: The Myth of Women's Masochism. New York, Dutton, 1985

Caplan PJ: The psychiatric association's failure to meet its own standards: the dangers of the self-defeating personality disorders category. Journal of Personality Disorders 1:178–182, 1987

Curtis R (ed): Self-Defeating Behaviors: Experimental Research, Clinical Impression, and Practical Implications. New York, Plenum, 1989

Fiester SJ: Self-defeating personality disorder: a review of data and recommendations for DSM-IV. Journal of Personality Disorders 5:194–209, 1991

Frances A: The DSM-III personality disorder section: a commentary. Am J Psychiatry 137:1050–1054, 1980

Freiman K, Widiger TA: Co-occurrence and diagnostic efficiency statistics. Unpublished raw data, Lexington, University of Kentucky, 1989

Fuller AK: Masochistic personality disorder: a diagnosis under consideration. Jefferson Journal of Psychiatry 4:7–21, 1986

Fuller AK, Blashfield RK: Masochistic personality disorder: a prototype analysis of diagnosis and sex bias. J Nerv Ment Dis 177:168–172, 1989

Herman JL, Schatzow E: Recovery and verification of memories of childhood sexual trauma. Psychoanalytic Psychology 4:1–14, 1987

Kaplan M: A woman's view of DSM-III. Am Psychol 38:786–792, 1983

Kass F: Self-defeating personality disorder: an empirical study. Journal of Personality Disorders 1:168–173, 1987

Kass F, Spitzer RL, Williams JBW: An empirical study of the issue of sex bias in the diagnostic criteria of DSM-III Axis II personality disorders. Am Psychol 38:799–801, 1983

Kass F, Mackinnon RA, Spitzer RL: Masochistic personality: an empirical study. Am J Psychiatry 143:216–218, 1986

Kass F, Spitzer RL, Williams JBW, et al: Self-defeating personality disorder and DSM-III-R: development of the diagnostic criteria. Am Psychol 146:1022–1026, 1989

Kernberg O: Severe Personality Disorder. New Haven, Yale University Press, 1984

Loranger AW: Personality Disorder Examination (PDE) Manual. Yonkers, NY, DV Communications, 1988

Millon T: Manual for the MCMI-II, 2nd Edition. Minneapolis, MN, National Computer Systems, 1987

Millon T, Tringone R: Co-occurrence and diagnostic efficacy statistics. Unpublished raw data, Miami, FL, University of Miami, 1989

Nurnberg GH, Siegel O, Prince R, et al: Axis II comorbidity of self-defeating personality disorder. Am J Psychiatry 148:1371–1377, 1991

Pfohl B: Discussion. Paper presented at the NIMH Conference on Personality Disorders, Williamsburg, VA, 1990

Reich J: Prevalence of DSM-III-R self-defeating (masochistic) personality disorder in normal and outpatient populations. J Nerv Ment Dis 175:52–54, 1987

Reich J: Criteria validity for DSM-III-R self-defeating personality disorder. Psychiatry Res 30:145–153, 1989a

Reich J: Familiality of self-defeating personality disorder. J Nerv Ment Dis 178:597–598, 1989b

Rosewater LB: A critical analysis of the proposed self-defeating personality disorder. Journal of Personality Disorders 1:190–195, 1987

Skodol A, Rosnick L, Kellman D, et al: Validating structured DSM-III-R personality disorder assessment with longitudinal data. Am J Psychiatry 145:1297–1299, 1988

Snell J, Rosenwald R, Robey A: The wife beater's wife. Arch Gen Psychiatry 11:107–112, 1964

Spitzer RL, Williams JBW, Kass F, et al: National field trial of the diagnostic criteria for self-defeating personality disorders. Am J Psychiatry 146:1561–1567, 1989

Spitzer RL, Williams JBW, Gibbon M, et al: User's Guide for the Structured Clinical Interview for DSM-III-R (SCID). Washington, DC, American Psychiatric Press, 1990

Sprock J, Blashfield RK, Smith B: Gender weighting of DSM-III-R personality disorder criteria. Am J Psychiatry 147:586–590, 1990

Stangl D, Pfohl B, Zimmerman M, et al: A structured interview for DSM-III personality disorder. Arch Gen Psychiatry 42:591–596, 1985

Walker L: Inadequacies of the masochistic personality disorder diagnosis for women. Journal of Personality Disorders 1:183–189, 1987

Widiger TA, Frances AJ: Controversies concerning the self-defeating personality disorder, in Self-Defeating Behaviors: Experimental Research, Clinical Impressions, and Practical Implications. Edited by Curtis R. New York, Plenum, 1989, pp 289–309

Williams JBW, Spitzer RL: The issue of sex bias in DSM-III. Am Psychol 38:793–798, 1983

Work Group to Revise DSM-III: DSM-III-R in Development (second draft). Washington, DC, American Psychiatric Association, August 1986

Chapter 37

Enduring Personality Change After Catastrophic Experience

M. Tracie Shea, Ph.D.

Introduction

ICD-10 has proposed a diagnostic category called "enduring personality change after catastrophic experience," with criteria including hostility and distrustfulness, social withdrawal, emptiness and/or hopelessness, an enduring feeling of being on edge or threatened, and severe estrangement (World Health Organization 1990) (Table 37–1). The purpose of this chapter is to provide a review of the literature to determine whether there is empirical support for inclusion of this diagnostic category in DSM-IV.

Statement of the Issues

1. Is there evidence of personality pathology after catastrophic events?
2. Is personality pathology after catastrophic experience characterized by specific types or patterns of maladaptive traits?
3. Does personality pathology occur in the absence of preexisting personality disorder or disturbance (i.e., is there evidence of personality change after catastrophic events)?
4. What is the relation of the proposed category to posttraumatic stress disorder (PTSD)?

I thank Alan Carver and Ali Kazim for their help in the preparation of this chapter.

Table 37–1.   Proposed diagnostic criteria for enduring personality change after catastrophic experience (ICD-10)

F62.0   Enduring personality change after catastrophic experience

A.   Evidence, (from the personal history or from key informants), of a definite and persistent change in a person's pattern of perceiving, relating to and thinking about the environment and one self, following exposure to catastrophic stress (i.e., concentration camp experience; torture; disaster; prolonged exposure to life-threatening situations).

B.   The personality change should be significant and represent inflexible and maladaptive features as indicated by the presence of **at least two of the following:**

   (1)   A permanent hostile or distrustful attitude toward the world in a person who previously was not showing any such traits

   (2)   Social withdrawal (avoidance of contacts with persons other than a few close relatives with whom he/she lives) which is not due to another current mental disorder like a mood disorder

   (3)   A constant feeling of emptiness and/or hopelessness, not limited to a discrete episode of mood disorder, and which was not present before the catastrophic stress experience; this may be associated with an increased dependency on others; inability to express negative or aggressive feelings; and prolonged depressive mood without any evidence of depressive disorder before the catastrophic stress exposure

   (4)   An enduring feeling of "being on edge" or being threatened without any external cause, as evidenced by an increased vigilance and irritability in a person who previously showed no such traits or hyper-alertness. This chronic state of inner tension and feeling threatened may be associated with a tendency to excessive drinking or use of drugs

   (5)   A permanent feeling of being changed or being different from others (estrangement). This feeling may be associated with an experience of emotional numbness.

C.   The change should cause either significant impairment in social or occupational functioning, or subjective distress to both the person and his family.

D.   The personality change should have developed after the catastrophic experience and there should be no history of a pre-existing adult personality disorder or trait accentuation, or personality or developmental disorders during childhood or adolescence, that could explain the current personality traits.

E.   The personality change must have been present **FOR AT LEAST THREE YEARS.** It is not related to episodes of other mental disorder, (except post-traumatic stress disorder) and cannot be explained by gross brain damage or disease.

F.   The personality change meeting the above criteria is often preceded by a post-traumatic stress disorder (F43.1). The symptoms of the two conditions can overlap and the personality change may be a chronic outcome of a post-traumatic stress disorder. However, an enduring personality change should not be assumed in such cases unless, in addition to at least two years of post-traumatic stress disorder there has been a further period of no less than two years during which the above criteria have been met.

Source.   World Health Organization 1990, pp. 106–107.

Significance of the Issues

Initially, stress disorders were conceptualized as short-term disturbances, with recovery to normal functioning over time. If the disturbance persisted, it was often attributed to preexisting character pathology. The first DSM (American Psychiatric Association 1952), for example, included a diagnosis called "gross stress reaction," believed to be characterized by quick recovery unless maintained by preexisting personality traits. The introduction of the diagnosis of PTSD in DSM-III (American Psychiatric Association 1980) among the anxiety disorders represented an important change in the conceptualization of stress reactions. The underlying assumption of this more recent formulation is that "normal" individuals may experience serious consequences after exposure to trauma, and such consequences may be long lasting.

The DSM-III-R (American Psychiatric Association 1987) criteria of the PTSD diagnosis include reexperiencing of the traumatic event, avoidance of stimuli associated with the trauma or numbing of general responsiveness, and persistent symptoms of arousal. As is described below, however, some studies have additionally emphasized long-term consequences of trauma on personality functioning. Permanent alteration in personality structure and functioning as a consequence of trauma is not currently diagnosable under any specific diagnostic category in DSM-III-R. The question here is whether and how such personality change might be covered in DSM-IV.

Methods

The boundaries of what might be considered "personality" versus "symptoms" overlap, and many studies report a mixture of both. The approach taken here was to be comprehensive and include studies that reported data or observations of personality-related features, even if the focus of the study was on psychiatric "symptoms" (usually of PTSD). Although the ICD-10 personality change diagnosis emphasizes "catastrophic" stress, this review does not attempt to define the boundaries of the severity of the traumatic experience and includes studies of traumatic events ranging in severity and duration. Finally, because the focus of this review is on personality change after catastrophic experience, the emphasis is on the effects of trauma in adults, and the emerging literature on the consequences of childhood trauma (i.e., physical and sexual abuse) on adult personality (e.g., Herman and van der Kolk 1987) is not included.

The literature reviewed here includes published articles, chapters, and books on consequences of traumatic stress. Whereas empirical studies are emphasized, relevant conceptual and theoretical articles are cited. Clinical case reports are not covered, although descriptive clinical reports based on large numbers of observations are included. Relevant studies were identified through a computer search (Medline, *Index Medicus*) of English language journal articles, using *trauma, catastrophic experience, stress,* and *personality* as index terms, and from bibliographies in published journal articles. Information was also sought from researchers working in the area of posttraumatic stress.

Results

A brief summary of the research is presented here. The literature covered is grouped in terms of three categories of trauma: 1) prolonged torture or victimization (primarily concentration camp and prisoner of war survivors), 2) combat, and 3) other traumatic events (usually natural or human-made disasters such as floods and fires).

Prolonged Torture/Victimization

The psychological aftereffects of the extreme form of traumatic stress induced by prolonged captivity, particularly of concentration camp survivors, and also prisoners of war, have been described in numerous clinical and empirical papers (e.g., Eitinger 1961). Highlights of the literature on prolonged torture and victimization, as it addresses personality change, are presented here.

In his review of the "survivor syndrome," Koranyi (1969) emphasized the characteristic clinical profile emerging from extensive studies of victims of the Nazi persecutions, as well as of survivors from other incidents of prolonged external stress, such as victims of Hiroshima. Based on these studies, and on his own observations of more than 1,000 cases, he concluded that extreme prolonged external stress is capable of producing a state of irreversible personality change (the survivor syndrome). Typical features include chronic depression, chronic anxiety, insomnia, nightmares, social withdrawal, reduced libido, severe apathy, irritability, temper outbursts, survivor guilt, rumination, and brooding. Koranyi also concluded that these features arise in the absence of a preexisting pathology, and that the presence of preexisting personality problems occurs among the ill survivors with the same frequency as in the general population. If preexisting problems did exist, they became obliterated or "buried under the uniform sameness of the syndrome" (p. 117).

Based on 149 randomly selected case records of concentration camp survivors, Krystal and Niederland (1968) described a postcaptivity personality emphasizing alterations of identity (i.e., persistent feelings of being "different from others and/or from one's previous self," feelings of "otherness," i.e., being of a different species).

Other features include depression, helplessness, disturbances of affect, masochism, and paranoia. They reported that, in the majority of cases (based on retrospective prepersecution histories), familial emotional disturbance and personal predisposition were ruled out.

Herman (1990) has also reviewed manifestations of prolonged, repeated trauma including childhood physical and sexual abuse and adult victimization. She cites three broad areas of disturbance that transcend simple PTSD: 1) symptomatic disturbances, which are more complex, diffuse, and tenacious; 2) characterological disturbances or personality changes, including deformations of relatedness and identity; and 3) vulnerability to repeated harm. The characterological changes include pathological changes in relationships, constriction in capacities for active engagement with the world, passivity, helplessness, and oscillations in relationships between intense attachment and terrified withdrawal. Also, pathological changes in identity are reported to occur, including loss or fragmentation of sense of self.

A few studies have used some type of formal assessment of survivors of concentration camps, and prisoners of war. Ursano et al.'s (1981) study is one of the rare studies that had pretrauma evaluations available, although only for a very small sample. Six Vietnam prisoners of war, all with extensive psychiatric/psychological evaluations before capture, were evaluated annually for 5 years after an average of 6 years in captivity characterized by extreme maltreatment, torture, and deprivation. An important conclusion from this study was that the presence of pretrauma psychiatric or personality disturbance was not necessary for the development of disturbances after the trauma, including character rigidity and decreased interpersonal relatedness.

Sutker et al. (1991) compared 22 Korean prisoners of war with 22 combat veterans 35 years after the trauma of captivity. Greater problems in adjustment and functioning were found in the prisoners of war, who were characterized by symptoms of suspiciousness, apprehension, confusion, isolation and detachment from others, guilt, and hostility. Clinical depression, somatic preoccupations, negative ruminations, and self-devaluation were also present.

Leon et al. (1981) assessed psychological adjustment in a group of 52 survivors of concentration camps and other survivors of World War II 30–40 years following captivity. They found, in contrast to other studies, that adjustment was within normal range. They reported little difference in adjustment between the survivors and 29 control subjects matched for age and cultural background. The few differences that did emerge suggested a tendency to act quickly, more wariness, and more restlessness among the male survivors and more suspiciousness among the female survivors compared with the control subjects. Dor-Shav (1978) also compared concentration camp survivors with control subjects matched for age and background, using standardized assessments. Survivors were found to manifest impoverishment and constriction of personality and appeared to be less accessible, less connected, and more labile. However, there were no differences between the groups on most of the variables assessed, and differences that did appear were not striking in magnitude.

Combat-Related Trauma

Although World War II was followed by studies and reports on effects of combat (commonly referred to as war neurosis), the Vietnam War has stimulated the largest literature on war trauma, particularly with regard to long-term effects of combat. This more recent literature is characterized by more formal assessments of symptoms and functioning and has also focused on the question of the relative contributions of preexisting psychopathology versus combat trauma to the development of PTSD and other symptoms and difficulties.

Studies of Axis II personality disorders in samples of Vietnam combat veterans, using self-report measures (Lindy et al. 1984; Sherwood 1990) or chart diagnoses (Faustman and White 1989), have reported particularly high rates of paranoid, schizoid, schizotypal, avoidant, antisocial, and borderline personality disorders. Other studies focusing specifically on antisocial personality disorder in treatment-seeking Vietnam veterans have reported rates ranging from 12% to 64% (Escobar et al. 1983; Sierles et al. 1986). Rates of impulsive violence have been reported for 42% to 56% of Vietnam veteran patient samples (Boman 1986; Yager 1976).

A few studies have investigated the relation of adult antisocial behavior in Vietnam veterans to preexisting personality (i.e., childhood antisocial behavior), as well as to combat, in an attempt to determine the relative influences of each. Two studies (Barrett et al. 1989; Resnick et al. 1989) have reported that both childhood behavior and exposure to combat show an independent relationship with adult antisocial behavior (Barrett et al. 1989; Resnick et al. 1989). However, Yager (1976) reported that adults who were violent after the Vietnam War were more likely to have a history of fighting in childhood and participating in violence in Vietnam, and Boman (1986) reported an absence of differences in post–Vietnam War violence among veterans with and without combat experience. In a separate review of this topic, Boman (1987) concluded that rates of drug addiction, alcoholism, violence, criminal convictions, and suicide are no different from those manifested by young men from similar socioeconomic backgrounds who have not been in military service.

Based on a large epidemiological sample, Helzer et al. (1987) reported that behavioral problems before the age of 15 years predicted 1) adult exposure to physical attack (i.e., being beaten or mugged) in the general population and to combat among Vietnam veterans and 2) the development of PTSD among those so exposed. Thus, those with childhood behavior problems were not only at higher risk for problems after combat but were also more likely to end up in combat.

In contrast to these findings are those from other studies showing a positive association between behavior difficulties and combat exposure, apparently not accounted for by preservice characteristics (Penk et al. 1981; Yager et al. 1984). Behavioral difficulties in the latter studies, however, did not include violence.

Finally, findings from the National Vietnam Veterans Readjustment Study (Kulka et al. 1988), which compared large and representative samples of Vietnam theater veterans, Vietnam-era veterans, and a matched sample of nonveterans, indicated that veterans exposed to high levels of war stress had higher rates of problems, including dissatisfaction with life, isolation, violent acts, and hostility. They also had higher rates of mental disorders.

Other Traumatic Events

There have been a number of studies on the effects of other kinds of traumatic events, including natural and man-made disasters. Most of these studies, however, focus exclusively on PTSD or other stress-related symptoms and do not report on personality variables (e.g., Green et al. 1985a, 1985b; McFarlane 1988a, 1988b, 1988c). An exception is a study reporting character change in survivors of the Buffalo Creek Disaster, a tidal wave of black mud resulting from the collapse of a dam, killing 125 people and leaving 4,000 homeless (Titchener and Kapp 1976). Disabling symptoms and changes in character structure, including interpersonal relationships and attitudes toward the self, were present in the majority of the 654 survivors 2 years after the event. Listlessness, apathy, pessimism, emptiness, hopelessness, isolation, and feelings of alienation were common features.

Leopold and Dillon (1963) found severe long-term reactions in the majority of 34 survivors of a maritime tanker explosion up to 4 years after the event. Common features included restlessness, depression, phobic reactions, feelings of isolation, paranoia, hostility, distrust, sleep disturbances, and gastrointestinal symptoms. The authors concluded that the nature of the accident itself was a more significant determinant of posttraumatic psychological illness than the preaccident personality and that, if untreated, such illness tends to worsen with time.

Discussion

There are a number of methodological limitations that must be considered in interpreting the research in this area. First is the use of retrospective assessment of pretrauma personality, which occurs for obvious reasons. Second, most of the studies cited were not designed to study personality change, instead the focus was usually on symptoms of traumatic stress. Consequently, there is little consistency among studies in the personality variables assessed or in the measures used. Third, many of the studies were based on treatment-seeking samples, which could select for personality dysfunction. Despite these limitations, it is possible to derive patterns from the available studies and on this basis to propose tentative conclusions. I now return to the originally posed questions:

1. *Is there evidence of personality pathology after catastrophic events?* There is consistent evidence of personality pathology after catastrophic events, in the form of numerous clinical descriptions and in studies using more standardized assessment methods.

2. *Is personality pathology after catastrophic experience characterized by specific types of maladaptive traits?* Despite the absence of assessment for a consistent domain of personality functioning/traits in different studies, certain patterns emerge across the diverse studies. Common features described include "isolation, withdrawal, and feelings of alienation; pervasive apathy, emptiness, and hopelessness; identity disturbance; problems with management of hostility and aggression; and distrust and suspiciousness." The findings reported in studies that assessed personality disorders converge with this pattern. The most frequent Axis II disorders reported include schizoid, schizotypal, and avoidant (reflecting the isolation and withdrawal), paranoid (reflecting the distrust and suspiciousness), and borderline and antisocial (reflecting the problems with hostility and aggression).

3. *Does personality pathology occur in the absence of preexisting personality disorder or disturbance (i.e., is there evidence of personality change after catastrophic events?* Different hypotheses can be posed to explain the findings of personality pathology after traumatic events. Personality pathology may precede the trauma and simply be exacerbated by the traumatic experience, function as a selector of those who end up in traumatic situations (e.g., combat), and/or develop as a consequence of the traumatic event. The last relationship is emphasized by the ICD-10 proposal.

It is important to distinguish between the concepts of preexisting personality disorder (or accentuated traits) and preexisting vulnerability. Recent conceptualizations of the etiology of PTSD emphasize an interaction of multiple factors including the stressor and the characteristics of the individual (e.g., Green et al. 1985a, 1985b). Although this model emphasizes the nature and intensity of the stressor as the primary etiological factor, the characteristics of the individual (e.g., the individual's coping style or the personal meaning of the event) will influence how the event is processed. Thus, a person with preexisting problems or a traumatic childhood might be more vulnerable to the effects of the stress (Green et al. 1985a, 1985b). However, such vulnerability does not necessarily represent a personality disorder and may not "explain" the posttraumatic symptoms or, similarly, the posttraumatic personality features.

Studies using treatment-seeking samples could result in an inflation of rates of personality disturbance in posttrauma populations due to what might actually be preexisting traits (i.e., those with preexisting personality problems might be more likely in general to develop symptoms and to seek treatment). However, the similarity of the profiles of individuals subjected to extreme stress, and the common finding of an absence of preexisting disturbance (at least as retrospectively assessed) argues against this possibility. Results from studies using samples not selected by treatment seeking have been mixed, with some reporting impaired personality functioning (e.g., Leopold and Dillon 1963; Titchner and Kapp 1976), and others finding little evidence of impairment (e.g., Leon et al. 1981). In the latter study, the question remains whether the findings are due to selectivity in the opposite direction (i.e., by choosing individuals who were functioning in society 30–40 years after concentration camp imprisonment and were willing to participate in the study).

The area that is most equivocal in terms of preexisting personality traits is the antisocial or violent behavior found in some studies of combat veterans. Studies to date suggest that, whereas combat may play a role in this for some individuals, many are likely to have a precombat history of antisocial behavior.

4. *What is the relationship of this proposed category to PTSD?* Given that both PTSD and the personality change category are defined as consequences of traumatic experience, their distinction and overlap are important to consider. There is some overlap in criteria, including increased vigilance and irritability and feelings of estrangement and emotional numbness. In a review of personality disorders and PTSD, Reich (1990) concluded that patients with PTSD, particularly if it is chronic, will have a tendency toward deleterious personality change. The literature reviewed here suggests that the symptoms described by the personality change criteria often occur within the context of other symptoms, including somatic, cognitive, and behavioral symptoms, many of which resemble the PTSD criteria items. The actual degree of overlap among these two diagnostic categories remains to be determined. Also to be determined is the relationship between the personality change criteria and the criteria recently proposed for disorders of extreme stress not otherwise specified (DESNOS) (Herman 1990).

Recommendations

To summarize, there are consistent reports of changes in personality features and functioning after severe trauma that persist for many years after the traumatic experience. It appears that different types of severe and prolonged trauma result in similar types of changes. The personality changes commonly reported include isolation and social withdrawal, pervasive apathy and hopelessness, identity disturbance, hostility, and suspiciousness; these often occur in the context of increased vigilance, hypersensitivity, and numerous somatic symptoms. The evidence suggests that such changes may occur in the absence of preexisting personality disturbance, although the absence of prospective assessments precludes conclusions regarding the influence of preexisting personality. It is likely that individual vulnerabilities interact with the nature and severity of the stressor in producing permanent changes in personality but that such changes can occur in individuals with normal adjustment and personality functioning in cases of severe trauma. Finally, it is clear that the current PTSD diagnosis does not capture the range of disturbance associated with more extreme and prolonged stress.

On this basis, it is the recommendation of the Axis II Work Group that the personality change after catastrophic experience diagnosis be considered for inclusion in the DSM-IV. Because the proposed criteria reflect enduring personality functioning, this category might be included on Axis II (similar to the ICD-10 placement). Alternatively, it might be considered as part of a larger category of stress-related disorders being considered for inclusion in DSM-IV.

Future research would be useful in determining the prevalence of the criteria in individuals experiencing severe trauma, the nature of the relationship between the proposed criteria and diagnosis and the PTSD and DESNOS criteria and diagnoses, and the relationship between the severity and duration of the trauma and the onset of the features described by the proposed criteria.

References

American Psychiatric Association: Diagnostic and Statistical Manual of Mental Disorders, First Edition. Washington, DC, American Psychiatric Association, 1952

American Psychiatric Association: Diagnostic and Statistical Manual of Mental Disorders, Third Edition. Washington, DC, American Psychiatric Association, 1980

American Psychiatric Association: Diagnostic and Statistical Manual of Mental Disorders, Third Edition, Revised. Washington, DC, American Psychiatric Association, 1987

Barrett DH, Resnick HS, Foy DW, et al: Antisocial behavior and post traumatic stress disorder in Vietnam veterans. Presented at the annual meeting of the American Psychological Association, New Orleans, LA, 1989

Boman B: Combat stress, post-traumatic stress disorder and associated psychiatric disturbance. Psychosomatics 27:567–573, 1986

Boman B: Antisocial behavior and the combat veteran: a review (with special reference to the Vietnam conflict). Medicine and Law 6:173–187, 1987

Dor-Shav NK: On the long range effects of concentration camp internment on Nazi victims: 25 years later. J Consult Clin Psychol 46:1–11, 1978

Escobar JI, Randolph ET, Puente G, et al: Post traumatic stress disorder in Hispanic Vietnam veterans: clinical phenomenology and sociocultural characteristics. J Nerv Ment Dis 171:585–596, 1983

Eitinger L: Pathology of the concentration camp syndrome preliminary report. Arch Gen Psychiatry 5:371–379, 1961

Faustman WO, White PA: Diagnostic psychopharmacological treatment characteristics of 536 inpatients with post-traumatic stress disorder. J Nerv Ment Dis 177:154–158, 1989

Green BL, Grace MC, Gleser GC: Identifying survivors at risk: long-term impairment following the Beverly Hills Supper Club fire. J Consult Clin Psychol 53:672–678, 1985a

Green BL, Lindy JD, Grace MC: Post traumatic stress disorder: toward DSM-IV. J Nerv Ment Dis 173:406–411, 1985b

Helzer JE, Robins LN, McEvoy L: Post traumatic stress disorder in the general population: findings of the epidemiologic catchment area survey. N Engl J Med 317:1630–1634, 1987

Herman JL: Complex PTSD: a syndrome in survivors of prolonged and repeated trauma. J Traum Stress 12:83–95, 1990

Herman JL, van der Kolk BA: Traumatic antecedents of borderline personality disorder, in Psychological Trauma. Edited by van der Kolk BA. Washington, DC, American Psychiatric Press, 1987, pp 111–126

Koranyi EK: A theoretical review of the survivor syndrome. Diseases of the Nervous System (Suppl) 30:115–118, 1969

Krystal H, Niederland WG: Clinical Observations of the Survivor Syndrome. New York, International Universities Press, 1968

Kulka RA: Executive Summary: Contractual Report of Findings From the National Vietnam Veterans Readjustment Study. Research Triangle Park, NC, November 7, 1988

Leon GR, Butcher JN, Kleinman M, et al: Survivors of the Holocaust and their children: current status and adjustment. J Pers Soc Psychol 41:503–516, 1981

Leopold RL, Dillon H: Psycho-anatomy of disaster: a long-term study of post-traumatic neuroses in survivors of a Marine explosion. Am J Psychiatry 120:913–921, 1963

Lindy JD, Grace MC, Green BL: Building a conceptual bridge between civilian trauma and war trauma: preliminary psychological findings from a clinical sample of Vietnam veterans, in PTSD: Psychological and Biological Sequelae. Edited by van der Kolk BA. Washington, DC, American Psychiatric Press, 1984, pp 105–123

McFarlane AC: Aetiology of post-traumatic stress disorders following a natural disaster. Br J Psychiatry 152:116–121, 1988a

McFarlane AC: Longitudinal course of post-traumatic morbidity: the range of outcomes and their predictors. J Nerv Ment Dis 176:30–39, 1988b

McFarlane AC: Phenomenology of post-traumatic stress disorder following a natural disaster. J Nerv Ment Dis 176:22–29, 1988c

Penk WE, Robinowitz R, Roberts WR, et al: Adjustment-differences among male substance abusers varying in degree of combat experience in Vietnam. J Consult Clin Psychol 49:426–437, 1981

Reich JH: Personality disorders and posttraumatic stress disorder, in Posttraumatic Stress Disorder: Etiology, Phenomenology, and Treatment. Edited by Wolf ME, Mosnaim AD. Washington, DC, American Psychiatric Press, 1990, pp 65–78

Resnick H, Foy DW, Donahue CP, et al: Antisocial behavior and post-traumatic stress disorder in Vietnam veterans. J Clin Psychol 45:850–866, 1989

Sherwood RJ: Adapted character styles of Vietnam veterans with post traumatic stress disorder. Psychol Rep 66:623–631, 1990

Sierles FS, Chen JJ, Messing ML, et al: Concurrent psychiatric illness in non-Hispanic outpatients diagnosed as having post-traumatic stress disorder. J Nerv Ment Dis 174:171–173, 1986

Sutker PB, Winstead DK, Galina ZH, et al: Cognitive deficits and psychopathology among former prisoners of war and combat veterans of the Korean conflict. Am J Psychiatry 148: 67–72, 1991

Titchener JL, Kapp FT: Family and character change at Buffalo Creek. Am J Psychiatry 133:295–299, 1976

Ursano RJ, Boydston JA, Wheatly RD: Psychiatric illness in U.S. Air Force Vietnam prisoners of war: a five year follow-up. Am J Psychiatry 138:310–318, 1981

World Health Organization: ICD-10 Chapter V. Mental and Behavioral Disorders. Diagnostic Criteria for Research. Geneva, Switzerland, World Health Organization, 1990

Yager J: Post-combat-violent behavior in psychiatrically maladjusted soldiers. Arch Gen Psychiatry 33:1332–1335, 1976

Yager J, Laufer R, Gallops MA: Some problems associated with war experience in men of the Vietnam generation. Arch Gen Psychiatry 41:327–333, 1984

Chapter 38

Personality Change Resulting From Another Mental Disorder

Joseph Triebwasser, M.D., and M. Tracie Shea, Ph.D.

Statement of the Issues

Among the diagnoses under consideration for DSM-IV is "personality change resulting from another mental disorder," a formulation corresponding to the provisional ICD-10 diagnosis "enduring personality change after psychiatric illness." We summarize the extant literature relevant to the proposed diagnosis. (See the *DSM-IV Options Book* [Task Force on DSM-IV 1991] for a text of the proposed DSM-IV entry.)

Significance of the Issues

There are both practical and theoretical advantages to eliminating unnecessary differences between the DSM-IV and the ICD-10 systems (Frances et al. 1990). However, potential concerns regarding the proposed diagnosis include: Is such a formulation consonant with current theoretical understandings of the interaction of mental disorder and personality? Do the available published data imply that the proposed diagnosis occurs with any frequency? What is the quality of these data, and how convincingly do they argue for or against the inclusion of the diagnosis?

Methods

Efforts were made to survey all articles, chapters, and books pertaining to the topic "personality change secondary to mental disorder." Relevant citations were found through a computer search (Paperchase), using the index terms *affective disorders, anxiety disorders, bipolar disorder, depression, panic disorder, personality,* and *person-*

ality disorders and through references cited in the articles identified. An empirical study was considered relevant if it assessed some aspect of personality after the resolution of a mood or anxiety disorder. Primary psychotic disorders were not included; although the ICD-10 authors state that a "diagnosis of schizophrenia does not preempt the diagnosis," outcome studies on schizophrenia have generally not focused on personality variables. The large literature on personality and substance abuse (Cox 1979; Pihl and Spiers 1978) was also felt to be beyond the scope of this review.

Results

Does Current Theory Support the Diagnosis?

Significant portions of the mental disorder literature have focused on the possibility of a cause-and-effect relationship between "mental disorder" and "personality." For most of this century, the dominant position has been that personality forms the background from which mental disorders emerge and the context in which they must be understood (Abraham 1927; Cohen et al. 1954; Keller and Shapiro 1982; O'Neill and Bornstein 1991; Sullivan 1949; Kraepelin, quoted in Wetzel et al. 1980). In the 1980s, a somewhat different viewpoint began to emerge that gave primacy not to character or personality but to mental disorders themselves (Cassano et al. 1983; Faravelli et al. 1986; Fennell and Campbell 1984; Matussek and Feil 1983; Waters and Calleia 1983). Two recent articles have offered synthetic reviews of these differing theoretical positions (Akiskal et al. 1983; Klein et al. 1993). Both reviews have included a construct that seems to correspond to the proposed DSM-IV diagnosis—Akiskal et al.'s "personality as a complication of affective illness" and Klein et al.'s "complication" or "scar" hypothesis.

Do Current Research Data Support the Diagnosis?

In the 15 articles that have studied personality scale scores of recovered depressive patients (Bech et al. 1980; Benjaminsen 1981; Boyce et al. 1989, 1990; Coppen and Metcalfe 1965; Duggan et al. 1990, 1992; Faravelli et al. 1986; Garside et al. 1970; Hirschfeld and Klerman 1979; Kendell and DiScipio 1968; Kerr et al. 1970; Perris 1971; Weissman et al. 1978; Wretmark et al. 1970), the dominant finding has been that these scales are heavily state-dependent, and that scores tend to normalize significantly with recovery from depression (Coppen and Metcalfe 1965; Garside et al. 1970; Wretmark et al. 1970), although at least two studies (Boyce et al. 1989; Kendell and DiScipio 1968) have found Eysenck Personality Inventory (EPI) scores to be fairly persistent despite remission. Interestingly, both these studies made use of what has come to be known as the Kendell and DiScipio instruction, in which subjects are told to respond to the EPI according to how they *usually* feel. (It should also be pointed out that neither of these studies used particularly rigorous criteria for recovery from the illness episode.) Duggan et al. (1992) followed up on Kendell and DiScipio's sample 18 years later and found that EPI scores had remained fairly stable over time and that a chronic and severe course of depression did not adversely affect follow-up EPI scores.

Two studies (Hirschfeld and Klerman 1979; Perris 1971) found persistently abnormal Maudsley Personality Inventory (MPI) scores in recovered depressive patients, but three other studies (Bech et al. 1980; Kerr et al. 1970; Weissman et al. 1978) found that recovered depressive patients had scores similar to or "healthier" than historical control subjects. Benjaminsen (1981) found that different subtypes of depressive patients had different postmorbid EPI scores, with neurotic and nonendogenous depressive patients tending to have persistently high N scores, whereas recovered endogenous depressive patients had normal N scores; E scores remained low in all subtype groups.

Discussion

There are several methodological obstacles to drawing conclusions from the relevant research findings about whether mental disorders can lead to lasting personality change. These problems include the studies' lack of premorbid personality assessment, uncertainty regarding remission of the index illness episode, and lack of adequate follow-up interval.

Almost all the studies reviewed here compare postmorbid personality findings with those of either control subjects, published norms, or the same patients during the index episode; they do not compare the postmorbid findings to prospectively obtained premorbid findings. The resulting data thus do not necessarily shed light on personality change caused by the mental disorder, because a recovered subject's abnormal personality traits may have been present before the episode as well (Matussek and Feil 1983). In fact, in interpreting personality scores of recovered populations, many authors make the assumption that such information provides a window onto the *premorbid* personality and therefore onto the reason the subject was vulnerable to the disorder in the first place (Boyce et al. 1990; Garside et al. 1970; Kendell and DiScipio 1968; Paykel and Weissman 1973).

The need for prospective data is especially important in view of an extensive literature that assumes that *most* individuals with mental disorders have preexisting personality abnormalities that predispose them to the disorder (Klein and Depue 1985; Kovacs and Beck 1978; O'Neill and Bornstein 1991). Research data on this topic are ambiguous: At least one older study suggested that certain personality traits place individuals at risk for the development of mental disorder (Nystrom and Lindegard 1975), whereas a more recent study showed surprisingly low correlation between personality features and the later development of depression (Hirschfeld et al. 1989). Wittenborn and Maurer (1977) found that "depressive" traits present in depressive patients at the 1-year follow-up had almost always been felt by the patients' relatives to have been present premorbidly (according to an interview during the index hospitalization). For certain patients, pathological traits described by relatives as having been present premorbidly were *not* present on recovery, thus implying that depression may have a beneficial effect on personality!

Some authors have commented on the need for studies with both premorbid and postmorbid data, although they have acknowledged the time and expense involved (Matussek and Feil 1983). Abnormal personality findings in subjects who later developed a mental disorder might, moreover, be difficult to interpret, because they might not represent personality per se but rather subclinical prodromal symptoms of the disorder itself. Several retrospective studies have suggested that such prodromal syndromes are fairly common in mania, depression, and panic disorder (Fava and Kellner 1991); these prodromal symptoms might be difficult to distinguish from character disturbance.

A second major obstacle toward drawing conclusions from the studies addressed in this review is the uncertainty regarding extent of recovery from the index episode. In the case of some studies, this uncertainty stems in part from the study design; either the recovery criteria are vague or unspecified (Kendell and DiScipio 1968; Perris 1971) or the postrecovery assessment is performed suspiciously early, for example, just before discharge from the hospital (Hamilton and Abramson 1983). Some studies assessed patients after a certain interval had elapsed from the index episode, but the extent of intervening symptoms or even episodes is unclear (Garside et al. 1970). Other studies judged patients "recovered" on the basis of moderately low scores on a depression scale but did not require a minimum duration for the remission, thus leaving the possibility that subjects had been depressed a short while before (Blackburn and Bishop 1983; Fennell and Campbell 1984).

Even studies with more rigorous inclusion criteria (e.g., Frank et al. 1987) leave room for doubt as to whether the subjects were truly recovered at the time of assessment. These studies inevitably rely on standardized rating scales that may not do justice to the full range of mental disorders, especially in the disorder's more attenuated forms. Patients with remitted depression continue to show some of the physiological abnormalities associated with depression (Hauri et al. 1974); one possible explanation for this is that even between episodes, depressive patients are, in some subclinical sense, still "disordered."

Recent findings have reinforced the idea that recovery from major mental disorders may be a relative concept. Goodnick et al. (1987) found that interepisode symptoms were common in patients with depression and bipolar disorder. Even "treatable" mental disorders may become chronic conditions with a high degree of relapse and failure to return to baseline (Keller et al. 1983; Kiloh et al. 1988; Lee and Murray 1988; Scott 1988; Winokur et al. 1969).

Doubts regarding the completeness of recovery of recovered subjects are especially troublesome in studies of personality, given the confounding effect that persistent symptoms may have on personality assessment. Researchers have repeatedly found "symptoms" difficult to differentiate from "personality" (Kerr et al. 1970; Parker and Brown 1982) and that the presence of an Axis I disorder has a confounding effect on measures of personality variables (Cochran and Hammen 1985; Liebowitz et al. 1979; Reich et al. 1986).

A further difficulty is related to the issue of the follow-up intervals of the studies reviewed. The *DSM-IV Options Book* (Task Force on DSM-IV 1991) specifies that the duration of the disturbance needs to have been at least 3 years. Of the studies reviewed here, only eight had a follow-up interval of even 2 years, and often the subjects were still symptomatic during at least part of this interval.

Recommendations

On both theoretical and empirical grounds, there seems to be room for skepticism regarding the concept "personality change resulting from another mental disorder." On a theoretical level, whereas some authors have advanced the idea that such change can occur, others have implied or stated that it is unlikely. Few robust, well-replicated findings regarding the extent of this phenomenon are to be found in the current research literature. Studies that seem to demonstrate lasting personality disturbances after mental disorders are often contradicted by other studies that fail to find such abnormalities. The findings that do emerge are often plagued by methodological difficulties or questions as to the wider applicability of the findings. This uncertainty in the research literature may reflect epistemological difficulties that would face the average clinician trying to apply the proposed diagnosis in daily practice.

In the light of these concerns, incorporating the proposed diagnosis into DSM-IV might be premature.

References

Abraham K: Selected Papers of Karl Abraham, M.D. New York, Brunner/Mazel, 1927
Akiskal H, Hirschfeld R, Yerevanian B: The relationship of personality to affective disorders. Arch Gen Psychiatry 40:801–810, 1983
Bech P, Shapiro R, Sihm R, et al: Personality in unipolar and bipolar manic-melancholic patients. Acta Psychiatr Scand 62:245–257, 1980

Benjaminsen S: Primary non-endogenous depressions and features attributed to reactive depression. J Affect Disord 3:245–259, 1981

Blackburn I, Bishop S: Changes in cognition with pharmacotherapy and cognitive therapy. Br J Psychiatry 143:609–617, 1983

Boyce P, Hadzi-Pavlovic D, Parker G, et al: Depressive type and state effects on personality measures. Acta Psychiatr Scand 81:197–200, 1989

Boyce P, Parker G, Hickie A, et al: Personality differences between patients with remitted melancholic and nonmelancholic depression. Am J Psychiatry 147:1476–1483, 1990

Cassano G, Maggini C, Akiskal H: Short-term, subchronic, and chronic sequelae of affective disorders. Psychiatr Clin North Am 6:55–67, 1983

Cochran S, Hammen C: Perceptions of stressful life events and depression: a test of attributional models. J Pers Soc Psychol 48:1562–1571, 1985

Cohen M, Baker G, Cohen R, et al: An intensive study of twelve cases of manic-depressive psychosis. Psychiatry 17:103–137, 1954

Coppen A, Metcalfe M: Effect of a depressive illness on MPI scores. Br J Psychiatry 111:236–239, 1965

Cox W: The alcoholic personality: a review of the evidence. Progress in Experimental Personality Research 9:89–148, 1979

Duggan C, Lee A, Murray R: Does personality predict long-term outcome in depression? Br J Psychiatry 157:19–24, 1990

Duggan C, Sham P, Lee A, et al: Does recurrent depression lead to a change in neuroticism? Psychol Med 22:28–37, 1992

Faravelli C, Ambonetti A, Pallanti S, et al: Depressive relapses and incomplete recovery from index episode. Am J Psychiatry 148:823–830, 1986

Fava G, Kellner R: Prodromal symptoms in affective disorders. Am J Psychiatry 148:823–830, 1991

Fennell M, Campbell E: The cognitions questionnaire: specific thinking errors in depression. Br J Clin Psychol 23:81–92, 1984

Frances A, Pincus H, Widiger T, et al: DSM-IV: work in progress. Am J Psychiatry 147:1439–1448, 1990

Frank E, Kupfer D, Jacob M, et al: Personality features and response to acute treatment in recurrent depression. Journal of Personality Disorders 1:14–26, 1987

Garside R, Kay S, Roy J, et al: MPI scores and symptoms of depression. Br J Psychiatry 116:429–432, 1970

Goodnick P, Fieve R, Schlegel A, et al: Inter-episode major and subclinical symptoms in affective disorder. Acta Psychiatr Scand 75:597–600, 1987

Hamilton E, Abramson L: Cognitive patterns and major depressive disorder: a longitudinal study in a hospital setting. J Abnorm Psychol 92:173–184, 1983

Hauri P, Chernik D, Hawkins D, et al: Sleep of depressed patients in remission. Arch Gen Psychiatry 31:386–391, 1974

Hirschfeld R, Klerman G: Personality attributes and affective disorders. Am J Psychiatry 136:67–70, 1979

Hirschfeld R, Klerman G, Lavori P, et al: Premorbid personality assessments of first onset of major depression. Arch Gen Psychiatry 46:345–350, 1989

Keller M, Shapiro R: "Double depression": superimposition of acute depressive episodes of chronic depressive disorders. Am J Psychiatry 139:438–442, 1982

Keller M, Lavori P, Lewis C, et al: Predictors of relapse in major affective disorder. JAMA 250:3299–3304, 1983

Kendell R, DiScipio W: Eysenck Personality Inventory scores of patients with depressive illnesses. Br J Psychiatry 114:767–770, 1968

Kerr T, Schapira K, Roth M, et al: The relationship between the Maudsley Personality Inventory and the course of affective disorders. Br J Psychiatry 116:1–19, 1970

Kiloh L, Andrews G, Neilson M: The long-term outcome of depressive illness. Br J Psychiatry 153:752–757, 1988

Klein D, Depue R: Obsessional personality traits and risk for bipolar affective disorder: an offspring study. J Abnorm Psychol 94:291–297, 1985

Klein M, Wonderlich S, Shea M: Models of relationship between personality and depression: toward a framework for theory and research, in Personality and Depression. Edited by Klein MH, Kupfer DJ, Shea MT. New York, Guilford, 1993, pp 1–54

Kovacs M, Beck A: Maladaptive cognitive structures in depression. Am J Psychiatry 135:525–533, 1978

Lee A, Murray R: The long-term outcome of Maudsley depressives. Br J Psychiatry 153:741–751, 1988

Liebowitz M, Stallone F, Dunner D, et al: Personality features of patients with primary affective disorder. Acta Psychiatr Scand 60:214–224, 1979

Matussek P, Feil W: Personality attributes of depressive patients: results of group comparisons. Arch Gen Psychiatry 40:783–790, 1983

Nystrom S, Lindegard B: Depression: predisposing factors. Acta Psychiatr Scand 51:77–87, 1975

O'Neill R, Bornstein R: Orality and depression in psychiatric inpatients. Journal of Personality Disorders 5:1–7, 1991

Parker G, Brown L: Coping behaviors that mediate between life events and depression. Arch Gen Psychiatry 39:1386–1391, 1982

Paykel E, Weissman M: Social adjustment and depression: a longitudinal study. Arch Gen Psychiatry 28:659–663, 1973

Perris C: Personality patterns in patients with affective disorders. Acta Psychiatr Scand Suppl 221:43–51, 1971

Pihl R, Spiers P: Individual characteristics in the etiology of drug abuse. Progress in Experimental Personality Research 8:93–95, 1978

Reich J, Noyes R, Coryell W, et al: The effect of state anxiety on personality measurement. Am J Psychiatry 143:760–763, 1986

Scott J: Chronic depression. Br J Psychiatry 153:287–297, 1988

Sullivan HS: The theory of anxiety and the nature of psychotherapy. Psychiatry 12:3–12, 1949

Task Force on DSM-IV: DSM-IV Options Book: Work in Progress. Washington, DC, American Psychiatric Association, 1991

Waters B, Calleia S: The effect of juvenile-onset manic-depressive disorder on the developmental tasks of adolescence. Am J Psychother 37:182–189, 1983

Weissman M, Prusoff B, Klerman G: Personality and the prediction of long-term outcome of depression. Am J Psychiatry 135:797–800, 1978

Wetzel R, Cloninger C, Hong B, et al: Personality as a subclinical expression of the affective disorders. Compr Psychiatry 21:197–205, 1980

Winokur TG, Clayton P, Reich T: Manic Depressive Illness. St. Louis, MO, CV Mosby, 1969

Wittenborn J, Maurer H: Persisting personalities among depressed women. Arch Gen Psychiatry 34:968–971, 1977

Wretmark G, Astrom J, Eriksson M: The Maudsley Personality Inventory as a prognostic instrument. Br J Psychiatry 116:21–26, 1970

Section V

Psychiatric System Interface Disorders

Introduction to Section V

Psychiatric System Interface Disorders (PSID)

Robert E. Hales, M.D.

The purpose of this introduction is to provide an overview of a number of important issues that faced the DSM-IV Work Group on Psychiatric System Interface Disorders (PSID). When the DSM-IV Task Force was being formed in 1988, it became apparent that a Work Group was needed to focus on those disorders that tended to overlap with other psychiatric disorders or that were of particular interest to other medical disciplines. Consequently, the acronym *PSID* was used to designate the DSM-IV Work Group that would be responsible for developing the diagnostic criteria, text, and literature reviews for the six categories of psychiatric disorders shown in Table 1.

Another important task of the PSID Work Group was to work closely with primary care specialties (family medicine, internal medicine, pediatrics, and obstetrics/gynecology) to determine how to make the DSM-IV more accessible and user friendly for these specialists. Jack D. Burke, M.D., and Jonathan F. Borus, M.D., spearheaded these efforts and, with the support of the National Institute of Mental Health, organized two meetings in Washington, D.C., that included representatives of the primary-care specialties and selected members of the DSM-IV Task Force. The primary care physicians provided consultation to the Task Force members concerning important diagnostic issues pertaining to several categories of disorder and provided input concerning the design of subsequent field trials investigating somatization disorder and mixed anxiety-depression.

The American Psychiatric Association's Office of Research, headed by Harold Pincus, M.D., then organized two planning meetings that involved official representatives from the major primary-care specialty societies to assist the American Psychiatric Association in developing a DSM-IV for Primary Care (DSM-IV–PC). This sub-Work Group, co-chaired by Thomas Wise, M.D., and Harold Pincus, M.D., is developing a DSM-IV–PC that is readily accessible to primary-care physicians and is compatible and totally consistent with the DSM-IV diagnostic criteria.

Table 1.   Psychiatric system interface disorders (DSM-III-R disorders revised)

Psychological factors affecting physical condition (PFAPC)
Somatoform disorders
Impulse control disorders not otherwise classified
Dissociative disorders
Adjustment disorders
Factitious disorders

This introduction does not focus on many of the important issues that have been discussed by the Primary Care sub-Work Group but rather summarizes some of the conclusions reached by the authors of the PSID Work Group Sourcebook chapters.

Somatoform Disorders

Because of the great diversity and complexity of the disorders falling within the somatoform disorders category, the work in this section was coordinated by several individuals in the PSID Work Group: C. Robert Cloninger, M.D., for somatization disorder; Ronald L. Martin, M.D., for conversion disorder, autonomic arousal disorder, and pseudocyesis; Steven King, M.D., for somatoform pain disorder; Katharine A. Phillips, M.D., for body dysmorphic disorder; David Barlow, Ph.D. and James Strain, M.D., for hypochondriasis; and Leslie Morey, Ph.D., and John E. Kurtz, Ph.D., for neurasthenia.

Somatization Disorder

The major problem with the DSM-III-R (American Psychiatric Association 1987) criteria for somatization disorder has been its complexity. Many clinicians find it difficult to remember the 35 possible symptoms from which 13 must be selected to make this diagnosis. As a result, clinicians often do not make systematic use of the full criteria, and patients often receive this diagnosis in error. The task for Cloninger et al. was either to reduce the total number of symptoms required to make the diagnosis or to regroup them in a different fashion. As Cloninger emphasizes in Chapter 39, although the grouping of symptoms in DSM-III-R was meant to assist the clinician in remembering the host of symptoms a patient could manifest, the assignment of symptoms to various groups was done in an arbitrary fashion. For instance, pain symptoms are included not only in the pain symptom group but also in the cardiopulmonary, sexual, and female reproductive symptom categories.

Another problem that the Somatization sub-Work Group identified was the specification in the DSM-III-R criteria that there could be no organic pathology or pathophysiological mechanism to explain the symptom. It was felt that this statement stigmatized patients and made the development of therapeutic plans with the psychiatrist difficult. Based on his comprehensive literature review and reanalysis of existing data compiled from patients with this disorder, Cloninger developed simplified diagnostic criteria. Instead of thirteen symptoms, the patient need only have eight symptoms, falling within four categories: pain related to at least four different sites, two gastrointestinal symptoms other than pain, one sexual reproductive symptom other than pain, and one symptom or deficit suggesting a neurologic disorder not limited to pain or a dissociative symptom. Extensive statistical analysis revealed satisfactory reliability and validity with this simplified schema. The results of a field trial further evaluating the reliability and validity of the simplified criteria will be presented in a later volume of the *DSM-IV Sourcebook.*

Conversion Disorder

Martin identified four important diagnostic issues for conversion disorder (Chapter 40). First, he questioned whether conversion disorder should include only "pseudo-neurological symptoms" (those suggesting a neurological disorder) and whether the symptoms should be confined to only sensory and involuntary motor function. If so, his sub-Work Group would need to develop a new diagnosis for cases with nonneurological symptoms (pseudocyesis) and for patients with symptoms that involve the autonomic nervous system (autonomic arousal disorder). Based on his extensive literature review, Martin concluded that it would be desirable to return the concept of conversion disorder to a more traditional and precisely defined concept limited to neurological symptoms involving only the special sensory and voluntary nervous system. As a result of this conclusion, it was proposed that a new disorder, "autonomic arousal disorder," focusing on symptoms attributed to autonomic arousal, be included in DSM-IV. This disorder would also be grouped in the somatoform disorders section. Because the ICD-10 (World Health Organization 1990) includes such an entity, it would make the DSM-IV criteria more compatible with the international classification system. Finally, it was proposed that, because of its rarity, pseudocyesis not be included as a disorder per se but be listed as an example of somatoform disorder not otherwise specified, along with neurasthenia and other selected conditions.

The second issue facing the Conversion Disorder sub-Work Group and the Dissociative Disorders sub-Work Group was whether conversion disorder should be grouped with the somatoform disorders or placed with the dissociative disorders. Conversion disorder was placed with the somatoform disorders section in DSM-III-R because of the shared characteristic of physical symptoms that are not intentionally produced. In his literature review, Martin concludes that conversion disorder should continue to be grouped with the somatoform disorders in DSM-IV but that it should also be cross-referenced with the dissociative disorders group because of the close association with the dissociative disorders in terms of pheno-menological, demographic, etiological, and possibly pathogenic relationships. Martin also recommends that patients with conversion disorders be carefully examined for dissociative symptoms and disorders and, conversely, that patients with a dissociative disorder be examined for conversion symptoms.

Finally, Martin recommends that the association with psychological factors be required for the diagnosis of conversion disorder but that this association not be necessarily etiological in nature. He further recommends that it be required that the conversion symptom or deficit should cause significant impairment in a person's social or occupational functioning, cause marked distress, or require medical attention or investigation. This change was proposed to limit the diagnosis to patients with clinically significant symptoms and thus to establish a threshold for the diagnosis.

Somatoform Pain Disorder

In their review of the somatoform pain disorder category (Chapter 41), King and Strain focused on the following questions: 1) Is somatoform pain disorder a valid and reliable diagnosis? 2) Are there factors that limit the clinical application of somatoform pain disorder? 3) To what extent can pain be considered a mental disorder? and 4) Are there alternative classification systems that may replace somatoform pain disorder?

Based on their review of the literature on these four issues, King and Strain have proposed a new and more broadly defined schema for pain. Somatoform pain disorder would be replaced by a new diagnostic category, "pain disorder." Further consideration would be given to separating pain disorder from the other somatoform disorders and creating a separate category from the somato-form disorders, in a similar manner to how sleep disorders are described in DSM-III-R. This alternative will probably not be instituted, because it would isolate pain from other disorders in which physical complaints are paramount. Pain disorder would have four subtypes: psychological type, secondary type due to a nonpsychiatric medical condition, combined type, and unspecified type. This new proposal would give the clinician much greater latitude to specify the factors presumed to be involved in the etiology or maintenance of the individ-ual's pain, include the possible differential diagnostic categories of pain disor-ders encountered in practice, delete from DSM-IV the unsubstantiated dualistic concept that pain associated with psychological factors is somehow different from that associated with other medical conditions, and eliminate what is often an impossible clinical judgment—whether the pain is in excess of what is expected.

The main criticisms of this new approach to pain disorders is that the secondary type may be seen as inappropriately broadening the concept of mental disorders to include virtually all individuals who exhibit significant pain, whether secondary to cancer or from psychological causes. The problem of secondary pain could probably be satisfied by coding the secondary type with an ICD-10 R code from outside the mental disorders section or by using another code. This problem is being investigated by the DSM-IV Task Force and should be solvable.

King and Strain's proposed diagnostic category is compatible with current theories of pain and broadens the concept to reflect the fact that the psychological state of patients is important in many more cases of pain than are currently being diagnosed using existing DSM-III-R criteria for somatoform pain disorder. Finally, the simplified and straightforward criteria proposed by King and Strain would make the classification of pain disorders more relevant to clinical practice and provide greater assistance to psychiatrists and other physicians who evaluate and treat patients with pain in a variety of clinical settings.

Hypochondriasis

Côté, O'Leary, Barlow, and Strain had an especially challenging task in conducting their literature review (Chapter 42), because hypochondriasis overlaps with other anxiety disorders (in particular, specific phobias) yet is placed within the somatoform disorders section. The reader will also notice some disparity between the literature review presented here and the possible options outlined in the *DSM-IV Options Book* (Task Force on DSM-IV 1991).

Côté et al. address three issues in their literature review. First, they examine the relationship between illness phobia and hypochondriasis and seek to determine whether a distinction exists between disease conviction and disease fear. The authors conclude that disease conviction is more consistent with a diagnosis of hypochondriasis, whereas illness phobia without disease conviction is more consistent with a diagnosis of specific phobia. They further conclude that the symptom of avoidance due to the fear of contracting a disease may be diagnosed as a "specific phobia, other type (contracting an illness)" or may occupy its own subtype of specific phobia, namely, illness type. In contrast, the major criterion for the diagnosis of hypochondriasis would be preoccupation with fears of *having* a disease or the idea that one *has* a serious disease.

The second issue they discussed was whether an unshakable conviction borders on a hypochondriacal delusion. Based on their review of the literature, they could make no firm recommendation concerning how to distinguish disease conviction in hypochondriasis from an unshakable belief in a delusion.

Finally, the authors address the issue of whether patients need to exhibit physical symptoms to receive the diagnosis of hypochondriasis. They found that, in the vast majority of the reports they studied, physical symptoms in hypochondriacal patients were quite important in making the diagnosis. Despite this conclusion, a proposed option for the DSM-IV is to eliminate the requirement that the fears concerning physical health be related to actual physical signs and symptoms. This change is supported by Côté et al.'s literature review, which showed that persistent worry about health can occur without somatic symptoms.

This change then leads to a consideration that was directly addressed in their review, namely, where should hypochondriasis be placed: within the somatoform disorders section or within the anxiety disorders section? Because many individuals with hypochondriasis frequently have comorbid anxiety disorders and because it may be difficult to distinguish hypochondriasis from generalized anxiety disorder or specific phobias, hypochondriasis may be more logically placed within the anxiety disorders section. At the same time, hypochondriasis may be more logically left within the somatoform disorders section because of the preoccupation of the individuals with bodily concerns and their frequent initial presentation in primary-care settings.

Body Dysmorphic Disorder

Phillips' and Hollander's literature review (Chapter 43) focused on four questions: 1) Is body dysmorphic disorder a discrete syndrome? 2) What is the relationship between body dysmorphic disorder and other psychiatric disorders? 3) What is the relationship between body dysmorphic disorder and a person's normal concern with appearance? and 4) Are there any data on the performance of structured assessment instruments for body dysmorphic disorder?

Although its status as a discrete disorder has been questioned, from their extensive review, Phillips and Hollander conclude that its historical classification, both in the European literature and DSM-III-R, together with preliminary empirical data support the inclusion of "body dysmorphic disorder" as a separate category in DSM-IV. Keeping body dysmorphic disorder as a separate syndrome would provide opportunities for much needed research on this disorder. The proposed DSM-IV exclusion criterion that specifies that the preoccupation is not better accounted for by another mental disorder (e.g., dissatisfaction with body shape and size in anorexia nervosa) emphasizes that, although body dysmorphic disorder may coexist with anorexia nervosa and other mental disorders, it should not be diagnosed if another disorder more accurately and comprehensively describes the person's condition. As to whether body dysmorphic disorder should remain classified with the somatoform disorders or be reclassified as a mood, psychotic, or anxiety disorder (in particular, as a subtype of obsessive-compulsive disorder), Phillips and Hollander believe that the data best support keeping body dysmorphic disorder as a separate entity within the somatoform disorders section.

Empirical evidence concerning its association with obsessive-compulsive disorder is still preliminary. Based on data concerning body dysmorphic disorder's boundary with no mental disorder, the authors conclude that the lack of a severity criterion for body dysmorphic disorder in DSM-III-R may have created excessive overlap with a person's normal concern with appearance. Their proposal to include the statement "the preoccupation causes significant impairment in social or occupational functioning or causes marked distress" would tend to prevent the overdiagnosis of this disorder and create a more homogeneous group for research purposes. Finally, although there are instruments to assess various aspects of appearance-related body image disturbance, only three are currently being used to diagnose body dysmorphic disorder per se, and an adequate database has not been established.

Phillips and Hollander conclude that there is a sharp contrast between body dysmorphic disorder's long and rich historical tradition and its almost nonexistent empirical base. Further research and inquiry are needed in regard to the phenomenology, course, associated symptoms, biological factors, family history, and treatment response of this disorder. In addition, its overlap with existing psychiatric disorders in other categories needs to be studied further.

Neurasthenia

In their literature review, Morey and Kurtz (Chapter 44) examined the historical use of the term *neurasthenia*, its relationship to the DSM-III-R diagnostic categories, and its compatibility with the *neurasthenia* category included in ICD-10. Based on their extensive review, they found that there is clearly a group of patients who present with fatigue and somatic weakness and who, on further study, also display symptoms of anxiety and depression. As they indicate in their chapter, although many of these patients may meet DSM-III-R criteria for dysthymia or other anxiety or depressive disorders, they did not believe that the anxiety or depressive syndromes would include all such patients. They conclude by recommending the inclusion of neurasthenia in DSM-IV because it would increase the compatibility of DSM-IV with ICD-10, improve the coverage of patients who satisfy these symptoms, and usefully combine a constellation of symptoms (somatic complaints and anxiety and depressive symptoms) that frequently appear together in such patients. Because there has been little systematic research concerning this disorder, because of the overlap between this disorder and various depressive and anxiety disorders, and because of the possibility of neurasthenia being used as a "wastebasket" diagnosis, the most likely outcome from further PSID Work Group and Task Force discussions will be to include neurasthenia as a subtype of undifferentiated somatoform disorder. Also, the proposed criteria set for neurasthenia that is outlined in the *DSM-IV Options Book* will probably be included in an appendix to the DSM-IV to encourage clinicians and investigators to study this condition further.

Dissociative Disorders

Cardeña, Lewis-Fernández, Bear, Pakianathan, and Spiegel address five issues in their literature review on the dissociative disorders (Chapter 45), three of which I briefly summarize. First, they propose the creation of a new diagnostic category, "trance and possession disorder," to enable the clinician to diagnose distressing and impairing instances of possession and trance that are not culturally sanctioned. Although trance and possession states are normal components of various religious ceremonies in many cultures, trance and possession disorder that produces distress and dysfunction is the most common dissociative disorder in non-Western cultures. In recognition of this frequency, ICD-10 has included a new category, "trance and possession disorders." Adding such an entity in DSM-IV would increase the compatibility with ICD-10 and would recognize the relative high frequency of this disorder in non-Western cultures. Although there are only a few databases that exist that include the symptoms of trance and possession disorder, unlike those for other dissociative conditions, Cardeña et al. provide descriptions of two syndromes with common dissociative components: *ataque de nervios* and possession. The authors conclude that, by proposing specific criteria for distress, impairment, and lack of indigenous sanction, they will respond to the argument that they are pathologizing ordinary non-Western cultural expressions. They also believe that this would enhance the diagnostic precision of this category while encouraging greater cultural sensitivity.

Second, Cardeña et al. propose the creation of a new diagnostic category, "secondary dissociative disorder due to a nonpsychiatric medical condition," to account for reports of common dissociative symptoms among people with complex partial seizures or other medical conditions. They extensively reviewed a number of case reports of patients who exhibit dissociative symptoms between seizures and found consistent support for the idea that patients with seizure disorders experience a greater number of dissociative phenomena than normal control subjects. They further found that patients with seizure disorders generally do not show the same frequency of symptoms or symptom profiles as patients with multiple personality disorder. Even though the majority of cases of multiple personality disorder occur without evidence of focal electrophysiological abnormalities, seizure activity is clearly related to dissociative phenomena in a substantial number of cases. For all these reasons, the authors believe that the literature justifies the creation of a new category, "secondary dissociative disorder due to a nonpsychiatric medical condition."

Finally, the authors propose a new diagnostic category, "acute stress reaction/brief reactive dissociative disorder." Their literature review focused on both a historical perspective and more recent findings from the aftermath of the San Francisco Bay Area earthquake of 1989, in which 25%–40% of the respondents experienced a variety of derealization and depersonalization symptoms. Based on their extensive literature review, they conclude that, when researchers investigate the presence of dissociative symptoms during or immediately after a traumatic event, they will find that a considerable number of the people interviewed will report alterations in consciousness, problems with everyday memory and attention, and other symptoms that, when extreme, may alter their personal and social functioning. Cardeñna et al. further believe that a strong dissociative component to the traumatic reaction seems well established and that the adoption of a new diagnostic category, "acute stress reaction/brief reactive dissociative disorder," should encourage greater clinical attention to a substantial number of people that may be affected by trauma. Adjustment disorders and posttraumatic stress disorder are not adequate diagnoses to use for individuals with acute and principally dissociative symptoms. Because there is no category in the DSM-III-R nosology for an acute and severe reaction to trauma, the "acute stress disorder/brief reactive dissociative disorder" category warrants serious consideration for inclusion in DSM-IV. For all these reasons, the authors urge the inclusion of this new category.

Factitious Disorders

An informal literature review on factitious disorder by Fagan and Plewes (for which a full Sourcebook chapter was not prepared) focused on two principal issues: revision of the diagnostic criteria for factitious disorder and a proposal for a new disorder, "factitious disorder by proxy." With regard to the first issue, Fagan and Plewes found that most individuals present with a mixed symptom pattern. DSM-III-R developed separate criteria sets for factitious disorder with physical symptoms and factitious disorder with psychological symptoms. However, because mixed cases are frequently encountered, Fagan and Plewes proposed merging the disorders into a single diagnostic category with one criteria set and three subtypes: predominantly psychological symptoms, predominantly physical symptoms, and combined physical and psychological symptoms if neither category predominates. The "not-otherwise-specified" category would consequently be eliminated. Most of their literature review consisted of analyzing either individual case reports or a small series of cases.

The other issue that they considered was how to include in DSM-IV those cases in which one individual produces factitious symptoms in another for the purpose of indirectly assuming the sick role. In most cases, the situation involves a parent who artificially creates physical symptoms in the child. From their review, they found over 68 presentations reported in the literature; however, no empirically controlled studies were found. Regardless, the substantial morbidity and mortality associated with this disorder appear to justify the addition of factitious disorder by proxy in DSM-IV.

A related issue considered by Fagan and Plewes was whether the diagnosis should be given to the person *inducing* the symptoms or to the individual *presenting* with the symptoms. They propose that the psychiatric diagnosis, "factitious disorder by proxy" should be given to the person who induces the symptoms. If there is evidence that the individual with the symptoms colluded in the intentional production of the symptoms, then he or she would receive the diagnosis of factitious disorder and the perpetrator would receive a diagnosis of factitious disorder by proxy. If an individual presents with physical signs or symptoms induced by a caregiver who has the diagnosis of factitious disorder by proxy and the individual did not collude with the caregiver in the production of symptoms, the individual would receive the diagnosis of induced factitious symptoms. This would not be a psychiatric disorder but would appear in the "other clinically significant conditions" section of DSM-IV.

Although there is general agreement concerning the changes proposed for factitious disorder, there is still much discussion in the child psychiatric community concerning the proposal for factitious disorder by proxy. The literature review and these proposals will undergo further careful review and consideration.

Impulse Control Disorders Not Elsewhere Classified

Five disorders are included in the section "impulse control disorders not elsewhere classified": intermittent explosive disorder, kleptomania, pyromania, pathological gambling, and trichotillomania. The literature reviews for these disorders are presented in Chapter 46 by Bradford, Geller, Lesieur, Rosenthal, and Wise. No substantial changes were proposed in the literature reviews for kleptomania and pyromania. Proposals concerning trichotillomania dealt mainly with placement: whether the disorder should be moved from the "impulse control disorders not elsewhere specified" section to the "disorders usually first diagnosed in infancy, childhood, or adolescence" section (because the onset is frequently during childhood or adolescence) or to the "anxiety disorders" section (because the patients frequently exhibit symptoms similar to obsessive-compulsive disorder). Additionally, because the literature review noted that hair pulling was a common associated feature of other mental disorders and selected nonpsychiatric medical conditions, it was proposed that an exclusion criterion be added.

Other impulse control disorders were suggested to the PSID sub-Work Group, but the members felt that they did not warrant inclusion in DSM-IV at this time.

Based on the literature review on pathological gambling, Wise et al. recommended some changes to the DSM-III-R criteria. The main change would be to increase the number of examples of maladaptive gambling behavior from which the clinician may select. The major concern with this change is that it would lower the threshold for making the diagnosis. At the same time, it was felt that this change, along with other text changes in the description of maladaptive gambling behavior, were necessary to distinguish social gamblers from those with a pathological condition. Other text and wording changes were based on their review of the literature.

Much of the attention of this sub-Work Group focused on the DSM-III-R category, "intermittent explosive disorder." Wise et al. found few cases in the psychiatric literature to support the diagnosis of intermittent explosive disorder with no known organic cause. They found that intermittent explosive disorder is a rare condition and that many of the patients who may have received this diagnosis would be more appropriately classified in the DSM-IV as having a secondary personality change, aggressive type. One of the major organic factors felt to be responsible for aggression in this population was traumatic brain injury. Other diagnostic tests such as an electroencephalogram, computerized tomography scan, magnetic resonance imaging, and neuropsychological testing usually provide additional evidence to substantiate this diagnosis. Many patients who have dementia, mental retardation, epilepsy, tumors, central nervous system infections, and intoxication with alcohol and other substances may have aggression as a significant component. However, these individuals would not be diagnosed with intermittent explosive disorder but would be diagnosed with their underlying condition.

Also, patients with antisocial personality disorder and borderline personality disorder may have periods of aggression. Other diagnoses that are commonly associated with aggression include delusional disorder, schizophrenia, and paranoid personality disorder. Some individuals with major depression may have irritable or angry episodes.

Although the PSID Work Group considered the elimination of "intermittent explosive disorder" as a category (with placement in the impulse control disorder not otherwise specified section), this alternative is not recommended, because it would preclude further study of this disorder in both clinical practice and research settings. From their literature review, Wise et al. found that intermittent explosive disorder is indeed a rare condition that should be infrequently diagnosed in the clinical setting. Whenever a patient does present with aggressive symptoms, other underlying nonpsychiatric causes or other psychiatric conditions should be considered first.

Adjustment Disorder

Strain, Wolf, Newcorn, and Fulop (Chapter 47) reviewed the literature on adjustment disorder. They identified two major issues: the lack of explicit operational criteria for the adjustment disorder diagnosis and the use of the disorder as a residual or "wastebasket" diagnosis for those cases that do not fulfill the criteria for another mental disorder. In addition, the adjustment disorder literature review addressed other possible classification schemes that may be considered for this category.

With regard to the lack of explicit operational criteria, Strain et al. recommend several changes in wording for the purpose of clarifying the diagnosis. However, these changes do not address directly the need for more explicit operational criteria. They propose field studies that would employ reliable and valid instruments to determine the exact specification and parameters for this diagnosis. In addition, analyses currently underway of data collected from the Western Psychiatric Institute and Clinic may provide valuable insights concerning the characteristics of patients who receive this diagnosis at different stages of their life.

The authors also recommend that the DSM-IV diagnosis of adjustment disorder should be changed to account for those situations in which a stressor is ongoing for more than 6 months. Additionally, clinicians who give this diagnosis to a patient should consider those situations in which the consequences of a stressful event could become stressors in their own right and should consider situations in which an individual might have prolonged symptoms in relation to a stressful event. Consequently, they recommended specifying adjustment disorder as "acute" for symptoms that persist for no longer than 6 months and "persistent or chronic" for symptoms that have persisted for 6 months or longer. Other proposals that Strain et al. are considering address the manner in which the relationship between the stressor and the adjustment reaction is defined.

The issue of whether adjustment disorder subtypes should be included in DSM-IV was also addressed. More information concerning the number of subtypes and whether they should be included will be obtained once the analysis of the data set from the Western Psychiatric Institute is completed. Additionally, Strain et al. considered a new subtype, "with suicidal behavior," for children, adolescents, or young adults who present with suicidal behavior in reaction to a stressor but who do not meet the diagnostic criteria for any other Axis I or Axis II disorder. Concern about adding a new subtype without documentation in the literature for its existence and that may preclude clinicians from further assessment to rule out other more severe psychiatric conditions was a major concern of the authors.

Finally, the entire question of placement of adjustment disorders was addressed in the literature review. Adjustment disorders could be included as part of a new section for "stress-related disorders." Other alternatives would be to place adjustment disorder subtypes among those disorders with which they share similar phenomenology. For instance, adjustment disorder with depressed mood would be placed within the mood disorder section, adjustment disorder with anxiety would be placed in the anxiety disorders section, and so forth. A final option would be to keep adjustment disorder as a separate section in DSM-IV, as it is treated in DSM-III-R.

Psychological Factors Affecting Physical Conditions

Stoudemire, Beardsley, Folks, Goldstein, Levenson, McNamara, Moran, and Niaura (Chapter 48) examined the diagnostic category, "psychological factors affecting physical condition" (PFAPC) by reviewing the historical background for the PFAPC category, identifying key diagnostic issues, and organizing extensive synopses of the literature for various psychophysiological conditions summarized elsewhere (Stoudemire and Hales 1991). They compiled an extensive literature review, based both on controlled study methodologies and empirically derived data, to support the concept that psychological factors influence many physical conditions. The task for Stoudemire et al.'s sub-Work Group was to determine which revisions to the diagnostic criteria for PFAPC could be made to facilitate a better understanding of the relationship between psychological factors and physical illness. From their review, they conclude that the diagnostic criteria for this category should be made more rigorous, be structured to denote the comorbid effects of Axis I and Axis II conditions, and in particular, that more specificity be applied to designate the types of psychological factors judged to adversely influence medical conditions. Additionally, they felt that proposed criteria should broaden the range of adverse relationships between the psychological and behavioral factors and medical conditions. They proposed that psychological or behavioral factors could adversely affect a nonpsychiatric medical condition in one of three ways: 1) these factors could influence the *course* of the medical condition, 2) these factors could lead to *noncompliance* with treatment recommendations, and 3) the factors could lead to *ignoring risk factors* known to cause or exacerbate the medical condition. Changes in the title of the disorder were made; however, the title remains somewhat cumbersome and difficult to remember. Whether the appropriate subtypes of psychological and behavioral factors have been identified and defined is also discussed.

A major change proposed by the PSID Work Group and the DSM-IV Task Force was to consider moving the category from the mental disorder section to a new section in the DSM-IV titled "other clinically significant problems that may be a focus of diagnosis or treatment." PFAPC would in effect cease to exist as a mental disorder if this proposal is adopted.

Although the category PFAPC has seldom been used in clinical settings or reported as such in the literature, meetings with representatives from general internal medicine, family medicine, and pediatrics, as well as psychiatrists working in medical settings, revealed that this disorder was of great importance to these clinicians. These groups urged that this disorder not be discarded and seemed in agreement with the general principles discussed in the review prepared by Stoudemire et al. Many of the details concerning the subtypes have stimulated discussion among other psychiatric groups for further review and revision.

Summary

The PSID Work Group held its first meeting in September 1988. Since this initial meeting, the size of the PSID Work Group has expanded to include 11 core members and 5 ex-officio members. Each of the members of the PSID Work Group has also consulted a wider group of advisers who have provided invaluable assistance to them in developing diagnostic criteria and text. The following chapters present the literature reviews for the disorders within the PSID Work Group's area of responsibility. The reader should keep in mind that this material represents a snapshot taken at this stage in the development of the DSM-IV and that many of the conclusions and recommendations presented in this section will undergo further review and modification in the months to come.

References

American Psychiatric Association: Diagnostic and Statistical Manual of Mental Disorders, 3rd Edition, Revised. Washington, DC, American Psychiatric Association, 1987

Stoudemire A, Hales RE: Psychological behavioral factors affecting medical conditions and DSM-IV: an overview. Psychosomatics 32:5–13, 1991

Task Force on DSM-IV: DSM-IV Options Book: Work in Progress. Washington, DC, American Psychiatric Association, 1991

World Health Organization: ICD-10 Chapter V. Mental and Behavioral Disorders. Diagnostic Criteria for Research. Geneva, Switzerland, World Health Organization, 1990

Chapter 39

Somatization Disorder

C. Robert Cloninger, M.D.

Statement of the Issues

The major issue regarding the DSM-III-R (American Psychiatric Association 1987) criteria for somatization disorder (SD) is that their complexity makes them difficult to remember and use in clinical practice and research. The criteria are valid but would be more useful if they were shorter and more easily remembered. A second issue is that the organic versus functional distinction in the wording of the DSM-III-R criteria might be taken to suggest that SD has no physiological or organic basis. The revision needs to allow for possible pathophysiological mechanisms that may be discovered in SD.

Significance of the Issues

Complexity

To make a diagnosis of SD, DSM-III-R requires impairment from at least 13 medically unexplained symptoms from 35 possible symptoms, including gastrointestinal, pain, cardiopulmonary, conversion or pseudoneurological, and sexual or reproductive. Assessment of all these symptoms is tedious and time consuming (Manu et al. 1989; Othmer and DeSouza 1985), so that systematic use of the full criteria is often neglected. Failure to use validated and reliable criteria leads to errors in diagnosis, which is unfortunate given the demonstrated utility of the diagnosis for outcome and treatment in psychiatry and primary health care (Guze 1967; Smith 1991; Woodruff et al. 1971). If diagnostic criteria could be developed that were short and easily remembered, this would facilitate more widespread acceptance and use of the diagnosis of SD.

Except for the polysymptomatic nature of SD, no symptom or group of symptoms is specifically required. Each of the 35 symptoms listed in DSM-III-R is given equal weight or significance. This contrasts with the original criteria for Briquet syndrome (BS), from which the DSM-III (American Psychiatric Association 1980) and DSM-III-R criteria for SD were derived. The criteria for BS require at least 1 symptom in at least 9 of 10 possible groups (Guze and Perley 1963). Likewise the abbreviated criteria for SD proposed for ICD-10 require symptoms to be distributed over at least two of four groups (gastrointestinal, cardiopulmonary, genitourinary, and skin and pain symptoms). However, the proposed ICD-10 (World Health Organization 1990) criteria exclude conversion or pseudoneurological symptoms from consideration altogether. The lack of specific requirements for the distribution of symptoms in a list of 35 symptoms means that patients with the same diagnosis may have different patterns of symptom distribution and may not share a single symptom, which may lead to inconsistent findings in research and in clinical practice. The grouping of symptoms in DSM-III-R was designed as a descriptive aid to memory, but assignment of symptoms to different groups was somewhat arbitrary. In particular, pain symptoms occur not only in the pain group but in every other group except conversions (e.g., abdominal pain, chest pain, pain during intercourse or menstruation).

Organicity

According to the DSM-III-R criteria, to count a symptom toward the diagnosis of SD, there can be "no organic pathology or pathophysiologic mechanism" to explain the symptom fully. Such a rigid distinction between organic and functional causation might wrongly suggest that SD has no underlying pathophysiology that is heritable or involuntary. This can contribute to the continued stigmatization of somatizers as weak-willed individuals who voluntarily make complaints for secondary gain according to the view of the general public and as excessively complaining patients by physicians. It may also reinforce attitudes by psychiatrists that are counterproductive to forming an effective therapeutic alliance with the patient (Cloninger 1986a). For DSM-IV, it is desirable to use language that makes it clear that SD is a disease with an identifiable pathophysiology.

Methods

Earlier reviews of the literature were consulted initially (Cloninger 1986a, 1986b; Guze 1967). This was supplemented by Medline searches for articles published between 1966 and March 1991 under several key words relevant to SD. This search identified 108 articles for *somatization disorder* and 55 articles for *Briquet syndrome*. These sources were reviewed for information about alternative diagnostic criteria or screening indices for SD. Second, to evaluate the grouping and weighting of symptoms, other Medline searches were carried out to identify epidemiological information about the relationship between somatization and specific groups of complaints. For example, *somatization and pain* yielded 78 articles with information on the relationship of somatization to the number, severity, and location of pain complaints and associated symptoms. Third, the organicity issue was evaluated by considering reviews of the inheritance and pathophysiology of SD and BS (Cloninger 1986b).

Results

Complexity

First, prior efforts to develop short criteria and screening indices for BS and SD were evaluated. More complete reviews of the validation of Guze's criteria for BS and simplification of those criteria to define SD in DSM-III are presented elsewhere (Cloninger 1986a, 1987). Guze described 59 symptoms in 10 groups as characteristic of BS and required at least 20 symptoms in 9 groups to make the diagnosis. The first effort to simplify and shorten the criteria set for BS identified clusters of 14 symptoms that discriminated patients with BS from those with other psychiatric disorders (Woodruff et al. 1973) and nonpsychiatric medical disorders (Reveley et al. 1977). No one symptom or sign was pathognomonic of BS, and no single cluster of symptoms identified even a majority of BS cases. Of the BS cases, 30% had the syndrome of back pain, abdominal pain, and suicidal thoughts with onset before age 26 years. Another 28% had the combination of recurrent vomiting and the conversion symptom ataxia. Most other cases had the onset of a complex illness before age 26 years with back pain, painful menstruation, and either sexual indifference or conversion symptoms. The recommended screening interview never gained widespread use.

Another effort was made to simplify the BS criteria for DSM-III (Cloninger 1987). Depressive symptoms and panic attacks were omitted from the criteria to avoid overlap with depressive and anxiety disorders. The remaining 37 symptoms that best discriminated persons with BS from others were retained. Requirements about the number of groups were dropped because the total number of somatization symptoms was highly correlated with the number of somatization groups (Cloninger 1987). The resulting criteria for SD were independently shown to be highly concordant with the BS criteria and slightly less time-consuming to apply (DeSouza and Othmer 1984; Swartz et al. 1987).

Nevertheless, the DSM-III criteria were still regarded as too time-consuming and cumbersome, and a screening test was developed (Othmer and DeSouza 1985) that was later incorporated into DSM-III-R. Seven symptoms were found that highly discriminated outpatients with SD from other psychiatric outpatients: vomiting, pain in extremities, shortness of breath when not exerting oneself, amnesia, difficulty swallowing, burning sensation in sexual organs or rectum, and painful menstruation. The presence of three of these seven symptoms was shown to have sensitivity of 73% for 30 outpatients with SD and specificity of 94% for 17 others without SD, for an overall accuracy of 81%. The suggested criterion in DSM-III-R was lowered to two symptoms to improve sensitivity as a screening test.

Meanwhile, studies in multiple community samples from the Epidemiologic Catchment Area (ECA) study (Regier et al. 1984) identified a naturally occurring cluster of somatic symptoms similar to SD. Using a multivariate classification technique called grade of membership analysis, they identified a group of respondents to the Diagnostic Interview Schedule (Robins et al. 1981) with poor overall health characterized by specific complaints of headache, painful urination, abdominal pain, pain during intercourse, vomiting when not pregnant, nausea, diarrhea, sexual difficulties, unusual spells, seizures, and amnesia (Swartz et al. 1986b). In further work, a screening index called the Somatic Symptom Index was developed to maximize predictive accuracy for SD. This index requires 5 of 11 symptoms as a screening threshold for SD (Swartz et al. 1986a). The 11 symptoms making up the Somatic Symptom Index are those that best differentiated 42 patients with SD from 14,750 others in the general population; these included abdominal gas, nausea, diarrhea, sickly feeling, abdominal pain, dizziness, chest pain, fainting spells, pain in extremities, vomiting, and weakness. This list shows that many different symptoms can be used to characterize SD, even in the same sample. Only two symptoms in the two proposed screening tests overlap: vomiting and pain in the extremities.

Some research has been done on the relative diagnostic accuracy of the proposed screening tests in independent samples. In one study of 100 outpatients with chronic fatigue syndrome, Othmer and DeSouza's index was found to have slightly greater sensitivity than the Somatic Symptom Index (Manu et al. 1989). On the other hand, when Othmer and DeSouza's screening test was applied in the ECA community sample, it had a sensitivity of only 70% (Swartz et al. 1987). In another sample of 196 general medical patients with multiple unexplained somatic complaints, DSM-III-R diagnoses of SD were compared to both screening tests through a range of possible symptom thresholds (Smith and Brown 1990). Positive predictive values ranged from 68% to 79%, and negative predictive values ranged from 72% to 81%. This suggests both tests are useful for preliminary screening but not for definitive diagnosis.

Organicity

The organic-functional distinction is considered in more detail in Volume 1 of the *Sourcebook* (Popkin and Tucker 1994). In DSM-III and DSM-III-R, headaches were excluded as possible criterion symptoms because they were to be coded on Axis III as physiologically explained. Common bodily pains and irritable bowel symptoms are highly associated with somatization and related psychopathology (Swartz et al. 1986b; Young et al. 1976). In epidemiological studies, the total number of pain complaints is more predictive of associated psychopathology (i.e., somatization and affective disturbance) (Dworkin et al. 1990) and utilization of health-care services (Von Korff et al. 1991) than the severity, persistence, site, or medical explanation of the complaint. In adoption studies, the number and diversity of common somatic complaints, such as headaches, backaches, abdominal pain, and gyneco-logical complaints, characterize heritable subgroups of somatoform disorders (Bohman et al. 1984; Cloninger et al. 1984). The importance of genetic factors in adoption studies of somatization disorder indicates that heritable pathophysiologi-cal mechanisms play a substantial role in the development of SD. Studies of brain function also indicate neurophysiological differences between patients with SD and others (Cloninger 1986b; James et al. 1989).

Discussion and Recommendations

Complexity

Available screening tests of SD do not have the predictive accuracy needed for definitive diagnostic criteria, but their content is informative. All systematic efforts at developing short criteria for SD have yielded symptom lists that included multiple bodily pains, gastrointestinal symptoms, conversion or pseudoneurologi-cal symptoms, and sexual or reproductive symptoms. Accordingly, the omission of conversion or pseudoneurological symptoms from the criteria proposed for ICD-10 is likely to lead to low concordance with longer criteria for SD and BS that have been validated by follow-up and family studies.

Given the limitations of short symptom lists for the diagnosis of SD, other strategies for improving clinical use of the diagnostic criteria had to be identified. Accordingly, I recommended that all symptoms be arranged into a few groups that are easily remembered and discriminate SD from other disorders: bodily pains, other gastrointestinal symptoms, sexual or reproductive symptoms other than pain, and symptoms suggesting a neurological disorder not limited to pain (con-version or dissociative symptoms). Diagnosis can then proceed by determining whether patients pass a predetermined threshold for number of symptoms from the examples listed in each group rather than by trying to preselect one or two specific symptoms from that cluster for all cases, as in the earlier screening indices. Instead of asking all questions of all patients, time-saving screening can be done by setting a minimum threshold for the number of symptoms required in each group. The requisite number of symptoms in each group can be determined empirically to maximize diagnostic concordance with the full SD and BS criteria; this calibration is being investigated in a DSM-IV field trial. To evaluate the feasibility of this strategy, I carried out analyses in a random sample of 500 psychiatric outpatients including 68 with SD. Empirically, it was found that patients with SD could be more simply characterized as patients with four or more bodily pains, two or more gastrointestinal complaints other than pain, at least one sexual or reproductive symptom, and at least one conversion or dissociative symptom. This definition agreed well with the full SD or BS criteria in the 500 outpatients whom I studied and described in other reports about SD (Cloninger et al. 1986). Cardiopulmonary symptoms were considered as a fifth group of symptoms but were found to be superfluous. In other words, if an individual does not have at least four bodily pain complaints, the diagnosis of SD is excluded, and no further questions need be asked. If they meet the first criterion (bodily pains), each of three additional criteria can be investigated in sequence until SD is either excluded at one step or the diagnosis is established by satisfying all four requirements. This stepwise screening was found to be timesaving in developing and testing assessment instruments for the DSM-IV field trials. In the general population, individuals with a single pain condition do not differ psychiatrically from those with no pain condition; those with pain at two or more sites are likely to have other psychiatric complaints (Dworkin et al. 1990). Patients with SD consistently have pain complaints at several sites. The robustness and generalizability of this screening and diagnostic procedure are being investigated in both psychiatric and primary-care samples in the DSM-IV field trials.

Organicity

The organicity issue is easily addressed. Headaches need not be automatically excluded from consideration. It is recommended that the criteria be revised to say "To count a symptom as significant, it must not be fully explained by a known nonpsychiatric medical condition, or the resulting complaints or impairment are in excess of what would be expected from physical examination or laboratory tests." This does not imply the absence of a discoverable pathophysiological mechanism or stigmatize patients with SD as falsifying or exaggerating their subjective experiences of pain and discomfort.

References

American Psychiatric Association: Diagnostic and Statistical Manual of Mental Disorders, 3rd Edition. Washington, DC, American Psychiatric Association, 1980

American Psychiatric Association: Diagnostic and Statistical Manual of Mental Disorders, 3rd Edition, Revised. Washington, DC, American Psychiatric Association, 1987

Bohman M, Cloninger CR, von Knorring AL, et al: An adoption study of somatoform disorders, III: cross-fostering analysis and genetic relationship to alcoholism and criminality. Arch Gen Psychiatry 41:872–878, 1984

Cloninger CR: Somatoform and dissociative disorders, in The Medical Basis of Psychiatry Edited by Winokur G, Clayton P. Philadelphia, PA, W.B. Saunders Company, 1986a, pp 123–151

Cloninger CR: A unified biosocial theory of personality and its role in the development of anxiety states. Psychiatric Developments 3:167–226, 1986b

Cloninger CR: Diagnosis of somatoform disorders: a critique of DSM-III, in Diagnosis and Classification in Psychiatry: A Critical Appraisal of DSM-III. Edited by Tischler GL. Cambridge, UK, Cambridge University Press, 1987, pp 243–259

Cloninger CR, Sigvardsson S, von Knorring A-L, et al: An adoption study of somatoform disorders, II: identification of two discrete somatoform disorders. Arch Gen Psychiatry 41:863–871, 1984

Cloninger CR, Martin RL, Guze SB, et al: Somatization in men and women: a prospective follow-up and family study. Am J Psychiatry 143:873–878, 1986

DeSouza C, Othmer E: Somatization disorder and Briquet's syndrome: an assessment of their diagnostic concordance. Arch Gen Psychiatry 41:334–336, 1984

Dworkin SF, von Korff M, LeResche L: Multiple pains and psychiatric disturbance: an epidemiologic investigation. Arch Gen Psychiatry 47:239–244, 1990

Guze SB: The diagnosis of hysteria: what are we trying to do? Am J Psychiatry 124:491–498, 1967

Guze SB, Perley MJ: Observations on the natural history of hysteria. Am J Psychiatry 119:960–965, 1963

James L, Gordon E, Kraiuhin C, et al: Selective attention and auditory event-related potentials in somatization disorder. Compr Psychiatry 30:84–89, 1989

Manu P, Lane TJ, Matthews DA, et al: Screening for somatization disorder in patients with chronic fatigue. Gen Hosp Psychiatry 11:294–297, 1989

Othmer E, DeSouza C: A screening test for somatization disorder (hysteria). Am J Psychiatry 142:1146–1149, 1985

Popkin MK, Tucker GJ: Mental disorders due to a general medical condition and substance-induced disorders: mood, anxiety, psychotic, catatonic, and personality disorders, in DSM-IV Sourcebook, Vol 1. Edited by Widiger TA, Frances AJ, Pincus HA, et al. Washington, DC, American Psychiatric Association, 1994, pp 243–276

Regier DA, Myers JK, Kramer M, et al: The NIMH Epidemiologic Catchment Area program: historical context, major objectives, and study populations characteristics. Arch Gen Psychiatry 41:934–941, 1984

Reveley MA, Woodruff RA Jr, Robins LN, et al: Evaluation of a screening interview for Briquet syndrome (hysteria) by the study of medically ill women. Arch Gen Psychiatry 34:145–149, 1977

Robins LN, Helzer JE, Croughan J, et al: National Institute of Mental Health Diagnostic Interview Schedule: its history, characteristics, and validity. Arch Gen Psychiatry 38:381–389, 1981

Smith GR Jr, Brown FW: Screening indexes in DSM-III-R somatization disorder. Gen Hosp Psychiatry 12:148–152, 1990

Smith RC: Somatization disorder: defining its role in clinical medicine. J Gen Intern Med 6:168–175, 1991

Swartz M, Hughes D, George L, et al: Developing a screening index for community studies of somatization disorder. J Psychiatr Res 20:335–343, 1986a

Swartz M, Blazer D, Woodbury M, et al: Somatization disorder in a US Southern community: use of a new procedure for analysis of medical classification. Psychol Med 16:595–609, 1986b

Swartz M, Hughes D, Blazer D, et al: Somatization disorder in the community: a study of diagnostic concordance among three diagnostic systems. J Nerv Ment Dis 175:26–33, 1987

Woodruff RA Jr, Clayton PJ, Guze SB: Hysteria: studies of diagnosis, outcome, prevalence. JAMA 215:425–428, 1971

Woodruff RA Jr, Robins LN, Taibleson M, et al: A computer assisted derivation of a screening interview for hysteria. Arch Gen Psychiatry 29:450–454, 1973

Von Korff M, Wagner EH, Dworkin SF, et al: Chronic pain and use of ambulatory health care. Psychosom Med 53:61–79, 1991

World Health Organization: ICD-10 Chapter V. Mental and Behavioral Disorders. Diagnostic Criteria for Research. Geneva, Switzerland, World Health Organization, 1990

Young SJ, Alpers DH, Norland CC, et al: Psychiatric illness and the irritable bowel syndrome: practical implications for the primary physician. Gastroenterology 70:162–166, 1976

Chapter 40

Conversion Disorder, Proposed Autonomic Arousal Disorder, and Pseudocyesis

Ronald L. Martin, M.D.

Statement of the Issues

In reviewing the DSM-III-R (American Psychiatric Association 1987) conversion disorder criteria during the process of developing the *DSM-IV Options Book* (Task Force on DSM-IV 1991), four diagnostic issues were identified: 1) the diagnostic boundaries of conversion disorder and the delimitation and taxonomic placement of a proposed autonomic arousal disorder and pseudocyesis, 2) the taxonomic placement of conversion disorder, 3) the psychological factors criteria for conversion disorder, and 4) the limitations on the diagnosis of conversion disorder—threshold parameters and preemptions by co-occurring disorders. Possible revisions to the criteria relative to these issues are considered individually from the perspectives of enhancing clinical utility, maintaining consistency with DSM-IV objectives and continuity with tradition, and obtaining compatibility with ICD-10 (World Health Organization 1992).

Methods

The existing literature was reviewed. Major texts and review articles were examined, and primary articles were obtained. Computerized searches were also performed for English language articles published between the years 1980 and 1991. Using the key words *conversion disorder* and *conversion-neurosis* with *diagnosis* (and synonyms), Medline yielded 39 articles, PsycInfo 28, and the National Library of Medicine's Elhill System 71. Additional searches using Medline with the key phrases *autonomic nervous system diseases* and *psychophysiologic disorders* with *mental ill-*

ness, yielded 53 review articles, and searches with the key words *pseudocyesis* and *pseudopregnancy* with *mental illness* yielded 14 articles. Bibliographies in articles obtained through these searches were also reviewed for relevant articles. The implications of this literature review were discussed with the Psychiatric Systems Interface Disorders Work Group.

Issue 1. Diagnostic Boundaries of Conversion Disorder and Delimitation and Taxonomic Placement of Proposed Autonomic Arousal Disorder and Pseudocyesis

Should conversion disorder be narrowed from the broadened DSM-III (American Psychiatric Association 1980) and DSM-III-R definition to include only "pseudoneurological" symptoms (i.e., those suggesting a neurological disorder)? If limited to pseudoneurological symptoms, should these be confined to symptoms affecting sensory or voluntary motor function, thus delimiting conversion from "dissociative" disturbances? If other symptoms subsumed under the DSM-III/ DSM-III-R definition are excluded, such as those involving the autonomic nervous system (e.g., "conversion" vomiting) or endocrine function (e.g., pseudocyesis), where should these symptoms be placed?

Significance

The question of whether to restrict the scope of conversion disorder in DSM-IV was suggested by a number of problems with the inclusive DSM-III/DSM-III-R delineation that broadened the traditional definition. The expansion was based on assumptions about underlying pathogenesis, abandoning any pretense of remaining atheoretical. The broadened definition has led to internal nosological inconsistency and has been of questionable clinical utility. If continued, disparity with ICD-10 would also result.

DSM-II (American Psychiatric Association 1968) characterized "hysterical neurosis, conversion type" as a neurosis "characterized by an involuntary psychogenic loss or disorder of function," affecting the "special senses or voluntary nervous system." DSM-III and DSM-III-R broadened the definition of conversion disorder to encompass disturbances that represented a "loss of, or alteration in, physical functioning that suggests physical disorder," as "an expression of a psychological conflict or need." Symptoms limited to pain or to a disturbance in sexual functioning were excluded.

As amplified in the DSM-III-R text, this definition included symptoms that "may involve the autonomic or endocrine system" in addition to classic conversion symptoms that suggest a neurological disorder. Inclusion of seemingly disparate symptoms under the rubric of conversion was justified on the basis of presumed shared underlying mechanisms. As stated in the text, vomiting "can represent revulsion and disgust"; pseudocyesis is "both a wish for, and a fear of, pregnancy." As admitted in the text, this deviated from the stated general objective of the DSM to avoid etiological or pathophysiological assumptions.

However, the expanded definition was not consistently used even within its source. DSM-III-R somatization disorder criteria included a symptom category designated "conversion or pseudoneurological symptoms," listing amnesia, difficulty swallowing, loss of voice, deafness, double vision, blurred vision, blindness, fainting or loss of consciousness, trouble walking, paralysis or muscle weakness, and urinary retention or difficulty in urinating. Thus, with the possible exception of fainting, all these symptoms were traditional conversion or dissociative symptoms suggesting neurological illness.

In DSM-III and DSM-III-R, symptoms involving the autonomic or endocrine system could also be included under "psychological factors affecting physical condition" (PFAPC), a category introduced to subsume the little-used DSM-II category "psychophysiological disorders," or could be included under Axis III as a "physical disorder" or "condition." Inclusion with conversion disorder required judgment that the symptom was "an expression of a psychological need or conflict," the evaluation of which has been shown to be difficult and of limited utility (Cloninger 1987; Lazare 1981; Watson and Buranen 1979).

Traditionally, *conversion* has been used to denote symptoms involving sensory or motor dysfunction, and *dissociative* has been used to denote symptoms involving integrative functions such as identity, memory, and consciousness. Yet, DSM-III-R listed amnesia and loss of consciousness as "conversion or pseudoneurological symptoms." Clarification of the demarcation of conversion and dissociative symptoms is significant, especially if, as is discussed in the section on issue 2, the dissociative disorders are maintained as a disorder grouping separate from the somatoform disorders.

If pseudoneurological symptoms differ from those involving autonomic or endocrine disturbances with respect to natural history and response to treatment, careful review is warranted from both clinical and research perspectives. If disparate conditions are combined, the clinical utility of conversion disorder would be compromised, and future research concerning conversion disorder would be severely hampered.

Finally, continuing with the broad definition of conversion would result in inconsistency with ICD-10, which, under a unified "dissociative (conversion) disorders" category, includes only pseudoneurological symptoms. Symptoms involving functions primarily under autonomic nervous system control are placed under "somatoform autonomic dysfunction," a category in the new ICD-10 "somatoform disorder" grouping. The psychiatric disorders section of ICD-10 does not include a specific category for symptoms of syndromes such as pseudocyesis involving endocrine function; therefore, such disturbances would not be included with the dissociative (conversion) disorders.

Results

Conversion disorder. The majority of conversion disorder patients in several studies had pseudoneurological symptoms. Folks et al. (1984) reported on 50 patients, all of whom had symptoms suggesting neurological illness; in descending order of frequency, these were spasms, weakness/paralysis, paresthesia/anesthesia, seizures, syncope/spells, visual disturbances, and coma/stupor. In a more recent report by Tomasson et al. (1991), nearly all of 51 conversion disorder patients had main complaints that were pseudoneurological. Two exceptions were patients with pseudocyesis.

Concerning the question of distinguishing dissociative from conversion symptoms, the literature reveals much theoretical discussion, but little empirical data. This is not surprising, because the question is one of definition. As is discussed in the section on issue 2, the literature does support an association between conversion and dissociative symptoms in that they co-occur, may have similar antecedents and underlying factors, and resemble one another in natural history and response to treatment. Some have argued that conversion requires a "dissociated" state of consciousness, but this has not been clearly demonstrated experimentally (Garcia 1990). As pointed out by Coons (1991), the two terms are not synonymous and can be differentiated phenomenologically according to the types of function affected.

As reviewed by Cloninger (1987), pseudoneurological conversion symptoms are generally similar to one another in natural history and response to treatment and differ on these parameters from disturbances involving the autonomic and endocrine systems (Table 40–1). Pseudoneurological conversion symptoms generally develop abruptly, are acutely debilitating, yet are transient. Patients with such symptoms often have had prior pseudoneurological symptoms. Many have somatization disorder. Although it does not necessarily account for their current conversion complaint, a high percentage of patients (17%–38%) have current or prior neurological disease (Ford and Folks 1985). Pseudoneurological conversion symptoms are notably responsive to a variety of treatments or remit spontaneously (Folks et al. 1984). Diagnostically, such symptoms mandate scrutiny for occult neurological disease, which will become manifest in from 25% to 50% of patients (Cloninger 1987; Gatfield and Guze 1962; Watson and Buranen 1979). The range of neurological disorders that have been reported to be initially misdiagnosed as pseudoneurological conversion disorders is broad. As reviewed in a recent report, these include drug-induced dystonic reactions, idiopathic dystonias, sensory seizures, basilar artery migraine, the on-off syndrome of Parkinson's disease, brain tumors, subdural hematoma, Guillain-Barre syndrome, Creutzfeldt-Jacob disease, paroxysmal kinesigenic choreoathetosis, Balint's syndrome, and spinal cord tumors (Jones and Barklage 1990). This list should be looked on as representative rather than exhaustive.

Proposed autonomic arousal disorder.   Symptoms that primarily implicate the functioning of the autonomic nervous system differ in a number of important ways from pseudoneurological symptoms (Cloninger 1987). Conversion vomiting, the DSM-III/DSM-III-R example of a conversion symptom involving the autonomic nervous system, is usually chronic yet not debilitating (Wruble et al. 1982). Response to treatment is inconsistent (Rosenthal et al. 1980). Diagnostically, patients must be scrutinized for nonpsychiatric gastrointestinal medical conditions and for eating disorders. Occult neurological possibilities are restricted primarily to a neurogenic motility disorder such as diabetic autonomic neuropathy (Abell et al. 1988; Ford et al. 1987).

Pseudocyesis.   Conversion disorder and pseudocyesis are similar in that they occur most frequently in medically unsophisticated persons. With greater sophistication of the general public, the occurrence of both syndromes may be declining (Cohen 1982). As with pseudoneurological conversion symptoms, pseudocyesis may develop abruptly. However, it is usually limited by the expected time of delivery or the induction of menses (Cloninger 1987; Small 1986). It also involves objective physical changes that mimic pregnancy. Most cases of pseudocyesis that have been

Table 40–1.   Comparison of proposed DSM-IV disorders

Disorder	Affected function	Degree of impairment	Usual course
Dissociative disorders	Cognition: identity, memory, consciousness	Major but temporary	Transient, may recur
Conversion disorder	Sensory, voluntary motor	Major but temporary	Transient, may recur
Autonomic arousal disorder	Physiological disturbances, involuntary motor	Minor, not debillitating	Chronic or recurrent
Pseudocyesis	Neuroendocrine changes	Major but temporary	Remitting, may recur

thoroughly worked up have shown measurable changes in endocrine hormone level (Cloninger 1987). However, these changes have been inconsistent from patient to patient. As reviewed by Whelan and Stewart (1990), hyperprolactinemia and persistent luteal activity occur in some but not all cases. As reviewed by Starkman et al. (1985), growth hormone, luteinizing hormone, and follicle-stimulating hormone abnormalities have also been observed. Similarity to a galactorrhea-amenorrhea-hyperprolactinemia syndrome has been suggested (Cohen 1982). Affected patients are not likely to have a history of pseudoneurological complaints or somatization disorder (Hardwick and Fitzpatrick 1981). Response to treatment is inconsistent. Diagnostically, patients with pseudocyesis must be differentiated from those with psychotic illness involving delusional pregnancy and those with an occult nonpsychiatric medical endocrine disorder (particularly hormone-secreting tumors) causing a pseudopregnancy.

As to whether conversion disorder and pseudocyesis share a psychological mechanism such as the expression of a psychological need or conflict in a physical symptom, the data are unclear. Psychological hypotheses on the etiology of pseudocyesis abound (Small 1986). Attention has also been directed toward the interpretation of pseudocyesis as a manifestation of an underlying depression (Brown and Barglow 1971; Rubman et al. 1989; Silber and Abdalla 1983).

Discussion

Conversion disorder.　First, the literature review demonstrated that, despite the broadening of the definition in DSM-III and DSM-III-R, *conversion* continues to be used in the pre–DSM-III "pseudoneurological" sense. This supports the option of returning to a narrower definition. The proposed criteria for conversion disorder as they appear in the *DSM-IV Options Book* are shown in Table 40–2. Another point in support of this option is the clinical benefit of isolating symptoms that, in a substantial number of cases, result from occult neurological disorders. Any loss of specificity in identifying such symptoms could delay accurate diagnosis and the institution of effective treatment to decrease potential morbidity and mortality.

Symptoms such as amnesia and loss of consciousness, although perhaps pseudoneurological, are not strictly physical but involve dysfunction in the "integrative functions of identity, memory, or consciousness." Such dysfunctions are described as the essential feature of the dissociative disorders. It is proposed that the dissociative disorders be retained as a separate category (*DSM-IV Options Book*, Task Force on DSM-IV, 1991, p. 13). It would appear that such symptoms would be better included there.

The nonpseudoneurological symptoms differed from the pseudoneurological conversion symptoms in that there were hints as to underlying pathophysiology.

Autonomic nervous system activity is involved in vomiting. Endocrine abnormalities are often present with pseudocyesis. On the other hand, the pseudoneurological symptoms do not conform to known patterns of innervation or endocrine involvement, and no pathophysiological explanation can yet be given.

Continuing with a broad definition of conversion disorder would also cause incongruity with ICD-10, where, although they are categorized as "dissociative disorders," the pseudoneurological symptoms are clearly separated from other symptoms involving alteration or loss of function, many of which are included under somatoform autonomic dysfunction. If symptoms implicating autonomic dysfunction and pseudocyesis are excluded from the DSM-IV conversion disorder, however, where should they be placed?

Proposed autonomic arousal disorder.   The proposed criteria for autonomic arousal disorder are shown in Table 40–3. The ICD-10 category somatoform autonomic dysfunction requires "symptoms of autonomic arousal that are attributed by the patient to a physical disorder of one or more" of the heart and cardiovascular system, esophagus and stomach, lower intestinal tract, respiratory system, and urogenital system. ICD-10 has specific requirements for symptoms in

---

Table 40–2.   Proposed DSM-IV criteria for conversion disorder

A. A development of a symptom or deficit suggestive of a neurological disorder affecting sensation (e.g., blindness, double vision, deafness, loss of touch or pain sensation) or voluntary motor function (e.g., aphonia, impaired coordination or balance, paralysis or localized weakness, difficulty swallowing, urinary retention, seizures).

B. Psychological factors are judged to be associated with the symptom(s) because of a temporal relationship between the initiation (or exacerbation) of the symptoms and stressors, conflicts, or needs.

C. The person is not conscious of intentionally producing the symptom (as in factitious disorder or malingering).

D. The symptom is not a culturally sanctioned response pattern and cannot, after appropriate investigation, be fully explained by a known nonpsychiatric medical condition.

E. The symptom is not limited to pain or to a disturbance in sexual functioning, and does not occur exclusively during the course of somatization disorder.

F. The symptom or deficit causes significant impairment in social or occupational functioning, or marked distress, or requires medical attention or investigation.

Specify if: single episode or recurrent

Specify if:

    acute (duration of less than 6 months)

    chronic (duration of 6 months or more)

each of two symptom groups, a requirement that is not included in the proposed DSM-IV criteria. Such symptoms would have been included in DSM-II under the little-used "psychophysiological disorders" class. As previously mentioned, DSM-III and DSM-III-R were ambiguous as to whether such symptoms were to be considered under conversion disorder or included in the PFAPC grouping, with the physical condition listed on Axis III. However, as Stoudemire et al. (1989) pointed out, PFAPC was rarely used by psychiatrists. In a study of 11,292 general psychiatric patients presenting for care, only 43 were diagnosed with a PFAPC (Mezzich 1989). It remains to be seen whether the newly proposed DSM-IV counterpart "psychological or behavioral factors affecting medical condition" will be better utilized.

The option was proposed to add a category similar to the ICD-10 somatoform autonomic dysfunction to capture such symptoms. The term *autonomic arousal disorder* is proposed. Inclusion in the somatoform disorders grouping makes *somatoform* in the title redundant. An alternative term that was considered was simply *autonomic function disorder*. *Autonomic* was retained in the title to give the category more specificity than the DSM-II "psychophysiological disorder."

The DSM-II category was characterized by physical symptoms involving "intense and sustained" physiological changes in response to emotional factors in a

Table 40–3. Proposed DSM-IV criteria for autonomic arousal disorder

A. The development of one or more persistent or recurrent symptoms, other than pain, attributable to autonomic arousal, in any of the following systems or organs:

    (1) cardiovascular system (e.g., palpitations, chest discomfort, fainting)

    (2) respiratory system (e.g., hyperventilation, dyspnea, hiccup)

    (3) gastrointestinal system (e.g., dry mouth, epigastric discomfort or burning, vomiting, aerophagia, diarrhea, frequent bowel movements)

    (4) urogenital system (e.g., frequent urination, dysuria)

    (5) skin (e.g., flushing, blushing)

B. Psychological factors are judged to be associated with the symptom(s) because of a temporal relationship between the initiation (or exacerbation) of the symptom(s) and stressors, conflicts, or needs.

C. After appropriate investigation, the disturbance cannot be explained by a known nonpsychiatric medical condition or pathophysiologic mechanism (e.g., effects of injury, medication, drugs, or alcohol) other than autonomic arousal.

D. Does not occur exclusively during the course of another mental disorder (e.g., somatization disorder, anxiety disorder, mood disorder, sexual disorders).

E. The symptom(s) cause significant impairment in social or occupational functioning, or cause marked distress.

"single organ system, usually under autonomic nervous system innervation" (p. 46). "Autonomic arousal disorder" implies a similar pathophysiology and thus can be seen as etiologically rather than descriptively based. The text will need to be explicit in qualifying such inferences, maintaining that the principal link between the syndromes included is that they involve functions that are primarily modulated by the autonomic nervous system. The definition should not deny the participation of the autonomic nervous system in certain symptoms, such as difficulty in swallowing and urinary retention, which involve voluntary motor function and are thus considered conversion symptoms.

Two potential autonomic arousal disorders that have been fairly well studied are psychogenic vomiting and the irritable bowel syndrome. Rosenthal et al. (1980), corroborating a determination of psychogenic vomiting on the basis of medically unexplained vomiting that was stress related, episodic, and exacerbated by emotional tension and anxiety, reported that one-third of the patients they studied showed an almost lifelong history of episodic stress-related vomiting. One-sixth were diagnosed with major depression, and two-thirds had various adjustment problems without major depression. High rates of anxiety and depression have been reported in patients with irritable bowel syndrome. Ford et al. (1987) reported that anxiety and depression were more common in irritable bowel patients than in those with serious, disabling gastrointestinal disorders. Conversely, Tollefson et al. (1991) reported that irritable bowel syndrome was more frequent in patients with anxiety and major depressive disorders than in control subjects. Patients with irritable bowel syndrome commonly have additional unexplained nongastrointestinal physical complaints, many of which are also attributable to autonomic arousal (Tollefson et al. 1991).

Why can such disturbances not simply be retained on Axis III as general medical conditions? Psychiatrists are consulted on such problems and are expected to provide suggestions for psychiatric or psychological management. Perhaps this could be addressed by an additional diagnosis of "psychological or behavioral factors affecting medical condition," but this would provide little specificity for communication or future studies. Another option is to relegate such symptoms to undifferentiated somatoform disorder, abandoning all hope for diagnostic precision.

If autonomic arousal disorder is adopted and it parallels the ICD-10 somatoform autonomic dysfunction, boundary issues with other disorders will result, particularly with somatization, anxiety, mood, and sexual disorders. The proposed criteria (see Table 40–3) specifically exclude patients whose symptoms occur exclusively during the course of one of these disorders.

As an example of how an autonomic arousal disorder category would be used, consider an individual who repeatedly experiences diarrhea and abdominal pain in psychologically stressful situations, symptoms for which there is no medical explanation other than irritable bowel syndrome. First, are the symptoms of sufficient severity to warrant a diagnosis? This is addressed in the proposed DSM-IV criteria by requiring that the symptoms "cause significant impairment in social or occupational functioning or cause marked distress." The next question is whether the disturbance was associated with psychological factors because of a "temporal relationship between the initiation (or exacerbation) of the symptom(s) and stressors, conflicts, or needs." Admittedly, these are difficult, subjective judgments. If such a relationship is apparent, a diagnosis of autonomic arousal disorder could be made after consideration of whether the disturbance was subsumed under a somatization, anxiety, mood, or sexual disorder diagnosis.

Pseudocyesis.   The proposed criteria for pseudocyesis are shown in Table 40–4. The literature review demonstrated that pseudocyesis was rare but definable as a discrete entity. Crucial to the diagnosis is not only the false belief of pregnancy, but also objective signs of pregnancy; endocrine changes are often detectable. However, the endocrine findings have been inconsistent, and thus, it cannot be said that a pathophysiological mechanism has been established. Pseudocyesis would thus still be included as a somatoform disorder rather than as an Axis III general medical condition. The fact that endocrine abnormalities are often present suggests the possibility of placing pseudocyesis under the category of psychological or behavioral factors affecting physical condition. Another possible placement would be to include pseudocyesis as an example of somatoform disorder not otherwise specified. This would appear preferable to establishing it as a separate category, given its rarity.

Recommendations

1. Restrict conversion disorder to symptoms suggesting neurological illness (i.e., pseudoneurological symptoms). Thus, symptoms attributed to autonomic nervous system dysfunction and pseudocyesis would be excluded. Symptoms included are those affecting sensory or voluntary motor system functions.

Table 40–4.   Proposed DSM-IV criteria for pseudocyesis (example under somatoform disorder not otherwise specified)

Pseudocyesis: A false belief of being pregnant associated with objective signs of pregnancy, which may include abdominal enlargement with inverted umbilicus, reduced menstrual flow, amenorrhea, subjective sensation of fetal movement, nausea, breast engorgement and secretions, and labor pains at the expected date of confinement. Endocrine changes may be present but the syndrome cannot be explained by a nonpsychiatric medical condition causing endocrine changes (e.g., hormone-secreting tumor).

Symptoms affecting the integrative functions of identity, memory, or consciousness would be delegated to the dissociative disorders. Loss of consciousness does include disturbance in motor function, and it is proposed that it be included as an example of a somatoform disorder not otherwise specified. However, it is also argued that alteration in integrative functions predominates over motor function changes so that it would be better to include loss of consciousness as a dissociative disorder not otherwise specified.

2. Include symptoms attributable to autonomic arousal as an autonomic arousal disorder grouped with the somatoform disorders. This recommendation is made with the realization that the validity of this disorder has not been empirically established. It is hoped that, with a more specific definition than would be obtained with the other options, systematic research would be encouraged that would help to clarify the optimal placement of such problems in the psychiatric taxonomy.

3. Include pseudocyesis as a somatoform disorder not otherwise specified, with criteria as shown in the *DSM-IV Options Book* (Task Force on DSM-IV 1991, p. I:13). The specific wording given in the Options Book criteria was adopted from a reference (Silber and Abdalla 1983) that seemed to represent a synthesis.

Issue 2. Taxonomic Placement of Conversion Disorder

Should conversion disorder continue to be grouped with the somatoform disorders or should it be placed with the dissociative disorders? Alternatively, should the dissociative disorders be placed with the somatoform disorders? Should the presumed linkage of conversion and dissociative disorders be acknowledged in some other way?

Significance

DSM-III and DSM-III-R placed conversion disorder with the somatoform disorders, a grouping based on a shared characteristic, physical symptoms that are not intentionally produced, "suggesting physical disorders for which there are no demonstrable organic or known physiologic mechanisms, and . . . the symptoms are linked to psychological factors or conflicts." A "dissociative disorders" category was established as an independent Axis I grouping. This separation departed from the traditional coupling of conversion and dissociation under the rubric of "hysteria." This union had its roots in antiquity, was made explicit by Janet (Nemiah 1991) and Freud (Ford and Folks 1985) in the late 19th and early 20th centuries, and was preserved in the 1968 DSM-II "hysterical neurosis; conversion, and dissociative types."

The DSM-III/DSM-III-R separation of conversion and dissociative disorders established inconsistency with the international nomenclature. ICD-9 (World Health Organization 1977) grouped conversion and dissociative disorders together under "hysteria." ICD-10, while adopting a "somatoform disorders" category, does not include conversion disorder with this grouping but with a fused "dissociative (conversion) disorders" category consisting of "dissociative amnesia," "dissociative fugue," "trance and possession disorders," "dissociative movement disorders," "dissociative convulsions," "dissociative anaesthesia and sensory loss," "mixed dissociative and conversion disorders," and "other dissociative and conversion disorders." Thus, retaining conversion disorder with the somatoform disorders in DSM-IV would result in inconsistency with the international system.

However, the clinical merits of continued placement with the somatoform disorders must be weighed against the problem of inconsistency with ICD-10. Conversion disorder clearly shares with the other somatoform disorders the essential clinical feature of "unintentional physical symptoms suggesting physical disorder," with the common diagnostic problem of excluding occult physical disorder (general medical condition in DSM-IV). Removing conversion disorder from the somatoform disorder class would seriously call into question the rationale for maintaining the grouping, thus having an effect on the overall structure of DSM-IV. At least in part, the pre–DSM-III taxonomic union of conversion and dissociation was grounded on an assumption about symptom formation based on shared antecedents and underlying psychological processes. The argument for restoring this fusion would be strengthened, although not necessarily mandated, by the empirical demonstration of such an etiological or pathogenetic linkage. Evidence for linkage with other somatoform disorders would also bear on this question.

Results

Except for sharing the essential somatoform characteristic of physical symptoms that suggest a general medical condition, conversion disorder appears to have little relationship to body dysmorphic disorder and hypochondriasis. The literature review supported an association between conversion disorder and multiple personality disorder among the dissociative disorders. In three recent series, conversion symptoms were found to occur in 40% to more than 70% of patients with multiple personality disorder (Coons et al. 1988; Putnam et al. 1986; Ross 1990). This has been attributed to an interpretation that conversion and dissociation have similar antecedents, with recent and remote physical and psychological trauma common to both, and shared underlying psychological and neurophysiological mechanisms (Kihlstrom 1992). Childhood sexual abuse rates as high as 83% have been reported in patients with multiple personality disorder (Putnam et al. 1986). Rates for conversion disorder patients per se were not identified in the studies reviewed, but a sexual abuse rate of more than 50% was reported in women with somatization disorder compared with just over 15% in control subjects with affective disorders in an interview study (Morrison 1989). A chart review study found a history of sexual abuse rate of 18% among somatization disorder patients compared with none in those with affective disorders (Coryell and Norton 1981). As is discussed later, conversion and somatization disorders are closely interrelated.

An association of conversion and dissociative disorders with certain other somatoform disorders is evident. In a study of 40 male "hysterics," conversion and dissociative symptoms coexisted in 10%, conversion and "psychogenic" pain in 48%, with 7% of the patients manifesting all three phenomena (Watson and Tilleskjor 1983). Thus, at least in this study, there was a stronger relationship between conversion and somatoform pain disorder than between conversion and dissociation. Unexplained pain is also frequently found in multiple personality disorder, as are other nonpseudoneurological symptoms of somatization disorder (Ross et al. 1989). As reviewed by Ross et al. (1989), "All investigators to date confirm a high rate of somatic symptoms in multiple personality disorder patients." Ross reported that 35% of multiple personality disorder patients also met criteria for somatization disorder. In addition, amnesia and urinary retention (dissociative and conversion symptoms, respectively), abdominal pain, vomiting, joint pain, and fainting were highly represented in the multiple personality disorder group.

It is evident that conversion disorder is related to somatization disorder. This is hardly surprising because conversion symptoms were part of the predecessor concepts of hysteria or Briquet's syndrome as defined in the Feighner criteria (Feighner et al. 1972) and, along with pain disorder symptoms, are included in the DSM-III, DSM-III-R, and the proposed DSM-IV criteria for somatization disorder. Among the various types of symptoms characterizing somatization disorder, conversion symptoms are prominent. In a study by Guze et al. (1971), more than 90% of patients with "definite" hysteria (i.e., somatization disorder) had at least one conversion symptom, almost 80% had several. Generalization of this finding to more recent studies is somewhat compromised by the fact that amnesia was included as a conversion symptom and the hysteria criteria were not identical to the DSM-III, DSM-III-R, or proposed DSM-IV somatization criteria. However, such problems are mitigated by the fact that most affected patients had multiple conversion symptoms (thus more than amnesia alone), and the hysteria diagnosis was found to be highly concordant with DSM-III somatization disorder (Cloninger et al. 1986).

Conversion symptoms were also common among patients with somatization disorder in a study of 65 somatization and 51 conversion patients (Tomasson et al. 1991). Although they did not receive an additional diagnosis because of DSM-III preemption rules, nearly 20% of somatization disorder patients also met inclusion criteria for conversion disorder. As a group, the 51 patients diagnosed with conversion disorder in this study resembled but were not indistinguishable from the group of somatization disorder patients. The majority (more than 75%) of conversion disorder patients, and nearly all somatization disorder patients were women. The age at onset (first medically unexplained symptom) occurred throughout the life span for conversion disorder patients, but mostly before the age of 21 for somatization patients. Somatization disorder was associated with substantially more impairment in other domains, with somatization patients more likely than conversion disorder patients to have a history of depression, attempted suicide, panic disorder, and divorce. Underscoring the interrelatedness of conversion and somatization disorder, of 32 patients originally diagnosed with conversion disorder, nearly 20% were diagnosed with somatization disorder when reexamined 4 years later (Kent et al. 1993).

Clinically, a somatization disorder diagnosis is useful in distinguishing patients with conversion symptoms from those with similar complaints but with occult general medical conditions (Cloninger 1987). As reviewed by Cloninger (1987), the only other factor shown to have equal utility is a past history of conversion symptoms.

In terms of underlying mechanisms, conversion and dissociation have traditionally been linked because of presumed psychological (particularly psychodynamic) similarities. Conversion is theorized to occur by the repression of an unacceptable thought or affect that is then somatically expressed. Similarly, repression is active in dissociation in which unacceptable mental contents are simply excluded from consciousness. In nonpsychodynamic terms, Kihlstrom (1992) argues that dissociation is intimately involved in conversion because, in addition to the physical symptom, there is a disconnection of the mental representation of the self from mental representation of the dysfunction. Although this is a plausible interpretation, it is not clear what observations would be needed to verify or refute it. Most of the available experimental evidence is based on the study of anecdotally identified patients with multiple personality disorder.

Discussion

The literature review suggests that conversion disorder is associated with at least multiple personality among the dissociative disorders in terms of co-occurrence, demographic similarities, phenomenology, and antecedent abuse. This may warrant recognition in the diagnostic schema. However, conversion disorder was also strongly related to certain somatoform disorders, namely, somatization disorder and pain disorders. The relationship with somatization disorder is particularly intriguing, because conversion disorder, pain disorder, and even dissociative disorder symptoms such as amnesia and unconsciousness are components of somatization disorder criteria. Yet, the etiological and pathogenetic interrelationships among these disorders remain unclear. In this regard, the reason for change in placement is not clear. Actually, it can be argued that dissociative disorders should be placed with the somatoform disorders. Changes in consciousness and in the integrative aspects of mental functioning, although not strictly physical symptoms, also suggest underlying general medical conditions. However, because dissociation symptoms are not strictly physical, this change would require modification of the definition of somatoform disorders.

It must also be remembered that DSM-IV is, for the most part, descriptive rather than etiological in its organization. In discussing the classification of dissociative and somatoform disorders, it has been argued that a classification system is most useful if it maintains a consistent frame of reference (Young 1990). Given the current differences of opinion, it may be best for it to maintain a system that is as phenomenologically based as possible, until clearer agreement on etiology is at hand.

Recommendations

It is recommended that conversion disorder continue to be grouped with the somatoform disorders in DSM-IV. However, given the evidence for an association with the dissociative disorders, there should be a cross-reference to this group in the text for conversion disorder. Phenomenological, demographic, and possibly etiological and pathogenetic relationships with dissociative disorders should be discussed in the DSM-IV text. Instruction should be given in the text that patients with conversion disorders be scrutinized for dissociative symptoms and disorders and likewise that patients with a dissociative disorder be examined for conversion symptoms.

Issue 3. Psychological Factors Criteria for Conversion Disorder

Should an association with psychological factors be required for a diagnosis of conversion disorder? If so, how is the relationship to be specified?

Significance

The DSM-III/DSM-III-R criterion B for conversion disorder requires that "psychological factors are judged to be etiologically related to the symptom because of a temporal relationship between a psychosocial stressor that is apparently related to a psychological conflict or need and initiation or exacerbation of the symptom." Two mechanisms explaining what a patient achieves from a conversion symptom were described in the DSM-III and DSM-III-R texts: 1) keeping an internal conflict or need out of awareness (primary gain) and 2) avoiding noxious activities or achieving environmental support (secondary gain). This description assumed a theoretical basis for conversion disorder that may not be firmly supported by the evidence.

The requirement for psychological factors may still be warranted, however, if such criteria are clinically useful, for example, in distinguishing symptoms attributable to physical disorders from those with no physical explanation.

Results

Lazare (1981) pointed out that, although "several psychological criteria are used to establish the diagnosis . . . there are few empirical data to confirm or refute these criteria." This void still exists. Evaluation of emotional stress, identification of primary or secondary gain, interpretation of a symptom as the symbolic expression of a repressed wish, or a dramatic or suggestible presentation have not been shown to be useful in distinguishing between conversion symptoms and symptoms with an organic explanation (Cloninger 1987; Watson and Buranen 1979). At times, the presumption of a psychological explanation may delay adequate diagnostic scrutiny to detect an underlying physical condition (Jones and Barklage 1990). Contemporary work demonstrates that recent and remote physical and emotional trauma are frequent in patients with conversion disorder, but, because such factors are also associated with somatization and dissociative disorders, they lack specificity. The criteria that have been shown to be helpful in distinguishing between apparent and actual conversion symptoms are descriptive rather than etiological. These include a past history of conversion symptoms and other unexplained somatic complaints and, in particular, a diagnosis of somatization disorder (Cloninger 1987; Folks et al. 1984).

Discussion

Considering the limitations of the "psychological factors" requirement, one option would be to eliminate such a criterion altogether. As defined by the DSM-III/DSM-III-R text, the somatoform disorders are "linked to psychological factors or conflicts." However, similar requirements for linkage to psychological criteria were not included in the DSM-III/DSM-III-R or in the proposed DSM-IV criteria for somatization disorder, hypochondriasis, and body dysmorphic disorder. At best, it appears that the requirement will be fulfilled based on the presumption of a relationship to psychological factors when no organic explanation can be rendered, rather than on positive evidence.

However, elimination of a psychological factor requirement would remove any semblance of a relationship to psychological factors. Although not particularly useful in diagnosis, such factors are important considerations in treatment. It can be argued, however, that, if they are to be included, they should not be defined with specificity. The recent data concerning the importance of psychological trauma in eliciting conversion symptoms (Ross 1990), although not necessarily incompatible with traditional explanations involving more intrapsychic mechanisms, underscore the fact that much more needs to be learned about underlying mechanisms before closure should be attempted.

Recommendations

It is recommended that the requirement for psychological factors be retained but that the etiological implications be lessened by rewording the criteria. Thus, "judged to be etiologically related to" would be changed to "judged to be associated with" (Table 40–2). The diagnostic process is to be carefully reviewed in the text with clinicians encouraged to scrutinize patients who present with conversion symptoms for a past history of conversion symptoms or somatization disorder. The text should strongly warn that perceived relationships to psychological factors should not reduce diagnostic scrutiny for an underlying physical condition.

Issue 4. Limitations on the Diagnosis of Conversion Disorder—Threshold Parameters and Preemptions by Co-occurring Disorders

If a threshold is incorporated, what parameters should be included, and how are they to be defined? Should conversion disorder be subsumed by any other diagnoses? If so, which ones?

Significance

The incorporation of threshold criteria for conversion disorder is significant in terms of preventing the diagnosis of trivial or inconsequential disturbances as mental disorders. For most diagnoses, DSM-III and DSM-III-R required that the disturbance reach a certain level on one of three parameters: 1) impairment in functioning (e.g., dementia, mania, schizophrenia), 2) implied distress or discomfort (depression, anxiety disorders), or 3) symptoms that led the person to receive medical care (somatization disorder). A specified duration of disturbance was often required, with disturbances of shorter duration relegated to "undifferentiated" or "not otherwise specified" categories. No such parameters were defined for conversion disorder. The only restrictions were that a symptom was "not a culturally sanctioned response pattern" and "not limited to pain or to a disturbance in sexual functioning." Additionally, although DSM-III/DSM-III-R criteria per se did not specify when conversion symptoms would be subsumed under another diagnosis, the text states that "Somatization Disorder and, more rarely, Schizophrenia may have conversion *symptoms*" and that a conversion disorder diagnosis should not be made if the symptoms are "due to" either somatization disorder or schizophrenia (DSM-III-R, American Psychiatric Association 1987, p. 259). Because conversion symptoms are part of the somatization disorder criteria, exclusion for that disorder may be warranted. However, exclusion on the basis of schizophrenia would not be justified unless conversion symptoms were shown to be a frequent concomitant.

Because apparent conversion disorder in many instances represents an occult organic disorder or is later seen to be an aspect of somatization disorder, the argument could be made that it is not a disorder at all but a symptom or, at most, a syndrome. Furthermore, whereas somatization disorder has been validated on the basis of follow-up and familial aggregation studies, this has not been the case with conversion disorder.

Results

Conversion symptoms appear to be common. It has been estimated that conversion symptoms occur in 20%–25% of the general population at some time in their lives (Lazare 1981), a figure similar to that reported in a randomly selected series of psychiatric outpatients (Guze et al. 1971). In the latter study, symptoms were "medically significant because they required treatment or interfered with the subject's normal life" (Guze et al. 1969, p. 584). This principle is more fully elucidated by Guze and colleagues in the Feighner criteria (Feighner et al. 1972), which specify that, to be scored positive, individual symptoms must either conform to these requirements or the examining physician must believe that, "because of its clinical importance, the symptom should be scored positive" (p. 58). An example of a conversion symptom was given: "a spell of blindness lasting only a few minutes that the patient minimizes . . . and which did not disrupt the patient's usual routine" (p. 58). Although not specifically mentioned, designation as "clinically important" would capture symptoms that mandate medical scrutiny regardless of a lack of impairment or patient concern.

Regarding preemptions, it does appear that conversion disorder is closely related to somatization disorder, which is frequently diagnosed as the more pervasive disorder when patients are reinterviewed (Kent et al. 1993). Conversion symptoms are not particularly frequent in schizophrenia (Cloninger 1987). Although patients with schizophrenia may present with somatic delusions, it is rarely difficult to distinguish these from conversion symptoms.

Data demonstrating longitudinal stability for conversion disorder do not exist as they do for somatization disorder (Cloninger et al. 1986). In fact, in two studies in which hysteria was defined on the basis of conversion symptoms, a lack of stability and familial aggregation were noted (Guze et al. 1969; Slater and Glithero 1965). In another study, a significant proportion of patients diagnosed with conversion disorder were later diagnosed with somatization disorder (Kent et al. 1993).

Discussion

To limit the diagnosis of conversion disorder to patients with clinically significant conversion symptoms, the option of adding a threshold criterion specifying "significant impairment in social or occupational functioning, or marked distress" is proposed (see Table 40–2). In addition, because patients may be less concerned with the implications of conversion symptoms than would be expected (the so-called *la belle indifférence*), consideration was given to including symptoms that mandate medical attention, regardless of the degree of impairment or distress. Thus, the addition of "requires medical attention or investigation" is proposed. Because a significant percentage of patients with apparent conversion symptoms will turn out to have an occult physical disorder, this addition would appear to be warranted.

Duration criteria were also considered. However, scrutiny for occult neurological illness may be indicated regardless of the duration of the disturbance. Medical scrutiny would also be warranted whether the disturbance was a single episode or recurrent. However, it is acknowledged that specification of these parameters may be useful as descriptors.

In terms of preemptions, conversion symptoms are part of the criteria for somatization disorder and, across time, conversion disorders may represent an incomplete manifestation of somatization disorder. Thus, it would appear that little would be gained by making an additional diagnosis of conversion disorder. DSM-III and DSM-III-R used the same rationale to exclude patients with schizophrenia. However, it does not appear that conversion symptoms are particularly frequent in schizophrenia (Cloninger 1987). Thus, it would be useful to note both diagnoses when they co-occur.

Acknowledging that the diagnosis of conversion disorder has not been validated by longitudinal or family studies, it is proposed that conversion disorder remain a "disorder." It is hoped that the more explicitly delimited definition will engender further research regarding its validity.

Recommendations

Including a requirement that "the symptom or deficit causes significant impairment in social or occupational functioning, or marked distress; or requires medical attention or investigation" is proposed (Table 40–2). A conversion disorder diagnosis will not be made if the symptom is subsumed under a diagnosis of somatization disorder. Although a similar preemption is not proposed for schizophrenia, the text should elaborate on the distinction between conversion symptoms and somatic delusions. Conversion disorder will remain a disorder, but discussion in the text will stress that such a diagnosis of conversion disorder should be seen clinically as tentative relative to scrutiny for underlying organic conditions or the more pervasive somatization disorder.

References

Abell TL, Chung KH, Malagelada J-R: Idiopathic cyclic nausea and vomiting—a disorder of gastrointestinal motility? Mayo Clin Proc 63:1169–1175, 1988

American Psychiatric Association: Diagnostic and Statistical Manual of Mental Disorders, 2nd Edition. Washington, DC, American Psychiatric Association, 1968

American Psychiatric Association: Diagnostic and Statistical Manual of Mental Disorders, 3rd Edition. Washington, DC, American Psychiatric Association, 1980

American Psychiatric Association: Diagnostic and Statistical Manual of Mental Disorders, 3rd Edition, Revised. Washington, DC, American Psychiatric Association, 1987

Brown E, Barglow P: Pseudocyesis: a paradigm of psychophysiological interaction. Arch Gen Psychiatry 24:221–229, 1971

Cloninger CR: Diagnosis of somatoform disorders: a critique of DSM-III, in Diagnosis and Classification in Psychiatry: A Critical Appraisal of DSM-III. Edited by Tischler GL. New York, Cambridge University Press, 1987, pp 243–259

Cloninger CR, Martin RL, Guze SB, et al: A prospective follow-up and family study of somatization in men and women. Am J Psychiatry 143:873–878, 1986

Cohen LM: A current perspective of pseudocyesis. Am J Psychiatry 139:1140–1144, 1982

Coons PM: Commentary: ICD-10 and beyond. Dissociation 3:216–217, 1991

Coons PM, Bowman ES, Milstein V: Multiple personality disorder: a clinical investigation of 50 cases. J Nerv Ment Dis 176:519–527, 1988

Coryell W, Norton SG: Briquet's syndrome (somatization disorder) and primary depression: comparison of background and outcome. Compr Psychiatry 22:249–256, 1981

Feighner JP, Robins E, Guze SB, et al: Diagnostic criteria for use in psychiatric research. Arch Gen Psychiatry 26:57–63, 1972

Folks DG, Ford CV, Regan WM: Conversion symptoms in a general hospital. Psychosomatics 25:285–295, 1984

Ford CV, Folks DG: Conversion disorders: an overview. Psychosomatics 26:371–383, 1985

Ford MJ, Miller PM, Eastwood J, et al: Life events, psychiatric illness, and the irritable bowel syndrome. Gut 28:160–165, 1987

Garcia FO: The concept of dissociation and conversion in the new edition of the International Classification of Diseases (ICD-10). Dissociation 3:204–208, 1990

Gatfield PD, Guze SB: Prognosis and differential diagnosis of conversion reactions: a follow-up study. Diseases of the Nervous System 23:1–8, 1962

Guze SB, Goodwin DW, Crane JB: Criminality and psychiatric illness. Arch Gen Psychiatry 20:583–591, 1969

Guze SB, Woodruff RA, Clayton PJ: A study of conversion symptoms in psychiatric outpatients. Am J Psychiatry 128:643–646, 1971

Hardwick PJ, Fitzpatrick C: Fear, folie, and phantom pregnancy: pseudocyesis in a fifteen-year-old girl. Br J Psychiatry 139:558–560, 1981

Jones JB, Barklage NE: Conversion disorder: camouflage for brain lesions in two cases. Arch Intern Med 150:1343–1345, 1990

Kent D, Tomasson K, Coryell W: Course and outcome of somatoform disorders: a four-year follow-up. Psychosomatics 34:293–297, 1993

Kihlstrom JF: Dissociation and conversion disorders, in Cognitive Science and Clinical Disorders. Edited by Stein DJ, Young J. Orlando, FL, Academic Press, 1992, pp 247–270

Lazare A: Conversion symptoms. N Engl J Med 305:745–748, 1981

Mezzich JE, Fabrega H, Coffman GA, et al: DSM-III disorders in a large sample of psychiatric patients: frequency and specificity of diagnoses. Am J Psychiatry 146:212–219, 1989

Morrison J: Childhood sexual histories of women with somatization disorder. Am J Psychiatry 146:239–241, 1989

Nemiah JC: Dissociation, conversion, and somatization, in American Psychiatric Press Review of Psychiatry, Vol 10. Edited by Tasman A, Goldfinger SM. Washington, DC, American Psychiatric Press, 1991, pp 248–260

Putman FW, Guroff JJ, Silberman EK, et al: The clinical phenomenology of multiple personality disorder: review of 100 recent cases. J Clin Psychiatry 47:285–293, 1986

Rosenthal RH, Webb WL, Wruble LD: Diagnosis and management of persistent psychogenic vomiting. Psychosomatics 21:722–730, 1980

Ross CA: Comments on Garcia's "The concept of dissociation and conversion in the new ICD-10." Dissociation 3:211–213, 1990

Ross CA, Heber S, Norton GR, et al: Somatic symptoms in multiple personality disorder. Psychosomatics 30:154–160, 1989

Rubman S, Goreczny AJ, Brantley PJ, et al: Pseudocyesis and depression: etiological and treatment considerations. J La State Med Soc 141:39–41, 1989

Silber TJ, Abdalla W: Pseudocyesis in adolescent females. J Adolescent Health Care 4:109–112, 1983

Slater ETO, Glithero C: A follow-up of patients diagnosed as suffering from "hysteria." J Psychosom Res 9:9–13, 1965

Small GM: Pseudocyesis: an overview. Can J Psychiatry 31:452–457, 1986

Starkman MN, Marshall JC, La Ferla J, et al: Pseudocyesis: psychologic and neuroendocrine interrelationships. Psychosom Med 47:46–57, 1985

Stoudemire GA, Strain JJ, Hales RE: Editorial. Psychosomatics 30:239–244, 1989

Task Force on DSM-IV: DSM-IV Options Book: Work in Progress. Washington, DC, American Psychiatric Association, 1991

Tollefson GD, Tollefson SL, Pederson M, et al: Comorbid irritable bowel syndrome in patients with generalized anxiety and major depression. Ann Clin Psychiatry 3:215–222, 1991

Tomasson K, Kent D, Coryell W: Somatization and conversion disorders: co-morbidity and demographics at presentation. Acta Psychiatr Scand 84:288–293, 1991

Watson CG, Buranen C: The frequency and identification of false positive conversion reactions. J Nerv Ment Dis 167:243–247, 1979

Watson CG, Tilleskjor C: Interrelationships of conversion, psychogenic pain, and dissociative disorder symptoms. J Consult Clin Psychol 51:788–789, 1983

Whelan CI, Stewart DE: Pseudocyesis—a review and report of six cases. Int J Psychiatry Med 20:97–108, 1990

World Health Organization: International Statistical Classification of Diseases, Injuries, and Causes of Death, 9th Revision. Geneva, Switzerland, World Health Organization, 1977

World Health Organization: The ICD-10 Classification of Mental and Behavioral Disorders: Clinical Descriptions and Diagnostic Guidelines. Geneva, Switzerland, World Health Organization, 1992

Wruble LD, Rosenthal RH, Webb WL: Psychogenic vomiting: a review. Am J Gastroenterol 77:318–321, 1982

Young WC: Comments on Dr. Garcia's article. Dissociation 3:209–210, 1990

Chapter 41

Somatoform Pain Disorder

Steven A. King, M.D., and James J. Strain, M.D.

Statement of the Issues

This review focuses on the following issues:

1. Is somatoform pain disorder a valid and reliable diagnosis?
2. Are there factors that limit the clinical application of somatoform pain disorder?
3. To what extent can pain be considered a mental disorder?
4. Are there alternative classification systems that may replace somatoform pain disorder?

Significance of the Issues

Each of the previous editions of the DSM has addressed the problem of pain and in so doing has sought to define the extent to which it might be considered a mental disorder. In DSM-II (American Psychiatric Association 1968), painful conditions caused by emotional factors were included in the "psychophysiological disorders." A new category specifically addressing pain, "psychogenic pain disorder," was introduced in DSM-III (American Psychiatric Association 1980). The essential features of this diagnosis were a complaint of pain, with evidence of psychological factors playing an etiological role, and either an absence of organic pathology to account for the pain or, if identifiable organic pathology was present, a degree of pain that was not consistent with the level of the physical findings. In DSM-III-R (American Psychiatric Association 1987), three major changes were made in this diagnosis: 1) the requirement that etiological psychological factors be present was eliminated; 2) the requirement that the pain not be due to another mental disorder was eliminated; and 3) instead of the pain itself being a criterion, "preoccupation with pain for at least 6 months" was required. In accordance with these changes, the category was renamed "somatoform pain disorder."

Despite this evolution in the DSM classification of pain, somatoform pain disorder has been the subject of criticism, and problems in its use have been identified (Blackwell et al. 1989; Dworkin and Burgess 1987)

Methods

A computer search for all journal articles published in English from 1966 through April 1991 was performed with Medline using the index term *pain* and each of the following terms: *DSM-III, DSM-III-R, mental disorders, taxonomy, classification, psychogenic,* and *somatoform.* In addition, all issues of the three major pain journals, *Pain, The Clinical Journal of Pain,* and *Journal of Pain and Symptom Management,* were reviewed for relevant articles. More than 2,000 references in English were identified. Where available, abstracts for the references were obtained and used to evaluate their relevance to the stated issues. Where there were an extensive number of articles on specific topics published over an extended period, review articles and those published during the last 5 years were read. Approximately 250 articles were reviewed.

We identified and reviewed 33 papers that described studies in which DSM-III criteria were applied to patients with pain. Of these, 6 appeared to use the same patient cohorts described in other papers and are therefore not included here (Chaturvedi 1987; Fishbain et al. 1988, 1989; Harrop-Griffiths et al. 1988; Hudson et al. 1984; Katon et al. 1988). The 27 remaining papers are listed in Table 41–1. As noted in the table, several of the studies only focused on specific diagnostic categories and did not seek to apply all the possible alternatives.

Only five articles in which DSM-III-R criteria were applied to patients with pain were found (Beitman et al. 1989; Gallagher et al. 1991; Parmalee et al. 1991; Schover 1990; Wulsin et al. 1991). It is unclear whether this scarcity reflects the limits of the usefulness of DSM-III-R criteria for this patient population or whether there has been insufficient time since its introduction for its application and for appropriate research to be performed.

Results

Is Somatoform Pain Disorder a Valid and Reliable Diagnosis?

None of the five articles that were identified as applying DSM-III-R to patients with pain employed the diagnosis of "somatoform pain disorder." Beitman et al. (1989)

Table 41–1.   DSM-III studies of patients with pain

Investigators	Patient population	DSM-III Axes I and II diagnoses	
Beitman et al. 1988	33 patients with chest pain with normal coronary arteries by cardiac catheterization	33% panic disorder 15% major depression	
Benjamin et al. 1988	106 patients at an outpatient pain clinic (91% had pain for >6 months)	33% major depression 15% hypochondriasis	
Bouckoms et al. 1985	62 patients with pain >6 months' duration admitted to an inpatient neurosurgery service	30% PFAPC 26% no diagnosis 24% major depression 11% personality disorder 5% somatoform disorder 5% dementia	
Chaturvedi and Michael 1986	203 patients with pain >3 months' duration and without identifiable organic pathology treated in an outpatient psychiatry department	43% dysthymic disorder 20% anxiety disorder 9% psychogenic pain disorder 8% conversion disorder 7% major depression	
Cormier et al. 1988	98 patients with chest pain who underwent cardiac testing	− cardiac tests	+ cardiac tests
		47% panic disorder	6%
		43% multiple phobias	12%
		39% major depression	8%
		20% no diagnosis	74%
		10% alcohol abuse/ dependence	6%
Fishbain et al. 1986	283 patients with pain >2 years' duration evaluated at pain clinic	59% personality disorder 43% adjustment disorder/anxious mood 38% conversion disorder 28% adjustment disorder/ depressed mood 23% dysthymic disorder 15% generalized anxiety disorder 15% alcohol and other drug dependence 13% adjustment disorder/work inhibition 10% intermittent explosive disorder 8% dementia 0.3% psychogenic pain	

(continued)

Table 41–1. DSM-III studies of patients with pain *(continued)*

Investigators	Patient population	DSM-III Axes I and II diagnoses
France et al. 1986[a]	44 patients with low back pain >6 months admitted to inpatient pain program	54% major depression
France et al. 1984	42 patients with low back pain >6 months with identifiable organic etiology admitted to inpatient pain program	52% major depression 24% dysthymic disorder 24% adjustment disorder/ depressed mood
France et al. 1987a	73 patients with chronic low back pain admitted to an inpatient pain program	47% major depression 7% dysthymic disorder
France et al. 1987b	39 patients with low back pain for >6 months	31% major depression other diagnoses were made but results not provided
France et al. 1988[a]	15 patients with low back pain for >6 months	40% major depression
Goldenberg 1986	82 patients with fibromyalgia/ fibromyositis in arthritis clinic	3% major depression 8% other unspecified disorders
Haley et al. 1985[a]	63 patients with chronic pain evaluated in pain clinic	49% major depression
Hudson et al. 1985	31 patients with fibromyalgia and pain >3 months in arthritis clinic	68% no diagnosis 26% major depression 6.4% somatization disorder
Jenkins 1991	25 patients with abdominal pain without organic cause referred to psychiatrist	28% major depression 24% psychogenic pain 20% conversion disorder
Katon et al. 1985	37 patients with pain >1 year in inpatient pain program	32% major depression 19% opioid dependence 16% somatization disorder
King and Strain 1989	167 general hospital inpatients with pain referred for psychiatric consultation	22% no disorder 16% adjustment disorder/ depressed mood 14% PFAPC 13% dysthymic disorder 10% opioid dependence 6% major depression 3% psychogenic pain
Kirmayer et al. 1988	20 patients with fibromyalgia treated by a rheumatologist	Only provided lifetime prevalence

Table 41–1. DSM-III studies of patients with pain *(continued)*

Investigators	Patient population	DSM-III Axes I and II diagnoses
Large 1986	50 patients with pain >6 months referred from pain clinic to psychiatrist	40% personality disorder 34% PFAPC 28% dysthymic disorder 8% psychogenic pain 8% somatization disorder 8% major depression
Love 1987[a]	68 patients with low back pain >6 months	25% major depression
Magni et al. 1984[a]	29 patients with pelvic pain >6 months (62% had + laparoscopy) (38% had − laparoscopy)	45% without organicity had major depression
Muse 1985	64 patients with pain >6 months seen in pain clinic	14% PFAPC 14% psychogenic pain 12% dysthymic disorder 11% generalized anxiety disorder 5% adjustment disorder/depressed mood 5% adjustment disorder/anxious mood
Reich et al. 1983	43 patients with chronic pain evaluated by a pain board	47% personality disorder 32% psychogenic pain 23% major depression 28% substance use disorder 19% PFAPC 14% adjustment disorder 14% V codes 12% somatization disorder
Remick et al. 1983	68 patients with atypical facial pain >6 months seen in pain clinic	26% no diagnosis 18% somatoform disorder 13% major depression 10% psychosis 8% adjustment disorder 7% personality disorder
Turner and Romano 1984	40 inpatients and outpatients with pain >6 months referred to a pain clinic	30% major depression

(continued)

Table 41–1. DSM-III studies of patients with pain *(continued)*

Investigators	Patient population	DSM-III Axes I and II diagnoses
Valdes et al. 1988[a]	41 patients diagnosed with psychogenic pain	Did not provide information on number of patients in cohort from which this subgroup was selected. Therefore, cannot determine what percentage of the patient population was diagnosed with this disorder
Walker et al. 1988	25 patients with pelvic pain >3 months (52% + laparoscopy) (48% − laparoscopy)	52% functional dyspareunia 32% phobias 28% inhibited sexual desire 28% inhibited sexual excitement 20% alcohol dependence or abuse 16% inhibited orgasm 12% drug dependence or abuse 8% panic disorder

Note. PFAPC = psychological factors affecting physical condition. DSM-III diagnoses show those found in >5% of the patient populations with the exception of psychogenic pain disorder.
[a]Patients were not evaluated for all DSM-III diagnoses.

examined the prevalence of panic disorder and major depression in chest pain patients with normal or near-normal coronary arteries by cardiac catheterization. They reported that 34% of the 94 patients met the criteria for panic disorder and 12% met the criteria for major depression. Schover (1990) only used DSM-III-R to evaluate mood and anxiety disorders in 48 male patients with genital pain in the absence of organic findings and diagnosed major depression in 27%. She did not employ the DSM-III-R pain-related diagnoses but rather used the terms *chronic nongenital pain* (50% of the patients studied) and *somatization disorder* (56%) without identifying the diagnostic criteria for either. Gallagher et al. (1991) observed a lifetime history of major depression in 41% of 84 female patients with temporomandibular pain and dysfunction syndrome. Parmelee et al. (1991) found a correlation between the presence and severity of pain and major depression among geriatric patients. Finally, Wulsin et al. (1991) studied 35 patients with atypical chest pain referred from an emergency room to a chest pain clinic and identified major depression in 23%, dysthymia in 17%, panic disorder in 31%, generalized anxiety disorder in 23%, and other anxiety disorders in 14%; 29% of the patients had various other Axis I disorders.

Because of the lack of relevant research on the use of somatoform pain disorder, the questions of its validity and reliability must be based to a certain degree on studies employing its DSM-III predecessor, "psychogenic pain disorder." In the studies that applied DSM-III to patients with pain, the diagnosis of psychogenic pain disorder was used infrequently (see Table 41–1). In the seven studies that employed this diagnosis, the following frequencies were reported: 9% of patients with pain for more than 3 months without identifiable organic pathology treated in an outpatient psychiatry department (Chaturvedi and Michael 1986); 0.3% of patients with pain for more than 2 years evaluated at a pain clinic (Fishbain et al. 1986); 24% of patients with abdominal pain without identifiable organic pathology referred to a psychiatrist (Jenkins 1991); 3% of general hospital inpatients with pain referred for psychiatric consultation (King and Strain 1989); 8% of patients with pain for more than 6 months referred from a pain clinic for psychiatric evaluation (Large 1986); 14% of patients with pain for more than 6 months seen in a pain clinic (Muse 1985); and 32% of patients with chronic pain evaluated by a pain board (Reich et al. 1983). In seven other studies where it is clear that psychogenic pain disorder was a diagnostic alternative, it was not used at all (Beitman et al. 1988; Benjamin et al. 1988; Bouckoms et al. 1985; Cormier et al. 1988; Hudson et al. 1985; Katon et al. 1985; Walker et al. 1988). An obvious problem in interpreting these results is the lack of uniformity in the patient populations, although there was great variability in the results even where the cohorts appeared to be similar.

One of the modifications in somatoform pain disorder that might increase its utilization in contrast to psychogenic pain disorder is the removal of the requirement that the "pain not be due to another mental disorder." Pain has been found to be a symptom of many other mental disorders (Dworkin and Caligor 1988; France and Krishnan 1988). Although it is possible that the modifications made in DSM-III-R might result in a change in its applicability to pain patients, it appears that many of the problems encountered in using psychogenic pain disorder still remain with somatoform pain disorder.

Are There Factors That Limit the Clinical Application of Somatoform Pain Disorder?

As noted earlier, whereas this diagnosis has apparently not yet been used in published research, the journal review process indicated that there are multiple problems that may markedly impair its employment:

1. Even when pain is a major part of the presenting picture, under the DSM-III-R classification system, it still may not be identified as such on Axis I. Although DSM-III-R requires the presence of "preoccupation with pain," it offers no guidance as to the meaning of this term, thereby leaving it open to individual interpretation.

2. As with the diagnosis of psychogenic pain disorder, there are problems in attempting to determine whether the pain is in "excess" of what would be expected.

The current literature indicates that there is no clear correlation between the level of pain and physical findings. For example, Gore et al. (1987) reported minimal correlation between radiological changes and the presence and severity of pain in patients who were evaluated 10 or more years after the initial onset of neck pain. Valkenburg and Haanen (1982) found that, even in the presence of spinal abnormalities of a severity sufficient to cause distress, pain is frequently absent. Therefore, pain remains a subjective report, with no criterion for ensuring the reliability or validity of the symptom picture or diagnosis.

It is suggested that the failure to identify underlying physical conditions that are etiologically related to the pain may occur because these conditions have not yet reached the threshold of clinical detection (e.g., subsyndromal) or because of deficiencies in the medical history or workup and perhaps inadequate training of physicians in the diagnosis of pain-related conditions (Gunn and Sola 1989; Hendler et al. 1982; Rosomoff et al. 1989). Furthermore, many of the therapies used for pain, such as medications, surgery, and extended periods of inactivity, can cause or exacerbate pain, further clouding its original etiology (King and Strain 1990; Osterweis et al. 1987). Because most patients with pain are not evaluated by mental health professionals until long after the onset of the pain, if they are evaluated at all, attempts to delineate the role of psychological factors and of nonpsychiatric medical conditions become more difficult, thus compounding the problems encountered in use of "somatoform pain disorder."

3. This diagnosis is not applicable to the majority of patients with chronic pain and the many patients with acute pain where both psychological factors and nonpsychiatric medical conditions are simultaneously involved in the development or maintenance of the pain, or to that group of patients who are reacting to their pain in a dysfunctional manner (Osterweis et al. 1987).

4. The diagnosis of somatoform pain disorder perpetuates the dualistic view that there is a difference between pain of organic origin and pain of psychological origin, a view that is unsupported by the literature. Attempts to find evidence for this by the use of psychological testing and neurochemical markers have generally failed (Main et al. 1991; Trief et al. 1987).

The use of somatoform pain disorder suggests that the pain it addresses is somehow different from pain for which there is an identifiable organic etiology. Unfortunately, this has often led to the belief that this pain is not "real," although it is clear that even when the etiological factors involved in the pain are psychological, the patient's perception of the pain is the same, and his or her suffering is as real. Thus, this diagnosis may unfairly stigmatize the patients to whom it is applied, prevent them from receiving appropriate treatment for their problems, and limit the involvement of mental health professionals, especially psychiatrists, in their care.

5. In DSM-III-R, there is no diagnostic category for acute pain. No single universal definition has yet been accepted for differentiating acute from chronic pain. In its classification system, the Subcommittee on Taxonomy of the International Association for the Study of Pain recommended that pain of greater than 3 months duration should be considered chronic (Merskey 1986). Others have suggested that the term *chronic pain* should not be defined by any specific time limit but rather should be used when the pain endures beyond the expected period for its resolution (Brena et al. 1984). However, from reviews of the literature, it appears that the definition most frequently employed is pain lasting 6 months or longer (Report of the Commission on the Evaluation of Pain 1987).

Although much research on pain has focused on the significance of psychological factors in the development and perpetuation of chronic pain, there is substantial evidence to support the role of these factors in acute pain and of psychologically based treatment modalities in its management, as discussed below (Chapman and Turner 1986).

To What Extent Can Pain Be Considered a Mental Disorder?

Although pain has not traditionally been considered a mental disorder, many current definitions of pain accept the primacy of psychological factors in the pain experience. The Subcommittee on Taxonomy of the International Association for the Study of Pain reported, "Activity induced in the nociceptor and nociceptive pathways by a noxious stimulus is not pain, *which is always a psychological state,* even though we may well appreciate that pain most often has a proximate physical cause" (Merskey 1986, p. S217, emphasis added). The Institute of Medicine Committee on Pain, Disability, and Chronic Illness Behavior stated, "The experience of pain is more than a simple sensory process. It is a complex perception involving higher levels of the central nervous system, emotional states, and higher order mental processes" (Osterweis et al. 1987, p. 13). Clearly there is a need to reassess the belief that, when an identifiable physiological process is playing a major role in pain, the recognition of psychological factors is of minimal importance in evaluation and treatment.

Reviews of the literature indicate that chronic pain has been found to be associated with virtually all Axis I diagnoses (Dworkin and Caligor 1988; France and Krishnan 1988). Whereas it is reported that mental disorders are more likely to be present when there is no identifiable physical etiology for the pain, they frequently occur even when there is organic pathology.

Much of the research on the association between pain and mental disorders has been devoted to the relationship between chronic pain and depression: the prevalence of depression in patients with chronic pain ranges from 10% to 100% (Romano and Turner 1985; Roy 1986/1987; Turner and Romano 1984). The exact nature of this association is the subject of controversy; it is unclear whether the depression is secondary to the pain, depression predisposes one to pain, or whether the two problems coexist either independently or as the result of common neurophysiological mechanisms (Blumer and Heilbronn 1982; Brown 1990; Feinmann 1985; Flor and Turk 1984; Gamsa 1990; Pilowsky 1988). In delineating this relationship, there is the additional problem of determining whether the most common symptoms of depression including sleep impairment, changes in appetite, anhedonia, and fatigue are due to the mood state, the pain, or the underlying physical illness, if one is identified. As indicated by Table 41–1, depression is the mental disorder most commonly found in patients with chronic pain.

The extent to which acute pain in association with an identifiable organic etiology should be considered a mental disorder is debatable. Beecher's (1946) observations on battlefield casualties, whose levels of pain were much less than expected given the severity of their wounds, indicate that psychological factors play a significant role in acute pain. Egbert et al. (1964) support this association with their findings that preoperative psychological preparation of a patient has a profound influence on postsurgical recovery, including the degree of pain described by the patient. Additionally, it is postulated that cultural factors and ethnicity may play significant roles in both acute and chronic pain (Zborowski 1969).

Are There Alternative Classification Systems That May Replace Somatoform Pain Disorder?

Many classification systems for pain have been proposed, but none has yet received widespread acceptance; most have concentrated on chronic pain and specific types of pain (e.g., most commonly back pain). A number of these taxonomical systems focus on the physical manifestations of pain (Merskey 1986; Olesen 1988). Those systems that do address the psychological aspects of the problem generally employ existing psychological instruments such as the Minnesota Multiphasic Personality Inventory (MMPI) (Hathaway and McKinley 1970) or have created new instruments to serve as the basis of classification (Costello et al. 1987; McNeill et al. 1986). Five classification systems for chronic pain have received the most attention in the literature, although none has been employed with any substantial frequency in published research.

The Subcommittee on Taxonomy of the International Association for the Study of Pain (Merskey 1986) proposed a five-axes classification system categorizing pain according to: I) anatomical region, II) organic system, III) temporal characteristics of pain and pattern of occurrence, IV) patient's statement of intensity and time since onset of pain, and V) etiology. This schema provides for comments on psychological factors on both the second axis, where psychiatric illness can be coded, and the fifth, where possible etiologies include "psychophysiological" and "psychological." It is important to note that the diagnosis of the psychiatric illness is based on current classification systems for mental disorders such as DSM-III-R.

Black (1975) described a "chronic pain syndrome," in which the patient suffers from "intractable, often multiple pain complaints, which are usually inappropriate to existing somatogenic problems; multiple physician contacts and many nonproductive diagnostic procedures; excessive preoccupations with the problem of pain; [and] an altered behavior pattern with some of the features of depression, anxiety, and neuroticism" (p.1000). Several of the difficulties encountered in the utilization of somatoform pain disorder are also encountered here. Furthermore, some of the factors described, such as the overuse of diagnostic procedures, may be related as much to limitations in training and knowledge about pain among medical professionals as to patient behavior.

Brena (1984) reported the development of the Emory Pain Estimate Model, which classifies patients based on both physical and psychological criteria. The behavioral rating includes the patient's activity, description of the pain, drug use, and MMPI scores; the physical assessment is based on the examination and diagnostic procedures. Using this model, the author divided patients with chronic pain into four classes. A significant concern with this model is its reliance on the MMPI, the validity of which is questioned for chronic pain patients (Main et al. 1991).

Turk and Rudy (1987) proposed the Multiaxial Assessment of Pain based on the West Haven–Yale Multidimensional Pain Inventory, a 52-question instrument. They identified three classes of patients whom they described as "dysfunctional," "interpersonally distressed," and "adaptive copers."

The Commission on the Evaluation of Pain (Report of the Commission on the Evaluation of Pain 1987) developed a method for classifying the disability status of patients with pain for the Social Security Administration. It described two groups of chronic pain patients, those with "competent coping" and those with "inability to cope," and subdivided these into "insufficient documented impairment" and "sufficient documented impairment." This system provides little information on the factors involved in the development and maintenance of the pain.

At this time, there does not appear to be any available diagnostic system for pain that is adaptable to the requirements of DSM-IV.

Discussion

Although the current literature does not provide any clear guidance as to how the problem of pain should be addressed in DSM-IV, there are apparent weaknesses in somatoform pain disorder that suggest that this diagnosis should be revised. In determining a more optimal approach for the classification of pain for DSM-IV, the following issues are regarded as essential: 1) that the problem of pain be coded when it is a significant part of the presenting picture, 2) that both acute and chronic pain be included, 3) that provision be made for the delineation of factors involved in either the onset or maintenance of the pain, and 4) that the diagnostic category not mandate training and knowledge about pain beyond that expected of the majority of DSM-IV users.

Two major options have been considered for classifying pain in DSM-IV. The first is that there be no separate diagnostic category for pain and that where there are psychological factors involved in the etiology or maintenance of the pain, they be identified by Axis I or II diagnoses, with the pain being classified on Axis III. An advantage of this approach is that it avoids the separation of pain into "psychogenic" and "organic" categories. However, it does not allow for any comment on the association between the psychological factors and the pain, if this can be discerned.

The second alternative is to adopt the conceptual framework of the DSM-III-R classification of sleep disorders as a template for the classification of pain in DSM-IV. Because both sleep disorders and pain are symptoms that can be related to many other disorders that are both psychological and nonpsychological, this is an important taxonomic parallel for pain. Thus, pain might be similarly classified as: "related to another mental disorder," "related to a known organic factor," or "not otherwise specified." In such a classification, two additional categories would be considered: "pain related to both another mental disorder or psychological factors *and* a known organic factor" and "pain related to psychological factors," where these factors are subthreshold for the diagnosis of another mental disorder.

The most significant criticism of this approach is that sleep disorders have generally been viewed as mental disorders, even when they are secondary to an organic condition, whereas there is no similarly accepted view for pain. Furthermore, the "sleep disorders" category was based on the abridgment of an existing diagnostic classification for sleep. None of the available systems for classifying pain can be so abridged for DSM-IV. Despite these concerns, this alternative with appropriate modifications was found to be the best, and recommendations based on this are described below.

Recommendations

The deficiencies in somatoform pain disorder lead to a proposal for a new, more broadly defined diagnostic schema for pain. The Psychiatric System Interface

Disorders Work Group has suggested that, in DSM-IV, somatoform pain disorder should perhaps be replaced by a new diagnostic category, "pain disorder." Because this category will extend beyond the traditional concepts of a somatoform disorder, the Work Group considered the option of creating a completely separate domain for pain similar to that used for the sleep disorders in DSM-III-R. However, to keep pain contiguous with other disorders in which physical complaints are paramount, the current proposal is that it should be retained under the somatoform disorders rubric for DSM-IV.

The criteria for this proposed new category are: (A) Pain in one (or more) anatomical site(s) is a major part of the clinical presentation; and, (B) The pain causes significant impairment in occupational or social functioning, or causes marked distress. The extent and nature of these qualifying statements is debatable. Although there is support for the inclusion of all pain, it was decided that there should be a "high threshold" before pain is considered to be a mental disorder.

Within the category of pain disorder, four subtypes are recommended:

1. Psychological type, where psychological factors are judged to account for the onset, severity, or exacerbation of the pain. If a nonpsychiatric medical condition is present, it is judged to play no more than a minor role in accounting for the pain.
2. Secondary type due to a nonpsychiatric medical condition, where a nonpsychiatric medical condition is present that accounts for the onset, severity, or exacerbation of the pain. If psychological factors are present, they play only a minor role in accounting for the pain.
3. Combined type, where both psychological factors and a nonpsychiatric medical condition are judged to play important roles in the onset, severity, or exacerbation of the pain.
4. Unspecified type.

Each subtype would be further specified as being acute (pain of less than 6 months duration) or chronic (pain of 6 months or greater duration). This division between acute and chronic is chosen because it is the one most commonly encountered in the literature. Furthermore, the proposed criteria for a number of other DSM-IV diagnoses, including "adjustment disorders," provide for specifying a similar period to differentiate between acute and chronic conditions.

A possible alternative to subtyping is to have each of these as a separate type. The decision to recommend subtyping is based on the belief that it is best to view pain as a single entity with multiple factors involved in its etiology and maintenance.

The optimal method for classifying pain secondary to a nonpsychiatric medical condition is controversial. To be consistent with ICD-10, which does not provide for identification of this type of pain in its mental disorders section, it is recommended that either it be classified in the "other clinically significant conditions" section of DSM-IV or that it be retained with the other pain subtypes for the sake of including a complete list of the diagnostic possibilities for pain and be accompanied by an explanatory statement noting that this particular subtype is not considered to be a mental disorder per se.

In summary, the proposed diagnostic category is compatible with current theories of pain and establishes the concept that the psychological state of patients is important in many more cases of pain than are identified by DSM-III and DSM-III-R diagnoses. Furthermore, it would 1) allow a greater opportunity for specification of the clinician's judgment of presumed etiological factors responsible for pain and thus provide for the development of treatment programs tailored to addressing them; 2) offer a clinically useful schema for differential diagnosis; 3) eliminate the requirement that the user attempt to correlate physical findings with pain, a difficult, if not impossible, task; and 4) include both acute and chronic pain. Thus, by directly addressing the important issues, this classification is more relevant to the clinical practice of medicine than somatoform pain disorder and provides greater assistance in the evaluation and treatment of patients with pain for the psychiatrist as well as for those in other disciplines of medicine.

References

American Psychiatric Association: Diagnostic and Statistical Manual of Mental Disorders, Second Edition. Washington, DC, American Psychiatric Association, 1968

American Psychiatric Association: Diagnostic and Statistical Manual of Mental Disorders, Third Edition. Washington, DC, American Psychiatric Association, 1980

American Psychiatric Association: Diagnostic and Statistical Manual of Mental Disorders, Third Edition, Revised. Washington, DC, American Psychiatric Association, 1987

Beecher HK: Pain in men wounded in battle. Ann Surg 123:98–105, 1946

Beitman BD, Mukerji V, Flaker G, et al: Panic disorder, cardiology patients, and atypical chest pain. Psychiatr Clin North Am 11:387–397, 1988

Beitman BD, Mukerji V, Lamberti JW, et al: Panic disorder in patients with chest pain and angiographically normal coronary arteries. Am J Cardiol 63:1399–1403, 1989

Benjamin S, Barnes D, Berger S, et al: The relationship of chronic pain, mental illness and organic disorders. Pain 32:185–195, 1988

Black RG: The chronic pain syndrome. Surg Clin North Am 55:999–1011, 1975

Blackwell B, Merskey H, Kellner R: Somatoform pain disorders, in Treatments of Psychiatric Disorders: A Task Force Report of the American Psychiatric Association. Washington, DC, American Psychiatric Association, 1989, pp 2120–2137

Blumer D, Heilbronn M: Chronic pain as a variant of depressive disease: the pain-prone disorder. J Nerv Ment Dis 170:381–394, 1982

Bouckoms AJ, Litman RE, Baer L: Denial in the depressive and pain-prone disorders of chronic pain. Clin J Pain 1:165–169, 1985

Brena SF: Chronic pain states: a model for classification. Psychiatr Ann 14:778–782, 1984

Brena SF, Crue BL, Stieg RL: Comments on the classification of chronic pain: its clinical significance. Bull Clin Neurosci 49:67–81, 1984

Brown GK: A causal analysis of chronic pain and depression. J Abnorm Psychol 99:127–137, 1990

Chapman CR, Turner JA: Psychological control of acute pain in medical settings. Journal of Pain and Symptom Management 1:9–20, 1986

Chaturvedi SK: A comparison of depressed and anxious chronic pain patients. Gen Hosp Psychiatry 9:383–386, 1987

Chaturvedi SK, Michael A: Chronic pain in a psychiatric clinic. J Psychosom Res 30:347–354, 1986

Cormier LE, Katon W, Russo J, et al: Chest pain with negative cardiac diagnostic studies: relationship to psychiatric illness. J Nerv Ment Dis 176:351–358, 1988

Costello RM, Hulsey TL, Schoenfeld LS: P-A-I-N: a four cluster MMPI typology for chronic pain. Pain 30:199–209, 1987

Dworkin SF, Burgess JA: Orofacial pain of psychogenic origin: current concepts and classification. Journal of the American Dental Association 115:565–571, 1987

Dworkin RH, Caligor E: Psychiatric diagnosis and chronic pain: DSM-III-R and beyond. Journal of Pain and Symptom Management 3:87–98, 1988

Egbert LD, Battit GE, Welch CD, et al: Reduction of postoperative pain by encouragement and instruction of patients. N Engl J Med 270:825–827, 1964

Feinmann C: Pain relief by antidepressants: possible modes of action. Pain 23:1–8, 1985

Fishbain DA, Goldberg M, Meagher BR, et al: Male and female chronic pain patients categorized by DSM-III psychiatric diagnostic criteria. Pain 26:181–197, 1986

Fishbain DA, Goldberg M, Labbe E, et al: Compensation and non-compensation chronic pain patients compared for DSM-III operational diagnoses. Pain 32:197–206, 1988

Fishbain DA, Goldberg M, Steele R, et al: DSM-III diagnoses of patients with myofascial pain syndrome (fibrositis). Arch Phys Med Rehabil 70:433–438, 1989

Flor H, Turk DC: Etiological theories and treatments for chronic back pain, I: somatic models and interventions. Pain 19:105–121, 1984

France RD, Krishnan KRR: Pain in psychiatric disorders, in Chronic Pain. Edited by France RD, Krishnan KRR. Washington, DC, American Psychiatric Press, 1988, pp 116–141

France RD, Krishnan KRR, Houpt JL, et al: Differentiation of depression from chronic pain with the dexamethasone suppression test and DSM-III. Am J Psychiatry 141:1577–1579, 1984

France RD, Krishnan KRR, Goli V, et al: Preliminary study of thyrotropin releasing hormone stimulation test in chronic low back pain patients. Pain 27:51–55, 1986

France RD, Krishnan KRR, Trainor M, et al: Chronic pain and depression, IV: DST as a discriminator between chronic pain and depression. Pain 28:39–44, 1987a

France RD, Urban BJ, Pelton S, et al: CSF monoamine metabolites in chronic pain. Pain 31:189–198, 1987b

France RD, Urban BJ, Krishnan KRR: CSF corticotropin-releasing factor-like immunoactivity in chronic pain patients with and without major depression. Biol Psychiatry 23:86–88, 1988

Gallagher RM, Marbach JJ, Raphael KG, et al: Is major depression comorbid with temporomanibular pain and dysfunction syndrome? A pilot study. Clin J Pain 7:219–225, 1991

Gamsa A: Is emotional disturbance a precipitator or a consequence of chronic pain? Pain 42:183–195, 1990

Goldenberg DL: Psychologic studies in fibrositis. Am J Med 81 (suppl 3a):67–70, 1986

Gore DR, Sepic SB, Gardner GM, et al: Neck pain: a long-term follow-up of 205 patients. Spine 12:1–5, 1987

Gunn CC, Sola AE: Chronic intractable benign pain (CIBP). Pain 39:364–365, 1989

Haley WE, Turner JA, Romano JM: Depression in chronic pain patients: relation to pain, activity, and sex differences. Pain 23:337–343, 1985

Harrop-Griffiths J, Katon W, Walker E: The association between chronic pelvic pain, psychiatric diagnoses, and childhood sexual abuse. Obstet Gynecol 71:589–594, 1988

Hathaway SR, McKinley JC: Minnesota Multiphasic Personality Inventory, Revised. Minneapolis, University of Minnesota, 1970

Hendler N, Uematesu S, Long D: Thermographic validation of physical complaints in "psychogenic pain" patients. Psychosomatics 23:283–287, 1982

Hudson JI, Pliner LF, Hudson MS, et al: The dexamethasone suppression test in fibrositis. Biol Psychiatry 19:1489–1493, 1984

Hudson JI, Hudson MS, Pliner LF, et al: Fibromyalgia and major affective disorder: a controlled phenomenology and family history study. Am J Psychiatry 142:441–446, 1985

Jenkins PLG: Psychogenic abdominal pain. Gen Hosp Psychiatry 13:27–30, 1991

Katon W, Egan K, Miller D: Chronic pain: lifetime psychiatric diagnoses and family history. Am J Psychiatry 142:1156–1160, 1985

Katon W, Hall ML, Russo J, et al: Chest pain: relationship of psychiatric illness to coronary arteriographic results. Am J Med 84:1–9, 1988

King SA, Strain JJ: The problem of psychiatric diagnosis for the pain patient in the general hospital. Clin J Pain 5:329–335, 1989

King SA, Strain JJ: Benzodiazepine use by chronic pain patients. Clin J Pain 6:143–147, 1990

Kirmayer LJ, Robbins JM, Kapusta MA: Somatization and depression in fibromyalgia syndrome. Am J Psychiatry 145:950–954, 1988

Large RG: DSM-III diagnoses in chronic pain: confusion or clarity. J Nerv Ment Dis 174:295–303, 1986

Love AW: Depression in chronic low back pain patients: diagnostic efficiency of three self-report questionnaires. J Clin Psychol 43:84–89, 1987

Magni G, Salmi A, de Leo D, et al: Chronic pelvic pain and depression. Psychopathology 17:132–136, 1984

Main CJ, Evans PJD, Whitehead RC: An investigation of personality structure and other psychological features in patients presenting with low-back pain: a critique of the MMPI, in Proceedings of the 6th World Congress on Pain. Edited by Bond MR, Charlton JE, Woolf CJ. Amsterdam, Netherlands, Elsevier Science Publishers, 1991

McNeill TW, Sinkora G, Leavitt F: Psychologic classification of low-back pain patients: a prognostic tool. Spine 11:955–959, 1986

Merskey HM: Classification of chronic pain. Pain Supp 3:S1–S226, 1986

Muse M: Stress-related, posttraumatic chronic pain syndrome: criteria for diagnosis, and preliminary report on prevalence. Pain 23:295–300, 1985

Olesen J: Classification and diagnostic criteria for headache disorders, cranial neuralgias and facial pain. Cephalalgia 8 (suppl 7):9–96, 1988

Osterweis M, Kleinman A, Mechanic D (eds): Pain and Disability. Washington, DC, National Academy Press, 1987

Parmelee PA, Katz IR, Lawton MP: The relation of pain to depression among institutionalized aged. J Gerontol 46:15–21, 1991

Pilowsky I: Affective disorder and pain, in Proceedings of the 5th World Congress on Pain. Edited by Dubner R, Gebhart GF, Bond MR. Amsterdam, Netherlands, Elsevier, 1988, pp 263–275

Reich J, Tupin JP, Abramowitz SI: Psychiatric diagnosis of chronic pain patients. Am J Psychiatry 140:1495–1498, 1983

Remick RA, Blasberg B, Campos PE, et al: Psychiatric disorders associated with atypical facial pain. Can J Psychiatry 28:178–181, 1983

Report of the Commission on the Evaluation of Pain: Publ No 64–031. Washington, DC, U.S. Department of Health and Human Services, Social Security Administration, Office of Disability, 1987

Romano JM, Turner JA: Chronic pain and depression: does the literature support a relationship. Psychol Bull 97:18–34, 1985

Rosomoff HL, Fishbain DA, Goldberg M, et al: Physical findings in patients with chronic intractable benign pain of the neck and/or back. Pain 37:279–287, 1989

Roy R: Measurement of chronic pain in pain-depression literature during the 1980s: a review. Int J Psychiatry Med 16:179–188, 1986–1987

Schover LR: Psychological factors in men with genital pain. Cleve Clin J Med 57:697–700, 1990

Trief PM, Elliott DJ, Stein N: Functional vs organic pain: a meaningful distinction? J Clin Psychol 43:219–226, 1987

Turk DC, Rudy TE: Towards a comprehensive assessment of chronic pain patients. Behav Res Ther 24:237–249, 1987

Turner JA, Romano JM: Self-report screening measures for depression in chronic pain patients. J Clin Psychol 40:909–913, 1984

Valdes M, Treserra J, Garcia L, et al: Psychogenic pain and psychological variables: a psychometric study. Psychother Psychosom 50:15–21, 1988

Valkenburg HA, Haanen HCM: The epidemiology of low back pain, in Symposium on Idiopathic Low Back Pain. Edited by White AA, Gordon SL. St. Louis, MO, CV Mosby, 1982, pp 9–22

Walker E, Katon W, Harrop-Griffiths J: Relationship of chronic pelvic pain to psychiatric diagnoses and childhood sexual abuse. Am J Psychiatry 145:75–80, 1988

Wulsin LR, Arnold LM, Hillard JR: Axis I disorders in ER patients with atypical chest pain. Int J Psychiatry Med 21:37–46, 1991

Zborowski M: People in Pain. San Francisco, CA, Jossey-Bass, 1969

Chapter 42

Hypochondriasis

Guylaine Côté, Ph.D., Tracy O'Leary, M.D.,
David H. Barlow, Ph.D., James J. Strain, M.D.,
Paul M. Salkovskis, Ph.D.,
Hilary M. C. Warwick, B.M., M.R.C.Psych.,
David M. Clark, Ph.D., Ronald Rapee, Ph.D., and
Steven A. Rasmussen, M.D.

Statement of the Issues

This chapter deals with three main issues related to clarifying the definition of hypochondriasis (HYP): 1) the relationship between HYP and illness phobia (IP), 2) whether "unshakable conviction" borders on hypochondriacal delusion, and 3) the necessity of requiring that physical symptoms be present to diagnose HYP. To address these issues, the results of three literature reviews are discussed: a review by Salkovskis et al. (1990) that mainly focuses on the separation of IP from HYP to make a nosological distinction between disease conviction and disease fear, a review by Rapee (1989) that discusses generalized anxiety disorder (GAD) with respect to boundary issues with somatoform and psychophysiological disorders, and a review by Rasmussen (1990) that discusses the relationship between HYP and obsessive-compulsive disorder (OCD). To consider the issue of differentiating hypochon-driacal delusions from unshakable convictions of illness/disease, reviews by Hollander (1989) on the relationship between body dysmorphic disorder and OCD and by Kozak and Foa (1991) on obsessions, overvalued ideas, and delusions in OCD are also considered. Finally, to address the issue regarding whether the presence of physical symptomatology is necessary for a diagnosis of HYP, papers by Adler (1989), Barsky and Wyshak (1990), Barsky et al. (1990), Kellner (1985, 1992), and Kellner et al. (1989, 1992) are cited.

Significance of the Issues

HYP and IP

DSM-III-R (American Psychiatric Association 1987) specifically states that the essential feature of HYP is "preoccupation with the fear of having, or the belief that one has, a serious disease, based on the person's interpretation of physical signs or sensations as evidence of physical illness." The inherent difficulty with this criterion lies in its failure to differentiate between a belief of having a disease and a fear of contracting a disease. Those individuals who fear contracting a disease but do not believe that they are ill have been diagnosed with HYP, along with those who believe they have an illness. The issue raises the question of whether disease conviction and IP represent two separate components of HYP.

Does Unshakable Conviction Border on Hypochondriacal Delusion?

This issue is addressed because of the difficulty researchers and clinicians have in making the distinction between a somatic delusion, from which the individual cannot even temporarily be dissuaded, and an unshakable conviction (which may wax and wane in intensity of belief). Confounding this topic is the paucity of empirical evidence and research in the area of hypochondriacal delusions. There has yet to be a systematic, empirical, nonanecdotal study that examines delusions in HYP. Review papers discuss the presence of hypochondriacal delusions in OCD and body dysmorphic disorder (Hollander 1989; Kozak and Foa 1991; Rasmussen 1990).

Necessity of Physical Symptoms in HYP

DSM-III-R states that the essential defining feature of all the somatoform disorders is the presence of physical symptoms that suggest a physical disorder and for which there is no conclusive, demonstrable organic basis. A firm assumption that the physical symptoms are tied to psychological factors must also be made to assign a somatoform diagnosis. According to the current diagnostic criteria for HYP, however, there must also be a preoccupation with the fear of having, or the belief that one has, a serious disease. Therefore, one may simply dread the prospect of contracting a disease, interpret innocuous bodily sensations such as fatigue as evidence for a disease (e.g., AIDS), and still receive a diagnosis of HYP. Some researchers argue that this phenomenon is better described as a variant of a simple phobia (IP; see Salkovskis et al. 1990) rather than as HYP. Another basic question is whether HYP should be considered a somatoform disorder and whether it is necessary to keep it within that diagnostic grouping on the basis of the presence of physical symptoms.

Methods

HYP and IP

Salkovskis et al. (1990) addressed whether HYP represents two separate categories: disease conviction and IP. Although the main issue addressed by Rapee's review (1989) was the discriminability of GAD from DSM-III-R somatoform disorders and from psychophysiological disorders, the author briefly discussed the issue relating to the distinction between disease conviction and disease fear.

Does Unshakable Conviction Border on Hypochondriacal Delusion?

To date, no systematic research has been done concerning HYP and the potential relationship between an unshakable disease conviction and a hypochondriacal/somatic delusion. Although the main issue covered by Rasmussen's (1990) review concerned the relation of HYP to the anxiety disorders, specifically OCD, Rasmussen also proposed a diagnostic decision tree that provides a categorization of beliefs into delusional or nondelusional to assist in making a diagnosis. In addressing this issue, we also examined reviews of empirical evidence by Kozak and Foa (1991) on overvalued ideas and delusions in OCD and by Hollander (1989) on the relationship between body dysmorphic disorder and OCD. Although these reviews do not directly answer the issue for HYP, they do provide some clarification of these concepts and aid in attempting to determine the nature of the conviction/belief. We also reviewed clinical and research literature on HYP to clarify the qualitative differences between disease conviction and somatic delusion.

Presence of Physical Symptoms in HYP

No systematic studies have been done to address the issue of whether or not a diagnosis of HYP should be given without concurrent physical symptoms. As it stands, DSM-III-R states that the disease conviction is based on a misinterpretation of physical sensations. Theoretically, these could range from innocuous, natural bodily fluctuations to the presence of a true organic disease. This makes it difficult to decide what physical symptoms or sensations can be subsumed under the general rubric and what types of sensations are most common in this disorder. To shed light on this issue, we reviewed several studies that discuss somatic symptoms and their relationship to HYP (Adler 1989; Barsky and Wyshak 1990; Barsky et al. 1990; Kellner 1985; Kellner et al. 1989, 1992; Rasmussen 1990).

Results

HYP and IP

The issue focused on whether disease conviction and IP represent two distinct categories of HYP. The review by Salkovskis et al. (1990) specifically addressed the preceding issue. In evaluating the evidence on the discriminability of GAD, HYP, and irritable bowel syndrome, Rapee (1989) briefly addressed the issue relating to the distinction between IP and HYP. These two reviews are summarized separately.

HYP, IP, and Other Anxiety Disorders

Method. The Salkovskis et al. (1990) literature review involved two parts. First, a review of available literature was presented. The authors mentioned the dearth of research and relevant literature related to HYP. Second, results from an investigation conducted by the authors were discussed. This investigation involved comparing several diagnostic groups with respect to cognitions, behaviors, attitudes, and fears of unexpected physiological changes. As part of this study, the group of patients with a DSM-III-R diagnosis of HYP were subdivided according to the level of disease phobia. Subjects completed a series of questionnaires including the following: 1) a version of a questionnaire measuring interpretations of ambiguous situations concerning panic attack sensations (e.g., "You notice that your heart is beating fast and pounding"), hypochondriacal sensations (e.g., "You notice lumps under the skin of your neck"), and external events (e.g., "A member of your family is late arriving home"); 2) a questionnaire measuring the behavior associated with the same ambiguous situations as above such as avoidance behavior, checking behavior, and minimal or no behavior change; 3) a set of scales measuring the frequency of a number of health-related behaviors, such as seeking reassurance and checking one's body for signs of illness; 4) the Chambless Agoraphobic Cognitions Questionnaire (Chambless et al. 1984); 5) the Fear Questionnaire (Marks and Mathews 1979); 6) the Beck Anxiety and Depression Inventories (Beck and Steer 1990; Beck et al. 1961) and the Spielberger State Anxiety Inventory (Spielberger et al. 1970); 7) a measure of hypochondriacal-related symptoms and behaviors; and 8) a questionnaire measuring fear of certain subtypes of unexpected symptoms: those increased by autonomic arousal associated with anxiety (e.g., heart pounding) and those not directly increased by anxiety (e.g., lumps under the skin).

Results. Control group comparisons and factor-analytic studies have affirmed the presence of two distinct dimensions of HYP: disease phobia and disease conviction (Kellner et al. 1987; Pilowsky 1967). However, it is uncertain whether these presentations represent separate syndromes. Demographic characteristics of the groups must be compared, along with the relative importance of factors such as avoidance and reassurance seeking. In some cases of HYP, the central feature seems to be a fear of contracting an illness as opposed to the belief that one has a disease. In these cases, the main behavioral feature is avoidance of internal and external anxiety-triggering stimuli. On the other hand, for cases in which the disease conviction component is stronger than the IP component, it would be predicted that reassurance seeking would be the prominent behavioral feature as opposed to avoidance. There is preliminary evidence that behavioral therapies based on principles of exposure may be effective in patients who show a phobic pattern of behavior (Warwick and Marks 1988), whereas treatments focusing on belief change may be more effective in patients with strong disease conviction (Salkovskis and Warwick 1986). It has been proposed that individuals who show a stronger component of fear of contracting a disease and for whom avoidance behavior is prominent are better classified as having simple phobia. However, diagnosis is more difficult than in other simple phobias, because general fears of illness are not always related to specific stimuli.

There is some support for making a distinction between disease conviction and disease phobia. The data indicate that almost all hypochondriacal patients show a high degree of disease conviction, although small subgroups with low disease conviction and high disease phobia, and vice versa, were noted. The authors attributed these findings to a sampling problem; patients who believe they have a disease are more likely to seek medical consultation than patients who are phobic of illness-related issues. A median split procedure was used to compare patients diagnosed with HYP with high versus low disease phobia and high versus low disease conviction. The results suggested that, unlike those patients who scored high on disease phobia, patients with high levels of disease conviction displayed higher scores on the core aspects of HYP such as misinterpretations of bodily sensations and checking behavior. Frequency of anxiety symptoms was associated with disease conviction. In addition, patients with high disease phobia had an early age at onset.

Discussion. Based on the foregoing observations, the authors concluded that the current definition of HYP probably incorporates two phenomenologically distinct entities: disease phobia and disease conviction. Salkovskis et al. (1990) suggested that the diagnostic criteria for HYP should require a disease conviction component. In addition, the authors suggested that the description of simple phobia be extended to incorporate fear of developing or being exposed to illnesses such as AIDS or cancer and avoidance of stimuli associated with such illnesses, provided the patient does not believe that she or he is currently suffering from the feared illness.

GAD: Boundary Issues With
Somatoform and Psychophysiological Disorders

The review by Rapee (1989) mainly focused on diagnostic issues relating to the discrimination of GAD, HYP, and irritable bowel syndrome.

Method. The method used involved two parts. First, *Psychological Abstracts* between 1970 and 1989 inclusive and *Index Medicus* between 1970 and 1989 inclusive were searched. *Hypochondriasis* was included as a key word. Also, any abstracts that referred to HYP-like disorders and another disorder of interest to the review were examined for possible relevance. Second, 12 clinics and laboratories around the world known to be involved in research into one of the three disorders were asked to supply unpublished and recently submitted data on the following issues: 1) medical record data, medical presentations; 2) comorbidity of GAD, somatoform disorders, and psychophysiological disorders; 3) mean number, type, and intensity of somatic symptoms associated with the disorders; 4) clinical features; 5) associated Axis II disorders; 6) questionnaire scores and physiological measures; and 7) treatment response.

Results and discussion. The primary conclusion relevant to the definition of HYP was that insufficient data exist to make any specific recommendations regarding the need to make changes in diagnostic criteria for enhancing the discriminability of GAD and HYP. No well-controlled studies have been conducted that compare GAD and HYP. However, Rapee (1989) concluded that clarification of the GAD and/or HYP diagnostic criteria would facilitate differential diagnosis. As one possible solution, the author referred to Pilowsky's (1967) identification of three basic factors in HYP: disease fear, bodily preoccupation, and disease conviction. Because GAD patients appear clinically to share the first two factors but perhaps not the third, Rapee (1989) suggested that disease conviction be made a central and defining characteristic of HYP. This is incorporated in the suggested DSM-IV A criterion: "Preoccupation with fears of having, or the idea that one has, a serious disease," which implies that conviction of illness is a core symptom of HYP.

Does Unshakable Conviction Border on Hypochondriacal Delusion?

This issue involves the possible boundary between an unshakable conviction and a hypochondriacal delusion. Rasmussen (1990), in his review of the boundary between HYP and OCD, offered a diagnostic decision tree that helps to specify the nature of a belief as delusional or nondelusional. Because there are no studies elucidating this issue specifically for HYP, we also examined reviews concerning delusions in OCD (Hollander 1989) and body dysmorphic disorder (Kozak and Foa 1991) to shed some light on the nature of delusions in psychopathology in general.

HYP and Its Relationship to OCD

Rasmussen's (1990) review primarily focused on whether HYP should be classified as an anxiety or as a somatoform disorder.

Method. The method was completed in two procedures. First, a Medline search of the psychiatric and psychological literature from 1970 to 1990 was done on the following topics: 1) all empirical studies of HYP, 2) all empirical studies of OCD and its relationship to hypochondriacal symptoms, 3) all empirical studies of panic disorder and its relationship to hypochondriacal symptoms, and 4) all empirical studies of depression and its relationship to hypochondriacal symptoms. By cross-referencing relevant articles from the above search, the time span was extended to 1960. Finally, the results of an unpublished treatment study of 575 patients meeting DSM-III-R criteria for OCD for at least 1 year from 20 geographically distinct sites were discussed. The OCD patients in the study had primary somatic obsessions, along with checking compulsions and the need to ask or confess. Excluded from the study were patients with a concurrent Axis I or II diagnosis, including panic disorder, major depression, Tourette's syndrome, or serious medical problems. The design involved a double-blind efficacy trial of clomipramine versus placebo, and patients were rated weekly using the Yale-Brown Obsessive Compulsive Scale (YBOCS) (Goodman et al. 1989) and the National Institute of Mental Health Global Obsessive Compulsive Scale (Kim et al. 1993). In examining these results, the YBOCS ratings of a comparison group of 415 patients with an unspecified diagnosis who had been examined at Rasmussen's Obsessive Disorders Clinic were used.

Results and discussion. Rasmussen cited evidence that resistance, conviction, and belief appear to lie on a continuum of severity in OCD; he hypothesized that the same continuum may hold true for HYP but cautions against making this assumption until research supports this impression.

Pertinent to this issue and based on current diagnostic nosology, Rasmussen outlined a diagnostic decision tree that forces the presence of a delusion to partly determine the official diagnosis given. After verification of severity and duration of the presenting complaint(s), the diagnostician must decide whether the somatic symptoms preoccupation, belief, and fear are of delusional intensity. If the symptom is delusional in nature and is accompanied by mood disturbance, according to Rasmussen, a diagnosis of major depression with psychotic features is most appropriate. The absence of mood disturbance, conversely, suggests delusional disorder, somatic type. The presence of a nondelusional belief, coupled with mood disturbance indicates major depression "with somatic features," and a nondelusional belief without mood disturbance must be further classified according to the presence or absence of anxiety. If anxiety is a major presenting feature, if an irrational fear of developing an illness is present but there is no history of spontaneous panic attacks, and if there are no obsessive-compulsive rituals, then a diagnosis of HYP may be made. A report of ritualizing, however, would lead to a diagnosis of OCD in Rasmussen's decision tree.

The major recommendation by Rasmussen (1990) in regard to this issue is that an irrational belief that the patient holds to be true is more aligned with delusional disorder or OCD with psychotic features. Also, concurrent checking rituals or resistance to feared thoughts/beliefs are most appropriately classified as OCD, not HYP. Finally, these checking rituals should not be limited only to numerous visits to the doctor. This recommendation to carefully distinguish other diagnoses that "border" on HYP from HYP is embodied in the proposed DSM-IV criterion E: "The preoccupation does not occur exclusively during the course of generalized anxiety disorder, obsessive-compulsive disorder, panic disorder, major depressive disorder, separation, anxiety, or another somatoform disorder." It also appears in the proposed criterion C: "The belief in A is not of delusional intensity, as in delusional disorder, somatic type, . . . and is not restricted to a circumscribed concern about appearance, as in body dysmorphic disorder."

Kozak and Foa (1991) conducted a literature search spanning the years 1983–1988. Key words used in the search included *overvalued ideation, delusion and OCD, OCD and schizophrenia,* and *OCD and psychosis.* The reviewers allude to the implication of delusions as viewed by DSM-III-R, that is, that they are usually fixed convictions that cannot be shaken, thereby equating the terms *unshakable conviction* and *delusion. Overvalued ideation,* on the other hand, is defined by the reviewers as an almost unshakable belief that can be acknowledged as potentially unfounded only after considerable discussion.

Although the strength of belief appears to be the determining factor in whether a conviction is really a delusion, the border remains highly ambiguous. Kozak and Foa (1991) cite McKenna's (1984) review on disorders with overvalued ideas, which appear to be associated with a strong affective response as well as a consistency between belief and action. Examples given by McKenna of these types of disorders are HYP, anorexia nervosa, querulous paranoid states, and morbid jealousy. The difficulty here lies in the fact that both overvalued ideas and delusions, according to Kozak and Foa, are perceived by the individual as sensible and valid. This definition depicts the two concepts as one and the same. Intuitively and clinically, however, this makes little sense. It seems that the reviewers follow the dichotomy of bizarre and nonbizarre delusions, the former indicating psychosis and the latter implying some semblance to intact reality testing. Overall, Kozak and Foa recommend using a continuum or dimension along which to place the strength of the fear/belief/conviction according to severity.

Hollander (1989), in examining the relationship between body dysmorphic disorder and OCD, also supports a dimensional system with the extremes of overvalued idea versus delusion for describing the strength of belief.

Kellner (1992) points out the pervasive difficulty in distinguishing delusional disorder, somatic type, from HYP. As a rule, Kellner states that one should assume a diagnosis of HYP based on the rarity of delusional disorder in clinical practice. In delusional disorder, somatic type, the delusion is most commonly circumscribed to convictions of having parasites or of emitting a foul odor. In HYP, the conviction is usually one of disease, such as heart disease, cancer, multiple sclerosis, or AIDS. Qualitatively, HYP and delusional disorder, somatic type, may be differentiated by the descriptive nature of the disease conviction in the majority of cases seen by mental health professionals. It was felt this degree of dimensionality regarding "overvalued idea versus delusion" would be difficult to specify in the DSM-IV options for the diagnosis of HYP at this time.

Presence of Physical Symptoms in HYP

This issue involves requiring that physical symptoms be present to make a diagnosis of HYP. There are no studies on this particular issue; however, several empirical studies on somatization and physical symptomatology in HYP may help to clarify this debate.

Kellner (1985) states that the presence of anxiety, depression, somatic symptoms, pain, a fear of disease, and conviction of disease comprise HYP. The intensity, severity, and interaction of any of the aforementioned features will vary on a case-by-case basis between and within individuals. Because anxiety and depression almost invariably have some manifestation of physical symptomatology, it seems likely that those same symptoms will often appear in HYP as well.

In a study investigating the relationship between hypochondriacal fears and anxiety, depression, and somatic symptoms, Kellner et al. (1992) administered several self-report scales to 100 general practice patients and 100 nonpsychotic outpatients. The scales included the Hypochondriacal Beliefs, Disease Phobia, and Hypochondriasis Subscales of the Illness Attitude Scales (Kellner 1985); the Hopkins Symptom Checklist-90 (HSCL) (Derogatis et al. 1974); an unspecified social questionnaire targeting demographic information and current life situation; and a scale consisting of factors 2 (disease fear) and 3 (disease conviction) of the Whiteley Index (Pilowsky 1967). The following independent variables were examined in a stepwise regression: age, four unspecified scales of the HSCL, depression, anxiety, phobic anxiety, and somatization. The results indicated that high self-ratings of somatic symptoms predicted high ratings on the Hypochondriacal Beliefs Scale. This finding held for all subjects except for female psychiatric patients, for whom anxiety was the predictor. Somatic symptoms did not, however, predict high scores on the Disease Phobia Scale. Rather, anxiety, phobic anxiety, and higher age appeared to predict the fear of disease. The authors concluded that patients who fear disease tend to be high in anxiety or phobic anxiety, whereas patients who falsely believe that they have a physical disease tend to report somatic symptoms of a greater number and severity.

The implication of these findings is that disease conviction is associated with concurrent physical symptomatology; the interaction of the two seems to be a reliable predictor of HYP. This relates to the issue concerning the distinction between disease phobia and disease conviction as well. Theoretically, one would not expect a preponderance of diffuse and unremitting physical symptoms in IP, because the DSM-III-R definition of simple phobia stipulates that exposure to the feared stimulus during some phase of the disturbance almost invariably provokes an immediate anxiety response. Therefore, the physical symptoms reported by one who fears disease (e.g., AIDS phobia) would typically be anxiety symptoms, such as tachycardia, sweating, and shortness of breath. It remains unclear what the characteristic physical symptoms of HYP are, because there are no studies that have addressed this topic using the DSM-III-R definition of HYP.

Kellner et al. (1989) examined depression, anxiety, and somatization in 21 psychiatric outpatients with a DSM-III diagnosis of HYP, comparing them to 21 nonpsychotic psychiatric outpatients matched by age and sex. Of these patients, 6 were diagnosed with unipolar major depression without melancholia, 5 had dysthymic disorder, 4 received a diagnosis of GAD, 4 were given a diagnosis of atypical depression, 2 had panic disorder, 1 was diagnosed as having agoraphobia with panic attacks, and 2 had adjustment disorders: 1 with depressed mood, and 1 with anxious mood. None of them had volunteered reports of hypochondriacal fears during the interview nor had any of them displayed conspicuous hypochondriacal behavior. When questioned, however, a few subjects in this group had expressed concerns about physical disease that were not their main complaints and were not judged to be significant by the interviewers. Self-rating scales included: the depression, anxiety, somatization, and anger/hostility scales of the HSCL; the Symptoms Rating Test (Kellner and Sheffield 1973), which measures state levels of anxiety, depression, and somatic symptoms; the Symptom Questionnaire (Kellner 1987), a state measure that assesses depression, anxiety, anger/hostility, and somatic symptoms; and the Illness Attitude Scales (Kellner 1985), which measures hypochondriacal and abnormal illness behavior. Two additional control groups (21 family practice patients and 21 employees) completed the same questionnaire battery with the exception of the HSCL. The two psychiatric groups were compared using the Wilcoxon paired two-sample test.

Results showed that the self-reported severity of somatic symptoms as reflected by scores on the somatization scale of the HSCL and the Symptom Rating Test were significantly higher in hypochondriacal patients than in the general psychiatric patients. In addition, hypochondriacal patients reported significantly more somatic symptoms than did the psychiatric group. In comparing all four groups, a two-way analysis of variance and a post-hoc multiple comparison test (Newman-Keuls) were employed. Results from these analyses indicated that somatic symptoms and anxiety were significantly greater in the hypochondriacal patients than in the other groups. Additionally, hypochondriacal patients had the highest scores of all groups in seven of the eight Illness Attitude Scales: illness worry, concern over pain, hypochondriacal beliefs, fear of death, disease phobia, bodily preoccupation, and treatment experience. The investigators argue that severe somatic symptoms are frequently reported in HYP and thus comprise an integral part of the nature of this disorder.

Barsky and Wyshak (1990) also conceptualize HYP primarily as a misinterpretation and consequent fear of somatic sensations. They go a step further, however, in asserting that hypochondriacal patients amplify all types of somatic sensations, from normal bodily fluctuations, to minor ailments, to sensations produced by emotional arousal, to serious organic disease processes. This amplification creates more severe and distressing physical sensations, which, when responded to with fear/anxiety, serve to intensify the sensations.

To test this hypothesis, a sample of 177 consecutive general outpatients at the Massachusetts General Hospital Clinic (none of whom had organic brain disease) were given a self-report battery that included the following measures: a sociodemographic questionnaire, the Whiteley Index (Pilowsky 1967), 11 symptoms taken from the somatization subscale of the HSCL, the hypochondriasis subscale of the Minnesota Multiphasic Personality Inventory (Hathaway and McKinley 1943), the Somatosensory Amplification Scale (SSAS) (Barsky et al. 1990), and an unspecified questionnaire assessing attitudes toward aging, health, medical care, beliefs about illnesses, and childhood history of family illness. Stepwise multiple regression was used to measure the proportion of variance accounted for by the independent/predictor variables, and product moment correlations were done to measure the association between two variables.

Results showed that amplification of somatic sensations accounted for the most variance in HYP (31%) and 12% of the variance in somatization, after sociodemographic variables had been taken into account. The zero-order correlation of HYP and amplification was .56. Although these results hold only for hypochondriacal symptoms and not for DSM-III-R HYP, the authors point out that their data support the DSM-III-R conceptualization of HYP as the misinterpretation of benign somatic symptoms and sensations as indicative of disease. Because the SSAS measures pathological symptoms and also bodily sensations such as noise, heat, and hunger, the authors proffer that hypochondriacal patients are more sensitive to, and intolerant of, physical sensations.

Adler (1989) conducted a study to assess the degree of overlap between anxiety and somatoform disorders, using measures of anxiety and somatic sensitivities, abnormal illness behaviors/beliefs, symptomatology, affect, and diagnostic comorbidity. The 68 subjects assessed were assigned to four groups: panic disorder (PD), somatoform disorder (SOM), irritable bowel syndrome, and medical illness–no mental disorder (MED).

Several important results were found. First, of 13 subjects with either HYP or SOM, 12 reported having 6 or more DSM-III-R GAD symptoms, with a mean of 11.6 DSM-III-R GAD symptoms. In addition, PD, HYP, and SOM subjects scored significantly higher on measures of anxiety and somatic sensitivities than MED subjects. The PD and SOM groups had significantly more self-reported somatic symptoms than the MED group, and no significant differences emerged between the PD and SOM group on this measure. The HYP subjects, however, reported significantly more symptoms than the PD subjects. In fact, the PD and SOM groups were not significantly different from each other on all but one measure of illness attitudes and behavior but scored significantly higher than the irritable bowel syndrome or MED groups. Supported by these findings, Adler postulated that panic disorder, HYP, and somatoform disorders are best conceptualized as dimensional manifestations of a separate class of disorders. The characteristics that the three disorders appear to share include anxiety, physical symptoms, anxiety sensitivity (a belief in the negative consequences of anxiety and somatic sensations), somatic sensitivity (a perceived heightened awareness of somatic events), and abnormal illness beliefs/behaviors. The author proposed a reclassification of these disorders into "abnormal illness response pattern," which would be based on the above characteristics as well as on the number and nature of symptoms (i.e., chronic versus acute) and perceived consequence/threat of those symptoms.

In summary, there appears to be a link between HYP and current physical symptomatology. Indeed, there may even be an amplification of a vast array of bodily sensations in HYP, as posited by Barsky and others. Although there was much debate on the necessity of basing the diagnosis of HYP on the person's interpretation of physical signs or sensations as evidence of physical disease (as specified in DSM-III-R), in view of the need for more studies it was proposed that the A criterion require only a "preoccupation with the fears of having, or the idea that one has, a serious disease."

Recommendations

HYP and IP

The DSM-IV Anxiety Disorders Work Group concurred with the suggestions proposed by Salkovskis et al. (1990) and Rapee (1989) and acknowledged that disease conviction is more consistent with a diagnosis of HYP, whereas IP without disease conviction is more consistent with a diagnosis of simple phobia. The importance of further revisions and specifications of the diagnostic criteria of HYP was recognized. A proposed option for DSM-IV HYP is that avoidance due to the fear of contracting a disease be diagnosed as a "specific phobia, other type (contracting an illness)," or possibly as its own subtype, "specific phobia, illness type."

Does Unshakable Conviction Border on Hypochondriacal Delusion?

Due to the lack of available evidence, no firm recommendation can be made concerning the categorization of disease conviction in HYP into unshakable belief and delusion. However, existing reviews on body dysmorphic disorder and OCD acknowledge that the intensity of belief is best described as lying on a continuum of severity: belief with insight, with overvalued ideas, and with delusions. Although this subtyping schema would probably make a diagnosis of delusional disorder, somatic type, much more stringent, it would also be in keeping with our understanding of the extremely low prevalence of delusional disorder to begin with.

Necessity of Physical Symptoms in HYP

Controversy surrounding this issue still exists, in that one option for HYP in DSM-IV includes eliminating the requirement that fears concerning physical health be related to physical symptomatology and sensations. Our review seems to point to the overwhelming preponderance of physical symptomatology in HYP patients and perhaps to the increased focus of attention or amplification of normal bodily fluctuations and sensations that typify individuals with this disorder.

Nevertheless, this preponderance of symptoms associated with HYP would seem to require qualification in at least two ways. First, individuals with IP do not seem to possess the symptoms they fear contracting (although they may present with some somatic symptoms associated with anxiety). Second, the presence of somatic symptoms may be sensitive to HYP with disease conviction (i.e., these physical symptoms may indicate the presence of HYP), but there is evidence that the presence of physical symptoms is not specific to HYP. Rather, self-focused attention on bodily sensations and consequent somatic amplification may be characteristic of a number of disorders, particularly certain anxiety disorders, as noted in the reviews. Nevertheless, in view of the need for additional studies confirming this finding, it was decided to propose the A criterion as noted above.

Summary

There is no question that additional retrospective studies are required to further delineate the specific criteria that would differentiate HYP from IP, GAD, and body dysmorphic disorder. One of the key issues remains, whether physical symptoms or accentuated body sensations are required to make the diagnosis of HYP. If it were to be a core (i.e., necessary) condition for the diagnosis of HYP, then it would mean persons with a conviction of illness, who remain preoccupied with this conviction despite medical workup and reassurance, and who meet the other criteria (e.g., no other major Axis I disorder, significant impairment in social or occupational functioning, or marked distress) would not qualify for the diagnosis of HYP. In view of the fact that it was important to be able to classify and diagnose this group of patients as well, it was decided not to require the presence of physical symptoms to make this diagnosis in the *DSM-IV Options Book* (Task Force on DSM-IV 1991) recommendations.

References

Adler CM: Somatic and anxiety sensitivities: an investigation of the phenomenological relationships between somatoform anxiety and psychophysiological disorders. Unpublished doctoral dissertation, Albany, NY, State University of New York at Albany, 1989

American Psychiatric Association: Diagnostic and Statistical Manual of Mental Disorders, Third Edition, Revised. Washington, DC, American Psychiatric Association, 1987

Barsky AJ, Wyshak G: Hypochondriasis and somatosensory amplification. Br J Psychiatry 157:404–409, 1990

Barsky AJ, Wyshak G, Klerman GL: The Somatosensory Amplification Scale and its relationship to hypochondriasis. J Psychiatr Res 24:323–334, 1990

Beck AT, Steer RA: Manual for the Beck Anxiety Inventory. San Antonio, TX, Psychological Corporation, 1990

Beck AT, Ward CH, Mendelson M, et al: An inventory for measuring depression. Arch Gen Psychiatry 4:561–571, 1961

Chambless DL, Caputo GC, Bright P, et al: Assessment of fear of fear in agoraphobics: the body sensation questionnaire and the agoraphobic cognitions questionnaire. J Consult Clin Psychol 52:1090–1097, 1984

Derogatis LR, Lipman RS, Rickels K, et al: The Hopkins Symptom Checklist (HSCL): a self-report symptom inventory. Behav Sci 19:1–15, 1974

Goodman WK, Price LH, Rasmussen SA, et al: The Yale-Brown Obsessive Compulsive Scale (Y-BOCS), I: development, use, and reliability. Arch Gen Psychiatry 46:1012–1016, 1989

Hathaway SR, McKinley JC: The Minnesota Multiphasic Personality Schedule. Minneapolis, University of Minnesota Press, 1943

Hollander E: Body dysmorphic disorder and its relationship to obsessive-compulsive disorder. Position paper for DSM-IV Work Group on OCD. New York, Department of Psychiatry, College of Physicians and Surgeons of Columbia University and the OCD Biological Studies Program, New York State Psychiatric Institute, 1989

Kellner R: Functional somatic symptoms and hypochondriasis: a survey of empirical studies. Arch Gen Psychiatry 42:821–833, 1985

Kellner R: A symptom questionnaire. J Clin Psychiatry 48:268–274, 1987

Kellner R: Diagnosis and treatments of hypochondriacal syndromes. Psychosomatics 33:278–289, 1992

Kellner R, Sheffield BF: A self-rating scale of distress. Psychol Med 130:102–105, 1973

Kellner R, Abbott P, Winslow WW, et al: Fears, beliefs, and attitudes in DSM-III hypochondriasis. J Nerv Ment Dis 175:20–25, 1987

Kellner R, Abbott P, Winslow WW, et al: Anxiety, depression, and somatization in DSM-III hypochondriasis. Psychosomatics 30:57–64, 1989

Kellner R, Hernandez J, Pathak D: Hypochondriacal fears and beliefs, anxiety, and somatization. Br J Psychiatry 160:525–532, 1992

Kim SW, Dysken MW, Kuskowski M, et al: The Yale-Brown Obsessive Compulsive Scale (Y-BOCS) and the NIMH Global Obsessive Compulsive Scale (NIMH-GOCS): a reliability and validity study. International Journal of Methods in Psychiatric Research 3:37–44, 1993

Kozak MJ, Foa EB: Obsessions, overvalued ideas, and delusions in obsessive-compulsive disorder. Review paper for the DSM-IV Work Group on OCD. Philadelphia, PA, Medical College of Pennsylvania, 1991

Marks IM, Mathews AM: Brief standard self-rating for phobic patients. Behav Res Ther 17:263–267, 1979

McKenna PJ: Disorders with overvalued ideas. Proc R Soc Med 29:325–336, 1984

Pilowsky I: Dimensions of hypochondriasis. Br J Psychiatry 113:89–93, 1967

Rapee RM: Generalized anxiety disorder boundary issues: GAD and somatoform disorders; GAD and psychophysiological disorders. Review paper for the DSM-IV subgroup on Generalized Anxiety Disorder. St. Lucia, Queensland, Australia, Department of Psychology, University of Queensland, 1989

Rasmussen SA: Hypochondriasis and its relationship to Obsessive-Compulsive Disorder. Position paper for DSM-IV Work Group on OCD. Providence, RI, Department of Psychiatry, Brown University School of Medicine, 1990

Salkovskis PM, Warwick HMC: Morbid preoccupations, health anxiety and reassurance: a cognitive behavioural approach to hypochondriasis. Behav Res Ther 24:597–602, 1986

Salkovskis PM, Warwick HMC, Clark DM: Hypochondriasis, illness phobia and other anxiety disorders. Review paper for the DSM-IV subgroup on Hypochondriasis. Oxford, UK, Department of Psychiatry, University of Oxford, Warneford Hospital, 1990

Spielberger CD, Gorsuch RL, Lushene RE: Manual for the State-Trait Anxiety Inventory. Palo Alto, CA, Consulting Psychologists Press, 1970

Task Force on DSM-IV: DSM-IV Options Book: Work in Progress. Washington, DC, American Psychiatric Association, 1991

Warwick HMC, Marks IM: Behavioural treatment of illness phobia. Br J Psychiatry 152:239–241, 1988

Chapter 43

Body Dysmorphic Disorder

Katharine A. Phillips, M.D., and Eric Hollander, M.D.

Statement of the Issues

This review focuses on the following issues:

1. Is body dysmorphic disorder (BDD) a discrete syndrome?
2. What is the relationship between BDD and other psychiatric disorders?
3. What is the relationship between BDD and no mental disorder (i.e., normal concern about appearance)?
4. Are there any data on the performance of structured assessment instruments for BDD?

Significance of the Issues

Although BDD has received little empirical study and is new to DSM-III-R (American Psychiatric Association 1987), it has long been described in the European, Russian, and Japanese literature under a variety of names, most commonly dysmorphophobia (Munro and Stewart 1991; Phillips 1991). Some of the major questions raised by this literature, and by the relatively little American literature, bear on issues relating to BDD's classification. In particular, some authors have questioned whether BDD is a discrete diagnostic entity (Finkelstein 1963; Fukuda 1977; Hay 1970, 1983). Others have suggested that BDD, although classified in DSM-III-R as a somatoform disorder, might be related to social phobia, mood disorder, obsessive-compulsive disorder (OCD), or psychotic disorders (in particular, delusional disorder) (Connolly and Gipson 1978; Hollander et al. 1989; Kasahara 1987; Lee 1987; Phillips 1991; Zaidens 1950). Still others have questioned whether BDD as currently defined is overly broad, overlapping excessively with normal concern about appearance (Fitts 1989). Despite more than a century of debate, these questions remain largely unresolved and are the focus of this review.

Methods

The psychiatric and psychological literatures were searched for all references related to BDD. This included a computer search with Medline of all English- and foreign-language journal articles published between 1966 and 1991 and with PsycLit and MEDLARS II of all articles published between 1974 and 1991, using index terms such as *body dysmorphic disorder, dysmorphophobia,* and *monosymptomatic hypochondriasis.* Additional articles and books were obtained from the bibliographies of these articles, and the *Index Medicus* was reviewed for 1991. This process produced approximately 160 references. Fifteen foreign-language articles (primarily Russian, French, Italian, German, and Japanese) were translated.

The review is based on those references that most directly inform the above-mentioned classification issues. This includes reports of phenomenology, comorbid disorders, age at onset and course, family history, and treatment response of BDD and possibly related disorders—features that, if shared by two disorders, suggest a close relationship between them. The review is limited by the finding that most of the identified literature consists of case reports and small case series; by the fact that, at the time of this search, only five articles had been published on BDD as defined by DSM-III-R; and by the literature's lack of clear, operationalized definitions of dysmorphophobia and other BDD precursors.

Results

Is BDD a Discrete Syndrome?

Although the literature generally implies that BDD is a discrete psychiatric disorder, several authors suggest that it is instead a nonspecific symptom that can occur in a variety of psychiatric syndromes (Finkelstein 1963; Fukuda 1977; Hay 1970, 1983)—or that it can be either (Barsky 1989; Yamada et al. 1978). Thomas (1984, 1990) highlights this distinction by differentiating between primary and secondary dysmorphophobia, the former being equivalent to the discrete disorder BDD and the latter a nonspecific symptom of a variety of underlying psychiatric syndromes such as schizophrenia, depression, monosymptomatic hypochondriasis, anorexia nervosa, and severe neurosis.

There are few empirical data to support these different views. However, preliminary evidence suggests that BDD may respond to serotonergic medications regardless of the "primary" or "secondary" nature of the symptoms, casting doubt on the validity of this distinction (Hollander et al. 1990a). Similarly, preliminary results from another study (Phillips et al. 1993) found that BDD may respond to treatment when comorbid disorders do not, which suggests that BDD is not simply a symptom of the comorbid disorders. This study also found that BDD tends to be chronic, regardless of the onset or resolution of accompanying disorders, and that patients often consider BDD their most severe and primary problem—findings suggesting that BDD is not simply a nonspecific symptom of other underlying syndromes. However, these data require confirmation.

A related question is whether BDD is a variant or subtype of another specific psychiatric disorder, such as OCD. This issue is discussed below.

What Is the Relationship Between BDD and Other Psychiatric Disorders?

Somatoform disorders. BDD's classification as a somatoform disorder reflects not only a concern with somatic complaints but also the fact that patients are often referred to consultation-liaison psychiatrists by plastic surgeons and other nonpsychiatrist physicians. In a more theoretical vein, it would seem that BDD might be related to hypochondriasis, in particular, given the similar focus on a somatic preoccupation in both disorders, in one case with having a physical disorder and in the other with a defect in appearance.

However, empirical evidence for an association between BDD and the somatoform disorders is lacking (Ross et al. 1987). For example, other somatoform disorders have not been described as comorbid with BDD or present in family members, although these reports did not systematically assess a broad range of comorbid disorders. The one study that has done so, using the Structured Clinical Interview for DSM-III-R (SCID) (Spitzer et al. 1989) in 30 patients with BDD, found low comorbidity with the somatoform disorders (Phillips et al. 1993).

Anorexia nervosa. BDD and anorexia nervosa also appear to have some features in common, most notably, an intense dislike of one's appearance and a marked disturbance in body image. However, it has been noted (Thomas 1987) that the disorders differ in that patients with BDD focus on one particular aspect of their appearance rather than their weight or overall appearance and that they actually look normal, whereas those with anorexia do not. Anorexia nervosa has been reported as comorbid with BDD in only a few case reports (Buvat and Buvat-Herbaut 1978; Hunecke and Bosse 1985) and had relatively low comorbidity with BDD in a preliminary study based on the SCID (Phillips et al. 1993). Other than their phenomenological similarities, there are few data to support a link between the two disorders.

Social phobia. In the Japanese and Korean literature (Kasahara 1987; Lee 1987), BDD is considered a subtype of a larger group of disorders (Taijin-Phobia in Japan) that closely resembles DSM's social phobia or avoidant personality disorder, reflecting a focus on BDD's interpersonal aspects. Similarly, Marks (1980) defined BDD as a social phobia, and other Western authors have noted in case reports that BDD's premorbid and comorbid features may include shyness or a reserved nature (Andreasen and Bardach 1977; Bezoari and Falcinelli 1977; Hay 1970; Liberman 1974; Marks 1987; Thomas 1984; Yamada 1978), social avoidance and isolation (Alliez and Robion 1969; Janet 1903; Liberman 1974; Vallat 1971; Zaidens 1950), introversion (Fukuda 1977), and avoidant personality disorder (de Leon et al. 1989). One data set (Phillips et al. 1993) found a surprisingly high comorbidity of BDD with social phobia as defined by DSM-III-R. The two disorders also have a similar early age at onset. However, whether social phobia and avoidant personality disorder are present in family members, have similar treatment response, or share other clinical features with BDD is unknown at this time.

Mood disorder.   The many case reports documenting the co-occurrence of BDD and depression suggest that depression may be the disorder most commonly associated with BDD (Alliez and Robion 1969; Bezoari and Falcinelli 1977; Bloch and Glue 1988; Braddock 1982; Campanella and Zuccoli 1968; de Leon et al. 1989; Hay 1970; Hollander et al. 1989; Liberman 1974; Marks and Mishan 1988; Riding and Munro 1975; Stekel 1949; Thomas 1984; Zaidens 1950). In Cotterill's (1981) series of 16 dysmorphophobic dermatology patients, 5 were depressed and 2 attempted suicide, making depression the most common associated disorder. Similarly, a study that used the SCID (Philips et al. 1993) found depression to be the disorder most frequently associated with BDD. In a case-control study (Hardy and Cotterill 1982), 5 of 12 dysmorphophobic dermatology patients were moderately or severely depressed, compared with none of the healthy or psoriatic control subjects and scored significantly higher as a group than control subjects on the Beck Depression Inventory (Beck 1978).

Case reports also document a family history of mood disorder in BDD probands (Andreasen and Bardach 1977; Bloch and Glue 1988; Braddock 1982; Campanella and Zuccoli 1968; Hay 1970; Jenike 1984), some of whom had no personal history of mood disorder. A study of five patients diagnosed with BDD by DSM-III-R criteria (Hollander et al. 1989) found mood disorder in the relatives of two. A study (Phillips et al. 1993) that blindly assessed family history of BDD probands found the morbid risk of major mood disorder among first-degree relatives to be similar to rates in relatives of mood-disorder probands. However, a family history of mood disorder in these two studies might reflect the presence of mood disorder rather than BDD in the probands, potentially weakening the evidence for a BDD-mood disorder link.

A link between BDD and mood disorder is also supported by the finding that

BDD may respond preferentially to antidepressant medication (Hollander et al. 1989; Phillips et al. 1993), although BDD's apparent poor response to electroconvulsive therapy (Braddock 1982; Corbella and Rossi 1967; Hay 1970; Hollander et al. 1989; Marks and Mishan 1988; Phillips et al. 1993; Thomas 1985b) weakens the evidence that BDD is a variant of, or related to, mood disorder.

OCD.   Several authors, including Morselli (1891), Janet (1903), and Kraepelin (1909), suggested that BDD is related to OCD. Hay (1970), using several psychometric scales, found dysmorphophobic subjects to be more "obsessoid" than control subjects, and Hardy and Cotterill (1982) found that both dysmorphophobic patients ($N = 12$) and psoriatic control subjects scored higher on the Leyton Obsessional Inventory than healthy control subjects, a finding of unclear significance. In case reports, OCD has been described as comorbid with BDD (Campanella and Zuccoli 1968; Corbella and Rossi 1967; Hay 1970; Hollander et al. 1989; Marks and Mishan 1988; Solyom 1985) and present in relatives of BDD probands (Hollander et al. 1989). A study that used the SCID (Phillips et al. 1993) found fairly high comorbidity with OCD. Other features that appear to be shared by BDD and OCD are early age at onset, an often chronic course, apparent high comorbidity with mood and anxiety disorders, substantial functional impairment, possible presumed etiology (Hollander et al. 1992), and possible preferential response to serotonergic medications (Hollander et al. 1989; Phillips et al. 1993). However, large-scale controlled studies are needed to confirm these apparent similarities.

In addition, BDD symptoms seem phenomenologically similar to obsessional thinking, in that they are persistent, intrusive thoughts that are difficult to resist. In addition, many patients have compulsive, ritualistic behaviors, such as frequent mirror checking or hair combing, that are designed to diminish their anxiety but may not be successful. However, several authors (de Leon 1989; McKenna 1984; Vitiello and de Leon 1990) have suggested that BDD symptoms are more akin to overvalued ideas than obsessions: the thoughts seem more natural than intrusive, are acquiesced to without much resistance, and are held with some conviction rather than regarded as senseless. Some authors (Hollander et al. 1990b) have suggested that overvalued ideas, and even delusions (see below), are also characteristic of some patients with OCD.

Psychotic disorders.   Many authors considered BDD a prodrome or variant of schizophrenia (Anderson 1964; Connolly and Gipson 1978; Korkina 1965; Yamada et al. 1978; Zaidens 1950). Schizophrenia has been found to coexist with BDD (Campanella and Zuccoli 1968; Connolly and Gipson 1978; Cotterill 1981; Hay 1970; Korkina 1965; Vaghina 1966; Yamada et al. 1978; Zaidens 1950) and to occur in relatives of BDD probands (Campanella and Zuccoli 1968; Cotterill 1981; de

Leon et al. 1989; Thomas 1984; Yamada et al. 1978), but one study (Phillips et al. 1993) found no personal or family history of schizophrenia as defined by DSM-III-R in 30 BDD patients assessed with the SCID (Spitzer et al. 1989). In addition, most reports suggest that BDD responds poorly to neuroleptics (Braddock 1982; Cotterill 1981; de Leon 1989; Hollander et al. 1989; Jenike 1984; Phillips et al. 1993; Thomas 1985b), although some suggest that, when delusional symptoms are present, BDD (or monosymptomatic hypochondriasis) may partially respond to the neuroleptic pimozide (Hollander et al. 1989; Riding and Munro 1975). Combined with the fact that earlier definitions of schizophrenia were overly broad by today's nosological standards, these data suggest that BDD is not a variant of schizophrenia.

What about a possible link with delusional disorder? BDD has been classified in the European literature as a type of monosymptomatic hypochondriasis (Bishop 1980; Munro and Chmara 1982), which is similar to delusional disorder, somatic type, in that it consists of a somatic delusion in the absence of other prominent psychotic symptoms. Although DSM-III-R specifies that BDD symptoms are not of delusional intensity, it also acknowledges that it is unclear whether BDD and delusional disorder can be distinguished or are variants of the same disorder. Many authors have argued for the latter view, stating that dysmorphophobia encompasses both nonpsychotic (or neurotic) and psychotic conditions (Campanella and Zuccoli 1968; Korkina 1965; Schachter 1971; Stekel 1949; Vaghina 1966; Vallat et al. 1971) or, similarly, that it may be variously expressed as a preoccupation, an obsession, an overvalued idea, or a frank delusion (Barsky 1989; Birtchnell 1988). In support of this view, it appears that nondelusional BDD symptoms may at times become delusional and vice versa (Hay 1970; Hollander et al. 1989; Phillips et al. 1993); it is unlikely that such patients have two different disorders. It can also be extremely difficult to distinguish delusional from nondelusional preoccupations (Barsky 1989; Braddock 1982; Brotman and Jenike 1985; Cotterill 1981; Phillips et al. 1993), making such differentiation somewhat arbitrary and unreliable. In addition, preliminary data (Phillips et al. 1993) suggest that patients with delusional BDD symptoms do not differ from those with nondelusional symptoms in terms of demographic features, associated features or psychopathology, course, or treatment response. In addition, although it has been suggested that BDD and delusional disorder should be distinguished because the latter may respond preferentially to pimozide (Munro and Stewart 1991; Riding and Munro 1975; Thomas 1985a;), it appears that BDD also sometimes partially responds to this treatment (usually in combination with serotonin reuptake blockers) (Hollander et al. 1989).

Although BDD's probable overlap with delusional thinking might seem to imply a link with psychosis, it is also compatible with a link with OCD, because a similar spectrum has been proposed for this disorder, with obsessions at the severe end being of delusional proportions (obsessive-compulsive psychosis) (Insel and

Akiskal 1986; Solyom et al. 1985). If BDD is related to OCD, BDD and delusional disorder, somatic type, might be similarly related along an obsessive-compulsive continuum from more to less insight, resistance, and dystonicity (Hollander et al. 1989; Sondheimer 1988), or, as suggested above, the single disorder BDD may in fact encompass the entire spectrum, subsuming both nondelusional and delusional thinking.

Koro. This non-DSM disorder, which consists of a complaint of genital retraction with fear of impending death, is phenomenologically similar to BDD in that it involves an imagined defect in appearance. However, in some other ways, the two disorders appear quite different: koro occurs far more frequently in men than in women, appears to have different associated features (primarily acute anxiety), tends to be of brief duration (whereas BDD is often chronic), may respond to reassurance, appears to be culture related (occurring primarily in Southeast Asia), and nearly always occurs as an epidemic. (Bernstein and Gaw 1990; Berrios and Morley 1984; Tseng et al. 1988). Thus, there is inadequate evidence to support the inclusion of koro within the BDD construct.

What Is the Relationship Between BDD and No Mental Disorder (i.e., Normal Concern With Appearance)?

Where to draw the line between normal and abnormal concerns (or symptoms) may be even less clear for BDD than for other psychiatric disorders, because concern with appearance is nearly universal, is influenced by cultural factors (Birtchnell 1988; Finkelstein 1963), and might even be considered a hallmark of normal adolescence. Indeed, a questionnaire survey that attempted to determine BDD's prevalence in a nonclinical population (Fitts et al. 1989) found that 70% of 258 college students were at least somewhat dissatisfied and 46% somewhat preoccupied with some aspect of their appearance, with 28% appearing to meet all criteria for BDD. Although the authors used an apparently unvalidated questionnaire and did not make clinical diagnoses, their findings do underscore the problem of how to differentiate normal from abnormal concern and raise the question of whether the DSM-III-R criteria are too broad and overlap excessively with normal concern.

The question of how to differentiate normal from abnormal concern also applies to the large number of patients who request plastic surgery or dermatological treatment to improve their appearance. Such differentiation may have important treatment implications, because the literature suggests that BDD patients often respond poorly to these nonpsychiatric treatments (Andreasen and Bardach 1977; Bezoari and Falcinelli 1977; Birtchnell 1988; Corbella and Rossi 1967; Fukuda 1977; Hollander et al. 1989; Ladee 1966; Phillips et al. 1993; Strian 1984). Two studies (Andreasen and Bardach 1977; Fukuda 1977) have estimated that 2% of individuals requesting plastic surgery have BDD, but there have been no large studies of BDD's prevalence in surgical or dermatological populations.

Despite the almost certain existence of a hazy area of overlap between normal and abnormal concern with appearance, there are clearly individuals who are so preoccupied, severely distressed, and substantially impaired by their concern about a minimal or nonexistent deformity that their symptoms should be distinguished from normal. However, as the above-mentioned study suggests, the DSM-III-R criteria, which lack an item requiring the presence of distress or impairment, may be too broad and overinclusive, potentially applying not only to persons with BDD but also to some with "normal" concerns.

Are There Data on Performance of Structured Assessment Instruments for BDD?

Although there are many instruments that assess various aspects of appearance-related body-image disturbance (Cash and Pruzinsky 1990), only three apply specifically to BDD. These consist of a BDD diagnostic questionnaire (E. Hollander, unpublished, 1991), a version of the Yale-Brown Obsessive Compulsive Scale modified to assess BDD (E. Hollander, unpublished, 1991), and a BDD diagnostic module (K. A. Phillips, unpublished, 1991). However, the performance of these instruments has not been adequately evaluated.

Discussion and Recommendations

Although BDD's status as a discrete disorder has been questioned, its historical classification as such in both the European literature and DSM-III-R combines with preliminary empirical data to support its separate status in DSM-IV. An important potential advantage of retaining BDD as a separate syndrome is the stimulation of much-needed research on the disorder. However, because the literature has also suggested that BDD may at times be secondary (i.e., a nonspecific symptom of another, underlying psychiatric disorder rather than a discrete disorder), it was proposed that DSM-IV (in a manner similar to DSM-III-R) state that BDD cannot occur exclusively during the course of another mental disorder, such as anorexia nervosa. Although this might discourage the assignment of multiple and possibly redundant diagnoses, it may be premature. First, it seems likely that BDD, as a discrete disorder, sometimes occurs only during the course of another disorder, such as anorexia nervosa; such co-occurrence seems inevitable, given BDD's apparent high comorbidity with other psychiatric disorders (Phillips et al. 1993). In addition, the proposed change implies a diagnostic hierarchy that is not supported by any empirical evidence. Finally, the proposal might lead to underdiagnosis and undertreatment of BDD.

It was therefore proposed that the DSM-III-R exclusion criterion "occurrence not exclusively during the course of anorexia nervosa or transsexualism" be changed to "The preoccupation is not better accounted for by another mental disorder (e.g., dissatisfaction with body shape and size in anorexia nervosa)," which, it is hoped, avoids the above-mentioned drawbacks of the DSM-III-R criterion.

Another question is whether BDD should remain classified with the somatoform disorders or be reclassified as a mood, psychotic, or anxiety disorder (in particular, as a type of OCD). The data appear to best support an association of BDD with OCD, as either a related but separate disorder or as an OCD subtype. However, the current empirical evidence is preliminary, making the association with OCD somewhat speculative. On balance, it seems that reclassification of BDD as a form of OCD or another nonsomatoform disorder would be premature at this time because there are no convincing data to support such a change or to clearly indicate to which section BDD should be moved.

Regarding BDD's relationship to its delusional counterpart (delusional disorder, somatic type), there is preliminary evidence that the disorders exist on a continuum, with a hazy area of overlap, and may even be the same disorder. A similar continuum between preoccupation, overvalued ideation, and delusional thinking may also exist for hypochondriasis and OCD, and it has therefore been suggested that the proposed subtyping scheme for OCD (i.e., with insight, with overvalued ideas, with delusions) be adopted for BDD. However, empirical support for this change is still inadequate at this time.

Finally, although there are few data addressing BDD's boundary with no mental disorder, it seems that DSM-III-R's lack of a severity criterion for BDD could be problematic, creating excessive overlap with normal concern with appearance. It was therefore proposed that the following criterion be added: "The preoccupation causes significant impairment in social or occupational functioning or causes marked distress." The potential advantages of this addition are the prevention of BDD's overdiagnosis and the creation of more homogeneous groups for research purposes.

The sharp contrast between BDD's long and rich historical tradition and its almost nonexistent empirical base is notable. All aspects of BDD need to be further researched, using standardized instruments in large clinical and nonclinical populations. Inquiry into BDD's phenomenology, course, associated psychopathology, biology, family history, and treatment response may help clarify how this disorder should be classified in DSM-V—as a somatoform, psychotic, mood, anxiety, or OCD-related disorder. In particular, BDD's relationship to OCD and delusional disorder needs further assessment not only to answer classification questions but also to shed light on the diagnosis and treatment of this distressing, impairing, and often secret disorder.

References

Alliez J, Robion M: Aspects psycho-pathologiques de la defiguration et leur relation avec la dysmorphophobie. Ann Med Psychol (Paris) 2:479–494, 1969

American Psychiatric Association: Diagnostic and Statistical Manual of Mental Disorders, 3rd Edition, Revised. Washington, DC, American Psychiatric Association, 1987

Anderson EW: Psychiatry. London, Bailliere, Tindall, & Cox, 1964

Andreasen NC, Bardach J: Dysmorphophobia: symptom or disease? Am J Psychiatry 134:673–676, 1977

Barsky AF: Somatoform disorders, in Comprehensive Textbook of Psychiatry, 5th Edition, Vol 1. Edited by Kaplan HI, Sadock BJ. Baltimore, MD, Williams & Wilkins, 1989, pp 1009–1027

Beck AT: Depression Inventory. Philadelphia, PA, Philadelphia Center for Cognitive Therapy, 1978

Bernstein RL, Gaw AC: Koro: proposed classification for DSM-IV. Am J Psychiatry 147:1670–1674, 1990

Berrios GE, Morley SJ: Koro-like symptoms in a non-Chinese subject. Br J Psychiatry 145:331–334, 1984

Bezoari M, Falcinelli D: Immagine del corpo e relazioni oggettuali: note sulla dismorfofobia. Rass Studi Psichiat 66:489–510, 1977

Birtchnell SA: Dysmorphophobia: a centenary discussion. Br J Psychiatry 153 (suppl 2):41–43, 1988

Bishop ER: Monosymptomatic hypochondriasis. Psychosomatics 21:731–747, 1980

Bloch S, Glue P: Psychotherapy and dysmorphophobia: a case report. Br J Psychiatry 152:271–274, 1988

Braddock LE: Dysmorphophobia in adolescence: a case report. Br J Psychiatry 140:199–201, 1982

Brotman AW, Jenike MA: Dysmorphophobia and monosymptomatic hypochondriasis (letter). Am J Psychiatry 142:1121, 1985

Buvat J, Buvat-Herbaut M: Dysperception de l'image corporelle et dysmorphophobies dans l'anorexie mentale: à propos de 115 cas des deux sexes, II: les dysmorphophobies dans l'anorexie mentale. Ann Med Psychol (Paris) 136:563–580, 1978

Campanella FN, Zuccoli E: In tema di dismorfofobia. Neuropsichiatria 24:475–486, 1968

Cash TF, Pruzinsky T (eds): Body Images: Development, Deviance, and Change. New York, Guilford, 1990

Connolly FH, Gipson M: Dysmorphophobia: a long-term study. Br J Psychiatry 132:568–570, 1978

Corbella T, Rossi L: La dysmorphophobie: ses aspects cliniques et nosographiques. Acta Neurol Belg 67:691–700, 1967

Cotterill JA: Dermatological non-disease: a common and potentially fatal disturbance of cutaneous body image. Br J Dermatol 104:611–619, 1981

De Leon J, Bott A, Simpson GM: Dysmorphophobia: body dysmorphic disorder or delusional disorder, somatic subtype? Compr Psychiatry 30:457–472, 1989

Finkelstein BA: Dysmorphophobia. Diseases of the Nervous System 24:365–370, 1963

Fitts SN, Gibson P, Redding CA, et al: Body dysmorphic disorder: implications for its validity as a DSM-III-R clinical syndrome. Psychological Reports 64:655–658, 1989

Fukuda O: Statistical analysis of dysmorphophobia in out-patient clinic. Japanese Journal of Plastic and Reconstructive Surgery 20:569–577, 1977

Hardy GE, Cotterill JA: A study of depression and obsessionality in dysmorphophobic and psoriatic patients. Br J Psychiatry 140:19–22, 1982

Hay GG: Dysmorphophobia. Br J Psychiatry 116:399–406, 1970

Hay GG: Paranoia and dysmorphophobia (letter). Br J Psychiatry 142:309–310, 1983

Hollander E: Body dysmorphic disorder questionnaires. Unpublished manuscripts, 1991

Hollander E, Leibowitz MR, Winchel R, et al: Treatment of body-dysmorphic disorder with serotonin reuptake blockers. Am J Psychiatry 146:768–770, 1989

Hollander E, Decaria C, Liebowitz MR, et al: Body-dysmorphic disorder (letter). Am J Psychiatry 147:817, 1990a

Hollander E, Neville D, Decaria C, et al: On dysmorphophobia misdiagnosed as obsessive compulsive disorder (letter). Psychosomatics 31:468–469, 1990b

Hollander E, Neville D, Frenkel M, et al: Body dysmorphic disorder: diagnostic issues and related disorders. Psychosomatics 33:156–165, 1992

Hunecke P, Bosse K: Dysmorphophobie als casus pro diagnosi. Z Hautkr 60:1986–1990, 1985

Insel TR, Akiskal HS: Obsessive-compulsive disorder with psychotic features: a phenomenologic analysis. Am J Psychiatry 143:1527–1533, 1986

Janet P: Les Obsessions et la Psychasthenie. Paris, Felix Alcan, 1903

Jenike MA: A case report of successful treatment of dysmorphophobia with tranylcypromine. Am J Psychiatry 141:1463–1464, 1984

Kasahara Y: Social phobia in Japan, in Social Phobia in Japan and Korea, Proceedings of the First Cultural Psychiatry Symposium between Japan and Korea. Seoul, Korea, The East Asian Academy of Cultural Psychiatry, 1987

Korkina MB: The syndrome of dysmorphomania (dysmorphophobia) and the development of psychopathic personality. Zh Nevropatol Psikhiatr 65:1212–1217, 1965

Kraepelin E: Psychiatrie, 8th Edition. Leipzig, Germany, JA Barth, 1909–1915

Ladee GA: Hypochondriacal Syndromes. Amsterdam, Netherlands, Elsevier, 1966

Lee SH: Social phobia in Korea, in Social Phobia in Japan and Korea, Proceedings of the First Cultural Psychiatry Symposium between Japan and Korea. Seoul, Korea, The East Asian Academy of Cultural Psychiatry, 1987

Liberman R: A propos des dysmorphophobies de l'adolescent. Revue de Neuropsychiatrie Infantile 22:695–699, 1974

Marks IM: Cure and Care of Neurosis: Theory and Practice of Behavioral Psychotherapy. New York, Wiley, 1980

Marks IM: Fears, Phobias, and Rituals. Oxford, UK, Oxford University Press, 1987

Marks I, Mishan J: Dysmorphophobic avoidance with disturbed bodily perception: a pilot study of exposure therapy. Br J Psychiatry 152:674–678, 1988

McKenna PJ: Disorders with overvalued ideas. Br J Psychiatry 145:579–585, 1984

Morselli E: Sulla dismorfofobia e sulla tafefobia. Bollettino della R. Accademia Medica di Genova 6:110–119, 1891

Munro A, Chmara J: Monosymptomatic hypochondriacal psychosis: a diagnostic checklist based on 50 cases of the disorder. Can J Psychiatry 27:374–376, 1982

Munro A, Stewart M: Body dysmorphic disorder and the DSM-IV: the demise of dysmorphophobia. Can J Psychiatry 36:91–96, 1991

Phillips KA: Body dysmorphic disorder: the distress of imagined ugliness. Am J Psychiatry 148:1138–1149, 1991

Phillips KA: Diagnostic module for body dysmorphic disorder. Unpublished manuscript, 1991

Phillips KA, McElroy SL, Keck PE, et al: Body dysmorphic disorder: 30 cases of imagined ugliness. Am J Psychiatry 150:302–308, 1993

Riding J, Munro A: Pimozide in the treatment of monosymptomatic hypochondriacal psychosis. Acta Psychiatr Scand 52:23–30, 1975

Ross CA, Siddiqui AR, Matas M: DSM-III: problems in diagnosis of paranoia and obsessive-compulsive disorder. Can J Psychiatry 32:146–148, 1987

Schachter M: Neuroses dysmorphiques (complexes de laideur) et delire ou conviction delirante de dysmorphie. Ann Med Psychol (Paris) 129:723–745, 1971

Solyom L, DiNicola VF, Phil M, et al: Is there an obsessive psychosis? Aetological and prognostic factors of an atypical form of obsessive-compulsive neurosis. Can J Psychiatry 30:372–379, 1985

Sondheimer A: Clomipramine treatment of delusional disorder-somatic type. J Am Acad Child Adolesc Psychiatry 27:188–192, 1988

Spitzer RL, Williams JBW, Gibbon M: Structured Clinical Interview for DSM-III-R (SCID). New York, New York State Psychiatric Institute, 1989

Stekel W: Compulsion and Doubt. Translated by Gutheil EA. New York, Liveright, 1949

Strian F: Die Dysmorphophobie als Kontraindikation kosmetischer Operationen. Handchir Mikrochir Plast Chir 16:243–245, 1984

Thomas CS: Dysmorphophobia: a question of definition. Br J Psychiatry 144:513–516, 1984

Thomas CS: Dysmorphophobia and monosymptomatic hypochondriasis (letter). Am J Psychiatry 142:1121, 1985a

Thomas CS: Dysmorphophobia or monosymptomatic hypochondriasis? (letter). Br J Psychiatry 146:672, 1985b

Thomas CS: Anorexia nervosa and dysmorphophobia (letter). Br J Psychiatry 150:406, 1987

Thomas CS: Body-dysmorphic disorder (letter). Am J Psychiatry 147:816–817, 1990

Tseng W, Kan-Ming M, Hsu J, et al: A sociocultural study of koro epidemics in Guangdong, China. Am J Psychiatry 145:1538–1543, 1988

Vaghina GS: Dysmorphophobia syndrome in the clinical treatment of schizophrenia. Zh Nevropatol Psikhiatr 66:1228–1234, 1966

Vallat JN, Leger JM, Destruhaut J, et al: Dysmorphophobie: syndrome ou symptome? Ann Med Psychol (Paris) 2:45–65, 1971

Vitiello B, de Leon J: Dysmorphophobia misdiagnosed as obsessive-compulsive disorder. Psychosomatics 31:220–222, 1990

Yamada M, Kobashi K, Shigemoto T, et al: On dysmorphophobia. Bull Yamaguchi Med Sch 25:47–54, 1978

Zaidens SH: Dermatologic hypochondriasis: a form of schizophrenia. Psychosom Med 12:250–253, 1950

Chapter 44

The Place of Neurasthenia in DSM-IV

Leslie C. Morey, Ph.D., and John E. Kurtz, Ph.D.

Statement and Significance of the Issues

The proposed ICD-10 (World Health Organization 1990) includes a syndrome called "neurasthenia" among the neurotic disorders. Also known as "fatigue syndrome," the salient feature of this disorder is the feeling of physical weakness or exhaustion and/or mental fatiguability in the absence of an identifiable organic basis. Other various somatic complaints and subcriterion levels of anxiety and depression may complement the clinical presentation of neurasthenia.

Efforts have been made in the last decade to increase the compatibility between ICD-10 and DSM-III-R (American Psychiatric Association 1987), used extensively by mental health workers in the United States. The DSM-III-R classification system does not contain the term *neurasthenia* or describe any syndrome whose main feature is the chronic feeling of mental or physical fatigue. Resolution of this discrepancy is important for the sake of global consistency in classification and diagnosis. Given that neurasthenia is the most commonly diagnosed mental disorder in the Soviet Union (Carson et al. 1988) and the most common nonpsychotic diagnosis in China (Kleinman 1982; Zhang 1989), identification of its parallel manifestations in the American classification scheme can give insight into the cultural forces that guide our understanding of nonpsychotic mental illnesses in general.

The purpose of this review is 1) to examine the historical use of this diagnostic term and determine why its importance has waxed and waned, 2) to determine its relationship to current North American diagnostic concepts, and 3) to discuss its viability within a classification scheme that is compatible with ICD-10.

Methods

A search of the psychiatric and psychological literature was conducted with Medline and *Psychological Abstracts* databases, with *neurasthenia* as the key word. The Medline search uncovered 63 references, including monographs; a survey of Psychological Abstracts back to 1927 produced 113 references from the journal literature. In addition, various historically important monographs and textbooks were reviewed to determine earlier uses of the term (e.g., Arieti 1959; Chrzanowski 1959; Laughlin 1967; Noyes and Kolb 1963).

Results

Historical Evolution

The lack of American recognition of neurasthenia is somewhat ironic because it was one of the few psychiatric terms of American origin that predated DSM-II (American Psychiatric Association 1968). Neurasthenia was originally identified by the neurologist George Miller Beard (1880) shortly after the end of the American Civil War. "A feeling of profound exhaustion" was but one of more than 50 symptoms, most of them somatic, according to Beard's original conception of neurasthenia (Ferraro 1954; Gosling 1987). An examination of case studies of neurasthenia in the late 19th century reveals that depressed, anxious/phobic, obsessive-compulsive, and most other neurotic individuals of the day were diagnosed as neurasthenics. It has been said that Beard's catchall diagnosis would account for the majority of the unfortunate individuals lodged between the extremes of those who were functioning "normally" and the institutionalized insane (Gosling 1987). Beard (1869) felt that the disease was the result of the mental overexertion common in the middle- and upper class members of society and that "both anemia and neurasthenia are most frequently met with in civilized, intellectual communities. They are part of the compensation for our progress and refinement" (p. 217).

Sigmund Freud was influential in narrowing the concept. He proposed that a large set of symptoms, including anxiety reactions, phobias, and obsessional ideas, be extracted from neurasthenia and associated with a new category, "anxiety neurosis" (Freud 1894/1953). The introduction of anxiety neurosis proved to be one of Freud's most significant accomplishments and has affected systems of psychiatric classification up to now. Neurasthenia was classified as an "actual neurosis," presumably having a physical as opposed to a psychological origin and being unsuitable for treatment with psychoanalysis.

More important for the present purposes are the clinical characteristics of neurasthenia that remained once those of the anxiety neurosis had been detached. Freud left for neurasthenia the symptoms "headache, spinal irritation, and dyspepsia with flatulence and constipation" (Freud 1894/1953). Not only is the syndrome without psychogenic etiology, but it has no psychological symptomatology. Freud does not mention fatigue as a symptom of either neurasthenia or the anxiety neurosis but instead sees it as contributing to the etiology of the latter. It is hard to see why anyone with the symptoms of neurasthenia as described by Freud would come to the attention of a psychiatrist. In comparison with the anxiety neuroses, Freud showed little interest in neurasthenia (despite the fact that he claimed to have suffered from it as a medical student) in terms of its etiology, course, prevalence, or prognosis.

Although Freud's common neuroses were widely accepted by the international psychiatric community, his concept of neurasthenia as an actual neurosis was a debatable topic throughout the first half of the 20th century. Ferraro (1954) observed that there was no clear consensus after Freud's redefinition of neurasthenia with regard to the etiology of such a "pleomorphic syndrome" or its position in psychiatric classification. The numerous viewpoints on neurasthenia from 1904 to 1950 as cited by Ferraro are summarized in Table 44–1. The perspectives of the principal psychiatric theorists of this time were divided between psychogenic and organic etiological theories, and definitions of the disorder were variously presented as neurosis, psychosis, or nonpsychiatric disease. Ferraro himself concluded that the removal of psychological elements (e.g., anxiety) from the definition of neurasthenia stripped it of any clinical meaning and that such a concept thus "should be denied a nosologic position in psychiatry" (Ferraro 1954, p. 312). A number of other psychiatrists of that period also dismissed neurasthenia as nonexistent; consequently, the diagnosis was less frequently assigned after the mid-20th century, and attention drifted away from the disorder in the United States.

The American Psychiatric Association introduced the first edition of the Diagnostic and Statistical Manual in 1952. Neurasthenia, by name, was not included in this edition, but was represented by the term *psychophysiologic nervous system reaction* (PNSR). PNSR was classified among the psychophysiological disorders and the clinical picture was comprised of "general fatigue" and "associated visceral complaints" (American Psychiatric Association 1952, p. 31). DSM-II reinstated the term *neurasthenia,* or *neurasthenic neurosis,* in the interest of international compatibility in psychiatric classification, specifically with respect to ICD-8 (Chatel and Peele 1970). The clinical description in DSM-II is similar to that of the original PNSR disorder in the first DSM, except that the condition is described in greater detail as being "characterized by complaints of chronic weakness, easy fatiguability, and sometimes exhaustion" (American Psychiatric Association 1968, pp. 40–41). The term is altogether absent in DSM-III (American Psychiatric Association 1980); a special appendix on changes in the third edition explains that the diagnosis was rarely used and hence not included. This conclusion is supported by the finding that inclusion of neurasthenia in the DSM-II system was a modification that was generally not welcomed by the American psychiatric community (Chatel and Peele 1970).

Table 44–1. Theoretical perspectives on neurasthenia (1904–1950)

Author	Date	Concept of neurasthenia
Krafft-Ebing	1904	"Neuropsychosis," psychogenic, not distinct from anxiety neurosis
Dubois	1910	Strongly psychogenic, amenable to rational psychotherapy
Kraepelin	1915	"Nervous exhaustion," possible internal toxin, nothing proved
Bleuler	1924	Two types: actual neurasthenia, of physical origin; pseudoneurasthenia, more common and psychogenic
Janet	1925	Precursor to psychasthenia, due to hereditary predisposition
Hertz	1928	"Weakness of nervous functions," many mental and somatic symptoms
Dejerine and Gauckler	?	"Psychoneurosis," emotional basis with somatic symptoms of anxiety
Wechsler	1930	Organic disease
Schilder	1930	Psychogenic conversion disorder
White	1935	"Psychoneurosis" caused by idleness, equal to hypochondriasis
Tanzi and Lugaro	?	"Obsessive psychosis," psychogenic
Strecker and Ebaugh	?	"Psychoneurosis," psychogenic
Muncie	1939	"Psychoneurosis," psychogenic
Noyes	1948	"Psychoneurosis," psychogenic
Weiss and English	1949	"Psychoneurosis," psychogenic
Henderson and Gillespie	1950	"Psychoneurosis," psychogenic
Brun	1950	"Functional organic hormopathy," "complex conditioning" psychic processes

Source. Adapted from Ferraro 1954.

One reviewer (Berger 1973) relates the fluctuating interest in neurasthenia to the divisive effects of large wars, especially as seen in the adjustment reactions of soldiers who must make the transitions from society to war and then back to society. Berger notes that neurasthenia returned to the attention of American psychiatry during the Vietnam War, during which participants were exposed to conflict both on the battlefield and at home. Beard's original formulation was also used to describe the adjustment reactions of veterans of the Civil War.

Neurasthenic Equivalent

Based on epidemiological studies of the prevalence of neurasthenia in countries where the diagnosis is accepted (e.g., Japan [Takahashi 1978]), it is reasonable to suspect that the population of neurasthenic patients in Asia and eastern Europe must have a North American equivalent. Kleinman (1982) examined 100 cases of neurasthenia in China and reported that 93 had some form of depressive disorder, with 87 of these cases meeting DSM-III criteria for major depressive disorder. The mean number of diagnoses per case was 2.5; 69 patients were diagnosed with an anxiety-related disorder, and 25 were assigned somatoform diagnoses (often involving dizziness, headaches, and/or chronic pain). Kleinman proposed that neurasthenia is, for the Chinese, an acceptable somatic manifestation of depression, anxiety, or other psychological difficulties. He stressed that, in considering the clinical presentations of mental illness in other countries, we must recognize these "culturally sanctioned idioms of distress and psychosocial coping" (Kleinman 1982, p. 119)

Zhang (1989) provided further detail about the comparability of neurasthenia to various North American nosological concepts. Zhang studied 40 Chinese patients who had been diagnosed as neurasthenic by two Chinese psychiatrists. These patients were assigned CATEGO (Wing et al. 1974) and DSM-III diagnoses on the basis of two structured interviews (Present State Examination [Wing et al. 1967]; Diagnostic Interview Schedule [Robins et al. 1981]). Additionally, a number of other self-report and rating scales were completed for these patients. This study reported five primary findings: 1) diagnoses for the patients were quite diverse, ranging from milder personality disorder to severe affective disorders; 2) most of the patients received either an anxiety disorder or affective disorder diagnosis; 3) the most prominent symptomatic features were anxiety and depression, and often a combination of both; 4) there was a group of neurasthenic patients who did not meet criteria for any disorder; and 5) the self-reports of patients tended to be more severe than assessments made by an objective interviewer. Zhang concluded that the term needed to be refined but that discarding it from psychiatric nosology would be premature.

Discussion

The task of identifying the American equivalent of neurasthenia would be facilitated by the introduction of operational criteria sets for all of the disorders in ICD-10. The proposed diagnostic guidelines specify two criteria that are necessary for a definite ICD-10 diagnosis of neurasthenia. The first is consistent with the historical concept: "either (a) persistent and distressing complaints of increased fatiguability after mental effort, or (b) persistent and distressing complaints of bodily weakness and exhaustion after minimal effort, accompanied by unpleasant physical sensations (e.g., muscular aches or pains), and inability to relax" (World Health Organization 1988, p. 119). The second criterion recognizes the problem of overlap in the historical concept: "the absence of symptoms of anxiety or depression sufficiently persistent and severe to fulfill the criteria for any of the more specific disorders in this classification" (World Health Organization 1988, p. 119). Of primary interest is the extent to which this exclusion criterion will deflate the incidence of neurasthenic cases in those countries that make frequent use of the diagnosis. In fact, the creators of the new guidelines predict that "many of the cases so diagnosed in the past would meet the current criteria for depressive disorder or anxiety disorder" (World Health Organization 1988, p. 119), a conclusion supported by the results of studies such as that of Zhang (1989). Until epidemiological studies that systematically apply this narrowed concept are completed, one can only speculate about the future of neurasthenia under ICD-10.

The proposed ICD definition, while providing reasonably detailed criteria, raises a number of potential problems. First, the use of the latter exclusion criterion makes certain assumptions about the superordinate position of depression and anxiety over neurasthenia in a hierarchy of psychopathology that may not be warranted (e.g., Foulds 1976). In fact, Foulds believed that anxiety and depression were very low (i.e., subordinate) in the hierarchy of mental disorder because of their wide prevalence and nonspecific nature as affective states. A second problem involves the purely somatic focus of the criteria. Earlier reviews (e.g., Ferraro 1954) concluded that a sole emphasis on somatic features in a definition of neurasthenia left the concept bereft of most of its clinical meaning. Furthermore, studies such as those by Kleinman (1982) and Zhang (1989) emphasize that both anxiety and depression are often a part of the clinical presentation and that these features are often sufficiently severe to meet DSM criteria. Thus, excluding these patients would substantially alter the meaning of the disorder as it is currently used in other countries. Furthermore, if these features of anxiety, depression, and somatic weakness constitute an empirically coherent syndrome (which remains to be demonstrated), it is not clear why this syndrome should be diagnostically subordinate to concepts such as major depression or anxiety disorder, which include quite heterogeneous groups of patients.

With respect to the inclusion of neurasthenia in DSM-IV, a consideration of the most likely candidates for overlap is warranted.

Affective Disorders

The index of selected symptoms in DSM-III-R cites 21 disorders that can be identified by the presence of a "decrease in energy or fatigue." If schizophrenia, organic and sleep disorders, and states relating to the use of psychoactive substances can be reasonably excluded, the remaining conditions are predominantly mood related: major depression, bipolar disorder, dysthymia, uncomplicated bereavement, adjustment disorder, and late luteal phase dysphoria. Of these, dysthymia is closest to the ICD-10 description of neurasthenia; the affective disturbance is insufficiently severe to warrant the diagnosis of major depression and chronic fatigue or lack of energy can be present.

The results of the Kleinman (1982) study in China have been replicated by others (Grauer 1984; Jun-mian 1987) who agree that actual depression is masked in the somatic presentations of most Chinese patients. These observations and the presence of fatigue symptoms in mood disturbances suggest that neurasthenia may be a depressive equivalent in countries where it is frequently diagnosed.

Anxiety Disorders

The neurasthenic syndrome as defined by ICD-10 may also include minor degrees of anxiety and its associated somatic symptoms. Some researchers see the disorder as merely "anxiety by another name" (Dalessio 1978). Similar physiological disturbances were found in patients with phobic and neurasthenic syndromes (Pankova and Keshokov 1982), and some current pharmacological literature coming out of eastern Europe claims successful treatment of the disorder with antianxiety medications (Zapletalek et al. 1981). Others have likened it to posttraumatic stress disorder or a "stress intolerance syndrome" that rises in incidence during times of war (Berger 1973).

Somatoform Disorders

Fatigue and weakness might be considered somatic symptoms, but neither is listed among the 35 somatic complaints common to somatization disorder in DSM-III-R. Classic descriptions of the neurasthenic syndrome point out that "an exaggerated degree of attention is paid to the bodily organs and their functions" (Noyes and Kolb 1963). Researchers in Austria (Guttel et al. 1977) point to an overactive autonomic system as the main feature accountable for the typical symptomatology of neurasthenia and hypochondriasis, and they conclude that the two syndromes are essentially redundant. The ICD-10 description differentiates "the patient's emphasis on fatiguability and weakness, and his concern about lowered mental and physical efficiency" (World Health Organization 1988, p. 119) from a preoccupation with bodily complaints and physical disease. Whether this is a valid distinction remains to be demonstrated; in Chinese samples, other somatic complaints including chronic pain and headaches are quite common (Kleinman 1986). More research is needed to determine the extent of somatic complaints and health concerns in the average case of neurasthenia. The little available evidence suggests that general somatic complaints are not necessarily common in these patients.

Personality Disorders

Some European researchers (Costantini et al. 1981; Verhaest and Pierloot 1981) support the view that neurasthenia is a wholly psychogenic personality disturbance with narcissistic features. This idea is not a new one. One American definition of the disorder remarks that "neurasthenic patients are typically narcissistic, self-centered, and manifest strong dependency needs" (Hinsie and Campbell 1976), and DSM-II included an allied personality disorder construct, "the asthenic personality."

Recommendations

The proposed ICD-10 has provided a reduced and clarified list of symptom descriptors for neurasthenia in an attempt to address apparent problems of differential diagnosis with other common and related mental disorders. This result leaves classification research with a new set of questions. Of primary interest is the potential change in the incidence or rate of diagnosis of neurasthenia that may result from the new, more stringent criteria. The authors of the ICD-10 section on neurasthenia suggest that there will be a residue of cases that are better described by the new guidelines than those of the other more common neurotic syndromes (World Health Organization 1988). Indeed, American physicians have historically recognized the widespread occurrence of fatigue in their patients, often distinguishable from those symptoms of affective origin, but the issue receives little attention in medical education (Laughlin 1967).

Furthermore, fatigue and weakness seem to play a role in a number of contemporary medical controversies. For example, recent years have seen a preoccupation with syndromes in which fatigue is a central feature, such as those putatively linked to the Epstein-Barr virus. The uncertain etiology of these conditions has led the Centers for Disease Control to provide diagnostic criteria for "chronic fatigue syndrome" without reference to specific etiology, in an attempt to improve clinical research on these vaguely defined problems (Holmes et al. 1988). Interestingly,

Kruesi et al. (1989) found a high prevalence of psychiatric disorder in patients meeting these criteria for chronic fatigue syndrome and reported that the psychiatric disorders tended to precede the fatigue rather than follow the onset of the syndrome. These trends suggest that individuals meeting historical criteria for neurasthenia may also be presenting to medical specialists as part of a heterogeneous group of patients complaining of fatigue. Delineation of specific and valid criteria for neurasthenia would help to address some of these issues, particularly with respect to increasing the coverage of the DSM-IV.

In conclusion, there seem to be recurring observations of a group of patients presenting with fatigue and somatic weakness who, on further investigation, also have prominent features of anxiety and depression. Although many of these patients probably would meet DSM-III/DSM-III-R criteria for anxiety disorders or depressive disorders (e.g., dysthymia), it is not clear that these syndromes would include all such patients or that these diagnoses capture the essence of this syndrome. Considering some of the criteria laid out by Frances et al. (1989) for making diagnostic changes in DSM-IV, there are a number of points in support of its inclusion. Clinical utility seems to have been demonstrated, given its prevalence in other countries, its historical use in the United States, and the current controversy surrounding related syndromes in other areas of medicine. However, the disorder has not been viewed favorably in the past, and care must be taken to insure that it does not become the "wastebasket" category that evoked these previous criticisms. Evidence of descriptive validity is sparse, but data such as those of Zhang (1989) suggest that there is a core of patients who are homogeneous in certain respects yet do not fall neatly into existing DSM-III-R categories. However, there is also evidence that many patients diagnosed as neurasthenic in countries where the disorder is prevalent will meet criteria for either a depressive or anxiety disorder in DSM-III-R. Finally, the external validity of the disorder is virtually unknown, and a variety of studies would need to be performed before this could be demonstrated. This research could be stimulated by including criteria for neurasthenia similar to those proposed for ICD-10 in an appendix to DSM-IV for diagnoses needing further study.

The inclusion of neurasthenia in ICD-10 provides a certain inducement for including a similar category in DSM-IV in the interest of compatibility. However, the proposed criteria in ICD-10 have certain weaknesses; in particular, the role of mixed anxiety and depression seems to be underemphasized in that definition. A focus on purely somatic elements seems to have been one factor in the demise of the construct in previous editions of DSM. If included in DSM-IV, an emphasis on the presence of chronic complaints of both anxiety and depression, of moderate severity, as well as on chronic complaints of fatigue and weakness might serve to make for a more restrictive diagnosis. This more narrowly defined concept, without the exclusion criteria that may serve as a problem with the ICD-10 definition, might serve to define a concept with greater clinical utility than previous incarnations of the disorder and provide a stimulus for the research needed to eventually document any inherent validity in the construct.

References

American Psychiatric Association: Diagnostic and Statistical Manual: Mental Disorders. Washington, DC, American Psychiatric Association, 1952

American Psychiatric Association: Diagnostic and Statistical Manual of Mental Disorders, 2nd Edition. Washington, DC, American Psychiatric Association, 1968

American Psychiatric Association: Diagnostic and Statistical Manual of Mental Disorders, 3rd Edition. Washington, DC, American Psychiatric Association, 1980

American Psychiatric Association: Diagnostic and Statistical Manual of Mental Disorders, 3rd Edition, Revised. Washington, DC, American Psychiatric Association, 1987

Arieti S: American Handbook of Psychiatry. New York, Basic Books, 1959

Beard GM: Neurasthenia, or nervous exhaustion. Boston Medical and Surgical Journal 80:217–221, 1869

Beard GM: A Practical Treatise on Nervous Exhaustion (Neurasthenia): Its Symptoms, Nature, Sequences and Treatment. New York, William Wood, 1880

Berger DM: The return of neurasthenia. Compr Psychiatry 14:557–562, 1973

Carson RC, Butcher JN, Coleman JC: Abnormal Psychology and Modern Life, 8th Edition. Glenview, IL, Scott, Foresman, 1988

Chatel JC, Peele R: A centennial review of neurasthenia. Am J Psychiatry 126:1401–1411, 1970

Chrzanowski G: Neurasthenia and hypochondriasis, in The American Handbook of Psychiatry. Edited by Arieti S. New York, Basic Books, 1959, pp 258–271

Costantini MV, de Leo D, Ferruzza E, et al: Sindrome neurastenica: riflessioni critiche sul problema nosografico attraverso uno studio di personalita: parte seconda. Rivista Sperimentale di Freniatria e Medicina Legale delle Alienazioni Mentali 105:1334–1348, 1981

Dalessio DJ: Hyperventilation, the vapors, effort syndrome. JAMA 239:1401–1402, 1978

Ferraro A: Nosological position of neurasthenia in psychiatry. J Nerv Ment Dis 119:299–314, 1954

Foulds GA: The Hierarchical Nature of Personal Illness. London, Academic Press, 1976

Frances AJ, Widiger TA, Pincus HA: The development of DSM-IV. Arch Gen Psychiatry 46:373–375, 1989

Freud S: On the grounds for detaching a particular syndrome from neurasthenia under the description "anxiety neurosis" (1894), in The Standard Edition of the Complete Psychological Works of Sigmund Freud. Translated by Strachey J. London, Hogarth Press, 1953

Gosling FG: Before Freud: Neurasthenia and the American Medical Community, 1870–1910. Urbana, University of Illinois Press, 1987

Grauer H: Geriatric depression in the West and the Far East. Psychiatr J Univ Ott 9:118–120, 1984

Guttel B, Schubert H, Zapotoczky H: Symptom constellations in neurotics. Nervenarzt 48:310–313, 1977

Hinsie LE, Campbell RJ: Psychiatric Dictionary, 4th Edition. New York, Oxford University Press, 1976

Holmes GP, Kaplan JE, Gantz NM, et al: Chronic fatigue syndrome: a working case definition. Ann Intern Med 108:387–389, 1988

Jun-mian X: Some issues in the diagnosis of depression in China. Can J Psychiatry 32:368–370, 1987

Kleinman A: Neurasthenia and depression: a study of somatization and culture in China. Cult Med Psychiatry 6:119–190, 1982

Kleinman A: Social Origins of Distress and Disease: Depression, Neurasthenia, and Pain in Modern China. New Haven, CT, Yale University Press, 1986

Kruesi MJ, Dale J, Straus SE: Psychiatric diagnoses in patients who have chronic fatigue syndrome. J Clin Psychiatry 50:53–56, 1989

Laughlin HP: The Neuroses. Washington, DC, Butterworths, 1967

Noyes AP, Kolb LC: Modern Clinical Psychiatry, 6th Edition. Philadelphia, PA, WB Saunders, 1963

Pankova OF, Keshokov AA: Some problem pertaining to vegetative-humoral regulation in patients with neuroses and neurotic development of personality. Zh Nevropatol Psikhiatr 82:1678–1684, 1982

Robins LN, Helzer JE, Croughan J, et al: National Institute of Mental Health Diagnostic Interview Schedule. Arch Gen Psychiatry 38:381–389, 1981

Takahashi T: (Onset ages of neuroses). Journal of Mental Health (Japan) 25:75–79, 1978

Verhaest S, Pierloot R: Psychodynamic features in neurasthenia or neurasthenic neurosis: a survey of the literature. Psychologica Belgica 21:181–194, 1981

Wing JK, Birley JLT, Cooper JE, et al: Reliability of a procedure for measuring and classifying 'Present Psychiatric State.' Br J Psychiatry 113:499–515, 1967

Wing JK, Cooper JE, Sartorius N: Description and Classification of Psychiatric Symptoms. Cambridge, UK, Cambridge University Press, 1974

World Health Organization: Draft of Chapter V. International Classification of Diseases, 10th Edition, 1988

World Health Organization: ICD-10 Chapter V. Mental and Behavioral Disorders. Diagnostic Criteria for Research. Geneva, Switzerland, World Health Organization, 1990

Zapletalek M, Libiger J, Hanus H, et al: Meclophenoxate and diazepam infusions in neurotic disorders. Act Nerv Super 23:194, 1981

Zhang MY: The diagnosis and phenomenology of neurasthenia: a Shanghai study. Cult Med Psychiatry 13:147–161, 1989

Chapter 45

Dissociative Disorders

Etzel Cardeña, Ph.D., Roberto Lewis-Fernández, M.D.,
David Bear, M.D., Isabel Pakianathan, M.D., and
David Spiegel, M.D.

Statement of the Issues

Systematic research on dissociative disorders has grown exponentially in the last decade, along with monographs, conferences, journals, and even specialized clinical and research centers (cf., Spiegel and Cardeña 1991). The considerable number of changes proposed in this review attest to the continuous growth of the relevant database and to greater sensitivity to issues such as cross-cultural dissociative phenomenology. The proposed modifications to the dissociative diagnostic categories include some minor changes for "dissociative amnesia" (called psychogenic amnesia in DSM-III-R [American Psychiatric Association 1987]), "depersonalization disorder," and "dissociative disorder not otherwise specified" (DDNOS), and more prominent changes in the definitions of "dissociative fugue" (called psychogenic fugue in DSM-III-R) and "multiple personality disorder" (MPD). The addition of three new categories has also been proposed: dissociative trance disorder, secondary dissociative disorder due to a nonpsychiatric medical condition, and acute stress (or brief reactive dissociative) disorder.

The specific issues discussed in this chapter are

1. The proposed change in the diagnosis of dissociative fugue from a previous definition requiring the assumption of a new identity to a definition requiring confusion about personal identity *or* assumption of a new identity (and the consequent deletion of DSM-III-R DDNOS example 6, which describes cases in which sudden unexpected travel and organized purposeful behavior with inability to recall one's past are not accompanied by the assumption of a new personal identity). It is also proposed that the terms *psychogenic amnesia* and *psychogenic fugue* be changed to *dissociative amnesia* and *dissociative fugue* to maintain conceptual concordance and for compatibility with ICD-10.

2. The proposal to change the name of MPD to "dissociative identity disorder" (DID) and to reinstate the criterion requiring amnesia for diagnosis.

3. The proposed creation of a new diagnostic category, "dissociative trance disorder," for instances of possession and trance states that are not culturally sanctioned and cause clinically significant distress and impairment.

4. The proposed creation of a new diagnostic category, "secondary dissociative disorder due to a nonpsychiatric medical condition," to describe the presence of common dissociative symptomatology among individuals with complex partial seizures and other medical conditions.

5. The proposed creation of a new diagnostic category, "acute stress disorder," to describe the usually transient but impairing dissociative, intrusive, avoidant, and hyperarousal symptoms experienced by some individuals exposed to natural or manmade disasters.

Significance of the Issues

A number of minor phrasing changes have been proposed to bring the two main diagnostic systems, DSM and ICD into greater lexical and conceptual concordance.

The significance of each of the proposed revisions is discussed in order:

1) DSM-III-R maintained a distinction between psychogenic fugue, which required the assumption of a new identity, and example 6 of DDNOS for cases in which sudden unexpected travel and organized purposeful behavior with inability to recall one's past are *not* accompanied by the assumption of a new personal identity. This distinction would be justified if the data supported the existence of two conceptually and empirically distinguishable syndromes, one characterized by the adoption of a new personal identity. Otherwise, understanding of dissociative fugue would be impaired by a too-restrictive criterion that might underrepresent the prevalence of the condition and unnecessarily multiply the number of diagnostic categories.

2) Precision in the diagnosis of MPD is particularly important given the varied manifestations of the syndrome, which may include presenting symptoms of headaches, depression, etc., and the controversy surrounding the diagnosis itself. The difficulty in accurate diagnosis of MPD is evidenced by a recent review of 100 cases from various sites in which it was found that patients had been given an average of 3.6 diagnoses over 6.8 years before the final MPD diagnosis was determined (Putnam et al. 1986). A later survey of 50 patients by Coons et al. (1988) found comparable figures of an average of 7.1 years and 2.3 other diagnoses before the diagnosis of MPD was made.

In their account of the revisions of the dissociative disorders for DSM-III-R,

Kluft et al. (1988) explained that amnesia had been eliminated as a diagnostic criterion for MPD because, although amnesia may be present in some form in at least the majority of patients with MPD, it is rarely investigated, and may even be denied on initial inquiry and only acknowledged much later. Additionally, amnesia may never be reported because many patients themselves may be unaware of the symptom (i.e., they are 'amnestic for amnesia'), and some may have developed false memories to cover up the gaps, or, if dissociation has occurred since early childhood, discontinuity of time may not be perceived by the patient as worth mentioning. Coons et al. (1988) also warn that MPD patients may be reluctant to discuss amnesia and may instead create fictitious memories for fear of being labeled as mentally ill (see also Kluft 1985). Finally, recent models of memory have proposed that memory may involve at least two different systems (i.e., implicit and explicit) and that certain amnestic phenomena may not be easily detected through traditional interview methods (cf., Squire and Zola-Morgan 1991).

Hence, a powerful reason to exclude amnesia as a defining criterion for MPD is that it may prevent the correct diagnosis of those individuals who do not initially report any amnestic problems and prevent them from receiving the appropriate treatment for their condition.

The opposing and also powerful argument is that exclusion of the amnesia criterion makes the MPD diagnosis too imprecise because it inappropriately blurs the distinction between less differentiated and more conscious ego states and MPD. Furthermore, amnesia has been thought of as an essential component in the development of MPD and is commonly reported when systematically evaluated for (see below); from this perspective, its exclusion would be conceptually suspect.

The Dissociative Disorders sub-Work Group also recommended deleting the word *full* from the DSM-III-R criterion that "at least two of these personalities or personality states recurrently take full control of the person's behavior" (p. 272). It was argued that the nature of dissociation is such that material kept out of conscious awareness still exerts an influence (Kihlstrom 1987; Kihlstrom and Hoyt 1990; Spiegel 1990). It was also pointed out that an "alter" may be experienced as exerting an influence through an internal voice rather than through complete control of the person. Therefore requiring "full" control would be unduly restrictive. Others opposed any weakening of the diagnostic criteria, feeling that the diagnosis is already applied too liberally. However, this risk would diminish with the reintroduction of the amnesia requirement noted above.

Finally, it was proposed by some members of the Task Force that the term *multiple personality disorder* be changed to *dissociative identity disorder* to stress that the nature of the condition is the lack of personal integration rather than the objective existence of various personalities within a single individual.

3) The experience of being possessed by some deity or spiritual entity and other

trance states (e.g., *ataque de nervios, amok*) is widespread throughout the world (Bourguignon 1976) and, in many instances, is eagerly sought by devotees as a means of expressing social tensions and ambiguities (Boddy 1989; Stoller 1989a) or as a form of transcendent experience (Cardeña 1989). These phenomena may typically occur within a ritual setting and be a normal component of religion. However, there are also other manifestations that occur outside of a ritual setting, are seemingly beyond the conscious control of the person, and cause marked impairment and/or distress. Up to this point, the categories described in the previous editions of DSM have been inadequate to characterize uncontrolled and impairing possession and trance manifestations, which may be the most prevalent dissociative disorders in non-Western settings and may be present among Western individuals as well (Cardeña 1992). For instance, Saxena and Prasad (1989) report that the majority of individuals with dissociative disorders (90%) seen in their clinic in India presented with forms of possession or simple dissociative disorders not covered by a specific diagnostic entity and hence were referred to as having "atypical dissociative disorders" (the DSM-III nomenclature for DDNOS).

The adoption of the new diagnostic entity "dissociative trance disorder" would be in accord with the new category in ICD-10 of "trance and possession disorders" and would give a more precise diagnosis to what may be the most prevalent dissociative disorders among a number of non-Western cultures and some immigrant groups to Western industrialized nations. Clinicians who may not be familiar with the "idioms of distress" (Nichter 1981) of a particular culture, including possession and trance phenomena, may be prone to diagnose these as manifestations of psychosis. The absence of a specific diagnostic entity for those instances of trance and possession behavior that are distressing, impairing, and not culturally sanctioned may hamper accurate diagnosis, treatment, and research.

Conversely, the adoption of "dissociative trance disorder" may be questioned on the grounds that the behavioral and experiential elements occurring in these syndromes cut across the diagnostic boundaries of DSM-IV, for instance, across affective, anxiety, dissociative, and somatoform categories. This argument could be made for the general phenomena subsumed under "trance and possession" and, even more strongly, for specific instances that may deviate from the prototypical definition.

A different problem is that the clinician might not be aware that a particular manifestation (e.g., possession during particular religious seasons) may be expected and culturally appropriate. This may happen because of the clinician's lack of cross-cultural knowledge or because of the patient's inability or disinclination to discuss matters of cultural and religious importance with someone from another culture. This risk would be diminished by including among the proposed diagnostic criteria the requirement that there be clinically significant distress or impairment.

4) The proposed new diagnostic category "secondary dissociative disorder due to a nonpsychiatric medical condition" would cover those individuals with seizure disorders and other nonpsychiatric conditions (e.g., electroencephalogram [EEG] dysrhythmias, Huntington's disease) who also present with impairing dissociative symptoms. Many reported symptoms of dissociation such as amnesias, blackouts, fugue states, depersonalization, derealization, dreamy states, unusual sensory perceptions, and hallucinations are also found among patients with seizure disorders (Blumer 1975; Litwin and Cardeña 1993). Mayeux et al. (1979) describe postictal episodes of aimless wandering and automatisms followed by amnesia and disorientation (poriomania), and Devinsky et al. (1989a) report a 6.3% incidence of autoscopic phenomena (out-of-body experiences or seeing one's double) among seizure patients, particularly those with temporal lobe conditions. Whereas the diagnosis of a complex partial seizure would almost certainly entail medical treatment of that condition, related dissociative symptomatology may go unheeded and untreated. The adoption of this category would sensitize clinicians to the possibility of dissociative symptomatology associated with seizure disorders and related conditions. Finally, it would bring the DSM and ICD systems into greater concordance because ICD-10 includes a category analogous to this one.

The main argument against this proposal is that the current evidence for an association between dissociative symptomatology and a seizure condition is considered by some to be inconclusive (Ross et al. 1989c). An alternative proposal would be to give other dissociative disorders as secondary diagnoses to the medical condition. Hence, a new diagnosis might seem unnecessary or premature at this stage.

5) The proposal to create a new diagnostic category, "acute stress disorder," is based on the observation that transient but impairing dissociative symptoms are a frequent by-product of exposure to trauma. There are a number of reasons to include this diagnosis in some way in DSM-IV. The definition of this disorder would be different from the current diagnosis of posttraumatic stress disorder (PTSD) in terms of duration (currently, a diagnosis of PTSD requires that at least 1 month elapse since the onset of disturbance) and symptom presentation. This category may help to describe cases that do not meet criteria for PTSD because of differences in onset, duration, and symptom presentation and that are more specific and severe than adjustment disorder.

No diagnostic category in DSM includes relatively short (up to 1 month) dissociative and anxiety reactions to a severe stressor. The main argument for the creation of this diagnosis is that, if dissociative and anxiety symptoms are prevalent after a disaster and can be socially and professionally impairing or severely distressing, the person should be diagnosed and treated without having to wait for a PTSD diagnosis 1 month after the traumatic incident. Indeed, the lack of recognition and treatment of the disorder during its inception or shortly thereafter could result in more long-lasting disorders. Other related diagnoses without the time constraints of PTSD such as "adjustment disorder" or "generalized anxiety disorder" have a constellation of symptoms that ignore dissociative phenomena. Finally, this diagnosis would be parallel to the new "acute stress reaction" diagnosis of ICD-10.

The main argument against the adoption of this category would be that dissociative and anxiety symptomatology may not be commonly encountered after trauma or that, when it lasts less than 1 month, its effects are negligible and do not constitute an impairing or distressing affliction.

Methods

Systematic reviews were obtained for the area of dissociation in general and for each of the dissociative categories. An initial computer search using the Medline database for the terms *dissociative disorders* and *dissociative neuroses,* from 1968 to 1988, produced approximately 100 nonoverlapping references. Additional computer searches were performed for the following terms: *MPD* or *multiple personality disorder* (approximately 40 references between 1980 and 1988), *depersonalization* (approximately 110 nonoverlapping references between 1972 and 1988), *psychogenic amnesia* and *psychogenic fugue* (24 nonoverlapping references from 1976 to 1988). Also, articles dealing with psychological reactions to *disasters* and relevant items from the PTSD literature were searched through Medline and PsycInfo databases and were complemented by review of bibliographies in articles and books. These original searches were supplemented by literature searches for the same terms using both Medline and PsycInfo databases for the years 1989 through the beginning of 1991. In addition, the main journals in the area (e.g., *American Journal of Psychiatry, Dissociation, Journal of Nervous and Mental Disease, International Journal of Clinical and Experimental Hypnosis*) and article and chapter bibliographies were systematically scanned for additional material.

The literature search focused on diagnostic and research issues. Drs. Spiegel and Cardeña and collaborators from the DSM-IV Dissociative Disorders sub-Work Group wrote comprehensive position papers on the following topics: MPD, depersonalization disorder, psychogenic fugue and amnesia (including dissociation and seizure disorders), Ganser's syndrome (a particular instance of DDNOS), prevalence of dissociative disorders, and acute stress disorder.

For the literature review concerning the proposed new category dissociative trance disorder, the cross-cultural psychiatrist Roberto Lewis-Fernández systematically scanned related articles and bibliographies and wrote a review of 132 references dealing with cross-cultural psychiatry in general and the syndromes of possession, *ataque de nervios,* and amok in particular. For the review of secondary dissociative disorder due to a nonpsychiatric medical condition, a clinical and research psychiatrist who specializes in seizure disorders, David Bear, surveyed the relevant literature up to the beginning of 1991 (nine items) and wrote a review on the prevalence of EEG abnormalities among patients diagnosed as having dissociative disorders and on the prevalence of dissociative disorders among patients with complex partial seizures.

All position papers were circulated among members of the Dissociative Disorders sub-Work Group, who provided critiques and additional data.

Results

Dissociative Fugue

Fugue states have been reported infrequently, but they have been carefully documented since the late 1800s, for instance, in the classic case of Ansel Bourne described by William James (1890/1923). Although the case described by James involved the adoption of an organized new identity, James himself did not assume that the assumption of such an identity was a defining symptom and thought of fugue as a form of long-lasting trance. In a similar fashion, Stengel (1941, in Loewenstein 1991) analyzed 36 cases of fugue and defined it as "states of altered or narrowed consciousness with the impulse to wander" (p. 255).

The current rarity of this diagnosis can be partly explained by its occurrence during very stressful circumstances such as war and its decrease during peacetime, although Loewenstein (1991) makes the point that our estimates of fugue may underrepresent the nonclassic presentation of fugue in which, for instance, adolescent runaways may escape from an abusive home during fugue-like periods and not come to the attention of clinicians.

In a recent review of the literature, Riether and Stoudemire (1988) concluded that the current DSM-III-R requirement that there be assumption of a new identity was overly restrictive. For instance, Fisher (1945) had distinguished three types of fugues: those with awareness of loss of personal identity, those with a change in identity, and those with only retrograde amnesia. This classification is supported by Bychowski (1958 and 1962, in Riether and Stoudemire 1988), who maintained that his fugue patients never actually forgot their identities but could alter their consciousness so as to be only vaguely aware of them.

Other authors illustrate the variety of manifestations of psychogenic fugue and agree that the current DSM-III-R definition of fugue is overly restrictive. Venn (1984) described a 15-year-old female, with a history of nightmares, hallucinations, fainting spells, and conversion reactions, who, after two specific incidents in which she had been rudely rejected by her peers, was found stuporous and eventually assumed a new identity (including changes in inflection, personality traits, etc.). On the other hand, Keller and Shaywitz (1986) wrote about a 16-year-old male found lying entangled in shrubbery along a state highway. He presented with amnesia, particularly for remote memory, and could not give any other information about himself other than his age. He did not present with any type of organized identity and remained confused about his personal history. It was eventually discovered that, in addition to behavioral problems in school, recent stressful events in his home had preceded the episode.

The current literature, then, supports the notion that during psychogenic fugue, various manifestations of amnesia and identity change are found. Restricting the diagnosis to the most extreme end of the continuum (i.e., total amnesia for a previous identity and the adoption of a new one) is not supported by data that show it to be of a different nature or prognosis than other manifestations of identity alterations during fugue.

A related issue is that various authors and two recent comprehensive reviews (Loewenstein 1991; Riether and Stoudemire 1988) have indicated a strong relation between severe stress and fugue.

MPD (DID)

The criterion of amnesia for the diagnosis of MPD was eliminated from DSM-III-R based on the argument that, although amnesia may indeed be a central feature of MPD (or DID as it is proposed that it be called in DSM-IV) for a number of reasons (e.g., lack of awareness of the deficit), it may not necessarily be a presenting symptom of MPD. The opposite viewpoint holds that patients with alternate identities without amnestic barriers (e.g., ego states) constitute a qualitatively distinct group of individuals from those with MPD and deserve a different diagnosis (e.g., P. M. Coons, personal communication, 1991). The sensitivity and specificity of the alternative definitions of MPD have not been directly evaluated, but there is considerable information about the rates of reported amnesia in various research projects.

Although aware of the difficulties in diagnosis, Coons (1984) has stated that amnesia should be considered a definite prerequisite for the diagnosis of MPD. In a recent study with 50 patients, Coons et al. (1988) used amnesia as a criterion for MPD and found that fugue was also present in about half of the patients. Amnesia was found to be localized (inability to recall all events in a circumscribed period) in 94% of the patients and selective (inability to recall some events in a specific period) in 6%; a high percentage (48%) of the amnestic periods lasted from 15 to 60 minutes.

In their review of 100 cases of MPD, Putnam et al. (1986) found that episodes of amnesia in some form had been reported by 98% of MPD patients, although amnesia had been a presenting symptom in only 57%. In a study using data from various centers, Ross et al. (1989c) reported that 95% of 236 MPD cases showed evidence of some type of amnesia. The incidence of amnestic symptoms in these studies is similar to that reported by Bliss (1980) in a survey of 14 MPD patients, 91% of whom had amnesia. In later research with 32 MPD patients and 38 possible MPD patients, Bliss (1984) found a higher prevalence of amnesia in females (85%) than males (64%). These studies are summarized in Table 45–1.

Although most of the previous studies have relied on therapists' reports to evaluate the presence of amnesia and hence do not necessarily provide the best estimate of the incidence of amnesia as a presenting symptom in MPD, other projects have included standardized questionnaires or semistructured interviews that could be used as part of a clinical evaluation. In an ongoing research project using the Dissociative Experiences Scale (DES) (Bernstein and Putnam 1986), F. W. Putnam (unpublished data, 1989) reports that all the MPD patients in his project ($N = 48$) had reported significant amounts of amnesia, which distinguished them from other diagnostic categories except for PTSD. With a different instrument, the Dissociative Disorders Interview Schedule (DDIS) (Ross et al. 1989a), Ross et al. (1989b) compared groups of 20 patients diagnosed with MPD, schizophrenia, panic disorder, or eating disorders. They found that, of 20 MPD patients, 13 (65%) satisfied criteria for a DSM-III-R diagnosis of psychogenic amnesia and 5 (25%) satisfied criteria for psychogenic fugue. These diagnoses of psychogenic amnesia and fugue among MPD patients significantly distinguished them from each of the other three clinical groups. In another study using the DDIS with 102 patients at four centers, Ross et al. (1990) (Table 45–2) reported that no MPD patient failed to endorse at least one amnesia item, with 82% endorsing three or more amnesia items. In a continuation of this research with 166 MPD patients, Ross

Table 45–1. Amnesia in multiple personality disorder: clinical reports

Study	Incidence of amnesia (%)
Bliss 1980	91
Bliss 1984[a]	
females	85
males	64
Putnam et al. 1986	98
Ross et al. 1989c	95

[a]Diagnosed and patients with suspected multiple personality disorder.

(1991) found that all of these patients endorsed at least one amnesia item. Finally, various projects using the Structured Clinical Interview for the Dissociative Disorders (SCID-D) (Steinberg et al. 1990), a semistructured, comprehensive interview protocol, have provided information about the incidence of amnesia symptoms among MPD patients, with the amnesia rated according to a scale where 1 = none, 2 = mild, 3 = moderate, and 4 = severe. Steinberg et al. (1990) found that 100% of the patients with MPD had severe amnesia symptoms. In a Dutch sample of 12 MPD patients, Boon and Draijer (1991) reported that all 12 had a severe rating (i.e., 4) on amnesia. Finally, in an ongoing project by M. Steinberg (unpublished data, 1991), two blind raters assessed the presence of amnesia among patients referred for MPD. Of 21 patients, none was assessed as lacking amnesia, and 20 of the 21 were found to have moderate or predominantly severe amnesia. These findings are summarized in Table 45–2.

Although no specific project has looked systematically at the sensitivity and specificity of amnesia for the diagnosis of MPD, the evidence strongly supports the position that, at least when using the relevant psychometric instruments (DES, DDIS, SCID-D), MPD patients will report at least mild and most likely moderate to severe amnestic syndromes. Hence, the evidence suggests that readopting the amnesia criterion for MPD would not produce false-negative diagnoses if a careful assessment of amnesia is done, and it would have the virtue of making the diagnosis more precise.

Dissociative Trance Disorder

The proposed diagnostic category dissociative trance disorder encompasses involuntary distressing and impairing alterations of consciousness that are characterized by possession or trance phenomenology and are not culturally sanctioned. The mere expression of possession or trance may serve many nonpathological func-

Table 45–2.   Amnesia in multiple personality disorder: standardized instruments

Study	Standardized instrument	Incidence of some form of amnesia (%)
Putnam, unpublished data, 1989	DES	100
Ross et al. 1990, 1991	DDIS	100
Steinberg et al. 1990	SCID-D	100 (severe)
Boon and Draijer 1991	SCID-D	100 (severe)
Steinberg et al. 1991	SCID-D	100 (95% moderate or severe)

Note.   DES = Dissociative Experiences Scale. DDIS = Dissociative Disorders Interview Schedule. SCID-D = Structured Clinical Interview for the Dissociative Disorders.

tions, including the expression of intense normal emotions, social protest by underprivileged groups, and/or religious functions. Some cases of these behaviors and experiences, however, occur outside of culturally sanctioned settings, are distressful and impairing, and come to the attention of the clinician, either because they have been recalcitrant to traditional treatments or because the patient may no longer have access to traditional healers in a mobile society (Ward 1989).

Although non-Western cultures make up 80% of the world and individuals from non-Western cultures make up one-third of the population of the United States, many of their indigenous syndromes have so far been included in the DSM nosology only as "atypical" or "not otherwise specified" variants of the dissociative disorders, despite the fact that they probably represent the most common examples of dissociative pathology in some non-Western cultures (e.g., in India [Adityanjee et al. 1989; Saxena and Prasad 1989]). The current proposal for the creation of a separate dissociative trance disorder category in DSM-IV is parallel to an equivalent category in ICD-10 and brings these indigenous syndromes into the professional nosology to facilitate treatment and research.

Although no research database exists for these syndromes that is equivalent to that for other dissociative disorders, we provide relevant descriptions of two syndromes with strong dissociative components: *ataque de nervios* and possession, although other manifestations such as *vimbuza* and amok may be considered dissociative in nature.

Ataque de nervios. *Ataque de nervios* ("attack of nerves" in Spanish) is a behavioral-experiential sequence indigenous to various Latin American cultures, including Puerto Rico, the Dominican Republic, Cuba, and Central America, that has received considerable attention in the last 30 years (e.g., De la Cancela et al. 1986; Guarnaccia et al. 1989; Lewis-Fernández 1994; Steinberg 1990).

A typical *ataque de nervios* is composed of the following elements:

1. Exposure to a stressful stimulus or situation, typically eliciting feelings of fear, grief, or anger and involving a person close to the subject, such as a spouse, child, family member, or friend. The severity of the stress ranges from mild-moderate (marital problems, disclosure of migration plans) to extreme (physical/sexual abuse, acute bereavement).

2. Initiation of the episode immediately on exposure to the stimulus or after a period of brooding or emotional "shock."

3. After the acute attack starts, there is a rapid evolution to an intense affective state characterized by an affect congruent with the stimulus (e.g., anger or fear), accompanied by all or some of the following:

a. Reported somatic perceptions and observable alterations such as trembling, chest tightness, difficulty breathing, heart palpitations, a sense of heat in the chest rising to the head, paresthesias of diverse location, "clouded or darkened vision" (*tener la vista nublada* or *opacada*), difficulty moving limbs, faintness, dizziness ("mareos").

b. Behaviors such as shouting, swearing, moaning, breaking objects, striking out at others or at self, attempting to harm self with nearest implement, falling to the ground, shaking with convulsive movements, lying "as if dead," etc.

4. Cessation of an episode may be abrupt or gradual, but it is usually rapid and often results from the ministration of others involving expressions of concern, prayers, or use of rubbing alcohol preparations (*alcoholado*). After the episode, there may be a return of ordinary consciousness and exhaustion.

5. Subsequent partial or total amnesia, and descriptions of the following during the acute episode: loss of consciousness, mind going blank, and /or general unawareness of surroundings.

Ataque de nervios is frequently associated with depression, anxiety, and suicidal ideation, is apparently more prevalent among females older than 45 with less than a high school education who are unmarried and out of the labor force. The precipitants of *ataque de nervios* range from family conflicts to natural disasters and its lifetime prevalence among Puerto Ricans is approximately 14% (Guarnaccia et al. 1993).

According to local convention, when *ataque de nervios* occurs as a response to experiences of severe stress, such as acute bereavement or marital abuse, it is considered a normal expression of suffering and a call for group support and concrete assistance. However, when it occurs spontaneously or after precipitants judged to be of insufficient severity, it may not be considered appropriate by the culture and may lead to referral for therapy.

Possession. *Possession* is an umbrella term encompassing multiple names and variations across the globe. Although possession has been studied more extensively among African-based and East Indian cultures, it is present in most cultures including modern societies (Bourguignon 1976; Crabtree 1985). Following Bourguignon (1976), we distinguish between the diagnosable entity of "possession trance," a state characterized by specific alterations in memory, behavior, and identity attributed to a spirit or other foreign influence, and "possession belief," which encompasses a range of reputed spiritual influences on human affairs, including healing and disease processes, independent of alterations in consciousness. The proposed new diagnosis refers exclusively to pathological forms of possession trance.

In most instances, radical alterations in embodied identity represent culturally accepted behavior, either as transcendent religious experiences (Cardeña 1989) or as expressions of sociocultural tensions (Boddy 1989; Stoller 1989a, 1989b). However, possession trance behaviors can also present as uncontrolled dissociative processes that are distressing, produce impairment, and lack cultural sanction (Freed and Freed 1964; Obeyesekere 1970; Ward 1989). Only the latter pathological forms of possession-trance can be given the diagnosis of dissociative trance disorder.

Although there has been a strong temptation to assume that possession is but MPD in a different cultural dressing, the etiological link of early abuse to multiplicity has not been established in possession, and these two phenomena also vary with regard to the nature and organization of, and control over, the alterations in consciousness (Adityanjee et al. 1989; Krippner 1987; Saxena and Prasad 1989; Walker 1972). A recent study of the related Western phenomenon of "channeling" found that "channelers" significantly differed from individuals with MPD in related dissociative diagnoses (e.g., amnesia), secondary features of MPD, and median scores in the DES (Hughes 1992).

Although it is proposed that they be included in DSM under the single category of dissociative trance disorder, indigenous syndromes falling under this rubric worldwide show some phenomenological variation. These local differences remain essential, particularly for distinguishing pathological conditions from culturally sanctioned ones and for conducting culturally appropriate treatment. A prototypical example of a possession-trance episode may be composed of most or all of the following elements:

1. Onset occurs in the context of subacute conflict or stress and shows considerable variation. It may be gradual and nonspecific (e.g., hot-cold flashes) or sudden and specific (i.e., involving a transition to an altered state of consciousness).

2. Behavior during the altered state consists of some or all of the following:

   a. Dramatic, semipurposeful movements (e.g., shaking of the body, flailing of the limbs, gyrating, falling to the ground) accompanied by guttural, incoherent verbalizations such as moaning or shrieking.

   b. Aggressive or violent actions directed at self or others including spitting, striking, suicidal or homicidal gestures, uncharacteristic derogatory comments or threats.

   c. Specific gestures, comments, or requests denoting the appearance of an unknown entity or of a known possessing personality as defined by 1) standard attributes of culturally recognizable figures or 2) attributes of living or deceased family members.

   d. A concluding stage after the possession episode, during which the individual may physically collapse and seem unaware of the environment. After "recovering" his or her original identity, the individual may appear dazed, exhausted, or confused about the situation and may report perceptual alterations as well as partial or total amnesia for the episode, although at least some reports of amnesia can be questioned (Frigerio 1989).

3. In all cases, this state is marked by the emergence of one or several personalities distinct from that of the individual. Most often, the individual displays only one possessing agent per episode, although in some cases, the ongoing possession may involve simultaneous multiple agents. Typically, these identities are regarded indigenously as originating outside the person, in contrast with MPD in which the identities are typically experienced as distinct inner selves.

4. Possession by the secondary personality(ies) is episodic, resulting in oscillations between the individual's own and the alternate identities. During transitions from one personality to another, the individual may experience a number of paresthesias and body image and sensory alterations, including dizziness and loss of equilibrium. States of consciousness may alternate continuously for minutes or even hours, and recurrent episodes of possession may last days, weeks, or even years.

5. The specific identities of the possessing personalities may frequently remain undisclosed for some time, requiring the active ministrations of family members and indigenous practitioners.

6. Outcome is variable and may vary from cessation after a single episode to prolonged and severe morbidity in the case of a pathological condition.

As with *ataque de nervios*, there is some evidence that pathological possession has a substantially higher prevalence among women of lower socioeconomic and educational status. Its precipitant is frequently some form of chronic conflict or subacute severe stress (Lewis-Fernández 1994).

The dissociative and pathological nature of some cases of possession, *ataque de nervios*, and other culture-bound syndromes have been amply described in the psychological and anthropological literature. The adoption of the new diagnostic category dissociative trance disorder would provide a sharper definition of the manifestations that qualify as genuine disorders, further differentiate the broad range of disturbances covered by DDNOS, and foster more focused research projects and treatment strategies.

In view of the argument that this new category may "pathologize" ordinary non-Western cultural expressions, we have proposed specific criteria requiring distress or impairment and lack of indigenous sanction to avoid this pitfall. Enhanced diagnostic specificity should foster greater cultural sensitivity. It is proposed that dissociative trance disorder be included in the appendix of DSM-IV for disorders requiring further study to allow for a period of evaluation as a new diagnostic entity.

Secondary Dissociative Disorder Due to a Nonpsychiatric Medical Condition

The proposal to introduce this new diagnostic category is based on a number of recent articles evaluating the presence of dissociative phenomena among patients with seizure conditions. Also relevant is the literature dealing with the presence of seizure disorders in patients with dissociative disorders.

We first review works dealing with the presence of dissociation among individuals with temporal lobe epilepsy and related conditions. We do not concentrate on the dissociative characteristics present during the seizure itself (Mayeux et al. 1979) or on substance-induced dissociative disorders (Good 1989) but rather on the general presence of dissociative symptomatology. Mesulam (1981) reported on 12 cases with probable temporal lobe epilepsy who also experienced dissociative phenomena, including alternate identities with and without amnesia, multiple episodes of altered states of consciousness, and the sense of supernatural possession. Schenk and Bear (1981) gave detailed descriptions of 3 of these patients whom they declared diagnosable as having MPD. They also agreed with Mesulam's conclusion that, overall, 12 of 23 (52%) female patients with temporal lobe epilepsy (13 of 40 female and male patients) also showed strong dissociative symptomatology (e.g., alternate identities with and without amnesia). Benson et al. (1986) described two case studies of epileptic patients in whom apparent dual personalities were the result of seizures. Lastly, in a conference paper, Drake (1986) described five patients with documented seizures, four of whom had different postictal personalities, whereas the fifth one, who had a toxic anticonvulsant level, reported four separate personalities. Although some of the case studies just reviewed are informally described as having MPD, other authors have pointed out that many of them did not fulfill diagnostic criteria for MPD and may instead be considered to have general dissociative phenomenology or other diagnoses such as transient delusional psychoses (Loewenstein and Putnam 1988; Ross et al. 1989b).

Loewenstein and Putnam (1988) compared the DES (Bernstein and Putnam 1986) scores of 12 patients with complex partial seizures, 9 MPD patients, and 36 PTSD patients. Although the median DES score of the epileptic patients was significantly lower than that of the MPD and PTSD patients (6.8, 47.5, and 28.75, respectively), the authors remarked that items dealing with depersonalization, derealization, and absorption differentiated the least between epileptic and MPD patients.

In a study using both the DES and the DDIS (Ross et al. 1989a), Ross et al.

(1989b) compared three unmatched groups of 20 patients, each diagnosed as having MPD, complex partial seizures, or other neurological problems such as Parkinson's disease. MPD patients differed significantly from the two other groups on all DSM-III dissociative disorder diagnoses and on the overall score on the Dissociative Experiences Scale (DES) (MPD mean score, 38.3; complex partial seizure patients, 6.7; neurological control subjects, 5.2). Nonetheless, of the 20 patients with complex partial seizures, 5 had received a diagnosis of psychogenic amnesia and the epileptic patients had more diagnoses of depersonalization than the neurological control subjects (although Table 1 of Ross et al. [1989b], p. 55, lists 0 individuals with depersonalization, this is a typo as the text suggests, and Ross corroborated with the first author).

Devinsky et al. (1989b), using the DES with 71 patients with epilepsy, 42 with MPD, and 34 normal control subjects, found that the median DES scores of the MPD patients (52.8) and of the epileptic patients (8.75) differed significantly, and that the median score of the epileptic patients also differed significantly from that of the control subjects (4.37). Within the epileptic group, patients with dominant hemisphere foci had significantly higher depersonalization subscale scores than those with nondominant foci.

Finally, in a study of patients with neurologically determined seizures ($N = 31$), Litwin and Cardeña (1993) found a high percentage of reports of trance-like episodes (77%) and a higher DES median score than that reported for non-pathological groups used in other studies. DSM-III-R diagnoses of dissociation for this sample were 29% with psychogenic amnesia, 16% with depersonalization, and 0% with fugue or MPD. It is also of interest that the DES score of epilepsy patients was almost half that of patients with nonorganic seizures ($n = 10$). These results are shown in Table 45–3.

Thus, results with the DES show that, although seizure patients do not have the extent of dissociation that MPD and PTSD patients do, they nonetheless have

Table 45–3.   Dissociative Experiences Scale scores of seizure patients and comparison groups

Study	Seizures	MPD	PTSD	NES	Controls
Loewenstein and Putnam 1988	6.8	47.5	28.75	—	—
Devinsky et al. 1989b	8.75	52.8	—	—	4.37
Ross et al. 1989b (means)	6.7	38.3	—	—	5.2
Litwin and Cardeña 1993	11.07	—	—	21.79	—

Note. MPD = multiple personality disorder. PTSD = posttraumatic stress disorder. NES = nonepileptic seizures.

a high incidence of amnesia and depersonalization symptoms.

A different issue is whether EEG abnormalities are a good diagnostic indicator of MPD. In their review of 100 cases, Putnam et al. (1986) found that only 10% of cases had diagnosed temporal lobe epilepsy, the same figure that Coons et al. (1988) found among their sample of 50 patients. Among the subset of Coons et al.' patients who underwent EEG evaluations, 7 of 30 (23%) showed abnormal EEGs. Finally, in a major study being conducted with more than 150 MPD patients, B. G. Braun (personal communication, 1992) has indicated a lack of association between MPD status per se and organic seizures. Although the rate of incidence of epilepsy in these studies is evidently not a reliable indicator of MPD diagnosis, a 10% incidence is still considerably higher than the base rate for epilepsy (a lifetime prevalence of about 0.5%) and suggests that a small subgroup of individuals with DID may also present EEG abnormalities.

Case studies relevant to this issue include the study by Devinsky et al. (1989a) with six MPD patients suspected of having seizure disorders as well. Although there were minor EEG abnormalities in three of the patients, none was found to have epilepsy. Coons et al. (1982) studied two patients with MPD and a control and found that one of the MPD patients showed abnormal EEG findings during waking. Cocores et al. (1984) did not find signs of abnormal EEGs in their case study of a patient with MPD, nor were signs of abnormal EEGs found in a number of previous case studies (Larmore et al. 1977; Ludwig et al. 1972). It is also of interest that there are clinical differences between the dissociative symptoms of epileptic patients and those of typical MPD patients. Epileptic patients tend to have dissociative symptoms that begin in adulthood rather than childhood and they typically lack a history of sexual or physical abuse in childhood (Kluft 1991; Mesulam 1981; Schenk and Bear 1981). In a related finding, Litwin and Cardeña (1993), using logistic regression analysis, found that one of the most important variables that significantly differentiated patients with epileptic and nonepileptic seizures was the presence and longer duration of reported physical and sexual abuse in the second group.

The articles reviewed show great variability in methodology and sample size but support the notion that patients with seizure disorders experience a greater number of dissociative phenomena (e.g., depersonalization, amnesia) than normal control subjects, although they do not generally show the same extent or symptom pattern as MPD patients. Hence, although the great majority of MPD cases occur without evidence of focal electrophysiological abnormalities, seizure activity is clearly related to some dissociative phenomena in a substantial number of cases, and the creation of a diagnosis of secondary dissociative disorder due to a nonpsychiatric medical condition is supported by the literature reviewed.

Acute Stress (or Brief Reactive Dissociative) Disorder

The proposal to include this new diagnostic category is based on a growing specialized literature on the presence of transient but impairing dissociative symptoms within populations exposed to different traumatic stimuli, symptoms that seem to be good predictors of long-term maladjustment.

Works by pioneers such as Janet, Prince, Breuer, Freud, and James described a link between trauma and dissociative phenomenology (Spiegel and Cardeña 1991). The long-term relationship between reported (and in some cases independently corroborated, e.g., Coons and Milstein 1986) early trauma and dissociative phenomenology has been supported by a number of reviews and articles on victimization and trauma (McCann et al. 1988; Spiegel et al. 1988; Terr 1991), incest (Gelinas 1983), dissociative phenomena among borderline patients (Herman et al. 1989; Ogata et al. 1990), disintegrated identity disorder (Coons and Milstein 1986; Putnam et al. 1986; Schultz et al. 1989; Spiegel 1984), pseudoseizure patients (Litwin and Cardeña 1993; Shen et al. 1990), and general psychiatric patients (Briere and Conte 1989; Chu and Dill 1990; Coons et al. 1989). Along the same lines, in an important study of trauma and dissociation among Cambodian refugees, Carlson and Rosser-Hogan (1991) found a significant correlation between the amount of reported trauma and scores on the DES (Bernstein and Putnam 1986). Although some form of relation between trauma and dissociation is amply supported by the evidence, the argument that trauma *causes* dissociation has a number of logical conundrums (Cardeña 1993) and tends to ignore the possibility of mediating variables such as general environmental disorganization (Nash et al. 1993).

Peritraumatic dissociative responses may not only be severe while they last but may also bring about long-term complications, as Lindemann's (1944) classic study of grief after the Coconut Grove fire suggested. More recently, in two retrospective studies, investigators have concluded that dissociative reactions significantly predict later PTSD. Brenmer et al. (1992) found that Vietnam veterans having PTSD reported significantly more dissociative symptomatology at the time of trauma and afterward than veterans without PTSD, even when controlling for difference in the level of combat, and found a significant correlation between PTSD (the Mississippi Scale for Posttraumatic Stress Disorder [Keane et al. 1984]) and dissociative (DES) symptoms. Marmar et al. (1992) obtained essentially the same results in a sample of 254 male Vietnam veterans and concluded that dissociative symptomatology at the time of stress is a significant and accurate predictor of later PTSD. In a careful longitudinal study of survivors of the Oakland/Berkeley Firestorm, it was shown that dissociative responses during or shortly after the fire not only brought about transient maladaptive responses but also significantly predicted later PTSD (Koopman et al., unpublished manuscript, 1993). This literature is consistent with two earlier studies showing that hypnotizability, a measure of formally elicited dissociation, is higher among veterans with PTSD (Spiegel et al. 1988; Stutman and Bliss 1985).

The literature on concurrent and transient dissociative reactions to traumatic events has had serious methodological limitations, including reliance on retrospective data collected months to years after the trauma, neglect of possible mediating variables, and lack of comparison groups. Nonetheless, the vast amount of the literature that has directly or indirectly addressed immediate and short-term dissociative reactions commonly shows three patterns of reaction: 1) an experience of detachment from oneself or the physical or social worlds, 2) alterations in perceptual experience, and 3) memory disturbances (e.g., amnesia, hypermnesia).

A sense of *detachment* from one's physical or psychological being (depersonalization) and/or from the surrounding social and physical environment (derealization) has been mentioned anecdotally by concentration camp and rape victims (e.g., Jaffe 1968; Rose 1986). Hillman (1981) and Siegel (1984) report that retrospective accounts of hostage victims frequently include experiences of temporal and spatial disorientation, alterations in body image and sensations, and depersonalization, whereas more than a third of tortured Norwegian seamen experienced social or psychological withdrawal (Weisaeth 1989b). With respect to war, Feinstein (1989), found that of 17 direct and indirect combatants in a bloody ambush, 41% showed markedly diminished interest in usual activities, and 24% expressed feelings of detachment or estrangement 1 week after the attack.

Noyes and Kletti (1977) studied 101 survivors of life-threatening events and reported that, during the ordeal, 72% had experienced feelings of unreality and an altered sense of time, 57% automatic movements, 56% lack of emotion, 52% a sense of detachment, 34% feeling detached from their bodies, and 30% derealization. An expanded analysis with 189 participants showed depersonalization and hyperalertness as factors that accounted for the most variance (Noyes and Slymen 1978–1979).

Madakasira and O'Brien (1987) found that, of 279 survivors of a series of tornadoes, 57% had experienced detachment, 45% diminished interest, and 35% diminished libido. Sloan (1988) found that 54% of the survivors of a crash landing reported feeling detached or estranged.

Among survivors of the Hyatt Regency Skywalk collapse, Wilkinson (1983) found that 36% reported inability to feel deeply about anything, 34% had a general loss of interest, and 29% felt detached. About one-third of survivors of the collapse of an oil rig also mentioned retrospectively an avoidance of activities and thoughts (A. Holen, unpublished data, 1991). About one-fourth of survivors of an industrial disaster who were in a high-stress group because they were more directly exposed to the trauma showed social withdrawal (Weisaeth 1989a). Finally, in a systematic survey conducted within a week of the Bay Area earthquake of 1989 with mildly affected individuals, Cardeña and Spiegel (1993) found that from 25% to 40% of respondents experienced various derealization and depersonalization symptoms, including the sense of being in unreal surroundings; feeling detached from people and activities; being at a distance from their emotions, thoughts, and feelings; and even feeling detached from their bodies. All of these symptoms had significantly decreased at a 4-month follow-up after cessation of trauma. Among children, psychological numbing and denial seems to occur more characteristically after long-standing repeated exposures to trauma (Terr 1991). These data are summarized in Table 45–4.

The data suggest that between one-fourth and three-fourths of traumatized individuals will experience a sense of unreality and detachment from their physical and psychological selves and/or from the social and material world and that there is some evidence that initial detachment or denial responses may increase the likelihood of later PTSDs (McFarlane 1986; Solomon et al. 1989), consistent with the high incidence of numbing and avoidance symptoms among PTSD populations.

Besides the changes in body image just mentioned, visual and auditory *perceptual alterations* have also been associated with severe stress, from concentration camps (Jaffe 1968) to childbirth (Farley et al. 1968). Terr (1979) reports that about a third of child kidnap victims experienced illusion and hallucinations and later a

Table 45–4. Percentage of trauma victims reporting detachment, disinterest, or a sense of unreality

Study	Detachment/ avoidance	Disinterest	Unreality
Noyes and Kletti 1977	52	—	72
Wilkinson 1983	29–36[a]	34	—
Madakasira and O'Brien 1987	57	45	—
Sloan 1988	54	—	—
Feinstein 1989	24	41	—
Weisaeth 1989a	38[a]	—	—
Weisaeth 1989b	32–38	—	—
A. Holen, unpublished data, 1991	33	—	—
Cardeña and Spiegel 1993: 1 week	28–40	40[a]	40
Cardeña and Spiegel 1993: 4 months	13	12	12

[a]Two percentages in the same category indicate that the author(s) had two or more categories for detachment/avoidance. The range of percentages for these categories is provided.

distorted sense of the sequence of events during and around the trauma. Siegel (1984) reports that adult hostage victims frequently experienced hallucinatory phenomena during captivity, including flashes of light, geometric patterns in the periphery of the visual field, and complex and realistic hallucinations. The literature on so-called near-death experiences also contains many reports of visual and other perceptual alterations in connection with an actual or perceived threat to one's life (Noyes and Kletti 1977). Finally, there is anecdotal (e.g., Hillman 1981; Valent 1984) and survey (Cardeña et al., in press) evidence of analgesia during or shortly after a disaster, probably mediated by the "stress-induced analgesia" associated with endorphins and other endogenous substances that may also mediate other perceptual alterations (Pitman et al. 1990).

With regard to short-term memory disturbances such as anterograde or retrograde amnesia after trauma, 61% of tornado victims reported some form of memory difficulties (Madakasira and O'Brien 1987), as did 79% of the survivors of an airplane crash landing (Sloan 1988), 44% of the Hyatt Regency victims, and one-fourth of the victims of an oil rig disaster (Cardeña et al., in press). The incidence of everyday problems with memory among those who experienced the Loma Prieta earthquake was 29% a week after the earthquake, a rate that decreased substantially after 4 months (Cardeña and Spiegel 1993). Table 45–5 summarizes these data.

Although few researchers have looked systematically at the effects of trauma on attentional processes, there is evidence that cognitive alterations such as difficulty concentrating and narrowing and automaticity of attention are frequent short-term (Cardeña and Spiegel 1993) and long-term (McFarlane 1986) effects of trauma.

Among children, Terr (1991) reports that single exposures to trauma may produce a detailed memory of the events (see also Dollinger 1985), whereas recurrent physical and/or sexual abuse may induce denial, amnesia, and other dissociative symptoms such as spontaneous "trance" episodes.

Table 45–5. Percentage of trauma victims reporting amnesia

Study	Percentage
Madakasira and O'Brien 1987	61
Sloan 1988	79
Wilkinson 1991	44
A. Holen, unpublished data, 1991	25
Cardeña and Spiegel 1993: 1 week	29
Cardeña and Spiegel 1993: 4 months	14

The presence of intrusive and detailed recollections for some aspects of trauma is not inconsistent with amnesia for the general context or peripheral aspects and is supported by laboratory research on attention and memory for highly emotional events (Christianson and Loftus 1987). For instance, 88% of the victims of the collapse of a skywalk (Wilkinson 1983), 92% of tornado survivors (Madakasira and O'Brien 1987), 61% of victims of an oil rig disaster (Holen 1991), and 39% of the Bay Area earthquake residents (Cardeña and Spiegel 1993) reported intrusive recollections. Recurrent dreams were found in 44% of tornado and 22% of earthquake victims (Cardeña and Spiegel 1993; Madakasira and O'Brien 1987). These results are summarized in Table 45–6.

The evidence consistently shows that whenever researchers investigate the presence of dissociative phenomenology during or shortly after a traumatic event, they find a substantial incidence of alterations in consciousness, problems with everyday memory and attention, and other phenomena that, when extreme, may alter everyday personal and social functioning. The presence of a strong dissociative component to traumatic reactions seems well established, but further research is required to determine the proportion and characteristics of the population likely to have impairment when confronted with traumatic events. Additional research is also warranted to determine coping responses that may predict good short- and long-term adjustment to trauma.

The adoption of the new diagnostic category of acute stress disorder should encourage greater clinical and research attention to the substantial number of people who may have acute and severe dissociative and anxiety reactions to trauma and bring the DSM nosology into greater accord with the ICD-10 diagnosis of acute stress reaction. It is proposed that the diagnosis of acute stress disorder be included in DSM-IV and be composed of dissociative, intrusion, avoidance, and hyperarousal symptoms occurring within 1 month of a stressor identical to that for PTSD. Because of this similarity to PTSD, it is proposed that acute stress disorder be included in the anxiety disorders section of DSM-IV.

Table 45–6.   Percentage of trauma victims reporting intrusive recollection after trauma

Study	Percentage
Wilkinson 1983	88
Madakasira and O'Brien 1987	92
A. Holen, unpublished data, 1991	61
Cardeña and Spiegel 1993: 1 week	39
Cardeña and Spiegel 1993: 4 months	17

Recommendations

The following description of the dissociative disorders represents the changes agreed to by the members of the Dissociative Disorders sub-Work Group and proposed for DSM-IV. Some minor phrasing changes may still occur after the writing of this chapter. Words in **bold** represent additions (including dissociative trance disorder, secondary dissociative disorder due to a nonpsychiatric medical condition, and acute stress disorder). Bracketed items represent deletions from DSM-III-R.

Dissociative Amnesia

Rationale: The DSM-III-R name "psychogenic amnesia" has been changed for ICD compatibility. The term *sudden* was removed from criterion A because it is unduly restrictive. The additional wording about the traumatic nature of the forgotten information is added for explanatory purposes and for compatibility with ICD-10.

A. The predominant disturbance is **one or more** episodes of [sudden] inability to recall important personal information, **usually of a traumatic or stressful nature,** that is too extensive to be explained by ordinary forgetfulness **or developmental age.**
B. The disturbance [is not due to] **does not occur exclusively as a symptom of dissociative identity disorder** and is not due to **substance-induced persisting amnestic disorder, substance intoxication, substance withdrawal, or a cognitive impairment disorder (e.g., amnestic disorder due to a nonpsychiatric medical condition).**

Dissociative Fugue

Rationale: The DSM-III-R name "psychogenic fugue" has been changed for ICD compatibility. Because DSM-III-R was unduly restrictive in requiring the "assumption of a new identity," criterion B has been broadened to include "confusion about personal identity."

A. The predominant disturbance is sudden, unexpected travel away from home or one's customary place of work, with inability to recall one's past.
B. **Confusion about personal identity or** assumption of new identity (partial or complete).
C. The disturbance [is not due to] **does not occur exclusively during the course of dissociative identity disorder** and is not due to **the direct effects of a substance (e.g., drugs of abuse, medication) or a general medical condition** (e.g., temporal lobe epilepsy).

DID (MPD)

Rationale: The suggested changes are 1) to change the name of the condition and reference to different "personalities," to clarify that the concept does not imply the objective existence of various personalities within one individual; 2) for the same reason, to replace the word *existence* in the first criterion with *presence*; 3) to restore criterion C, which was a part of the DSM-III criteria set and was eliminated from DSM-III-R. It is reinstated now to increase the precision and threshold of the diagnosis and because it is central to the construct of the condition. The term *full* was deleted from the criterion that a personality state take control of the person's behavior, because it was felt that dissociative phenomena may occur with less than full control, for example, in the case of auditory hallucinations that may represent the intrusion of one personality state into another.

A. The [existence within the person] **presence** of two or more distinct [personalities] **identities** or personality states (each with its own relatively enduring pattern of perceiving, relating to, and thinking about the environment and self).

B. At least two of these [personalities] **identities** or personality states recurrently take [full] control of the person's behavior.

C. **Inability to recall important personal information that is too extensive to be explained by ordinary forgetfulness.**

D. **The disturbance is not due to a substance-induced disorder (e.g., blackouts or chaotic behavior during alcohol intoxication). In children, the symptoms are not attributable to imaginary playmates or other fantasy play.**

Depersonalization Disorder

Rationale: There are only minor wording changes.

A. **Persistent or recurrent experiences of feeling detached from, and as if one is an outside observer of, one's mental processes or body (e.g., feeling like an automaton).** [Persistent or recurrent experiences of depersonalization as indicated by either (1) or (2):

   (1)   an experience of feeling detached from, and as if one is an outside observer of, one's mental processes or body

   (2)   an experience of feeling like an automaton or as if in a dream]

B. **During the depersonalization experience, reality testing remains intact.**

C. **The depersonalization** [is sufficiently severe and persistent to cause] **causes significant impairment in social or occupational functioning, or causes marked distress.**

D. The depersonalization experience [is the predominant disturbance and is not a symptom of another disorder] **does not occur exclusively in association with another disorder** such as schizophrenia, **dissociative identity disorder, or panic disorder,** [or agoraphobia without history of panic disorder but with limited symptom attacks of depersonalization] **and is not due to a substance-induced disorder (e.g., substance intoxication).**

Dissociative Trance Disorder

Rationale: Possession and trance states are common and normal components of religious and other ceremonies in many cultures. However, dissociative trance disorder (leading to distress and dysfunction) is also the most common dissociative disorder reported in non-Western culture. DSM-III mentioned trance-like states as an example of atypical dissociative disorder. DSM-III-R expanded the example and provided a definition of trance. ICD-10 has included a new category, dissociative trance disorders, within the dissociative disorders.

A. Either (1) or (2):
   (1)   trance, i.e., temporary marked alteration in the state of consciousness or loss of customary sense of personal identity, associated with at least one of the following:
      (a) narrowing of awareness of immediate surroundings, or unusually narrow and selective focusing on environmental stimuli
      (b) stereotyped behaviors or movements that are experienced as being beyond one's control
   (2)   possession trance, i.e., a single or episodic alteration in the state of consciousness, characterized by the replacement of the customary sense of personal identity by a new identity. This is attributed to the influence of a spirit, power, deity or other person and is associated with at least one of the following:
      (a) stereotyped and culturally determined behaviors or movements that are experienced as being controlled by the possessing agent
      (b) full or partial amnesia for the event
B. The trance or possession state is not a normal part of a broadly accepted collective cultural or religious practice.
C. The trance or possession state causes significant impairment in social or occupational functioning or causes marked distress.
D. Not occurring exclusively during the course of a psychotic disorder (including mood disorder with psychotic features and brief reactive psychosis) or dissociative identity disorder (multiple personality disorder), and is not due to substance-induced disorder (e.g., substance intoxication) or a secondary dissociative disorder.

Secondary Dissociative Disorder Due to a Nonpsychiatric Medical Condition

Rationale: This category has been proposed but not accepted for DSM-IV and is included in ICD-10. It is supported by studies that suggest an elevated prevalence of dissociative symptoms in individuals with complex partial seizures and that dissociative symptoms accompanying complex partial seizures are not associated with a history of physical and sexual trauma.

A. Amnesia, fugue, depersonalization, derealization, or other dissociative symptoms.

B. There is evidence from the history, physical examination, or laboratory findings that a general medical condition (e.g., complex partial seizure or drug toxicity) is etiologically related to the dissociative symptoms.

C. The dissociative symptoms cause significant impairment in social or occupational functioning, or cause marked distress.

D. Does not meet criteria for a secondary cognitive impairment disorder (i.e., due to a general medical condition).

DDNOS

Rationale: DSM-III-R example 6 is deleted because it is now covered by the revised definition of dissociative fugue. Example 1 has been altered to reflect the suggested change in definition for dissociative identity disorder (multiple personality disorder). Example 4 would be listed only if dissociative trance disorder is not included as a separate disorder, and it would similarly require the presence of significant impairment and/or dysfunction.

This category is for disorders in which the predominant feature is a dissociative symptom (i.e., a disturbance or alteration in the normally integrative functions of identity, memory, or consciousness), but the criteria are not met for a specific dissociative disorder.

Examples:

(1) Cases similar to **dissociative identity disorder** but failing to meet full criteria for this disorder. Examples include cases in which (a) **not more than one personality state is sufficiently distinct,** [to meet the full criteria for dissociative identity disorder (multiple personality disorder) (b) a second personality never assumes complete executive control]; or (b) **amnesia for important personal information does not occur.**

(2) Derealization unaccompanied by depersonalization, [only in adults] **except in childhood.**

(3) States of dissociation that occur in people who have been subjected to periods of prolonged and intense coercive persuasion (e.g., brainwashing, thought reform, or indoctrination while the captive of terrorists or cultists).

(4) Dissociative trance or possession phenomena: single or episodic alterations in the state of consciousness that are indigenous to particular locations and cultures. Dissociative trance involves narrowing of awareness of immediate surroundings or stereotyped behaviors or movements that are experienced as being beyond one's control. Possession trance involves replacement of the customary sense of personal identity by a new identity, attributed to the influence of a spirit, power, deity, or other person and associated with stereotyped "involuntary" movements or amnesia. Examples include *amok* (Indonesia), *bebainan* (Indonesia), *benzi mazurazura* (Southern Africa), *latah* (Malaysia), *pibloktoq* (Artic), *phii pob* (Thailand), *vimbuza* (Nigeria), *ataque de nervios* (Latin America), and *possession (India, Africa, Caribbean). The dissociative trance disorder is not a normal part of a broadly accepted collective cultural or religious practice.*

(5) Loss of consciousness, stupor, or coma not attributable to a general medical condition.

(6) Ganser's syndrome: the giving of "approximate answers" to questions, commonly associated with dissociative amnesia or fugue. [other symptoms such as amnesia, disorientation, perceptual disturbances, fugue and conversion symptoms

(6) *Cases in which sudden unexpected travel and organized purposeful behavior with inability to recall one's past are not accompanied by the assumption of a new personal identity.]*

Acute Stress Disorder

Rationale: This is a proposed new diagnosis, parallel to one included in ICD-10 (as acute stress reaction), which may help to describe cases that do not meet the criteria for PTSD (because of differences in onset, duration, and symptom presentation) and that are more specific and severe than adjustment disorder.

A. The person has been exposed to a traumatic event in which both of the following have been present:
   (1) the person has experienced, witnessed, or been confronted with an event or events that involve actual or threatened death or serious injury or a threat to the physical integrity of oneself or others
   (2) the person's response involved intense fear, helplessness, or horror
B. Either while experiencing or immediately after experiencing the distressing event, the individual has at least three of the following dissociative symptoms:

(1) subjective sense of numbing, detachment, or absence of emotional responsiveness

(2) a reduction in awareness of one's surroundings (e.g., "being in a daze")

(3) derealization

(4) depersonalization

(5) dissociative amnesia

C. The traumatic event is persistently reexperienced in at least one of the following ways: recurrent images, thoughts, dreams, illusions, flashback episodes, or a sense of reliving the experience or distress on exposure to reminders of the traumatic event.

D. Marked avoidance of stimuli that arouse recollections of the trauma (e.g., thoughts, feelings, conversations, activities, places, or people)

E. Marked symptoms of anxiety or increased arousal (e.g., difficulty sleeping, irritability, poor concentration, hypervigilance, exaggerated startle response, and motor restlessness).

F. The disturbance causes clinically significant distress or impairment in social, occupational, or other important areas of functioning, or the individual is prevented from pursuing some necessary task, such as obtaining necessary medical or legal assistance or mobilizing personal resources by telling family members about the traumatic experience.

G. The symptoms last for a minimum of 2 days and a maximum of 4 weeks and occur within 4 weeks of the traumatic event.

H. Not due to the direct effects of a substance (e.g., drugs of abuse, medication) or a general medical condition and is not merely an exacerbation of a preexisting Axis I or Axis II disorder.

References

Adityanjee, Raju GS, Kandewal SK: Current status of multiple personality disorder in India. Am J Psychiatry 146:1607–1610, 1989

American Psychiatric Association: Diagnostic and Statistical Manual of Mental Disorders, 3rd Edition, Revised. Washington, DC, American Psychiatric Association, 1987

Benson DF, Miller B, Signer SF: Dual personality associated with epilepsy. Arch Neurol 43:471–474, 1986

Bernstein EM, Putnam FW: Development, reliability, and validity of a dissociation scale. J Nerv Ment Dis 174:727–735, 1986

Bliss EL: Multiple personalities: a report of 14 cases with implications for schizophrenia and hysteria. Arch Gen Psychiatry 37:1388–1397, 1980

Bliss EL: A symptom profile of patients with multiple personalities including MMPI results. J Nerv Ment Dis 172:197–201, 1984

Blumer D: Temporal lobe epilepsy and its psychiatric significance, in Psychiatric Aspects of Neurological Disorders. Edited by Benson DF, Blumer D. New York, Grune & Stratton, 1975

Boddy J: Wombs and Alien Spirits. Madison, University of Wisconsin Press, 1989

Boon S, Draijer N: Diagnosing dissociative disorders in the Netherlands: a pilot study with the Structured Clinical Interview for DSM-III-R Dissociative Disorders. Am J Psychiatry 148:458–462, 1991

Bourguignon E: Possession. San Francisco, CA, Chandler & Sharp, 1976

Brenmer JD, Southwick S, Brett E, et al: Dissociation and posttraumatic stress disorder in Vietnam combat veterans. Am J Psychiatry 149:328–332, 1992

Briere J, Conte J: Amnesia in adults molested as children: testing theories of repression. Paper presented at the 97th Annual Convention of the American Psychological Association, New Orleans, LA, 1989

Cardeña E: The varieties of possession experience. Association for the Anthropological Study of Consciousness Quarterly 5:1–17, 1989

Cardeña E: Trance and possession as dissociative disorders. Transcultural Psychiatric Research Review 29:283–297, 1992

Cardeña E: Dissociation and trauma: how are they linked? Invited address at the 101st Annual Convention of the American Psychological Association, Toronto, August 1993

Cardeña E, Spiegel D: Dissociative reactions to the Bay Area earthquake. Am J Psychiatry 150:474–478, 1993

Cardeña E, Holen A, McFarlane A, et al: A multi-site study of acute-stress reaction to a disaster, in DSM-IV Sourcebook, Vol 4. Edited by Widiger TA, Frances AJ, Pincus HA, et al. Washington, DC, American Psychiatric Press (in press)

Carlson EB, Rosser-Hogan R: Trauma experiences, posttraumatic stress, dissociation, and depression in Cambodian refugees. Am J Psychiatry 148:1548–1551, 1991

Christianson SA, Loftus EF: Memory for traumatic events. Applied Cognitive Psychology 1:225–239, 1987

Chu J, Dill D: Dissociative symptoms in relation to childhood physical and sexual abuse. Am J Psychiatry 147:887–892, 1990

Cocores JA, Bender AL, McBride E: Multiple personality, seizure disorder, and the electroencephalogram. J Nerv Ment Dis 172:436–438, 1984

Coons PM: The differential diagnosis of multiple personality. Psychiatr Clin North Am 7:51–67, 1984

Coons PM, Milstein V: Psychosexual disturbances in multiple personality: characteristics, etiology and treatment. J Clin Psychiatry 47:106–110, 1986

Coons PM, Milstein V, Marley C: EEG studies of two multiple personalities and a control. Arch Gen Psychiatry 39:823–825, 1982

Coons PM, Bowman ES, Milstein V: Multiple personality disorder: a clinical investigation of 50 cases. J Nerv Ment Dis 176:519–527, 1988

Coons PM, Bowman ES, Pellow TA: Post-traumatic aspects of the treatment of victims of sexual abuse and incest. Psychiatr Clin North Am 12:325–337, 1989

Crabtree A: Multiple Man: Explorations in Possession and Multiple Personality. New York, Praeger, 1985

De la Cancela V, Guarnaccia PJ, Carrillo E: Psychosocial distress among Latinos: a critical analysis of ataque de nervios. Humanity and Society 10:431–447, 1986

Devinsky O, Feldmann E, Burrowes K, et al: Autoscopic phenomena with seizures. Arch Neurol 46:1080–1088, 1989a

Devinsky O, Putnam F, Grafman J, et al: Dissociative states and epilepsy. Neurology 39:835–840, 1989b

Dollinger SJ: Lightning-strike disaster among children. Br J Med Psychol 58:375–383, 1985

Drake ME: Epilepsy and multiple personality: clinical and EEG findings in 15 cases. Epilepsia 27:635, 1986

Farley J, Woodruff RA, Guze SB: The prevalence of hysteria and conversion symptoms. Br J Psychiatry 114:1121–1125, 1968

Feinstein A: Posttraumatic stress disorder: a descriptive study supporting DSM-III-R criteria. Am J Psychiatry 146:665–666, 1989

Fisher C: Amnestic states in war neurosis: the psychogenesis of fugue. Psychoanal Q 14:437–468, 1945

Freed SA, Freed RS: Spirit possession as illness in a North Indian village. Ethnology 3:152–171, 1964

Frigerio A: Levels of possession awareness in Afro-Brazilian religions. Association for the Anthropological Study of Consciousness Quarterly 5:5–11, 1989

Gelinas DJ: The persisting negative effects of incest. Psychiatry 46:312–332, 1983

Good MI: Substance-induced dissociative disorders and psychiatric nosology. J Clin Psychopharmacol 9:88–93, 1989

Guarnaccia PJ, Rubio-Stipec M, Canino G: *Ataques de nervios* in the Puerto Rican Diagnostic Interview Schedule: the impact of cultural categories on psychiatric epidemiology. Culture, Medicine and Psychiatry 13:275–295, 1989

Guarnaccia PJ, Canino G, Rubio-Stipec M, et al: The prevalence of *Ataques de nervios* in the Puerto Rico disaster study: the role of culture in psychiatric epidemiology. J Nerv Ment Dis 181:159–167, 1993

Herman JL, Perry JC, van der Kolk BA: Childhood trauma in borderline personality disorder. Am J Psychiatry 146: 490–495, 1989

Hillman RG: The psychopathology of being held hostage. Am J Psychiatry 138:193–1197, 1981

Hughes DJ: Differences between trance channeling and multiple personality disorder on structured interview. Journal of Transpersonal Psychology 24:181–192, 1992

Jaffe R: Dissociative phenomena in former concentration camp inmates. Int J Psychoanal 49:310–312, 1968

James W: The Principles of Psychology. New York, Holt, 1890/1923

Keane T, Malloy P, Fairbank J: The empirical development of an MMPI subscale for the assessment of combat-related post-traumatic stress disorders. J Consult Clin Psychol 52:888–891, 1984

Keller R, Shaywitz BA: Amnesia or fugue state: a diagnostic dilemma. Developmental and Behavioral Pediatrics 7:131–132, 1986

Kihlstrom JF: The cognitive unconscious. Science 237:1445–1452, 1987

Kihlstrom JF, Hoyt I: Repression, dissociation, and hypnosis, in Repression and Dissociation. Edited by Singer JL. Chicago, IL, University of Chicago Press, 1990, pp 181–208

Kluft RP: Making the diagnosis of multiple personality disorder (MPD). Direct Psychiatry 23:1–10, 1985

Kluft RP: Multiple personality disorder, in American Psychiatric Press Review of Psychiatry, Vol 10. Edited by Tasman A, Goldfinger SW. Washington, DC, American Psychiatric Press, 1991, pp 161–188

Kluft RP, Steinberg M, Spitzer RL: DSM-III-R revisions in the dissociative disorders: an exploration of their derivation and rationale. Dissociation 1:39–46, 1988

Koopman C, Classen C, Cardeña E, et al: The development of a state measure of dissociative reactions to trauma. Unpublished manuscript, Palo Alto, CA, Stanford University, 1993

Krippner S: Cross-cultural approaches to multiple personality disorder: practices in Brazilian spiritism. Ethos 15:273–295, 1987

Larmore K, Ludwig AM, Cain RL: Multiple personality: an objective case study. Br J Psychiatry 131:35–40, 1977

Lewis-Fernández R: The role of culture in the configuration of dissociative states: a comparison of Puerto Rican *ataque de nervios* and Indian "possession syndrome," in Dissociation: Culture, Mind and Body. Edited by Spiegel D. Washington, DC, American Psychiatric Press, 1994, pp 123–167

Lindemann E: Symptomatology and management of acute grief. Am J Psychiatry 101:141–148, 1944

Litwin RG, Cardeña E: Dissociation and reported trauma in organic and psychogenic seizure patients. 101st Annual Convention of the American Psychological Association, Toronto, 1993

Loewenstein RJ: Psychogenic amnesia and psychogenic fugue: a comprehensive review, in American Psychiatric Press Review of Psychiatry, Vol 10. Edited by Tansman A, Goldfinger S. Washington, DC, American Psychiatric Press, 1991, pp 189–222

Loewenstein RJ, Putnam FW: A comparative study of dissociative symptoms in patients with complex partial seizures, multiple personality disorder and posttraumatic stress disorder. Dissociation 1:17–23, 1988

Ludwig AM, Brandsma JM, Wilbur CB, et al: The objective study of a multiple personality. Arch Gen Psychiatry 26:298–310, 1972

Madakasira S, O'Brien K: Acute posttraumatic stress disorder in victims of a natural disaster. J Nerv Ment Dis 175:286–290, 1987

Marmar CR, Weiss DS, Schlenger WE, et al: Peritraumatic dissociation and post-traumatic stress in male Vietnam theater veterans. 8th Annual Meeting of the International Society for Traumatic Stress Studies, Los Angeles, CA, October 1992

Mayeux R, Alexander MP, Benson F, et al: Poriomania. Neurology 29:1616–1619, 1979

McCann IL, Sakheim DK, Abrahamson DJ: Trauma and victimization: a model of psychological adaptation. Counseling Psychologist 16:531–594, 1988

McFarlane AC: Posttraumatic morbidity of a disaster. J Nerv Ment Dis 174:4–14, 1986

Mesulam MM: Dissociative states with abnormal temporal lobe EEG. Arch Neurol 38:176–181, 1981

Nash MR, Hulsey TL, Sexton MC, et al: Long-term sequelae of childhood sexual abuse: perceived family environment, psychopathology and dissociation. J Consult Clin Psychol 61, 276–283, 1993

Nichter M: Idioms of distress: alternatives in the expression of psychosocial distress. Culture, Medicine and Psychiatry 5:379–408, 1981

Noyes R, Kletti R: Depersonalization in response to life-threatening danger. Compr Psychiatry 18:375–384, 1977

Noyes R, Slymen DJ: The subjective response to life-threatening danger. Omega 9:313–321, 1978–1979

Obeyesekere G: The idiom of demonic possession: a case study. Social Science and Medicine 4:97–111, 1970

Ogata S, Silk K, Goodrich S, et al: Childhood sexual and physical abuse in adult patients with borderline personality disorder. Am J Psychiatry 147:1008–1013, 1990

Pitman RK, Orr SP, van der Kolk BA, et al: Analgesia: a new dependent variable for the biological study of posttraumatic stress disorder, in Posttraumatic Stress Disorder: Etiology, Phenomenology, and Treatment. Edited by Wolf ME, Mosnaim AD. Washington, DC, American Psychiatric Press, 1990, pp 140–147

Putnam FW, Guroff JJ, Silberman EK, et al: The clinical phenomenology of multiple personality disorder: review of 100 recent cases. J Clin Psychiatry 47: 285–293, 1986

Riether AM, Stoudemire A: Psychogenic fugue states: a review. South Med J 81:568–71, 1988

Rose DS: "Worse than death": psychodynamics of rape victims and the need for psychotherapy. Am J Psychiatry 143:817–824, 1986

Ross CA: Differentiating MPD and DDNOS. Paper presented at the 8th International Conference on Multiple Personality/Dissociative States, Chicago, IL, 1991

Ross CA, Heber S, Norton GR, et al: The dissociative disorders interview schedule: a structured interview. Dissociation 2:169–189, 1989a

Ross CA, Heber S, Norton R, et al: Differences between multiple personality disorder and other diagnostic groups on structured interview. J Nerv Ment Dis 177:487–491, 1989b

Ross CA, Heber S, Norton R, et al: Multiple personality disorder: an analysis of 236 cases. Can J Psychiatry 34:413–418, 1989c

Ross CA, Miller SD, Reagor P, et al: Structured interview data on 102 cases of multiple personality disorder from four centers. Am J Psychiatry 147; 147:596–601, 1990

Saxena S, Prasad K: DSM-III subclassifications of dissociative disorders applied to psychiatric outpatients in India. Am J Psychiatry 146:261–262, 1989

Schenk L, Bear D: Multiple personality and related dissociative phenomena in patients with temporal lobe epilepsy. Am J Psychiatry 138:1311–1316, 1981

Schultz R, Braun BG, Kluft RP: Multiple personality disorder: phenomenology of selected variables in comparison to major depression. Dissociation 2:45–51, 1989

Shen W, Bowman ES, Markand ON: Pseudoseizures. Neurology 40:1478–1479, 1990

Siegel RK: Hostage hallucinations. J Nerv Ment Dis 172:264–272, 1984

Sloan P: Post-traumatic stress in survivors of an airplane crash landing: a clinical and exploratory research intervention. J Traumatic Stress 1:211–229, 1988

Solomon Z, Mikulincer M, Benbenistry R: Combat stress reactions: clinical manifestations and correlates. Military Psychology 1:35–47, 1989

Spiegel D: Multiple personality as a post-traumatic stress disorder. Psychiatr Clin North Am 7:101–110, 1984

Spiegel D: Hypnosis, dissociation and trauma: hidden and overt observers, in Repression and Dissociation. Edited by Singer JL. Chicago, IL, University of Chicago Press, 1990, pp 82–104

Spiegel D, Cardeña E: Disintegrated experience: the dissociative disorders revisited. J Abnorm Psychol 100:366–378, 1991

Spiegel D, Hunt T, Dondershine EH: Dissociation and hypnotizability in posttraumatic stress disorder. Am J Psychiatry 145:301–305, 1988

Squire LR, Zola-Morgan S: The medial temporal lobe system. Science 253:1380–1386, 1991

Steinberg M: Transcultural issues in psychiatry: the ataque and multiple personality disorder. Dissociation 3:287–289, 1990

Steinberg M, Rounsaville B, Ciccheti DV: The structured clinical interview for DSM-III-R dissociative disorders: preliminary reports on a new diagnostic instrument. Am J Psychiatry 147:76–82, 1990

Stoller P: Stressing social change and Songhay possession, in Altered States of Consciousness and Mental Health. A Cross-Cultural Perspective. Edited by Ward CA. Newbury Park, CA, Sage, 1989a, pp 267–284

Stoller P: Fusion of the worlds. Chicago, IL, University of Chicago Press, 1989b

Stutman RK, Bliss E: Posttraumatic stress disorder, hypnotizability, and imagery. Am J Psychiatry 142:741–743, 1985

Terr LC: Children of Chowchilla: a study of psychic trauma, in The Psychoanalytic Study of the Child. Edited by Solnit AJ, Eissler R, Freud A, et al. New Haven, CT, Yale University Press, 1979, pp 1543–1550

Terr LC: Childhood traumas: an outline and overview. Am J Psychiatry 148:10–20, 1991

Valent P: The Ash Wednesday bushfires in Victoria. Med J Aust 141:291–300, 1984

Venn J: Family etiology and remission in a case of psychogenic fugue. Family Process 23:429–435, 1984

Walker SS: Ceremonial Spirit Possession in Africa and Afro-America. Leiden, Netherlands, EJ Brill, 1972

Ward CA: Possession and exorcism: psychopathology and psychotherapy in a magico-religious context, in Altered States of Consciousness and Mental Health. A Cross-Cultural Perspective. Edited by Ward CA. Newbury Park, CA, Sage, 1989, pp 125–144

Weisaeth L: The stressors and the post-traumatic stress syndrome after an industrial disaster. Acta Psychiatr Scand Suppl 355:25–37, 1989a

Weisaeth L: Torture of a Norwegian ship's crew. Acta Psychiatr Scand Suppl 355:63–72, 1989b

Wilkinson CB: Aftermath of a disaster: the collapse of the Hyatt Regency Hotel skywalks. Am J Psychiatry 140:1134–1139, 1983

Chapter 46

Impulse Control Disorders

John Bradford, M.D., Jeffrey Geller, M.D.,
Henry R. Lesieur, Ph.D., Richard Rosenthal, M.D.,
and Michael Wise, M.D.

Statement and Significance of the Issues

Intermittent Explosive Disorder (IED)

DSM-III-R (American Psychiatric Association 1987) contains the following commentary about IED: "This category has been retained in DSM-III-R despite the fact that many doubt the existence of a clinical syndrome characterized by episodic loss of control that is not symptomatic of one of the disorders that must be ruled out before the diagnosis of Intermittent Explosive Disorder can be made" (p. 321). IED remains a controversial diagnosis, despite the fact that aggressive and explosive behaviors are commonly encountered in society and by clinicians. Because doubts exist about whether IED is a separate disorder or merely a symptom of other disorders, the DSM-IV sub-Work Group on Impulse Control Disorders Not Elsewhere Classified conducted an extensive literature review.

Kleptomania

Systematic studies of kleptomania are lacking and the differentiation between shoplifting for gain and kleptomania is often confused in case reports and studies. Recent reported associations between kleptomania and other psychiatric disorders needed investigation so that DSM-IV might clarify these relationships. Three issues were examined in recommending changes to the DSM-III-R kleptomania criteria. One of the most important was the distinction between kleptomania, an exceedingly rare condition, and shoplifting, which is very common. Shoplifting is an important sociolegal problem that causes the loss of millions of dollars annually. The impact of shoplifting is so great that, if all shoplifting were to cease, it is estimated that retail prices would drop 20% (Rawlins 1978). Shoplifting and kleptomania are associated, but kleptomania is rarely seen (Arieff and Bowie 1947;

Bradford and Balmaceda 1983; Cameron 1964; Gibbens 1981; Gibbens and Prince 1962; Gibbens et al. 1971; Kahn and Martin 1977; Meyers 1970; Money 1983). The second issue was to review the research foundation for kleptomania's diagnostic criteria. The third and more recent issue is the reported association between kleptomania and several other psychiatric disorders, such as mood disorders, obsessive-compulsive disorder, and eating disorders.

Pyromania

In the first DSM (American Psychiatric Association 1952), pyromania was classified as an obsessive-compulsive reaction. Although pyromania remained a focus of attention in the 1950s, it was apparently rejected as a specific mental disorder in the 1960s and was entirely excluded from DSM-II (American Psychiatric Association 1968). In the 1970s, several authorities cited pyromania as a distinct impulse disorder, and it was returned to the standard psychiatric taxonomy by its inclusion in DSM-III (American Psychiatric Association 1980) and DSM-III-R. The preparation of DSM-IV necessitates a review of the scientific basis for the diagnostic criteria for pyromania. What is the prevalence of the diagnosis of pyromania using DSM-III and DSM-III-R criteria, and is there anything in the literature to support either expanding or narrowing the diagnostic criteria?

Pathological Gambling

The diagnostic criteria for pathological gambling in DSM-III-R were specifically modeled after those for psychoactive substance dependence. Although this marked a significant departure from DSM-III, the criteria were not tested except with regard to the cutoff point (Lesieur 1988a). Issues that need to be addressed include: How well do specific criteria discriminate between pathological and social gamblers? Are there other criteria that would better accomplish this? Was there anything lost in the shift from DSM-III? What is the experience of the individual therapist who attempts to use DSM-III-R? Are the criteria clear and objective? Are they useful in difficult diagnostic situations? Does the accompanying text adequately describe the disorder? Finally, most of the research on pathological gambling has been done in the past 4–5 years. Is the comparison with substance dependence and addiction still valid?

Lesieur (1988a) noted that several of the DSM-III-R items possessed less-than-adequate discriminative value. Specifically, social gamblers could answer in the affirmative without necessarily having gambling problems. Due to time limitations, there was no attempt to replace them with alternative criteria.

When DSM-III-R was a year old, Rosenthal (1989) interviewed a dozen of the most influential experts in pathological gambling, selected for their involvement in evaluating gamblers and in training others in this area. They represented all the major gambling treatment programs in the United States. These clinicians voiced dissatisfaction with the new criteria and expressed a preference for a compromise between DSM-III and the newer DSM-III-R criteria. They complained that several of the criteria were too ambiguous and subjective. For example, item 5 was a compound sentence, the two halves of which could be answered independently. Items 7, 8, and 9 had too much overlap. The criteria offered little help in diagnosing difficult cases.

Rosenthal found that the biggest criticism was how much had been left out. Several clinicians and academicians attributed this to the need to have the criteria conform to those for psychoactive substance dependence. The general feeling was that pathological gambling was in fact an addiction, but clinicians were unable to specify or agree on what should be added to the diagnostic criteria to make it distinct from substance dependence. Everything pointed to the need for a more definitive study, a survey that would compare DSM-III and DSM-III-R criteria as well as other possible items for inclusion.

It was also noted that there was a great disparity between epidemiological and treatment surveys (Ciarrocchi and Richardson 1989; Lesieur 1988b; Sommers 1988; Volberg and Steadman 1988, 1989). For example, females, nonwhites, and individuals less than 30 years old tend to be underrepresented in treatment and in Gamblers Anonymous. Jewish individuals are overrepresented in Gamblers Anonymous and in treatment (Ciarrocchi and Richardson 1989; Custer and Custer 1978; Lesieur 1988b; Nora 1984), but not in survey findings (Sommers 1988; Volberg and Steadman 1988, 1989). There are also differences from one geographic area to another, notably in the type of gambling. Because DSM-III criteria may have a middle-class bias (Lesieur 1984, 1987), it was entirely possible that generalizations were made that were only true for limited groups or subgroups of pathological gamblers. In particular, there was a need to ensure that the criteria applied equally well to females and males.

Furthermore, the term *problem gambler* was appearing in the literature with greater frequency. Problem gambling is a more inclusive application applied to all patterns of gambling behavior that may compromise, disrupt, or damage family, personal, or vocational pursuits. Problem gambling includes but is not limited to pathological gambling. The National Council on Compulsive Gambling recently recognized this and changed its name to the National Council on Problem Gambling. Different types of problem gamblers have been described by Custer (1982), Abt et al. (1985), and Rosenthal (1989).

With greater public education and awareness of gambling as a disorder, many individuals who have gambling problems but who are not pathological gamblers will be requesting consultation. Pathological gamblers will also be seeking help in earlier stages of the disorder. It will therefore be even more essential to tighten the criteria to clearly distinguish pathological from other high-frequency gamblers.

IED

Method

The initial approach to the literature review included an automated Medline search using the terms *rage, violence, aggression, explosive, episodic dyscontrol, agitation,* and *combative behavior.* This produced such a large number of references that an alternate strategy was used. Articles were selected that primarily discussed the diagnosis of explosive personality, IED, or episodic dyscontrol. References at the end of each article provided additional references for review. This pyramid-style approach was repeated until a sufficient body of literature on episodic violent behavior (EVB) was collected. In addition, experts in IED were asked to submit reference lists for review.

Only English-language books and journal articles were reviewed; references ranged from 1937 to 1991. Included in the review were 258 articles and 30 books. References were examined in which patients met the DSM-III-R criteria for IED. Patients were not included in the data if, by definition, they were excluded from an IED diagnosis in DSM-III-R (e.g., by a diagnosis of antisocial or borderline personality disorder). Each article was reviewed by two independent reviewers and results were compared to ensure reliable data collection. The reviewer recorded the presence of EVB in the patients studied and noted the diagnostic criteria that were used.

Specific patient data were recorded, including sex, history of a psychotic disorder, history of attention-deficit/hyperactivity disorder (ADHD), antisocial personality disorder, other personality disorders, alcohol abuse/pathological intoxication, psychosis, other psychoactive substance intoxication, abnormal neuropsychological testing, history of a learning disorder, electroencephalogram (EEG) abnormalities, history of seizures, prodromal symptoms, abnormal head computed tomography, history of head trauma, history of other neurological abnormality, genetic abnormality, family history of EVB, history of legal problems/prison, and remorse.

We found 51 articles that included patients diagnosed with IED, episodic dyscontrol (EDC), or explosive personality. Several authors, specifically Bach-y-rita, Elliot, and Mattes, may have used the same patients for more than one article. Therefore, to be conservative and to avoid counting patients more than once in this review, data from 45 articles (842 patients) were collected for analysis.

Results

Patients with EVB were diagnosed using at least five different sets of diagnostic criteria. Most authors simply used the occurrence of the outburst itself as sufficient for diagnosis, with little information available in the text to determine the characteristics associated with the behavior of the patient. The sex distribution of persons with EVB was 80% male (667 of 819 patients). DSM-III criteria were used to diagnose 19% of patients. The majority of patients (60%) were diagnosed as episodic dyscontrol, with miscellaneous diagnoses accounting for another 15%. Together, non-DSM, non-ICD diagnoses accounted for 75% of the patients in our review. Only Felthous et al. (1991) used DSM-III-R criteria for IED.

Table 46–1 shows the characteristics of patients with EVB. The first column lists the number of patients positive for a test or characteristic relative to all patients tested for that characteristic and the percentage represented by the first figure. The column labeled "% examined" indicates the percentage of patients who were "evaluated" by a test or for a characteristic out of the total population (842 patients).

Table 46–1. Features reported in the diagnosis of 842 individuals with episodic violent behavior (EVB)

Feature	n yes/Total N (%)[a]	Examined (%)[b]
History of seizures	215/733 (29)	87
History of legal problems	216/621 (35)	74
History of head trauma	182/617 (30)	73
Attention-deficit/hyperactivity disorder	262/582 (45)	69
Other psychoactive substance intoxication	82/547 (15)	65
History of other neurological abnormality	350/539 (65)	64
History of psychotic disorder	33/527 (6)	62
Antisocial personality disorder	15/445 (3)	53
Alcohol abuse/pathological intoxication	238/417 (57)	50
Abnormal electroencephalogram	202/368 (55)	44
Family history of episodic violent behavior	109/264 (41)	31
Prodromal symptoms	77/202 (38)	24
Other personality disorders (Axis II)	39/168 (23)	20
Abnormal neuropsychological testing	97/167 (58)	20
Remorse present	96/153 (63)	18
Genetic abnormality	4/151 (2.6)	18
History of a learning disorder	38/99 (38)	12
Abnormal head computed tomography scan	16/98 (16)	12

[a]Number of patients positive for a test or characteristic relative to all patients tested for that characteristic and the percentage of patients tested for that characteristic who were positive.
[b]Percentage of patients who were evaluated by a test or for a characteristic out of the total population of 842 patients.

Despite the prominence of certain findings, these features were not reported in a large number of cases. Most often neglected were neuropsychological testing and systematic evaluation of personality. Neuropsychological testing was abnormal in 58% of patients tested but was performed in only 20% of cases. No author evaluated personality in a systematic fashion. This is a critical omission, because antisocial personality disorder and borderline personality disorder (BPD) are exclusion criteria for a DSM-III-R IED diagnosis. Some authors mentioned that BPD had been excluded in their patients, but no information was given about how this was done.

Patients with EVB frequently had neurological abnormalities, but EEGs were performed for fewer than half the patients, and computed tomography results were reported only for 12%. When remorse, which is part of the ICD-9-CM (U.S. Department of Health and Human Services 1979) diagnostic criteria, was recorded, it was found in 63% of patients; however, it was reported on in only 18% of all cases. Even though alcohol use was associated with violent outbursts in 57% of cases where it was investigated, alcohol intake was not evaluated in 425 of 842 patients (50%). No studies were found in which toxicological analyses of urine or blood samples were performed at the time of the violent episode.

Discussion

The diagnostic classification of individuals who exhibit EVB has undergone considerable change (Table 46–2). Currently, two DSM-III-R diagnoses are available to the clinician who wants to classify a patient with EVB. These are IED and organic personality syndrome (OPS), explosive type. IED has several inclusion criteria and numerous exclusion criteria, whereas OPS requires the presence of a specific organic factor that is judged to be etiologically related to the violence.

This literature review found that many, if not most, of the patients with EVB had evidence of CNS dysfunction. Where examined, a significant percentage of patients had abnormal EEGs (55%), neurological examinations (65%), and neuropsychological tests (58%); a history of learning disability (38%); ADHD (45%); seizures (29%); or head trauma (30%). Unfortunately, these tests of CNS function were frequently unreported and may not have been performed. When the patient does have evidence of CNS dysfunction, it is often difficult to establish a clear cause-and-effect relationship between the CNS dysfunction and the EVB, which is necessary to meet DSM-III-R criteria for OPS, explosive type.

When 842 cases of EVB documented in the literature were carefully reviewed using DSM-III-R criteria for IED, 17 possible patients were found. Mattes (1990) reported 4 patients diagnosed with IED (4 of 51 patients or 8%) that were without any evidence of organicity; he did not perform a systematic personality analysis. Felthous et al. (1991), after an extensive evaluation process, reported 13 patients with IED; however, they did not perform neuropsychological testing or systematic personality assessment. Given the percentage of patients with EVB who have Axis II disorders (23%) or abnormalities on neuropsychological testing (58%), a finding that all 17 patients would meet DSM-III-R criteria for IED seems unlikely.

Authors usually diagnose IED when EVB occurs and do not use any other diagnostic criteria. Some authors use their own criteria for studies of violent patients or prefer to use the EDC (Menninger 1963) diagnosis and criteria. The variation in diagnostic criteria may be partially due to the many revisions in

Table 46–2. Historical perspective: the diagnosis of episodic violent behavior

Year	Method	Diagnosis
1952	First DSM	Passive-aggressive personality, aggressive type
1955	ICD-7	Immature personality, aggressiveness subtype
1956	Menninger 1963	Episodic dyscontrol
1960	Menninger 1963	Dyscontrol: chronic, repetitive; episodic, impulsive; disorganized, episodic
1968	DSM-II	Explosive personality
1970	Monroe 1970	Episodic behavioral disorders
1970	Mark and Erwin 1970	Dyscontrol syndrome
1977	ICD-9	Explosive personality exclude: dyssocial, hysterical
1979	ICD-9-CM	Intermittent explosive disorder: recurrent, significant; not due to any other mental disorder; disproportionate to stressor; regret, self-reproach (remorse)
1980	DSM-III	Intermittent explosive disorder: several, discrete, serious; disproportionate to stressor; no other impulsivity, aggression Exclude: schizophrenia, antisocial personality disorder, conduct disorder Isolated explosive disorder
1987	DSM-III-R	Intermittent explosive disorder: several, discrete, serious; disproportionate to stressor; no other impulsivity, aggression Exclude: psychosis, organic personality syndrome, antisocial or borderline personality disorder, conduct disorder, intoxication Organic personality syndrome, explosive type: recurrent, disproportionate; specific organic factors, etiologically related; no attention-deficit/hyperactivity disorder in child, adolescent; no delirium, dementia

classification of EVB since the first DSM (Table 46–2).

To date, the reports of Mattes (1990) and Felthous et al. (1991) are the most thorough and most comprehensive. We refer readers to these articles with the caveat that both reports are incomplete. This is also true of the review that we performed. Additional factors that could have been considered, but were not, include age at onset, suicidality, history of birth trauma, mental retardation, amnesia during violence, pattern of onset/remission, and social impairment. Family history of violence could also include specifically witnessing domestic violence and physical abuse.

Recommendations

Ideally, future individual case reports of patients with EVB would include data on all features listed in Table 46–1, as well as factors omitted in this review that were mentioned previously as important for research in this area.

Aspects of DSM-III-R criteria for IED that require further clarification are

1. The requirement that there are no signs of generalized impulsiveness or aggressiveness between violent episodes (criterion C). This criterion is not required by ICD-9-CM. Its inclusion in DSM-III-R may have been another attempt to eliminate Axis II character pathology from the IED group.
2. The requirement for "several discrete episodes" of violence (criterion A) does not establish a threshold for IED (e.g., several each day versus several each month). Guidelines similar to those for panic disorder might be considered, although data to establish this criterion are lacking.
3. Should the time between the provocation and the loss of control be limited? This question was raised by Felthous et al. (1991).

As a result of this review, several options are under consideration for DSM-IV:

1. Retain IED, without modification, in DSM-IV. This would stabilize the diagnostic criteria (which have changed significantly in every previous DSM). This would allow clinicians to become better aware of IED's diagnostic criteria and to perform research using these criteria.
2. Eliminate IED as a disorder, and list it as an example of an impulse disorder not otherwise specified. This would allow clinicians to diagnose IED using only the occurrence of EVB and no other diagnostic criteria, which is what they did in 75% of the cases reviewed. This would mean no criteria would exist for research or reporting purposes and that the diagnoses of IED would become equivalent to reporting the occurrence of EVB.

From this literature survey, we conclude that EVB is a relatively common clinical symptom that is associated with a wide variety of organic and psychiatric disorders. EVB is usually found in patients with CNS dysfunction. If DSM-III-R's IED exists as a distinct diagnostic disorder, like pyromania and kleptomania, it appears to be a rare entity.

Kleptomania

Method

A detailed comprehensive literature review of kleptomania was completed. This initially covered the period from 1966 until 1989; a further review was completed in January 1991. Literature before 1966 was selectively reviewed. A number of case reports were reviewed but were not reported in detail because they were anecdotal. There was not a consistent method of documenting phenomenology and the diagnostic criteria for kleptomania as opposed to shoplifting per se (Chiswick 1976; Coid 1984; Cunningham 1975; Davis 1979; Fishbain 1987; Singer 1978).

Results

There are a number of studies of shoplifters that provide the empirical basis for what we know about kleptomania (Table 46–3). To summarize, shoplifting is common and is associated with significant psychiatric morbidity. Kleptomania is rare among shoplifters and is found in fewer than 5% of admitted shoplifters. Several studies fail to report the incidence of kleptomania among shoplifters. Kleptomania has a significant association with major mood, anxiety, and eating disorders (Gibbens et al. 1971; McElroy et al. 1989, 1991a, 1991b).

Discussion and Recommendations

There is a lack of systematic research on kleptomania; therefore, it is recommended that the DSM-III-R diagnostic criteria be retained. The committee did consider minor changes to the criteria and in the end rejected them. Until additional studies are completed, the validity of the existing criteria is assumed to be appropriate. Future research on kleptomania should concentrate on clinical characteristics, associated conditions (e.g., obsessive-compulsive disorder and mood and eating disorders), and the effectiveness of a variety of treatment options including the response to selective serotonin reuptake inhibitors.

Pyromania

Method

The English-language literature, including psychiatric, medical, and arson literatures for the period 1980–1990, was reviewed. The psychiatric literature review included works on adult and child firesetting. Where relevant, literature predating 1980 was consulted.

Results

An examination of the English-language psychiatric literature on adult firesetters, in which each paper reported on at least five cases (Table 46–4), indicates that the diagnosis of pyromania is rarely made when DSM-III or DSM-III-R criteria have been applied. The arson literature applies the diagnosis of pyromania much more readily (Pisani 1982; Witkin-Lanloil 1981). In the latter literature, however, it is not

Table 46–3.　Frequency of kleptomania among shoplifters

Study	N	Clinical features
Arieff and Bowie 1947	338	93% female; 70% some psychiatric disorder; sample was 1.8% of total group of shoplifters arrested during the period of study; kleptomania only in 3.8% of total sample
Gibbens and Prince 1962	776	69% female; depression common; higher-than-average psychiatric hospital admission; 0% kleptomania
Ordway 1962	85	43% depressed (first DSM) unknown percentage kleptomania
Cameron 1964	873	Only females in study; 1.4% depressed; <1% kleptomania
Medlicott 1968	50	52% female; 28% depressed, all female; all had some psychiatric disorder; 8% kleptomania
Gillen 1976	48	100% female; 100% psychiatric disorder; <5% kleptomania
Bradford and Balmaceda 1983	50	62% female; 42% depressed; 4% kleptomania
Cupchik and Atcheson 1983	24	71% female; unknown percentage kleptomania
Silverman and Brener 1988	34	100% female; unknown percentage kleptomania; shoplifters were compared with agoraphobic, depressive patients; shoplifters had high levels of psychosocial stress (e.g., marital discord)

Table 46–4. English-language literature on pathological firesetting in adults, 1980–1990

Study	Source	N	Sex M	Sex F	Age (mean or range)	Pyromania	Schizophrenia	Affective Disorder	Personality Disorders	Alcohol	MR	Other
Bradford 1982	University forensic service	34	26	8	30.3	0	2	0	18	3	5	OBS (4), paranoia (1), neurosis (7), sexual deviation (2), adjustment disorder (4). One individual with features of pyromania
Hill et al. 1982	University forensic service	38	38	0	26	0	8	0	25	6	7	Sexual deviation (1)
Koson et al. 1982	Maximum security state hospital	26	26	0	17–56	0	6	2	5	6	5	Substance abuse (1), no disorder (1)
Pascoe 1983	Court	45	34	11	18% over 30	0	0	0	0	0	0	Psychotic (15)
Yesavage et al. 1983	Court	27	26	1	24	0	5	0	2	0	11	Anxiety disorder (4), OBS (2), epilepsy (1), sexual perversion (1), no diagnosis (1)
Geller 1984	State hospital	13	6	7	18–63	0	6	2	2	0	3	
Harris and Rice 1984	Maximum security state hospital	13	13	0	28.9	0	10	0	2	0	2	OBS (1)
Molnar et al. 1984	Arrest records	217	189	28	27.33	0	0	0	0	0	0	Psychotic (22), history of substance abuse (114)

(continued)

Table 46–4. English language literature on pathological firesetting in adults, 1980–1990 (*continued*)

Study	Source	N	Sex M	Sex F	Age (mean or Range)	Pyro-mania	Schizo-phrenia	Affective Disorder	Person-ality Disorders	Alcohol	MR	Other
Taylor and Gunn 1984	Prison	28	28	0	?	0	9	0	0	0	0	Mixed psychiatric disorder (9), no disorder (10)
Virkkunen 1984	University hospital	59	59	0	30.1	15	0	0	32	0	0	Intermittent explosive disorder (22)
Zeegers 1984	University hospital	17	16	1	17–75	0	0	0	2	0	7	Neurosis (8)
Geller and Bertsch 1985	State hospital	35	22	13	21–60	0	18	5	5	2	3	Schizoaffective disorder (2)
Harmon et al. 1985	Court	27	0	27	17–62	0	7	1	9	0	0	Substance abuse (3), psychotic (1), paranoid disorder (1), impulse disorder (1), adjustment disorder (1), no diagnosis (3). States no woman met DSM-III criteria for pyromania
Prins et al. 1985	Parole	113	113	0	?	0	0	0	0	0	0	"26 acted at least in part as a result of emotional or intellectual difficulties"
Virkkunen 1985	University hospital	10	10	0	27.3	10	0	0	0	0	0	Anxiety disorder (4), adjustment disorder (2), conduct disorder (3)
Bradford and Dimock 1986	University forensic service	59	48	11	28.3	0	6	5	17	16	6	

Study	Setting											
Jacobson et al. 1986	University hospital	12	5	7	23.6	0	4	3	5	0	0	All cases are of self-incineration
Prins 1986, 1987	Unknown	8	7	1	16–50	0	0	0	1	0	4	No diagnosis (3)
Roy et al. 1986; Virkkunen et al. 1987, 1989a, 1989b; Linnoila et al. 1989	University forensic service prison	22	22	0	19–44	0	0	21	20	20	0	Intermittent explosive disorder (15)
Geller 1987	State	6	3	3	24–57	0	2	1	1	1	1	
Jackson et al. 1987	Maximum security hospital	18	18	0	26.8	0	0	0	12	0	2	MR and personality disorder (4)
O'Sullivan and Kelleher 1987	Psychiatric hospitals jails	54	41	13	15–46+	0	21	4	16	4	4	No disorder (5). Two individuals had some features of pyromania
Rodenhauser and Khamis 1988	Maximum security forensic hospital	34	34	0	?	0	0	0	26	0	0	Psychotic (21)
Quinsey et al. 1989	Maximum security hospital	26	26	0	28.15	0	0	0	18	0	0	Psychotic (8)
Rice and Harris 1990	Maximum security hospital	243	243	0	28.7	0	74	0	122	0	0	Undiagnosed (47)

Note. OBS = organic brain syndrome. MR = mental retardation.

clear that DSM-III or DSM-III-R criteria have been used.

The child psychiatric literature also reveal few cases of pyromania (Heath et al. 1985; Jacobson 1985a, 1985b; Kazdin and Kolko 1986; Kolko and Kazdin 1989; Kolko et al. 1985; Kuhnley et al. 1982; Showers and Pickrell 1987; Stewart and Culver 1982; Strachan 1981). As found in the adult literature, most of the firesetters are male. Most of the cases are diagnosed as having conduct disorder, attention-deficit/hyperactivity disorder, or adjustment disorders. In only one study was the diagnosis of pyromania applied to any childhood firesetters. Heath et al. (1985) found that 2 of 32 firesetters (6.25%) from a sample of 204 child psychiatric outpatients met the criteria for pyromania. The consistent observation that most children with firesetting histories have multiple, significant problems may partially explain the infrequency with which pyromania is diagnosed in children. The arson literature, on the other hand, uses the diagnosis of pyromania in children with much greater frequency than the psychiatric literature (Mercilliott 1983; Wooden and Berkey 1984).

Discussion and Recommendations

There is little in the literature that argues for changing the DSM-III-R diagnostic criteria for pyromania, with one minor exception. Criterion E, which lists exclusion criteria, does not include mania. There are reports in the psychiatric literature (Geller 1984; Gunderson 1974), commentary in the arson literature (O'Connor 1987), and clinical experiences that indicate that firesetting can occur as a component of a manic episode. Hence, it is recommended that a manic episode be included in criterion E.

Future research needs to focus on 1) increasing the effective use of DSM criteria by those in the arson investigation field to determine whether rates of pyromania are truly different in the populations observed in psychiatric and arson studies or whether that difference is due to the application of alternative criteria, 2) understanding what accounts for the marked frequency of firesetting in persons with serious and persistent mental illness, 3) joint research by investigators who have focused on child and adult firesetters because these have historically been distinct enterprises, 4) follow-up studies of child and adolescent firesetters to determine which, if any, become adults who are best diagnosed as having pyromania.

Pathological Gambling

Method

Three different methodological procedures were used in investigating pathological gambling. First, all published material that was available to the authors was reviewed. This included systematic searches of *Index Medicus, Science Citation and Social Science Citation Index, Psychological Abstracts,* and papers presented at international conferences on gambling and risk taking, as well as conferences of the National Council on Problem Gambling.

Second, members of the National Council on Problem Gambling (NCPG) who attended its annual conference in Iowa in 1989 were invited to participate in the construction of a questionnaire to examine the diagnostic criteria for pathological gambling. The questionnaire included DSM-III, DSM-III-R, and other suggested criteria. Questions were asked in different ways to see which wording would best discriminate between pathological gamblers and control subjects. The questionnaire was pretested by members of the NCPG and revised.

Treatment professionals in eight states then distributed questionnaires to their patients and to Gamblers Anonymous members. Participating in the study were 221 (164 male) pathological gamblers and 54 (30 male) substance-dependent control subjects (control subjects were "social gamblers"; none gambled rarely or never). The majority of the subjects were from Nevada, California, and New Jersey, and the rest were from Iowa, Montana, New York, Ohio, and Virginia.

After the survey data were analyzed, the resulting criteria, along with the preliminary descriptive text, were presented at the 8th International Conference on Risk and Gambling in London in August 1990. As at the Iowa conference, individuals in the audience were asked for both verbal and written comments on the criteria. These people included experts on pathological gambling from the United States, the Netherlands, Germany, Spain, the United Kingdom, Australia, New Zealand, Canada, and other countries.

Results and Discussion

The results of the survey were subject to item analysis to determine which items discriminated between self-described compulsive gamblers and control subjects. In addition, the data for males and females were examined independently. The status of the DSM-III-R criteria was as follows: Item 1 was maintained but reworded to better discriminate between social and pathological gamblers. The reworded form was chosen by none of the control subjects and 94% of self-identified pathological gamblers. Item 2 of DSM-III-R was chosen by 20% of the control subjects. Gambling longer than intended seems to be fairly common. Because other items discriminated better, this criterion was dropped. Item 3 was retained but reworded. This item was chosen by 8% of the control subjects and 89% of self-identified pathological gamblers. Items 4 and 6 were combined. These items were highly collinear. Item 5 was retained but reworded to better discriminate. This was chosen by 10% of control subjects and 98% of self-identified pathological gamblers. Items

7, 8, and 9 were reformulated as a result of extensive critiques and suggestions by therapists to use the DSM-III wording.

A new set of criteria emerged that represented a compromise between DSM-III and DSM-III-R. With the exception of item 7 (illegal acts), each item was selected by at least 83% of self-identified compulsive gamblers. None of the new items was selected by more than 10% of the substance-dependent control subjects. These criteria represent a combination of DSM-III (criteria 6–9) and DSM-III-R (criteria 1–3 and 5) and the addition of "escape" (criterion 4), which has recently been recognized as important for compulsive gamblers, slot and poker machine players in particular (Lesieur and Blume 1991). "Dimensions" for each of the criteria are 1) progression and preoccupation, 2) tolerance, 3) withdrawal and loss of control, 4) escape, 5) chasing, 6) lies/deception, 7) illegal acts, 8) family/job disruption, and 9) financial bailout. The proposed wording seems to answer the critiques of DSM-III-R. These items and their frequency of occurrence were used as discriminator variables in Table 46–5.

A cutoff point of four or more items was created based on the sample used for the generation of the findings. The results along with the cutoff point are included in Table 46–6.

The resulting set of criteria was then sent to treatment professionals who were asked to conduct field trials. Approximately 30 clinicians have responded in writing. Although the comments have been overwhelmingly favorable, a number of specific suggestions have been made. Each of them was given serious consideration, and many have been incorporated. When they have not, it has been because of lack of supporting data, because other items discriminated better, or because they would have weakened the comprehensibility of the existing criteria. However, some minor changes were incorporated in the criteria. Further changes suggested by the DSM-IV Task Force were also examined, and some were accepted. The revised proposed criteria are listed below:

Maladaptive gambling behavior as indicated by at least four of the following:

1. Preoccupied with gambling (e.g., preoccupied with reliving past gambling experiences, handicapping or planning the next venture, or thinking of ways to get money with which to gamble)
2. Needs to gamble with significantly increasing amounts of money to achieve the desired excitement
3. Restless or irritable when attempting to cut down or stop gambling
4. Gambles as a way of escaping from problems or relieving dysphoric mood (e.g., feelings of helplessness, guilt, anxiety, depression)
5. After losing money gambling, often returns another day to get even ("chasing" one's losses)

Table 46–5. Proposed DSM-IV criteria cross-tabulated by three different indicators of pathological gambling in a sample of compulsive gamblers and substance abusers

Proposed DSM-IV criterion	Self-identification A			Self-identification B		Ever have gambling treatment?	
	Social (%)	Problem gambler (%)	Compulsive gambler (%)	No problem (%)	Compulsive (or problem) gambler (%)	No (%)	Yes (%)
1. Preoccupation	3.1	42.8	97.4	9.1	96.5	12.0	93.7
2. Tolerance	12.5	71.4	89.2	14.9	89.7	20.3	87.4
3. Withdrawal	8.3	57.1	89.7	9.8	91.1	13.7	88.3
4. Escape problems	4.1	42.9	90.7	6.1	91.1	11.8	87.8
5. Chase losses	14.4	78.6	98.5	18.4	98.0	24.4	95.7
6. Lies/deception	3.1	78.6	94.8	8.0	94.1	12.8	91.7
7. Illegal acts	1.0	35.7	67.2	3.5	68.1	7.6	65.7
8. Family/job	3.1	38.5	90.2	4.4	90.6	6.0	88.9
9. Financial bailout	2.2	64.3	88.1	8.3	86.2	12.4	84.5
10. Loss of control	7.2	42.9	82.0	12.3	80.9	15.3	78.7

Note. *Self-identification A*—Do you believe that you are a social gambler, professional gambler, or compulsive gambler? Answer categories included social gambler, problem gambler, compulsive gambler, professional gambler, or other (specify)—results for first three only.
Self-identification B—Do you believe that you are (or were) a compulsive gambler (or have a gambling problem)? Answer categories: yes, no.
Ever have gambling treatment?—Yes = positive answer to either of the following: Have you ever been to Gamblers Anonymous for help with a gambling problem? or Have you ever been to a therapist for help with a gambling problem?

Table 46–6. Proposed DSM-IV criteria cross-tabulated by three different indicators of pathological gambling in a sample of compulsive gamblers and substance abusers

Score on DSM-IV	Self-identification A			Self-identification B		Ever have gambling treatment?	
	Social (%)	Problem gambler (%)	Compulsive gambler (%)	No problem (%)	Compulsive (or problem) gambler (%)	No (%)	Yes (%)
0	74	7	0	71	0	66	2
1	12	7	0.5	10	0.5	11	0.5
2	8	0	0	7	0	6	0.5
3	2	0	1.5	3	0.5	3	0.5
Cutoff point							
4	1	29	1	3.5	1.5	4	1
5	1	21	1.5	2	3	3	3
6	0	7	7	2	6	1	7
7	1	7	14	1	15	2	14
8	0	7	25	0	24	0	24
9	0	14	49	0	50	3	47
Total (%)	99	99	99.5	99.5	100.5	99	99.5
N	97	14	195	114	204	119	207

Note. Self-identification A—Do you believe that you are a social gambler, pathological gambler, or compulsive gambler? Answer categories included social gambler, problem gambler, compulsive gambler, professional gambler, or other (specify)—results for first three only.
Self-identification B—Do you believe that you are (or were) a compulsive gambler (or have a gambling problem)? Answer categories: yes, no.
Ever have gambling treatment?—Yes = positive answer to either of the following: Have you ever been to Gambler's Anonymous for help with a gambling problem? or Have you ever been to a therapist for help with a gambling problem?
Correlation with self-identification B. $r = .92$ ($P < .001$).
Correlation with self-identification B. $r = .85$ ($P < .001$).
Pearson correlations with self-identification A not statistically appropriate. However, they are highly associated, as can be observed from the table.

6. Lies to family members or others to conceal the extent of involvement with gambling
7. Illegal acts (e.g., forgery, fraud, theft, or embezzlement) are committed to finance gambling
8. Has jeopardized or lost a significant relationship, job, educational, or career opportunity because of gambling
9. Reliance on others (or institutions) to provide money to relieve a desperate financial situation caused by gambling

Comparisons between pathological gambling and psychoactive substance dependence have been made. Although money is important to the pathological gambler, most will say that they are seeking "action," an aroused, euphoric state comparable to the high derived from cocaine or other drugs (Anderson and Brown 1987; Blaszczynski et al. 1986; Brown 1987; Dickerson 1979; Lesieur 1984). The desire to remain in action is so intense that many gamblers will go for days without sleep, without eating, and even without going to the bathroom. Some describe a rush, characterized by sweaty palms, rapid heartbeat, and nausea, that is also experienced during a period of anticipation.

A review of the literature has made it clear that a number of issues have been laid to rest. Progression and preoccupation (Custer 1982; Lesieur and Custer 1984; Walker 1989) and loss of control and disregard for consequences (Lesieur and Rosenthal 1991) clearly exist among pathological gamblers in ways that approximate the same conditions among psychoactive substance-dependent individuals.

Features that appear in the literature but on which further research is needed include tolerance and withdrawal. Tolerance has been discussed particularly with regard to racetrack, sports, and casino betters (Custer and Milt 1985; Lesieur 1984) because gamblers state that they could not get excited by small bets once they were making large wagers. Further investigation is needed relative to slot and poker machine gambling. Self-reported withdrawal symptoms (both psychological and psychosomatic) have been the subject of several studies (Meyer 1989; Wray and Dickerson 1981), and the survey conducted for DSM-IV provided further support for the existence of withdrawal symptoms (Rosenthal and Lesieur 1992).

In addition to the above phenomena, trance-like or dissociative states and blackouts among pathological gamblers are well described by clinicians and have been the subject of some research (Browne 1989; Jacobs 1988; Kuley and Jacobs 1988). However, the exact nature of these phenomena need further investigation.

As the literature review and survey demonstrate, features resembling those described for psychoactive substance dependence have been documented for pathological gambling. These traits, when combined, effectively discriminate between pathological gamblers and control subjects.

One problem remains with the diagnostic criteria as proposed. The old "loss of control" criterion (item 4) in DSM-III-R was tested in the survey and was found to be highly correlated with other items and was removed. However, several clinicians from the United States, Austria, and Germany desired to reinsert loss of control as a diagnostic criterion. The wording they suggested puts more emphasis on the repeated unsuccessful attempts to control gambling. It would read as follows: "10. Made repeated unsuccessful attempts to control, cut back, or stop gambling."

This represents an improvement on the DSM-III-R wording. We believe that if field trials were made including this new wording, clinicians would favor its inclusion. Item analysis for a slightly different version of loss of control is included in Tables 46–5 and 46–7. The arguments for inclusion are strong. Loss of control is a theoretically significant element of behavioral dependence on gambling and is recounted in numerous articles (Browne 1989; Dickerson et al. 1990; Griffiths 1990) as central to the phenomenon.

Recommendations

Additional field trials will be conducted to test the proposed criteria and to examine criterion 10 (loss of control) for possible inclusion and see how it would affect the cutoff point. Clinicians should address the potential benefits and drawbacks of this inclusion.

Research into common features between pathological gambling and psychoac-

Table 46–7.   Item analysis of DSM–IV criteria

| | DSM–IV classification | | | |
| | Not a pathological gambler | | Pathological gambler | |
DSM–IV criterion	n yes/N^a	%	n yes/N^a	%
1. Preoccupation	0/103	0.0	206/219	94.1
2. Tolerance	8/103	7.8	197/222	88.7
3. Withdrawal	6/102	5.9	192/221	86.9
4. Escape problems	2/104	1.9	192/220	87.3
5. Chase losses	10/104	9.6	217/222	97.1
6. Lies/deception	2/103	1.9	202/220	91.8
7. Illegal acts	0/104	0.0	145/222	65.3
8. Family/job	1/103	1.0	190/220	86.4
9. Financial bailout	1/99	1.0	187/220	85.0
10. Loss of control	8/104	7.7	173/221	78.3

[a]The numerical base varies for each question because not all respondents answered all questions.

tive substance dependence points to many similarities. It is suggested that this be more clearly recognized in DSM-IV. Further study should be encouraged to examine points of divergence as well as similarities. Areas for further research include the nature of the rush, cravings, blackouts and dissociative states, and withdrawal phenomena.

References

Abt V, Smith JF, Christiansen EM: The Business of Risk. Lawrence, KS, University of Kansas, 1985

American Psychiatric Association: Diagnostic and Statistical Manual: Mental Disorders. Washington, DC, American Psychiatric Association, 1952

American Psychiatric Association: Diagnostic and Statistical Manual of Mental Disorders, 2nd Edition. Washington, DC, American Psychiatric Association, 1968

American Psychiatric Association: Diagnostic and Statistical Manual of Mental Disorders, 3rd Edition. Washington, DC, American Psychiatric Association, 1980

American Psychiatric Association: Diagnostic and Statistical Manual of Mental Disorders, 3rd Edition, Revised. Washington, DC, American Psychiatric Association, 1987

Anderson G, Brown RIF: Some applications of reversal theory to the explanation of gambling and gambling addictions. Journal of Gambling Behavior 3:179–189, 1987

Arieff AJ, Bowie CG: Some psychiatric aspects of shoplifting. Journal of Clinical Psychopathology 8:565, 1947

Blaszczynski AP, Winter SW, McConaghy N: Plasma endorphin levels in pathological gambling. Journal of Gambling Behavior 2:3–14, 1986

Bradford JMW: Arson: a clinical study. Can J Psychiatry 27:188–193, 1982

Bradford JMW, Balmaceda R: Shoplifting: is there a specific psychiatric syndrome? Can J Psychiatry 28:248–254, 1983

Bradford J, Dimock J: A comparative study of adolescents and adults who willfully set fires. Psychiatr J Univ Ottawa 11:228–234, 1986

Brown RIF: Models of gambling and gambling addiction as perceptual filters. Journal of Gambling Behavior 3:224–236, 1987

Browne BR: Going on tilt: frequent poker players and control. Journal of Gambling Behavior 5:3–21, 1989

Cameron MB: Department Store Shoplifting: The Booster and the Snitch. New York, Free Press, 1964

Chiswick D: Shoplifting, depression and an unusual intracranial lesion. Med Sci Law 16:266–268, 1976

Ciarrocchi J, Richardson R: Profile of compulsive gamblers in treatment: update and comparison. Journal of Gambling Behavior 5:53–65, 1989

Coid J: Relief of diazepam-withdrawal syndrome by shoplifting. Br J Psychiatry 145:552–554, 1984

Cunningham C: Absent mind versus guilty mind in cases of shoplifting. Med Leg J 43:101–106, 1975

Cupchik W, Atcheson JD: Shoplifting: an occasional crime of the moral majority. Bull Am Acad Psychiatry Law 11:343–354, 1983

Custer RL: An overview of compulsive gambling, in Addictive Disorders Update. Edited by Carone PA, Yolles SF, Kieffer SN, et al. New York, Human Sciences Press, 1982, pp 107–124

Custer RL, Custer LF: Characteristics of the recovering compulsive gambler: a survey of 150 members of Gamblers Anonymous. Paper presented at the 4th Annual Conference on Gambling, Reno, NV, December 1978

Custer RL, Milt H: When Luck Runs Out. New York, Facts on File Publications, 1985

Davis H: Psychiatric aspects of shoplifting. South African Medical Journal 43:101–106, 1979

Dickerson MG: FI schedules and persistence at gambling in the UK betting office. J Appl Behav Anal 12:315–323, 1979

Dickerson M, Walker M, England SL, et al: Demographic, personality, cognitive and behavioral correlates of off-course betting involvement. Journal of Gambling Studies 6:165–182, 1990

Felthous AR, Bryant SG, Wingerter CB, et al: The diagnosis of intermittent explosive disorder in violent men. Bull Am Acad Psychiatry Law 19:71–79, 1991

Fishbain DA: Kleptomania as risk taking behaviour in response to depression. Am J Psychother 41:598–603, 1987

Geller J: Arson: an unforeseen sequela of deinstitutionalization. Am J Psychiatry 141:504–508, 1984

Geller JL, Bertsch G: Fire-setting behavior in the histories of a state hospital population. Am J Psychiatry 142:464–468, 1985

Gibbens TCN: Shoplifting. Br J Psychiatry 138:346–347, 1981

Gibbens TCN, Prince J: Shoplifting. London, The Institute for the Study and Treatment of Delinquency, 1962

Gibbens TCN, Palmer C, Prince J: Mental health aspects of shoplifting. BMJ 3:612–615, 1971

Gillen RS: A study of woman shoplifters. South Australian Clinics 11:173–176, 1976

Griffiths MD: The acquisition, development, and maintenance of fruit machine gambling in adolescents. Journal of Gambling Studies 6:193–204, 1990

Gunderson JG: Management of manic states: the problem of fire-setting. Psychiatry 37:137–146, 1974

Harmon RB, Rosner R, Wiederlight M: Women and arson: a demographic study. J Forensic Sci 30:467–477, 1985

Harris GT, Rice ME: Mentally disordered firesetters: psychodynamic versus empirical approaches. Int J Law Psychiatry 7:19–34, 1984

Heath GA, Hardesty VA, Goldfine PE, et al: Diagnosis and childhood firesetting. J Clin Psychol 41:571–575, 1985

Hill W, Langevin R, Paitich D, et al: Is arson an aggressive act or a property offence? a controlled study of psychiatric referrals. Can J Psychiatry 27:648–654, 1982

Jackson HF, Hoe S, Glass C: Why are arsonists not violent offenders? International Journal of Offender Therapeutics and Criminology 31:143–151, 1987

Jacobs DF: Evidence for a common dissociative-like reaction among addicts. Journal of Gambling Behavior 4:27–37, 1988

Jacobson RR: Child firesetters: a clinical investigation. J Child Psychol Psychiatry 26:759–768, 1985a

Jacobson RR: The subclassification of child firesetters. J Child Psychol Psychiatry 26:769–775, 1985b

Jacobson R, Jackson M, Berelowitz M: Self-incineration: a controlled comparison of inpatient suicide attempts: clinical features and history of self-harm. Psychol Med 16:107–116, 1986

Kahn K, Martin JCA: Kleptomania as a presenting feature of cortical atrophy. Acta Psychiatr Scand 56:168–172, 1977

Kazdin AE, Kolko DJ: Parent psychopathology and family functioning among childhood firesetters. J Abnorm Child Psychol 14:315–329, 1986

Kolko DJ, Kazdin AE: The children's firesetting interview with psychiatrically referred and nonreferred children. J Abnorm Child Psychol 17:609–624, 1989

Kolko DJ, Kazdin AE, Meyer EC: Aggression and psychopathology in childhood firesetters: parent and child reports. J Consult Clin Psychol 53:377–385, 1985

Koson DF, Dvoskin J: Arson: a diagnostic study. Bull Am Acad Psychiatry Law 10:39–49, 1982

Kuhnley EJ, Hendren RL, Quinlan DM: Firesetting by children. Journal of the American Academy of Child Psychiatry 2:560–563, 1982

Kuley NB, Jacobs DF: The relationship between dissociative-like experiences and sensation seeking among social and problem gamblers. Journal of Gambling Behavior 4:197–207, 1988

Lesieur HR: The Chase: Career of the Compulsive Gambler. Cambridge, MA, Schenkman Books, 1984

Lesieur HR: Gambling, pathological gambling and crime, in Handbook on Pathological Gambling. Edited by Galski T. Springfield, IL, Charles C Thomas, 1987, pp 87–110

Lesieur HR: Altering the DSM-III criteria for pathological gambling. Journal of Gambling Behavior 4:38–47, 1988a

Lesieur HR: Report on pathological gambling in New Jersey, in Report and Recommendations of the Governor's Advisory Commission on Gambling. Trenton, NJ, Governor's Advisory Commission on Gambling, 1988b, pp 103–165

Lesieur HR, Blume SB: When lady luck loses: the female pathological gambler, in Feminist Perspectives on Treating Addictions. Edited by van den Bergh N. New York, Springer, 1991, pp 181–197

Lesieur HR, Custer RL: Pathological gambling: roots, phases, and treatment. Annals of the American Academy of Political and Social Sciences 474:146–156, 1984

Lesieur HR, Rosenthal RJ: Pathological gambling: a review of the literature (prepared for the American Psychiatric Association Task Force on DSM-IV Committee on Disorders of Impulse Control Not Elsewhere Classified). Journal of Gambling Studies 7:5–40, 1991

Linnoila M, DeJong J, Virkkunen M: Family history of alcoholism in violent offenders and impulsive firesetters. Arch Gen Psychiatry 46:613–616, 1989

Mark V, Erwin F: Violence and the Brain. New York, Harper & Row, 1970

Mattes JA: Comparative effectiveness of carbamazepine and propranolol for rage outbursts. Journal of Neuropsychiatry 2:159–164, 1990

McElroy SL, Keck PE, Pope HG, et al: Pharmacological treatment of kleptomania and bulimia nervosa. J Clin Psychopharmacol 9:358–360, 1989

McElroy, SL, Hudson, JI, Pope HG, et al: Kleptomania: clinical characteristics and associated psychopathology. Psychol Med 21:93–108, 1991a

McElroy Sl, Pope HG, Hudson JI, et al: Kleptomania: a report of 20 cases. Am J Psychiatry 148:652–657, 1991b

Medlicott RW: Fifty thieves. N Z Med J 67:183–188, 1968

Menninger K: The Vital Balance. New York, Viking, 1963

Mercilliott F: Juvenile fire setters. Fire and Arson Investigator 34:3–12, 1983

Meyer G: Gluckspieler in Selbsthilfegruppen: Erste Ergebnisse einer Empirischen Unter-suchung. Hamburg, Germany, Neuland, 1989

Meyers TJ: A contribution to the psychopathology of shoplifting. J Forensic Sci 13:295–310, 1970

Molnar G, Keitner L, Harwood BT: A comparison of partner and solo arsonists. J Forensic Sci 29:574–583, 1984

Money J: Medicoscientific nonjudgementalism incompatible with legal judgementalism: a model case report: kleptomania. Med Law 2:361–375, 1983

Monroe RR: Episodic Behavior Disorder. Cambridge, MA, Harvard University Press, 1970

Nora R: Profile survey on pathological gamblers. Paper presented at the 6th National Conference on Gambling and Risk Taking, Atlantic City, NJ, December 1984

O'Connor JJ: Practical Fire and Arson Investigation. New York, Elsevier, 1987

O'Sullivan GH, Kelleher MJ: A study of firesetters in the southwest of Ireland. Br J Psychiatry 151:818–823, 1987

Ordway JA: "Successful" court treatment of shoplifters. Journal of Criminal Law, Criminol-ogy and Political Science 53:344–347, 1962

Pascoe H: Edmonton's arson epidemic: February 1980. Med Law 2:173–180, 1983

Pisani AL Jr: Identifying arson motives. Fire and Arson Investigator 32:18–30, 1982

Prins H: Dangerous Behavior, the Law, and Mental Disorder. London, Tavistock, 1986

Prins H: Up in smoke—the psychology of arson. Med Leg J 55:69–84, 1987

Prins H, Tennet G, Trick K: Motives for arson (fire raising). Med Sci Law 25:275–278, 1985

Quinsey VL, Chaplin TC, Upfold O: Arsonists and sexual arousal to fire setting: correlation unsupported. J Behav Ther Exp Psychiatry 20:203–209, 1989

Rawlins V: Antishoplifting Manual. Canadian Police College. Department of the Solicitor General, Ottawa, Canada, 1978

Rice ME, Harris GT: Firesetters admitted to a maximum security psychiatric institution: characteristics of offenders and offenses. Penetanguishene Mental Health Centre Re-search Report 7:1–27, 1990

Rodenhauser P, Khamis HJ: Relationships between legal and clinical factors among forensic hospital patients. Bull Am Acad Psychiatry Law 16:321–332, 1988

Rosenthal RJ: Pathological gambling and problem gambling: problems in definition and diagnosis, in Compulsive Gambling: Theory, Research and Practice. Edited by Shaffer H, Stein SA, Gambino B, et al. Lexington, MA, Lexington Books, 1989, pp 101–125

Rosenthal RJ, Lesieur HR: Self-reported withdrawal symptoms and pathological gambling. American Journal on Addictions 1:150–154, 1992

Roy A, Virkkunen M, Guthrie S, et al: Indices of serotonin and glucose metabolism in violent offenders, arsonists and alcoholics. Ann NY Acad Sci 487:202–220, 1986

Showers J, Pickrell E: Child firesetters: a study of three populations. Hosp Community Psychiatry 38:495–501, 1987

Silverman G, Brener N: Psychiatric profile of shoplifters (letter). Lancet 2:157, 1988

Singer BA: A case of kleptomania. Bull Am Acad Psychiatry Law 6:414–422, 1978

Sommers I: Pathological gambling: estimating prevalence and group characteristics. Int J Addict 23:477–490, 1988

Stewart MA, Culver KW: Children who set fires: the clinical picture and a follow-up. Br J Psychiatry 140:357–363, 1982

Strachan JG: Conspicuous firesetting in children. Br J Psychiatry 138:26–29, 1981

Taylor PJ, Gunn J: Violence and psychosis. BMJ 288:1945–1949, 1984

US Department of Health and Human Services: The International Classification of Diseases, 9th Revision, Clinical Modification. Washington, DC, US Department of Health and Human Services, 1979

Virkkunen M: Reactive hypoglycemic tendency among arsonists. Acta Psychiatr Scand 69:445–452, 1984

Virkkunen M: Urinary free cortisol secretion in habitually violent offenders. Acta Psychiatr Scand 72:40–44, 1985

Virkkunen M, Nuutila A, Goodwin FK, et al: Cerebrospinal fluid monoamine metabolite levels in male arsonists. Arch Gen Psychiatry 44:241–247, 1987

Virkkunen M, DeJong J, Linnoila M: Psychobiological concomitants of history of suicide attempts among violent offenders and impulsive firesetters. Arch Gen Psychiatry 46:604–606, 1989a

Virkkunen M, DeJong J, Bartko J, et al: Relationships of psychological variables to recidivism in violent offenders and impulsive firesetters. Arch Gen Psychiatry 46:600–603, 1989b

Volberg RA, Steadman HJ: Refining prevalence estimates of pathological gambling. Am J Psychiatry 145:502–505, 1988

Volberg RA, Steadman HJ: Prevalence estimates of pathological gambling in New Jersey and Maryland. Am J Psychiatry 146:1618–1619, 1989

Walker MB: Some problems with the concept of "gambling addiction": should theories of addiction be generalized to include excessive gambling? Journal of Gambling Behavior 5:179–200, 1989

Witkin-Lanloil G: "All pyros are psychos"—but they split into three types of disorders. Fire and Arson Investigator 32:13–16, 1981

Wooden WS, Berkey ML: Children and Arson. New York, Plenum, 1984

Wray I, Dickerson M: Cessation of high frequency gambling and 'withdrawal' symptoms. Br J Addict 76:401–405, 1981

Yesavage JA, Benezech M, Ceccaldi P, et al: Arson in mentally ill and criminal populations. J Clin Psychiatry 44:128–130, 1983

Zeegers M: Criminal fire-setting: a review and some case studies. Med Law 3:171–176, 1984

Chapter 47

Adjustment Disorder

James J. Strain, M.D., Dennis Wolf, M.D.,
Jeffrey Newcorn, M.D., and George Fulop, M.D.

Statement of the Issues

The primary issues for the adjustment disorder (AD) diagnosis are 1) the lack of explicit operational criteria and 2) the possible use of the diagnosis as a residual, "wastebasket" for cases that do not fulfill the criteria for other mental disorder diagnoses.

Significance of the Issues

In reviewing the diagnosis of AD in terms of how it might be altered in DSM-IV, two fundamental issues emerge. First, because the diagnosis lacks behavioral or operational criteria, what is the effect of this imprecision on the reliability and validity of the diagnosis in various settings? The second issue involves the classification of syndromes that do not fulfill the criteria for a major mental illness but may present with serious symptomatology that requires intervention and/or treatment. This symptomatology by default may then itself be viewed as subthreshold, because it is categorized in a subthreshold diagnosis. AD is thus designed as a means for classifying psychiatric conditions that are clinically significant but whose symptom profile is as yet insufficient to meet the more specifically operationalized criteria for the major syndromes. Such conditions are deemed to be in excess of a normal reaction to the stressor in question, involve impairment in vocational or interpersonal functioning, and are not just psychosocial problems (V codes) requiring medical attention (e.g., noncompliance with treatment).

However, the essential requirements for any psychiatric disorder in DSM-III-R

We thank Mirjami Easton for assistance in the development of this manuscript.

are "painful symptomatology" or impairment of functioning (American Psychiatric Association 1987, p. xxii). The imprecision of the AD diagnostic criteria is immediately apparent in its DSM-III-R description: "1) a maladaptive reaction, 2) to a psychosocial stressor, 3) that remits when the stressor remits, or an adaptation has taken place, but in any case within six months." Difficulties are inherent within each of these three diagnostic elements. In contrast to other DSM-III disorders, the AD criteria include no clear and specific profile (or list) of symptoms that collectively comprise a psychiatric (medical) syndrome or disorder. The V codes, a problem level of diagnoses, are understandably devoid of a symptom-based diagnostic schema.

First, it is unclear how the concept of the "maladaptive reaction" can or should be operationalized. Social, vocational, and relationship dysfunctions that are qualitatively or quantitatively unspecified lend themselves neither to reliability nor to validity. The criteria imply that a differentiation between an "abnormal" and "normal" state exists, but there are no guidelines to assess issues of culture, age, sex, religion, geography, etc. For example, uncomplicated bereavement is not considered an AD even though it is associated with a stressor and frequently with significant psychosocial dysfunction and psychological symptomatology. Yet, loss of a body part, which might also lead to bereavement, could qualify as a stressor and produce sufficient dysfunction to warrant the diagnosis of AD.

Second, no criteria or guidelines are offered in DSM-III-R to quantify stressors for the AD or assess their effect or meaning for a particular individual at a given time, nor is the assessment of stress linked by an algorithm to Axis IV. An objectively overwhelming stress could have little impact on one individual, whereas a minor one could be regarded as catastrophic by another. A recent minor stress superimposed on a previous underlying (major) stress may have a significant impact, not operating independently, but by its additive effect (Rahe 1990). The measurement of the severity of the stressor, and its temporal and causal relationship to demonstrable symptoms, is often uncertain and at times impossible.

The time course and chronicity of both stressors and symptoms need further exploration. Both may exceed the 6-month limitation that is specified in DSM-III-R (3 months according to DSM-III criteria). If an individual originally identified as having an AD has a duration of distress greater than 6 months, is the diagnosis dropped or a new one assigned (as directed by DSM-III-R)? Does an HIV patient with an AD at 5 months 29 days receive a different diagnosis at 6 months and 14 days?

Although the diagnosis of AD is not scientifically rigorous because it is confounded by its current conceptual framework, it is this imprecision that also makes the diagnosis so useful to psychiatry. Because a wide latitude exists in assigning this diagnosis, clinicians have a "legitimate" nomenclature for those patients who require treatment and are receiving continuing care, although they fail to qualify for the strict criteria of one of the better-defined major syndromes. Although it could be argued that employing such an imprecise diagnosis is evidence of sloppiness or an insufficient effort to pursue an evaluation, it is often difficult to identify an emerging illness in its early stages. In such instances the AD diagnosis serves as a temporary diagnosis that can be modified with information gained from longitudinal evaluation and treatment. Important psychiatric treatment takes place with patients who do not qualify for a diagnosis of a major syndrome.

Even serious symptomatology (e.g., suicidal behavior) that does not appear to be related to a major mental disorder needs treatment and a diagnosis under which it can be placed. It has been suggested that suicide could be a subtype of AD, because there are subtypes of AD with work inhibition, physical symptoms, etc. Although AD is regarded as a subthreshold diagnosis, this does not necessarily imply the presence of subthreshold symptomatology within its domain.

Finally, the issue of boundaries between the major syndromes—depression not otherwise specified, anxiety not otherwise specified, and AD—remains problematic. How often are the major syndromes associated with a stressor? How different are the symptom profiles of depression and anxiety not otherwise specified? Further investigations are required to demonstrate the boundaries between the subthreshold and minor/major disorders.

Methods

A Medline search yielded 500 citations from 1966 to June 1990 using the search strategy *adjustment disorder, subthreshold diagnoses, transitional diagnoses,* and eliminating articles that were case reports and letters, or were not in English. Articles were also eliminated if 1) they did not evaluate a sample of patients or 2) they were commentaries or reviews. Articles that addressed an issue that was judged to be relevant to the understanding of AD (e.g., minor depression) were also included.

Accordingly, 110 articles remained for extensive review by the faculty in the Department of Psychiatry at the Mount Sinai School of Medicine (New York City). Sixty-eight articles addressed the relationship of stress to psychiatric illness (mostly depression), although they did not specifically discuss AD; 33 of the most important are referenced (Akiskal et al. 1978; Benjaminsen 1981; Breslau and Davis 1987; J. D. Brown and Siegel 1988; G. W. Brown et al. 1986; Byrne 1984; Cohen 1981; Copeland 1984; Dohrenwend et al. 1978; Escobar 1987; Garvey et al. 1984; Glass 1985; Green et al. 1985; Hirschfeld and Cross 1982; Hirschfeld et al. 1985; Holmes and Rahe 1967; Horowitz et al. 1980, 1987; Klerman et al. 1979; Lindy et al. 1987; McMiller et al. 1987; Monroe 1982; Paykel and Tanner 1976; Paykel et al. 1969, 1984; Perris

1984; Perris et al. 1982; Rundell et al. 1989; Snyder et al. 1989; Tennant 1983; Ursano 1987; Winokur 1985; Wynne 1975). Sixteen reports focused on the use of the DSM-III diagnostic system; 10 are referenced (Fabrega et al. 1987; Gordon et al. 1985; Koenigsberg et al. 1985; Mezzich et al. 1989; Rey et al. 1988; Schrader et al. 1986; Spitzer and Williams 1979; Williams 1985a, 1985b; Zimmerman et al. 1987). Eight articles evaluated the use of rating scales or biological markers specifically for AD (Checkley et al. 1984; De Leo et al. 1985, 1986; Lesser et al. 1983; Maes et al. 1986; Perris et al. 1984; Rupprecht et al. 1988; Zilberg et al. 1982). The evaluation of treatment response of disorders thought to be brought on by stress was reviewed (De Leo 1985; Garvey et al. 1984; Imlah 1985; Jefferson 1985). Six studies provided background information on the development of the concept of the relationship of stress to psychiatric illness (J. D. Brown and Siegel 1988; Depue and Monroe 1986; Dew et al. 1987; Fabrega et al. 1987; Miller 1988; Vinokur and Caplan 1986). Finally, a number of papers directly evaluated the use of the AD diagnosis with patients in database studies (Andreasen and Hoenk 1982; Andreasen and Wasek 1980; Andreasen and Winokur 1979; Blazer et al. 1988; Fabrega et al. 1987; Looney and Gunderson 1978; Popkin et al. 1983, 1988).

Of the articles reviewed, 75% were in refereed journals, 51% were from sources in the United States, and 66% were published since 1980. DSM-III criteria were used to make the diagnoses in only 35% of the citations, whereas previous versions of DSM or other diagnostic taxonomies were used in the remainder.

Results

Symptom Characteristics and Their Frequency

AD is a commonly used diagnosis in diverse settings. Andreasen and Wasek (1980) report that 5% of an inpatient and outpatient sample at the University of Iowa were labeled AD. Fabrega et al. (1987) observed that 2.3% of a sample of patients presenting to the Western Psychiatric Institute and Clinic (University of Pittsburgh) Diagnostic and Evaluation Center walk-in clinic were judged to meet criteria for AD with no other diagnosis on Axis I or Axis II. However, a total of 20.5% had the diagnosis of AD when patients with other Axis I diagnoses (Axis I comorbidities) were also included. In general hospital psychiatric consultation populations, Popkin et al. (1988) diagnosed AD in 11.5% of patients, and Snyder and Strain (1990) diagnosed AD in 21.5% of patients.

Only a few studies evaluated patients for the presence of symptoms considered essential to the diagnosis (Andreasen and Hoenk 1982; Andreasen and Wasek 1980;

Andreasen and Winokur 1979; Fabrega et al. 1987; Looney and Gunderson 1978). Andreasen and Wasek (1980) used a chart review method and reported that more adolescents experienced acting out and behavioral symptoms than adults, who had significant depressive symptomatology (63.8% of adolescents had depressive symptoms versus 87.2% of adults). Anxiety symptoms were frequent at all ages.

Mezzich et al. (1981) and Fabrega et al. (1987) used a semistructured assessment, the Initial Evaluation Form, to evaluate for 64 symptoms currently present in three cohorts: specific diagnoses (SD), AD, and not ill (NI) (Fabrega et al. 1987). Vegetative, substance-use, and characterological symptoms were greatest in SD, intermediate with AD, and least in NI. The symptoms of mood and affect, general appearance, behavior, disturbance in speech and thought pattern, and cognitive functioning had a similar distribution: greatest in SD, intermediate with AD, and least in NI. Those diagnosed with AD were significantly different from NI with regard to more "depressed mood" and "low self-esteem" ($P < .0001$). AD and NI had minimal pathology of thought content and perception. On the item suicide indicators, 29% of AD versus 9.0% of NI had a positive response. The three cohorts did not differ on the frequency of Axis III disorders.

Maladaptation

As mentioned earlier, assessment of the "maladaptive" component of the diagnosis is also problematic. Furthermore, the patient's functional status evaluation (Axis V) is not linked via an algorithm to the AD construct in DSM-III-R. With the exception of the Fabrega et al. (1987) and Mezzich et al. (1981) studies, little attention has been paid to the discreet assessment of the patient's functional status. Fabrega et al. (1987) state that both subjective symptoms and decrement in social function can be considered maladaptive and that the severity of either of these is subject to great individual variation. Although the authors demonstrated higher levels of psychopathology in patients identified with AD than in those with NI, using data from Axis V and their "new" Axis VI (an additional and more specific functional status Axis on the Initial Evaluation Form), they could not conclude that the level of psychopathology correlates with impaired functioning. Axis VI assesses current functioning from "superior" to "markedly impaired" in three domains: occupational, with family, and with other individuals and groups (Mezzich et al. 1981). The degrees of impairment are clearly defined.

Although Andreasen and Wasek (1980) observed symptom characteristics of other psychiatric illnesses in the AD cohort and argued for the subtyping of AD on the basis of the predominant symptom picture, they did not report assessing maladaptation.

Stress

More information is available regarding the criterion of the "psychosocial stressor," although its definition was poorly specified in the majority of studies reviewed. The intuitively attractive concept that psychiatric disorders are precipitated by stress has been discussed for centuries. In more modern times, Wynne (1975) summarized the DSM-II designation of "transient situational disturbance," emphasizing that an "overwhelming stressor" was not required, although data were not cited to support this contention. Based on Wynne's suggestions, the criteria for AD were changed for DSM-III, in part by dropping the requirement for an overwhelming stressor.

The literature is replete with reports regarding the impact of life events on illness and psychosocial functioning. Major contributions have been made by investigators doing life events research: J. D. Brown and Siegel (1988), G W. Brown et al. (1986), Dohrenwend et al. (1978), and Paykel et al. (1969). Limitations of the current construct of stress for research have been described (Cohen 1981). Holmes and Rahe (1967) attempted to assign relative values to specific stressors, but there has been much concern about their methodology and results (Cohen 1981). Other life events scales (Dohrenwend et al. 1978; Paykel et al. 1971; Tennant 1983) have also been shown to be inconsistent in their ability to link stress and illness. Many authors have cautioned that the vulnerability of the individual (e.g., ego strengths, support system, underlying personality disorders, the timing and concatenation of the stress[es], the issue of control over the stressor, and the desirability of the event) need to be assessed to ascertain the importance of the situation for the individual. Axis IV of DSM-III was included to allow the clinician to assess the presence of stress in the multiaxial diagnoses of psychiatric disorders, but it has been confounded by low reliability (Rey et al. 1988; Spitzer and Williams 1979; Zimmerman et al. 1987).

Hirschfeld (1981) and Winokur (1985) discuss both sides of the controversy regarding "neurotic" (related to a stressor) and "endogenous" (not stressor related) depression. Several studies indicate that it is difficult to demonstrate a significant temporal link between the onset of an identified stressor and the occurrence of depressive illness (Akiskal et al. 1978; Andreasen and Winokur 1979; Benjaminsen 1981; Garvey et al. 1984; Hirschfeld 1981; Paykel and Tanner 1976; Winokur 1985).

The chronological relationship between the stressor and symptoms has been less extensively examined. Depue and Monroe (1986) and Rahe (1990) state that the model of a single stressor impinging on an undisturbed individual to cause symptoms at a single point in time is insufficient to account for the many presentations of stress and illness in the clinical situation. As stated before, it is difficult to account for the confounding circumstances presented by underlying chronic illness, personality disorder, the maintenance of stress, etc., all of which have an impact on the meaning of the stress to the individual. Additionally, Depue and Monroe (1986) and Skodol et al. (1990) identified significant methodological problems in evaluating the quality, quantity, and timing of both stressors and symptoms.

Currently, there is no documented research with representative patient groups to support or refute either the criterion requiring that the onset of symptoms occur within 3 months of the onset of the stressor (DSM-III) or the limitation requiring that symptoms persist for no longer than 6 months after the occurrence of the stressor as prescribed by DSM-III-R.

Andreasen and Wasek (1980) describe the differences between the types of stressors seen in adolescents and those seen in adults; respectively, 59% and 35% of the precipitants had been present for 1 year or more and 9% and 39% for 3 months or less. Fabrega et al. (1987) report that their AD group had significantly greater registration of stressors compared with the SD and NI cohorts. There was a significant difference in the number and severity of stressors reported to be relevant to the clinical request for evaluation: the group with AD were overrepresented in the "higher-stress" categories compared with the SD and NI patients. Popkin et al. (1988) report that 68.6% of the cases in their consultation cohort were judged to have their medical illness as the primary psychosocial stressor. Finally, Snyder and Strain (1990) observed that the assessment of stressors on Axis IV was significantly higher ($P < .0001$) for consultation patients with AD compared with those diagnosed with other disorders.

With regard to the long-term outcome of AD, Andreasen and Hoenk (1982) suggest that the prognosis is good for adults, whereas in adolescents many major psychiatric illnesses are likely to eventually occur. At the 5-year follow-up, 71% of adults were completely well, whereas 8% had an intervening problem, and 21% had developed a major depressive disorder or alcoholism. In contrast, at the 5-year follow-up, only 44% of the adolescents were without a psychiatric diagnosis, 13% had an intervening illness, and 43% went on to develop major psychiatric morbidity (schizophrenia, schizoaffective disorders, major depression, bipolar disorders, substance abuse, and personality disorders). In contrast to the adults, the chronicity of the illness and the presence of behavioral symptoms in the adolescents were the strongest predictors for major pathology at the 5-year follow-up. The number and type of symptoms were less useful than the length of treatment and chronicity of symptoms as predictors of future outcome.

J. E. Mezzich, J. Newcorn, and J. J. Strain (personal communication, 1992) are currently examining the 5-year outcome of their patients. With regard to short-term outcome, it has been found that AD and major depression diagnoses remain stable, with repeated observations over the length of hospital stay for patients on medical/surgical units (Snyder et al. 1989).

Both J. E. Mezzich (personal communication, 1991) and J. J. Strain (personal communication, 1991) found that many of the subtypes of AD were infrequently used (e.g., "with mixed emotional features"), whereas "with physical complaints," "with withdrawal," and "with work" (or "academic inhibition") were DSM-III-R categories and therefore have had insufficient time to be observed.

Adjustment Disorder as a Diagnostic Construct

The usefulness of the AD diagnosis in identifying subthreshold syndromes was addressed by Fabrega et al. (1987). They report that the diagnosis of an AD defines a level of psychopathology that is intermediate between no illness and that of a major psychiatric diagnosis, and is a distinct entity for an acute evaluation. The studies of Looney and Gunderson (1978), Andreasen and Winokur (1979), Andreasen and Wasek (1980), and Andreasen and Hoenk (1982) support the validity of AD with regard to long-term follow-up observations. Although Looney and Gunderson (1978) and Andreasen and Winokur (1979) warn of the imprecise clinical diagnostic practices that may arise from having a "wastebasket" category available, Andreasen and Winokur (1979) argue that it remains a frequently used diagnosis. Looney and Gunderson (1978), writing before DSM-III, favored the use of "transient situational disorder" when the diagnosis is unclear, to indicate that a disorder does indeed exist. Furthermore, they state that it is useful in some populations (e.g., adolescents and military personnel) to avoid stigmatizing the patient when a more serious disorder exists. Andreasen and Winokur (1979) and Andreasen and Wasek (1980) share this point of view.

Discussion

This review indicates that only a little literature has been published concerning the evaluation of the reliability, validity, and clinical utility of the diagnosis of AD. However, the available information does allow us to make some inferences and indicates some directions for further investigation.

The issue of operational diagnostic criteria remains problematic. There appears to be a dichotomy between having rigorous criteria that enhance greater specification of the illness and more formal research, and having relatively "loose" criteria that offer the clinician latitude in identifying disorders that are poorly defined and incipient but in which psychological dysfunction in excess of normal is present. To facilitate more rigorous diagnosis, it would be essential to have more precise criteria for 1) symptom profiles, 2) maladaptation, 3) how stressors impinge on the experience of individuals with and without a predisposition to psychiatric illness, 4) reliable and valid assessment measures, and 5) the characteristic time course of a poorly defined illness. Such an effort would not only enhance research, but offer opportunities to obtain meaningful data about prognosis and treatment outcomes rather than leave a vague diagnosis more usable for nondescript patients (M. Kline, personal communication, 1992).

No investigator has been able to account satisfactorily for the effect of chronic or recurring stressors, nor has the issue of chronic symptoms lasting months to years after the onset of the stressor been sufficiently examined. An especially complicated issue is the relationship between the underlying personality structure and both the response and timing of symptom occurrence. Whether to attribute symptoms to the underlying personality organization or to assign an additional diagnosis to account for the presence of symptoms in a particular setting remains an unresolvable theoretical issue.

Further study of diagnostic criteria is required to identify symptom profiles that may differentiate AD from SD and NI cohorts. The studies of Looney and Gunderson (1978) and Andreasen and Wasek (1980) were done with psychiatric inpatients, whereas Fabrega et al. (1987) evaluated outpatients who presented to a walk-in psychiatric clinic. Popkin et al. (1988) and Snyder et al. (1989, 1990) report on consultation patients from general hospital populations. However, in most of these studies, the symptoms and their outcome were evaluated by individuals who also formulated the diagnosis, so that assessments of the symptom characteristics, stressors, maladaptation, and diagnostic formulation were not independent of each other.

Because a community sample may differ from patient data in terms of maladaptation, stressor criterion, and chronicity, an important contribution to the criteria and eventual diagnosis of AD is the symptom characteristics and profiles from such a sample. However, the Epidemiologic Catchment Area (ECA) investigations did not include AD (Regier et al. 1984). Blazer et al. (1988) in the Duke portion of the ECA cohort demonstrated a subthreshold diagnostic group (type I) that had significant depressive symptoms but did not reach the criterion for a psychiatric disorder. The Diagnostic Interview Schedule (Robins et al. 1981) did not have an inventory for the AD category, so it is not possible to know whether some of these type I patients would qualify for the AD nomenclature. Because the frame of reference for the grade of membership method used by the Duke group was only a symptom profile, it differs significantly in approach from the DSM-III-R, which does not include symptoms.

In addition, instruments need to be perfected that more clearly define these criteria, especially in the areas of stress and maladaptation. Even the current diagnostic screening scales such as the Hamilton Depression Scale (Hamilton 1967) and the Spielberger anxiety scale (Spielberger 1968) are confounded by the difficulty that besets the diagnosis of depression and anxiety disorders in the medically ill (Endicott 1984; Strain 1978). However, studies employing surveys (Eaton et al.

1981) in a primary-care setting suggest an ability to differentiate patients with major and minor illness from those who are not ill.

Studies in which adequate symptom checklists are rated independently from the establishment of the diagnosis would help clarify the threshold between major and minor depression and anxiety, as well as serve as a guide for setting a cutoff point for AD. Although the upper threshold is established by the criteria for the major syndromes, the lower threshold between AD and problem/normality is undesignated with operational criteria and illustrates the difficulty of the "boundary issue" described earlier. The careful examination of associated demographic and treatment outcome variables would also assist in a more specific description of the boundaries between diagnoses. Andreasen and Wasek (1980) observed that, in their AD cohorts, 21.6% of the adolescents' fathers and 11.8% of the adults' fathers had problems with alcohol.

As discussed earlier, regardless of whether greater precision can be achieved in making this diagnosis and distinguishing it from other disorders or normal behavior, AD remains a diagnosis of great utility in clinical settings. AD serves as a "refuge" for poorly defined psychiatric morbidity and affords a flexible diagnosis for the clinical finding encountered. There is a danger that it could be overused as a "wastebasket" for subthreshold clinical findings. AD is a vehicle for both temporizing with a diagnosis and cataloging poorly defined disorders.

There are several possible classification schemas for AD:

1. AD could be subsumed under the respective major disorder within which the majority of the symptoms seem to fall, usually mood, conduct, or anxiety, or within the specific category of "not otherwise specified" within that major syndrome. For example, AD with depressed mood could be classified as a depressive disorder not otherwise specified.
2. Alternatively, the disorder could be described in a category of stress-related disorders.
3. AD could be collapsed into the V-code section, which includes clinical problems that are a focus of attention or treatment but that are not major illnesses with specified symptoms. This would put AD conceptually into the "life problems" category similar to bereavement.
4. AD could remain as a distinct diagnostic entity. Regardless of their position on the diagnostic tree, subthreshold syndromes can encompass significant psychopathology that must not only be recognized but also treated. Cross-sectionally, AD may appear to be the incipient phase of an emerging major syndrome. Consequently, although impeded by problems of reliability and validity, AD serves an important diagnostic function in the practice of psychiatry wherever it is eventually categorized or placed.

The proposition that the AD diagnosis could be merged into other illness categories (e.g., spectrum diagnoses, stress disorders, V codes) has not been discussed in the literature. AD with depressed mood is conceptually inappropriate as a depression not otherwise specified, because it is a diagnosis related to a precipitant (i.e., stress) and is therefore part of a different theoretical construct than the other non-stress-related atheoretical depressive disorders. The theoretical position of the affective disorders and the relevance of stressors to their etiology would need to be reconsidered. Similar conceptual issues arise with regard to a stressor in the etiology of the anxiety disorders.

Although it might be argued that AD could be placed in a new category of "stress response syndromes," the literature does not offer any data to support such a grouping. In the extreme, the AD concept could be eliminated altogether, with the advantage of maintaining the atheoretical approach of DSM-III-R. However, posttraumatic stress disorder, the organic mental disorders, and the conversion disorders also mandate a theoretical underlying etiology and therefore deviate from the atheoretical schema of DSM-III-R.

Eliminating AD would also have major implications for medical reporting, reimbursement for treatment, and communication with other physicians, who may wonder why a patient is undergoing mental health treatment from a psychiatrist without a designated psychiatric morbidity.

Research is needed to discern whether clearer characterization of the disorder will continue to support its use in its current form. Based on the guidelines that recommended changes for DSM-IV should be based on scientifically derived data, no clear evidence exists at present to support databased amendments. Neither is there compelling evidence to support eliminating the AD category as it now stands and identifying subthreshold syndromes under the diagnoses that represent the predominant symptoms of the patient. As discussed above, the use of a spectrum disorder approach is problematic.

Recommendations

The recommended criteria for AD, as they appear in the *DSM-IV Options Book* (Task Force on DSM-IV 1991), are listed below:

A. The development of emotional or behavioral symptoms in response to an identifiable psychosocial stressor(s), which occurs within 3 months of the onset of the stressor(s).
B. These symptoms or behaviors are clinically significant as evidenced by either of the following:

(1) there is marked distress that is in excess of what would be expected from exposure to the stressor

(2) there is significant impairment in social or occupational (academic) functioning

C. The stress-related disturbance does not meet the criteria for any specific Axis I disorder and is not merely an exacerbation of a preexisting Axis I or Axis II disorder.

D. Does not represent uncomplicated bereavement

Options for criterion E (duration of symptoms):

Option E1: DSM-III-R (strict duration requirement of 6 months): The maladaptive reaction has persisted for no longer than 6 months.

Option E2: A broader definition that allows for enduring stressors: The symptoms do not persist for more than 6 months after the termination of the stressor (or its consequences).

Option E3: No duration (adjustment disorder can last indefinitely): Omit

Specify:

Acute: if the symptoms have persisted for no longer than 6 months

Persistent/Chronic: if the symptoms have persisted for 6 months or longer

Specify type:

Option #1: retain DSM-III-R types

With anxiety

With depressed mood

With disturbance of conduct

With mixed disturbance of emotions and conduct

With mixed emotional features

With physical complaints

With withdrawal

With work (or academic) inhibition

Not otherwise specified

Option #2: add new subtype

With suicidal behavior: if criteria not met for other subtypes of adjustment disorder

In summary, the issues of diagnostic rigor and clinical utility seem at odds. Field studies that would employ reliable and valid instruments (e.g., depression or anxiety rating scales, stress assessments, and length of disability, treatment outcome, family patterns) would allow more exact specification of the parameters of the diagnosis. Identification of the time course, remission or evolution to another diagnosis, and the evaluation of stressors (characteristics, duration, and nature of adaptation to stress) would enhance understanding of the concept of a stress-response illness.

Currently, analyses are under way to examine the data from the Western Psychiatric Institute and Clinic for 1980–1988 for the characteristics of those patients who were given the diagnosis of AD compared to others. This analysis examines three cohorts: children and youth, adults, and the elderly. It may be that the characteristics of a mental disorder vary over the life cycle; that certain developmental epochs are associated with one symptom profile versus another; that the effect of the stressor may vary; and, the assessment of functioning must be "measured" according to the demands of the developmental stage: school (youth), work (adults), self-care and maintenance (elderly). In addition, a subset of the sample that was originally investigated is being reevaluated at the 5-year follow-up to examine the stability of the diagnosis and the outcome of the patient's original symptoms and functioning (J. E. Mezzich, J. Newcorn, and J. J. Strain, unpublished data, 1992).

Finally, Newcorn and Strain (1992) have reviewed the child and youth literature to assess the need for changes in the AD criteria for children in DSM-IV. They have observed that AD is a diagnosis that is commonly used in this age group (up to 70% of all diagnoses in many in- and outpatient settings), that it may be an early stage or prodromata of another evolving mental disorder, and that it is often associated with severe symptomatology (e.g., suicidal behavior) and therefore requires separate definition and analysis from that diagnosis used in adults. It may be that AD is the first mental disorder to be considered not only from epidemiological and phenomenological dimensions but also along the developmental lines of the evolving human organism.

Other diagnoses may also vary along the developmental schema from birth to senescence. Illnesses such as major depressive disorders, organic mental disorders, sexual dysfunctions, eating disorders, etc., may all need to be recast in another hierarchy to incorporate the stage of the life cycle extant at the time of the assessment. Considerations such as the normal variations across developmental epochs would improve the validity and reliability of DSM with regard to children and youth, the elderly, and the medically ill (Strain 1981). It would be a taxonomy tempered by the vicissitudes of development and medical illness. Such an effort may also make the DSM more useful to child psychiatrists, pediatricians, geriatricians, geriatric psychiatrists, and primary-care physicians, who currently feel that their patients too often do not conform to psychiatry's lexicon.

References

Akiskal HS, Bitar AH, Puzantian VR, et al: The nosological status of neurotic depression: a prospective three- to four-year follow-up examination in light of the primary-secondary and unipolar-bipolar dichotomies. Arch Gen Psychiatry 35:756–766, 1978

American Psychiatric Association: Diagnostic and Statistical Manual of Mental Disorders, 3rd Edition, Revised. Washington, DC, American Psychiatric Association, 1987

Andreasen NC, Hoenk PR: The predictive value of adjustment disorders: a follow-up study. Am J Psychiatry 139:584–590, 1982

Andreasen NC, Wasek P: Adjustment disorders in adolescents and adults. Arch Gen Psychiatry 37:1166–1170, 1980

Andreasen NC, Winokur G: Secondary depression: familial, clinical, and research perspectives. Am J Psychiatry 136:62–66 , 1979

Benjaminsen S: Stressful life events preceding the onset of neurotic depression. Psychol Med 11:369–378, 1981

Blazer D, Swartz M, Woodbury M, et al: Depressive symptoms and depressive diagnoses in a community population: use of a new procedure for analysis of psychiatric classification. Arch Gen Psychiatry 45:1078–1084, 1988

Breslau N, Davis GC: Posttraumatic stress disorder: the stressor criterion. J Nerv Ment Dis 175:255–264, 1987

Brown GW, Bifulco A, Harris T, et al: Life stress, chronic subclinical symptoms and vulnerability to clinical depression. J Affect Disord 11:1–19, 1986

Brown JD, Siegel M: Attributions for negative life events and depression: the role of perceived control. J Pers Soc Psychol 54:316–322, 1988

Byrne DG: Personal assessments of life-event stress and the near future onset of psychological symptoms. Br J Med Psychology 57:241–248, 1984

Checkley SA, Glass IB, Thompson C, et al: The GH response to clonidine in endogenous as compared with reactive depression. Psychol Med 14:773–777, 1984

Cohen F: Stress and bodily illness. Psychiatr Clin North Am 4:269–286, 1981

Copeland JRM: Reactive and endogenous depressive illness and five-year outcome. J Affect Disord 6:153–162, 1984

De Leo D: S-adenosyl-L-methionine (SAMe) in clinical practice: preliminary report on 75 minor depressives. Curr Ther Res 37:658–661, 1985

De Leo D, Pellegrini C, Serraiotto L: Adjustment disorders and suicidality. Psychol Rep 59:355–358, 1985

De Leo D, Pellegrini C, Serraiotto L, et al: Assessment of severity of suicide attempts: a trial with the dexamethasone suppression test and 2 rating scales. Psychopathology 19:186–191, 1986

Depue RA, Monroe SM: Conceptualization and measurement of human disorder in life stress research: the problem of chronic disturbance. Psychol Bull 99:36–51, 1986

Dew MA, Bromet EJ, Schulberg HC: A comparative analysis of two community stressors' long-term mental health effects. Am J Community Psychol 15:167–184, 1987

Dohrenwend BS, Krasnoff L, Askenasy AR, et al: Exemplification of a method for scaling life events: the PERI life event scale. J Health Soc Behav 19:205–229, 1978

Eaton WW, Regier DA, Locke BZ: The Epidemiologic Catchment Area Program of the National Institute of Mental Health. Public Health Rep 96:319–325, 1981

Endicott J: Measurement of depression in patients with cancer. Cancer 53:287–300, 1984

Escobar J: Commentary: posttraumatic stress disorder and the perennial stress-diathesis controversy. J Nerv Ment Dis 175:265–266, 1987

Fabrega H Jr, Mezzich JE, Mezzich AG: Adjustment disorder as a marginal or transitional illness category in DSM-III. Arch Gen Psychiatry 44:567–572, 1987

Garvey MJ, Schaffer CB, Tuason VB: Comparison of pharmacological treatment response between situational and non-situational depressions. Br J Psychiatry 145:363–365, 1984

Glass RM: Situational and neurotic-reactive depression. Arch Gen Psychiatry 42:1126–1127, 1985

Gordon RE, Jardiolin P, Gordon KK: Predicting length of hospital stay of psychiatric patients. Am J Psychiatry 142:235–237, 1985

Green BL, Lindy JD, Grace MC: Posttraumatic stress disorder: toward DSM-IV. J Nerv Ment Dis 173:406–411, 1985

Hamilton M: Development of a rating scale for primary depressive illness. Br J Clin Psychol 6:278–296, 1967

Hirschfeld RMA: Situational depression: validity of the concept. Br J Psychiatry 139:297–305, 1981

Hirschfeld RMA, Cross CK: Epidemiology of affective disorders. Arch Gen Psychiatry 39:35–46, 1982

Hirschfeld RMA, Klerman GL, Andreasen NC, et al: Situational major depressive disorder. Arch Gen Psychiatry 42:1109–1114, 1985

Holmes TH, Rahe RH: The social readjustment rating scale. J Psychosom Res 11:213–218, 1967

Horowitz MJ, Wilner N, Kaltreider N: Signs and symptoms of posttraumatic stress disorder. Arch Gen Psychiatry 37:85–92 , 1980

Horowitz MJ, Weiss DS, Marmar C: Commentary: diagnosis of posttraumatic stress disorder. J Nerv Ment Dis 175:267–268, 1987

Imlah NW: An evaluation of alprazolam in the treatment of reactive or neurotic (secondary) depression. Br J Psychiatry 146:515–519, 1985

Jefferson JW: Biologic treatment of depression in cardiac patients. Psychosomatics 26 (suppl):31–36, 1985

Klerman GL, Endicott J, Spitzer R, et al: Neurotic depression: a systematic analysis of multiple criteria and meanings. Am J Psychiatry 136:57–61, 1979

Koenigsberg HW, Kaplan RD, Gilmore MM, et al: The relationship between syndrome and personality disorder in DSM-III: experience with 2,462 patients. Am J Psychiatry 142:207–212, 1985

Lesser IM, Rubin RT, Finder E, et al: Situational depression and the dexamethasone suppression test. Psychoneuroendocrinology 8:441–445, 1983

Lindy JD, Green BL, Grace MC: Commentary: the stressor criterion and posttraumatic stress disorder. J Nerv Ment Dis 175:269–272, 1987

Looney JG, Gunderson EKE: Transient situational disturbances: course and outcome. Am J Psychiatry 135:660–663, 1978

Maes M, de Ruyter M, Hobin P, et al: The dexamethasone suppression test, the Hamilton Depression Rating Scale and the DSM-III depression categories. J Affect Disord 10:207–214, 1986

McMiller P, Ingham JG, Kreitman NB, et al: Life events and other factors implicated in onset and in remission of psychiatric illness in women. J Affect Disord 12:73–88, 1987

Mezzich JE, Dow JT, Rich CL, et al: Developing an efficient clinical information system for a comprehensive psychiatric institute, II: initial evaluation form. Behav Research Methods Instrum 13:464–478, 1981

Mezzich JE, Fabrega H Jr, Coffman GA, et al: DSM-III disorders in a large sample of psychiatric patients: frequency and specificity of diagnoses. Am J Psychiatry 146:212–219, 1989

Miller TW: Advances in understanding the impact of stressful life events on health. Hosp Community Psychiatry 39:615–622, 1988

Monroe SM: Life events and disorder: event-symptom associations and the course of disorder. J Abnorm Psychol 91:14–24, 1982

Newcorn J, Strain JJ: Adjustment disorders in children and adolescents: a review of pertinent issues and defining characteristics in anticipation of DSM-IV. J Am Acad Child Adolesc Psychiatry 31:318–326, 1992

Paykel ES, Tanner J: Life events, depressive relapse and maintenance treatment. Psychol Med 6:481–485, 1976

Paykel ES, Myers JK, Dienelt MN, et al: Life events and depression: a controlled study. Arch Gen Psychiatry 21:753–760, 1969

Paykel ES, Prusoff BA, Uhlenhuth EH: Scaling of life events. Arch Gen Psychiatry 25:340–347, 1971

Paykel ES, Rao BM, Taylor CN: Life stress and symptom pattern in out-patient depression. Psychol Med 14:559–568, 1984

Perris H: Life events and depression, part 2: results in diagnostic subgroups, and in relation to the recurrence of depression. J Affect Disord 7:25–36, 1984

Perris H, von Knorring L, Perris C: Genetic vulnerability for depression and life events. Neuropsychobiology 8:241–247, 1982

Perris H, von Knorring L, Oreland L, et al: Life events and biological vulnerability: a study of life events and platelet MAO activity in depressed patients. Psychiatry Res 12:111–120, 1984

Popkin MK, Mackenzie TB, Callies AL: A consultation-liaison outcome evaluation system (CLOES), I: consultant-consultee interaction. Arch Gen Psychiatry 40:215–219, 1983

Popkin MK, Callies AL, Colon EA: The treatment and outcome of adjustment disorders in medically ill inpatients. NIMH Conference, Pittsburgh, PA, June 1988

Rahe RH: Psychosocial stressors and adjustment disorder: Van Gogh's life chart illustrates stress and disease. J Clin Psychiatry 51 (suppl):13–24, 1990

Regier DA, Myers JK, Kramer M: The NIMH Epidemiologic Catchment Area (ECA) Program: historical context, major objectives, and study population characteristics. Arch Gen Psychiatry 41:934–941, 1984

Rey JM, Stewart GW, Plapp JM, et al: DSM-III Axis IV revisited. Am J Psychiatry 145:286–292, 1988

Robins LN, Helzer JE, Croughan J, et al: National Institute of Mental Health Diagnostic Interview Schedule: its history, characteristics, and validity. Arch Gen Psychiatry 38:381–389, 1981

Rundell JR, Ursano RJ, Holloway HC, et al: Psychiatric responses to trauma. Hosp Community Psychiatry 40:68–74, 1989

Rupprecht R, Barocka A, Beck G, et al: Pre- and post-dexamethasone plasma ACTH and beta-endorphin levels in endogenous and nonendogenous depression. Biol Psychiatry 23:531–535, 1988

Schrader G, Gordon M, Harcourt B: Usefulness of DSM-III Axes IV and V. Am J Psychiatry 143:904–907, 1986

Skodol AE, Dohrenwend BP, Line BG, et al: The nature of stress: problems of measurement, in Stressors and the Adjustment Disorders. Edited by Noshpitz JD, Coddington RD. New York, Wiley, 1990, pp 78–94

Snyder S, Strain JJ: Diagnostic instability in psychiatric consultations. Hosp Community Psychiatry 41:10–13, 1990

Snyder S, Strain JJ, Wolf D: Differentiation of major depression and adjustment disorder with depressed mood in the medical setting. Gen Hosp Psychiatry 12:159–165, 1989

Spielberger C: The State-Trait Anxiety Inventory. Palo Alto, CA, Consulting Psychologists Press, 1968

Spitzer RL, Williams JBW: DSM-III field trials, II: initial experience with the multiaxial system. Am J Psychiatry 136:818–820, 1979

Strain JJ: Psychological Interventions in Medical Practice. New York, Appleton-Century-Crofts, 1978

Strain JJ: Diagnostic considerations in the medical setting. Psychiatr Clin North Am 4:287–300, 1981

Task Force on DSM-IV: DSM-IV Options Book: Work in Progress. Washington, DC, American Psychiatric Association, 1991

Tennant C: Editorial: life events and psychological morbidity: the evidence from prospective studies. Psychol Med 13:483–486, 1983

Ursano RJ: Commentary: posttraumatic stress disorder: the stressor criterion. J Nerv Ment Dis 175:273–275, 1987

Vinokur A, Caplan RD: Cognitive and affective components of life events: their relations and effects on well-being. Am J Community Psychol 14:351–371, 1986

Williams JBW: The multiaxial system of DSM-III: Where did it come from and where should it go? I. Its origins and critiques. Arch Gen Psychiatry 42:175–180, 1985a

Williams JBW: The multiaxial system of DSM-III: Where did it come from and where should it go? II: empirical studies, innovations, and recommendations. Arch Gen Psychiatry 42:181–186, 1985b

Winokur G: The validity of neurotic-reactive depression: new data and reappraisal. Arch Gen Psychiatry 42:1116–1122, 1985

Wynne LC: Adjustment reaction of adult life, in Comprehensive Textbook of Psychiatry, 2nd Edition. Edited by Freedman AM, Kaplan HI, Sadock BJ. Baltimore, MD, Williams & Wilkins, 1975, pp 1609–1618

Zilberg NJ, Weiss DS, Horowitz MJ: Impact of Event Scale: a cross-validation study and some empirical evidence supporting a conceptual model of stress response syndromes. J Consult Clin Psychol 50:407–414, 1982

Zimmerman M, Pfohl B, Coryell W, et al: The prognostic validity of DSM-III Axis IV in depressed patients. Am J Psychiatry 144:102–106, 1987

Chapter 48

Psychological Factors Affecting Physical Condition (PFAPC)

Alan Stoudemire, M.D., Gale Beardsley, M.D.,
David G. Folks, M.D., Michael G. Goldstein, M.D.,
James Levenson, M.D., M. Eileen McNamara, M.D.,
Michael Moran, M.D., and Raymond Niaura, Ph.D.

Introduction

In this chapter, we summarize the work of the subcommittee of the Psychiatric Systems Interface Disorders Work Group, who examined the diagnostic category psychological factors affecting physical condition (PFAPC) for revision in DSM-IV. We review the methodology of this subcommittee's work, discuss the historical background of the PFAPC category, identify the key diagnostic issues involved, present synopses of the literature reviews, and set forth options for revisions to the PFAPC category.

Statement of the Issues

Although it is generally well established that psychological factors may affect physical conditions, the precise types of psychological factors that are involved, the specific types of illnesses they may affect, and at what point in the course of certain physical illnesses they appear to be operative are issues that remain largely unresolved and that are the source of ongoing research. Nevertheless, there is an extensive tradition in the psychiatric literature of examining psychological variables that may affect physical illnesses and of recognizing that psychological factors are potentially important in the pathogenesis, exacerbation, and perpetuation of many physical disorders. From the standpoint of classification, such relationships were recognized in the diagnostic nomenclature in earlier versions of the DSM system using "psychophysiologic" terminology (see DSM-II, American Psychiatric Association 1968). In DSM-III (American Psychiatric Association 1980), a substantial change was effected in which the term *psychophysiologic* was abandoned and the category "psychological factors affecting physical condition" adopted.

Problems with the PFAPC category have subsequently become evident, however, because the diagnosis is rarely used clinically, and almost no clinical research has been generated using this term. We explore the possible problems with the PFAPC category and outline several options for its revision in DSM-IV. The major options for revision that are considered are

1. Allow the category to stand as it is, without significant changes.
2. Discard the category altogether or use other psychiatric diagnoses whenever possible in the context of medical illness (such as adjustment disorders).
3. Revise the category with more specific diagnostic criteria.
4. Select an alternative name for the category.

Significance of the Issues

A few historical comments are needed to explain the significance and original development of the category "psychological factors affecting physical condition" in DSM-III. In a background paper for the development of the PFAPC concept, Looney et al. (1978) proposed abandoning the DSM-II term *psychophysiologic* and based this recommendation on the following points:

1. The DSM-II term *psychophysiologic* was rarely used as a diagnosis.
2. The clinical decision of whether a patient's condition was psychophysiologic or "organic" was arbitrary and idiosyncratic.
3. The term *psychophysiologic* decreased collaboration between specialists, particularly between internists and psychiatrists.
4. The psychophysiologic terminology perpetuated simplistic and unicausal ideas about disease etiology.
5. The term *psychophysiologic* was often used as a last resort when previous efforts at medical diagnosis and treatment had failed.
6. The DSM-II system was deficient because it referred only to causation and did not address how psychological factors might perpetuate or exacerbate a physical problem.
7. No clear operational criteria defined the DSM-II system.
8. The DSM-II classification of psychophysiologic disorders was inadequate for methodological purposes in research.

The DSM-III PFAPC category that was proposed and subsequently adopted was believed to offer significant advantages over the DSM-II psychophysiologic terminology because it integrated psychological contributions to medical illness into the multiaxial diagnostic system. PFAPC was considered to be a category and not a diagnosis per se. Hence, if a clinician believed that psychological factors were significant in the patient's condition, this observation could be noted on Axis I by using the PFAPC category and then on Axis III by noting the physical disorder involved. The medical disorder noted on Axis III could be any of the traditional "psychosomatic" disorders, any disorder that would have been a psychophysiologic disorder in DSM-II, or any other physical condition that the clinician believed was influenced by psychological factors. By broadening the scope beyond the DSM-II psychophysiologic disorders, it was believed that the new category would enlarge the range of psychological and behavioral factors considered to contribute to the onset or exacerbation of physical illnesses (Linn and Spitzer 1982).

Despite this rationale, there is little evidence to suggest that PFAPC has fared any better than its DSM-II psychophysiologic predecessor. Although there has been a considerable upsurge in interest in the relationships between psychological and behavioral factors in the etiology and course of physical disorders, almost no studies in either the medical or psychiatric literature using the term *PFAPC* have been generated. Fewer than 10 articles have been published in the past 10 years that used the term *PFAPC* in their title or as a substantial component of their content; no articles were found that used it as a basis for empirical research.

The reasons behind the paucity of use of PFAPC are unclear. The lack of research is especially perplexing because the DSM-III multiaxial system attempted to provide a concrete way to identify the physical disorder or symptoms that the psychological factors had initiated or exacerbated. Perhaps the wording of the PFAPC category was too cumbersome, or perhaps the problem arose from the lack of specific criteria for identifying the types of psychological factors involved. Given that PFAPC may not have fulfilled its intended purpose, a review of the category and its placement in the DSM classification system seemed timely.

Methods

Survey

The paucity of the use of PFAPC both in clinical and research settings presented obvious reasons for considering revision of the category or eliminating it entirely from DSM-IV. In an effort to solicit the opinion of academicians, a survey of more than 85 leaders in consultation-liaison psychiatry, psychosomatic medicine, and general hospital psychiatry was conducted. Individuals were selected based on evidence of scholarly publications and membership on editorial boards in areas of study relevant to this category or as officers or board members of prominent professional organizations.

The survey was conducted in two phases. The first consisted of an 11-item "yes/no/no opinion" brief survey designed to elicit general opinion as to matters relevant to PFAPC such as whether the category was deemed valid or useful, whether changes were considered necessary for DSM-IV, whether a return to a separate psychophysiologic category was needed, whether a change in name was required, whether a subcategorization scheme for PFAPC would be useful, and how individuals actually used the term clinically. The response rate to this survey, with one follow-up request to individuals who did not respond to the first questionnaire, was 60%. A second questionnaire was also mailed to individuals who had participated in the first phase, requesting expanded comments and suggestions regarding PFAPC, including recommendations for proposals and revisions; these comments were circulated and considered in the subcommittee's work.

Literature Review

A major component of the methodology involved a review of the literature on the relationship between psychological factors and physical illness. The purposes of the literature review were as follows:

1. To document the existing literature that would confirm that psychological factors affect physical illness.
2. To better delineate the specific *types* of psychological factors that could affect specific types of physical illness.
3. To identify at what phase of physical illness evidence existed for psychological factors to actually have some effect on the course of a physical illness.

A survey of the more recent literature that focused on empirical studies was simplified by two strategies. First, the work of the reviewers was distributed on a subspecialty basis (i.e., cardiology, gastroenterology, endocrine, dermatology, pulmonary, immunology, rheumatology, neurology, oncology, and nephrology). In addition, a review of "lifestyle risk factors," focusing primarily on cigarette smoking and obesity, was also conducted. Second, review efforts primarily focused on reports that employed systematic research methodology, preferably involving controlled studies rather than anecdotal case reports and theoretical papers.

Individual committee members were responsible for technical aspects of the literature review in their given area. All of the literature reviews involved Medline searches of the psychiatric/medical literature focusing on the relationship between psychological, psychiatric, and behavioral factors and medical conditions affecting the predisposition, onset, exacerbation, perpetuation, maintenance, or relapse of physical illnesses.

The key psychologically related factors selected for review included topics such as anxiety, depression, stress, personality factors, interpersonal factors, psycho-physiologic variables, habits, lifestyle factors, and nonspecific psychological/affective factors. Studies of comorbid Axis I/Axis II psychiatric factors and their relevance to physical conditions were also examined. Alcoholism, substance abuse, and eating disorders were not considered because it was believed this would overlap with the work of other DSM-IV review committees and that these disorders were generally outside the range of the intended parameters of the PFAPC category.

Results

Itemized Survey Results

As may be seen from Table 48–1, no general consensus emerged from the survey regarding the usefulness of PFAPC, although it was apparent that the majority of the respondents (85%) believed the PFAPC category was valid or useful (item 1), indicating PFAPC had a significant face validity. More than half (54%) of the respondents, however, believed that changes in definition, terminology, or diagnostic criteria were necessary for the category in DSM-IV; this sentiment was reflected in item 5, where 52% felt that changes in diagnostic criteria for PFAPC were necessary to enable better categorization of patients where psychological factors were deemed to affect a physical condition. Approximately 56% of the respondents did not feel that PFAPC provided sufficiently for the diagnostic classification of patients where psychological-behavioral factors contributed to physical disorders (item 3), and 36% did not feel PFAPC accurately described the spectrum of patients that the category attempted to cover in DSM-III-R (item 6). About 42% felt an alternate title was needed (item 7). There was no clear-cut trend toward returning to *psychophysiologic* as a primary or secondary term, although a surprising 19% currently classified patients with psychophysiologic-psychosomatic symptoms under somatoform disorders, contrary to specific recommendations in DSM-III-R. Based on this brief item-based survey, it was apparent that, although the majority of experts believed that PFAPC was valid and useful, arguing against the total abandonment of the category, most of the respondents believed that some form of revision in the diagnostic criteria was needed.

Table 48–1. Results of brief questionnaire

In respect to the DSM-III-R category psychological factors affecting physical condition (PFAPC), please reply specifically to any or all of the following inquiries:

1. Do you think the PFAPC is a valid and useful diagnostic category?
84%	Yes
16%	No
0%	No opinion

2. Do you feel that changes in either the definition, terminology, or diagnostic criteria are necessary for PFAPC?
54%	Yes
46%	No
0%	No opinion

3. Do you think DSM-III-R as a whole sufficiently provides for the diagnostic classification of patients where psychological-behavioral factors contribute to the onset, exacerbation or perpetuation of physical-medical disorders?
44%	Yes
56%	No
0%	No opinion

4. Would you be in favor of a separate diagnostic category for patients with psycho-physiological symptoms?
47%	Yes
49%	No
2%	No opinion
2%	Subcategory

5. Do you feel that changes in the diagnostic criteria for PFAPC are necessary to enable you to better categorize patients where psychological factors affect their physical condition?
52%	Yes
40%	No
6%	No opinion
2%	Subcategory

6. Do you think the term *psychological factors affecting physical condition* accurately describes the spectrum of patients that this category of DSM-III attempts to cover?
62%	Yes
36%	No
2%	No opinion

7. Would you be in favor of an alternate title other than PFAPC for this diagnostic category?
42%	Yes
42%	No
16%	No opinion

Table 48–1.   Results of brief questionnaire *(continued)*

8. Where do you currently classify patients with psychophysiologic-psychosomatic symptoms in DSM-III-R?
    19%   Somatoform disorders
    63%   PFAPC
    18%   Other

9. Do you think that psychophysiologic symptoms-syndromes should be included under the somatoform disorders or under PFAPC?
    21%   Somatoform disorders
    62%   PFAPC
    17%   Other

10. Do you think that sufficient scientific evidence exists to justify listing specific types of personality profiles or characteristics as being risk factors for psychophysiologic disorders or for the development or exacerbation of certain physical disorders?
    18%   Yes
    80%   No
    2%   No opinion

11. Would you be in favor of subcategories that would list certain psychophysiologic systems by organ system under this category (cardiovascular, gastrointestinal, urological, etc.)?
    49%   Yes
    51%   No
    0%   No opinion

Literature Review Synopses

Only brief synopses of the results of the literature reviews are presented in this chapter, highlighted for issues relevant to proposed revisions in PFAPC for DSM-IV. (Expanded versions of these literature reviews have been published elsewhere as a series of review articles in the journal *Psychosomatics*: Beardsley and Goldstein 1993 [endocrine]; Folks and Kinney 1992a [dermatology]; Folks and Kinney 1992b [gastrointestinal]; Goldstein and Niaura 1992; Niaura and Goldstein 1992 [cardiovascular]; Levenson and Bemis 1991 [cancer]; Levenson and Glocheski 1991 [renal disease]; McNamara 1991 [neurological]; and Moran 1991 [pulmonary and rheumatological]).

Endocrine literature (Beardsley and Goldstein 1993).   Research that has explored the relationship between psychological factors and the onset, exacerbation, and perpetuation of endocrine diseases has focused primarily on three diseases: diabetes mellitus, Graves' disease, and Cushing's disease. The effects of psychological factors on other endocrine disorders have received only scant attention.

Several conclusions were drawn from the literature search. First, with respect to diabetes mellitus, there is insufficient evidence to support the position that psychological factors directly affect the onset of illness (Cobb and Rose 1973; Gendel and Benjamin 1946; Helz and Templeton 1990; Robinson and Fuller 1985). Although some retrospective studies suggest a relationship between stressful life events and the course of diabetes mellitus, most of these studies are methodologically flawed. A recent study of the effects of laboratory-induced stress found there was no difference in measures of glycemic control in both patients with diabetes mellitus and control subjects (Kemmer et al. 1986). However, there is evidence suggesting that temperament influences glycemic control in diabetic children and adolescents (Rovet and Ehrlich 1988). A prospective study found that self-esteem, perceived competence, social functioning, and behavioral symptoms predicted compliance behaviors in children with recent onset of diabetes (Jacobson et al. 1987). Two studies found that stress had a direct effect on metabolic control of diabetes when the effect of compliance was controlled (Hanson et al. 1987; Linn et al. 1983). These findings need to be confirmed in subsequent studies before firm conclusions can be drawn.

Studies that have reported a link between psychological factors and the onset and course of Graves' disease have been methodologically flawed, and there is no good evidence that psychological characteristics of patients predispose them to develop Graves' disease or any other thyroid disorder (Weiner 1977). There is also insufficient evidence to suggest that psychological factors affect the course of Graves' disease.

With respect to Cushing's disease, there are no controlled studies in humans that show a relationship between psychological factors and onset and course of the disease. Finally, there is also a paucity of research on psychological factors affecting other endocrine disorders. Recommendations for future research in this area include use of prospective designs, well-defined subject populations, and meaningful control groups. The development and use of laboratory paradigms to assess the physiological reactivity of the endocrine system to psychological challenges may help to elucidate the psychophysiologic mechanisms that may underlie the relationships between psychological factors and endocrine disease (Beardsley and Goldstein 1993).

Dermatological literature (Folks and Kinney 1992a). The traditional clinical approach to dermatological illness implies that psychological factors are prominent in patients with dermatological conditions (Van Moffaert 1982). However, the literature contained only a few systematic studies of dermatological conditions with respect to psychological factors. Moreover, the importance of psychological factors is unclear because of the heterogeneity of many cutaneous disorders and the presumptive diagnostic approach that is commonly applied.

The existing literature supports the notion that urticaria, pruritus, neurotic excoriations, and factitial disorders, as well as a number of specific dermatoses, are significantly associated with psychological factors (Engel 1985). A number of psychotropic medications are also known to impact the etiology, pathogenesis, or clinical outcome of dermatological cases, the most noteworthy of which is the interplay between lithium preparations and psoriasis (Gupta et al. 1987).

The review yielded 436 citations between 1979 and 1989 that showed an association between psychological factors and dermatological conditions. We identified articles that met the criteria of rigorous research design or review methodology or that reported clinical experience in detail. The contributions of these articles were mostly responsible for advancing the existing knowledge about psychological factors and dermatological conditions.

The outcome of the literature review resulted in the identification of a number of dermatological symptoms or syndromes that appear to be significantly affected by psychological factors (e.g., pruritus, hyperhidrosis, urticaria, acne, and atopic dermatitis). Specific disease categories were not well represented, although psoriasis (Gupta et al. 1989), chronic urticaria (Fava et al. 1980), and atopic dermatitis (Faulstich and Williamson 1985) were often the subject of specific inquiry and appeared to be significantly associated with psychological factors.

Recent studies of psychological factors and their association with dermatological conditions have strengthened some of the concepts regarding the influence of stressors, mood, psychosocial factors, personality or lifestyle factors, and psychobiological mechanisms. Specifically, anxiety disorders, depression, and bipolar illness, together with maladaptive coping styles and personality factors (i.e., hostility, perfectionism, and low self-esteem) have been shown to significantly affect dermatological conditions in a variety of ways. Future studies are needed to confirm the significance of these factors.

A diagnostic and nosological schemata is needed that would better link temporal and psychosocial relationships, and psychobiological mechanisms associated with dermatological conditions. Moreover, pharmacological influences affecting the cause, course, or outcome of dermatological disorders deserve specific inquiry using rigorous research design. The current database is largely descriptive and presumptive at best, with the exception of the well-established relationship between lithium compounds and psoriasis. A clinical and research diagnostic format that considers psychological factors in a more systematic fashion would represent the logical next step in the future approach to dermatological conditions and associated psychological factors.

Gastrointestinal literature (Folks and Kinney 1992b). Alexander (1950, 1987) identified several emotional factors believed to affect gastrointestinal disturbances of appetite and eating, swallowing, digestion, and elimination. A diagnostic and nosological approach is needed that more clearly delineates the association between psychological factors and gastrointestinal conditions. Such a system would enable investigators to improve their research designs, and clinicians could more effectively document the nature and significance of psychological factors. Eating disorders are now considered a separate nosological category but a number of gastrointestinal conditions (e.g., irritable bowel syndrome, ulcerative colitis, and peptic ulcer disease) continue to be strongly implicated as having associated psychological factors.

A review of the literature resulted in 336 citations published between 1979 and 1989 regarding gastrointestinal conditions and psychological factors. Among these abstracts, 112 articles were selected for full review to identify those that met the criteria for either rigorous research design or review techniques, or detailed reporting of clinical experiences.

The outcome of this review suggested that certain psychological factors are indeed prominent and are frequently associated with gastrointestinal conditions. Two conditions, irritable bowel syndrome (Creed and Guthrie 1987; Walker et al. 1990) and peptic ulcer disease (Feldman et al. 1986), illustrate that a significant association may exist. Ulcerative colitis remains controversial in that, although systematic studies fail to show a significant association with psychological factors, such factors are often a focus of treatment (Arapakis et al. 1986; North et al. 1986). Psychiatric disturbances (e.g., anxiety, depression, and somatization) and lifestyle factors (e.g., alcohol abuse and tobacco use, self-destructive behaviors, and resistance to preventive medicine and rehabilitation approaches) are often reported as having an impact on gastroenterological disorders. Also, psychophysiologic reactions mediated through neuroendocrine or immunological systems now represent a new area of scientific and clinical inquiry.

To develop a clinical and research approach to clinical populations that takes into account the possible relationship between psychological factors and gastrointestinal conditions, more data must be collected on specific illness categories. This database might then enable investigators to formulate some practical generalizations regarding gastroenterological illness. New research pertaining to the psychological aspects of gastrointestinal disorders, particularly the etiological and pathophysiological relationships, remains a difficult area of investigation. Sampling methods, heterogeneity of illness categories, and confounding influences on the physical condition itself remain controversial.

A diagnostic and nosological system that considers psychological stressors, psychological influences on well-being and lifestyle, and outcome from therapeutic interventions would likely improve our future conceptualization of gastroenterology and increase our knowledge base as to what psychological factors operate. The relative influence of coping style and psychosocial support are also possible areas for future investigation.

Lifestyle risk factors literature (Goldstein and Niaura 1992).   Literature that focused on the relationship between behavioral or lifestyle factors and the onset, exacerbation, or perpetuation of physical conditions was reviewed. The literature on cigarette smoking (Fielding 1985; Kannel 1987; U.S. Department of Health and Human Services 1983, 1984, 1989) and obesity (Foster and Burton 1985; Garfinkel 1985; Kral 1985; National Institute of Health 1985; Wadden and Stunkard 1985) clearly demonstrates that these lifestyle factors affect the onset, exacerbation, and perpetuation of physical conditions and illnesses. Moreover, there is strong evidence that reduction or elimination of smoking (Rosenberg et al. 1985; U.S. Department of Health and Human Services 1983) leads to improved health outcomes and some evidence that reduction in obesity also reduces morbidity (National Institutes of Health 1985). Other lifestyle factors that have been associated with negative health outcomes include a sedentary lifestyle (Leon et al. 1987; Paffenbarger et al. 1986), a diet high in cholesterol and fats and low in fiber (U.S. Preventive Services 1989; U.S. Department of Health and Human Services 1988a), sexual practices that increase the risk of HIV infection (Darrow et al. 1987; Winkelstein et al. 1987), sun and other ultraviolet light exposure (U.S. Preventive Services 1989), and not using safety restraints when riding in a motor vehicle (Osray et al. 1988).

However, both obesity and smoking are not just simple behaviors or groups of behaviors. These factors are actually complex composites with biological, social, psychological, and behavioral determinants. Cigarette smoking is also an addiction to nicotine for most smokers (U.S. Department of Health and Human Services 1988b). Obesity has strong genetic and physiological determinants (Elliot et al. 1987). Thus, obesity and cigarette smoking can also be conceptualized as specific conditions or disorders, themselves. Nicotine dependence is currently a diagnostic category in DSM-III-R, although obesity is not. The other lifestyle factors that have been associated with negative health outcomes are more clearly behaviors. Therefore, inclusion of such behavioral factors as "psychological factors" in the PFAPC category seems warranted.

Cardiovascular disease literature (Goldstein and Niaura 1992; Niaura and Goldstein 1991).   The review of the literature on psychological factors affecting cardiovascular disease focused on three problems: coronary artery disease (CAD), sudden death (including serious ventricular arrhythmias), and hypertension. Literature for this review was identified from recent review articles and computerized literature searches. Only controlled studies were included in the review.

Several conclusions can be drawn from the results of the literature search. First, there is strong epidemiological evidence that the type A behavior pattern (TABP) is a possible risk factor for the *development* of CAD (French-Belgian Cooperative Group 1982; Haynes et al. 1980; Rosenman et al. 1975). Hostility (defined here as a personality trait) is the subcomponent of TABP that is most related to risk of CAD. In patients with CAD, hostility also predicts CAD morbidity and mortality (Barefoot et al. 1983, 1989; K. A. Matthews et al. 1977; Shekelle et al. 1983). Moreover, several studies have demonstrated that psychological treatment of TABP improves clinical outcome of CAD (Nunes et al. 1987). Cardiovascular reactivity, a correlate of TABP and its subcomponents, may contribute to the development of CAD, although the strongest evidence for this comes from primate studies (Krantz and Manuck 1984; Manuck and Krantz 1986). There is also strong evidence that patients with a major depressive disorder are at increased risk for cardiovascular morbidity and mortality (Avery and Winokur 1976; Carney et al. 1988; Murphy et al. 1987), but more research is needed to establish a relationship between depressive and anxiety symptoms and the development and progression of cardiovascular disease.

There is good evidence that silent myocardial ischemia may be precipitated by both physical and mental stress (Deanfield et al. 1984; Rozanski et al. 1988; Selwyn and Ganz 1988) and some evidence to suggest a connection between sudden death and acute disturbing life-events (Fricchione and Vlay 1986; Reich et al. 1981; Tavazzi et al. 1986). There is also good evidence that job strain affects the risk for cardiovascular disease (Alfredsson et al. 1985; Karasek et al. 1982; Lacroix and Haynes 1987) and that low levels of social support may compound this risk (Johnson and Hall 1988).

With respect to hypertension, there is considerable evidence suggesting that blood pressure reactivity is a risk factor for the development of hypertension (Pickering and Gerin 1988) and some evidence to suggest that blood pressure reactivity is a risk factor for the progression of this disease (Shapiro 1988). There is also evidence linking personality traits or coping style with both pressor reactivity and hypertension, but almost all the research is retrospective or cross-sectional in design (Houston 1986; Shapiro 1988). The relationship between psychological factors and the maintenance of hypertension is indirectly supported by evidence demonstrating the effectiveness of behavioral interventions on blood pressure control (Glasgow et al. 1989; Patel et al. 1985).

Oncology literature (Levenson and Bemis 1991). This review focused on two hypotheses: 1) that cancer onset and progression are affected by psychosocial variables, and 2) that psychological factors affect the immune system, which in turn can contribute to cancer onset and progression. Psychosocial variables examined include affective states, coping/defensive styles and personality traits, stressful life events, and the impact of psychosocial interventions on cancer outcome.

Literature was identified from reviews (Fox 1983; Holland 1989; Spiegel and Sands 1990) supplemented by *Index Medicus* and computer searches through 1989. Only reasonably well-controlled studies were included. There is both epidemiological (Shekelle et al. 1981) and clinical (Greer et al. 1979) evidence that depressive states are associated with an increased risk of cancer onset and/or progression, although a larger number of studies have not supported this relationship (Cassileth et al. 1985; Zonderman et al. 1989). Bereavement has also been considered a possible risk factor. Although most studies have not supported this, interest has been kindled by the finding that bereavement is associated with a decrement in immune function (Holland 1989; Irwin et al. 1987a). A number of studies have linked personality characteristics with cancer outcome (Temoshok et al. 1985), although again there are important negative studies (Cassileth et al. 1985; Persky et al. 1987). A number of human studies have shown increased incidence of stressful life events preceding the onset of cancer, but an equivalent number have failed to find any association (Fox 1983). One study found a relationship between stress and cancer recurrence (Ramirez et al. 1989). Some studies have documented improvement in medical and psychosocial outcome in cancer patients receiving group therapy (Fawzy et al. 1990; Grossarth-Maticek et al. 1984; Spiegel et al. 1989). Evidence of the effects of psychological factors on the immune system that in turn contribute to cancer onset and progression remains patchy (Holland 1989), but a relationship between psychosocial variables and immune function has been demonstrated in patients with cancer (Levy et al. 1987).

Nephrology literature (Levenson and Glocheski 1991).　Most psychiatric studies of end-stage renal disease have focused on the prevalence of psychiatric disorders (mainly depression) or on a comparison of the quality of life accompanying the different treatment options (e.g., hemodialysis, peritoneal dialysis, transplantation). There have been a few studies of the influence of psychological factors on the course of end-stage renal disease, nearly all focused on depression or noncompliance. There have been essentially no studies of chronic renal failure before the end stage. Literature for this review was derived from standard references in psychonephrology (Levy 1981, 1983) supplemented by computer searches covering 1984–1990. Only studies using well-established assessment measures were included.

Estimates of the prevalence of depression vary greatly because of differences in definitions and criteria used and variable potential confounding factors (Levenson and Glocheski 1991). In general, patients receiving renal transplants had better psychosocial outcomes than those receiving hemodialysis, whereas there is disagreement as to whether there are differences in quality of life on hemodialysis versus continuous ambulatory peritoneal dialysis (CAPD). All of these modality comparison studies must be interpreted with caution because patients have never been randomly assigned.

Most of the studies of the effects of psychological factors on outcome have focused on depression. Depression has been shown in at least one study to be a better predictor of (shorter) survival in dialysis patients than age or pathophysiological variables (Burton et al. 1986). This and other studies provide support for the diagnostic category "psychiatric factors affecting physical condition" (Levenson and Glocheski 1991), although negative studies have also appeared (Devins et al. 1990).

Other outcome studies have focused on the impact of noncompliance (Cummings et al. 1982; Manley and Sweeney 1986; Reiss et al. 1986). Because of methodological limitations, conclusions that one can draw from these studies are limited. The effects of noncompliance on dialysis patients' outcomes are well recognized by clinicians but have not been sufficiently characterized empirically.

There is only one published psychosocial intervention outcome study on end-stage renal disease. Patients who participated in a support group lived longer than nonparticipants, even after controlling for 13 psychosocial and physiological covariates, but this is a naturalistic, nonrandomized study (Friend et al. 1986).

Neurological illness literature (McNamara 1991).   Despite variations in methodology and changing conceptual organization, the convergence of a number of studies over decades firmly supports the association of neurological illness with certain psychological factors and significant psychiatric disorders. This review, focused on the incidence of depression, summarized the evidence from studies in four major neurological diseases: stroke, multiple sclerosis, Parkinson's disease, and epilepsy. Some observations hold true across all four disease categories. Earlier studies tended to frame questions in purely psychological terms. Factors such as loss of self-esteem, guilt, and social isolation were examined for their impact on rehabilitation and prognosis. More recent investigators have tended to focus on the depression that subsumes these factors rather than on the individual psychological components.

Older studies in the literature contain a tacit assumption that psychiatric characteristics existed independently of and were impervious to the changes in the brain produced by neurological illness. More modern research has largely dropped this posture and instead seeks, with some early success, to understand the association of psychiatric and neurological illness in terms of common pathophysiology.

■   **Stroke.**   Estimates of the incidence of depression, strongly defined by DSM-III or the Hamilton Rating Scales (Hamilton 1967), range from 26% to 48%

(Robinson and Price 1982; Robinson et al. 1984). Further, the presence of depression has been shown to be associated with poorer outcome (Robinson and Price 1982; Robinson et al. 1986). Although there are suggestive case reports and small series, there is as yet a lack of literature to show that treatment of depression improves outcome, because there is no consensus on a safe and successful method of treatment (Mayberg et al. 1988; Reding 1986).

- Multiple sclerosis. Using Research Diagnostic Criteria (Spitzer et al. 1978), Joffe et al. (1987) reported a 42% incidence of depression in a series of 100 patients. Numerous other, less detailed studies support this finding (Whitlock and Siskind 1980). Preliminary work has linked depression to both the onset and exacerbation of multiple sclerosis (Dalos et al. 1983; Homer et al. 1987), although there is some contradiction in the literature as to how depression is related to functional impairment (Schiffer 1987).

- Parkinson's disease. Depression is common in Parkinson's disease, with a prevalence of 28%–35% or higher in carefully designed studies (Mayeux et al. 1981). Low serotonin levels, a direct result of the disease, may be partly responsible (Mayeux et al. 1984, 1986). The degree of depression of motor impairment at any given time is clearly linked to mood state, and affective and cognitive dysfunction account for significant functional disability (Cantello et al. 1986; Santamaria et al. 1986).

- Epilepsy. Patients with seizures have a rate of suicide at least five times that of the general population (W. S. Matthews and Barbas 1981). Depression is common in epileptic patients, with several causes postulated, including psychological, biochemical, and anatomical etiologies, all of which have some research support (Levin et al. 1988; Mendez et al. 1986; Robertson 1989). Despite the bulk of this literature, most of the work remains preliminary.

There is a large and active body of research on the interplay of neurological and psychiatric illness. For each of the major disease categories reviewed, there is clear support for the common association of depression. Most studies have also found that depression may affect the onset, course, and prognosis of the neurological symptoms as well, stressing the importance of identifying these psychiatric factors.

Pulmonary, immunological, and rheumatological literature (Moran 1991). The review of this literature focused on three illnesses (asthma, chronic obstructive pulmonary disease [COPD], and rheumatoid arthritis) and on a number of human and animal studies within immunology. Literature was identified from recent review articles and from computerized searches. Although the paucity of controlled studies was considered a problem, it also reflected the state-of-the-art in the arenas under study.

Anxiety and stress reactions are seen as playing provocative and maintenance roles in the worsening of asthma symptoms (Tieramaa 1979, 1981). Certain defense or coping styles, especially those that have "alexithymic" or somatothymic attributes, may lead to poor awareness of symptoms, a decreased ability to report them, and thus what may appear to be noncompliance with treatment (Hudgel et al. 1982; Sharma and Nandkumar 1980). Depression may have a quite direct and pernicious effect on the asthma patient, both by affecting the ability to comply with treatment and through autonomic mechanisms (Bengtsson 1984; Friedman 1984; Knapp and Mathe 1985; Mathe and Knapp 1969; Schiavi et al. 1951).

The work on COPD emphasizes the necessity for long-term adaptive skills in both the patient and the patient's family (Agle and Baum 1977; Clark and Cochrane 1970). Thus, coping style and interpersonal disturbances play a role in the patient's perception of symptoms and in compliance (Dudley et al. 1980; Sandhu 1986). Anxiety can lead the patients to erroneously interpret their inner states as being due to pulmonary-based dyspnea; this misinterpretation can result in inappropriate or excessive use of medications (Burns and Howell 1969).

Most of the clinical research on rheumatoid arthritis centers on personality types that are associated with the most severe forms of rheumatoid arthritis (Gardiner 1980; Moos 1964; Polley et al. 1970). The difficulty in interpreting these studies involves distinguishing the psychological results of a chronic illness from the psychological antecedents of that illness (Moos 1964). Nevertheless, there is some consensus concerning the power of personality traits and coping styles to adversely affect the course of the disease. Rehabilitative efforts are also undermined by certain personality types, as is the case for COPD patients (Polley et al. 1970).

Many workers have studied stress and its effects on the immune system, and there seems to be little doubt that many immunological parameters are changed by induction of stress and probably by depressive affect (Irwin et al. 1987b; Melnechuk 1988). There are two problems with the studies reviewed. First, there is little uniformity in the types of stress induced (stress is poorly defined in many studies). The second concern is lack of consistency across studies in the timing of the immunological measurements from the point of stress induction. Because some of the perturbations induced in the immune system may be focal and potentially short-lived, certain interrelationships that could have been detected may have remained undetected (Calabrese et al. 1987; Irwin et al. 1987b; Melnechuk 1988).

Discussion

As might be predicted, an impressive body of literature, much of it based on controlled study methodologies and empirically derived data, supports the influence of psychological factors in many physical conditions. The literature in this area is still maturing in respect to methodological sophistication, and the study of psychological, psychiatric, and behavioral factors affecting physical illness is becoming more rigorous. The overall task of this committee, however, was to evaluate how revisions in the diagnostic criteria for PFAPC and its positioning in the DSM system could possibly facilitate the understanding of the relationship between psychological factors and physical illness.

First, it seems that, for purposes of both clinical and research communication, diagnostic criteria for the category should be made more rigorous if the category is to have true meaning. This would require more specificity in the diagnostic criteria as to the *types* of psychological factors involved, with the option for the clinician to designate at what phase of the patient's condition the psychological factor in question was deemed to be operative.

From the standpoint of achieving greater specificity as to the types of psychological factors involved, based on the literature review, six potential areas emerged in which psychologically related factors could affect physical illness. These areas would include formal Axis I or Axis II disorders, as well as subsyndromal emotional or psychological symptoms such as anxiety, depression, or other more nonspecific psychological phenomena (e.g., hostility, anger, or apathy). Other potential areas included the tendency for severe physiological reactions to stress, personality traits, coping, or defensive styles; behavior patterns such as high-risk health habits, noncompliance, smoking, and overeating; interpersonal dysfunction in marital or family sphere; and cultural factors affecting compliance with treatment. Based on the identification of these areas, subcategories were developed for consideration and are summarized in Table 48–2. As noted in the proposed revised criteria for PFAPC in Table 48–2, the subcategorization scheme allows the clinician to designate the primary psychological factor believed to be affecting the patient's physical condition, or, if one specific factor does not appear to predominate, the presence of "mixed" factors can be noted. If a defined Axis I disorder (e.g., major depression) is involved, this may be noted as well.

A clear conceptual departure from DSM-III and DSM-III-R (American Psychiatric Association 1987) relates to the definition of what constitutes a "psychological factor." In DSM-III-R, psychological factors were defined in regard to the individual's response to environmental stimuli. In the proposed revision, a much broader array of comorbid psychological, psychiatric, behavioral, and psychosocial factors may be designated as affecting physical conditions. Hence, the emphasis is placed on psychiatric, psychological, and behavioral *comorbidity* as it affects the course of medical illness rather than traditional psychophysiologic-based reactivity to stressful environmental stimuli. The existing literature that has examined possible relationships among psychological, behavioral, and physical disorders supports

Table 48–2. Proposed diagnostic criteria for psychological and behavioral factors (specify type of factors) affecting nonpsychiatric medical condition (as of February 13, 1991)

A. Psychological or behavioral factors adversely affect a nonpsychiatric medical condition (coded on Axis III) in one of the following ways:

    1. the factors influence the course of the nonpsychiatric medical condition (e.g., there is a close temporal association between the psychological or behavioral factors and the development, exacerbation, recovery, or stabilization of the medical condition).

    2. the factors lead to noncompliance with treatment recommendations (e.g., individual with denial of illness refusing to take medication).

    3. the factors lead to ignoring risk factors known to cause or exacerbate the medical condition.

Specify the nature of the psychological or behavioral factors (if more than one factor is present, indicate the most prominent):

F59.00   *Psychological symptoms* affecting nonpsychiatric medical condition (i.e., Axis I conditions or subthreshold anxiety and depression)

F59.01   *Personality trait* affecting nonpsychiatric medical condition (e.g., DSM-IV personality disorder or traits)

F59.02   *Defense or coping style* affecting nonpsychiatric medical condition (e.g., denial of illness, type A behavioral traits)

F59.03   *Physiologic stress reaction* affecting nonpsychiatric medical condition (e.g., exacerbation of ulcer)

F59.04   *Lifestyle factors* affecting nonpsychiatric medical condition (e.g., overeating, risk-taking sexual behavior)

F59.05   *Noncompliance* with treatment regimen affecting nonpsychiatric medical condition (e.g., refusal to take medication or lack of cooperation in taking medication; inability to understand nature of illness)

F59.06   *Cultural factors* affecting nonpsychiatric medical condition (e.g., cultural values leading to refusal or delay in seeking treatment)

F59.07   *Interpersonal disturbance* affecting nonpsychiatric medical condition (e.g., marital conflict)

F59.08   *Mixed psychological or behavioral factors* affecting nonpsychiatric medical condition

F59.09   *Unspecified psychological or behavioral factors* affecting nonpsychiatric medical condition

an emphasis on co-morbidity relationships rather than a primary psychophysiologic model (Keitner et al. 1991; Saravay et al. 1991; Wells et al. 1989).

Other Special Issues: The Problem of Noncompliance

A significant consideration for PFAPC relates to the issue of noncompliance. The issue of noncompliance was left in limbo in DSM-III-R by being relegated to a V code. The V-code description for noncompliance in DSM-III designated that the category could "be used when the focus of attention or treatment is noncompliance with medical treatment that is apparently not due to a mental disorder" (p. 360). Examples included noncompliance due to denial of illness, noncompliance due to religious beliefs, and decisions based on personal value judgments about the advantages and disadvantages of proposed treatments. The category for noncompliance in DSM-III-R was not to be used if the noncompliance was due to a mental disorder, such as schizophrenia or a psychoactive substance use disorder (American Psychiatric Association 1987). Hence, perhaps the single greatest psychologically and behaviorally determined factor that affects response to physical treatment, namely, medical noncompliance, was left in limbo in DSM-III-R, because only compliance problems *not* due to a mental disorder could be coded in the V code. No provision was made for medical noncompliance due to psychiatric and psychological factors. We agree with Skodol's conclusion that "the PFAPC category should be used in cases of non-compliance in which the clinician's judgment is that the non-compliance is due to a mental disorder" (Skodol 1989, p. 328) and incorporated noncompliance in the proposed revision.

Lifestyle Factors

Another matter of special importance to PFAPC relates to how certain lifestyle habits (overeating) and substance use disorders (nicotine addiction, alcohol dependence/abuse) should be categorized. Because adequate provision was already made for diagnosing nicotine addiction, alcohol-related syndromes, and eating disorders in the DSM, it was considered to be redundant to include these diagnoses under PFAPC. Although behavioral and lifestyle factors such as nicotine dependence, alcohol dependence, and other substance use disorders obviously affect physical conditions, there are a number of other behavioral and lifestyle factors that might affect health that were not accounted for by the DSM-III-R system. Such factors include sedentary lifestyles, a diet high in cholesterol and fats and low in fiber, sexual practices that increase risk of HIV infection and other venereal diseases, excessive exposure to sunlight, failure to use safety belts, and other risk-taking behaviors with acute and long-term deleterious health effects. Although these types of behaviors are not necessarily "psychiatric" disorders, they account for *major* "psychological" factors that affect health in the United States (Stoudemire and Hales 1991). Thus, it was proposed that these lifestyle and behavioral factors be included under the rubric of PFAPC.

Recommendations

The original options for revision of the PFAPC category noted in the first part of this report are now considered in more detail.

Option 1: Allow the category to stand as is without change: Based on this review of PFAPC, it is evident that some changes are needed in this category. This is reflected in the opinion of the experts surveyed and the almost nonexistent use of the category for clinical and research purposes. The primary issue revolved around *how* it should be changed.

Option 2: Discard the category: Primarily on theoretical grounds, a few experts recommended discarding the diagnosis, but this was a minority opinion. The option to utilize an "adjustment disorders" category, particularly a proposed category of "adjustment disorder with pathological denial," was also recommended. The PFAPC category, however, should embrace a much *broader* array of psychological, psychiatric, and behavioral factors, and not all situations in which such an interaction exists between psychological and behavioral factors would comprise an adjustment disorder as defined in DSM-III-R. Hence, relying on the adjustment disorders category to denote relationships with psychological factors and physical conditions did not appear to be a viable solution.

Option 3: Retain and revise the category with more specific diagnostic criteria: There was considerable support for improving the category with more rigorous diagnostic criteria. Although the details of the types of psychological factors that would be coded in the subcategorization scheme were subject to debate, it was felt that a more systematized approach to diagnosis would bring greater rigor to this category and result in it being more clinically useful, especially to primary-care providers.

Option 4: Select an alternative name for the category: Because the term *PFAPC* was considered cumbersome by many experts, it was proposed that another term be chosen for the category that would be more efficient. To embrace the broadest range of factors that could potentially affect physical health, the term *psychological and behavioral factors affecting medical condition* was proposed. In using the diagnosis, clinicians would then select from the subcategories of psychological/behavioral factors the items they considered most predominant. Hence, if a patient's denial of illness was interfering with medical treatment, item 59.02 (see Table 48–2) would be selected, and the clinician would write "defense or coping style affecting medical condition."

Placement of PFAPC in the DSM-IV Text

Along with several other conditions and syndromes that are not formal "mental disorders" as such, consideration is being given to placing the PFAPC category in a separate section of the DSM-IV text titled "other clinically significant conditions that may be a focus of diagnosis and treatment." Other syndromes and conditions included in this section would be sleep disorders and pain syndromes. Several clinicians and researchers have been concerned that this will relegate the PFAPC category to the equivalent of the former V codes and may jeopardize reimbursement and formal recognition of these conditions as being legitimate conditions for psychiatric treatment. The placement of PFAPC in the DSM-IV system and particularly in the "other clinically significant conditions" section of the manual remains a source of concern to many.

Conclusion

It remains to be seen whether the currently proposed modifications for the PFAPC category in DSM-IV will result in greater utility and broader application of this category in clinical practice and research settings. It is hoped, however, that as conceptually problematic as the issue of relating psychological and physical factors remains, the new criteria will result in enhanced recognition of and interest in such interactions.

References

Agle DP, Baum GL: Psychological aspects of chronic obstructive pulmonary disease. Med Clin North Am 61:749–758, 1977

Alexander F: Psychosomatic Medicine. New York, WW Norton, 1950

Alexander F: Psychosomatic Medicine: Its Principles and Applications. New York, WW Norton, 1987

Alfredsson L, Spetz CL, Theorell T: Type of occupation and near-future hospitalization for myocardial infarction and some other diagnoses. Int J Epidemiol 14:378–388, 1985

American Psychiatric Association: Diagnostic and Statistical Manual of Mental Disorders, 2nd Edition. Washington, DC, American Psychiatric Association, 1968

American Psychiatric Association: Diagnostic and Statistical Manual of Mental Disorders, 3rd Edition. Washington, DC, American Psychiatric Association, 1980

American Psychiatric Association: Diagnostic and Statistical Manual of Mental Disorders, 3rd Edition, Revised. Washington, DC, American Psychiatric Association, 1987

Arapakis G, Lyketsos CG, Gerolymatos K, et al: Low dominance and high intropunitiveness in ulcerative colitis and irritable bowel syndrome. Psychother Psychosom 46:171–176, 1986

Avery D, Winokur G: Mortality in depressed patients treated with electroconvulsive therapy and antidepressants. Arch Gen Psychiatry 33:1129–1037, 1976

Barefoot JC, Dahlstrom WC, Williams RB: Hostility, CHD incidence and total mortality: a 25-year follow-up study of 255 physicians. Psychosom Med 45:59–63, 1983

Barefoot JC, Dodge KA, Peterson BL, et al: The Cook-Medley hostility scale: item content and ability to predict survival. Psychosom Med 51:46–57, 1989

Beardsley G, Goldstein MG: Psychological factors affecting physical condition: endocrine disease literature review. Psychosomatics 34:12–19, 1993

Bengtsson U: Emotions and asthma I. European Journal of Respiratory Diseases (suppl) 136:123–129, 1984

Burns BH, Howell JBL: Disproportionately severe breathlessness in chronic bronchitis. Q J Med 38:277–294, 1969

Burton HJ, Kline SA, Lindsay RM, et al: The relationship of depression to survival in chronic renal failure. Psychosom Med 48:261–258, 1986

Calabrese JR, Kling MA, Gold PW: Alterations in immunocompetence during stress, bereavement, and depression: focus on neuroendocrine regulation. Am J Psychiatry 144:1123–1134, 1987

Cantello R, Gilli M, Riccio A, et al: Mood changes associated with "end-of-dose deterioration" in Parkinson's disease: a controlled investigation. J Neurol Neurosurg Psychiatry 49:1182–1190, 1986

Carney RM, Rich MW, Freedland KE, et al: Major depressive disorder predicts cardiac events in patients with coronary artery disease. Psychosom Med 50:627–633, 1988

Cassileth BR, Lusk EJ, Miller DS, et al: Psychological correlates of survival in advanced malignant disease? N Engl J Med 312:1551–1555, 1985

Clark RJH, Cochrane GM: Effect of personality on alveolar ventilation in patients with chronic airways obstruction. BMJ 1:273–275, 1970

Cobb S, Rose RM: Hypertension, peptic ulcer and diabetes in air traffic controllers. JAMA 224:489–492, 1973

Creed F, Guthrie E: Psychological factors in the irritable bowel syndrome. Gut 28:1307–1318, 1987

Cummings K, Becker M, Kirscht J, et al: Psychosocial factors affecting adherence to medical regimens in a group of hemodialysis patients. Med Care 20:567–580, 1982

Dalos NP, Rabins PV, Brook BR, et al: Disease activity and emotional state in multiple sclerosis. Ann Neurol 13:573–577, 1983

Darrow WW, Echenberg DF, Jaffe HW, et al: Risk factors for human immunodeficiency virus (HIV) infection in homosexual men. Am J Public Health 77:479–483, 1987

Deanfield JE, Kensett M, Wilson RA, et al: Silent myocardial ischemia due to mental stress. Lancet 2:1001–1004, 1984

Devins GM, Mann J, Mandin H, et al: Psychosocial predictors of survival in end-stage renal disease. J Nerv Ment Dis 178:127–133, 1990

Dudley DL, Glaser EM, Jorgenson B, et al: Psychosocial concomitants to rehabilitation in chronic obstructive pulmonary disease, part 1: psychosocial and psychological considerations. Chest 77:413–420, 1980

Elliot DL, Goldberg L, Girard DE: Obesity: pathophysiology and practical management. J Gen Intern Med 2:188–198, 1987

Engel WD: Dermatologic disorders, in Psychosomatic Illness Review. Edited by Dorfman W, Cristofar L. New York, Macmillan, 1985, pp 146–161

Faulstich ME, Williamson DA: An overview of atopic dermatitis: toward a biobehavioral integration. J Psychosom Res 29:415–417, 1985

Fava GA, Perini GI, Santonastaso P, et al: Life events and psychological distress in dermatologic disorders: psoriasis, chronic urticaria and fungal infections. Br J Med Psychol 53:277–282, 1980

Fawzy FI, Cousins N, Fawzy WW, et al: A structured psychiatric intervention for cancer patients, I: changes over time in methods of coping and affective disturbance. Arch Gen Psychiatry 47:720–725, 1990

Feldman M, Walker P, Green JL, et al: Life events, stress and psychosocial factors in men with peptic ulcer disease: a multidimensional case-controlled study. Gastroenterology 91:1370–1379, 1986

Fielding JE: Smoking: health effects and control (first of two parts). N Engl J Med 313:491–498, 1985

Folks DB, Kinney FC: The role of psychological factors in dermatologic conditions. Psychosomatics 33:45–54, 1992a

Folks DG, Kinney FC: The role of psychological factors in gastrointestinal conditions: a review pertinent to DSM-IV. Psychosomatics 33:257–270, 1992b

Foster WR, Burton BT: Introduction: health implications of obesity. Ann Intern Med 103:981–982, 1985

Fox BH: Current theory of psychogenic effects on cancer incidence and prognosis. Journal of Psychosocial Oncology 1:17–31, 1983

French-Belgian Cooperative Group: Ischemic heart disease and psychological patterns: prevalence and incidence studies in Belgium and France. Adv Cardiol 29:25–31, 1982

Fricchione GL, Vlay SC: Psychiatric aspects of patients with malignant ventricular arrhythmias. Am J Psychiatry 143:1518–1526, 1986

Friedman MS: Psychological factors associated with pediatric asthma death: a review. J Asthma 21:97–117, 1984

Friend R, Singletary Y, Mendell N, et al: Group participation and survival among patients with end-stage renal disease. Am J Public Health 76:670–672, 1986

Gardiner BM: Psychological aspects of rheumatoid arthritis. Psychol Med 10:159–163, 1980

Garfinkel L: Overweight and cancer. Ann Intern Med 103:1034–1036, 1985

Gendel BR, Benjamin JE: Psychogenic factors in the etiology of diabetes. N Engl J Med 234:556–560, 1946

Glasgow MS, Engel BT, D'Lugoff BC: A controlled trial of a standardized behavioral stepped treatment for hypertension. Psychosom Med 51:10–26, 1989

Goldstein MG, Niaura R: Psychological factors affecting physical condition: cardiovascular disease literature review, I: coronary artery disease and sudden death. Psychosomatics 33:134–145, 1992

Greer S, Morris T, Pettingale KW: Psychological response to breast cancer: effect on outcome. Lancet 2:785–787, 1979

Grossarth-Maticek R, Schmidt P, Veter H, et al: Psychotherapy research in oncology, in Health Care and Human Behavior. Edited by Steptoe A, Mathews A. London, Academic Press, 1984

Gupta MA, Gupta AK, Haberman HF: Psoriasis and psychiatry: an update. Gen Hosp Psychiatry 9:157–166, 1987

Gupta MA, Gupta AK, Kirkby S, et al: A psychocutaneous profile of psoriasis patients who are stress reactors. Gen Hosp Psychiatry 11:166–173, 1989

Hamilton M: Development of a rating scale for primary depressive illness. British Journal of Social and Clinical Psychology 6:278–296, 1967

Hanson CL, Henggeler SW, Burghen GA: Social competence and parental support as mediators of the link between stress and metabolic control in adolescents with insulin dependent diabetes mellitus. J Consult Clin Psychol 55:529–533, 1987

Haynes SG, Feinleib M, Kannel WB: The relationship of psychosocial factors to coronary heart disease in the Framingham study, III: eight-year incidence of coronary heart disease. Am J Epidemiol 111:37–58, 1980

Helz JW, Templeton B: Evidence of the role of psychosocial factors in diabetes mellitus: a review. Am J Psychiatry 147:1275–1282, 1990

Holland JC: Behavioral and psychosocial risk factors in cancer: human studies, in Handbook of Psychooncology. Edited by Holland JC, Rowland JH. New York, Oxford University Press, 1989, pp 705–726

Homer WG, Hurwitz T, Li DKB, et al: Temporal lobe involvement in multiple sclerosis patients with psychiatric disorders. Arch Neurol 44:187–190, 1987

Houston BK: Psychological variables and cardiovascular and neuroendocrine reactivity, in Handbook of Stress, Reactivity, and Cardiovascular Disease. Edited by Matthews KA, Weiss SM, Detre T, et al. New York, Wiley, 1986, pp 207–229

Hudgel DW, Cooperson DM, Kinsman RA: Recognition of added resistive loads in asthma: the importance of behavioral styles. Am Rev Respir Dis 126:121–125, 1982

Irwin M, Daniels M, Weiner H: Immune and neuroendocrine changes during bereavement. Psychiatr Clin North Am 10:449–465, 1987a

Irwin M, Daniels M, Bloom ET, et al: Life events, depressive symptoms, and immune function. Am J Psychiatry 144:437–441, 1987b

Jacobson AM, Hauser ST, Wolfsdorf JI, et al: Psychological predictors of compliance in children with recent onset of diabetes mellitus. J Pediatr 110:805–811, 1987

Joffe RT, Lippert GP, Gray TA, et al: Mood disorder and multiple sclerosis. Arch Neurol 44:376–378, 1987

Johnson JV, Hall EM: Job strain, work place social support, and cardiovascular disease: a cross-sectional study of a random sample of the Swedish working population. Am J Public Health 78:1336–1342, 1988

Kannel WB: New perspectives on cardiovascular disease. Am Heart J 114:213–219, 1987

Karasek RA, Theorell TG, Schwartz J, et al: Job, psychological factors and coronary heart disease: Swedish prospective findings and U.S. prevalence findings using a new occupational inference method. Adv Cardiol 29:62–87, 1982

Keitner GI, Ryan CE, Miller IW, et al: 12-Month outcome of patients with major depression and comorbid psychiatric or medical illness (compound depression). Am J Psychiatry 148:345–350, 1991

Kemmer FW, Bisping R, Steingruber HJ, et al: Psychological stress and metabolic control in patients with type I diabetes mellitus. N Engl J Med 314:1078–1084, 1986

Knapp PII, Mathe AA: Psychophysiologic aspects of bronchial asthma: a review, in Bronchial Asthma: Mechanisms and Therapeutics. Edited by Weiss EB, Segal MS, Stein M. Boston, MA, Little, Brown, 1985, pp 914–931

Kral JG: Morbid obesity and related health risks. Ann Intern Med 103:1043–1047, 1985

Krantz DS, Manuck SB: Acute psychophysiologic reactivity and risk of cardiovascular disease: a review and methodologic critique. Psychol Bull 96:435–464, 1984

Lacroix AZ, Haynes SG: Gender differences in the stressfulness of workplace roles: a focus on work and health, in Gender and Stress. Edited by Barnett R, Baruch G, Biener L. New York, Free Press, 1987, pp 96–121

Leon AS, Connett J, Jacobs DR, et al: Leisure-time physical activity levels and risk of coronary heart disease and death: the Multiple Risk Factor Intervention Trial. JAMA 258:2388–2395, 1987

Levenson JL, Bemis C: The role of psychological factors in cancer onset and progression. Psychosomatics 32:124–132, 1991

Levenson JL, Glocheski S: Psychological factors affecting end-stage renal disease. Psychosomatics 32:382–389, 1991

Levin R, Banks S, Berg B: Psychosocial dimensions of epilepsy: a review of the literature. Epilepsia 209:805–816, 1988

Levy NB (ed): Psychonephrology 1: Psychological Factors in Hemodialysis and Transplantation. New York, Plenum, 1981

Levy NB (ed): Psychonephrology 2: Psychological Problems in Kidney Failure and Their Treatment. New York, Plenum, 1983

Levy S, Herberman R, Lippman M, et al: Correlation of stress factors with sustained depression of natural killer activity and predicted prognosis in patients with breast cancer. J Clin Oncol 5:348–353, 1987

Linn L, Spitzer RL: DSM-III, implications for liaison psychiatry and psychosomatic medicine. JAMA 247:3207–3209, 1982

Linn MW, Linn BS, Skyler JS, et al: Stress and immune function in diabetes mellitus. Clin Immunol Immunopathol 27:223–233, 1983

Looney JG, Lipp MR, Spitzer RL: A new method of classification for psychophysiologic disorders. Am J Psychiatry 135:304–308, 1978

Manley M, Sweeney J: Assessment of compliance in hemodialysis adaptation. J Psychosom Res 30:153–161, 1986

Manuck SB, Krantz DW: Psychophysiologic reactivity in coronary heart disease and essential hypertension, in Handbook of Stress, Reactivity, and Cardiovascular Disease. Edited by Matthews KA, Weiss SM, Detre T, et al. New York, Wiley, 1986, pp 11–34

Mathe AA, Knapp PH: Decreased plasma free fatty acids and urinary epinephrine in bronchial asthma. N Engl J Med 281:234–238, 1969

Matthews KA, Glass DC, Rosenman RH, et al: Competitive drive, pattern A, and coronary heart disease: a further analysis of some data from the Western Collaborative Group Study. Journal of Chronic Diseases 30:489–498, 1977

Matthews WS, Barbas G: Suicide and epilepsy: a review of the literature. Psychosomatics 22:515–524, 1981

Mayberg HS, Robinson RG, Wond DF, et al: PET imaging of cortical S2 serotonin receptors after stroke: lateralized changes and relationship to depression. Am J Psychiatry 145:937–943, 1988

Mayeux R, Stern Y, Rosen J, et al: Depression, intellectual impairment, and Parkinson's disease. Neurology 31:645–650, 1981

Mayeux R, Stern Y, Cote L, et al: Altered serotonin metabolism in depressed patients in Parkinson's disease. Neurology 34:642–646, 1984

Mayeux R, Stern Y, Williams JB, et al: Clinical and biochemical features of depression in Parkinson's disease. Am J Psychiatry 143:757–759, 1986

McNamara ME: Psychological factors affecting neurological conditions: depression and stroke, multiple sclerosis, Parkinson's disease, and epilepsy. Psychosomatics 32:255–267, 1991

Melnechuk T: Emotions, brain, immunity, and health: a review, in Emotions and Psychopathology. Edited by Clynes M, Panksepp A. New York, Plenum, 1988, pp 88–107

Mendez MF, Cumming JL, Benson F: Depression in epilepsy. Arch Neurol 43:766–770, 1986

Moos RH: Personality factors associated with rheumatoid arthritis: a review. Journal of Chronic Diseases 17:41–55, 1964

Moran MG: Psychological factors affecting pulmonary and rheumatologic diseases. Psychosomatics 32:14–23, 1991

Murphy JM, Monson PR, Olivier DC, et al: Affective disorders and mortality: a general population study. Arch Gen Psychiatry 44:473–480, 1987

National Institutes of Health Consensus Development Panel on the Health Implications of Obesity. Health implications of obesity: National Institutes of Health Consensus Development Conference Statement. Ann Intern Med 103:1073–1077, 1985

Niaura R, Goldstein MG: Psychological factors affecting physical condition: cardiovascular disease literature review, II: coronary artery disease, sudden death, and hypertension. Psychosomatics 33:146–155, 1992

North CS, Clouse RE, Spitznagel EL, et al: The relation of ulcerative colitis to psychiatric factors: a review of findings and methods. Am J Psychiatry 147:974–981, 1986

Nunes EV, Frank KA, Kornfeld DS: Psychologic treatment for the type A behavior pattern and for coronary heart disease: a meta analysis of the literature. Psychosom Med 48:159–173, 1987

Osray EM, Turnbull TL, Dunne M, et al: Prospective study of the effect of safety belts on morbidity and health care costs in motor vehicle accidents. JAMA 252:2571–2575, 1988

Paffenbarger RS Jr, Hyde RT, Wing AL, et al: Physical activity, all-cause mortality, and the longevity of college alumni. N Engl J Med 314:605–613, 1986

Patel C, Marmot MG, Terry DJ, et al: Trial of relaxation in reducing coronary risk: four year follow-up. BMJ 290:1102–1106, 1985

Persky VW, Kempthorne-Rawson J, Shekelle RP: Personality and risk of cancer: 20-year follow-up of the Western Electric Study. Psychosom Med 49:435–449, 1987

Pickering TG, Gerin W: Ambulatory blood pressure monitoring and cardiovascular reactivity for the evaluation of the role of psychosocial factors and prognosis in hypertensive patients. Am Heart J 116:665–672, 1988

Polley HF, Swenson WN, Steinhilber R: Personality characteristics of patients with rheumatoid arthritis. Psychosomatics 11:45–49, 1970

Ramirez AJ, Craig TK, Watson JP, et al: Stress and relapse of breast cancer. BMJ 298:291–293, 1989

Reding R: Antidepressants after stroke. Arch Neurol 43:762–765, 1986

Reich P, DeSilva RA, Lown B, et al: Acute psychological disturbances preceding life-threatening ventricular arrhythmias. JAMA 246:233–235, 1981

Reiss D, Gonzalez S, Kramer N: Family process, chronic illness, and death. Arch Gen Psychiatry 43:795–804, 1986

Robertson MM: The organic contribution to depressive illness in patients with epilepsy. J Epilepsy 2:189–230, 1989

Robinson N, Fuller JH: Role of life events and difficulties in the onset of diabetes mellitus. J Psychosom Res 29:583–591, 1985

Robinson RG, Price TR: Post-stroke depressive disorders: a follow-up of 103 patients. Stroke 13:635–641, 1982

Robinson RG, Star LB, Price TR, et al: A two year longitudinal study of mood disorders following stroke, prevalence and duration at 6 months follow-up. Br J Psychiatry 144:256–262, 1984

Robinson RG, Bolla-Wilson K, Kaplan E, et al: Depression influences intellectual impairment in stroke patients. Br J Psychiatry 148:541–547, 1986

Rosenberg L, Kaufman DW, Helmrich SP, et al: The risk of myocardial infarction after quitting smoking in men under 55 years of age. N Engl J Med 313:1511–1514, 1985

Rosenman RH, Brand RJ, Jenkins CD, et al: Coronary heart disease in the Western Collaborative Group Study: final follow-up experience of eight and one-half years. JAMA 233:872–877, 1975

Rovet J, Ehrlich RM: Effect of temperament on metabolic control in children with diabetes mellitus. Diabetes Care 11:77–82, 1988

Rozanski A, Bairey CN, Krantz DS, et al: Mental stress and the induction of silent myocardial ischemia in patients with coronary artery disease. N Engl J Med 318:1005–1012, 1988

Sandhu HS: Psychosocial issues in chronic obstructive pulmonary disease. Clin Chest Med 7:642–649, 1986

Santamaria J, Tolosa E, Valles A: Parkinson's disease with depression: a possible subgroup of idiopathic parkinsonism. Neurology 36:1130–1133, 1986

Saravay SM, Steinberg MD, Weinschel B, et al: Psychological comorbidity and length of stay in the general hospital. Am J Psychiatry 148:324–329, 1991

Schiavi R, Stein M, Sethi BB: Respiratory variables in response to a pain-fear stimulus and in experimental asthma. Psychosom Med 13:254–261, 1951

Schiffer RB: The spectrum of depression multiple sclerosis. Arch Neurol 44:596–599, 1987

Selwyn AP, Ganz P: Myocardial ischemia in coronary disease. N Engl J Med 318:1058–1060, 1988

Shapiro AP: Psychological factors in hypertension: an overview. Am Heart J 116:632–637, 1988

Sharma S, Nandkumar VK: Personality structure and adjustment pattern in bronchial asthma. Acta Psychiatr Scand 61:81–88, 1980

Shekelle RB, Raynor WJ Jr, Ostfeld AM, et al: Psychological depression and 17-year risk of death from cancer. Psychosom Med 43:117– 125, 1981

Shekelle RB, Gale M, Ostfield A, et al: Hostility, risk of coronary heart disease and mortality. Psychosom Med 45:109–114, 1983

Skodol AE: Problems in Differential Diagnosis: From DSM-III to DSM-III-R in Clinical Practice. Washington, DC, American Psychiatric Press, 1989

Spiegel D, Sands SH: Psychological influences on metastatic disease progression, in Progressive States of Malignant Neoplastic Growth. Edited by Kaiser HE. Dordrecht, Netherlands, Martinus Nijhoff, 1990, pp 246–284

Spiegel P, Bloom JR, Kraemer HC, et al: Effects of psychosocial treatment on survival of patients with metastatic breast cancer. Lancet 2:888–891, 1989

Spitzer RL, Endicott J, Robins E: Research Diagnostic Criteria: rationale and reliability. Arch Gen Psychiatry 35:773–782, 1978

Stoudemire A, Hales RE: Psychological and behavioral factors affecting medical conditions and DSM-IV: an overview. Psychosomatics 32:5–13, 1991

Tavazzi L, Zotti AM, Rondanelli R: The role of psychologic stress in the genesis of lethal arrhythmias in patients with coronary artery disease. Eur Heart J 7 (suppl A):99–106, 1986

Temoshok L, Heller BW, Sagebiel RW, et al: The relationship of psychosocial factors to prognostic indicators in cutaneous malignant melanoma. J Psychosom Res 29:139–153, 1985

Tieraamaa E: Psychic factors and the inception of asthma. J Psychosom Res 23:253–262, 1979

Tieraamaa E: Psychosocial factors, personality, and acute-insidious onset asthma. J Psychosom Res 25:43–49, 1981

U.S. Department of Health and Human Services: The Health Consequence of Smoking: Cardiovascular Disease: A Report of the Surgeon General (Publ No DHHS-PHS-84-50204). Rockville, MD, U.S. Department of Health and Human Services, Public Health Service, Office on Smoking and Health, 1983

U.S. Department of Health and Human Services: The Health Consequence of Smoking: Cancer: A Report of the Surgeon General. Rockville, MD, U.S. Department of Health and Human Services, Public Health Service, Office on Smoking and Health, 1984

U.S. Department of Health and Human Services: The Surgeon General's Report on Nutrition and Health (Publ No DHHS-PHS-88-50210). Washington, DC, U.S. Government Printing Office, 1988a

U.S. Department of Health and Human Services: The Health Consequence of Smoking: Nicotine Addiction: A Report of the Surgeon General. Rockville, MD, U.S. Department of Health and Human Services, Public Health Service, Office on Smoking and Health, 1988b

U.S. Department of Health and Human Services: The Health Consequence of Smoking: Reducing the Health Consequences of Smoking: 25 Years of Progress: A Report of the Surgeon General. Rockville, MD, U.S. Department of Health and Human Services, Public Health Service, Office on Smoking and Health, 1989

U.S. Preventive Services Task Force Guide to Clinical Preventive Services. Baltimore, MD, Williams & Wilkins, 1989

Van Moffaert M: Psychosomatics for the practicing dermatologist. Dermatologica 165:73–87, 1982

Wadden TA, Stunkard AJ: Social and psychological consequences of obesity. Ann Intern Med 103:1062–1067, 1985

Walker EA, Roy-Byrne PP, Katon WJ: Irritable bowel syndrome and psychiatric illness. Am J Psychiatry 174:565–572, 1990

Weiner H: Psychobiology and Human Disease. New York, Elsevier, 1977

Wells KB, Stewart A, Hays RD, et al: The functioning and well-being of depressed patients: results from the medical outcome study. JAMA 262:914–919, 1989

Whitlock FA, Siskind MM: Depression as a major symptom of multiple sclerosis. J Neurol Neurosurg Psychiatry 43:861–865, 1980

Winkelstein W, Lyman DM, Padian N, et al: Sexual practices and risk of infection by the human immunodeficiency virus: the San Francisco men's health study. JAMA 257:321–325, 1987

Zonderman AB, Costa PT Jr, McCrae RR: Depression as a risk for cancer morbidity and mortality in a nationally representative sample. JAMA 262:1191–1195, 1989

Section VI

Sexual Disorders

Introduction to Section VI

Sexual Disorders

Chester W. Schmidt, Jr., M.D., Raul C. Schiavi, M.D.,
Leslie R. Schover, Ph.D., R. Taylor Segraves, M.D., and
Thomas N. Wise, M.D.

The purpose of this introduction is to provide an executive summary of the proceedings and results of the DSM-IV Work Group on Sexual Disorders, to address any proposals/options that were not covered by a literature review, and to address any inconsistencies between the recommendations of the literature review and the *DSM-IV Options Book* (Task Force on DSM-IV 1991). Issues identified for each criteria set are reviewed, and the rationale of the recommended changes for DSM-IV is discussed.

Methods

The recommendations incorporated in the *DSM-IV Options Book* were derived from literature review papers developed for diagnostic terms within the sexual disorders section. These papers were constructed as follows: 1) a statement of the issues identified for each diagnosis, 2) an elaboration of the significance of those issues, 3) a description of the methods used to study the issues raised, 4) a summary of the results of the studies, 5) a discussion developing the rationale that led to the recommendations, and 6) a statement of the specific recommendations being made. Literature reviews were designed to compile available data on each of the diagnostic issues identified. Reviews included Medline search, Psychological Abstracts, and PsycInfo. Journals reviewed by hand included *Archives of Sexual Behavior, Journal of Sex Research, Journal of Sex and Marital Therapy, British Journal of Sexual Medicine, American Journal of Psychiatry, Journal of Nervous and Mental Disease, Psychosomatic Medicine, Journal of Sex Education and Therapy,* and *Marriage and the Family.* Some unpublished data sets were also used. The initial diagnostic issues were developed during a series of meetings of the Sexual Disorders Work Group. Members of the Work Group then worked on their individual sections and, over a series of months, developed the papers following the format described above.

In general, the Work Group found limited published data supporting the current diagnoses and criteria sets. In addition, the reviews revealed that investigators frequently do not use the criteria sets in DSM-III-R (American Psychiatric Association 1987) in their research methodology. As a result, the Work Group, following the mandate of the DSM-IV Task Force that recommended changes in DSM-IV must be data based, has suggested relatively few major changes for the sexual disorders section of DSM-IV. Several recommendations are made for the purpose of enhancing the compatibility of DSM-IV with ICD-10 (World Health Organization 1990). In addition, it is proposed that a new criterion be added to the criteria sets for all sexual dysfunctions: "The disturbance causes marked distress or interpersonal difficulty." The purpose of this new criterion is to establish the clinical significance of the dysfunction. This addition is not supported by a literature review but is being added at the recommendation of the DSM-IV Task Force with the agreement of the Sexual Disorders Work Group. Finally, it is proposed that two new criteria sets be added to the section on sexual dysfunctions: secondary sexual dysfunction due to a nonpsychiatric medical condition and substance-induced sexual dysfunction. The rationale for this addition is described in the chapter by Popkin and Tucker (1994) on mental disorders due to a general medical condition and substance-induced disorders in the first volume of the *DSM-IV Sourcebook*.

Historical Perspective

In DSM-II (American Psychiatric Association 1968), psychological problems associated with menstruation, micturition, and psychosexual problems were grouped together as psychophysiological genitourinary disorders. Before DSM-III (American Psychiatric Association 1980), clinicians employed various diagnostic systems for psychosexual disorders including those of Masters and Johnson (1970), who described a four-stage model of excitement, plateau, orgasm, and resolution, and Kaplan (1974a), who described a biphasic model of excitement and orgasm. The response cycle was modified when Kaplan (1974b) introduced a three-stage model of desire, excitement, and orgasm. DSM-III incorporated an amalgam of these concepts, creating separate diagnoses for inhibited sexual excitement, inhibited sexual desire, and inhibited orgasm. The assumption of male-female similarities in sexual response also played a major role in DSM-III and DSM-III-R. DSM-III-R was modified by the addition of a sexual aversion disorder, and inhibited sexual excitement was subdivided into female arousal disorder and male erectile disorder, partially abandoning the theoretical model of male-female similarities. The point of this historical review is to highlight the diagnostic turmoil and progress in this new arena of psychiatric inquiry and to stress the relative "newness" of the terminology and the theoretical assumptions that underlie the bases for the development of the criteria sets.

Sexual Dysfunctions

Sexual Desire Disorders

Hypoactive sexual desire disorder. Three issues associated with the criteria set for hypoactive sexual desire disorder are addressed by Schiavi in Chapter 49:

1. Is there empirical evidence that may assist in the formulation of more precise diagnostic criteria for this dysfunction?
2. Are there data that may permit operationalizing this diagnosis such as frequency criteria for fantasy, desire, and behavior?
3. Is there evidence for the formation of subcategories of patients with hypoactive sexual desire disorder?

Reviews revealed a paucity of empirical information on sexual desire disorders. Only a few investigators have focused on the topic, and even fewer studies have used DSM-III or DSM-III-R criteria for subject selection. The Sexual Disorders Work Group supports Schiavi's recommendation that there be no changes in the current criteria set for hypoactive sexual desire disorder aside from the additions of the new criterion C ("Not due to a substance-induced [i.e., drugs, medication] or a secondary sexual dysfunction") and the new criterion D ("The disturbance causes marked distress or interpersonal difficulty"). This recommendation is based on the concern that the field might be thrown into confusion with changes in criteria sets that are not supported by data. Future research might focus on defining the criteria to include the seeking out of sexual cues (or awareness of sexual cues) and developing operational criteria for frequency of sexual desire or activity, both of which would have the merit of providing objective diagnostic guidelines and of being more congruent with ICD-10.

Sexual aversion disorder. The issue identified was, "Is there systematic, empirically gathered information on the clinical utility, validity, and reliability of broader versus narrower criteria for sexual aversion disorder?" Based on the findings of only two data-oriented studies, the evidence does not support narrowing the diagnosis of sexual aversion disorder to include individuals with aversions limited to one or a few components of sexual interaction. The only recommendation is the addition of criterion C, "The disturbance causes marked distress or interpersonal difficulty."

Sexual Arousal Disorders

Female sexual arousal disorder. The issues raised by Segraves in Chapter 50 focused on the existing criteria set, which includes a combination of objective and subjective symptoms. Segraves was concerned about the vagueness of the criteria set and the extent of clinical judgment required to make a diagnosis. He noted that requiring either subjective or objective symptoms presupposes two response systems that are correlated and constitute part of the same syndrome. The literature reviews produced scant support for determining whether the subjective and objective criteria are part of the same syndrome. A second literature review was carried out in which the issue was restated to ask whether there is research evidence to support the existing diagnosis and criteria set. Again, Segraves found limited data, with the best data coming from an unpublished data set. Based on the available data, he proposed three alternative recommendations: 1) deletion of the term, 2) retention of the term as is, and 3) modification of the diagnostic term to agree with ICD-10. Segraves recommended retention of the diagnostic term as is to limit further research confusion with the hope that investigators would tackle the challenge and develop empirically based data to support diagnostic criteria sets. The Work Group, however, supported the elimination of the subjective component of the DSM-III-R criteria so that the DSM-IV criteria would be compatible with the terminology in ICD-10. Thus, the Work Group recommends that the subjective component, "persistent or recurrent lack of subjective sense of sexual excitement and pleasure in a female during sexual activity" be eliminated from the criteria set. Criterion A would then read "persistent or recurrent inability to attain or maintain an adequate lubrication swelling response of sexual excitement until completion of sexual activity." For compatibility with ICD-10, it is recommended that the words "partial or complete" be removed, the word "failure" be changed to "inability," and the word "adequate" be added to the phrase "adequate lubrication swelling response." The DSM-IV Task Force also recommended that an expanded criterion B ("Does not occur exclusively during the course of another Axis I disorder [other than a sexual dysfunction] such as major depressive disorder, and is not due to a substance-induced [i.e., drugs, medication] or secondary sexual dysfunction") and a new criterion C ("The disturbance causes marked distress or interpersonal difficulty") be added.

Male erectile disorder. In Chapter 51, Segraves identifies two issues in this criteria set: 1) the diagnosis may be made on the basis of either objective or subjective symptoms, and 2) the definition of the objective criterion is made broad by using the terms *persistent, recurrent partial,* and *complete* failure. The concern about the objective and subjective symptoms was the same as noted for female arousal disorder. The broad definition of erectile failure raises questions about the ability of investigators to select homogeneous sets and subsets for studies. Literature reviews found no evidence that the subjective criterion is ever used to make the diagnosis of the disorder. In addition, there was no data set to support a more precise definition of the disorder with regard to the issue of genital failure. Literature reviews were also completed to address the issues of duration and frequency criteria. The reviews did not produce data sufficient to make specific recommendations. Segraves therefore recommended no change in the criteria. He pointed out that further changes might create confusion for future investigators. The Work Group, however, believed Segraves's work supported the proposed option to return to the DSM-III wording by deleting the subjective criterion. They also recommended narrowing the objective criteria to conform to ICD-10. The DSM-IV Task Force recommended that an expanded criterion B and a new criterion C be added as they were for female sexual arousal disorder.

Orgasm Disorders

Female orgasmic disorder (inhibited female orgasm). In Chapter 52, Schover identified three issues associated with this diagnostic term: 1) the name of the disorder, which suggests it is the result of psychological inhibition; 2) the circular reasoning of the criteria set (i.e., that one may only be able to judge the correctness of the diagnosis by the success of the treatment plan it generates); and 3) whether there are subtypes of orgasmic disorders. Literature reviews revealed that *orgasmic disorder* and *orgasmic dysfunction* were the terms used most frequently in recent years to specify orgasm phase disorder. The assumption of a psychological inhibition of the reflex as causal to the disorder was not supported by literature reviews. Few studies used the term *inhibited female orgasm.* On the basis of the reviews and to be compatible with ICD-10, the name "female orgasmic disorder" was recommended. With regard to the existing criteria, Schover's reviews suggested that the criteria should take into account evidence of the range of sexual stimulation that triggers orgasm and the fact that women's ability to reach orgasm increases with both age and sexual experience. These findings led to Schover's recommendation (supported by the Work Group) that certain wording in criterion A be deleted and that the following wording for criterion A be adopted: "Persistent or recurrent delay in, or absence of, orgasm following a normal sexual excitement phase. Women exhibit wide variability in the type or intensity of stimulation that triggers orgasm. The diagnosis of female orgasmic disorder should be based on the clinician's judgment that the woman's orgasmic capacity is less than would be reasonable for her age, sexual experience, and the adequacy of sexual stimulation she receives." This new criterion acknowledges that skilled clinical judgment is required to differentiate situational orgasm problems from normal female functioning. With regard to subtyping, evidence from a variety of research sources was inadequate to justify subtyping of female orgasmic disorders beyond the dimensions of lifelong versus acquired and generalized versus situational. Schover suggested a subtyping scheme that divides the subtypes into stimulation-specific categories (i.e., women who are totally inorgasmic [generalized], and the situational categories of inorgasmic except with solo masturbation, inorgasmic with noncoital caressing from a partner, or inorgasmic only in coitus). Based on that recommendation, the Work Group proposed that a subtyping scheme be added to the criteria set, as shown in the *DSM-IV Options Book,* that specifies generalized or situational with the stimulation-specific categories as recommended above. Criterion B is to be modified with the addition of "not due to a substance-induced or secondary sexual dysfunction," and criterion C ("The disturbance causes marked distress or interpersonal difficulty.") will be added, both at the recommendation of the Task Force.

Male orgasmic disorder (inhibited male orgasm).   Schover noted the same problem with regard to the concept of the term *inhibition* as discussed in the section on female orgasm disorders. As a result of a discussion between the Sexual Disorders Work Group and the DSM-IV Task Force, the recommendation was made to change the name of this disorder to male orgasmic disorder to make it compatible with ICD-10 and with the way clinicians and researchers identify the disorder in the literature. It is also recommended that criterion A be shortened by deleting a number of explanatory phrases that the DSM-IV Task Force suggested would be best addressed in the text. This would also make criterion A compatible with ICD-10. As with the other dysfunctions, criterion B is to be expanded by adding "and not due to a substance-induced or secondary sexual dysfunction" and a new criterion C ("The disturbance causes marked distress or interpersonal difficulty.") is to be added, paralleling changes in the criteria for female orgasmic disorder.

Premature ejaculation.   No issues were identified with this criteria set, and literature reviews revealed no specific problems to be addressed. A new criterion B ("The disturbance causes marked distress or interpersonal difficulty") is to be added to be consistent with the criteria sets for all the sexual dysfunctions.

Sexual Pain Disorders

Dyspareunia.   The only issue noted by Schiavi in Chapter 53 was the fact that a criterion excluding pain during intercourse due to a physical condition or another

Axis I disorder was left out of DSM-III-R. The recommendation to expand the exclusion criterion was supported by a literature review. It is therefore recommended that a new criterion C be added, "Not due to a substance-induced (i.e., drugs, medication) or a secondary sexual dysfunction" and that criterion B be modified by adding "and is not better accounted for by another Axis I disorder (e.g., somatization disorder)." A new criterion D ("The disturbance causes marked distress or interpersonal difficulty") is to be added to be consistent with all the other criteria sets for sexual dysfunctions.

Vaginismus. No issues were identified, and no literature review was performed. It is recommended that criterion B be expanded by adding substance-induced and secondary sexual dysfunction as exclusion factors and that a new criterion C ("The disturbance causes marked distress or interpersonal difficulty") be added for consistency with the other sexual dysfunction criteria sets.

New Criteria Sets

The DSM-IV Task Force has also recommended two important options, the inclusion of criteria sets for secondary sexual dysfunction due to a nonpsychiatric medical condition and for substance-induced sexual dysfunction in the section on sexual dysfunctions. The inclusion of these criteria sets would facilitate the differential diagnosis of sexual dysfunctions and enhance compatibility with ICD-10.

Sexual Dysfunction Not Otherwise Specified

The proposed changes in the wording of the examples listed under sexual dysfunction not otherwise specified are the result of editorial changes recommended by the DSM-IV Task Force and recommendations made by Segraves in the chapters on the arousal disorders. The first proposed change is editorial: the introductory statement would read, "This category includes disorders with symptoms of a sexual dysfunction that do not meet criteria for any specific sexual dysfunction." Based on Segraves's recommendation, the first example would now read, "No (or substantially diminished) subjective erotic sensation despite otherwise normal arousal and orgasm." The addition of the term *arousal* is a consequence of the recommended changes in the section on arousal disorders, which eliminated the subjective components of arousal from those criteria sets. Because of the introduction of criteria sets for substance-induced sexual dysfunction and secondary sexual dysfunction, it is recommended that the following example be added to the list under sexual dysfunction not otherwise specified: "Situations in which the clinician has concluded that a sexual dysfunction is present but is unable to determine whether it is primary, secondary, or substance-induced." This option was recommended by the DSM-IV Task Force and was supported by the Sexual Disorders Work Group.

Paraphilias

The literature review of the paraphilias by Wise and Schmidt (Chapter 54, this volume) did not identify any issues except in the instance of transvestic fetishism. A criteria set is also proposed for telephone scatalogia because of the increased frequency of this diagnosis. An issue was identified in the wording of the examples for sexual disorder not otherwise specified, namely, the concept of "sexual addiction."

Transvestic Fetishism

Wise and Schmidt found that gender dysphoria is a common comorbid condition with transvestic fetishism. This raised the question as to whether individuals with transvestic fetishism and gender dysphoria have two disorders, a paraphilia and a gender identity disorder, or whether they have a paraphilia with a particular subtype. Literature reviews revealed that gender dysphoria associated with transvestic fetishism is usually of mild to moderate intensity and waxes and wanes over the course of the disorder. Individuals who exhibit gender dysphoria and are transvestic seek surgical reassignment and make efforts to live in the cross gender in an inconsistent manner. The recommended option was that these individuals be given one diagnosis, transvestic fetishism, with the subtype "with gender dysphoria." This option would allow the clinician to note the presence of a subthreshold level of gender dysphoria in these individuals. If, however, the full criteria are met for gender identity disorder, that diagnosis would take precedence. To implement this option, it is recommended that a C criterion be added, "Does not occur exclusively during the course of gender identity disorder" and that the option to specify "with gender dysphoria" if the person is distressed with gender role or gender identity be included in the criteria set.

Telephone Scatalogia

The literature review revealed that telephone scatalogia is being diagnosed with increased frequency. However, because the literature consists only of descriptive, anecdotal reports and no systematic studies, the option recommended by the DSM-IV Task Force and the Sexual Disorders Work Group is that this new criteria set be proposed for inclusion in the appendix for new disorders needing further study to stimulate additional research.

Sexual Disorders Not Otherwise Specified

The diagnosis of sexual disorder not otherwise specified is for those disorders that are not classifiable in any of the specific categories in the sexual disorders section. Three examples are listed under sexual disorder not otherwise specified. In the second example, the term *nonparaphilic sexual addiction* is used. The concept of sexual addiction has recently received considerable attention so that a literature review was carried out to test the scientific validity of the concept. The results of the review revealed abundant clinical evidence of sexual activity that can be characterized as *excessive*. However, there are no scientific data to support the concept that high-frequency sexual behavior can be considered addictive in the sense that the term *addiction* is conceptually, historically, and currently used in medicine. For this reason, the Sexual Disorders Work Group recommends that the term *nonparaphilic sexual addiction* be deleted and that the example now read, "Distress about a pattern of repeated sexual conquests involving a succession of people who exist only as things to be used."

References

American Psychiatric Association: Diagnostic and Statistical Manual of Mental Disorders, 2nd Edition. Washington, DC, American Psychiatric Association, 1968

American Psychiatric Association: Diagnostic and Statistical Manual of Mental Disorders, 3rd Edition. Washington, DC, American Psychiatric Association, 1980

American Psychiatric Association: Diagnostic and Statistical Manual of Mental Disorders, 3rd Edition, Revised. Washington, DC, American Psychiatric Association, 1987

Kaplan H: The New Sex Therapy, Active Treatment of Sexual Dysfunctions. New York, Brunner/Mazel, 1974a

Kaplan H: Disorders of Sexual Desire. New York, Brunner/Mazel, 1974b

Masters W, Johnson V: Human Sexual Inadequacy. Boston, MA, Little, Brown, 1970

Popkin MK, Tucker GJ: Mental disorders due to a general medical condition and substance-induced disorders: mood, anxiety, psychotic, catatonic, and personality disorders, in DSM-IV Sourcebook, Volume I. Edited by Widiger TA, Frances AJ, Pincus HA, et al. Washington, DC, American Psychiatric Association, 1994, pp 243–276

Task Force on DSM-IV: DSM-IV Options Book: Work in Progress. Washington, DC, American Psychiatric Association, 1991

World Health Organization: ICD-10 Chapter V: Mental and Behavioral Disorders: Diagnostic Criteria for Research. Geneva, Switzerland, World Health Organization, 1990

Chapter 49

Sexual Desire Disorders

Raul C. Schiavi, M.D.

Statement of the Issues

Sexual desire disorders include two diagnostic entities: hypoactive sexual desire (HSD) and sexual aversion disorder. The following issues were addressed in this review:

Hypoactive Sexual Desire Disorder

1. Is there empirical evidence that may assist in the formulation of more precise diagnostic criteria for this dysfunction?
2. Are there data that may permit the operationalization of this diagnosis such as frequency criteria for fantasy, desire, and behavior?
3. Is there evidence for the formation of subcategories of HSD?

Sexual Aversion Disorder

Is there systematic, empirically based information on the clinical utility, validity, and reliability of a "broader" versus a "narrower" definition of sexual aversion disorder?

Significance of the Issues

Hypoactive Sexual Desire Disorder

HSD, in contrast to other sexual dysfunctions, lacks psychophysiological correlates that may help to define it. The diagnosis is based primarily on subjective criteria; frequency of sexual behavior by itself is not a specific indicator of desire (or lack of), because it may be influenced by partner pressure or other motivational states. The DSM-III-R (American Psychiatric Association 1987) diagnosis adequately reflects the appetitive component involved in this dysfunction, but the diagnostic criteria rely almost exclusively on clinical judgment. Insufficient precision in the subjective characterization of the dysfunction and lack of quantitative criteria may account at least in part for the discrepant prevalence rates in clinical samples, ranging from 1% to 55%. The DSM-III-R criteria are clinically applicable, but their relative vagueness may lead to the diagnosis of a heterogeneous group of patients with possibly divergent biological and psychological characteristics. An operational definition of HSD may permit a more reliable acquisition of information and be more useful for research purposes. On the other hand, validity may not be enhanced by an operational definition that will, by necessity, be arbitrary due to the paucity of age- and sex-related normative information on sexual desire in the population at large.

Sexual Aversion Disorder

Sexual aversion disorder appeared for the first time as a diagnostic entity in DSM-III-R. There are differences of opinion as to whether hypoactive sexual desire and sexual aversion differ quantitatively on a continuum of sexual desire, with sexual aversion representing the most severe deficiency, or whether the diagnostic entities are categorically different. Although the DSM-III-R diagnostic criteria encompass "all or almost all genital sexual contact," in some therapy programs, this diagnosis appears to be applied to patients with aversion/avoidance limited to specific sexually related behaviors.

Methods

A review was conducted to identify empirical information by searching all published articles that included 1) explicit diagnostic criteria for inhibited sexual desire (ISD) (DSM-III, American Psychiatric Association 1980) or for hypoactive sexual desire disorder and sexual aversion disorder (DSM-III-R), 2) descriptive diagnostic information indicative of a sexual desire disorder, or 3) a statement that the study focused on patients with sexual desire or sexual aversion disorders even though the criteria used were not made explicit. This search did not include theoretical or speculative contributions or clinical reviews or articles that assessed the psychological or biological determinants or correlates of sexual desire as a separate dimension from sexual dysfunction.

The review is based on 1) a Medline computer search from 1966 to August 1989 with the terms *hypoactive, inhibited and low sexual desire, libido, inhibited sexual desire, aversion with sex, phobic disorders,* and *psychosexual dysfunction;* 2) a PsycInfo computer search from 1966 to August 1989 with the terms *hypoactive, low, inhibited or lack of sexual desire, sexual function, sexual disturbances, sex therapy, sex drive,* and *sexual aversion;* and 3) the issues of the following journals published between 1988 and 1990: *American Journal of Psychiatry, Journal of Nervous and Mental Disease, Psychosomatic Medicine, Archives of Sexual Behavior, Journal of Sex and Marital Therapy, Journal of Sex Research, Journal of Behavioral Medicine, Journal of Sex Education and Therapy,* and *Journal of Marriage and the Family.* No attempt was made to incorporate unpublished data sets into this review.

Results

Hypoactive Sexual Desire Disorder

We identified eight articles stemming from five independent investigations. Methodological features, sample characteristics, and a brief summary of the findings are presented below.

Schover and LoPiccolo (1982)

Methodological features.   The diagnostic criteria used in this study were 1) a low frequency of sexual activity (less than once/2 weeks unless patient complies with spouse's pressure for sex) and 2) "a subjective lack of desire for sexual activity; desire here includes sexual dreams and fantasies, attention to erotic materials, awareness of wishes for sexual activity, noticing attractive potential partners, and feelings of frustration if deprived of sex." Patients with sexual aversion were included in the study. Sex desire problems were classified as global versus situational and lifelong versus not lifelong.

The method of data collection involved obtaining an intake and sexual history and the Sex History Form (a multiple-choice questionnaire). Information was obtained from the patient and spouse. The study was conducted in a sexual dysfunction clinic.

The following selection procedure was employed: potential subjects included all 747 couples who had an intake interview between 1974 and 1981 at a sex therapy clinic. Two senior clinicians reviewed each file and rediagnosed subjects in terms of the multiaxial problem-oriented diagnostic system of Schover et al. (1982).

Sample characteristics.   The groups were defined as couples seeking help in which one spouse had a diagnosis of either low sexual desire or aversion to sex; 152 couples were studied. The percentages of those with low desire dysfunction that was lifelong were 17% for males, 39% for females, and 11% for females with aversion to sex. The percentages of those with dysfunctions that were global were 40% for males,

58% for females, and 48% for females with aversion to sex.

"Interrater reliability was informally checked during the course of rediagnosing spouses in all past clinic cases with the new multiaxial problem-oriented system" (Schover and LoPiccolo 1982, p. 181). Of the 152 couples, 38% were diagnosed as having low desire in the husbands, 49% as having low desire in the wives, and 18% as experiencing female aversion to sex. There were no males with a diagnosis of sexual aversion. The mean age for husbands in the study was 36.6 years (SD 7.6) and for the wives was 32.8 years (SD 7.6). Comorbid diagnoses were not evaluated.

Results. Couples were treated for 15–20 weekly sessions of conjoint behavioral sex therapy. Of all patients evaluated at intake, 38% did not enter sex therapy. Of those who began, 79% completed posttherapy questionnaires, and 67% provided follow-up data at 3 months. There were significant positive changes after treatment in marital adjustment, overall sexual satisfaction, frequency of intercourse and masturbation, and patterns of initiation of sexual activity. "Sex therapy was equally successful for male-centered versus female-centered problems, for low sex desire versus aversion to sex, and for global or lifelong dysfunctions versus the more recent or situational ones" (Schover and LoPiccolo 1982, p. 179). Although therapeutic improvement was statistically significant, it was of modest clinical importance.

Nutter and Condron (1983)

Methodological features. The diagnostic criteria used in this study were not described. Data were collected using a demographic questionnaire and a sexual fantasy scale. The source of information was the patient. The study was conducted in a sexual dysfunction clinic. The selection procedures used were not specified.

Sample characteristics. The group was defined as women who sought help for sexual problems and had at least occasional fantasies during sex. The study involved 25 patients with ISD and 30 control subjects. No data on reliability were collected. All subjects were women, with a mean age of 34.5 years. Comorbid diagnoses were not evaluated.

Results. Women with inhibited sexual desire reported less fantasizing during sexual activity and less general daydreaming than the control group. The content of fantasies did not differ between groups. There were no differences in masturbatory frequency or frequency of orgasms during masturbation, but the women with ISD did have fewer coital orgasms than the control subjects.

Nutter and Condron (1985)

Methodological features. The diagnostic criteria used in this study were not described. Data were collected using a demographic questionnaire and a sexual fantasy scale. The source of information was the patient. The study was conducted in a sexual dysfunction clinic. The selection procedure used was not specified.

Sample characteristics. The group was defined as men who sought help for sexual problems and had at least occasional fantasies during sex. The study involved 13 patients with ISD, 20 patients with erectile dysfunction, and 37 control subjects. No data on reliability were collected. All subjects were men, with a mean age of 43.6 years. Comorbid diagnoses were not evaluated.

Results. The study compared the responses of 37 men who reported a satisfying sex life with those of 33 men who came to a sex clinic complaining of either erectile dysfunction or ISD. It was reported that the frequency of sexual fantasies in the ISD group was significantly lower than in the control and/or erectile dysfunction groups. The content of fantasy was similar. The frequency of masturbation was greater in the ISD males.

Stuart et al. (1987)

Methodological features. The diagnostic criteria used in this study were at least three of the following: a lifelong history of phobic avoidance of sex, low level of initiation or sexual receptivity, low frequency of sexual activity, a consistent negative reaction to sexual activity, verbal expression of a lack of interest in sex, significant decrease in libido from a past norm of engaging in sex for reasons other than desire, and partner complaint. The diagnosis included the specification of whether the problem was primary or secondary and global or situational.

Two investigators independently reviewed the patients' case records and agreed with one another on the diagnostic assignments of 88 of the 92 respondents in the ISD and non-ISD groups. The source of information was the patient. The study was conducted at a sexual dysfunction clinic. The selection procedure was sequential.

Sample characteristics. The initial group was defined as married women who presented to a sex clinic for a sexual problem during a 27-month period. The study involved 59 subjects with ISD (66% of the initial sample) and 31 subjects who expressed normal sexual desire. All subjects were women, with a mean age of 36 years (SD 9.3). Twenty-seven of the women with ISD received a second sexual dysfunction diagnosis.

Results. This was a multidimensional study. The ISD group was compared with 31 women who expressed normal desire, 21 of whom had normal sex functioning and 10 of whom had sexual dysfunctions. There were no group differences in prolactin and testosterone (single sample), Minnesota Multiphasic Personality Inventory (MMPI) scales (Hathaway and McKinley 1970), age, education, income, religious preference, or dimensions of past sexual behavior. The women with ISD scored lower on the Dyadic Adjustment Scale (Spanier 1976) and reported more dissatisfaction with several aspects of their marriage (lower level of emotional closeness, love and romantic feelings, and attractiveness toward spouse). Behaviorally, the ISD group initiated sex less frequently, refused sex more, enjoyed sex less, and only engaged in sex to please husbands rather than for pleasure. There were no group differences with regard to mean monthly frequency of sexual intercourse. Discriminant analysis identified two factors that distinguished ISD from non-ISD groups: 1) feelings of romantic love and 2) satisfaction with one's own ability to listen. No information was provided on the relation between primary/secondary and global/situational characteristics and the results obtained.

Crenshaw (1987)

Methodological features. DSM-III diagnostic criteria for ISD were used. No specification as to lifelong/acquired, global/situational was made. Data were collected by clinical interview and self-report inventory. The source of information was the patient and partner. The study was done in a sexual dysfunction clinic. The selection procedures were sequential.

Sample characteristics. The group was defined as patients seeking pharmacological treatment for sexual dysfunctions. The study involved 60 subjects: 50 were patients with ISD or sexual aversion, the remainder presented with arousal/ inorgasmic problems as the primary dysfunction. No data on reliability were collected. The age range of the patient group was 27–63 years, and 60% of the subjects were male. Thirty patients had more than one sexual dysfunction.

Results. This was a double-blind, placebo-controlled study of bupropion treatment of sexual dysfunctions. "Ratings by the patient of sexual desire and ratings by the patient and clinician of global improvement showed treatment with bupropion to be superior to treatment with placebo" (Crenshaw 1987, p. 247). Measures of sexual activity failed to demonstrate a therapeutic effect of bupropion relative to the placebo.

Schreiner-Engel and Schiavi (1986)

Methodological features. DSM-III diagnostic criteria for ISD global were used and operationally defined as 1) reported frequency of all sexual activity twice per month or less over at least the previous 6 months and 2) a corresponding lack of subjective desire for engaging in any sexual behavior. In addition, the following selection criteria were required: ages 25–55 years in men and 21–45 years in women, married for at least 1 year, healthy, on no drugs or medication, and free from major psychopathology (classifiable as a DSM-III Axis I disorder).

Data were collected by clinical interviews and self-report inventories. The source of information was the couple. The study was done in a sexual dysfunction clinic. The selection procedures were sequential evaluations.

Sample characteristics. The groups were defined as 438 individuals and couples who were evaluated in a sexual dysfunction clinic between April 1982 and March 1985, 395 of whom were found to have sexual dysfunctions. Of 88 patients who complained of insufficient sexual desire, 58 subjects (35 men and 23 women) were diagnosed as having ISD according to DSM-III criteria (14.7% of all patients identified as having sexual dysfunctions). Of these subjects, 45 did not meet the study's selection criteria; among the 13 remaining eligible clinic couples, 5 consented to participate in the study. During the same period, 240 men and women called to volunteer for the study. After a preliminary screening over the phone, 96 couples were evaluated by interview. Of these, 41 met selection criteria and agreed to participate in the investigation. The total number of subjects who participated included 46 ISD subjects and 36 nondysfunctional control subjects. No data on reliability were gathered. The study involved 22 men and 24 women, with the mean age of the men 44.0 years (range 27–54) and of the women 33.3 years (range 27–40). There were 21 control men with a mean age of 44 years (range 27–54) and 15 control women with a mean age of 34 years (range 26–45). None of the subjects with ISD or the control subjects met criteria for a current Research Diagnostic Criteria (RDC) diagnosis of anxiety, affective, or psychotic disorders.

Results. The men and women with ISD had a markedly elevated lifetime prevalence of affective disorders. The proportion of individuals with ISD who had histories of major and/or intermittent depression alone was almost twice as high as that of control subjects. Additionally, the initial episode of the depressive disorder almost always coincided with or preceded the onset of the ISD. Significantly more women with ISD than control subjects also had severe premenstrual symptoms.

Schiavi et al. (1988)

Methodological features.   See Schreiner-Engel and Schiavi (1986).

Sample characteristics.   For the definition of the group, see Schreiner-Engel and Schiavi (1986). Seventeen men with ISD and 17 nondysfunctional control subjects participated in this aspect of the investigation. Among the 17 men with ISD, there were 6 men without problems of sexual arousal and 11 with secondary erectile impotence. No data on the reliability of diagnosis were gathered. All the subjects were male, with mean age for those who were potent being 44 years (range 31–55), and for those who were impotent being 43 years (range 28–53). For information on comorbidity, see Schreiner-Engel and Schiavi (1986).

Results.   The total group of men with ISD had significantly lower plasma testosterone (measured hourly through the night) than control subjects, and there was a positive relationship between testosterone and frequency of sexual behavior. There were no differences in free testosterone, prolactin, luteinizing hormone (LH), and estradiol between the ISD and control groups. The nocturnal penile tumescence (NPT) parameters of men with ISD with secondary impotence were consistently and significantly lower than the nondysfunctional men.

Schreiner-Engel et al. (1989)

Methodological features.   See Schreiner-Engel and Schiavi (1986).

Sample characteristics.   For the definition of the group, see Schreiner-Engel and Schiavi (1986). Seventeen women with ISD and 13 nondysfunctional control subjects completed the endocrine phase of the study. No data on the reliability of diagnosis were gathered. All the subjects were female, with a mean age of 33.4 years (range 27–39). For information on comorbidity, see Schreiner-Engel and Schiavi (1986).

Results.   The gonadal hormones of the women with ISD fluctuated normally over the menstrual cycle, were within normal limits for each cycle phase, and were never significantly different from those of control subjects. Testosterone, non–sex hormone–binding globulin testosterone, and prolactin did not differentiate the women with the most from the least severe ISD parameters (e.g., frequency of fantasy, masturbation, and female-initiated coitus) or women with lifelong from those with acquired ISD.

Sexual Aversion Disorder

Sexual aversion was considered as a separate diagnostic category in the previously reviewed study by Schover and LoPiccolo (1982). We could only identify one additional data-oriented article that specifically focused on this disorder (Murphy and Sullivan 1981). However, evaluation of this article does not provide convincing evidence that the subjects met criteria for this dysfunction.

Murphy and Sullivan (1981)

Methodological features. The diagnostic criterion used was "an unwillingness to become involved in sexual activity with an avoidance of any touching or communication that might lead to sexual involvement" (Murphy and Sullivan 1981, p. 16).

Data were collected from an intake and sexual history using the Sexual Response Questionnaire for Women, the State-Trait Anxiety Inventory (Spielberger et al. 1970), the Tennessee Self-Concept Scale (Fitts 1965), and a Social-Sexual History Questionnaire (the Sexual Response Questionnaire for Women and the Social-Sexual History Questionnaire are described in the article but no references are provided). The source of information was the patients. The study was done in a sexual dysfunction clinic and a gynecologist's office. The selection procedure was not stated.

Sample characteristics. The groups were defined as subjects seeking help for sexual difficulties. Twenty "sexually aversive" patients and 35 "nonaversive" control subjects participated in the study. No data on reliability were gathered. All subjects were women. The mean age was not given for the aversive group. The mean age of the total group ($N = 55$) was 31.4 years (range 20–58). No data were given on comorbid diagnoses.

Results. The two groups differed significantly on anxiety and self-concept measures. "Sexually aversive" women reported anxiety and had difficulties with identity and self-acceptance to a significantly higher degree than control subjects. There were also differences between groups in response to the Social Sexual History Questionnaire (statistical analysis not done).

Discussion

This review underlines the paucity of empirical information on sexual desire disorders. Few investigators have focused on this topic, and even fewer studies have used DSM-III or DSM-III-R criteria for subject selection. Specific characteristics of the dysfunctions (i.e., lifelong/acquired, generalized/situational) are frequently omitted in the presentation of results. On the basis of available knowledge, there is little that can be stated with any degree of certainty about these dysfunctions.

Recommendations

It may be worth considering for a future DSM to further define HSD criteria to include the seeking out of sexual cues (or awareness of sexual cues) as proposed in ICD-10. In addition, several investigators and clinicians include as an operational criterion for HSD a frequency of sexual desire and/or activity of less than once every 2 weeks (or twice per month or less). Although this criterion is arbitrary and does not take into account possible age-related changes in sexual desire, it has the merit of providing an objective guideline and of being congruent with ICD-10. However, there are no data derived from systematic research that support changing the DSM-III-R criteria for sexual desire disorders. No basis exists for forming diagnostic subcategories other than the present distinctions of lifelong/acquired and generalized/situational. There is also no evidence to support narrowing the diagnosis of sexual aversion disorder to include individuals with aversions limited to one or a few components of the sexual interaction.

References

American Psychiatric Association: Diagnostic and Statistical Manual of Mental Disorders, 3rd Edition. Washington, DC, American Psychiatric Association, 1980
American Psychiatric Association: Diagnostic and Statistical Manual of Mental Disorders, 3rd Edition, Revised. Washington, DC, American Psychiatric Association, 1987
Crenshaw TL: The pharmacological modification of psychosexual dysfunction. J Sex Marital Ther 13:239–252, 1987
Fitts WH: Manual: Tennessee Self-Concept Scale. Nashville, TN, Counselor Recordings and Tests, 1965
Hathaway SR, McKinley JC: Minnesota Multiphasic Personality Inventory, Revised. Minneapolis, University of Minnesota, 1970
Murphy C, Sullivan M: Anxiety and self-concept correlates of sexually aversive women. Sexuality and Disability 4:15–26, 1981
Nutter DE, Condron MK: Sexual fantasy and activity patterns of females with inhibited sexual desire versus normal controls. J Sex Marital Ther 9:276–282, 1983
Nutter DE, Condron MK: Sexual fantasy and activity patterns of males with inhibited sexual desire and males with erectile dysfunction versus normal controls. J Sex Marital Ther 11:91–98, 1985

Schiavi R, Schreiner-Engel P, White D, et al: Pituitary-gonadal function during sleep in men with hypoactive sexual desire and in normal controls. Psychosom Med 50:304–318, 1988

Schover LR, LoPiccolo J: Treatment effectiveness for dysfunctions of sexual desire. J Sex Marital Ther 8:179–197, 1982

Schover LR, Friedman C, Weilers M, et al: The multi-axial problem-oriented diagnostic system for the sexual dysfunctions: an alternative to DSM-III. Arch Gen Psychiatry 39:614–619, 1982

Schreiner-Engel P, Schiavi RC: Lifetime psychopathology in individuals with low sexual desire. J Nerv Ment Dis 174:646–651, 1986

Schreiner-Engel P, Schiavi RC, White D, et al: Low sexual desire in women: the role of reproductive hormones. Hormones and Behavior 23:221–234, 1989

Spanier G: Measuring dyadic adjustment: new scales for assessing the quality of marriage and similar dyads. J Marriage Fam 38:15–29, 1976

Spielberger CD, Gorsuch RL, Lushene RE: Manual: State-Trait Anxiety Inventory. Palo Alto, CA, Consulting Psychologists Press, 1970

Stuart FM, Hammond DC, Pett MA: Inhibited sexual desire in women. Arch Sex Behav 16:91–106, 1987

Chapter 50

Female Sexual Arousal Disorder

R. Taylor Segraves, M.D.

Issue 1

Statement of the Issue

Female sexual arousal disorder is defined in DSM-III-R (American Psychiatric Association 1987) as 1) persistent or recurrent partial or complete failure to attain or maintain the lubrication-swelling response of sexual excitement until completion of the sexual activity or 2) persistent or recurrent lack of a subjective sense of sexual excitement and pleasure in a female during sexual activity.

These diagnostic criteria may be problematic in at least two major ways: 1) the vagueness or extent of clinician judgment required to make this diagnosis and 2) the combination of subjective and objective criteria for the same diagnostic entity in the absence of data that these two response systems are correlated and constitute part of the same syndrome.

The original goal of this project was thus to assess whether sufficient data are available in the literature to 1) operationally define this syndrome and 2) assess whether subjective and objective data sets are part of the same syndrome.

Significance of the Issue

A more precise definition of the syndrome might permit a cleaner delineation of a homogeneous group of patients and thus facilitate clinical generalizations and replication of research findings.

Method

Medline and PsycInfo (knowledge index) searches were performed using *female sexual arousal disorder, female sexual arousal, desire disorder, frigidity and sexual excitement,* and *inhibited sexual excitement* as key words.

Results

In both databases, no articles were indexed by the diagnostic term *female sexual arousal disorder*. The other key words elicited many references, none of which were specific to the research questions asked. A considerable research literature addresses the question of covariance between the vasocongestive response and subjective sexual arousal (e.g., Rosen and Beck 1988). The literature to date appears inconsistent, and the research has not been conducted in patients with symptoms diagnosed as female sexual arousal disorder.

Discussion

The paucity of literature concerning female sexual arousal disorder can perhaps best be appreciated in historical context. In DSM-II (American Psychiatric Association 1968), psychological problems associated with menstruation, micturition, and psychosexual problems were grouped together as psychophysiological genitourinary disorders. Before DSM-III (American Psychiatric Association 1980), clinicians employed various diagnostic systems for the psychosexual disorders (Kaplan 1974; Moore 1989). Masters and Johnson (1966) described four stages of sexual response, including excitement, plateau, orgasm, and resolution. However, they described three female disorders: dyspareunia, vaginismus, and orgasmic dysfunction (primary and secondary). This system was modified by Kaplan (1974) with the subdivision of general sexual unresponsiveness as a separate category from orgasmic dysfunction. The system was further modified when Kaplan (1977, 1979) introduced a three-stage model of desire, excitement, and orgasm. DSM-III then incorporated these concepts with separate diagnoses for inhibited sexual excitement, inhibited sexual desire, and inhibited orgasm. The assumption of similarities in male and female sexual response also played a major role in DSM-III and DSM-III-R. DSM-III-R was further modified by the addition of a sexual aversion disorder. Inhibited sexual excitement was subdivided into female sexual arousal disorder and male erectile disorder, partially abandoning the theoretical model of male-female similarities.

The point of this historical review is to highlight the diagnostic turmoil or progress in this new arena of psychiatric inquiry and to stress that what we now call female sexual arousal disorder may have been previously diagnosed as frigidity, orgasmic dysfunction, or general sexual unresponsiveness. What previously was classified as inhibited sexual excitement may now be diagnosed as hypoactive sexual desire disorder (inhibited sexual desire in DSM-III).

Issue 2

Statement of the Issue

Based on the literature review concerning issue 1, the original question was modified, because it was determined that a meaningful question to address at this point was whether there is sufficient evidence for retaining the diagnostic entity female sexual arousal disorder. Part of the motivation for retaining female sexual arousal disorder appears to be theoretical, based on the triphasic model and the assumption of similarity between the two sexes (i.e., something to match male erectile disorder).

Methodology

In view of the negligible yield from the computerized searches, a search of the clinical literature (which is often found in books and unindexed) was undertaken to find evidence of clinical utility for female sexual arousal disorder.

Results

In a number of major texts concerning treatment of sexual dysfunction, the diagnostic term *female arousal disorder* is not mentioned or is mentioned only cursorily (Moore 1989). Major texts not mentioning this diagnosis or not having differential treatment plans for it include Arentewicz and Schmidt (1983), Farber (1985), Nadelson and Marcotte (1983), Leiblum and Peruin (1980), LoPiccolo and LoPiccolo (1978), Kaplan (1974), and Bancroft (1983).

In a review of 22 studies concerning the prevalence of psychosexual disorders, Nathan (1986) could not find one study concerning the prevalence of female arousal disorder. In a review of the treatment of sexual disorders, LoPiccolo and Stock (1986) did not discuss this syndrome. Kaplan (1984) and Meyer et al. (1985) both briefly discussed this diagnosis. Kaplan commented that female arousal disorder appears to be an infrequently encountered diagnosis.

It is clear that decreased vaginal lubrication may be associated with estrogen deficiency states or with certain chronic diseases (Schover and Jensen 1988) or with insufficient foreplay (Nathan 1986); however, it is unclear how commonly this diagnosis occurs in women in good health who receive adequate foreplay.

The only information concerning diagnosis of this disorder is from a recent multisite pharmacological study of desire, arousal, and orgasm disorders. In this study of 532 women, only 8% had female arousal disorder. Of the female arousal disorder group, 74% were coded as having decreased subjective and physiological arousal (Segraves and Segraves 1991).

Discussion

A major question to be addressed by future research is whether female sexual arousal disorder exists as a discrete entity or whether it appears primarily as a secondary diagnosis in women having desire-phase or orgasm-phase disorders. The existing database does not allow us to make this determination.

Recommendation for DSM-IV

There appear to be three major alternatives concerning the diagnostic category female sexual arousal disorder for DSM-IV: 1) deletion, 2) retention, or 3) modification to agree fully with ICD-10 (World Health Organization 1990).

One could argue that this diagnosis should be deleted on the grounds that there is minimal evidence that this diagnosis exists as a discrete syndrome and that there is minimal evidence to support its clinical utility. The literature review supports this recommendation.

A second alternative would be to retain the diagnosis in its current form on the grounds that there has been insufficient time to judge its status. The accompanying DSM-IV text would address this issue. The rationale for retaining the diagnostic criteria unchanged is as follows.

In DSM-III, the diagnosis of female arousal disorder was made solely on the basis of failure of genital response. This was modified in DSM-III-R to include both subjective and objective criteria. A revision of the criteria back to the previous definition would create unnecessary confusion without supporting evidence. The text should address the issue of the uncertainty concerning the diagnostic criteria.

The third alternative would be to seek full compatibility with ICD-10. In ICD-10, the corresponding diagnosis is failure of genital response. This diagnosis is made solely on the report of insufficient vaginal lubrication. Note that this definition of female arousal disorder essentially reverts back to the DSM-III form. The advantage of this modification would be compatibility between the sexes and between DSM-IV and ICD-10.

The Work Group recommends that criterion A read, "Persistent or recurrent inability to attain or maintain an adequate lubrication-swelling response of sexual excitement until completion of the sexual activity." A second recommendation is that the concept of a lack of subjective sense of sexual excitement and pleasure be retained for at least research purposes by including the concept as an example of sexual dysfunction not otherwise specified, 302.70. The proposed wording would be "No (or substantially diminished) subjective erotic sensation despite otherwise normal arousal and orgasm."

The scientific study of sexual disorders is in its infancy. The field is struggling to find acceptable theoretical models and consistent ways of defining clinical syndromes. In my opinion, any unnecessary modification of the current diagnostic system would be a disservice to the field. I recommend that the diagnosis of female sexual arousal disorder be retained, with the text specifying the lack of information concerning the existence and definition of this syndrome.

References

American Psychiatric Association: Diagnostic and Statistical Manual of Mental Disorders, 2nd Edition. Washington, DC, American Psychiatric Association, 1968

American Psychiatric Association: Diagnostic and Statistical Manual of Mental Disorders, 3rd Edition. Washington, DC, American Psychiatric Association, 1980

American Psychiatric Association: Diagnostic and Statistical Manual of Mental Disorders, 3rd Edition, Revised. Washington, DC, American Psychiatric Association, 1987

Arentewicz G, Schmidt G: The Treatment of Sexual Disorders. New York, Basic Books, 1983

Bancroft J: Human Sexuality and Its Problems. Edinburgh, Churchill Livingstone, 1983

Farber M: Human Sexuality: Psychosexual Aspects of Disease. New York, Plenum, 1985

Kaplan HS: The classification of the female sexual dysfunction. J Sex Marital Ther 1:124–138, 1974

Kaplan HS: Hypoactive sexual desire. J Sex Marital Ther 3:3–9, 1977

Kaplan HS: Disorders of Sexual Desire. New York, Brunner/Mazel, 1979

Kaplan HS: The New Sex Therapy. New York, Brunner/Mazel, 1984

Leiblum SR, Peruin LA: Principles and Practice of Sex Therapy. New York, Guilford, 1980

LoPiccolo J, LoPiccolo L: Handbook of Sex Therapy. New York, Plenum, 1978

LoPiccolo J, Stock WE: Treatment of sexual dysfunction. J Consult Clin Psychol, 54:158–167, 1986

Masters WH, Johnson VE: Human Sexual Response. Boston, MA, Little, Brown, 1966

Meyer JK, Schmidt CW, Wise TN: Clinical Management of Sexual Disorders. Baltimore, MD, Williams & Wilkins, 1985

Moore C: Female arousal disorder and inhibited female orgasm, in Treatments of Psychiatric Disorders, Vol 3. Washington, DC, American Psychiatric Association, 1989, pp 2279–2290

Nadelson CC, Marcotte DB: Treatment Intervention in Human Sexuality. New York, Plenum, 1983

Nathan SG: The epidemiology of the DSM-III psychosexual dysfunction. J Sex Marital Ther 12:267–281, 1986

Rosen RC, Beck JG: Patterns of Sexual Arousal. New York, Guilford, 1988

Schover LR, Jensen SB: Sexuality and Chronic Illness. New York, Guilford, 1988

Segraves RT, Segraves KB: Diagnosis of female arousal disorder. Sexual and Marital Therapy 6:9–13, 1991

World Health Organization: ICD-10 Chapter V: Mental and Behavioral Disorders: Diagnostic Criteria for Research. Geneva, Switzerland, World Health Organization, 1990

Chapter 51

Male Erectile Disorder

R. Taylor Segraves, M.D.

Issue 1

Statement of the Issue

In DSM-III-R (American Psychiatric Association 1987), male erectile disorder can be diagnosed if *either* of the following criteria are met: 1) persistent or recurrent partial or complete failure in a male to attain or maintain erection until completion of the sexual activity; 2) persistent or recurrent lack of subjective sense of sexual excitement and pleasure in a male during sexual activity. By definition, a male with erectile failure and a male with normal erectile function but decreased subjective pleasure would receive the same diagnosis of male erectile disorder. This definition of male erectile disorder appears to deviate from the standard clinical usage of this term.

Significance of the Issue

The definition of male erectile disorder in DSM-III-R appears not to have been accepted by many members of the scientific and clinical community. The existence of varying definitions for the same syndrome can lead to considerable confusion in both the clinical and research literature.

Method

The literature concerning the diagnosis of male erectile disorder was reviewed in the following manner: 1) Medline search from 1986 to 1991, 2) PsycInfo search from 1974 to 1991, 3) review of author's personal reprint files, and 4) search for relevant articles from 1980 to 1991 in *Archives of Sexual Behavior, Journal of Sex and Marital Therapy, Journal of Sex Education and Therapy,* and *British Journal of Sexual Medicine.*

Results

No evidence was found in the literature to suggest that these two states are part of the same diagnostic entity. In numerous publications discussing the diagnosis and treatment of erectile disorder (e.g., Ansari 1976; Cooper 1981; Everaerd and Dekker 1985; Gillan 1987; Hawton 1982; Heiman and LoPiccolo 1983; Johnson 1965a; Reynolds 1977; Schmidt 1983; Whitehead and Mathews 1977; Wright et al. 1977), the diagnosis of male erectile disorder is based on objective criteria alone. Not one author was found who used the subjective criteria to make the diagnosis of male erectile disorder.

Discussion

The available evidence suggests that the DSM-IV definition of male erectile disorder be modified so that it simply specifies erectile failure. This change would essentially delete the DSM-III-R modification of this definition and revert back to the DSM-III (American Psychiatric Association 1980) definition. This redefinition would be roughly compatible with the ICD-10 definition (World Health Organization 1990), which specifies failure of the genital response. This change in definition would also be compatible with current usage of this diagnosis by the scientific and clinical community.

ICD-10 includes a category for lack of sexual enjoyment. This category might subsume men with lack of pleasurable sexual arousal but who achieve normal erections. However, there is no evidence that men exist who have decreased sexual arousal in the absence of desire or orgasm dysfunction. The current evidence does not support the inclusion of such a diagnosis for men with decreased subjective arousal.

Recommendation

I therefore recommend that male erectile disorder be diagnosed solely by failure of the genital response.

Issue 2

Statement of the Issue

The objective criteria for the diagnosis of male erectile disorder, "persistent or recurrent partial or complete failure in a male to attain or maintain erection until completion of the sexual activity," is quite broad and encompasses a possibly heterogeneous group of patients. Certain criteria sets might be considered that would more precisely delineate this diagnostic entity. Logical criteria to consider might include the duration of the disorder and the frequency of erectile failure that is necessary to reach diagnostic criteria.

Significance of the Issue

More precise diagnostic criteria might help clinicians and clinical investigators to delineate a clinical population for which treatment approaches can be generalized.

Method

Computerized database searches similar to those described for issue 1 were performed.

Results

Duration criteria. Studies have indicated that certain cases of male erectile disorder will spontaneously remit without formal treatment (Nathan 1986; Segraves et al. 1982, 1985), and it is commonly assumed that many males experience idiopathic transient erectile failure that remits without medical intervention. For research purposes, certain investigators have arbitrarily set a 3-month duration as a protocol requirement to enter studies of erectile disorder (Segraves et al. 1987). Other investigators have used a 6-month criterion (Hatch et al. 1987), or a 1-year criterion (Everaerd and Dekker 1985). These criteria have been arbitrarily chosen because there is no precise information on the duration of transient erectile difficulties in the normal population. Similarly, there is minimal information concerning the relationship between duration of erectile dysfunction and the likelihood of spontaneous remission. Other work has indicated that chronicity of the complaint (with chronicity variously defined) may portend a less favorable prognosis (Cooper 1969, 1981; Johnson 1965b; Segraves et al. 1982).

Frequency criteria. DSM-III-R does not specify the frequency at which erectile failure must occur in order to meet diagnostic criteria. Various criteria have been arbitrarily used in the literature. For example, some clinicians diagnose secondary impotence if the patient's failure to achieve erections exceeds 25% of coital opportunities (Masters and Johnson 1970; Nagler et al. 1985). Investigators have often arbitrarily chosen 50% (Segraves et al. 1987) and 75% (Munjack et al. 1984) failure rates. The significance of the failure to specify the frequency of erectile failure in the diagnosis of male erectile disorder can perhaps best be appreciated by realizing that one of the largest treatment outcome studies to date (Arentewicz and Schmidt 1983) used criteria for erectile dysfunction that were virtually identical to those in DSM-III-R. In this study, 36% of the men with erectile dysfunction had successful erections in 50% or more of coital attempts. Of these men, 22% achieved erections in 75% of coital attempts. It should also be noted that 56% of this sample of men with erectile failure had successful coitus at least five times a month.

Discussion

The problem with this diagnostic ambiguity is obvious. The solution unfortunately is not so clear. We simply lack the data to meaningfully specify duration or severity criteria. To my knowledge, there is no sound evidence relating severity or duration of this difficulty to treatment outcome or preferred treatment approach.

There appear to be two major options: the current vague criteria could be maintained in DSM-IV, allowing future research to more clearly delineate diagnostic parameters, or one could arbitrarily set criteria such as a 50% failure rate for at least 6 months duration.

Recommendation

It is recommended that we retain the current imprecise criteria because we lack sufficient information to meaningfully modify these criteria.

References

American Psychiatric Association: Diagnostic and Statistical Manual of Mental Disorders, 3rd Edition, Revised. Washington, DC, American Psychiatric Association, 1987
Ansari JMA: Impotence prognosis (a controlled study). Br J Psychiatry 128:194–198, 1976
Arentewicz G, Schmidt G: The Treatment of Sexual Disorders. New York, Basic Books, 1983
Cooper AJ: Disorder of sexual potency in the male: a clinical and statistical study of some factors related to short-term prognosis. Br J Psychiatry 115:709–719, 1969
Cooper AJ: Short-term treatment in sexual dysfunction: a review. Compr Psychiatry 22:206–217, 1981
Everaerd W, Dekker J: Treatment of male sexual dysfunction: sex therapy compared with systematic desensitization and rational emotive therapy. Behav Res Ther 1:13–25, 1985
Gillan P: Sex Therapy Manual. Oxford, UK, Blackwell Scientific Publications, 1987
Hatch JP, DeLapena LM, Fisher J: Psychometric differentiation of psychogenic and organic erectile disorders. Journal of Urology 138:781–783, 1987
Hawton K: The behavioral treatment of sexual dysfunction. Br J Psychiatry 140:94–101, 1982
Heiman JR, LoPiccolo J: Clinical outcome of sex therapy. Arch Gen Psychiatry 40:443–449, 1983
Johnson J: Androgyny and disorders of sexual potency. BMJ 3:572–573, 1965a
Johnson J: Prognosis of disorders of sexual potency in the male. J Psychosom Res 9:195–200, 1965b
Masters WH, Johnson VE: Human Sexual Inadequacy. Boston, MA, Little, Brown, 1970
Munjack DJ, Schlaks A, Sanchez UC, et al: Rational-emotive therapy in the treatment of erectile failure: an initial study. J Sex Marital Ther 10:170–175, 1984

Nagler HM, White RD, Blaivas JG: Impotence: diagnosis and treatment, in Human Sexuality: Psychosexual Effects of Disease. Edited by Farber M. New York, Macmillan, 1985, pp20240–263

Nathan SG: The epidemiology of the DSM-III psychosexual dysfunctions. J Sex Marital Ther 12:167–281, 1986

Reynolds BS: Psychological treatment models and outcome research for erectile dysfunction: a critical review. Psychol Bull 84:1218–1238, 1977

Schmidt CW: Common male sexual disorders: impotence and premature ejaculation, in Clinical Management of Sexual Disorders. Edited by Meyer JK, Schmidt CW, Wise TN. Baltimore, MD, Williams & Wilkins, 1983, pp 173–187

Segraves KA, Segraves RT, Schoenberg HW: Use of sexual history to differentiate organic from psychogenic impotence. Arch Sex Behav 16:125–137, 1987

Segraves RT, Knopf J, Camic P: Spontaneous remission in erectile impotence. Behav Res Ther 20:89–91, 1982

Segraves RT, Camic R, Ivanoff J: Spontaneous remission in erectile dysfunction. Behav Res Ther 23:203–204, 1985

Whitehead A, Mathews A: Attitude change during behavioural treatment of sexual inadequacy. Br J Soc Psychol 16:275–281, 1977

World Health Organization: ICD-10 Chapter V. Mental and Behavioral Disorders. Diagnostic Criteria for Research. Geneva, Switzerland, World Health Organization, 1990

Wright J, Perreault R, Mathieu M: The treatment of sexual dysfunction: a review. Arch Gen Psychiatry 34:881–890, 1977

Further Reading

Abel GG, Becker JU, Cunningham-Rathner J, et al: Differential diagnosis of impotence in diabetics. Neurourology and Urodynamics 1:57–69, 1982

Alarie P, Eltrami E: Organicity in cases of male erectile dysfunction referred to sexual therapy, in Emerging Dimension of Sexology. Edited by Segraves RT, Haeberle EJ. New York, Praeger, 1984, pp 101–112

Bancroft J: Human Sexuality and Its Problems. Edinburgh, Churchill Livingstone, 1983

Barlow DH: Causes of sexual dysfunction: the role of anxiety and cognitive interference. J Consult Clin Psychol 54:140–148, 1986

Beck JG, Barlow DH: Current conceptualizations of sexual dysfunction: a review and an alternative perspective. Clinical Psychology Review 4:363–378, 1984

Beck JG, Barlow DH: The effects of anxiety and attentional focus on sexual responding, 1: physiological patterns in erectile dysfunction, 2: cognitive and affective patterns. Behav Res Ther 24:9–26, 1986

Cole M: Sex therapy: a critical appraisal. Br J Psychiatry 147:337–351, 1985

Cooper AJ: Outpatient treatment of impotence. J Nerv Ment Dis 149:337–359, 1969

Eysenck HJ: Sex and Personality. Austin, University of Texas Press, 1976

Frank E, Anderson C, Rubinstein D: Frequency of sexual dysfunction in normal couples. N20Engl J Med 299:111–115, 1978

Glover J: Factors affecting the outcome of treatment of sexual problems. British Journal of Sexual Medicine 7:28–31, 1983

Graber B, Kline-Graber G: Research criteria for male erectile failure. Journal of Sex and Marital Therapy 7:37–48, 1981

Kaplan HS: The New Sex Therapy. New York, Brunner/Mazel, 1984

Kockott G, Feil W, Revenstorf D, et al: Symptomology and psychological aspects of male sexual inadequacy: results of an experimental study. Arch Sex Behav 9:457–475, 1980

Levine SB: The psychological evaluation and therapy of psychogenic impotence, in Diagnosis and Treatment of Male Erectile Dysfunction. Edited by Segraves RT, Schoenberg HW. New York, Plenum, 1985, pp 87–104

Montague DK: The evaluation of the impotent male, in Management of Male Impotence. Edited by AH Bennett. Baltimore, MD, Williams & Wilkins, 1982, pp 52–60

Nettelbladt P, Uddenberg N: Sexual dysfunction and sexual satisfaction in 58 married Swedish men. J Psychosom Res 23:141–147, 1979

Schiarr RC: Psychological determinants of erectile disorders. Sexuality and Disability 4:86–92, 1981

Schiavi RC, Fisher C, White D, et al: Pituitary-gonadal function during sleep in men with erectile impotence and normal controls. Psychosom Med 46:239–254, 1984

Schover LR, Friedman JM, Weiler SJ, et al: Multiaxial problem-oriented system for sexual dysfunctions. Arch Gen Psychiatry 39:614–619, 1982

Segraves RT. Male erectile disorder, in Treatments of Psychiatric Disorders, Vol 3. Edited by Karasu TB. Washington, DC, American Psychiatric Association, 1989, pp 2318–2329

Segraves RT, Schoenberg HC: Diagnosis and treatment of erectile problems: current status, in Diagnosis and Treatment of Erectile Disturbances. Edited by Segraves RT, Schoenberg HW. New York, Plenum, 1985, pp 1–22

Segraves RT, Schoenberg HW, Zarins CK, et al: Discrimination of organic from psychogenic impotence with the DSF1. J Sex Marital Ther 7:230–238, 1981

Spitzer RL, Williams JBW: Introduction, in Diagnostic and Statistical Manual of Mental Disorders, 3rd Edition, Revised. Washington, DC, American Psychiatric Association, 1987

Vansteenwegen A, Luyens M, Daelemans S: Outcome of ten years of residential and outpatient sex therapy: an exploratory and comparative study, in Emerging Dimensions of Sexology. Edited by Segraves RT, Haeberle EJ. New York, Praeger, 1984, pp 133–144

Chapter 52

Female Orgasm: Proposals Regarding Name, Criteria, and Subtyping

Leslie R. Schover, Ph.D.

Statement of the Issues

In this chapter, revisions to the DSM-III-R (American Psychiatric Association 1987) name *inhibited female orgasm* and to the diagnostic criteria for this disorder are considered. Empirical evidence for the subtyping of the disorder is also discussed. The question of subtyping for inhibited female orgasm entails examining several related research questions: Are there physiological subtypes of female orgasm, so that one type may be inhibited and another not? Are there specific antecedents in terms of personality or behavior that discriminate between women with subtypes of inhibited orgasm disorder? Does subtyping explain some variance in treatment outcome?

Significance of the Issues

Changing the name from *inhibited female orgasm* to *female orgasmic disorder* would be helpful because the new term would be more consonant with the research literature and with ICD-10 (World Health Organization 1990). Deletion of the word *inhibited* also avoids use of the concept of *psychological inhibition* of orgasm, a term that assumes a certain theoretical view of causation that has no empirical support.

The current DSM-III-R definition may also be circular, in that one may only be able to judge the correctness of the diagnosis by the success of the treatment plan it generates. The debate on whether lack of orgasm from intercourse constitutes a disorder remains open. Other clinical judgments entailed in making this diagnosis are equally controversial. The clinician needs general guidelines to apply in situational cases rather than specific instructions that are only relevant to coital inorgasmia and have little empirical grounding.

In DSM-III-R, inhibited female orgasm is a very broad diagnostic category comprising either persistent delay or total absence of orgasm during any type of sexual stimulation. This lack of specificity means that the diagnosis could apply to a woman who had never experienced an orgasm; to someone who was easily orgasmic in masturbation but not with a partner; or to a woman who consistently required a longer than average duration of coital thrusting to reach orgasm, even though she had consistent orgasm with brief clitoral stimulation by a partner. The use of the lifelong versus acquired and generalized versus situational modifiers may help researchers and clinicians communicate and compare outcomes; but could more specificity in subtyping be obtained?

Two schemes for subtyping inhibited female orgasm have been proposed in published studies. The multiaxial, problem-oriented diagnostic system (MAPODS) for sexual dysfunctions (Schover et al. 1982) divides female orgasmic dysfunctions into categories based on the type of stimulation that does produce an orgasm. It assumes that the severity of the disorder is measured in the intensity of stimulation a woman requires. Thus, a woman could receive one of the following diagnoses (each modified as lifelong versus not lifelong): inorgasmic, inorgasmic except for vibrator or mechanical stimulation, inorgasmic except for masturbation, inorgasmic except for partner manipulation (noncoital), coitally inorgasmic, or infrequently coitally orgasmic. A mere delay in the time to reach orgasm is not included as a dysfunction.

Derogatis et al. (1989) have proposed four subtypes based on multivariate analysis of the Derogatis Sexual Functioning Inventory (DSFI) profiles for 76 women: low-desire inorgasmia, histrionic/marital conflict, psychiatric disorder, and constitutional. These subtypes depend on the presence of other sexual dysfunctions, the degree of psychological distress and mood disturbance, and the presence of physical factors. Because no data on interrater reliability, concurrent or predictive validity, or cross-validation are available for either subtyping system, I examine the issue of subtypes without preconceptions as to the best system.

Methods

Materials for this review were gathered by a computer Medline search using a number of key words with *female*. These include *orgasm, orgasmic dysfunction, inorgasmia, sex disorders, psychosexual dysfunction,* and *frigidity.* The search was limited to English-language publications of studies with human subjects from 1983 through 1989. The search generated 101 references. Issues of *Archives of Sexual Behavior, Journal of Sex and Marital Therapy,* and *Journal of Sex Research* were reviewed for 1982 through 1989. Recent textbooks were also consulted where relevant (Arentewicz and Schmidt 1983; Rosen and Beck 1988).

Results

Changing the Name of the Disorder

Changing the name "inhibited female orgasm" to "female orgasmic disorder" would conform more closely to ICD-10, which has a combined category of "orgasmic dysfunction" for men and women. A review of all relevant literature gleaned from the methods described above revealed that *orgasmic disorder* or *orgasmic dysfunction* was the most frequent term used in recent years to specify orgasm-phase problems in women (25 articles). The next most common term was *anorgasmia* or *inorgasmia* (16 articles). One article used the term *preorgasmic,* but three used the DSM-III-R term *inhibited female orgasm.*

On a theoretical level, the term *inhibited female orgasm* assumes that an orgasm is psychologically inhibited by anxiety, as Kaplan (1974) comments, "because it has acquired symbolic meaning, or because its intensity frightens the woman, or because unconscious conflicts are evoked by erotic feelings. Other deeply rooted factors may be involved as well" (p. 384).

Kaplan goes on to compare the "overcontrol" of the orgasmic reflex to constipation. Although the inhibition hypothesis of etiology is interesting, it has no empirical basis. Kaplan's clinical speculations in 1974 have not been tested by research.

As Kaplan (1974) herself notes, her theory is inconsistent with data showing that sex therapy is more effective for the most extreme, generalized forms of the disorder than for women who are orgasmic in some situations and merely want to have orgasms triggered by less intense or prolonged stimulation (De Amicis et al. 1985; Heiman and LoPiccolo 1983; LoPiccolo and Stock 1986). A number of surveys, beginning with Kinsey et al. (1953), have suggested that women's capacity to reach orgasm increases with sexual experience both in terms of orgasmic consistency and response to a wider range of stimulation techniques (Freese and Levitt 1984; Newcomb 1984; Newcomb and Bentler 1983; Raboch and Bartak 1983; Schoty et al. 1984). These data are consistent with a view of orgasmic capacity as dependent on women learning skills to achieve high sexual arousal or to trigger the orgasm reflex. The data do not support a model of psychological inhibition preventing orgasm. No clear personality correlates that apply to a majority of women with orgasmic problems have been found (Derogatis et al. 1989; Heiman and Grafton-Becker 1989). Barlow et al. (Cranston-Cuebas and Barlow 1990; Rosen and Beck 1988) have also completed a series of studies on sexual arousability in men demonstrating that anxious thoughts during sex act more as distracters than as inhibitors. These findings may also apply to female sexual dysfunction.

Is Difficulty Reaching Coital Orgasm a Disorder?

According to DSM-III-R, inhibited female orgasm can be diagnosed in a subset of women who are orgasmic with some types of stimulation but not with vaginal intercourse. The clinician must judge whether the lack of coital orgasm is within the normal range of female sexual responsiveness or represents psychopathology (Morokoff 1989; Wakefield 1987b). Similar judgments must be made in other situations. If a woman can reach orgasm during intercourse, but only after 20 minutes of thrusting, is she "normal" or "disordered"? What if she needs direct clitoral manipulation to reach orgasm, but she and her partner do not regard this as a problem? Should she be given a diagnosis if this pattern is uncovered as part of an evaluation?

The "normal" range of orgasmic consistency for women is determined by societal values. Some nonhuman female primates seem to have orgasms, at least under laboratory conditions (Heiman and Grafton-Becker 1989). Expectations about women's orgasmic capacity vary cross-culturally, from a total lack of orgasms among Irish women from the Isle of Inis Beag, where female sexual pleasure is considered sinful, to a universal experience of multiple orgasms in women of traditional Mangaian culture in Polynesia, where sexual skills are explicitly taught (Morokoff 1978).

In our own society, the ability to reach orgasm during intercourse is currently valued highly. Estimates of women's ability to have coital orgasms are based on surveys. Most such studies focus on samples that are better educated and more liberal politically than the population at large. Two of the most representative samples were 1,044 women surveyed by Hunt (1974) in the United States and 225 40-year-old Danish women interviewed by Garde and Lunde (1984) in the late 1970s. In the American study, 53% of women had coital orgasms on all or almost all attempts, with another 40% coitally orgasmic from one- to three-quarters of the time. The Danish group included 19% who were always coitally orgasmic and 61% who were often or almost always orgasmic. In both cases, 10% or fewer women were rarely or never coitally orgasmic. Very similar results were seen in 92 American women who comprise the normative sample for the Sex History Form (Schover and Jensen 1988), of whom 42% were coitally orgasmic on at least 90% of tries. Another 50% reached orgasm in intercourse from 25% to 75% of the time. These figures are far more favorable than the 30% of women in the Hite report who were regularly orgasmic with intercourse (Hite 1976). The discrepancy is probably due to the unusual sample that Hite recruited and her biased questionnaire. Hite's sample consisted of readers of selected women's magazines and included women of higher education and more liberal and feminist sexual attitudes than in the general population. Yet, it is the Hite estimate that seems to be most frequently quoted and that has influenced our view of regular coital orgasms for women as the exception rather than the rule.

Previous definitions of orgasmic disorder may also have exaggerated its prevalence by ignoring the fact that many women do not experience adequate clitoral stimulation through self-touch or a partner's caress and thus have not had the opportunity to reach orgasm (Wakefield 1987b). Morokoff (1978) also notes that some women labeled as inorgasmic with diagnostic systems prior to DSM-III-R primarily had unrecognized deficits in desire or subjective sexual arousability. Thus, in the past, far more women than men were diagnosed as having an orgasmic disorder. Definitions used in DSM-III-R and now proposed for DSM-IV eliminate much of this gender bias.

Are There Physiological Subtypes of Female Orgasm?

The controversy over the normalcy of coital orgasm began with the Freudian theory of the superiority of orgasms produced by vaginal stimulation to those achieved by clitoral caressing. Masters and Johnson (1966) stated that there was no anatomical difference in the physiological markers of orgasm, no matter what type of stimulation triggered the reflex. Kaplan (1974) further asserted that inability to reach orgasm from vaginal stimulation alone was a normal variant of female sexuality and should not be classified as a dysfunction. Others have tried to resurrect a typology of coital versus noncoital orgasm but without any impressive empirical evidence to support such a distinction (Rosen and Beck 1988).

The most recent of these typologies was that proposed by Ladas et al. (1982). They asserted, based on subjective reports and not on physiological measures, that women who ejaculate fluid at orgasm from stimulation of the upper anterior vaginal wall have a different type of orgasm in terms of vaginal muscle contractions. They assert that such orgasms result from stimulation of the autonomic nerves in the uterine and cervical region as opposed to the pudendal nerve stimulation that mediates clitoral orgasms. Not only have their more testable observations not been replicated (Rosen and Beck 1988), but their hypothesis about innervation would equate coital orgasm with the emission phase of male orgasm without subsequent ejaculation. Men's subjective pleasure at emission is certainly not analogous to the ecstatic and fulfilling experience of G spot orgasm described by Ladas et al. Furthermore, the pudendal nerve does innervate the outer third of the vagina and thus would be stimulated during penile-vaginal intercourse.

A recent pilot study of sensory thresholds to electrical stimulation on the vulva and in the vagina found a mildly sensitive area on the anterior wall and a high degree of variability on the clitoris (Weijmar Schultz et al. 1989). Overall, the vagina was not highly sensitive. Subjects included 60 healthy women. The technology used has not been validated before. Thus, empirically based evidence for a physiological difference in types of orgasm does not exist.

Are There Personality or Behavioral Correlates of Subtypes of Orgasmic Disorder?

Although orgasms from different types of stimulation do not have different physiological characteristics, perhaps women who have difficulty reaching orgasm from different types of stimulation (currently specified in the generalized versus situational modifier) could be distinguished by history, current behavior, or personality.

In terms of personality, Loos et al. (1987) found that volunteers from the community who reported themselves as consistently orgasmic during intercourse attributed their success to stable, internal ability as men often do. Woman low in coital orgasm consistency blamed their failure on themselves and attributed successes to external causes. Such a cognitive strategy could interfere with a woman's learning to be more easily orgasmic. Orgasmic consistency with other types of stimulation was not investigated, however.

Kilmann et al. (1984) compared self-reports of sexual behavior for couples with a woman partner who had problems reaching coital orgasm with that in couples without sexual dysfunction. In the dysfunctional couples, both partners were more dissatisfied with the variety of their sexual behaviors. Women reported below-average sexual pleasure ratings. Men were not accurate in their beliefs about the wives' sexual preferences and also were dissatisfied with their own sexual pleasure.

Another study verified through factor analysis that orgasmic responsiveness in situations of coital stimulation, noncoital stimulation from a partner, and solo masturbation can be distinguished (Newcomb and Bentler 1983). There was also a generalized orgasmic responsiveness factor, however, that correlated highly with each subscale. Women who were more easily and frequently orgasmic overall had first coitus at an earlier age, more lifetime sexual partners, and a higher frequency of masturbation and intercourse. Ability to reach orgasm during masturbation was a better predictor of coital orgasm than of orgasm with noncoital partner stimulation, contrary to models espoused in sex therapy.

Earlier age at first intercourse was also correlated with ease of reaching orgasm in two other samples (Newcomb 1984; Raboch and Bartak 1983). Women's orgasmic ability overall, with coitus alone and with varying stimulation sites, also increases with age (Freese and Levitt 1984; Schoty et al. 1984). Women who masturbate more frequently are also more likely to reach orgasm during intercourse (Newcomb 1984; Newcomb and Bentler 1983), but use of clitoral versus vaginal stimulation during masturbation does not seem to predict ability to have coital orgasm (Leff and Israel 1983; Schoty et al. 1984).

The natural history of female orgasmic disorder should be studied. These data suggest that in young, inexperienced women, orgasm is less frequent and depends on a narrow type of stimulation. As women learn more about their sexual responsiveness, they may become more reliably orgasmic with a wider variety of stimuli. The specific hypothesis that clitoral stimulation in masturbation is the strongest stimulus, followed by clitoral stimulation by a partner, and then by vaginal penetration and thrusting is not clearly supported, however.

One other approach to subtyping female orgasmic disorder on a personality dimension has been taken by Derogatis et al. (1986, 1989). In two separate papers, they present statistical analyses of DSFI profiles for women seen at a sex therapy clinic and given a DSM-III (American Psychiatric Association 1980) diagnosis of inhibited female orgasm. The first effort split the women into two groups based on whether they reported using a sexual fantasy theme of homosexual sex. Not surprisingly, women who had such fantasies also reported more frequent sexual activity and fantasies, as well as more liberal sexual attitudes. This arbitrary grouping does not seem of high value for diagnosis or treatment planning, however. A later case series (whether consecutive referrals were included is unspecified) was analyzed using hierarchical cluster techniques. Again the women were all diagnosed with inhibited female orgasm, and the data were from the DSFI. Four subtypes were identified. One group of women also had low sexual desire. A second group exhibited "histrionic" traits and marital conflict. A high rate of concurrent psychiatric disorders was seen in the third group, and the fourth group of women were better adjusted but had medical problems and lifelong difficulty reaching orgasm. Although these groupings are of interest, they need to be cross-validated on other samples before more confidence can be placed in them. Their usefulness in planning treatment also remains to be tested. Although Derogatis et al. (1989) report concurrent rates of psychiatric disorders and the lifelong versus acquired nature of the orgasmic disorder, they do not mention the global versus situational dimension.

Subtypes of Orgasmic Disorder and Sex Therapy Outcome

A number of sex therapy outcome studies have included patients with female orgasmic disorder. Fewer studies have distinguished between success of treatment for women with subtypes of the dysfunction. This section reviews those outcome studies that report results separately for lifelong versus acquired disorders or global versus situational disorders. A related issue is the generalizability of improved orgasmic capacity from one type of stimulation to another (i.e., solo masturbation to noncoital stimulation by a partner to coitus).

As LoPiccolo and Stock (1986) have pointed out, most studies have divided orgasmic disorders into primary versus secondary categories. This confounds the more precise dimensions of generalized versus situational and lifelong versus acquired specified in DSM-III-R, because a primary disorder is lifelong and generalized, whereas a secondary one is acquired but may be either generalized or situational across types of stimulation or different partners. There is consensus that primary inorgasmia can be successfully treated in a variety of sex therapy formats (Andersen 1983; LoPiccolo and Stock 1986). LoPiccolo and Stock (1986) report that of 150 women with lifelong, generalized orgasmic disorder treated in their sex therapy clinic, 95% became orgasmic in masturbation, 85% with partner noncoital stimulation, and 40% during intercourse. Outcome with secondary orgasmic dysfunction has been less successful. Heiman and LoPiccolo (1983) compared 1-year follow-up for 25 couples with a primary female orgasmic dysfunction versus 16 with a secondary dysfunction. Changes in the frequency of orgasm were significant only for the primary group, although the secondary group made nonsignificant gains in coital orgasm frequency. A 3-year follow-up of a smaller number of couples treated in the same clinic revealed a similar pattern (De Amicis et al. 1985). Sexual satisfaction showed an enduring improvement, but actual frequency of orgasm from various types of stimulation regressed to pretreatment levels in both groups. The incompleteness of the sample reached for long-term follow-up mitigates the results, however.

In a small study of 11 couples, Kilmann et al. (1987) found that women who had experienced coital orgasm at least once made greater gains in marital happiness from sex therapy in a group format than did coitally inorgasmic women. Actual improvements in coital orgasm frequency did not differ between the two groups, however. In a longer-term follow-up of 38 of 66 women treated in groups for secondary orgasmic dysfunction, this group found that coital orgasmic frequency increased over time to 34% on the average, with higher frequencies for masturbation (87%) and oral sex with a partner (53%). The greatest gains were for young women with functional partners, initially low sexual frequency, and high couple conflict about sex (Milan et al. 1988).

Wakefield (1987a) and Nairne and Hemsley (1983) have reviewed data on the success of groups for primarily inorgasmic women in fostering orgasmic capacity with partner stimulation. They point out the limited success of such treatment in promoting consistent orgasms with partner stimulation. The studies cited above suggest that even for women who are already occasionally orgasmic with a partner, various formats of sex therapy have better success in promoting orgasms through masturbation than from partner caress or intercourse. In the more recent literature, significant gains in coital orgasm or at least orgasm with a partner have been reported by some investigators (Kuriansky et al. 1982; Milan et al. 1988), but nonsignificant generalization has occurred in other studies (Andersen 1981; Cohen-Huston and Wheeler 1983). Such a variety of specific behavioral techniques have been used that no conclusions can be drawn about any one modality and its effectiveness in generalizing orgasms from masturbation to partner stimulation.

Discussion

The literature suggests that *female orgasmic disorder* would be a more effective diagnostic title than *inhibited female orgasm*. This name change (suggested also for the male diagnosis) would bring DSM-IV into better conformity with current clinical usage and with ICD-10. The assumption that psychological "inhibition" of a reflex is causal in this disorder cannot be supported empirically.

This lack of proof also is a relevant reason to eliminate labeling coital inorgasmia as a disorder only when a "psychological inhibition" is present. Furthermore, diagnosing a disorder retrospectively on the basis of the success of sex therapy is clearly problematic. Close to two-thirds of women in Western society are coitally orgasmic with reasonable frequency. Thus, the small percentage who never or very rarely have coital orgasms are statistical outliers. To justify a diagnosis of situational orgasmic disorder of any type, however, a woman should have had adequate learning experiences and currently be exposed to skilled stimulation yet have a persistently poor ability to reach orgasm. Rather than using arbitrary diagnostic criteria based only on the site of sexual stimulation that a "normal" woman needs, the clinician should base a diagnosis of female orgasmic disorder on the woman's age and sexual experience and the adequacy of the stimulation her partner gives (in terms of duration, intensity, and accurate response to her feedback). We need more representative normative samples of women, with more detailed information on the type, duration, and site(s) of stimulation that lead to orgasm. Given our current knowledge, our diagnostic criteria must remain flexible, with room for clinical judgment. A patient's own degree of distress and wish to increase her orgasmic capacity should also be considered, because we as clinicians may be imposing a standard of sexual performance based on societal mores rather than on biology.

Although the most promising subtyping schema currently would be to divide the disorder into stimulation-specific categories (i.e., women who are totally inorgasmic [generalized], and the situational categories of inorgasmic except with solo masturbation, inorgasmic except with noncoital caressing from a partner, or inorgasmic only in coitus), evidence from a variety of sources is inadequate to justify the subtyping of female orgasmic disorder beyond the dimensions of lifelong

versus acquired and generalized versus situational. Physiological data do not support a distinction between orgasms resulting from different sites of stimulation.
Personality correlates of generalized versus situation-specific deficits in orgasmic
capacity have not been appropriately studied yet. It does seem that women's ability
to reach orgasm increases with age and sexual experience and that women often
learn over time to become orgasmic with a wider range of types of stimulation. This
raises a question for the future about the very classification of orgasmic disorder as
a psychiatric problem. Age-appropriate norms for orgasmic capacity in healthy
women are not currently available but could be useful clinically in deciding when
to label difficulty reaching orgasm as a problem

Data from therapy outcome studies confirm that it is relatively easy, in clinical
samples, to teach women to masturbate to orgasm but more difficult to produce
enduring changes in women's ability to reach orgasm from manual, oral, or coital
stimulation by a partner.

In conclusion, the situation-specific subtyping of female orgasmic disorders
has some potential heuristic and clinical utility, but more information is needed
before incorporating it into a system such as DSM-IV.

Recommendations

Based on the results of this literature review, the following recommendations are
made for DSM-IV:

The name of this disorder and of the male parallel diagnosis should be changed
to "female orgasmic disorder" and "male orgasmic disorder."

Criterion A should be revised, deleting material about inability to reach orgasm
during intercourse and replacing it with the following:

> Women exhibit wide variability in the type or intensity of stimulation that triggers
> orgasm. The diagnosis of situational female orgasmic disorder should be based on
> the clinician's judgment that the woman's orgasmic capacity is less than would be
> reasonable for her age, sexual experience, and the adequacy of sexual stimulation
> she receives.

Rather than labeling coital inorgasmia as a disorder only if "psychological inhibition" is present, any situational form of female orgasmic disorder will be diagnosed
only if a woman's orgasmic capacity is not consonant with her expectations and when
these are realistic in the clinician's judgment. The addition of criterion C, "The
disturbance causes marked distress or interpersonal difficulty," ensures that the clinician takes the woman's own goals for her sexual function into account.

Subtyping of female orgasmic disorder on the basis of personality or physiological typologies cannot be justified based on current empirical data and should not be included in DSM-IV. Subtypes will likely be coded as generalized or situational, however. The generalized form of the disorder is used when a woman is currently inorgasmic in all situations. Situational subtypes are defined by the situations in which a woman reaches orgasm (e.g., with self- or vibrator stimulation only, with partner noncoital stimulation but not during intercourse, or only with a particular partner). Because the same subtypes will be used for male orgasmic disorder, concerns expressed by Wakefield (1987b) as to gender bias will be addressed. He felt that the prevalence of female orgasmic disorder was inflated because of the inclusion of difficulty in achieving coital orgasm and that only global and lifelong female orgasmic disorder could be considered comparable to male orgasmic disorder.

Future research is needed to address several issues. We need age-related norms for women's capacity to reach orgasm from various types of sexual stimulation. We need more information about typologies of situational orgasmic disorder: Do personality styles predict women's orgasmic capacity across sexual situations? Are some situation-specific orgasmic disorders more amenable than others to respond to current sex therapy techniques? Are there any biological differences in women's ease of reaching orgasm within or across sites of stimulation?

References

American Psychiatric Association: Diagnostic and Statistical Manual of Mental Disorders, 3rd Edition. Washington, DC, American Psychiatric Association, 1980

American Psychiatric Association: Diagnostic and Statistical Manual of Mental Disorders, 3rd Edition, Revised. Washington, DC, American Psychiatric Association, 1987

Andersen BL: A comparison of systematic desensitization and directed masturbation in the treatment of primary orgasmic dysfunction in females. J Consult Clin Psychol 49:568–570, 1981

Andersen BL: Primary orgasmic dysfunction: diagnostic considerations and review of treatment. Psychol Bull 93:105–136, 1983

Arentewicz G, Schmidt G: The Treatment of Sexual Disorders. New York, Basic Books, 1983

Cohen-Huston AL, Wheeler KA: Preorgasmic group treatment: assertiveness, marital adjustment, and sexual function in women. J Sex Marital Ther 9:296–302, 1983

Cranston-Cuebas MA, Barlow DH: Cognitive and affective contributions to sexual functioning, in Annual Review of Sex Research, Vol 1. Edited by Bancroft J, Davis CM, Weinstein D. Lake Mills, IA, Society for the Scientific Study of Sex, 1990, pp 119–161

De Amicis LA, Goldberg DC, LoPiccolo J, et al: Clinical follow-up of couples treated for sexual dysfunction. Arch Sex Behav 14:467–489, 1985

Derogatis LR, Fagan PJ, Schmidt CW, et al: Psychological subtypes of anorgasmia: a marker variable approach. J Sex Marital Ther 12:197–210, 1986

Derogatis LR, Schmidt CW, Fagan PJ, et al: Subtypes of anorgasmia: a mathematical taxonomy. Psychosomatics 30:166–173, 1989

Freese MP, Levitt, EE: Relationships among intravaginal pressure, orgasmic function, parity factors, and urinary leakage. Arch Sex Behav 13:261–268, 1984

Garde I, Lunde K: Influence of social status of female sexual behaviour: a random sample study of 40-year-old Danish women. Scand J Prim Health Care 1:5–10, 1984

Heiman JR, Grafton-Becker V: Orgasmic disorders in women, in Principles and Practice of Sex Therapy: Update for the 1990s. Edited by Leiblum SR, Rosen RC. New York, Guilford, 1989, pp 51–88

Heiman JR, LoPiccolo J: Clinical outcomes of sex therapy: effects of daily versus weekly treatment. Arch Gen Psychiatry 40:443–449, 1983

Hite S: The Hite Report: A Nationwide Study of Female Sexuality. New York, Dell, 1976

Hunt M: Sexual Behavior in the 1970s. New York, Dell, 1974

Kaplan HS: The New Sex Therapy. New York, Brunner/Mazel, 1974, pp 384, 398–400

Kilmann PR, Mills KH, Caid C, et al: The sexual interaction of women with secondary orgasmic dysfunction and their partners. Arch Sex Behav 13:41–49, 1984

Kilmann PR, Milan RJ, Boland JP, et al: The treatment of secondary orgasmic dysfunction II. J Sex Marital Ther 13:93–105, 1987

Kinsey AC, Pomeroy W, Martin C, et al: Sexual Behavior in the Human Female. Philadelphia, PA, WB Saunders, 1953

Kuriansky JB, Sharpe L, O'Connor D: The treatment of anorgasmia: long-term effectiveness of a short-term behavioral group therapy. J Sex Marital Ther 8:29–43, 1982

Ladas AK, Whipple B, Perry JD: The G Spot. New York, Holt, Rinehart & Winston, 1982

Leff JJ, Israel M: The relationship between mode of female masturbation and achievement of orgasm in coitus. Arch Sex Behav 12:227–236, 1983

Loos VE, Bridges CF, Critelli JW: Weiner's attribution theory and female orgasmic consistency. Journal of Sex Research 23:348–361, 1987

LoPiccolo J, Stock WE: Treatment of sexual dysfunction. J Consult Clin Psychol 54:158–167, 1986

Masters WH, Johnson VE: Human Sexual Response. New York, Bantam Books, 1966, pp 65–67

Milan RJ, Kilmann PR, Boland JP: Treatment outcome of secondary orgasmic dysfunction: a two-to-six year follow-up. Arch Sex Behav 17:463–480, 1988

Morokoff P: Determinants of female orgasm, in Handbook of Sex Therapy. Edited by LoPiccolo J, LoPiccolo L. New York, Plenum, 1978, pp 147–165

Morokoff P: Sex bias and POD (letter). Am Psychol 44:73–75, 1989

Nairne KD, Hemsley DR: The use of directed masturbation training in the treatment of primary anorgasmia. Br J Clin Psychol 22:283–294, 1983

Newcomb MD: Sexual behavior responsiveness, and attitudes among women: a test of two theories. J Sex Marital Ther 10:272–286, 1984

Newcomb MD, Bentler PM: Dimensions of subjective female orgasmic responsiveness. J Pers Soc Psychol 44:862–873, 1983

Raboch J, Bartak V: Coitarche and orgiastic capacity. Arch Sex Behav 12:409–413, 1983

Rosen RC, Beck JG: Patterns of Sexual Arousal: Psychophysiological Processes and Clinical Applications. New York, Guilford, 1988, pp 134–157, 280–284

Schoty MJ, Ephross PH, Plaut SM, et al: Female orgasmic experience: a subjective study. Arch Sex Behav 13:155–164, 1984

Schover LR, Jensen SB: Sexuality and Chronic Illness: A Comprehensive Approach. New York, Guilford, 1988, p 133

Schover LR, Friedman JM, Weiler SJ, et al: Multiaxial problem-oriented system for sexual dysfunctions. Arch Gen Psychiatry 39:614–619, 1982

Wakefield JC: The semantics of success: do masturbation exercises lead to partner orgasm? J Sex Marital Ther 13:3–14, 1987a

Wakefield JC: Sex bias in the diagnosis of primary orgasmic dysfunction. Am Psychol 42:464–471, 1987b

Weijmar Schultz WCM, van de Wiel HBM, Klatter JA, et al: Vaginal sensitivity to electric stimuli: theoretical and practical implications. Arch Sex Behav 18:87–96, 1989

World Health Organization: ICD-10 Chapter V. Mental and Behavioral Disorders. Diagnostic Criteria for Research. Geneva, Switzerland, World Health Organization, 1990

Chapter 53

Sexual Pain Disorders

Raul C. Schiavi, M.D.

Statement of the Issues

Dyspareunia

The following issues regarding dyspareunia were examined:

1. Is it appropriate to use the sexual dysfunction diagnosis of dyspareunia when the pain is clearly due to genital pathology (e.g., vaginal infections, endometriosis)?
2. Is it appropriate to diagnose dyspareunia in patients who meet criteria for another Axis I disorder such as somatization disorder?

Vaginismus

There are no issues that require examination concerning the diagnostic category of vaginismus.

Significance of the Issues

The diagnostic criteria for dyspareunia in DSM-III (American Psychiatric Association 1980) included the following statement: "B. The disturbance is not caused exclusively by a physical disorder and is not due to lack of lubrication, functional vaginismus, or another Axis I disorder." In DSM-III-R (American Psychiatric Association 1987), this statement was changed, and the proviso that this disturbance should not be caused exclusively by a physical disorder or be due to another Axis I disorder was eliminated. However, these exclusions remained part of the required criteria for vaginismus.

Methods

A review was conducted to identify empirical information on both dyspareunia and vaginismus due to the close association between these two disorders. The review was based on a Medline and a PsycInfo (Psychological Abstracts) computer search from 1966 to September 1989. The following journals published between 1988 and 1990 were also reviewed for pertinent articles: *American Journal of Psychiatry, Journal of Nervous and Mental Disease, Psychosomatic Medicine, Archives of Sexual Behavior, Journal of Sex and Marital Therapy, Journal of Sex Research, Journal of Behavioral Medicine, Journal of Sex Education and Therapy, American Journal of Obstetrics and Gynecology,* and *Obstetrics and Gynecology.*

Results

The Medline search identified 106 articles under the heading of *dyspareunia* and 59 under the term *vaginismus*. The PsycInfo search identified 101 articles under the headings of *dyspareunia* or *vaginismus*. Most of the articles are case reports, clinical reviews concerning a wide range of organic conditions, or discussions about assessment and therapeutic management. Data-based, systematic investigations of dyspareunia as a sexual dysfunction are extremely few, are mainly focused on the prevalence of the disorder (Bachman et al. 1989; Osborn et al. 1988), and are not directly related to the two issues raised above.

Discussion

Although the review of the literature has not contributed relevant information, it seems that it would be conceptually more consistent with other disorders, as well as diagnostically more accurate, to return to the DSM-III criteria. The criteria for dyspareunia should explicitly exclude patients in whom the problem is solely due to medical conditions or to other Axis I disorders. Exclusion of patients with dyspareunia primarily caused by organic pathology will also make DSM-IV criteria more consistent with ICD-10 nomenclature.

Recommendations

The proposed diagnostic criteria for dyspareunia are

A. Recurrent or persistent genital pain in either a male or a female before, during, or after sexual intercourse.
B. Disturbance is not caused exclusively by lack of lubrication or vaginismus and is not better accounted for by another Axis I disorder (e.g., somatization disorder).

C. Not due to a substance-induced (i.e., drugs, medication) or a secondary sexual dysfunction.
D. The disturbance causes marked distress or interpersonal difficulty.

References

American Psychiatric Association: Diagnostic and Statistical Manual of Mental Disorders, 3rd Edition. Washington, DC, American Psychiatric Association, 1980

American Psychiatric Association: Diagnostic and Statistical Manual of Mental Disorders, 3rd Edition, Revised. Washington, DC, American Psychiatric Association, 1987

Bachman GA, Leiblum SR, Grill J: Brief sexual inquiry in gynecologic practice. Obstet Gynecol 73:425–427, 1989

Osborn M, Hawton K, Gath D: Sexual dysfunction among middle-aged women in the community. BMJ 296:959–962, 1988

Chapter 54

Paraphilias

Thomas N. Wise, M.D., and Chester W. Schmidt, Jr., M.D.

T he task of the sub-Work Group on Paraphilias of the DSM-IV Work Group on Sexual Disorders was to review the DSM-III-R (American Psychiatric Association 1987) diagnostic categories of paraphilias to identify diagnostic issues that should be considered. No issues were identified with regard to the diagnoses of exhibition-ism, pedophilia, sexual masochism, sexual sadism, voyeurism, or frotteurism. Specific issues were raised with regard to the diagnoses of fetishism, transvestic fetishism, telephone scatologia, and the term *sexual addiction* in sexual disorders not otherwise specified. The issues associated with each of these diagnoses are addressed in this chapter.

Methods

Literature reviews were conducted to compile all available data on each of the diagnoses and associated issues. Literature within the English language or extracted translations from Medline and Psychological Abstracts literature searches were collected. In addition, a literature search was done by computerized database using both Medline and PsycInfo using the key words *fetish, transvestic fetishism, paraphilia, telephone scatologia, sexual addiction, sexual compulsivism*, etc. The specific journals focusing on sexuality and sex research were reviewed by hand. Journals included the *Archives of Sexual Behavior, The Journal of Sex Research, The Journal of Sex in Marital Therapy*, and *The British Journal of Sexual Medicine*. Books on specific topics associated with the issues raised for the various diagnostic categories were also reviewed and are included in the bibliography. When possible, studies were cataloged with respect to the number of subjects, the average age of the subjects, the source of the study cohort, the diagnostic criteria used, the presence of comorbid psychiatric disorders, whether other paraphilias were noted, therapeutic issues, and whether phallometry was used.

Transvestic Fetishism

Statement of the Issue

In DSM-III (American Psychiatric Association 1980), transvestic fetishism is sharply differentiated from transsexualism. In fact, the diagnostic criteria for transvestic fetishism excludes criteria for gender identity disorder of adolescents or adults, nontranssexual type, or transsexualism. The text indicates that in the rare incidences in which transvestic fetishism evolves into transsexualism, the diagnosis of transvestic fetishism should be changed to transsexualism. In ICD-9 (World Health Organization 1978), the diagnostic criteria for transvestism specifically excludes transsexualism. In ICD-10 (World Health Organization 1990), the diagnostic guidelines will suggest that fetishistic transvestism be distinguished from transsexualism. It will further note that a history of fetishistic transvestism is commonly reported as an earlier phase by transsexuals and probably represents a stage in the development of transsexualism in such cases.

Because transvestic fetishism and gender dysphoria are now recognized as common comorbid conditions, the question arises whether individuals with transvestic fetishism and gender dysphoria should be diagnosed as transvestic fetishism, gender dysphoric type, or as gender identity disorder or receive two diagnoses—transvestic fetishism and gender identity disorder.

Significance of the Issue

Although the exact prevalence and incidence of transvestic fetishism is not known, it is estimated that 50% of the applicants for sexual reassignment have been transvestic in the past. Clinically, it is also common for individuals with transvestic fetishism to report episodic gender dysphoria. This review considers the emergence of gender dysphoria in the course of transvestic fetishism because of the common association between the two conditions that is now recognized.

Since the first report of sexual reassignment surgery in 1931, there have been numerous follow-up reports (Lothstein 1982; Lundstrom et al. 1984). Although retrospective reviews of the outcome of sexual reassignment surgery have been cautiously favorable, even the most optimistic reports suggest that 10%–15% of such patients have a poor outcome (Kuiper and Cohen-Kettenis 1988). Hunt and Hampson (1980) followed 17 males sexually reassigned to females and found their Minnesota Multiphasic Personality Inventory (MMPI) scores showed no change. However, the patients did report improved economic functioning and interpersonal relationships. On the other hand, Lindermalm et al. (1986) noted that overall sexual adjustment was rarely changed at long-term follow-up of 13 patients and that 30% of their sample felt surgery was a mistake. With such results, it is important to develop selection criteria that will help predict those who are most likely to have the best treatment outcome following surgery (Blanchard et al. 1989).

Results

Meyer (1974) described various clinical variants of gender dysphoric individuals who seek sexual reassignment. The individuals described included the transvestic applicant whose gender dysphoric state was fostered by aging or loss of a significant other. In the ensuing 15 years, other studies indicate that many individuals requesting sexual reassignment surgery are, in fact, fetishistically aroused by the idea of wearing female clothes (Dixen et al. 1984). Shore (1984) presents a case report on an individual who is best understood as a fetishistic transvestite and who became gender dysphoric and requested surgical reassignment but either retreated from the procedure or was disappointed following reversible surgery. Levine's reports on "Ruth" also seem to fit this category (Levine 1984; Levine and Shumaker 1983). Wise's (1979) report on therapy with an aging transvestite illustrates the intense gender dysphoria that can occur in the fetishistic transvestite in a setting of loss or physical illness. Wise and Meyer (1980) described the clinical characteristics of a group of transvestic applicants for sexual reassignment and found that they became gender dysphoric in settings of loss, retirement, forced intimacy, or the onset of an Axis I disorder. A study of distressed transvestites reported that those who were gender dysphoric also cross-dressed at an earlier age and had more bisexual experiences than the non–gender dysphoric transvestites (Fagan et al. 1988). Earlier, Buhrich (1977) found that there appeared to be syndromes of "nuclear" and "marginal transvestites." They studied members of an Australian Club for cross-dressers and partitioned those individuals that considered surgical reassignment from those that were primarily interested in fetishistic cross-dressing (Buhrich and McConaghy 1977a, 1977b). The gender dysphoric subset, termed "marginal" transvestites, had more homosexual experience, cross-dressed more frequently, and began cross-dressing at an earlier age than the "nuclear" transvestic group. Two studies using phallometric methods found that heterosexual cross-dressers of various diagnostic categories tended to have fetishistic arousal (Blanchard et al. 1986; Buhrich 1977). Even those heterosexual cross-dressers who stated they never had fetishistic arousal responded with arousal when given transvestic stimuli. Gender dysphoria and fetishistic behavior have been found to be far from mutually exclusive (Blanchard et al. 1985). Many heterosexual cross-dressers simultaneously report gender dysphoria and fetishistic arousal. One study has demonstrated the social desirability factors that distort the self-report of fetishistic arousal in individuals in gender dysphoria clinics (Blanchard et al. 1985). A recent study reports that gender dysphoric individuals are often hesitant and ambivalent even if offered sexual reassignment surgery. The ambivalent individuals have a tendency to be older, more often married, and more often financially secure (Kockott and Fahrner 1987). These individuals may be the gender dysphoric fetishistic transvestites reported by many other authors.

Discussion

The literature review reveals the frequent association of transvestic fetishism and gender dysphoria. The development of gender dysphoria in transvestic fetishists may be associated with specific losses and with the development of Axis I disorders such as depression. In other instances, the development of the gender dysphoria cannot be specifically associated with a stressor. Clinically, the presence of gender dysphoria may either be progressive and continuous over time or, in other instances, episodic and best characterized as a waxing and waning of the gender dysphoria and the press for surgical reassignment. The literature does not appear to be sufficiently developed to support the statements that transvestic fetishism and transsexualism are mutually exclusive or that transvestic fetishism may represent a stage in the development of transsexualism in those cases in which both transvestic fetishism and gender dysphoria are reported. The one fact that emerges from the literature is that transvestic fetishism and gender dysphoria are commonly associated and that the interrelationships of the two conditions are not well understood.

Recommendations

Diagnostic nomenclature is needed to highlight the clinical instance of patients with transvestic histories who are now gender dysphoric and may be requesting surgical reassignment. We recommend adding a gender dysphoric subtype to the existing diagnosis of transvestic fetishism. The addition of this recommended subtype would reflect a clinical reality and augment the collection of data, thus enhancing both research and treatment.

A subcommittee of the Work Group on childhood disorders has also reviewed the issues and our recommendation. This subcommittee found our proposal to be problematic because "many such individuals appear to lose the transvestic arousal as the gender dysphoria develops." They point out that subtyping transvestic fetishists as gender dysphoric could then require a change of diagnosis to gender identity disorder when fetishistic arousal diminished or disappeared. The subcommittee recommends that fetishistic arousal should not be an exclusion criteria for gender identity disorder. Individuals who currently experience erotic arousal in association with cross-dressing as well as gender dysphoria would receive two diagnoses—gender identity disorder and transvestic fetishism.

We believe there may be clinical instances when the two diagnoses are appropriate. However, there are other instances when the gender dysphoria is either mild to moderate or waxes and wanes to a sufficient degree that the patient does not consistently seek surgical reassignment or make efforts to live in the cross-gender role. In those clinical instances, an additional diagnosis of gender identity disorder would seem inappropriate. Our preference remains the addition of the gender dysphoric subtype to transvestic fetishism.

Fetishism

Statement of the Issue

The purpose of the review was to determine whether there is any need to change the present DSM-III-R diagnostic criteria or text for fetishism.

Significance of the Issue

The literature review was performed to determine whether there were new data regarding fetishistic objects and behaviors that would warrant changes in DSM-IV.

Results

The majority of current reports are single case studies. An exception is Chalkley and Powell's (1983) report of 48 cases of sexual fetishism in individuals referred primarily by the court. They report that these individuals often had multiple fetishes and comorbid diagnoses, including depression, anxiety, neurosis, and personality disorder. Abel et al. (1988) reviewed 561 nonincarcerated paraphilics and found the majority of the individuals in his sample had multiple paraphilic behaviors including fetishism, voyeurism, and exhibitionism. Three fetishes or fetishistic-like behavior have received recent attention. Enema irrigation has been reported as a preferred erotic stimulus (Agnew 1982; Denko 1976). A recent report from the *Journal of the American Medical Association* described enema irrigation in conjunction with bondage and noted serious medical side effects such as opportunistic infection due to eradication of the normal intestinal flora (Sorvillo et al. 1989). Erotic attraction to amputees has been described (Dixon 1983).

Discussion

The literature review revealed little additional information regarding the age at onset, incidence, and prevalence of fetishism. Some of the published data come from surveys of magazine subscribers and underground networks. The reliability of these data sources is questionable.

Recommendations

The literature review indicates there are not sufficient data to change the current diagnostic criteria for fetishism.

Telephone Scatologia (Lewdness)

Statement of the Issue

This paraphilia, telephone scatalogia, is listed in DSM-III-R under paraphilia not otherwise specified (302.90). The list of examples are paraphilias that do not meet the criteria for any of the specific categories separately listed as paraphilias. The frequency of occurrence of this particular paraphilia might warrant removal from the list of examples with placement as a specific category of paraphilia with defined diagnostic criteria.

Significance of the Issue

The development of a specific category of telephone scatalogia with its own diagnostic criteria will stimulate research. The frequency of occurrence may be at least as great as, if not greater than, that of frotteurism, which is listed as a specific paraphilia with its own criteria set in DSM-III-R.

Results

Of the 12 reports found that discussed telephone scatologia, only 1 employed a large population. Murray and Bevan (1968) surveyed a group of college undergraduates and found that 90% of the females and 73% of the males had received lewd phone calls. The majority of the phone calls were directly obscene or characterized by heavy breathing. The study was merely a survey, and the content of the phone calls was not further described. Other reports are either single case reports or small sample reports. Dalby (1988) reviewed four obscene phone callers who were all referred from the court system. Of note was the finding that one individual was also transvestic. Saunders et al. (1986) reviewed 63 adolescent sexual offenders and found that only one was an obscene phone caller. Other reports described either behavioral or psychodynamic treatment approaches for the single cases presented. Another indication that obscene phone calling may be common are reports from college counseling services that discuss management of the obscene phone call (Clark et al. 1986). These reports do not describe case material but emphasize the frequency of phone calls reported to counseling services and counseling telephone hot lines (Walfish 1983).

The literature review suggests the obscene phone caller may also have other paraphilias. Alford et al. (1980) described an obscene phone caller who was also an exhibitionist, whereas in one case Dalby (1988) reported transvestic behavior. These single case reports suggest that obscene phone calling is a repetitive, desired stimulus associated with sexual arousal and orgasmic release. The disorder is found primarily in males. The age at onset appears to be during adolescence.

Discussion

The incidence and prevalence of telephone scatologia cannot be cited but appear to be relatively common, as evidenced by reports from telephone counseling services and college counseling literature that cite obscene phone calls as a problem that needs to be addressed by their services. The literature on the subject is obviously sparse. The development of research on this paraphilia would be enhanced by calling greater attention to the disorder and by providing specific diagnostic criteria.

Recommendations

It is proposed that telephone scatologia be specifically denoted as a paraphilia within DSM-IV, with the following diagnostic criteria:

1. Over a period of at least 6 months, recurrent and intense sexual urges and sexually arousing fantasies are aroused by calling a nonconsenting individual and either overtly verbalizing erotic or obscene language or silently fantasizing such material while on the telephone.
2. The individual has acted on these urges or is markedly distressed by them.
3. This is not an episodic behavior undertaken with a group of peers during latency or adolescence.

Sexual Addiction

Statement of the Issue

DSM-III-R currently includes the term *sexual addiction* in the second example of sexual disorder not otherwise specified (302.90, p. 296). The example is "distress about a pattern of repeated sexual conquests or other forms of nonparaphilic sexual addiction, involving a succession of people who exist only as things to be used." The concept of sexual addiction, whether paraphilic or nonparaphilic, has been popularized in a series of books and articles that have no scientific database. The issue is whether this concept is sufficiently supported scientifically to be included in DSM-IV.

Significance of the Issues

DSM-III-R acknowledges the concept of sexual addiction. The scientific interests in excessive sexual behavior has been heightened by the AIDS epidemic and recognition that certain individuals engage in sexual activities with extraordinary frequency. Scientific support for the concept of sexual addiction would have important impact on research and treatment. For these reasons the concept was considered by the Work Group.

Results

The literature review revealed few database studies. There are several single case reports, but most of the literature consists of position papers that either support or attack the concepts of sexual addiction, sexual compulsivity, and sexual impulsivity. Quadland (1985) reported on 30 gay and bisexual men who defined themselves as being sexually compulsive and who sought treatment for that problem. Carnes (1987) has written an influential book, *The Sexual Addiction*, in which he attempts to define the concept of sexual addiction and offers treatment approaches for the disorder. The book consists of case histories of individuals with a wide variety of paraphilic disorders, a common theme in all cases being high sex drive. No database studies are included in the book. Carnes has not empirically demonstrated that "sexual addiction" is distinctly different from the paraphilias currently within the diagnostic nomenclature. Levine and Troiden (1988) reviewed the cultural changes over the past three decades that have minimized the guilt regarding sexual activity that is not directly procreative. Quadland and colleagues (Quadland 1985; Quadland and Shattle 1987) reported on individuals with problems in what they call "sexual control" and have conceptualized the problem to be that of sexual compulsivity. Barth and Kinder (1987) have suggested impulse control disorder not otherwise specified be used diagnostically for the clinical phenomenon of excessive sexual behaviors. Coleman (1988) has developed an interesting rationale for considering the concept of sexual compulsivity rather than sexual addiction. A recent study reported that there are individuals who continue to practice sexual behavior with a high risk of infection with HIV and appear unable to control their sexual impulses (Richwald et al. 1988). It has also been shown that certain organic lesions can foster hypersexuality (Harvey 1988; Myers and Carrera 1989).

Discussion

There is abundant clinical evidence of sexual activity that can be characterized as "excessive." However, the concept of sexual addiction is troublesome in that the term *addiction* has a specific meaning associated with physiological processes of withdrawal. In addition, there is no scientific database to support the concept of excessive sexual behavior as being in the realm of an addiction. Competing concepts of compulsivity or impulsive control disorders are intriguing possibilities but lack database support. The whole issue of excessive sexual behavior is worthy of scientific study, but the interests of research are not served by restricting the focus of these efforts to a process of addiction. To illustrate the confusion on the subject, it is important to note that ICD-10 will include a disorder titled "excessive sexual drive" under the section on sexual dysfunctions. The clinical description associated with the disorder states that both men and women may occasionally complain of excessive sexual drive as a problem in its own right, usually during late teenage years or early adulthood. The clinical description then includes nymphomania and satyriasis as associated conditions. As to whether these two conditions are non-paraphilic in nature and should be placed within the clinical descriptor for this newly defined condition is open to question.

Recommendations

There is insufficient scientific data to support the inclusion of the term *sexual addiction* in DSM-IV. Research should begin to empirically study individuals who engage in excessive sexual behavior. The phrase containing the term *sexual addiction* in example 2 of sexual disorder not otherwise specified (302.90) should be eliminated. We suggest that example 2 read, "Distress about a pattern of repeated sexual conquests involving a succession of people who exist only as things to be used."

References

Abel GG, Becker JV, Cunningham-Rathner J, et al: Multiple paraphilic diagnoses among sex offenders. Bull Am Acad Psychiatry Law 16:153–168, 1988

Agnew J: Klismaphilia: a physiological perspective. Am J Psychother 36:554–566, 1982

Alford GS, Webster JS, Sanders SH: Covert aversion of two interrelated deviant sexual practices: obscene phone calling and exhibitionism. a single case analysis. Behavior Therapy 11:15–25, 1980

American Psychiatric Association: Diagnostic and Statistical Manual of Mental Disorders, 3rd Edition. Washington, DC, American Psychiatric Association, 1980

American Psychiatric Association: Diagnostic and Statistical Manual of Mental Disorders, 3rd Edition, Revised. Washington, DC, American Psychiatric Association, 1987

Barth RJ, Kinder BN: The mislabeling of sexual impulsivity. J Sex Marital Ther 13:15–23, 1987

Blanchard R, Clemmensen LH, Steiner BW: Social desirability response set and systematic distortion in the self-report of adult male gender patients. Arch Sex Behav 14:505–516, 1985

Blanchard R, Racansky IG, Steiner BW: Phallometric detection of fetishistic arousal in heterosexual male crossdressers. Journal of Sex Research 22:452–462, 1986

Blanchard R, Steiner BW, Clemmensen LH, et al: Prediction of regrets in postoperative transsexuals. Can J Psychiatry 34:43–45, 1989

Buhrich N: Transvestism in history. J Nerv Ment Dis 165:64–66, 1977

Buhrich N, McConaghy N: Clinical comparison of transvestism and transsexualism: an overview. Aust N Z J Psychiatry 11:83–86, 1977a

Buhrich N, McConaghy N: The clinical syndromes of femmiphilic transvestism. Arch Sex Behav 6:397–412, 1977b

Carnes P: The Sexual Addiction. Minneapolis, MD, Compcare, 1987

Chalkley AJ, Powell GE: The clinical description of 48 cases of sexual fetishism. Br J Psychiatry 142:292–295, 1983

Clark SP, Borders LD, Knudson ML: Survey of telephone counselor's responses to sexual and sexually abusive callers. American Mental Health Counselors Association Journal 8:73–78, 1986

Coleman E: Definition, etiology and treatment considerations, in Chemical Dependency and Intimacy Dysfunction. Edited by Coleman E. New York, Haworth, 1988

Dalby JT: Is telephone scatologia a variant of exhibitionism? International Journal of Offender Therapy and Comparative Criminology 32:45–49, 1988

Denko JD: Klismaphilia, application of the erotic enema. Am J Psychother 30:236–255, 1976

Dixen JM, Maddever H, VanMaasdam J, et al: Psychosocial characteristics of applicants evaluated for surgical reassignment. Arch Sex Behav 13:269–276, 1984

Dixon D: An erotic attraction to amputees. Sexuality and Disability 6:3–19, 1983

Fagan PJ, Wise TN, Schmidt CE: The distressed transvestite: psychometric characteristics. J Nerv Ment Dis 176:626–632, 1988

Harvey NS: Serial cognitive profiles in levodopa-induced hypersexuality. Br J Psychiatry 153:833–836, 1988

Hunt DD, Hampson JL: Followup of 17 biologic male transsexuals after sex reassignment surgery. Am J Psychiatry 137:432–438, 1980

Kockott G, Fahrner E: Transsexuals who have not undergone surgery: a followup study. Arch Sex Behav 16:511–522, 1987

Kuiper B, Cohen-Kettenis P: Sex reassignment surgery: a study of 141 Dutch transsexuals. Arch Sex Behav 17:439–457, 1988

Levine MP, Troiden RR: The myth of sexual compulsivity. Journal of Sex Research 25:347–363, 1988

Levine SB: Letter to the editor. Arch Sex Behav 13:287–289, 1984

Levine SB, Shumaker RE: Increasingly Ruth: toward understanding sex reassignment. Arch Sex Behav 12:247–261, 1983

Lindermalm G, Korlin D, Uddenberg N: Long term follow-up of "sex change" on 13 male-to-female transsexuals. Arch Sex Behav 15:187–210, 1986

Lothstein LM: Sex reassignment surgery: historical, bioethical and theoretical issues. Am J Psychiatry 139:417–426, 1982

Lundstrom B, Pauly I, Walinder J: Outcome of sex reassignment surgery. Acta Psychiatr Scand 702:289–294, 1984

Meyer JK: Clinical variants among sex reassignment applicants. Arch Sex Behav 3:527–558, 1974

Murray FS, Bevan LC: A survey of nuisance telephone calls. Psychological Record 18:107–109, 1968

Myers WC, Carrera F: Carbamazepine-induced mania with hypersexuality in a nine year old boy. Am J Psychiatry 146:400, 1989

Quadland, MC: Compulsive sexual behavior: definition of a problem and an approach to treatment. J Sex Marital Ther 11:121–132, 1985

Quadland MC, Shattle WD: AIDS, Sexuality and Sexual Control. Binghamton, NY, Haworth, 1987, pp 277–298

Richwald GA, Kyle GR, Gerber MM, et al: Sexual activities in bathhouses in Los Angeles County: implications for AIDS prevention education. Journal of Sex Research 25:169–180, 1988

Saunders E, Award GA, White G: Male adolescent sexual offenders: the offender and the offense. Can J Psychiatry 31:542–549, 1986

Shore ER: The former transsexual: a case study. Arch Sex Behav 13:277–285, 1984

Sorvillo F, Mascola L, Kilman L: Bondage, dominance, irrigation and "aeromonas hydrophilia": California dreaming. JAMA 261:697–698, 1989

Walfish S: Crisis telephone counselor's views of clinical interaction situations. Community Ment Health J 19:219–226, 1983

Wise TN: Psychotherapy of an aging transvestite. J Sex Marital Ther 5:368–373, 1979

Wise TN, Meyer JK: The border area between transvestism and gender dysphoria: transvestitic applicants for sex reassignment. Arch Sex Behav 9:327–341, 1980

World Health Organization: Mental Disorders: Glossary and Guide to Their Classification in Accordance with the Ninth Revision of the International Classification of Diseases. Geneva, World Health Organization, 1978

World Health Organization: ICD-10 Chapter V. Mental and Behavioral Disorders. Diagnostic Criteria for Research. Geneva, Switzerland, World Health Organization, 1990

Further Reading

Anonymous: Nature and management of transvestism. Lancet 1:919–921, 1974

Bak RC: Fetishism. J Am Psychoanal Assoc 1:285–298, 1953

Ball JRB: A case of hair fetishism, transvestitism, and organic cerebral disorder. Acta Psychiatr Scand 44:249–254, 1968

Beatrice JA: Psychological comparison of heterosexuals, transvestites, preoperative transsexuals, and postoperative transsexuals. J Nerv Ment Dis 173:358–365, 1985

Benjamin H: Transvestism and transsexualism in the male and female. Journal of Sex Research 3:107–127, 1967

Bentler PM, Prince C: Psychiatric symptomatology in transvestites. J Clin Psychol 26:434–435, 1970

Blakemore CB, Thorpe JG, Barker JC, et al: The application of a faradic aversion conditioning in a case of transvestism. Behav Res Ther 1:29–34, 1963

Blanchard R: Nonhomosexual gender dysphoria. Journal of Sex Research 24:188–193, 1988

Blanchard R: The classification and labeling of nonhomosexual gender dysphorias. Arch Sex Behav 18:315–334, 1989

Blanchard R, Clemmensen LH, Steiner BW: Gender reorientation and psychosocial adjustment in male-to-female transsexuals. Arch Sex Behav 12:503–509, 1983

Blanchard R, Clemmensen LH, Steiner BW: Heterosexual and homosexual gender dysphoria. Arch Sex Behav 16:139–152, 1987

Blanchard R, Steiner BW, Clemmenson LH, et al: Prediction of regrets in postoperative transsexuals. Can J Psychiatry 34:43–45, 1989

Bond IK, Evans DR: Avoidance therapy: its use in two cases of underwear fetishism. Can Med Assoc J 96:1160–1162, 1967

Boots: The feelings of a fetishist. Psychiatr Q 10:742–758, 1957

Bourget D, Bradford J: Fire fetishism, diagnostic and clinical implications: a review of two cases. Can J Psychiatry 32:459–462, 1987

Brantley JT, Wise TN: Anti-androgenic treatment of a gender dysphoric transvestite. J Sex Marital Ther 11:109–112, 1985

Brierly H: Transvestism. New York, Pergamon, 1979

Buckner HT: The transvestic career path. Psychiatry 33:381–389, 1970

Buhrich N: A case of familial heterosexual transvestism. Acta Psychiatr Scand 55:199–201, 1977

Buhrich N: Motivation for crossdressing in heterosexual transvestism. Acta Psychiatr Scand 57:145–152, 1978

Buhrich N: Psychological adjustment in transvestism and transsexualism. Behav Res Ther 19:407–411, 1981

Buhrich N, Beaumont T: Comparison of transvestism in Australia and America. Arch Sex Behav 10:269–279, 1981

Buhrich N, McConaghy N: Transvestite fiction. J Nerv Ment Dis 163:420–427, 1976

Buhrich N, McConaghy N: Can fetishism occur in transsexuals? Arch Sex Behav 6:223–235, 1977

Buhrich N, McConaghy N: Pre-adult feminine behaviors of male transvestites. Arch Sex Behav 14:413–419, 1985

Bullough VL: Transvestites in the middle ages. American Journal of Sociology 79:1381–1394, 1973

Burgess AW, Hazelwood RR: Autoerotic asphyxial deaths and social network response. Am J Orthopsychiatry 53:166–170, 1983

Cautela JR: Behavioral analysis of a fetish: first interview. Journal of Behavioral and Experimental Psychiatry 17:262–265, 1986

Cavenar JO, Spaulding JG, Butts NT: Autofellatio: a power and dependency conflict. J Nerv Ment Dis 165:356–360, 1977

Chambers WM, Janzen WB: The eclectic and multiple therapy of a shoe fetishist. Am J Psychother 30:317–326, 1976

Clark DF: Fetishism treated by negative conditioning. Br J Psychiatry 109:404–407, 1963

Cliffe MJ: Paradoxical psychotherapy in a case of transvestism. Br J Med Psychol 60:283–285, 1987

Coles P: Nine months therapy with a transvestite. Psychoanalytic Psychotherapy 2:155–166, 1986

Coltart NE: The treatment of a transvestite. Psychoanalytic Psychotherapy 1:65–79, 1985

Croughan JL, Saghir M, Cohen R, et al: A comparison of treated and untreated male crossdressers. Arch Sex Behav 10:515–528, 1981

Davenport CW: A follow-up study of 10 feminine boys. Arch Sex Behav 15:511–517, 1986

Denson R: Undinism: the fetishization of urine. Can J Psychiatry 27:336–338, 1982

Dietz PE, Evans B: Pornographic imagery and prevalence of paraphilia. Am J Psychiatry 139:1493–1495, 1982

Epstein AW: Fetishism: a study of its psychopathology with particular reference to a proposed disorder in brain mechanisms as an etiologic factor. J Nerv Ment Dis 130:107–119, 1960

Everaerd W: A case of apotemnophilia: a handicap as sexual preference. Am J Psychother 37:285–293, 1983

Fagan PJ, Wise TN, Derogatis LR, et al: Distressed transvestites: psychometric characteristics. J Nerv Ment Dis 176:626–631, 1988

Freund K, Steiner BW, Chan S: Two types of cross-gender identity. Arch Sex Behav 11:49–63, 1982

Gebhard PH: Fetishism and sadomasochism. Science and Psychoanalysis 15:71–80, 1969

Gershman L: Case conference: a transvestite fantasy treated by thought-stopping, covert sensitization and aversive shock. Journal of Behavioral and Experimental Psychiatry 1:153–161, 1970

Glynn JD, Harper P: Behavior therapy in transvestism. Lancet 1:619, 1961

Golosow N, Weitzman EL: Psychosexual and ego repression in the male transsexual. J Nerv Ment Dis 149:328–336, 1968

Graves RW, Allison EJ, Bass AW, et al: Anal eroticism: two unusual rectal foreign bodies and their removal. Southern Medical Journal 76:677–678, 1983

Green R: Sexual Identity Conflict in Children and Adults. New York, Basic, 1974

Green R: The significance of feminine behavior in boys. J Child Psychol Psychiatry 16:341–344, 1975

Green R: Transsexualism: a research note. Archives of Sexual Behavior 7:383–384, 1978

Greenacre P: Certain relationships between fetishism and faculty development of the body image. Psychoanal Study Child 8:79–98, 1953

Greenberg DF: Why was the berdache ridiculed? Journal of Homosexuality 11:179–189, 1985

Hazelwood, RR, Burgess AW, Groth A: Death during dangerous autoerotic practice. Soc Sci Med 15E:129–133, 1981

Hoenig J, Kenna JC: The nosological position of transsexualism. Arch Sex Behav 3:273–287, 1974

Jones K: The effect of stilboestrol in two cases of male transvestism. Journal of Mental Science 106:1080–1081, 1960

Junginger J: Summation of arousal in partial fetishism. J Behav Ther Exp Psychiatry 19:297–300, 1988

Krueger DW: Symptom passing in a transvestite father and three sons. Am J Psychiatry 135:739–742, 1978

Lambley P: Treatment of transvestism and subsequent coital problems. J Behav Ther Exp Psychiatry 5:101–102, 1974

Lavin NI: Behavior therapy in a case of transvestism. J Nerv Ment Dis 133:346–353, 1961

Lazare A: Hidden conceptual models in clinical psychiatry. N Engl J Med 288:345–351, 1973

Lebegue BJ: Paraphilias in pornography. Australian Journal of Sex, Marriage, and Family 6:33–36, 1985

Lotherstein LM: The aging gender dysphoria (transsexual) patient. Arch Sex Behav 8:431–444, 1979

Lukianowicz N: Survey of various aspects of transvestism in the light of our present knowledge. J Nerv Ment Dis 128:36–64, 1959

MacDonald IJ: Behavior therapy in a case of transvestism. Lancet 1:889–890, 1961

Malitz S: Another report on the wearing of diapers and rubber pants by an adult male. Am J Psychiatry 122:1435–1437, 1966

Marks IM: Phylogenesis and learning in the acquisition of fetishism. Danish Medical Bulletin 19:307–310, 1972

Marks IM, Gelder MG: Transvestism and fetishism: clinical and psychological changes during faradic aversion. Br J Psychiatry 113:711–729, 1967

Marks IM, Rachman S, Gelder MG: Methods for assessment of aversion treatment in fetishism with masochism. Behav Res Ther 3:253–258, 1965

Marshall WL: A combined treatment approach to the reduction of multiple fetish-related behaviors. J Consult Clin Psychol 42:613–616, 1974

McHugh PR, Slavney PR: The perspectives of psychiatry. Baltimore, MD, Johns Hopkins University Press, 1983

McSweeney AJ: Fingernail fetishism: report of a case treated with hypnosis. American Journal of Clinical Hypnosis 15:139–143, 1972

Miller BL, Cummings JL, McIntyre H, et al: Hypersexuality or altered sexual preference following brain injury. J Neurol Neurosurg Psychiatry 49:867–873, 1986

Mitchell W, Falconer MA, Hill D: Epilepsy with fetishism relieved by temporal lobectomy. Lancet 1:626–630, 1952

Money J, Ehrhardt AA: Man and Woman, Boy and Girl. Baltimore, MD, Hopkins Press, 1972

Money J, Jobaris R, Furth G: Apotemnophilia: two cases of self-demand amputation as a paraphilia. Journal of Sex Research 13:115–125, 1977

Munroe RL, Munroe RH: Male transvestism and subsistence economy. J Soc Psychol 103:307–308, 1977

Nagler SH: Fetishism: a review and a case study. Psychiatr Q 10:713–741, 1957

Nanda S: The Hijras of India: cultural and individual dimensions of an institutionalized third gender role. Journal of Homosexuality 11:35–54, 1985

Newcomb MD: The role of perceived relative parent personality in the development of heterosexuals, homosexuals, and transvestites. Arch Sex Behav 14:147–164, 1985

Newman LE, Stoller R: Nontranssexual men who seek sex reassignment. Am J Psychiatry 131:437–441, 1973

O'Gorman EC: A retrospective study of epidemiological and clinical aspects of 28 transsexual patients. Arch Sex Behav 11:231–236, 1982

Oversey L, Person E: Transvestism: a disorder of the sense of self. International Journal of Psychoanalytic Psychotherapy 2:219–236, 1976

Person E, Oversey L: Transvestism: new perspectives. J Am Acad Psychoanal 6:301–323, 1978

Prince V, Bentler PM: Survey of 504 cases of transvestism. Psychological Reports 31:903–917, 1972

Raymond M, O'Keefe K: A case of pinup fetishism treated by aversion conditioning. Br J Psychiatry 111:579–581, 1965

Resnick H: Eroticized repetitive hangings: a form of self-destructive behavior. Am J Psychother 26:4–21, 1972

Rosenblum S, Faber M: The adolescent sexual asphyxia syndrome. Journal of the American Academy of Child Psychiatry 17:546–558, 1979

Segal MM: Transvestism as an impulse and a defense. Int J Psychoanal 46:209–217, 1966

Serber MA: The "as if" personality and transvestism. Psychoanal Rev 60:605–612, 1973

Stoller RJ: Transvestites' women. Am J Psychiatry 124:333–339, 1967

Stoller RJ: The term "transvestism." Arch Gen Psychiatry 24:230–237, 1971

Stoller RJ: Male transsexualism: uneasiness. Am J Psychiatry 130:536–539, 1973

Stoller RJ: Sex and Gender, Vol 2. New York, Aronson, 1974

Stoller RJ: Does perversion exist? The Johns Hopkins Medical Journal 134:43–57, 1974

Stoller RJ: Sexual excitement. Arch Gen Psychiatry 33:899–909, 1976

Strzyzewsky J, Zierhoffer M: Aversion therapy in a case of fetishism with transvestitic component. Journal of Sex Research 3:163–167, 1967

Van Kammen DP, Money J: Erotic imagery and self-castration in transvestism/transsexualism: a case report. Journal of Homosexuality 2:359–366, 1977

Ward NG: Successful lithium treatment of transvestism associated with manic depression. J Nerv Ment Dis 161:204–206, 1975

Winick C: A content analysis of sexually explicit magazines. Journal of Sex Research 21:206–210, 1984

Wise TN: Coping with a transvestitic mate: clinical implications. J Sex Marital Ther 11:293–300, 1985

Wise TN: Fetishism—etiology and treatment: a review from multiple perspectives. Compr Psychiatry 26:249–257, 1985

Wise TN, Meyer JK: Transvestism: previous findings and new areas for inquiry. J Sex Marital Ther 6:116–128, 1980

Wise TN, Dupkin C, Meyer JK: Partners of distressed transvestites. Am J Psychiatry 138:1221–1224, 1981

Zavitzianos G: Fetishism and exhibitionism in the female and their relationship to psychopathy and kleptomania. Int J Psychoanal 52:297–305, 1971

Zavitzianos G: The perversion of fetishism in women. Psychoanal Q 51:405–425, 1982

Index

Page numbers printed in **boldface** *type refer to tables or figures.*